Levitt and Tapley's

TECHNOLOGICAL BASIS OF RADIATION THERAPY

Clinical Applications

Third Edition

Levitt and Tapley's

TECHNOLOGICAL BASIS OF RADIATION THERAPY

Clinical Applications

Third Edition

Edited by

Seymour H. Levitt, M.D.
Professor and Head
Department of Therapeutic Radiology-Radiation Oncology
University of Minnesota Hospital
Minneapolis, Minnesota

Roger A. Potish, M.D.
Professor
Department of Therapeutic Radiology-Radiation Oncology
University of Minnesota Hospital
Minneapolis, Minnesota

Faiz M. Khan, Ph.D.
Professor and Director
Radiation Physics Section
University of Minnesota Hospital
Minneapolis, Minnesota

Carlos A. Perez, M.D.
Director
Mallinckrodt Institute of Radiology
Washington University Medical Center
St. Louis, Missouri

LIPPINCOTT WILLIAMS & WILKINS
A **Wolters Kluwer** Company
Philadelphia • Baltimore • New York • London
Buenos Aires • Hong Kong • Sydney • Tokyo

Editor: Charles W. Mitchell
Managing Editor: Grace E. Miller
Marketing Manager: Peter Darcy
Production Editor: June Choe

351 West Camden Street
Baltimore, Maryland 21201–2436 USA

Rose Tree Corporate Center
1400 North Providence Road
Building II, Suite 5025
Media, Pennsylvania 19063–2043 USA

Printed in the United States of America

First Edition 1985
Second Edition 1992

Library of Congress Cataloging-in-Publication Data

Levitt and Tapley's technological basis of radiation therapy :
clinical applications / [edited by] Seymour H. Levitt
. . . [et al.].—3rd ed.
p. cm.
Includes bibliographical references and index.
ISBN 0-683-30123-3
1. Cancer—Radiotherapy. I. Levitt, Seymour H. II. Tapley,
Norah duV., 1921– .
[DNLM: 1. Neoplasms—radiotherapy. 2. Radiotherapy—methods.
3. Radiotherapy Planning. Computer-Assisted—methods. QZ 269 L6658
1999]
RC271.R3L48 1998
616.99′40642—dc21
DNLM/DLC
for Library of Congress 98-3836
CIP

The publishers have made every effort to trace the copyright holders for borrowed material. If they have inadvertently overlooked any, they will be pleased to make the necessary arrangements at the first opportunity.

To purchase additional copies of this book, call our customer service department at **(800) 638-0672** or fax orders to **(800) 447-8438.** For other book services, including chapter reprints and large quantity sales, ask for the Special Sales department.

Canadian customers should call **(800) 665-1148**, or fax **(800) 665-0103.** For all other calls originating outside of the United States, please call **(410) 528-4223** or fax us at **(410) 528-8550.**

Visit Williams & Wilkins on the Internet: **http://www.wwilkins.com** or contact our customer service department at **custserv@wwilkins.-com**. Williams & Wilkins customer service representatives are available from 8:30 am to 6:00 pm, EST, Monday through Friday, for telephone access.

99 00 01 02 03
1 2 3 4 5 6 7 8 9 10

Dedication

I dedicate this third edition to my wife, Solveig, and my children, Mary Jeanne, Jennifer Gaye, and Scott Hayden, who have been and continue to be my inspiration. I also dedicate this edition in memoriam to Norah duVernet Tapley, M.D., and Drs. Gilbert and Mary Fletcher.

Seymour H. Levitt

To my wife, Kathy, and daughters, Dara, Yasmine, and Rachael, for their love and patience.

Faiz M. Khan

To my wife, Susie, and to our staff, as well as to our patients, all of whom have contributed unselfishly to my professional growth.

Carlos A. Perez

To my wife, Jane, and children, Willie, Robby, and Annie, for their patience and inspiration.

Roger A. Potish

Preface

Several important advances in radiation therapy have occurred since the last edition of this book was published in 1992. Improvements in treatment planning with the greater use and availability of three-dimensional conformal therapy, intensity modulated radiation, and high-dose rate brachytherapy are increasing the ability of radiation therapy to enhance clinical outcomes. As these methods become more refined, so too does the possibility of truly optimizing the use of radiation therapy by fulfilling its basic tenets of accurate localization, adequate dosage, and reproducibility of the daily treatment fields.

New chapters covering these advances in treatment planning are included in this revised edition, and chapters included from the previous edition have been updated to reflect any modifications in treatment. We made some changes to the chapters in Part II: Practical Clinical Applications to better focus or broaden the discussion of specific tumor sites. As before, the chapters are written by experts who have vast experience in the treatment of cancer patients.

We hope this book will help radiation oncologists, and other professionals in the field, provide the highest quality of care to their patients. The information in this book is meant to augment and help guide clinical decision making in the use of radiotherapy to treat various cancer types. We trust that the readers of this book will evaluate these recommendations based on their own knowledge and experience.

As in the previous two editions, we wish to acknowledge the advice, guidance, and friendship of Gilbert H. Fletcher who aided in the inception and creation of the past editions. His influence on the field of radiation oncology is evident here in these pages as it is in the practice of radiation oncology throughout the world.

We are very grateful to the contributors of the chapters for this edition, and our editorial and secretarial staffs, especially Mary Beth Nierengarten, Editor at the University of Minnesota, and Charles Mitchell, Senior Editor, and Grace Miller, Managing Editor at Williams & Wilkins, who, with their valuable contributions and dedication, made this publication possible.

Contributors

Ron Allison, M.D.
Associate Professor of Radiation Oncology
State University of New York at Buffalo
Buffalo, New York

Hassan Aziz, M.D.
Clinical Professor
Department of Radiation Oncology
State University of New York
Health Science Center of Brooklyn
Brooklyn, New York

Ellen Bellairs, M.D.
Cancer Care Center
Pomona Valley Hospital
Pomona, California

J. Daniel Bourland, Ph.D.
Assistant Professor
Department of Radiation Oncology
Wake Forest University School of Medicine
Winston-Salem, North Carolina

Frank J. Bova, Ph.D.
Professor
Department of Radiation Oncology
University of Florida
Gainesville, Florida

Thomas A. Buchholz, M.D.
Assistant Professor
Department of Radiation Oncology
University of Texas
M.D. Anderson Cancer Center
Houston, Texas

K. S. Clifford Chao, M.D.
Assistant Professor of Radiology
Radiation Oncology Center
Washington University School of Medicine
St. Louis, Missouri

Kwan H. Cho, M.D., M.Sc.
Assistant Professor
Department of Radiation Oncology
University of Minnesota Hospital and Clinic
Minneapolis, Minnesota

Joseph Cirrone, M.D.
Assistant Professor
Department of Radiation Oncology
State University of New York
Health Science Center of Brooklyn
Brooklyn, New York

William A. Dezarn, Ph.D.
Research Fellow
Department of Radiation Oncology
Wake Forest University School of Medicine
Winston-Salem, North Carolina

Kathryn E. Dusenbery, M.D.
Associate Professor
Department of Radiation Oncology
University of Minnesota
Minneapolis, Minnesota

Bahman Emami, M.D., F.A.C.R.
Professor and Chairman
Department of Radiotherapy
Loyola University of Chicago
Maywood, Illinois

Gary A. Ezzell, Ph.D.
Coordinator, Radiation Oncology Physics
Gershenson Radiation Oncology Center
Karmanos Cancer Institute
Assistant Professor
Department of Radiation Oncology
Wayne State University
Detroit, Michigan

Russell L. Gerber, M.S.
Radiation Oncology Center
Mallinckrodt Institute of Radiology
Washington University School of Medicine
St. Louis, Missouri

Bruce J. Gerbi, Ph.D.
Associate Professor
Department of Therapeutic Radiology-Radiation Oncology
University of Minnesota
Minneapolis, Minnesota

Mary V. Graham, M.D.
Assistant Professor of Radiology in Radiation Oncology
Mallinckrodt Institute of Radiology
Washington University School of Medicine
St. Louis, Missouri

Perry W. Grigsby, M.D., M.B.A., F.A.C.R.
Professor of Radiology
Department of Radiation Oncology
Washington University School of Medicine
St. Louis, Missouri

Leonard L. Gunderson, M.D.
Professor of Oncology
Mayo Medical School
Rochester, Minnesota

Michael G. Haddock, M.D.
Assistant Professor of Oncology
Mayo Medical School
Rochester, Minnesota

Eric J. Hall, D.Phil., D.Sc., F.A.C.R.
Higgins Professor of Radiation Biophysics
Center for Radiological Research
College of Physicians & Surgeons
Columbia University
New York, New York

Walter A. Hall, M.D.
Associate Professor
Departments of Neurosurgery and Radiation Oncology
University of Minnesota Hospital and Clinic
Minneapolis, Minnesota

David H. Hussey, M.D., F.A.C.R.
Professor and Director
Department of Radiation Oncology
University of Iowa
Iowa City, Iowa

Faiz M. Khan, Ph.D.
Professor and Director
Radiation Physics Section
University of Minnesota Hospital
Minneapolis, Minnesota

Chung Kyu Kim Lee, M.D.
Professor
Department of Therapeutic Radiology-Radiation Oncology
University of Minnesota Medical School
Minneapolis, Minnesota

Seymour H. Levitt, M.D.
Professor and Head
Department of Therapeutic Radiology-Radiation Oncology
University of Minnesota Hospital
Minneapolis, Minnesota

Daniel A. Low, Ph.D.
Assistant Professor
Division of Radiation Oncology
Mallinckrodt Institute of Radiology
Washington University School of Medicine
St. Louis, Missouri

Mark G. Marshall, M.S.
Assistant Professor
Department of Radiation Oncology
Wake Forest University Baptist Medical Center
Winston-Salem, North Carolina

James A. Martenson, Jr., M.D.
Associate Professor of Oncology
Mayo Medical School
Rochester, Minnesota

Alvaro A. Martinez, M.D.
Department of Radiation Oncology
William Beaumont Hospital
Royal Oak, Michigan

Marsha D. McNeese, M.D.
Associate Professor
Department of Radiation Oncology
University of Texas
M.D. Anderson Cancer Center
Houston, Texas

William M. Mendenhall, M.D.
Professor
Department of Radiation Oncology
University of Florida
Gainesville, Florida

Jeff M. Michalski, M.D.
Assistant Professor of Radiology
Department of Radiology/Radiation Oncology
Mallinckrodt Institute of Radiology
Washington University School of Medicine
St. Louis, Missouri

Rodney R. Million, M.D.
Professor Emeritus
Department of Radiation Oncology
University of Florida
Gainesville, Florida

Jatinder R. Palta, Ph.D.
Professor and Chief of Physics
Department of Radiation Oncology
University of Florida
Gainesville, Florida

James T. Parsons, M.D.
Professor
Department of Radiation Oncology
University of Florida
Gainesville, Florida

Carlos A. Perez, M.D.
Director
Mallinckrodt Institute of Radiology
Washington University Medical Center
St. Louis, Missouri

Roger A. Potish, M.D.
Professor
Department of Therapeutic Radiology-Radiation Oncology
University of Minnesota Hospital
Minneapolis, Minnesota

James A. Purdy, Ph.D., F.A.C.R.
Professor and Associate Director
Radiation Oncology Center
Mallinckrodt Institute of Radiology
Washington University School of Medicine
St. Louis, Missouri

Donald M. Roback, Ph.D.
Assistant Professor
Department of Therapeutic Radiology-Radiation Oncology
University of Minnesota
Minneapolis, Minnesota

Marvin Rotman, M.D.
Professor and Chairman
Department of Radiation Oncology
State University of New York
Health Sciences Center at Brooklyn
Brooklyn, New York

Alan R. Schulsinger, M.D.
Assistant Professor
Department of Radiation Oncology
SUNY Health Science Center at Brooklyn
Brooklyn, New York

Edward G. Shaw, M.D.
Professor and Chairman
Department of Radiation Oncology
Bowman Gray School of Medicine
Winston-Salem, North Carolina

Joseph Simpson, M.D., Ph.D., F.A.C.R.
Associate Professor of Radiology
Radiation Oncology Center
Mallinckrodt Institute of Radiology
Washington University School of Medicine
St. Louis, Missouri

Chul K. Sohn, M.D.
Assistant Professor
Department of Radiation Oncology
SUNY Health Science Center at Brooklyn
Brooklyn, New York

Judith Anne Stitt, M.D., M.S.
Professor, Department of Human Oncology
University of Wisconsin-Madison
Madison, Wisconsin

Eric A. Strom, M.D.
Assistant Professor of Radiation Oncology
University of Texas
M.D. Anderson Cancer Center
Houston, Texas

Bruce Robert Thomadsen, Ph.D.
Assistant Professor
Department of Medical Physics and Human Oncology
University of Wisconsin-Madison
Madison, Wisconsin

Roby C. Thompson, M.D.
Professor and Head
Department of Orthopedic Surgery
University of Minnesota Hospital & Clinic
Minneapolis, Minnesota

Vinceno Valentini, M.D.
Department of Radiation Oncology
Catholic University
Rome, Italy

Gordon Watson, M.D., Ph.D.
Assistant Professor
Department of Radiation Oncology
Wake Forest University School of Medicine
Winston-Salem, North Carolina

Contents

Part I: Basic Concepts in Treatment Planning

CHAPTER 1
Basic Clinical Parameters 3
Gilbert H. Fletcher (Deceased)

CHAPTER 2
Clinical Principles and Applications of Chemoirradiation 14
Joseph Cirrone, Hassan Aziz, Marvin Rotman

CHAPTER 3
Fundamentals of Treatment Planning in Radiation Oncology 30
Carlos A. Perez, James A. Purdy

CHAPTER 4
The Simulation Process in the Determination and Definition of the Treatment Volume and Treatment Planning 52
Bruce J. Gerbi

CHAPTER 5
Complex Field Arrangements: Field Shaping and Separation of Adjoining Fields 64
Faiz M. Khan

CHAPTER 6
Electron Beam Therapy 72
Faiz M. Khan, Marsha D. McNeese

CHAPTER 7
Treatment Aids for External Beam Radiotherapy 86
Donald M. Robach, Faiz M. Khan

CHAPTER 8
Three-Dimensional Treatment Planning and Conformal Therapy 104
James A. Purdy, Bahman Emami, Mary V. Graham, Jeff Michalski, Carlos A. Perez, Joseph Simpson

CHAPTER 9
Intensity Modulated Radiation Therapy 128
Daniel A. Low, James A. Purdy, Carlos A. Perez, K. S. Clifford Chao, Russell L. Gerber

CHAPTER 10
Stereotactic Radiosurgery and Radiotherapy 147
Kwan H. Cho, Bruce J. Gerbi, Walter A. Hall

CHAPTER 11
Brachytherapy: Rules of Implantation and Dose Specification 173
Faiz M. Khan

CHAPTER 12
Radiobiology of Low and High Dose Rate Brachytherapy 184
Eric J. Hall

CHAPTER 13
The Physics of High Dose Rate Brachytherapy 200
Gary A. Ezzell

CHAPTER 14
Clinical Applications of Low Dose Rate and High Dose Rate Brachytherapy 210
Judith Anne Stitt, Bruce Robert Thomadsen

Part II: Practical Clinical Applications

CHAPTER 15
Central Nervous System Tumors 223
Gordon Watson, Mark G. Marshall, William A. Dezarn, J. Daniel Bourland, Edward G. Shaw

CHAPTER 16
Head and Neck Cancer 269
James T. Parsons, Jatinder R. Palta,
William M. Mendenhall, Frank J. Bova, Rodeny R. Million

CHAPTER 17
Breast Cancer 301
Marsha McNeese, Eric A. Strom, Thomas A. Buchholz,
Seymour H. Levitt, Faiz M. Khan

CHAPTER 18
Carcinoma of the Lung and Esophagus 315
Mary V. Graham

CHAPTER 19
Cancers of the Colon, Rectum, and Anus 335
James A. Martenson Jr., Michael G. Haddock,
Leonard L. Gunderson

CHAPTER 20
Bladder Cancer 349
Alan R. Schulsinger, Ron Allison, Chul K. Sohn,
Vinceno Valentini, Marvin Rotman

CHAPTER 21
Low-Dose Rate-Brachytherapy for Carcinoma of the
Cervix 363
Kathryn E. Dusenbery

CHAPTER 22
Technical Aspects of Radiation Therapy
for Endometrial Carcinoma 387
Perry W. Grigsby, K. S. Clifford Chao

CHAPTER 23
Carcinoma of the Vulva 403
Ellen Bellairs, Roger A. Potish

CHAPTER 24
Carcinoma of the Vagina 417
Carlos A. Perez

CHAPTER 25
Prostate 435
Carlos A. Perez, Jeff M. Michalski, Alvaro A. Martinez

CHAPTER 26
Testicular Cancer 467
David H. Hussey

CHAPTER 27
Extremity Soft Tissue Sarcoma in Adults 481
Kathryn E. Dusenbery, Roby C. Thompson

CHAPTER 28
Total Body Irradiation in Conditioning Regimens
for Bone Marrow Transplantation 499
Kathryn E. Dusenbery, Bruce J. Gerbi

CHAPTER 29
Hodgkin's Disease 519
Chung Kyu Kim Lee

PART I

Basic Concepts in Treatment Planning

Chapter 1

Basic Clinical Parameters

Gilbert H. Fletcher*

Three generic tissue types are 1) early responding normal tissue, such as the epithelial surfaces and the hemoleukopoietic system; 2) slowly (late) responding normal tissues, such as spinal cord, kidney, and dermis; and 3) tumors, which as a general class can be considered analogous to acutely responding normal tissues. The concepts regarding the radiation response of these tissues have changed through the decades, leading to the development of a variety of treatment techniques with conflicting results (1). Some aspects of the parameters most directly connected with clinical practice are discussed in this chapter.

SURVIVAL FRACTION CURVE

In 1956, Puck and Marcus showed that in tissue cultures, the same proportion, not the same number, of mammalian cells (squamous cell carcinoma of the cervix in their experiment) is killed with each incremental dose of irradiation (2). The corollary is that higher doses are needed for the eradication of a tumor cell population as the number of clonogens increases. The survival fraction methodology gave the basis for a quantitative instead of a morphologic approach to radiobiology, which up to that time had been essentially radiopathology.

TWO-COMPONENT SURVIVAL FRACTION CURVES

In skin reaction experiments, one supraclavicular area of patients with lung cancer was irradiated with one exposure, whereas another supraclavicular area was irradiated with two exposures separated by no less than 6 hours. Results showed no increment, i.e., no recovery, with fraction sizes less than 200 rad (Table 1.1) (3). Dutreix and colleagues concluded that the experimental data were compatible with a two-component model of cell killing involving 1) single lethal events and 2) accumulation of sublethal events. The total cell kill is the sum of the two components. An x-ray beam produces lethal lesions by both single-hit and multihit mechanisms. The biophysical basis for single-hit or multihit killing is not established, but it is simplest to consider it in terms of how an electron loses its energy after being ejected by a photon. The rate of deposition of energy by a charged particle is inversely proportional to its energy. Hence, along its track, the electron initially is sparsely ionizing, but as it loses its energy through collisions and scattering, it becomes more densely ionizing. The dense ionization at the end of the track is presumed to be sufficient to induce irreversible single-hit injury without requiring additional accumulation of ionization injury from other electron tracks. Because of the predominance of single-hit lethal effects up to 200 rad, the presence of molecular oxygen is not as important as with large fractions, a possible explanation for why treatment in hyperbaric tanks with conventional fractionation did not show any superiority of results (4).

LINEAR QUADRATIC EQUATION

The two-component survival fraction curve is best represented by a linear quadratic equation, in which D is the dose:

$$\text{Survival fraction is } S = e^{-(\alpha D + \beta D2)}.$$

Figure 1.1 shows that the curve has an initial, essentially linear region before beginning to bend. The downward bending results from the accumulation of sublethal lesions, which interact to become lethal. When the dose per fraction or the dose rate is low enough, cell killing resulting from accumulation of sublethal injuries is insignificant, because of continuous or repeated repair during the overall duration of exposure(s); then, essentially all cell killing results from single-hit injury.

*Deceased.

Table 1.1. Increments for Two Exposures Separated by 6 Hours to Produce Same Skin Reactions as One Exposure

	100		265		410	
	200	200	400	530	600	820
	100		265		410	
Increment	0		130		220	

Two exposures of 100 rad produce the same reaction as one exposure of 200 rad, whereas for larger fractions of 400 rad and 600 rad, an increment is needed.

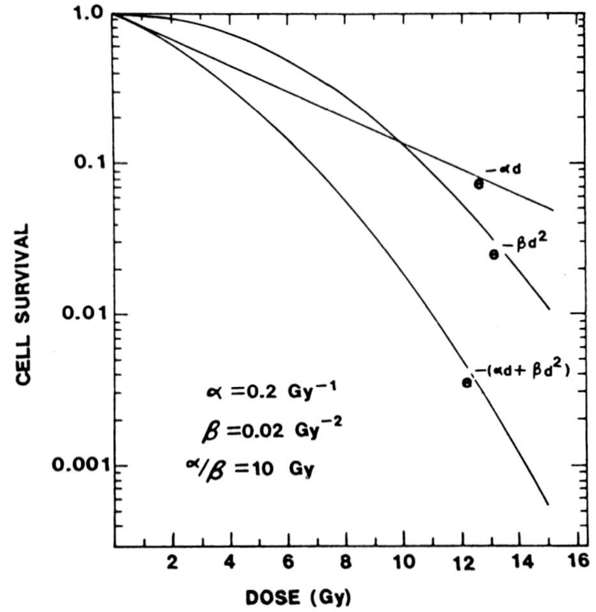

Figure 1.1. Model dose-survival curves for mammalian cells. Experimentally determined curve (lowest curve) is product of two mechanisms, single-hit injury described by essentially linear region ($e^{-\alpha d}$) and multihit or cumulative injury described by continuously bending curve ($e^{-\beta d2}$). Rate at which survival curve bends from initial essentially linear region depends on the ratio (α/β) of coefficients for single-hit and multihit killing; the lower the value, the sooner and more steeply the curve bends. (Reprinted with permission from Withers HR. Biologic basis of radiation therapy. In: Perez CA, Brady LW, eds. Principles and Practices of Radiation Oncology. Philadelphia, J.B. Lippincott, 1987.)

This equation describes logarithmic cell killing by two coefficients, α for single-hit killing (i.e., a linear function of dose) and β for multihit killing (i.e., a function of the square of the dose) (Figure 1.1). The α/β ratio can be determined from multifraction experiments. The value is high for acutely responding tissues, e.g., 10 Gy, and is low for late-responding tissues, e.g., 2 to 4 Gy. This implies that the cell killing that underlies acute radiation responses is more the result of single hits and irreparable mechanisms than is the case for the target cells for late injury. The α/β ratio merely describes the relative susceptibility of tissues to single-hit and multihit killing (5).

Acute Reactions

In the kilovoltage era, one was constantly aware of the reactions of the skin and mucosa because they were the limiting factors to treatment. Coutard showed that there were increasing degrees of moist desquamation of the skin depending on the level of stem cell depletion in the epithelium and damage to the dermis (6). When cell kill is not total, polycyclic recovery occurs from the periphery and also from islands in the area of moist desquamation. When all the cells have been killed and damage to the dermis is severe, there is a long period of recovery and the epithelium regrows linearly along the edges of the denuded area. The skin, as it heals, is already atrophied, a consequential damage of very severe acute reaction.

With megavoltage, the reactions of the mucosa (upper respiratory and digestive tracts, bladder, and intestines) are a limiting factor. Coutard observed that the faster the same dose is given, the sooner the mucositis appears, the stronger it is, and the longer it takes to heal (Figure 1.2) (6). The four degrees of mucositis are redness, studded exudate, confluent exudate with a pink substrate, and, when damage to the underlying tissues occurs, a thick yellowish membrane. The fourth degree is rarely, if ever, seen in present day practice. If it is, as in some accelerated fractionation schemes, the mucositis takes a long time to heal.

Late Effects

Late effects are produced by the killing of target cells that are different from those producing acute reactions. It is generally believed that the target cells for the late se-

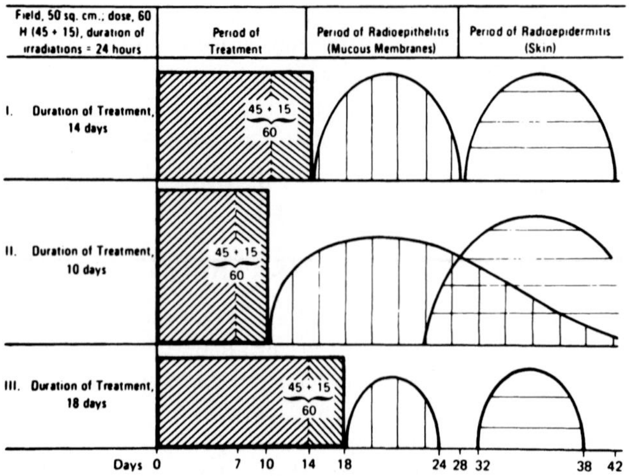

Figure 1.2. Evolution of mucous membrane and cutaneous lesions of normal epithelium in therapy of squamous epitheliomas of hypopharynx and larynx. The whole is composed of three equal periods of 2 weeks each or 6 weeks. 45 H is given to one side of neck; 15 H to other side (1 H = 100 roentgens). (Reprinted with permission from Coutard H. Roentgentherapy of epitheliomas of the tonsillar region, hypopharynx, and larynx from 1920–1926. AJR 1932;28:313.)

quelae turn over slowly and, therefore, do not show significant regeneration during the course of a conventionally fractioned regimen. Attention has been directed primarily to specific complications, such as bone necrosis and bowel obstruction. Fibrosis has been underestimated; it has been poorly appreciated that fibrosis manifesting after a latency period never ceases to increase and can eventually be very severe. For instance, in the protracted irradiation of advanced breast cancer by irradiation alone, severe fibrosis, eventually manifesting as skin ulceration, has developed 10 or 15 years after treatment (Figure 1.3) (7). If the latency period is long (i.e., fibrosis is detectable only after several years), the problem will not be severe. If the fibrosis develops early, perhaps 2 to 3 years after treatment, the problem will eventually be severe. The latency period and the progression of late effects have been quantified (8,9).

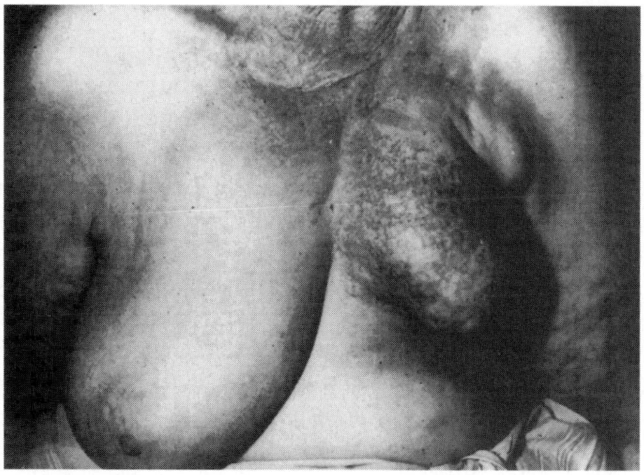

Figure 1.3. A 51-year-old woman presented in 1968 with tumor of left breast that was at least 10 cm in diameter with skin fixation. Biopsy results revealed adenocarcinoma. Tumor was treated with cobalt 60, 6000 rad in 8 weeks, 5 fractions per week, followed by boost to breast mass of 3000 rad with 12 MeV electrons. During treatment, patient had only mild erythema. She developed progressive fibrosis (this photograph, taken at 10 years follow-up) and eventual ulceration in 1981, which was removed in 1982. Patient had no evidence of disease in 1987. This case is a striking example of dissociation between acute reactions and late effects and progression of late damage. (Reprinted with permission from Spanos WJ, Montague ED, and Fletcher GH. Late complications of radiation only for advanced breast cancer. Int J Radiat Oncol Biol Phys 1980;6:1473.)

Dissociation of Acute Reactions and Late Effects

The cell survival curve in acutely responding tissues has a longer initial linear region (single-hit cell killing kinetics), whereas the curve for slowly responding tissues is "curvier" (Figure 1.4) (10). Thus, the α/β ratio is greater for acutely responding tissues (10 to 25 Gy) than for late responding tissues (1 to 3 Gy). Consequently, there is relatively less fractionation effect in acutely responding than in late-responding tissues. If tumors, as a general class, are analogous to acutely responding normal tissues, repair of sublethal injury as a result of fractionation of dose should spare tumor cells to about the same extent as acutely responding normal tissues. Data seem to indicate that at least 6 hours are necessary for repair of accumulated sublethal damage in late effect tissues. Few data at doses per fraction less than 2 Gy are available, but they suggest that further preferential sparing of late injury may be possible through the use of doses per fraction less than 2 Gy.

With increasing fraction size, the total dose to produce equal late effects must be diminished considerably more than is needed to produce equivalent acute reactions (Figure 1.5) (11). This fact has not been taken into account in the schemes of hypofractionation used in the past. In the treatment of subclinical melanoma, a total dose of 30 Gy delivered in 3 weeks with 60 Gy per fraction does not produce a late effect because it is much smaller than the

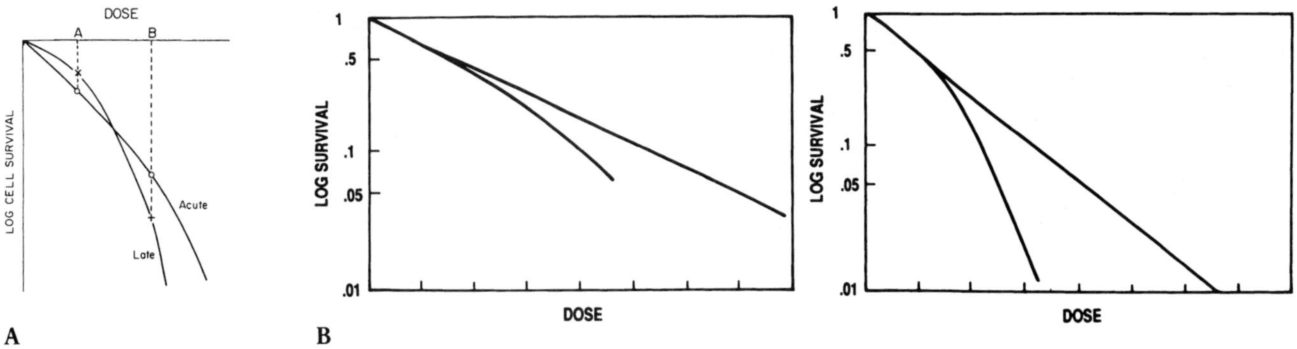

A B

Figure 1.4. **A.** Hypothetic survival curves of target cells for acute and late effects in normal tissues exposed to x-rays. **B.** Linear region of curve for acute reactions (left) is longer than for late effects (right). Therefore, α/β ratio in $S = e^{-(\alpha D + \beta D^2)}$ is greater for acute effects than for late effects, resulting in a greater rate of change in late-responding tissues with change in dose. At dose A, survival of target cells is higher in late effects than in acute-effects tissues, whereas at dose B, reverse is true. Therefore, increasing dose per fraction from A to B will result in relatively greater increase in late rather than acute injury. (Modified from Fowler JR. Fractionation and Therapeutic gain. *In* Biological Basis of Radiotherapy. Edited by Steel GG, Adams GE, Peckham MJ. Amsterdam, Elsevier Science Publishers, 1983.)

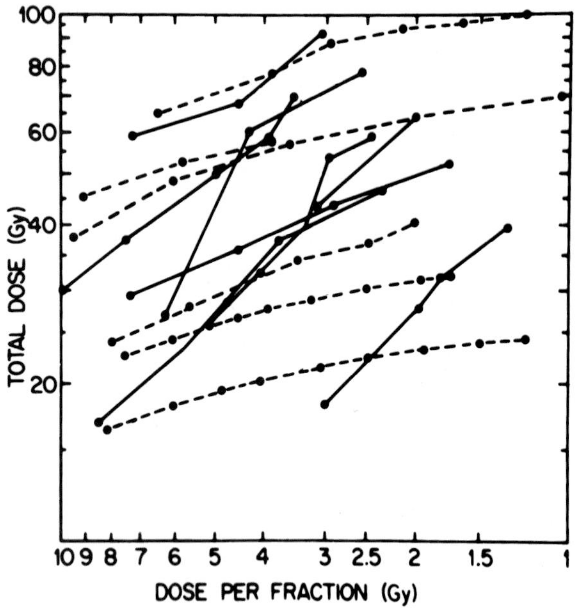

Figure 1.5. Total dose for isoeffect as a function of dose per fraction. Curves describing late isoeffects *(solid lines)* have steeper slopes than those for early isoeffects *(dashed lines).* (Reprinted with permission from Thames HD, Withers HR, Peters LJ, Fletcher GH. Changes in early and late radiation responses with altered dose fractionation: Implications for dose-survival relationships. Int J Radiat Oncol Biol Phys 1982;8:219.)

conventional 50-Gy dose delivered in 5 weeks with 2 Gy per fraction.

Isoeffect Formulas

Since the 1920s, radiotherapists have tried to develop formulae to calculate the equivalent of total doses with varying overall treatment times. The best known is the Strandqvist formula (12), which shows no advantage to protracting treatment times because the lines for various degrees of skin reaction, necrosis, and cure of skin cancer are parallel. Clinical applications of the formula, however, have led to horrendous complications.

The importance of fraction size was appreciated in the early 1960s (13) when a label on the nominal single dose (NSD) formula was used to correlate total dose, number of fractions, and overall treatment times (14);

$$\text{NSD (rets)} = D\,N^{-0.24}\,T^{-0.11}$$

in which D is total dose in rad, N is number of fractions, and T is overall treatment time in days. Every one of the assumptions of the NSD formula can be challenged.

1. The recovery exponent for skin damage was obtained on mild skin reactions and not on connective tissue damage. The recovery exponent of 0.33 for skin was obtained by assuming 1 day for a single exposure, whereas the recovery exponent of 0.22 for skin cancer was obtained by assuming 0.35 of a day for a single exposure.
2. Like normal tissues, tumors respond to cell kill by accelerated repopulation.
3. The NSD concept does not take into account that the survival fraction curve has two components and results from single-hit lethal events and accumulation of sublethal events. The total cell kill is the addition of the two components. Up to 2 Gy per fraction, single lethal events predominate.
4. The NSD concept does not differentiate between acute and late effects. If the dose per fraction increases, a slight diminution of total dose is needed to produce equivalent acute reactions, whereas a greater diminution is required to produce the same late effects.

The use of the NSD formula and its derivatives, like time dose factor (TDF) and cumulative radiation effect (CRE), has often resulted in excessive late complications. Recently, the fractionation response for different schemes of early- and late-responding tissues has been compared in terms of α/β ratios.

If 76 Gy is given (two times a day) with 1.2 Gy per fraction, the total dose equivalent with the conventional 2 Gy per day can be calculated by using the following formula (15,16):

$$Dx = Dr\,\frac{\alpha/\beta + dr}{\alpha/\beta + dx}$$

in which Dr is total dose with 1.2 Gy two times a day, Dx is total dose with 2 Gy, dr is 1.2 Gy, and dx is 2 Gy, with α/β appropriate to the tissue for which the isoeffective dose is required. For acute reactions, an α/β of 10 is assumed.

$$Dr = 76\,\frac{10 + 1.2}{10 + 2} = 69\text{ Gy}$$

For late effects, an α/β of 3 is assumed.

$$Dx = 76\,\frac{3 + 1.2}{3 + 2} = 63\text{ Gy}$$

The therapeutic ratio is enhanced because the equivalent dose is higher for acute reactions and for tumors than for late effects.

These calculations do not factor in other radiobiologic parameters and must be considered an approximation. The development of formulae for calculating isoeffective doses while taking into consideration various radiobiologic parameters is rapidly evolving.

UNCONVENTIONAL FRACTIONATION

What is "conventional" fractionation? A conventional scheme would be 1.8 to 2 Gy per fraction 5 days per week.

Hyperfractionation. In such schemes, fractional doses smaller than 2 Gy are given two or three times daily to achieve an increase in the total dose in the same overall time. Because of the sigmoid response curve, a higher dose should increase the control rate. Acute reactions can be stronger, but late effects should not be increased because the doses per fraction are small.

Accelerated Fractionation. The overall treatment time in this scheme is shortened by using doses per fraction of slightly less than conventional size two to three times per day. Various strategies are shown in Figure 1.6 (17).

Accelerated Hyperfractionation. If possible, improving the therapeutic ratio by combining both a decrease in dose per fraction and a shortening of overall treatment duration is desirable. The limitation of accelerated hyperfractionation is acute toxicity, because both strategies independently increase acute reactions.

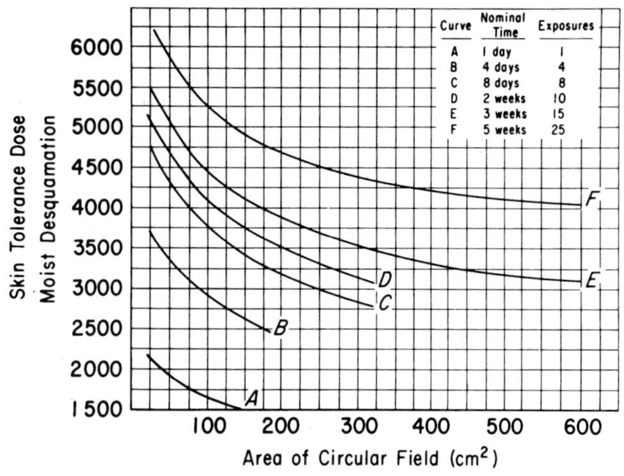

Figure 1.7. Relationship between dose and size of area irradiated (healthy skin in an "average" site) to produce moist desquamation for various overall treatment times (daily irradiation at about 50 R per minute for each exposure with radiation of half-value layer 1.5 mm Cu). (From Paterson R. The Treatment of Malignant Disease by Radium and X-rays. Baltimore, Williams & Wilkins, 1949.)

TOLERANCE AS FUNCTION OF VOLUME OF TISSUE IRRADIATED

Because a daily observation when using kilovoltage x-rays was that the dose the skin could tolerate was a function of the area irradiated, diminishing sharply as the area increased, the relationship of volume irradiated and tolerance was clear. Graphs correlating dose-time-area, like that by Paterson (Figure 1.7), were a working tool (18). Because of the absence of skin reaction with megavoltage irradiation, the relationship of complications with volume irradiated is no longer as strongly appreciated.

In cancer of the cervix, the use of extended fields to L_4 or T_{12} has shown dramatically that there is a strong relationship between volume irradiated and tolerance (19). With the "box" technique for pelvic irradiation, the volume receiving a high dose is approximately 2000 cm (20), whereas with parallel opposed portals to L_4 or more to T_{12}, it is between 6000 and 7000 cm (20). When lymphangiography or lymphadenectomy demonstrated involvement of the external iliac, obturator, or hypogastric nodes, the common iliac nodes were included as a matter of policy in the irradiation field. When the common iliac or low paraaortic nodes were involved, the treatment portals were extended to the diaphragm. A review of the records of patients who had extended field irradiation showed that the rate of severe complication was high compared with use of the technique in which portals are limited to 15 × 15 cm. If used injudiciously, the increase in complication rate may outweigh the improvement in tumor control probability.

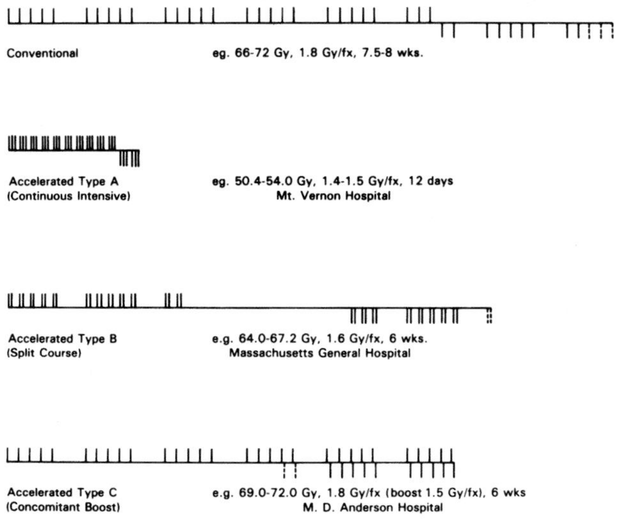

Figure 1.6. Comparison of conventional and three prototypical accelerated fractionation schedules. Bars above line denote large field treatment; bars below line denote boost field treatment; dotted bars represent treatments omitted in lower ranges of total dose. (Reprinted with permission from Peters LJ, Ang KK, Thames HD Jr. Accelerated fractionation in the radiation treatment of head and neck cancer: A critical comparison of different strategies. Acta Oncol 1988;27:185.)

TUMOR KINETICS

Many tumor cell divisions take place before a tumor mass becomes clinically detectable. Through several mechanisms, cells are continually lost from the proliferative cell population; the proportion of new cells lost during each cell cycle is called the cell loss factor (CLF) (21). A palpable tumor mass consists of clonogenic and nonclonogenic tumor cells and stroma, the proportions varying with different histologic types and, within the same histologic type, from tumor to tumor.

Theoretically, anaplastic tumors should have a fast cycling cell population and probably have both a higher proportion of clonogens and a more rapid increase in their number, but the clinical setting must be considered. For instance, large neck nodes originating from the undifferentiated squamous cell carcinomas of the nasopharynx are systematically controlled with doses that do not exceed 70 Gy in 7 weeks. Nodes of the same size from an undifferentiated squamous cell carcinoma of the base of the tongue would not be systematically controlled with the same doses. No reason for the difference in the radiation response has been established, but it is a clinical fact. Therefore, differentiation per se may not provide a guide for determining a more efficient irradiation scheme for a mass.

Kinetic data obtained from human tumors by using radioisotope labeling techniques are shown in Table 1.2 (8). Because of the CLF, the actual volume doubling time is considerably greater than the potential doubling time, which is the time it would take for the tumor cell population to double if no cell loss occurred. During the past 10 years, repopulation has been determined to be a major obstacle to cure by irradiation. Before that time, the hypoxic cells were considered the predominant obstacle to radiocurability. An accelerated regenerative response has been demonstrated in some experimental tumor systems. For the squamous cell carcinomas of the upper respiratory and digestive tracts, 70 to 80% of recurrences appear by 1 year, and in excess of 90% by 2 years. For some anatomic sites, this interval is even shorter. Depending on the CLF value, calculations of the time to recurrence imply a potential doubling time as short as 4 days. For treatment times between 4 and 8 weeks, the exponent for T was found to be 0.30 to 0.40 for the squamous cell carcinomas of the oropharynx (Figure 1.8) (22). Results of studies of the response of pulmonary metastases to irradiation indicate that a regenerative response is triggered (23,24). This accelerated growth response possibly is caused in part by a diminution of the CLF, i.e., cells that otherwise would have stopped cycling keep on cycling, producing new clonogenic cells. The data also suggest that, in at least some tumors, regeneration begins within the time of a conventional course of radiotherapy. Treatments should not be prolonged by using 1.8 Gy per day, unless patients are fragile and/or large volumes are irradiated, as in most pharynx tumors. Split courses should be avoided.

These data are well established for the squamous cell carcinomas of the upper respiratory and digestive tracts. No data are available for the adenocarcinomas and other histologic types that would suggest that accelerated repopulation occurs within the treatment period.

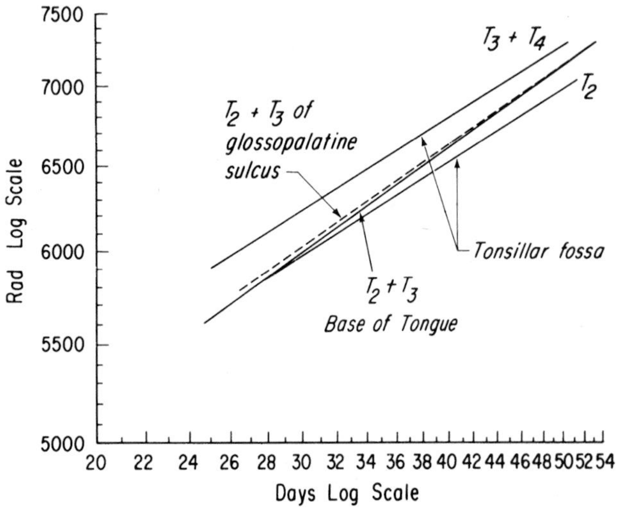

Figure 1.8. Hand-drawn exclusion lines with most of failures below. Slopes are 0.30 for tonsillar fossa, 0.35 for glossopalatine sulcus, and 0.38 for base of the tongue squamous cell lesions. (Reprinted with permission from Fletcher GH, Shukovsky LJ. Isoeffect exponents for the production of dose-response curves in squamous cell carcinomas treated between 4 and 8 weeks. J Radiol Electrol 1976;57:825.)

Table 1.2. Growth Kinetics of Selected Human Solid Tumors (Median Values)

Histology	No. Patients	Potential Doubling Time (Days)	Volume Doubling Time (Days)	Cell Loss Factor (%)
Burkitt's lymphoma	19	1.2	2.8	69
Undifferentiated carcinoma of lung	22	3.8	79.0	95
Squamous cell carcinoma	198	4.1	58.0	93
Adenocarcinoma				
Gastrointestinal tract	72	3.7	95.0	96
Breast	138	24.0	105.0	78
Melanoma	45	11.0	54.0	80

(Reprinted with permission from Thames HD, Peters LJ, Withers HR, Fletcher GH. Accelerated fractionation vs. hyperfractionation: Rationales for several treatments per day. Int. J. Radiat. Oncol. Biol. Phys. 1983;9:127.)

TUMOR DOSE

Subclinical Disease

Subclinical disease consists of aggregates of cancer cells that cannot be seen or felt in accessible areas. These aggregates are not necessarily microscopic.

Clinical data on the effectiveness of doses of irradiation on subclinical disease were obtained in squamous cell carcinomas of the upper respiratory and digestive tracts and adenocarcinomas of the breast by electively irradiating clinically negative lymphatic areas that were surgically undisturbed. A dose of 50 Gy delivered in 25 fractions of 2 Gy in 5 weeks eradicates in excess of 90% of the occult deposits (Table 1.3) (25,26).

Table 1.3. Tumor Control Probability Correlated with Irradiation Dose and Volume of Cancer

Dose	Squamous Cell Carcinoma of the Upper Respiratory and Digestive Tracts	Adenocarcinoma of the Breast
50 Gy*	>90% subclinical 60% T1 lesions of nasopharynx 50% 1–3 cm neck nodes	>90% subclinical
60 Gy*	90% T1 lesions of pharynx and larynx 50% T3 and T4 lesions of tonsillar fossa	
70 Gy*	90% 1–3 cm neck nodes 70% 3–5 cm neck nodes 90% T2 lesions of tonsillar fossa and supraglottic larynx 80% T3 and T4 lesions of tonsillar fossa	90% clinically positive axillary nodes, 2.5 to 3 cm†
70–80 Gy (8–9 wk)		65% 2–3 cm primary 30% >5 cm primary
80–90 Gy (8–10 wk)		56% >5 cm primary
80–100 Gy (10–12 wk)		75% >5–15 primary

* 10 Gy in five fractions each week.
† Control rate is corrected for the percentage of nodes that would be positive histologically had dissection of the axilla been done.
(Reprinted with permission from Fletcher GH, Shukovsky LJ. The interplay of radiocurability and tolerance in the irradiation of human cancers. J. Radiol. Electrol. 1975;56:383.)

Gross Cancer

As a first approximation, the number of malignant clonogens is a function of the size of a tumor mass. In Table 1.3, doses giving a high control rate are correlated with increasing volume of cancer (27). Because tolerance is a function of the volume irradiated, the delivery of high doses necessitates the use of the shrinking field technique (Figure 1.9) (28).

The clinical variety and the extensions of the primary tumor are paramount determining factors in its radiocurability. For instance, infiltrative and ulcerative tumors of the base of the tongue and tumors of the anterior faucial pillar and retromolar trigone that have penetrated the masseter muscle or the pterygoid space are incurable by irradiation, no matter the scheme used.

Postoperative Setting

In a postoperative setting, the status of the margins must be considered (Figure 1.10) (29,30). When cancer is found at the margins of resection, the amount of residual tumor is greater than when the margins are clear. Table 1.4 shows that there are more local recurrences after surgery with unsatisfactory margins of resection than when margins are satisfactory (clear for 5 mm) (31).

The density of clonogenic infestation can be estimated by the incidence of failures after a surgical procedure. If multiple levels of nodes are involved in the surgical specimen after a radical neck dissection, the failure rate is higher than if a single level is involved (32). Recurrences after a radical neck dissection are more frequent when nodes are clinically and histologically positive than when nodes are clinically or histologically negative (Table 1.5) (33). Clinically and histologically positive nodes are likely to have a broken capsule, and the presence in the surgical specimen

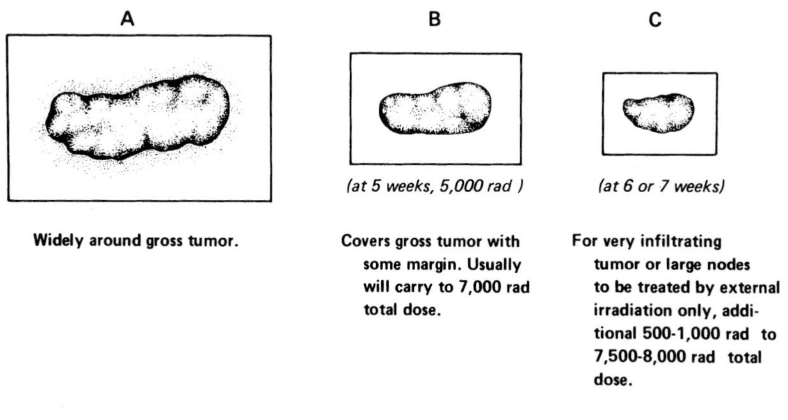

A
B
C
(at 5 weeks, 5,000 rad)
(at 6 or 7 weeks)
Widely around gross tumor.
Covers gross tumor with some margin. Usually will carry to 7,000 rad total dose.
For very infiltrating tumor or large nodes to be treated by external irradiation only, additional 500-1,000 rad to 7,500-8,000 rad total dose.

Figure 1.9. Shrinking field technique. (Reprinted with permission from Fletcher GH. Textbook of Radiotherapy. 3rd Ed. Philadelphia, Lea & Febiger, 1980.

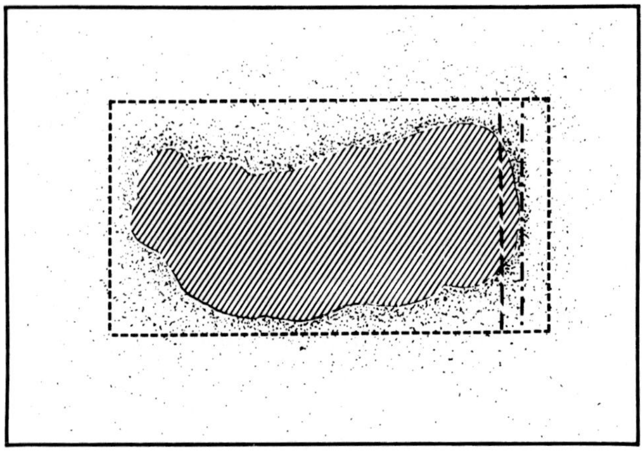

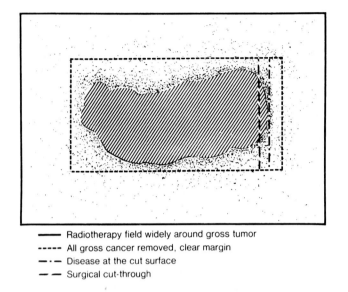

—— Radiotherapy field widely around gross tumor
----- All gross cancer removed, clear margin
—·— Disease at the cut surface
— — Surgical cut-through

Figure 1.10. Three discontinuous lines show three possibilities after surgical excision: 1) clear margin exists between gross disease and planes of resection; 2) disease is at margins of resection, although all gross disease seems to have been resected; and 3) gross disease is within margins of resection. (Reprinted with permission from Fletcher GH. Combined surgery and radiation therapy. *In* Modern Radiation Oncology: Classic Literature and Current Management 12:720, 1984.)

Table 1.4. Recurrence at the Primary Site After Multimethod Treatment in Stages III or IV Squamous Cell Carcinoma of the Head and Neck

Surgery Only 1960–1970		Surgery + Postop Irradiation 1975–1980	
Satisfactory Margins	Unsatisfactory Margins	Satisfactory Margins	Unsatisfactory Margins
39%	73%	2%	10.5%

(Reprinted with permission from Vikram B, Strong EW, Shah JP, Spiro R. Failure at the primary site following multimodality treatment in advanced head and neck cancer. Head Neck 1984;6:720.)

Table 1.5. Recurrences After Radical Neck Dissection According to Clinical or Histologic Staging and Doses of Irradiation

Staging	≤45 Gy	>45 Gy
N0 (clinical OR histologic)	20%	0%
N + (clinical AND histologic)	50%	20%

(Reprinted with permission from Arriagada R, Eschwege F, Cachin Y, Richard JM. The value of combining radiotherapy with surgery in the treatment of hypopharyngeal and laryngeal cancers. Cancer 1983;51:1819.)

Table 1.6. Breast Cancer: Percentage of Local-Regional Failures with 50 Gy Given Electively to Subclinical Deposits

Supraclavicular area after radical mastectomy (consecutive patients with axilla histologically positive)	1.5%
Chest wall and peripheral lymphatics after radical mastectomy (87% of patients with histologically positive axilla and a mean number of 9.8 of positive nodes in patients with positive nodes). No adjuvant chemotherapy.	9%
Chest wall and peripheral lymphatics after simple mastectomy and dissection of the lateral axilla for AJC stage III and IV, excluding inflammatory carcinoma and positive supraclavicular nodes	13%

(Reprinted with permission from Fletcher GH. Implications of the density of clonogenic infestation in radiotherapy. Int. J. Radiat. Oncol. Biol. Phys. 1986;12:1675.)

of disease in connective tissue is associated with a high failure rate in the radically dissected neck (34).

In breast cancer, the incidence of local-regional failures is a function of the advancement of disease in the breast and the axilla. When 50 Gy was given electively after radical mastectomy, an increased failure rate was found in association with increasing advancement of the local-regional disease (Table 1.6) (34). After resection of rectal or sigmoid cancers, the failure rate increases with increasing penetration of the bowel wall, the highest rate noted if disease has been peeled off from surrounding structures (35). In soft tissue sarcomas, the local recurrence rate with conservative excision and postoperative irradiation is higher in tumors that are undifferentiated and located in the fleshy parts than in those that are well-differentiated and located on the wrists or ankles (36). Even if all gross cancer has been removed, higher doses are needed in large undifferentiated soft tissue sarcomas than in small well-differentiated sarcomas.

Postoperatively, and for that matter after complete response following chemotherapy, residual clonogenic cells accelerate their growth, and dose adjustments should be made depending on the cycling time of the clonogens of a particular tumor. Squamous cell carcinomas of the upper respiratory and digestive tracts have a short cycling time, and so postoperative irradiation should not be delayed. Adenocarcinomas of the breast, except of the inflammatory type, have a slow cycling time. If both chemotherapy and irradiation are planned after mastectomy, the irradiation can probably be given within a few months after the operation, during interruption of the chemotherapy.

Dose adjustment in the postoperative setting depends on the volume of tissue irradiated. In the neck, 60 to 70 Gy can be delivered postoperatively to selected areas, but in breast cancer, these doses cannot be given on the chest wall because the volume of tissue irradiated is too large.

With doses in excess of 50 Gy, the incidence of fibrosis of the chest wall, rib fractures, and pneumonitis are prohibitive. The same dose limitation applies to irradiation combined with surgery in tumors of the pelvis. A small volume, however, may be boosted to doses greater than 50 Gy when the probability of residual disease is high (e.g., disease has extended to adjacent structures).

CLINICAL TREATMENT PLANNING

Clinical treatment planning comes before physical treatment planning. The first step is to decide to use primary irradiation or primary surgical intervention with postoperative irradiation if indicated. Then, the target volume to cover is determined, which in addition to the primary tumor (how generous the margins are to be), includes clinically positive nodes and clinically negative lymphatic areas to be irradiated electively. Control of a tumor mass that has developed in a short time or of a recurrence appearing shortly after a surgical procedure requires giving a high dose in a short time. Certain clinical data strongly suggest that in selected cases of squamous cell carcinoma of the upper respiratory and digestive tracts, 70 to 80 Gy delivered in 6 weeks using twice-a-day fractionation instead of 70 Gy in 7 to 7½ weeks with one daily treatment is advantageous. In inflammatory breast cancer, shortening the overall treatment time has proven effective (20).

The growth rate of a tumor mass is a useful indicator of the total number of clonogens to be sterilized, because it reflects the rate at which new clonogens are added to the tumor during a treatment lasting several weeks (37). The regression rate during treatment must be assessed cautiously; the total tumor dose must not be diminished too much if the regression rate is fast. The status at the end of treatment correlates better with prognosis if all of the tumor has clinically disappeared at the end of treatment (38).

Head and Neck

A 1.8 Gy fraction (i.e., 9 Gy per week) is not used unless large volumes are irradiated or the patient is fragile or elderly. Also, protracting the treatment by using a split course is not recommended because the accelerated repopulation that occurs in head and neck squamous cell carcinoma is now well known (39). Between 4 and 8 weeks, the potential doubling time is probably 4 days. If 1.8 Gy fractions are used, an extra 5 Gy should be given in two or three fractions.

The clinical variety, irrespective of the treatment scheme, must be very carefully considered when choosing primary irradiation for treatment and also in irradiation treatment planning. How generous the coverage should be for the primary tumor is based on the natural history of the tumor. For instance, in tumors of the pharyngeal walls, margins are very generous because of skipped areas.

Effective elective irradiation of clinically negative lymphatic areas requires only 50 Gy with 2 Gy per fraction. The areas covered depend on the location of the primary tumor and its aggressiveness. Data are available for each anatomic site (28). Determining the dose for clinically positive lymph nodes involves following the same guidelines for determining doses for the primary (see Table 1.3), while keeping in mind that lymph nodes from the tonsillar fossa and nasopharynx primaries are more radiocurable than those from other anatomic sites. In postoperative treatment, the timing and rate of recurrence must be considered. Irradiation of tumors of the pyriform sinus is started as soon as possible because recurrences appear early, by which time one is dealing with gross cancer (Figure 1.11) (37). If the patient already has a clinically detectable recurrence, accelerated fractionation is used (Figure 1.12) (30). The dose depends on the number of indications for postoperative irradiation (40). Positive or close margins, T_3 or T_4, multiple nodes involved, or extracapsular extension create a high risk situation for which the dose is 65 to 70 Gy in 6.5 to 8 weeks.

Breast Tumor

Gross cancer in breast carcinomas is not treated, except for recurrences on the chest wall after radical mastectomy; 50 Gy is then delivered to the whole chest wall and, with

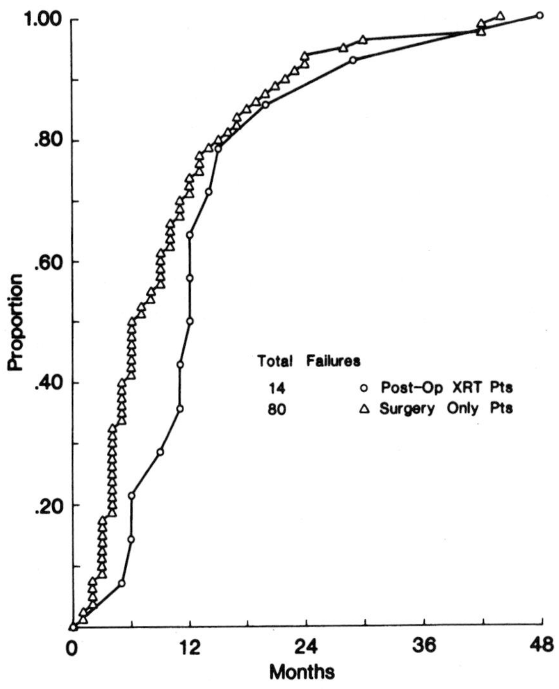

Figure 1.11. Cumulative rate of failure above clavicles (pyriform sinus). Almost one-half of failures in surgery-only group occurred by 6 months. (Reprinted with permission from Fletcher GH. Keynote address: The scientific basis of the present and future practice of clinical radiotherapy. Int J Radiat Oncol Biol Phys 1983;6:1073.)

small fields, as much as 65 or 70 Gy is given to gross masses. For primary advanced cancer, the first step in treatment is chemotherapy, possibly followed by mastectomy; irradiation is used for residual subclinical disease.

As an adjuvant to radical, modified radical, or simple mastectomy or to conservation surgery, 5000 rad to the chest wall and peripheral lymphatics is well-tolerated. After radical or simple mastectomy for advanced disease with a high proportion of involved axillary nodes, the local-regional failure rate is still in excess of 10% (Table 1.6). Giving more than 50 Gy in 5 weeks may be considered, but because very large areas of skin and thoracic cage are irradiated, 60 Gy in 6 weeks results in skin atrophy, rib fractures, and fibrosis of the anatomic structures of the shoulder that produces marked limitation of motion.

Pelvic Tumors

Squamous Cell Carcinoma of the Cervix

In cancers of the cervix, because of the T-shaped arrangement of the radioactive sources, a precipitous falloff of dose occurs from the radioactive sources to the outer

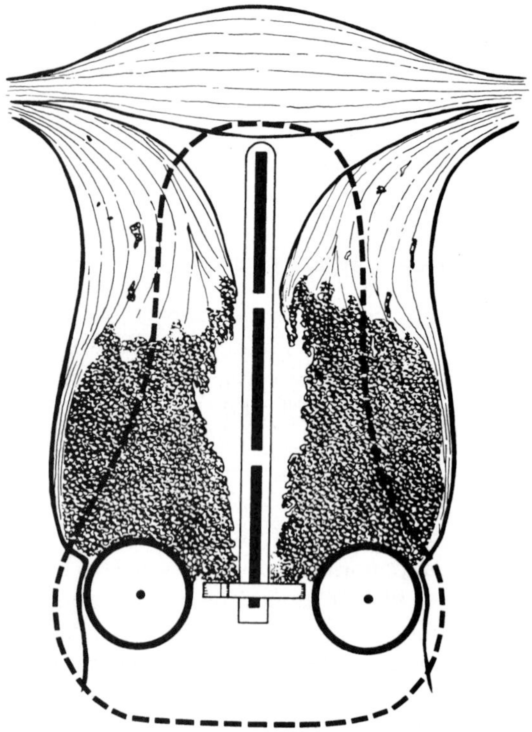

Figure 1.13. Squamous cell carcinoma of cervix involving lower uterine segment, producing a "barrel-shaped" lesion. Before intracavitary x-ray therapy is initiated, the lesion must be made to shrink so radioactive sources will be closer to peripheral margin of disease.

pelvic structures. The distance from the sources to the periphery of the disease is the main obstacle to adequate irradiation. This problem is exemplified best in the expanding tumors of the endocervix (Figure 1.13). To ensure effective brachytherapy, the expanding mass must be shrunk by external irradiation. The intracavitary applications deliver huge doses in the vicinity of the cervix, up to 300 Gy. The usual radiobiologic parameters used in external beam irradiation treatment alone are not applicable.

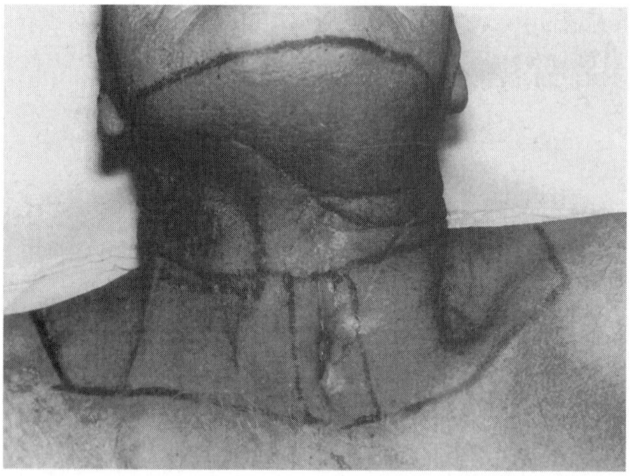

Figure 1.12. Patient with T4 lesion of right pyriform sinus and 6.5-cm mass in right side of the neck underwent laryngo-partial pharyngectomy and right radical neck dissection with reconstruction with deltopectoral flap in 1983. Tumor was attached to the carotid artery, but carotid was not removed because of previous bilateral endarterectomy. Pathologic examination revealed squamous cell carcinoma of right pyriform sinus. Because of a fistula, postoperative irradiation was delayed 6 weeks. Through parallel opposed portals, upper neck received 63 Gy in 7 weeks (1.8 Gy/fraction) and, through anterior appositional portals, lower neck received 52.2 Gy (2 Gy/fraction) in 5 weeks with cobalt 60 and 7 MeV. During treatment, mass developed in right side of the neck. Biopsy of the mass revealed squamous cell carcinoma. Concomitant boost of 20 Gy (10 $\times$ 2 Gy) was given to mass through small field with 7-MeV electron beam 4 hours after first treatment, bringing total dose to the mass to 83 Gy in 7 weeks. Patient died in 1988 of lung cancer with no evidence of disease above the clavicles. (Reprinted with permission from Fletcher GH. Implications of the density of clonogenic infestation in radiotherapy. Int J Radiat Oncol Biol Phys 1986;12:1675.)

References

1. Fletcher GH. Regaud lecture perspectives on the history of radiotherapy. Radiother Oncol 1988;12:253.
2. Puck TT, Marcus PI. Action of x-rays on mammalian cells. J Exp Med 1956;103:653.
3. Dutreix J, Wambersie A, Bounik, C. Cellular recovery in human skin reactions. Application to dose, fraction number, overall time relationship in radiotherapy. Eur J Cancer 1973;9:159.
4. Palcic B, Skarsgard LD. Reduced oxygen enhancement ratio at low doses of ionizing radiation. Radiat Res 1984;100:328.
5. Withers HR. Biologic basis of radiation therapy. In: Perez CA, Brady LW, eds. Principles and Practices of Radiation Oncology. Philadelphia: JB Lippincott, 1987.
6. Coutard H. Roentgentherapy of epitheliomas of the tonsillar re-ion, hypopharynx and larynx from 1920–1926, AJR 1932;28:313.
7. Spanos WJ, Montague ED, Fletcher GH. Late complications of radiation only for advanced breast cancer. Int J Radiat Oncol Biol Phys 1980;6:1473.

8. Bentzen SM, Overgaard M, Thames HD. Fractionation sensitivity of a functional endpoint: Impaired shoulder movement after post-mastectomy radiotherapy. Int J Radiat Oncol Biol Phys 1989;17:531-7.
9. Turesson I. The progression rate of late radiation effects in normal tissue and its impact on dose-response relationships. Radiother Oncol 1989;15:217-26.
10. Fowler JR. Fractionation and therapeutic gain. In: Steel GG, Adams GE, Peckham MJ, eds. The Biological Basis of Radiotherapy. Amsterdam, Elsevier Science, 1983.
11. Thames HD, Withers HR, Peters LJ, Fletcher GH. Changes in early and late radiation responses with altered dose fractionation: Implications for dose-survival relationships. Int J Radiat Oncol Biol Phys 1982;8:219.
12. Strandqvist M. Studien uber die Kumulative Wirkung der Rontgenstrahlen bei Fraktionierung. Acta Radiol Suppl (Stockh.) 1944;55:1.
13. Fowler JF, Stern BE. Dose-time relationships in radiotherapy and the validity of cell survival curve models. Br J Radiol 1963;36:163.
14. Ellis F. Fractionation in radiotherapy. In: Deeley TJ, Wood J, eds. Modern Trends in Radiotherapy. London, Butterworths, 1967.
15. Thames HD, Peters LJ, Withers HR, Fletcher GH. Accelerated fractionation vs. hyperfractionation: Rationales for several treatments per day. Int J Radiat Oncol Biol Phys 1983;9:127.
16. Withers JR, Thames HD, Peters LJ. A new isoeffect curve for change in dose per fraction. Radiother Oncol 1983;1:187.
17. Peters LJ, Ang KK, Thames HD, Jr. Accelerated fractionation in the radiation treatment of head and neck cancer: A critical comparison of different strategies. Acta Oncol 1988;27:185.
18. Paterson R. The Treatment of Malignant Disease by Radium and X-rays. Baltimore, Williams & Wilkins, 1949.
19. El Senoussi MA, Fletcher GH, Borlase BC. The correlation of radiation and surgery parameters with complications in the extended field technique for carcinoma of the cervix. Int J Radiat Oncol Biol Phys 1979; 5:927.
20. Barker JL, Nelson AJ, III, Montague ED. Inflammatory carcinoma of the breast. Radiology 1976; 121:173.
21. Steel G. Cell loss from experimental tumours. Cell Tissue Kinet 1968; 1:193.
22. Fletcher GH, Shukovsky LJ. Isoeffect exponents for the production of dose-response curves in squamous cell carcinomas treated between 4 to 8 weeks. J Radiol 1976; 57:825.
23. Malaise EP, Charbit A, Chavaudra N, et al. Change in volume of irradiated human metastases. Investigation of repair of sublethal damage and tumour repopulation. Br J Cancer 1972; 26:43.
24. vanPeperzeel HA. Effects of single doses of radiation on lung metastases in man and experimental animals. Eur J Cancer 1972;8:665.
25. Fletcher GH. Elective irradiation of subclinical disease in cancers of the head and neck. Cancer 1972; 29:1450.
26. Fletcher GH. Subclinical disease. Lucy Wortham James Lecture. Cancer 1984;33:1274.
27. Fletcher GH, Shukovsky LJ. The interplay of radiocurability and tolerance in the irradiation of human cancers. J Radiol 1975;56:383.
28. Fletcher GH. Textbook of Radiotherapy. 3rd Ed. Philadelphia, Lea & Febiger, 1980.
29. Fletcher GH. Combined surgery and radiation therapy. In: Modern Radiation Oncology: Classic Literature and Current Management 1984;12:720–751.
30. Fletcher GH. Implications of the density of clonogenic infestation in radiotherapy. Int J Radiat Oncol Biol Phys 1986;12:1675.
31. Vikram B, Strong EW, Shah JP, Spiro R. Failure at the primary site following multimodality treatment in advanced head and neck cancer. Head Neck 1984;6:720.
32. Strong EW. Preoperative irradiation and radical neck dissection. Surg Clin North Am 1969;49:271.
33. Arriagada R, Eschwege F, Cachin Y, Richard JM. The value of combining radiotherapy with surgery in the treatment of hypopharyngeal and laryngeal cancers. Cancer 1983;51:1819.
34. Cachin Y. Les modalities et la valeur pronostique de l'envahissement ganglionnaire cervical dans les carcinomas des voies aerodigestives superieures. Vie Med Can Fr 1972;1:48.
35. Withers HR et al. Elective radiation therapy in the curative treatment of cancer of the rectum and rectosigmoid colon. In: Stroehlein J, Romsdahl MM, eds. Gastrointestinal Cancer. New York, Raven, 1981.
36. Lindberg RD, Martin RG, Romsdahl MM, Barkley HT, Jr. Conservative surgery and postoperative radiotherapy in 300 adults with soft tissue sarcomas. Cancer 1981;47:2391.
37. Fletcher GH. Keynote address: The scientific basis of the present and future practice of clinical radiotherapy. Int J Radiat Oncol Biol Phys 1983;6:1073.
38. Barkley HT, Jr, Fletcher GH. The significance of residual disease after external irradiation of squamous cell carcinomas of the oropharynx. Radiology 1977;124:493.
39. Parsons JT, Bova FJ, Million RR. A reevaluation of split course technique for squamous cell carcinoma of the head and neck. Int J Radiat Oncol Biol Phys 1980;6:1645.
40. Amdur RJ, et al. Postoperative irradiation for squamous cell carcinoma of the head and neck: An analysis of treatment results and complications. Int J Radiat Oncol Biol Phys 1988;16:1.

Chapter 2

Clinical Principles and Applications of Chemoirradiation

Joseph Cirrone, Hassan Aziz, and Marvin Rotman

INTRODUCTION

In a substantial number of cancer patients, local tumor control remains a major problem. Several trials of high Linear Energy Transfer (LET) radiation (1), electron-affinic (misonidazole) compounds (2), and hyperthermia (3) failed to show significant benefits with respect to local control of a variety of tumors. In order to achieve better local tumor control, chemotherapy has been combined with irradiation. Ideally, the selected drugs for combined treatment should have established anticancer action against the tumor being treated as well as an ability to radiosensitize the tumor cells. An increased radiosensitivity may be achieved as a result of the inhibition of repair of sublethal and potentially lethal irradiation damage in tumor cells (including hypoxic cells), or by synchronization of cells in a radiosensitive phase of the cell cycle. In this chapter, the mechanism of action of specific drugs when used concomitantly with irradiation will be discussed, along with their toxicity and a brief summary of the clinical responses achieved in a variety of malignancies.

Biologic Basis of Combined Modality Therapy

In combined modality therapy, several biologic factors appear to enhance local tumor response (Table 2.1). Combined modality treatment may prevent emergence of resistant clones of tumor cells: cells resistant to one modality may be sensitive to another. Drug resistance that may arise because of changes in certain drug-activating enzymes may not apply to irradiation. However, cross resistance between radiation and chemotherapy is not uncommon (4).

Chemotherapy, given in relatively small amounts, can enhance the effect of radiation (5). The mechanism of radiosensitization may involve synchronization of the cell cycle by accumulating tumor cells into a radiation sensitive phase such as G2/M (e.g., Paclitaxel). In addition, oxygenation of hypoxic cells may occur (Mitomycin) or there may be inhibition of repair of sublethal or potentially lethal damage with drugs such as Cis-Platinum and Adriamycin (6,7). Concomitant chemotherapy and irradiation may inhibit or slow the rate of repopulation of tumor cells, thus increasing the effectiveness of the treatment (8).

Various methods of sequencing chemotherapy and irradiation have been employed. In the experience at SUNY-Health Science Center at Brooklyn, concomitant, continuous infusion chemotherapy and irradiation have produced the greatest cell kill with the least toxicity. Most chemotherapeutic agents are active only against cells in the deoxyribonucleic acid (DNA)- synthetic phase of the cell cycle. Since the synthetic phase is only a small portion of the cell cycle in most epithelial tumors, and most chemotherapeutic agents have short biologic half-lives (9), bolus administration significantly reduces the likelihood of exposure to drugs at the critical phase of the cell cycle. Continuous drug infusion overcomes this problem because it avoids the short-lived peak concentrations of drugs. Further, by avoiding these high concentrations, it produces less toxicity than bolus administration. Sequential administration of drugs appears to reduce toxicity, but can induce faster doubling time of the tumor. Alternating chemotherapy and radiation may reduce the risk to normal tissue as has been suggested by Looney (10). Such an approach might also be less effective for tumor control.

DRUGS USED WITH IRRADIATION

Chemotherapeutic agents used concomitantly with irradiation include 5-Fluorouracil (5-FU), Cis-Platinum

Table 2.1. Biologic Basis of Combined Modality Therapy

- Prevention of emergence of resistant tumor clones
- Radiosensitization of tumor cells
- Inhibition of tumor cell repopulation
- Reduced toxicity in normal tissues

(CDDP, Cisplatin), Doxorubicin (Adriamycin), Paclitaxel (Taxol), Mitomycin-C, Hydroxyurea, and Camptothecins (Table 2.2).

5-Fluorouracil (5-FU)

The effect of 5-Fluorouracil (5-FU), a cell cycle-specific antimetabolite, as a radiosensitizer has been known for more than 40 years, though the exact mechanisms of its synergistic activity are not fully understood (11). Heidelberger et al (12) and others (13,14,15) showed that when suboptimal doses of 5-FU and radiation were combined, greater tumoricidal effects were seen in experimental animals. As a result of in vitro experiments (16,17), it was suggested that the timing of therapy plays an important role in optimizing the radiosensitizing effect. The greatest benefit was seen when 5-FU was given from 5 minutes up to 8 hours after the dose of irradiation. Concurrent continuous infusion of 5-FU avoids peak concentrations of the drug, decreasing the myelotoxicity seen with bolus administration; however, the incidence of diarrhea and mucositis is increased, requiring close monitoring during treatment.

Cisplatinum (CDDP, Cisplatin)

When Cisplatin and radiation were used concomitantly, there was considerable enhancement of cell killing (18,19). Two mechanisms of radiation enhancement have been suggested (20,7): The first, applicable in hypoxic or oxygenated cells, occurs at the time of irradiation and involves formation of free radicals with altered binding of platinum to DNA. The second inhibits repair of sublethal damage and may be the most important effect of concomitant Cisplatin and radiation therapy. When Cisplatin is used with hyperfractionated irradiation, a further enhancement of radiation damage can be achieved (21,22). In addition, a decrease in the side effects of nausea and nephrotoxicity may be seen with continuous infusion Cisplatin. Carboplatin, a Cisplatin analog that can be given in higher doses with less toxicity, appears to have similar radiosensitizing effects.

Table 2.2. Outline of Common Chemotherapy Agents Used with Radiation

Agent	Mechanism of Action	Radiosensitizing Effect	Treatable Tumors Sites	Side Effect Profile
5-Fluorouracil (5-FU)	Binds Thymidylate Synthetase Inhibits DNA Synthesis.	Inhibits repair of sublethal damage.	Gastrointestinal Head and Neck Bladder Cervix	Myelotoxicity Mycotoxicity Mucositis Diarrhea
Cis-platinum (CDDP)	Crosslinking of DNA Bases inhibits DNA Synthesis.	Inhibits repair of potentially lethal and sublethal damage.	Gyn Head and Neck Bladder Lung (non-small cell and small cell)	Nephrotoxicity Nausea Peripheral Neuropathy
Doxorubicin (Adriamycin)	Inhibits mitochondrial cellular respiration leading to topoisomerase II activation and fragmentation of DNA.	Inhibits repair of single strand DNA breaks.	Soft tissue Sarcoma Hepatoma	Cardiomyopathy Radiation recall (Hypersensitivity reaction)
Paclitaxel (Taxol)	Stabilization of microtublar elements - Inhibits microtubular function during interphase and mitosis.	Synchronizes cells in G2/M phase of cell cycle (radiosensitive phase).	Central Nervous System Breast Lung (non-small cell) Ovary Head and Neck	Myelosuppression Hypersensitivity Sensory Neuropathy
Mitomycin-C (MMC)	Crosslinking of DNA Bases Inhibits DNA Synthesis.	Enhanced radiosensitivity in hypoxic environment.	Anal	Myelosuppression Hemolytic Uremic Syndrome (HUS)
Hydroxyurea (HU)	Inhibits ribonucleotide reductase during DNA Synthesis.	Increased tumor cell kill during S-phase of cell cycle (radioresistant phase).	Central Nervous System Cervix Head and Neck	Myelosuppression
Camptothecin (Topotecan) (Irinotecan)	Inhibition of Topoisomerase I during DNA Synthesis.	Inhibition of Sublethal and Potentially Lethal Damage. Assist Radiation Induced Cell Death (Apoptosis).	Colon Head and Neck Lung	Myelosuppression (Neutropenia) Diarrhea

Doxorubicin (Adriamycin)

Several factors may be involved where adriamycin is used as a radiosensitizer. Although the mechanisms are not well understood (23,24), adriamycin is an inhibitor of mitochondrial and tumor cell respiration, which reduces oxygen consumption by the cells in the outer layer of the tumor. This provides more oxygen to centrally located anoxic cells. It has also been shown that Adriamycin inhibits the enzymatic repair of irradiation-induced single-strand breaks of DNA (25). Despite the observation that the combination can be well-tolerated (23,26), its concomitant use with irradiation was avoided because it was thought to be cardiotoxic and was associated with enteritis and esophagitis. Infusion of doxorubicin over 48 to 96 hours decreased cardiac injury (27), as did a 96-hour continuous infusion with a dose not exceeding 60 mg/m^2 per cycle (28). Five-day continuous infusions have also shown decreased cardiac toxicity when compared to bolus administration (29). The radiosensitizing effect is greatest when the drug is given during or just after radiation (30).

Paclitaxel (Taxol)

A microtubular inhibitor, Paclitaxel, acts by stabilizing microtubules at low concentrations and preventing mitosis by blocking cells in the G2/M phase of the cell cycle. This portion of the cell cycle is radiosensitive, which may lead to greater radiosensitivity when the drug is combined with irradiation. Steren and associates (31) showed that treatment with Taxol 48 hours before the administration of radiation had a greater sensitizing effect than treatment only 24 hours before. Common toxicities associated with Taxol are neutropenia, hypersensitivity reactions, and neurosensory changes.

Mitomycin-C

Although Mitomycin-C is classified as an antibiotic, its mechanism of action mimics that of an alkylating agent. Activation of Mitomycin-C occurs when the drug is enzymatically reduced, enabling it to cross-link with DNA and inhibit DNA synthesis. The drug is more toxic to hypoxic cells (32) and because hypoxic cells are radioresistant, especially in necrotic tumors, concomitant infusion of Mitomycin-C may act as a sensitizer of these cells. Preclinical studies revealed supra-additive cell kill when the drug was administered 15 minutes or 24 hours prior to irradiation (33,34). When given after radiation, only an additive effect resulted (34). Mitomycin-C has been used primarily in the treatment of gastrointestinal tumors. In the Radiation Therapy Oncology Group (RTOG) anal carcinoma study, the addition of Mitomycin-C to 5-FU enhanced local control and survival. In a prospective randomized trial comparing radiation and Mitomycin-C to radiation alone in head and neck cancer, a significant increase in locoregional control in the combined modality arm with no increase in toxicity was revealed (35).

The major toxicity attributed to this drug is dose-limiting myelosuppression. Mitomycin-C has also been implicated in the development of Hemolytic Uremic Syndrome (HUS), which consists of microangiopathic hemolytic anemia, thrombocytopenia, and renal failure.

Hydroxyurea

Hydroxyurea is an antimetabolite that functions by inhibiting ribonucleotide reductase, which impairs DNA synthesis and causes cell death. This activity primarily occurs during the S phase of the cell cycle. S phase cells are usually radioresistant and in this phase hydroxyurea shows increased cell kill when combined with irradiation (36,37,38). Currently, clinical studies with 5-FU, Hydroxyurea, and irradiation in cervical, central nervous system (CNS), and head and neck cancers are ongoing.

Camptothecins

Camptothecins (Topotecan, Irinotecan) are a new class of antineoplastic agents that cause cytotoxicity through inhibition of topoisomerase I. This occurs during the S phase of the cell cycle and causes breakage in the DNA during replication. Preclinical trials suggest that camptothecins may potentiate radiation-induced cell death (39). Postulated mechanisms of action between camptothecins and irradiation include inhibition of sublethal or potentially lethal damage repair after radiotherapy as shown in two human melanoma cell lines (40). This increases the proportion of cells in the S phase by slowing the rate of progression with radiation and increasing sensitivity to the drug (41). Hennequin (41) also showed supra-additivity of cell killing in HeLa cells and V-79 fibroblast cell lines following concomitant exposure to camptothecin and low dose rate radiation.

Camptothecins are active against colon, ovarian, lung, esophageal, and head and neck cancers. Clinical trials combining camptothecins and radiation therapy are currently underway for advanced lung, head and neck, and colon cancers, especially in recurrent disease. The major dose limiting toxicities reported are myelosuppression and diarrhea.

CLINICAL EXPERIENCE

Advanced carcinomas of the gastrointestinal tract, head and neck, lung, cervix, and urinary bladder have been treated with combined modality therapy. Experience in combined modality therapy with advanced soft tissue sarcomas and mesotheliomas is limited and anecdotal. A variety of drug and dose delivery and sequencing methods have been used; however, concomitant use of infusion therapy with radiation continues to show the most encouraging results.

Carcinomas of the Gastrointestinal Tract

Carcinoma of the Anus Until recently, abdominoperineal resection has been the standard treatment for carcinoma of the anus (Table 2.3). Unimpressive survival statistics of 30 to 60%, high local recurrence rates of 25 to 40%, and associated severe morbidity have led to the call for improved therapeutic options (42,43). As a result of radiation sensitivity of the perineum and perianal tissues, the use of radiation therapy was difficult to advocate in all but the most superficially infiltrating tumors. Nigro (44) used a small radiation dose of 3,000-3,500 cGy, concomitant 5-FU infusion and Mitomycin-C bolus which successfully ablated large infiltrating anal cancers. Nigro (45) also reported using this schema as a neoadjuvant treatment prior to definitive abdominoperineal resection or local excision. Local control rates of 85% and a 5-year survival rate of 80% were reported.

From those early reports, other investigators who used progressively higher doses of radiation and 5-FU, with or without Mitomycin-C, showed that larger, more infiltrating tumors could be successfully treated and that the use of abdominoperineal resection could be reserved for radiation failures. Cummings (46) treated these patients with continuous radiation (5,000 cGy at 250 cGy per fraction) with concomitant infusion of 5-FU and bolus administration of Mitomycin-C. As the complication rate was high, a split course technique of 2,400 cGy (200 cGy per fraction in each split course of radiation), 5-FU infusion of 1,000 mg/m^2/day for 4 days, and bolus administration of Mitomycin-C at 10 mg/m^2 during each course was used. Local control for tumors larger than 5 cm was reported to be 90% and 5-year survival was 76% (47). To reduce morbidity, John and colleagues (48) used a shrinking field technique and a low dose of radiation (5,000-5,500 cGy) to produce a complete response rate of 86% for T3 and T4 tumors.

Sischy's group (49) reported preliminary results from an RTOG trial. Results were evaluated for tumors that were either smaller or larger than 3 cm in diameter. The local control of tumors smaller than 3 cm was 84% at 8 months, and for tumors greater than 3 cm in diameter, it was 62%. The disease-free survival at 2 years was 77% and 53%, respectively. This study showed that the rate of complete response is dependent on tumor size and adequacy of the treatment. This protocol employed a total of 4,080 cGy concomitantly with two 96-hour infusions of 5-FU. Byfield (50) concluded that if the infusion period is reduced by 24 hours (from 120 to 96), cell kill will be reduced by at least one log. Byfield then recommended multiple 120-hour 5-FU infusions, and a radiation dose of 5,000 cGy, dependent upon the tumor size.

In a randomized trial, the European Organization for Research and Treatment of Cancer (EORTC), Roelofsen (51) reported the results of combined treatment where radiation alone (6,000-6,500 cGy) was compared to radiation plus 5-FU (75 mg/m^2 for 5 days [days 1-5 and 29-33]) and Mitomycin-C (15 mg/m^2 on day 1) for patients with T3 and T4 or T1-2, N1-3 disease. Results with combined modality therapy fared better at 77% versus 53% ($p<0.01$). For small tumors of the anus, the difference was not so obvious. The RTOG and the Eastern Cooperative Oncology Group (ECOG), in an intergroup trial (52), confirmed the efficacy of Mitomycin-C with a 75% survival of 4 years in the 5-FU, Mitomycin-C, and radiation group of patients versus 51% in the 5-FU and radiation group alone.

Carcinoma of the Rectum Major advances in multimodality therapy, specifically for Stages II and III rectal adenocarcinoma are expected to improve survival rates over the next decade (53). Reports from the Gastrointestinal Tumor Study Group (GITSG), the North Central Cancer Treatment Group (NCCTG), and the National Surgical Adjuvant Breast

Table 2.3. Treatment of Carcinoma of Anus with Chemotherapy and Radiation

Reference	No. of Patients	Treatment	CR Rate	Survival (%)
Nigro et al (44) (1974)	28	3000 cGy/3wk + 5-FU infusion × 5d at 1000 mg/m^2/d and mitomycin-C bolus on d1 at 15 mg/m^2 (pre-op).	74% at surgery increased to 85% APR	80% at 5 yrs
Cummings et al (46) (1983)	31	5000 cGy/4wk or 2500 cGy/2wk at 5-FU infusion × 4 d at 1000 mg/m^2/d with bolus mitomycin-C 10mg/m^2/d1.	90%	76%
John et al (48) (1987)	22	3060 cGy to entire pelvis/3.5 wk + 900–1000 cGy additional to lower pelvis and primary with 5-FU infusion × 4d at 1000 mg/m^2/dx^2 with mitomycin-C bolus at 15 mg/m^2 on d1.	86% for T3/T4 tumors	
Sischy et al (49) (1989)	29	4000–4500 cGy 4–5 wks and 5-FU infusion × 4 d at 1000 mg/m^2/d × 2 with mitomycin-C bolus on d1 at 10mg/m^2 (1000–1500 cGy Boost RT added).	89%	85%
Roelofsen et al (51) (1995)		6000–6500 cGy with 5-FU (75 mg/m2) day 1–5, 29–33 mmc 15 mg/m2 day.	RT alone 53% RT/CT 77%	

and Bowel Project (NSABP) have shown improved local control and survival with postoperative external irradiation, 5-FU, and Methyl-CCNU chemotherapy in resectable carcinoma of the rectum. (54,55,56).

Preoperative concomitant infusional 5-FU has been used in the treatment of advanced carcinomas of the rectum (13). In a series of 64 patients with ulcerated tumors in the lower third of the rectum, 4 cm in diameter or larger, no tumor was found in 12.5% of surgical specimens after treatment, as outlined below. Only 26.5% had positive nodes after treatment with 4,000 cGy/4.5 weeks of preoperative irradiation with courses 5-FU infusion (96 hours) beginning on days 2 and 28 of radiation, and 10 mg/m^2 of Mitomycin-C. In advanced disease, one would expect 40% of patients to have positive nodes. The reported overall disease-free 5-year survival rate was 64%.

Rich and associates (57) used a protracted 30-day 5-FU infusion concomitantly with radiation therapy for patients with advanced residual or recurrent rectal cancer. 5-FU (300 mg/m^2/day) was administered throughout the course of radiotherapy. Results from this study were promising, and it is currently being compared to standard therapy as an RTOG protocol.

Randomized trials are currently being conducted to determine the value of both preoperative and postoperative combined modality therapy. Preoperative therapy may improve resectability, local control rates, and in some cases preservation of the sphincter. On the other hand, postoperative therapy may allow the adjustment of therapy according to surgical and pathologic findings (58).

Carcinoma of the Esophagus Results of single modality therapy for carcinoma of the esophagus have been disappointing (Table 2.4) (59,60). Usually, at the time of presentation, the cancer is locally advanced and has spread hematogenously. Doggett and colleagues from Stanford University (61) reported that in 58% of patients who died, the tumor was confined to the esophagus and/or the regional nodes in the epigastric region. This supports the belief that local and regional failure remains an important component of poor survival.

Studies from Leichman (62) and the Southwest Oncology Group (63) showed that 3,000 cGy, 5-FU infusion, and bolus administration of Cisplatin or Mitomycin-C preoperatively could produce complete response rates of 25%. In the latter study, 80% of the patients who had evidence of tumors in the surgical specimen died of distant metastasis. Patients who had no residual tumor had a survival rate of 60%, which suggests the futility of surgery in advanced cases. Richmond and associates (64) further confirmed these results in a three-arm study: irradiation alone was compared with irradiation and infusion chemotherapy and with irradiation together with infusion chemotherapy and surgery. The median survivals were 5, 12, and 14 months respectively, and revealed no significant benefit of the addition of surgery to radiation with infusion chemotherapy. In later trials, higher doses of radiation with 5-FU infusion and bolus administration of Cisplatin and Mitomycin-C were used with curative intent.

John (65) treated three groups of clinical Stage II and III patients with progressively more intense radiation and chemotherapy, which led to improved local control and survival. This work did much to set the stage for other investigators to use multidrug chemotherapy and more intense radiotherapy in the treatment of esophageal cancer.

Coia et al (66,67) reported that 57 patients (out of a series of 90) with Stage I and II disease were treated curatively. The remainder of patients with Stage III and IV disease were treated palliatively. All patients received 6,000 cGy, along with two courses of 96-hour 5-FU infusion and

Table 2.4. Treatment of Carcinoma of the Esophagus with Chemotherapy and Radiation Therapy

Reference	No. of Patients	Treatment	CPR	Survival
Leichman et al (62) (1984)	55	3000 cGy/3 wk 5-FU infusion × 4d at 1000 mg/m^2/d × 2 with mitomycin at 15 mg/m^2 on d1 or Cisplatin at 100 mg/m^2 on day 1, 19 (pre-op).	25%	60%–2 yrs
John et al (65) (1989)	21	3000–5040 cGy/3.5–5.5 wk 5-FU infusion × 4d on wk 1, 4, 8, 12 at 1000 mg/m^2/d with mitomycin bolus alt with Cisplatin 75 mg/m^2 wk 4, 12 and mitomycin 10 mg/m^2 wk 1, 9.	77%	15 mos median survival
Coia et al (66) (1991)	30	6000 cGy × 6–7 wk 5-FU infusion at 1000 mg/m^2/d × 2 and mitomycin bolus at 10 mg/m^2/d^2.	—	24 mos. median survival. 91% 2yr. OS Stage I 33% 2yr. OS Stage II
Forastiere et al (69) (1990)	43	3750 cGy/3 wk or 4500 cGy at 150 Cgy BID/3 wk with Cisplatin 20 mg/m^2/d infusion d1–5 and 17–21 and 5-FU continuous infusion 300 mg/m^2/d × 21d vinblastine bolus 1 mg/m^2/d d1–4 and 17–20 (pre-op, transhiatal Esophagectomy day 42).	24%	median survival >26 mos. 59% 2yr. OS.
Al-Sarraf et al (72) (1997)	61	5000 cGy/5 wk with 5-FU infusion day 1–4 at 1000 mg/m^2/d and 4 wk later with Cisplatin 75 mg/m^2/d and d1 each 5-FU.	—	14.1 mos median survival. 27% 5yr survival rate. (6% RT alone group)

Mitomycin-C. The 2-year survival for squamous cell carcinoma in the curative group was 57%, compared to 38% for adenocarcinoma. Two-year survival was 91% for Stage I patients and 33% for Stage II. Good palliation for those who were not treated for cure was obtained; median survival in this group was 8 months. In contrast, Keane and colleagues (68) studied a series of 35 patients with advanced unresectable esophageal carcinomas. A curative dose of radiation therapy (continuous or split course) and concomitant 5-FU infusion (1,000 $mg/m^2/day \times 1$ or 2) with Mitomycin-C bolus (10 mg/m^2) was administered. A complete response rate of 48% and a 2-year survival rate of 28% were reported. Patients who responded later died of their disease.

Other promising results were reported by Forastiere and Rich. Forastiere and colleagues (69) used hyperfractionated radiation with intensive infusional chemotherapy in a preoperative, neoadjuvant setting in a series of 43 patients and achieved a 20 to 25% complete response rate at surgery, a median survival of 29 months and a 2-year survival rate of 59%. Rich (70) used 6,000 cGy over 6.5 weeks on 12 patients, along with protracted infusion of 5-FU at 300 $mg/m^2/day$ concomitantly with radiation. A median survival of 24 months was reported.

The most significant study was reported by Herskovic and colleagues for RTOG (71). In a prospective clinical trial from 1986 to 1990, 125 patients were randomized to determine whether concomitant 5-FU and bolus administration of Cisplatin were superior to radiation alone. At 12 months, the radiation alone group had a survival rate of 33%, while the combined modality therapy group had a survival rate of 50%. At 2 years, survival of the radiation therapy group was 7%, and for the combined radiation and chemotherapy group 37%. Although side effects were higher in the combined modality group, they were outweighed by the survival advantage. A recent 5-year follow-up report of these patients by Al-Sarraf and colleagues (72) confirmed the benefit of a combined modality group. Five-year survival rate for the radiation therapy alone group was 0% and 27% for the combined modality group.

Burmeister and associates (73) reported on 137 patients treated with irradiation (6,000 cGy) plus two courses of Cisplatin and 5-FU; the 2-year survival rate was 54%.

Although the overall survival of patients with esophageal carcinoma remains inadequate, new therapies combining concomitant radiation therapy and chemotherapy promise a better quality of life through maintenance of a functioning esophagus, while not adversely affecting survival. Further studies are needed on the optimal dose of radiation and on the optimal selection and concentrations of drugs.

Carcinoma of the Pancreas

Resectable Pancreatic Cancer Less than 25% of patients who present with pancreatic cancer are eligible for curative surgery. Locoregional recurrence after the Whipple procedure is as high as 50% with median survivals of 10 to 20 months (74). In an attempt to prevent recurrence and improve survival, postoperative radiation therapy has been used with or without chemotherapy. GITSG (75) reported on a randomized trial where patients who were treated with surgery alone were compared to patients who were adjuvantly treated with 5-FU infusion and radiation therapy. Twenty of the 49 patients received radiation therapy (2,000 cGy) in two split courses over 2 weeks, each separated by an interval of 2 weeks. These patients concomitantly received intravenous bolus injection of 5-FU (500 $mg/m^2/day$) for the first 3 days of each course of radiation. Two-year disease-free survival for the surgery alone group was 15% compared to 42% for the combined modality therapy group.

Unresectable Pancreatic Cancer Since the 1960s, radiation therapy along with 5-FU chemotherapy have been the standard of care for unresectable pancreatic carcinoma. Childs and associates (76) and Moertel and colleagues (77) determined that 5-FU combined modality therapy was superior to radiation therapy alone. Smith and colleagues (78) (1983) conducted a phase II trial to test combined chemotherapy treatment of Streptozotocin, Mitomycin-C, and 5-FU (SMF), plus 5-FU against irradiation alone. This study also showed that radiation therapy alone was inferior to combined modality therapy. A GITSG study (79) showed that by using combination SMF and 5-FU during the fifth and last 3 days of irradiation, it was better than SMF alone (41% versus 19% 1-year survival). This confirmed the basis of chemoirradiation in the treatment of pancreatic carcinoma.

Another GITSG study (80) undertook a phase III trial with three arms: high dose double split course of radiation therapy (6,000 cGy) and intravenous bolus of 5-FU chemoirradiation where 5-FU was given with split course radiation (6,000 cGy or 4,000 cGy). The high dose radiation therapy alone arm was abandoned because of poor results. Median survival rates for the chemoirradiation arms were 36.5 weeks with 4,000 cGy and 49.4 weeks with 6,000 cGy. However, the toxicity from the 6,000 cGy chemoirradiation group was severe.

Gunderson and associates (81) used electron boost intraoperative radiation therapy (2,000 cGy) at the time of surgical exploration. The remainder of the treatment consisted of 4,500 to 5,000 cGy given with external beam irradiation along with concomitant 5-FU intravenous bolus (500 $mg/m^2/day$) given during the first 3 days of weeks 1 and 5 of external therapy. Forty-nine patients were entered into the trial and results were compared to those of patients who received only external therapy and 5-FU without electron boost intraoperative radiation therapy. There was an increase in the local control rate from 48% to 82% at 1 year. There was no increase in the median survival rate because patients failed distally in the abdomen and liver.

To combat these patterns of failure, Komaki and colleagues (82) at the Medical College of Wisconsin designed a protocol combining pancreatic radiotherapy (6,120 cGy in 34 fractions), prophylactic liver radiotherapy (23,400 cGy in 13 fractions), and a single course of concomitant 5-FU chemotherapy (500 mg/m^2/day) on days 1 through 3 of pancreatic irradiation. There was considerable improvement in the disease-free survival, which was 47% at 2 years. The median survival of 60 weeks was better than the conventional GITSG regimen (1988).

Rich (83) reported on the results of a study of protracted infusion of 5-FU (250 to 300 mg/m^2/day) during the entire course of radiation therapy (5,500 cGy). Fifteen patients received 1 to 2 g/day of intraperitoneal 5-FU infusion for 5 days, followed by external beam radiotherapy and intravenous 5-FU treatment. A 35% survival rate and 32% local control rate were evident at 22 months. Toxicity, however, was considerable.

Recently, Gemcitobine has been used in the treatment of unresectable pancreatic carcinoma. The current series (84) are promising for their combined use with irradiation.

Hepatic Metastasis (Carcinoma of the Colon) The liver is a common site of metastasis from colon carcinoma. At diagnosis, approximately 10% of patients present with hepatic metastasis, but ultimately the liver will be involved in as many as 70% of patients (85). In more than half the patients that die of advanced disease, the liver is the only site of metastasis (86). Untreated patients have a poor prognosis (87), with a median survival of 6 to 20 weeks. Treatment options for hepatic metastasis are varied and are dependent on several factors. These factors include the overall condition of the patient, number and size of the lesions, and control of primary and other metastatic disease. Treatment options include surgical resection, systemic chemotherapy, intra-arterial chemotherapy, and radiation therapy alone or with infusional chemotherapy. These treatments may be used with hopes of prolonging survival or for palliation of symptoms.

While radiation remains a major therapy for patients with multiple metastases, single modality therapy results have been disappointing. Using radiotherapy alone can give adequate palliation for painful hepatic metastases, but produces an average survival rate of no longer than 4.5 months (88,89). RTOG showed there was no benefit with the use of the radiosensitizer misonidazole (90). Sullivan (91) and Lokich and colleagues (92) obtained response rates of 59 to 62% with intra-arterial infusion of 5-FU or 5-fluro-2′-deoxyuridine (FUDR) with radiation. In the Lokich series, 50% of the patients developed thrombosis at the catheter site. The Central Oncology Group showed there was no benefit of hepatic artery infusion over intravenous infusion of 5-FU, although others have shown a benefit with intra-arterial infusion.

At the SUNY-Health Science Center at Brooklyn, Rotman (93) reported on the use of split course radiation with systemic continuous infusion of 5-FU. A series of 27 patients were treated with external radiation (2,700 to 3,200 cGy to the whole liver in five daily fractions of 150 to 200 cGy) and concomitant intravenous 5-FU (25 mg/kg/day) over 5 days during weeks 1, 3, and 5. No complete objective response was achieved, as evidenced by pre- and post-treatment liver scanning and liver function tests. Partial responses, however, were obtained in 56% of the patients. The median survival of these patients was 45 weeks. Thirty-five percent of the patients with disease confined only to the liver had a median survival of 49 weeks; patients with multiple organ or lung involvement had a median survival of only 25 weeks. Karnofsky performance status appeared to be an important prognostic indicator: Patients with scores of more than 60 had median survivals of 49 weeks; patients with scores of less than 60 had median survivals of 27 weeks. Toxicity from this protocol was limited. These results suggest that hepatic irradiation with concomitant administration of 5-FU infusion can be administered safely in patients with hepatic metastasis.

Carcinoma of the Head and Neck

Historically, surgery and radiation therapy have been the primary definitive therapies for head and neck carcinoma. Although the use of chemotherapy has produced impressive results, it has not translated clinically into significantly prolonged survivals. In most patients, at the time of diagnosis, the disease is still confined to the locoregional area even though it is advanced.

Fletcher and associates (94), in a randomized trial for advanced squamous cell carcinoma of the head and neck, showed that bolus 5-FU with radiation increased acute and late toxicity and did not increase survival. Lo and colleagues (95) used 5-FU infusion concomitantly with radiotherapy, which showed an increase in 5-year survival. Adelstein and colleagues (96), Byfield and colleagues (97), Hahn and colleagues (98), Kaplan and colleagues (99), Keane and colleagues (100), and Murthy and colleagues (101) all reported higher than expected complete response and survival rates in the treatment of advanced tumors of the head and neck with continuous and split course radiation and concomitant 5-FU with various combinations of Cisplatin and Mitomycin-C.

Choi et al, at the SUNY-Health Science Center at Brooklyn (102), treated advanced or recurrent carcinomas of the paranasal sinuses or nasopharynx with Cisplatin infusion (5 to 7 mg/m^2/day) for 2 weeks with hyperfractionated radiation (125 cGy/fraction) twice a day. Cycles were repeated two to three times with rest periods of 1 to 2 weeks. A complete response rate of 91% and 2-year overall survival of 67% was reported. Five-year survival was 58%.

For the treatment of unresectable carcinoma of the head and neck, Taylor and colleagues (103) used bolus Cisplatin and 5-FU infusion concomitantly with radiation. Treatment was given every other week for seven cycles. On day 1 of each cycle, Cisplatin (60 $mg/m^2/day$) was administered by intravenous bolus and 5-FU (800 $mg/m^2/day$) was administered by 120-hour intravenous infusion from days 1 to 5. The total dose of radiation was 7,000 cGy. They reported a complete response rate of 55% and a median survival of 37 months. For unresectable disease, Harrison and associates (104) used conventional and hyperfractionated radiation with Cisplatin. They reported a complete response rate of 64%. At present, concomitant radiotherapy, Taxol, 5-FU, and Hydroxyurea are being used in the treatment of advanced or recurrent carcinomas of the head and neck with some success. In addition, the concurrent use of Taxol and Carboplatin with radiation is being studied in the treatment of advanced carcinomas of the head and neck (105). Preliminary results of phase I trials of intensive radiotherapy and prolonged continuous infusion of Taxol for the treatment of solid tumors have been reported with acceptable toxicity (106,107). There has been further progress in the treatment of advanced carcinoma of the head and neck. Concurrent radiation with Taxol and 5-FU and hydroxyurea have been used with encouraging results (108). Preliminary results of a phase I trial using prolonged Taxol infusion with irradiation have been reported. Since toxicity was acceptable, dose escalation is being tested.

Gynecologic Cancers

Cervical Cancer It is estimated that 60% of patients who die of cervical cancer have local treatment failure. Paunier and colleagues (109) demonstrated that with local control of disease, the rate of distant metastasis is low, 2.5 to 17%. The rate rises to 35 to 75% with local failure. Even though radiation therapy has been the conventional treatment for locally advanced carcinoma of the cervix, earlier attempts to achieve better control rates with the radiosensitizer misonidazole or hyperbaric oxygen have failed. In addition, attempts to increase survival by increasing the dose of radiation have been met with a high rate of toxicity.

Several investigators have used the successful treatment of anal cancer as a model for the treatment of advanced cervical cancer. Initial studies by Thomas' group at Princess Margaret Hospital (110) used concomitant radiation therapy and 5-FU with Mitomycin-C bolus, and reported a complete response rate of 74% with a 15-month disease-free survival rate of 59%. Ludgate and colleagues (111) treated 38 patients with bulky Stage IIB through IVA disease with two cycles of 5-FU infusion (1,000 $mg/m^2/day$ on days 2 to 5 and 21 to 24 of radiation) and a single bolus of Mitomycin-C (10 mg/m^2 on the first day) concurrently with irradiation. Complete responses were reported in 70% of the patients, with 3-year overall survival rates of 55%.

John and associates (112) treated advanced cervical carcinoma with 5-FU infusion, irradiation, and Cisplatin. A 100% complete response rate in a small series of patients was reported. Eighty percent were still alive and free of disease at 28 months. Perez and Associates (113) revealed no significant improvement in pelvic tumor control or disease-free survival in patients with squamous cell carcinoma of the cervix treated with chemotherapy and irradiation. Perez recommended that patients with locally advanced squamous cell carcinoma (stage IB>4cm—IVA) of the cervix should be considered for randomized trials, such as the RTOG trial comparing pelvic and para-aortic irradiation (best arm of RTOG protocol 79-20) with pelvic irradiation and three concomitant chemotherapy cycles of cisplatin and 5-FU.

Other Gynecologic Cancers Other recurrent or advanced gynecologic tumors have been treated with 5-FU infusion and radiotherapy, however, the studies were small. Evans and associates (114) reported 46% of patients with advanced carcinoma of the vagina or vulva treated in this fashion were disease-free at 29 months. In other studies, Grigsby and associates (115) and Perez and associates (113) treated small numbers of patients with endometrial and vulvar carcinomas with similar techniques. In all studies, patients with endometrial cancer did not survive longer than 12 months. From these results, it would appear that cancer of the vulva may be more responsive to concomitant chemotherapy and radiation.

Lung Cancer

Non-Small Cell Lung Cancer The traditional approach for the treatment of locally advanced unresectable non-small cell lung carcinoma has been radiation therapy alone or with chemotherapy in addition to irradiation, providing modest benefits. Aziz and colleagues (116) of the SUNY-Health Science Center at Brooklyn treated two groups of patients with advanced, inoperable non-small cell carcinoma of the lung in a phase II trial. The first group of 8 patients received low dose Cisplatin (5.7 $mg/m^2/day$) and the second group of 12 patients received intermediate dose Cisplatin (20 $mg/m^2/day$) during the course of radiotherapy. Both groups of patients received the Cisplatin infusion at a slow, constant rate in 14-day cycles. The total dose of radiation ranged from 4,200-6,000 cGy at 160-180 cGy/fraction. The treatment cycles were repeated after a 1- or 2-week break to allow for recovery of the hematopoietic system. Complete responses were reported in 25% of the low dose group; 37.5% achieved partial response. For patients receiving the intermediate dose, 41.5% achieved complete and partial response. Those with a complete response had improved survivals over partial or non-responders. Three out of five patients reporting complete response from the intermediate dose group were alive after 1 year. There were no reported treatment interruptions secondary to nausea, vomiting, renal, or hematologic toxicity. In an RTOG trial (117) with similar treatment, the rate of complete response was 25% in the low dose group and 41.5% in the intermediate dose group. Perhaps a greater complete response can be obtained with a higher dose of Cisplatin.

Schaake-Koning and associates (118) used concomitant Cisplatin bolus (35 mg/m^2) weekly with radiation therapy versus radiation therapy alone. A significant difference of overall survival in the concomitant therapy arm was reported (16% versus 2%). Severe Cisplatin-induced emesis was the limiting factor for 25% of the patients receiving the drug.

Reports by Dillman and associates (119) and Sause and associates (120) have confirmed the benefit of a combined modality approach with treatment for non-small cell lung cancers. Dillman used neoadjuvant chemotherapy with Cisplatin and Vinblastine followed by radiation therapy on day 50 to 6,000 cGy over 6 weeks. The 3-year overall survival rate was 23% for the chemotherapy and irradiation group, with median survival of 14 months compared to 11% for the radiation alone group, with median survival of 10 months.

Dautzenberg and colleagues (121) studied adjuvant chemotherapy and radiation versus radiation alone and reported no difference in overall survival in patients who had surgery, but less metastatic progression in the patients who had chemotherapy. The Non-Small Cell Lung Cancer Collaborative Group (122), in an analysis of studies, found some small benefits to chemotherapy. Byhardt (123) suggested that the small benefits would lead to increased toxicity and cost, and decrease the quality of life.

Current protocols combining new chemotherapeutic agents, such as Paclitaxel, Carboplatin, Topotecan, Gemcitabine, and Navelbine with standard radiation therapy (124), hyperfractionation (125), or stereotactic radiosurgery show promising results in the treatment of locally advanced non-small cell lung carcinoma.

Small Cell Carcinoma Small cell lung cancer differs from non-small cell lung cancer by its sensitivity to chemotherapy and radiotherapy and its propensity for early dissemination. Controversy exists over the use and benefit of concomitant chemotherapy and radiotherapy for the treatment of limited stage small cell lung cancer. Complete response rates with the use of chemotherapy alone have been reported to be 50% (126); however, the 3-year survival rate is only 5 to 15% (127). Eighty percent of patients treated with chemotherapy relapse in the chest, and some die of local disease without evidence of dissemination (128). Single institution studies have shown mixed results in comparing thoracic radiation to chemotherapy. Pignon (129), in a meta-analysis, reported a modest 5% increase in 2- and 3-year survival rates, and a 25 to 30% increase in local tumor control in limited stage disease when patients were treated with both radiation and chemotherapy. In these analyses, combined modality therapy had increased hematologic, mucosal, skin, and pulmonary toxicity over chemotherapy alone. Murray and colleagues (130) and Perry and colleagues (131) reported advantages to early and late introduction of radiation. Subsequent chemotherapy dose intensity may be compromised by introducing radiation therapy early. However, early radiation may effectively treat chemoresistant clones before they metastasize outside the local field (130). New approaches, including hyperfractionation and high dose therapy with stem cell or marrow rescue, continue to be tested because local recurrence rates still exceed 50% at 3 years.

Urinary Bladder

In 1997, it was estimated that 11,700 deaths occurred from cancer of the urinary bladder (Table 2.5) (132). Although progress has been made through surgery and radiation therapy, the management of deeply invasive bladder carcinoma remains a challenge to the oncology team. Survival rates of only 25 to 30% have been reported for surgical or radiation therapy alone (133,134,135). The use of preoperative irradiation increases survival rates to 40 to 45% (136,137,138). Treatment of these carcinomas with radical cystectomy, with or without radiation, means loss of bladder and sexual function. In view of these factors, better, alternative methods of therapy have been studied.

In the studies using preoperative radiation therapy, patients with a complete response at the time of surgery fared better than those whose bladders still contained tumor (137,138,139). Using the radiosensitizer Misonidazole or high LET radiation in an attempt to improve the complete response rate was not successful.

Stein and Kaufman (140) and Woodruff and colleagues (141) reported using bolus 5-FU and irradiation in bladder cancer. In the first study using concomitant continuous infusion chemotherapy and irradiation, Rotman and colleagues (142) at the SUNY-Health Science Center at Brooklyn reported on the results of concomitant continuous infusion 5-FU (with or without bolus Mitomycin-C) and irradiation for locally advanced bladder carcinomas. Twenty-two of the 25 patients had transitional cell carcinoma. The remaining three had squamous cell carcinoma. Median age was 72 years. The cancers were staged by the Jewitt-Marshall staging system: Stage A (1 patient), Stage B1 (7 patients), Stage B2 (9 patients), Stage C (6 patients), Stage D (2 patients). Ninety-two percent of the patients had a high tumor grade (III or IV), while the rest had grade II disease. Over half of the bladder was involved in 26% of the patients, hydronephrosis was present in 32% of the patients, and residual tumor was present at the beginning

Table 2.5. Treatment of Muscle Invasive Carcinoma of the Bladder with Chemotherapy and Radiation Therapy

Reference	No. of Patients	Treatment	CR Rate	Survival (%)
Rotman et al (142) (1990)	25	4000–4500 cGy/4.5–5wk to pelvis + 2000–2500 cGy boost to bladder, 5-FU infusion 120 hr, 1000 mg/m^2/d × 2 or 3 wk 1, 4, 7 of rt. Mitomycin-C bolus (25 mg/m^2) on d1. Intravesicular mitomycin-C. (no TURBT performed initially).	63.6% within 6 mos	62% at 5 yrs (80% Stage A and B1) (40% Stage B2, C, D)
Russell et al (143) (1988)	14	4000 cGy/5wk to pelvis, 5-FU infusion 96 hr at 1000 mg/m^2/dx^2, if CR then RT to 6000 cGy, if no CR then cystectomy.	57% with 3 wk 2 pts no tumor at cystectomy. Total CR 71%	93% median FY 7 mos
Kaufman et al (146) (1993)	53	Initial TURBT then 2 cycles MCV chemotherapy (methotrexate, cisplatin, vinblastine) then 4500 cGy/5 wks combined with bolus Cisplatin wk 1, 4. If CT by cystoscopy bolus Cisplatin and 1980 cGy to bladder. If no CR then radial cystectomy.	Initial CR rate 53% with 89% functioning bladders.	45% at 4 yrs NED 58% at 4 yrs functioning bladders
Eapen et al (149) (1989)	25	400 cGy/4 wk to pelvis with intraarterial cisplatin 60–120 m^2/m^2 3 wk prior to RT × 1 then 2× during RT. 5 pts then received cystectomy and 20 pts received an addition of 20Gy/2 wk to bladder.	93%	90% at 2 yrs
Arcangeli et al (150) (1996)	34	Initial TURBT then 2 cycles of MCV chemotherapy followed by RT, 50Gy Fx TID for 4.5 wks. Concomitant infusion with 5-FU 180–220 mg/m^2/day and cisplatin 4–6 mg/m^2/day.		

of therapy in 63% of the patients. The treatment protocol consisted of pelvic radiotherapy (4,000-4,500 cGy in 4 to 4.5 weeks) followed by boost to the bladder (2,000-2,500 cGy in 2 to 2.5 weeks). Concomitant chemotherapy was administered via infusion of 5-FU (25 mg/kg/day) over 120 hours during weeks 1, 4, and 7 or weeks 2, 5, and 8. Five patients received Mitomycin-C bolus (10 mg/m^2) on day 1. Twenty-two patients were evaluated by cystoscopy and biopsy. In 6 months, 64% of patients showed complete response. Patients who were not complete responders received additional therapy with either transurethral resection of bladder tumor (TURBT), intra-vesicular bacillus Calmette-Guérin (BCG), or intra-vesicular Mitomycin-C. This therapy increased the complete response rate to 86%. The 5-year survival for Stages A and B1 was 80%, and for Stages B2, C, and D was 40%. Acute and chronic toxicity was minimal. Eighty-one percent of the patients developed diarrhea by the second week of treatment, 18% developed mucositis, while another 18% complained of anorexia. All symptoms were reversible. No patients showed myelodepression. Chronic toxicity was infrequent with three patients developing an irritable bladder and one patient developing chronic diarrhea. Advantages to this approach are its superiority to single modality therapy and preservation of the bladder. This study has provided future direction for the management of high stage, high grade carcinoma of the bladder.

In a similar study, Russell and associates (143) treated 33 patients preoperatively with radiotherapy to the whole pelvis (4,000 cGy in 5 weeks) along with two 96-hour infusions of 5-FU in weeks 1 and 3 or radiotherapy. At 3 weeks of treatment, 57% of the patients had a complete response. Radiation (4,400-6,000 cGy) was given to complete treatment. Incomplete and non-responders had cystectomy. The final complete response rate was 71%.

The two studies outlined above show that it is not uncommon to obtain a delayed complete response even 6 months after therapy is completed. The decision to do cystectomy should be clearly delayed for that 6-month period.

In a study sponsored by the National Bladder Cancer Group (144), 70 patients not eligible for surgery with stage T2-T4b disease were treated with Cisplatin (70 mg/m^2) and radiation therapy (6,400 cGy). Survival at 4 years was 64% for stage T2 and 24% for stage T4. In a phase II RTOG trial

(145) 48 patients with stages T2-4, N0-2, or NXM0 were treated with pelvic radiation (4,000 cGy in 4 weeks) and Cisplatin (100 mg/m^2 on days 1 and 22 of radiation). Patients who had a complete response had 2,400 cGy or boost dose of radiation with a similar Cisplatin dose. Patients with residual tumor after the initial treatment had cystectomy. Sixty-seven percent obtained a complete response and 64% survived 3 years. Forty percent had tumor-free bladders.

Kaufman and associates (146) reported on a phase II study of 53 patients with muscle invading bladder cancer. The protocol consisted of initial transurethral resection of the bladder tumor followed by two cycles of Methotrexate (30 mg/m^2 on days 1, 15, and 22), Cisplatin (70 mg/m^2 on day 2), and Vinblastine (3 mg/m^2 on days 2, 15, and 22 over a 28-day cycle) (MCV). After the two cycles were completed, patients were evaluated with cystoscopy. Forty-three percent of patients had positive tumor site biopsy results. Radiotherapy (4,500 cGy in 5 weeks) was then combined with Cisplatin bolus (70 mg/m^2/day) on day 22 before radiation. Patients were again evaluated by cystoscopy. Only 26% had positive tumor site biopsies. Complete responders received 2,480 cGy as a boost dose. All other patients had cystectomy. At the initial evaluation, 53% of the patients had complete responses and 89% had functioning bladders. At the 4-year follow-up point, 45% of patients were alive with no evidence of disease and 58% had functioning bladders free of invasive disease. Distant metastases, however, were reported in 42% of the patients. Housset and colleagues (147) showed that when 5-FU and Cisplatin are given together with radiation, a complete response rate of 74% can be obtained. Sauer and associates (148) reported an even better complete response rate of 85% when radiotherapy and Cisplatin infusion are administered together. Unfortunately, this result did not translate into survival benefits.

An intergroup phase III trial is underway to confirm the benefit of organ preservation as reported above. It is hoped that the use of Methotrexate, Vinblastine, Doxorubicin, and Cisplatin, along with the use of 5-FU and radiotherapy, will play an important role in eliminating micrometastases and increase survival. Eapen et al (149) has utilized bilateral hypogastric arteries for infusing cis-platinum. Cis-platinum was infused 3 weeks prior to irradiation and also concomitantly during the first week of irradiation. A complete response rate of 90% was obtained among patients with advanced bladder carcinoma. Arcangeli et al (150) have also reported on phase I and II trials where patients with invasive bladder carcinoma were treated with or without two cycles of MCV, followed by concomitant infusion of cis-platinum and 5-FU infusion given with irradiation. Irradiation consisted of three 100 cGy fractions/day for a total dose of 5000 cGy in 4.5 weeks. If required, a further dose of 2000 cGy was given for residual dose. A complete response of 91% was obtained in a series of 34 patients.

Carcinoma of the Breast

In the treatment of breast cancer, many patients receive chemotherapy combined with radiation after conservative surgery. A review of studies of combined chemotherapy and radiation for early stage breast cancer produces conflicting data making it difficult to determine if treating patients with each modality separately would affect survival or recurrence. Lara-Jimenez and associates (151) studied postmastectomy patients in a randomized trial and compared radiation followed by chemotherapy, chemotherapy with six cycles of cyclophosphamide-methotrexate-5-fluorouracil (CMF) followed by radiation, and a sandwich approach of three cycles of chemotherapy, radiation, and three additional cycles of chemotherapy. Patients treated with the sandwich approach fared the best. Harris and Recht (152) retrospectively studied node-positive patients treated with adjuvant chemotherapy and radiation therapy. A 5-year local recurrence rate of 28% was obtained if radiation was administered more than 16 weeks after surgery. Only 5% had a 5-year local recurrence rate if surgery was performed less than 16 weeks after surgery.

In addition, an increased risk of acute skin reactions and radiation pneumonitis, and a decrease in long-term cosmetic results were reported when methotrexate was given concurrently with radiation therapy (152). The use of concurrent radiation and Adriamycin may increase cardiac toxicity (153). It may be necessary to omit these drugs during the radiation treatment. Currently, the question of proper timing of chemotherapy and radiation for the adjuvant treatment of breast cancer remains under investigation.

Soft-Tissue Sarcoma

Historically, surgical resection has been the traditional therapeutic modality for control of soft-tissue sarcomas. Because of the introduction of multimodality therapy, almost 80% of patients with sarcomas of the extremity are candidates for limb sparing procedures. The cure rate for osteosarcoma has increased from 20% to almost 60% because of the advent of adjuvant chemotherapy (154) since radiotherapy does not play a role in the initial treatment. On the other hand, conservative surgery and pre- or post-operative radiation produce local tumor control rates equal to amputation (155). However, more than 50% of patients with tumors larger than 5 cm will eventually die of metastasis. Thus far, the addition of chemotherapy to the treatment regimen has been of marginal benefit and is still controversial.

Sordillo and colleagues (156) published one of the first reports on the benefits of combining Adriamycin which was administered 90 minutes before radiation for the treatment of soft-tissue sarcomas. Twenty-one percent of the patients received a complete response, while 41% received a partial response. The persistence of tumors outside the radiation port necessitated the combined treatment modality.

At the SUNY-Health Science Center at Brooklyn and Long Island College Hospital, Rosenthal and associates (29) treated 9 patients with locally advanced, unresectable, nonextremity soft-tissue sarcomas in a phase II trial with a combination of Adriamycin and radiation. Adriamycin (12 mg/m^2/day) was administered via continuous 5-day infusion in three or four cycles. During each cycle, concomitant irradiation was administered in 5 daily fractions of 100-180 cGy. Three weeks of rest followed each cycle to allow for hematopoietic recovery since the most common side effect was moderate bone marrow depletion. Four patients received a complete response, two of whom have been free of disease for more than 5 years.

Turner and colleagues (157) successfully treated a patient with a 25x8 cm pleomorphic soft-tissue sarcoma of the popliteal fossa using the SUNY protocol. The patient received six cycles of continuous infusion Adriamycin (12 mg/m^2/day) concomitantly during radiation (total dose of 5,400 cGy). The response was excellent, with minimum long term toxicity and no evidence of disease after 7 years.

TOXICITY OF COMBINED MODALITY THERAPY

One of the problems with combined modality therapy is that it can cause damage to normal tissue cells. This damage may occur as a result of cumulative effects of each modality in the same tissues or effects on different tissues on the same organ. The effect of combined modality therapy may result in enhanced toxicity, dependent upon the tissues involved, the route of administration of the drugs, timing, and radiation dose and fractionation.

Bone Marrow Toxicity

In a study by Kovacs and associates (158), the changes in the hematopoietic system after radiotherapy and chemotherapy were investigated. Adriamycin produced immediate and prolonged bone marrow depression. In contrast, 5-FU and Cyclophosphamide demonstrated their effect on bone marrow more immediately. Drugs that affect the more primitive stem cells may cause bone marrow depression for a longer duration than chemotherapeutic agents that affect more mature cells. The concomitant use of chemotherapy and radiation could promote enhancement of bone marrow suppression.

Cardiac Toxicity

It has been well-documented that Adriamycin is cardiotoxic. Cardiac damage from radiation is caused by diffuse interstitial fibrosis and decrease in capillaries about 3 months posttherapy. This leads to ischemia and secondary myocardial fibrosis. The combined effects of both treatment modalities result in injury to different target cells.

Fajardo et al (159) noted a synergistic effect on cardiac damage in rabbits when radiation and Adriamycin were administered together. Bellingham (160) performed cardiac biopsies on patients who had received a total dose of 90 to 445 mg/m^2 of Adriamycin and 4,600 to 5,700 cGy of radiation. The Adriamycin had been given 6 to 14 years after the radiation. Histopathologic changes were significantly higher for the radiated group. It was concluded that prior radiation potentiated the cardiac damage due to Adriamycin.

To limit the incidence of cardiotoxicity, investigators have made various suggestions. Administering Adriamycin by continuous infusion may reduce the rate of cardiac toxicity (161,29). Decreasing the dosage of each modality by 25 to 50% has been proposed by Mayer and associates (162). Using cardioprotective agents such as ICRF-187 may be helpful in reducing cardiac toxicity as per Speyer and associates (163). Finally, several other chemotherapeutic agents with less cardiac toxicity have been developed. These include Epirubicin and Mitoxantrone.

Small and Large Bowel Toxicity

The most serious toxicity from multimodality therapy is to the small bowel. Toxicities to the small bowel include hemorrhage, diarrhea, small bowel obstruction, and small bowel perforation or fistula. In a GITSG trial for advanced rectal carcinoma (54), the incidence of small bowel complications was higher in the combined modality therapy group, with two deaths related to small bowel toxicity. In a study from the North Central Cancer Therapy Group (164), improved radiation techniques were used (four field technique versus two field technique) and severe bowel injury occurred in less than 5% of the patients in both the single modality and combined modality arms.

After radiotherapy for carcinoma of the rectum, cervix, endometrium or prostate, large bowel injury may occur from a few months to several years later. Endarteritis obliterans with the development of telangiectasia, fibrosis, and strictures may be found. Surgery may be required for rectal ulceration, large bowel obstruction, and bleeding. Improved techniques of radiation with hyperfractionation in combined modality treatment may provide a reduction in the rate of large bowel injury.

CONCLUSIONS

Several sequencing strategies are available for the use of chemotherapy and radiation therapy in the combined modality treatment of advanced malignant disease. The experience with continuous concomitant infusion of various chemotherapeutic agents has been very encouraging. The radiosensitization effect obtained with this type of therapy appears to be at its maximum with tolerable toxicity. In addition, the treatment increases locoregional control which consequently increases survival. Combined modality therapy has allowed for organ sparing in the treatment of anal, esophageal, head and neck, bladder, and rectal carcinomas. In the most advanced cases, combined modality treatment may produce effective palliation.

The treatment technique, fractionation size of radiation, and scheduling of chemotherapy infusion or bolus needs to be refined further to obtain the optimal result. Further work also needs to be done to ascertain the specificity of certain drugs against given tumors. Randomized trials will be required to answer these questions, and others concerning long-term toxicity.

References

1. Griffin TW, Wambersie A, Lavamore GE et al. High Let heavy particle trials. Int J Radiat Oncol Biol Phys 1988;14:583.
2. Fazekas JT, Pajak TF, Marcial VA, et al. The RTOG randomized trial 79-15. Misonidazole adjuvant to radiation therapy in advanced head and neck squamous cell cancers. Proc Am Soc Oncol 1984;3:185.
3. Perez CA, Pajak T, Emami B, et al. Randomized phase III study comparing irradiation and hyperthermia with irradiation alone in superficial measurable tumors. Final Report by the RTOG. Am J Clin Oncol 1991;14:133-141.
4. Sklar MD. The ras oncogenes increase the intrinsic resistance of NIH3T3 cells to ionizing radiation. Science 1988;239:645-647.
5. Fu K. Biological basis for the interaction of chemotherapeutic agent and radiation therapy. Cancer 1985;55:2123-2130.
6. Dewit L. Combined treatment of radiation and cis-diamminedichloroplatinum (II): A review of experimental and clinical data. Int J Radiat Oncol Biol. Phys. 1987;13:403-426.
7. Douple EB. Platinum radiation interactions. NCI Monogr 1988;6: 315-319.
8. Withers HR, Taylor JMG, Maciejewski B. The hazard of accelerated tumor clonogen repopulation during radiotherapy. Acta Oncol 1988;27:131-146.
9. Chabner B. Pharmacologic Principles of cancer treatment. Philadelphia: Saunders, 1982.
10. Looney WB, Alternating Chemotherapy and Radiotherapy. NCI Monogr 1988;6:85-94.
11. Bagshaw MA. Possible role of potentiator in radiation therapy. Am J Roentgenol 1961;85:822-833.
12. Heidelberger C, Greishbach L, Montag BJ, et al. Studies in fluorinated pyrimidine. II. Effects on transplanted tumors. Cancer Res 1958;18:305-317.
13. Haghbin M, Sischey B, Hinson J, et al. Combined modality preoperative therapy in poor prognostic rectal adenocarcinoma. Radiother Oncol 1988;13(1):75-81.
14. Van Paperzeel HA. Effects of single doses of radiation on lung metastases in man and experimental animals. Eur J Cancer 1972;8:665-675.
15. Vermund H, Hodgett J, Ansfield FJ. Effects of combined radiation and chemotherapy in transplanted tumors in mice. Am J Roentgenol 1961;85: 559-567.
16. Byfield JE, Barone R, Mendelsohn J, et al. Infusional 5-Fluorouracil and x-ray therapy for non-resectable esophageal cancer. Cancer 1980;45: 703-708.
17. Vietti J, Eggerding F, Valeriote F. Combined x-radiation and 5-fluorouracil in survival of transplanted leukemic cell. J Natl Cancer Inst 1971;47:865-870.
18. Wodinsky I, Swiniarski J, Kensler CJ, et al. Combination radiotherapy and chemotherapy for P388 lymphocytic leukemia in vivo. Cancer Chemother 1974;Rep.4(1):73-97.
19. Zak M, Drabnik J. Effects of cis-dichlorodiammine platinum (II) on the post-irradiation lethality in mice after irradiation with x-rays. Strahlentherapie 1971;142:112-115.
20. Coughlin CT, Richmond RC. Biologic and clinical developments of cisplatin combined with radiation: Concepts, utility, projections for new trials and the emergence of carboplatin. Semin Oncol 1989;16-S6:31.
21. Dritschillo A, Kellman A, et al. The effect of cisplatinum on the repair of radiation damage in plateau phase Chinese hamster (V-79) cells. Int J Radiat Oncol Biol Phys 1979;5:1345-1349.
22. Lelieveld P, Scoles MA, Brown JM, et al. The effect of treatment in fractionated schedules with the combination of irradiation and six cytotoxic drugs on the RIF-1 tumor and normal mouse skin. Int J Radiat Oncol Biol Phys 1985;11:111-121.
23. Byfield JE, Lee YC, Tu L. Molecular interactions between Adriamycin and x-ray damage in mammalian tumor cells. Cancer 1977;19:186-193.
24. Durand R. Adriamycin: A possible indirect radiosensitizer of hypoxic tumor cells. Radiology 1979;119:217-222.
25. Watering W, Byfield JE, Lagasse L, et al. Combination Adriamycin and radiation therapy in gynecologic cancer. Gynecol Oncol 1974; 2:518-526.
26. Rowley R, Bacharach M, Hopkins NA, et al. Adriamycin and irradiation effects upon an experimental solid tumor resistant to therapy. Int J Radiat Oncol Biol Phys 1977;5:1291-1295.
27. Benjamin RS, Riggs CE Jr, Bachus NR, et al. Pharmacokinetics and metabolism of adriamycin in man. Clin Pharmacol Ther 1973;14: 592-600.
28. Legha S, Benjamin R, Mackay B, et al. Reduction of doxorubicin cardiotoxicity by prolonged continuous infusion. Ann Intern Med 1982;96:133-139.
29. Rosenthal CJ, Rotman, Bhutiani I, et al. Concomitant radiation therapy and doxorubicin by continuous infusion in advanced malignancy. A phase I and II study. Evidence of synergistic effect in soft tissue sarcomas and hepatomas. In: Rosenthal CJ, Rotman M, eds. Clinical Applications of Continuous Infusion Chemotherapy and Concomitant Radiation Therapy. New York: Plenum Press, 1986.
30. Schaeffer J, El-Mahdi AM, Combination adriamycin-radiation treatment of pulmonary tumors in mice. Oncology 1981;38:35-39.
31. Steren A, Sevin BU, Perras J, et al. Taxol as a radiation sensitizer: A flow cytometric study. Gynecol Oncol 1981;50(1):89-93.
32. Rockwell S. Use of hypoxia directed drugs in the therapy of solid tumors. Semin Oncol 1992;19(11): 29-40.
33. Seiman DW, Keng PC. Responses of tumor cell sub-population to single-modality and combined modality therapies. WCI Monograph 1988;6:101-105.
34. Gran C, Overgaard J. Radiosensitizing and cytotoxic properties of mitomycin-C in a C3H mouse mammary carcinoma in vivo. Int J Radiat Oncol Biol Phys 1991;20:265-269.
35. Weissberg JB, Son YH, Papac RH, et al. Randomized clinical trial of mitomycin-C as an adjunct to radiotherapy in head and neck cancer. Int J Radiat Oncol Biol Phys 1989;17:3-9.
36. Flam RJ, Kufe DW. Inhibition of DNA excision repair and the repair of x-ray induced DNA damage by cytosine arabinoside and hydroxyurea. Pharmacol Ther 1985;31:165-176.
37. Schlisky RL. Biochemical Pharmacology of chemotherapeutic drugs used as radiation enhancers. Semin Oncol 1992;4(11):2-7.
38. Sinclair WL. The combined effect of hydroxyurea and x-rays on Chinese hamster cells in-vitro. Cancer Res 1968;28:198-206.
39. Mattern MR, Hoffman GA, McCabe FL, et al. Synergistic cell killing by ionizing radiation and topoisomerase I inhibitor topotecon (SK& F 104864). Cancer Res 1991;51:5813-5816.
40. Ng CE, Bussey AM, Raaphorst GP. Inhibition of potentially lethal and sublethal damage repair by camptothecin and etoposide in human melanoma cell lines. Int J Radiat Oncol Biol Phys 1994;66:49-57.
41. Hennequin C, Giocanti N, Balosso J, et al. Interaction of ionizing radiation with the topisomerase I poison camptothesin in growing V-79 and HeLa cells. Cancer Res 1994;54:1720-1728.
42. Beahrs OH. Management of squamous cell carcinoma of the anus and adenocarcinoma of the anus and the lower rectum (editorial). Int J Radiat Oncol Biol Phys 1985;11:1741-1742.
43. Rotman M, Aziz H. Carcinoma of the Anus. Int J Radiat Oncol Biol Phys 1987;13:465-466.
44. Nigro ND, Vaitkevicius VK, Considine B, et al. Combined therapy for the anal canal: A preliminary report. Dis Colon Rectum. 1974; 17:354-356.
45. Nigro ND. An evaluation of combined therapy for squamous cell cancer of the anal canal. Dis Colon Rectum 1984;27:763.

46. Cummings BJ, Harwood AR, Keane TJ. Anal canal carcinoma: Improving the therapeutic ratio with combined radiation and chemotherapy. Int J Radiat Oncol Biol Phys 1983;9:110.
47. Cummings BJ, Keane T, Harwood A, Thomas G. Combined modality therapy with 5-fluorouracil, mitomycin-C and radiation therapy. In: Rosenthal CJ, Rotman M, eds. Clinical Applications of Continuous Infusion Chemotherapy and Concomitant Radiation Therapy. New York: Plenum, 1986;133-147.
48. John M, Flam M, Lovalvo L, et al. Feasibility of non-surgical definitive management of anal canal carcinoma. Int J Radiat Oncol Biol Phys 1987;13:299-303.
49. Sischy B. The use of radiation therapy combined with chemotherapy in the management of squamous cell carcinoma of the anus and marginally resectable adenocarcinoma of the rectum. Int J Radiat Oncol Biol Phys 1985;11:1587-1593.
50. Byfield JE. Useful interactions between 5-fluorouracil and radiation in man: 5-fluorouracil as a radiosensitizer: In: Hill BT, Bellamy AS, eds. Anti-tumor Drug Radiation Interaction. Boca Raton: CRC Press, 1990;87.
51. Roelofsen F, Bosset J, Eschwege F, et al. Concomitant Radiotherapy and Chemotherapy superior to radiotherapy alone in the treatment of locally advanced anal cancer: Results of a phase III randomized trial of the EORTC Radiotherapy and Gastrointestinal Cooperative Groups. Proc ASCO 1995;14:194.
52. Flam MS, John M, Pajak T, et al. Radiation (RT) and 5-Fluorouracil (5-FU) vs. radiation, 5-FU, mitomycin-C (MMC) in the treatment of anal carcinoma. Results of a phase III randomized RTOG/ECOG intergroup trial. Proc ASCO 1995;14:443.
53. Steele GD, Augenlicht LH, Begg CB, et al. National Institute of Health Consensus Development Conference: Adjuvant Therapy for Patients with Colon and Rectal Cancer. JAMA 1990;264,1444-1450.
54. Gastrointestinal Tumor Study Group: Prolongation of disease-free interval in surgically treated rectal carcinoma. N Engl J Med 1985; 312:1465.
55. O'Connell MJ, Martenson JA, Wieland HS, et al. Improving Adjuvant Therapy for Rectal Cancer by Protracted infusion fluorouracil with radiation therapy after curative surgery. N Engl J Med 1994;331:502-507.
56. Fisher B, Wolmark N, Rockette H, et al. Post operative adjuvant chemotherapy or radiation therapy for rectal cancer. Results from NSABP Protocol R-01. J Natl Cancer Inst 1988;80,21-29.
57. Rich TA, Weiss DR, Meis C, et al. Sphincter preservation in patients with low rectal cancer treated with radiation therapy with or without local excision or fulguration. Radiology 1985;156:527-531.
58. Pahlman L, Glimelius B. Pre-or post-operative radiotherapy in rectal and recto-sigmoid carcinoma: Report from a randomized multicenter trial. Ann Surg 1990;211:187-195.
59. Earlam R, Cunha-Melo, Jr. Esophageal squamous cell carcinoma: A critical review of surgery. Br J Surg 1980;67:384.
60. Newaishy GA, Read GA, Duncan W, et al. Results of radical radiotherapy of squamous cell carcinoma of the esophagus. Clin Radiol 1982;33:347-352.
61. Doggett RLS, Grernsey J, Bagshaw M. Combined radiation and surgical treatment of carcinoma of the thoracic esophagus. Rad Ther Oncol 1970;5:147-154.
62. Leichman L, Steiger Z, Seydel HG, et al. Preoperative chemotherapy and radiation therapy for patients with cancer of the esophagus: A potentially curative approach. J Clin Oncol 1984;2:75-79.
63. Leichman L, Steiger Z, Sydel HG, Vaitkevicus VK. Combined preoperative chemotherapy and radiation therapy for cancer of the esophagus. The Wayne State University, South West Oncology Group and Radiation Therapy Oncology Group experience. Semin Oncol 1984; 11:178-185.
64. Richmond J, Seydel HG, Bac Y, Lewis J, Burdakin J, Jacobson G, et al. Comparison of three strategies for esophageal cancer within a single institution. Int J Radiat Oncol Biol Phys 1987;11:1617-1620.
65. John MJ, Flam MS, Mowry PA, et al. Radiotherapy alone and chemoradiation for non metastatic esophageal carcinoma. Cancer 1989;63: 2397-2403.
66. Coia LR, Engstrom PF, Paul AR. Long term results of infusional 5-FU, mitomycin-C and radiation as primary treatment of esophageal carcinoma. Int J Radiat Oncol Biol Phys 1991;20(1):29.
67. Coia LR, Esophageal Preservation: The management of esophageal cancer with concomitant radiation and chemotherapy. Endoscopy 1993;25:664-669.
68. Keane TJ, Harwood AR, Rider WD, et al. Concomitant radiation and chemotherapy for squamous cell carcinoma of the esophagus (abstract), Int J Radiat Oncol Biol Phys 1984;10:89.
69. Forastiere A, Orringer MB, Perez-Tamayo C, Urba SG, Husted S, Takasugi BJ, Zahurak M. Concurrent Chemotherapy and Radiation Therapy followed by Transhiatal Esophagectomy for Loco-Regional Cancer of the Esophagus. J Clin Oncol 1990;8:119-127.
70. Rich T. Protracted (Continuous 5-Fluorouracil) infusion with concomitant radiation therapy. Indications and results. In: Rotman M, Rosenthal CJ, eds. Concomitant Continuous Infusion Chemotherapy and Radiation. Berlin Springer-Verlag 1991;181.
71. Herskovic A, Martz K, Al-Sarraf M, Leichman L, Brindle J, Vaitkevicius V, Cooper J, Byhardt R, Davis L, Emani B. Combined chemotherapy and radiotherapy compared with radiotherapy alone in patients with cancer of the esophagus. N Engl J Med 1992;326:1593-8.
72. Al-Sarraf M, Martz K, Herskovic A, Brindle JS, Vaitkevicius VK, Cooper J, Byhardt R, Davis L, Emami B, Progress Report of Combined Chemoradiotherapy versus Radiotherapy alone in Patients with Esophageal Cancer. An Intergroup Study. J Clin Oncol 1997; 15:277-284.
73. Burmeister BH, Denham JN, O'Brien M, et al. Combined modality therapy for esophageal carcinoma: Preliminary results from a large Australian multicenter study. Int J Radiat Oncol Biol Phys 1995;32(4) 997-1006.
74. Tepper JE, Nardi GE, Suit HD, et al. Carcinoma of the pancreas: Review of MFH experience from 1963 to 1973. Cancer 1976;37:1519.
75. Gastrointestinal Tumor Study Group: Further evidence of effective adjuvant combined radiation and chemotherapy following curative resection of pancreatic cancer. Cancer 1987;59:2006.
76. Childs DS, Jr, Moertel CG, Holbrook MA, et al. Treatment of malignant neoplasms of gastrointestinal tract with a combination of 5-FU and radiation therapy. A randomized double-blind study. Radiology 1965;84:843-848.
77. Moertel CG, Reitmeier RJ, Childs DS, et al. Advanced gastrointestinal cancer. Mayo Clin Proc 1964;39:767.
78. Smith FP, Stablein D, Korsmeyer S, et al. Combination chemotherapy for locally advanced pancreatic cancer: Equivalence to external beam irradiation and implication of future management. J Clin Oncol 1983;1:413.
79. Gastrointestinal Tumor Study Group: Treatment of locally unresectable carcinoma of the pancreas: Comparison of combined-modality (chemotherapy plus radiotherapy) to chemotherapy alone. J Natl Cancer Inst 1988;80(10):751-755.
80. Gastrointestinal Tumor Study Group: Therapy of locally unresectable pancreatic carcinoma. A randomized comparison of high dose (6000 rads) radiation alone, moderate dose radiation (4000 rads + 5-fluorouracil), and high dose + 5-fluorouracil. Cancer 1981;48: 1705.
81. Gunderson LL, Martin JK, Kvols LK, et al. Intraoperative and external beam radiation + 5-FU for locally advanced pancreatic cancer. Int J Radiat Oncol Biol Phys 1987;13:319.
82. Komaki R, Hanson R, Cox JD, et al. Phase I and II study of prophylactic hepatic irradiation with local irradiation and systemic chemotherapy for adenocarcinoma of the pancreas. Int J Radiat Oncol Biol Phys 1988;15:1447.
83. Rich T, Byrd M. Protracted 5-FU infusion in gastro-intestinal tumors. Neoadjuvant Chemotherapy J 1986;683-689.
84. Lawrence TS, Chang EY, Hahn TM, Hertel LW, Shewach DS. Radiosensitization of pancreatic cancer cells by 2'2'-difluoro 2'-deoxycytidine. Int J Radiat Oncol Biol Phys 1996;34(4): 867-72.
85. Welch JP, Donaldson GA. The clinical correlation of an autopsy study of recurrent colo-rectal cancer. Ann Surg 1979;189:496.
86. Cady B, McDermott MW. Major hepatic resection for metachronous metastases from colon cancer. Ann Surg 1985; 201-204.
87. Jaffe BM, Donegan WL, Watson F, et al. Factors influencing survival in patients with untreated hepatic metastases. Surg Gynecol Obst 1968;127:1.
88. Prasad B, Lee MS, Hendrickson FR. Radiation of hepatic metastases. Int J Radiat Oncol Biol Phys 1977;2:129-132.
89. Sherman DM, Weiselbaum R, Order SE, Cloud L, Trey C, Piro AJ. Palliation of hepatic metastases. Cancer 1978;41:2013-2017.

90. Leibel SA, Pajak TF, Order SE, et al. Hepatic metastases: Results of treatment and identification of prognostic factors. RTOG Report (abstract). Int J Radiat Oncol Biol Phys 1985 (suppl. I),6-117.
91. Sullivan R. Systemic and arterial infusion chemotherapy for metastic liver cancer. Int J Radiat Oncol Biol Phys 1976;1:973-976.
92. Lokich J, Kinsella T, Perri J, Malcolm A, Clouse M. Concomitant hepatic radiation and intraarterial fluorinated pyrimidine therapy: Correlation of liver scan, liver function tests and plasma CEA with tumor response. Cancer 1981;48:2569-2574.
93. Rotman M, Kuruvilla A, Choi K, et al. Response of colorectal hepatic metastases to concomitant radiotherapy and intravenous infusion of 5-FU. Int J Radiat Oncol Biol Phys 1987;12:2179-2189.
94. Fletcher GH, Suit HD, Howe CD, et al. Clinical method of testing radiation sensitizing agents in squamous cell carcinoma. Cancer 1963;16:355-363.
95. Lo TC, Wiley AL, Jr, Ansfield FJ, et al. Combined radiation therapy and 5-Fluorouracil for advanced squamous cell carcinoma of the oral cavity and orophorynx: A randomized study. Am J Roentgenol 1976;126:229-235.
96. Adelstein DJ, Sharon VM, Earle AS. Chemo-radiation therapy as initial management in patients with squamous cell carcinoma of the head and neck. Cancer Treat Rep 1986;70:761-767.
97. Byfield JE, Sharp TR, Frankel SS, et al. Phase I, II trial of 5-day infused 5-fluorouracil and radiation in advanced cancer of the head and neck. J Clin Oncol 1984;2:406-413.
98. Hahn SS, Kim JA, Constable WE. Concomitant chemotherapy and radiotherapy for advanced squamous cell carcinoma of the head and neck. Int J Radiat Oncol Biol Phys 1984;10:191.
99. Kaplan MJ, Hahn SS, Johns ME, et al. Mitomycin and fluorouracil with concomitant radiation therapy in head and neck cancer. Arch Otolaryngol 1985;111:220.
100. Keane TJ, Harwood AR, Beale FA, Cummings BJ, Payne DG, Ravlinson E. A pilot study of mitomycin-C and 5-Fluorouracil infusion combined with split course radiation therapy for advanced carcinomas of the larynx and hypopharynx. J Otolaryngol 1985;15:286-288.
101. Murthy AK, Taylor WSG, Showel J, et al. Treatment of advanced head and neck cancer with concomitant radiation and chemotherapy. Int J Radiat Oncol Biol Phys 1987; 13:1807-1813.
102. Choi K, Rotman M, Aziz H, Stark R, Rosenthal CJ, Marti J. Locally advanced paranasal sinus and nasopharyngeal cancers: Effects of hyperfractionated radiation and concomitant continuous infusion cisplatin. In: Rotman M, Rosenthal CJ, eds. Medical Radiology. Berlin: Springer, 1991;197-204.
103. Taylor SG, Murthy AK, Cardarelli DD, et al. Combined simultaneous cisplatin/5-FU infusion chemotherapy and split course radiation in advanced head and neck cancer. J Clin Oncol 1989;17:846.
104. Harrison L, Pfister D, Foss D, et al. Concomitant chemotherapy radiotherapy followed by hyperfractionated radiation therapy for advanced unresectable head and neck cancer. Int J Radiat Oncol Biol Phys 1991;21:703-708.
105. Forastiere A, Newberg D, Taylor S, et al. Phase II evaluation of Taxol in advanced head and neck cancer: An Eastern Cooperative Group Trial. Proceedings of ASCO 1993;12:277.
106. Ettinger D. Overview of Paclitaxel (Taxol) in advanced lung cancer. Semin Oncol 1993;20:46-49.
107. Tishler R, Schiff P, Geard C, Hall E. Taxol: A novel radiation sensitizer. Int J Radiat Oncol Biol Phys: 1992;22:613-617.
108. Haraf DF, Stenson K, Witt ME, et al. Concomitant Radiotherapy, Paclitaxel, 5-Fluorouracil, and Hydroxyurea in patients with advanced or recurrent head and neck cancer. Semin Radiat Oncol 1997;7-51:34-38.
109. Paunier J, Delclos L, Fletcher GH. Causes, time of death, and sites of failure in squamous cell carcinoma of the uterine cervix on intact uterus. Radiology 1967;88:555-562.
110. Thomas G, Dembo A, Beale F, et al. Concurrent radiation, mitomycin-C and 5-fluorouracil in poor prognoses carcinoma of the cervix: Preliminary result of phase I, II study. Int J Radiat Oncol Biol Phys. 1984;10:1785-1790.
111. Ludgate SM, Crandon AJ, Hudson CN, et al. Synchronous 5-fluorouracil, mitomycin-C, and radiation therapy in the treatment of locally advanced carcinoma of the cervix. Int J Radiat Oncol Biol Phys 1988; 15:893-899.
112. John M, Kook K, Flam M, et al. Preliminary results of concomitant radiotherapy and chemotherapy in advanced cervical carcinoma. Gynecol Oncol 1987;28:101-110.
113. Perez CA, Grigsby PW, Chao CKS. Chemotherapy and irradiation in locally advanced squamous cell carcinoma of the uterine cervix. A review. Seminars in Radiat Oncol 1997; 45-65.
114. Evans LS, Kersh CR, Constable WC, et al. Concomitant 5-Fluorouracil, mitomycin-C and radiotherapy for advanced gynecological malignancies. Int J Radiat Oncol Biol Phys 1988;15:901.
115. Grigsby P, Graham M, Perez C. et al. Prospective phase I/II study of definitive radiotherapy and chemotherapy for advance gynecologic malignancies. Am J Clin Oncol 1996;19(1):1-6.
116. Aziz H, Rosenthal J, Potters L, Nuthakki M, Rotman M. Non-small cell carcinoma of the lung. In: Rotman M, Rosenthal CJ, eds. Medical Radiology. Berlin: Springer, 1991; pp 223-228.
117. Perez CA, Stanley H, Rubin P, et al. A prospective randomized study of various irradiation doses and fractionation schedules in the treatment of inoperable non-oat cell carcinoma of the lung. Cancer 1980; 45:2744-2753.
118. Schaake-Koning C, van den Bogaert W, Dalesio O, et al. Effects of concomitant cisplatin and radiotherapy in inoperable non-small cell lung cancer. N Engl J Med 1992;326:563-565.
119. Dillman RO, Seagren SL, Propert KR et al. A randomized trial of induction chemotherapy plus high dose radiation versus radiation alone in stage III non-small cell lung cancer. N Engl J Med 1990; 323:940-945.
120. Sause WT, Scott C, Taylor S, et al. Radiation Therapy Oncology Group (RTOG) 88-08 and Eastern Cooperative Oncology Group (ECOG) 4588. Preliminary results of a phase III trial in regionally advanced, unresectable non-small cell lung cancer. J Natl Cancer Inst 1995;87:198-205.
121. Dautzenberg B, Chastang C, Arriagada R, et al. (for the GETCB Groupe d'Etude et de Traitement des Cancers Bromchiques): Adjuvant radiotherapy versus combined sequential chemotherapy followed by radiotherapy in the treatment of resected non-small cell lung carcinoma: a randomized trial of 267 patients. Cancer 1995;76: 779-786.
122. Faber PL. Current status of neoadjuvant therapy for non-small cell lung cancer. Chest: 1994:106,6:355-359.
123. Byhardt RW, Scott CB, Ettinger DS, et al. Concurrent hyperfractionated irradiation and chemotherapy for unresectable non-small cell lung cancer: Results of Radiation Therapy Oncology Group 90-15. Cancer 1995;75(9):2337-2344.
124. Choy H, Akerley W, Safran H, et al. Preliminary analysis of Paclitaxel, Carboplatin, and concurrent radiation in the treatment of patients with advanced non-small cell lung cancer. Sem Radiat Oncol 1997; 7-51:15-18.
125. Komaki R, Scott C, Lee JS, et al. Impact of adding concurrent chemotherapy to hyperfractionated radiotherapy for locally advanced non-small cell lung cancer (NSCLC). Comparison of RTOG 83-11 to RTOG 91-06. Am J Clin Oncol 1997;20:435-440.
126. Hong WK, Nicaise C, Lawson R, et al. Etoposide combined with cyclophosphamide plus vincristine compared with doxorubicin plus cyclophosphamide plus cincristine and with high dose cyclophosphamide plus vincristine in the treatment of small cell carcinoma of the lung: A randomized trial of the Bristol Lung Cancer Study Group. J Clin Oncol 1989;7:450-456.
127. Osterlind K, Hansen M, Dombernowsky, P. Mortality and morbidity in long term survival patients treated with chemotherapy with or without radiation for small cell lung cancer. J Clin Oncol 1986;4: 1044-1052.
128. Ward P, Payne D. Does thoracic irradiation improve survival and local control in limited stage small cell carcinoma of the lung? A meta-analysis. J Clin Oncol 1992;10:890-895.
129. Pignon JP, Arrigada R, Ihde DC, et al. A meta analysis of thoracic radiotherapy for small cell lung cancer. N Engl J Med 1992;327:1618-1624.
130. Murray N, Coy P, Pater JL, et al. Importance of timing for thoracic irradiation in the combined modality treatment of limited stage small cell lung cancer. The National Institute of Canada Clinical Trial Group. J Clin Oncol 1993;11:336-344.
131. Perry MC, Eaton WL, Propert KJ, et al. Chemotherapy with or without radiation in limited small cell carcinoma of the lung. N Engl J Med 1987;316:912-918.

132. Parker S, Tong T, Bolden S, Wingo P. Cancer Statistics 1997;47:5-10.
133. Duncan W, Quilty PM. The results of 963 patients with transitional cell carcinoma of the urinary bladder primarily treated with radical megavoltage x-ray therapy. Radiother Oncol 1986;11:2043.
134. Goffinet DR, Schneider MJ, Glatstein EJ, et al. Bladder Cancer: Results of radiation therapy in 384 patients. Radiology 1992;153:771-782.
135. Montie JE, Straffon RA, Stewart BH. Radical cystectomy without radiation therapy for carcinoma of the bladder. J Urol 1984;131:477.
136. Anderstrom C, Johansson S, Nilsson S, et al. A prospective randomized study of pre-operative radiation with cystectomy or cystectomy alone for invasive bladder carcinoma. Eur Urol 1983;9:142.
137. Bloom HJG, Hendry WF, Wallace DM, et al. Treatment of T3 bladder cancer: Controlled trial of pre-inoperative radiotherapy and radical cystectomy versus radical radiotherapy: Second report and review (for the Clinical Trials Group. Institute of Urology) Br J Urol 1982; 54:136.
138. Whitmore WF, Jr, Batata MA, Hilaris BS, et al. A comparative study of two pre-operative radiation regimens with cystectomy for bladder cancer. Cancer 1977;40:1077.
139. Hope-Stone HF, Oliver RTD, England HR, et al. T3 bladder cancer: Salvage rather than elective cystectomy after radiotherapy. Urology 1984;24:315.
140. Stein JJ, Kaufman JJ. Treatment of carcinoma of the bladder with special reference to the use of pre-operative radiation combined with 5-Fluorouracil. AJR 1968;10:519-529.
141. Woodruff MW, Murphy WT, Hopson JM. Further observation of the use of combination 5-FU and supervoltage radiation therapy in the treatment of advanced carcinoma of the bladder. J Urol 1963;90: 747-758.
142. Rotman M, Aziz H, Porrazzo M, Choi KN, Silverstein M, Rosenthal CJ, Laungani G, Macchia R. Treatment of advanced transitional cell carcinoma of the bladder with irradiation and concomitant 5-fluorouracil infusion. Int J Radiat Oncol Biol Phys 1990;18:1131-1137.
143. Russell KJ, Boileau MA, Ireton R, et al. Transitional cell carcinoma of the urinary bladder: Histological clearance with combined 5-FU and radiation therapy. Preliminary results of a bladder preservation study. Radiology 1988;167:845-850.
144. Shipley WV, Provt Jr, JR, Eienstein AB, et al. Treatment of invasive bladder cancer by cisplatin and irradiation in patients unsuited for surgery. A high success rate in clinical stage T2 tumors in a National Bladder Cancer Group trial. JAMA 1987;258:931.
145. Tester W, Caplan R, Heaney J, et al. Neoadjuvant combined modality program with selective organ preservation for invasive bladder cancer: Results of Radiation Therapy Oncology Group Phase II Trial 8802. J Clin Oncol 1996;14:119-126.
146. Kaufman DS, Shipley WV, Griffin PP, et al. Selective bladder preservation by combination treatment of invasive bladder cancer. N Engl J Med 1993;329:1377-1382.
147. Housset M, Maulard C, Chretien Y, et al. Combined radiation and chemotherapy for invasive transitional cell carcinoma of the bladder: A prospective study. J Clin Oncol 1993;11(11)2150-2157.
148. Sauer WT, Schrott KM, Dunst J, et al. Preliminary results of treatment of invasive bladder carcinoma with radiotherapy and cisplatinum. Int J Radiat Oncol Biol Phys 1988;15:871-875.
149. Eapen L, Stewart D, Danjoix D, et al. Intra-arterial cisplatin and concomitant radiation for locally advanced bladder cancer. J Clin Oncol 1989;7:230-233.
150. Arcangeli G, Tririndelli-Danesi D, Mecozzi A, Saracino B, Cruciani E. Combined Hyperfractionated Irradiation and Protracted Infusion Chemotherapy in Invasive Bladder Cancer with Conservative Intent (abstract). Phase I Study. Int J Radiat Oncol Biol Phys 1996;36:314.
151. Lara-Jimenez P, Garcia-Puch J, Pedvaza V. Adjuvant combined modality treatment in high-risk cancer patients. Ten year results (abstract). Proceedings of the 5th EORTC Breast Cancer Working Conference A293,1991.
152. Harris JR, Recht A. How to combine adjuvant chemotherapy and radiation therapy. Recent results. Cancer Res 1993;127:129-136.
153. Buzzoni R, Bonadonna G, Valagussa P, et al. Adjuvant chemotherapy with doxorubicin plus cyclophosphamide, methotrexate, and fluorouracil in the treatment of resectable breast cancer with more than three positive axillary nodes. J Clin Oncol 1991;9:2134-2140.
154. Link MP, Goorin AM, Miser AW, et al. The effect of adjuvant chemotherapy on relapse-free survival in patients with osteosarcoma of the extremity. N Engl J Med 1986; 314:1600-1606.
155. Spiro IJ, Rosenberg AE, Springfield D, et al. Combined surgery and radiation therapy with adriamycin and radiation in sarcomas and other malignant tumors. J Surg Oncol 1982;21:23-26.
156. Sordillo P, Magill G, Schauer P, Vikram B, Kim J, Hilaris B. Preliminary trial of combination therapy with adriamycin and radiation in sarcomas and other malignant tumors. J Surg Oncol 1982;21:23-26.
157. Turner S, Shetty R, Gandhi H, et al. Combination of radiation with concomitant continuous adriamycin infusion in a patient with partially excised pleomorphic soft tissue sarcoma of the lower extremity. In: Rosenthal CJ, Rotman M, eds. Clinical Applications of Continuous Infusion Chemotherapy and Concomitant Radiation Therapy. New York: Plenum, 1986⊥.183-188.
158. Kovacs C, Evans M, Hooker J, et al. Long term consequences of chemotherapeutic agents on hematopoiesis: Development of altered radiation tolerances. NCI Monogr 1988;6:45.
159. Fajardo LF, Stewart JR. Pathogenesis of radiation-induced myocardial fibrosis. LaG Invest 1973;29:244-257.
160. Bellingham ME. Endomyocardial changes in anthracycline treated patients with or without irradiation. Front Radiat Oncol 1979;13:67-81.
161. Legha S, Benjamin R, Mackay B, et al. Reduction of Doxorubicin cardiotoxicity by rolonged continuous infusion. Ann Intern Med 1982;96:133-139.
162. Mayer EG, Poulter CA, Aristizabal SA. Complication of irradiation related to apparent drug potentiation by Adriamycin. Int J Radiat Oncol Biol Phys 1976;1:1179.
163. Speyer JL, Green MD, Kramer E, et al. Protective effect of the bispiprazinedone (ICRF-187) against doxorubicin-induced cardiac toxicity in women with advanced breast cancer. N Engl J Med 1988; 319:745.
164. Krook JE, Moertel CG, Gunderson LL, et al. Effective surgical adjuvant therapy for high risk rectal carcinoma. N Engl J Med 1991;324: 709-715.

Chapter 3

Fundamentals of Treatment Planning in Radiation Oncology

Carlos A. Perez and James A. Purdy

Irradiation is an effective modality in the treatment of many patients with cancer. It can completely eradicate the tumor in the irradiated volume; it can also provide palliative relief to patients with incurable cancer. The success of radiation therapy depends on the delivery of an adequate dose to the entire tumor volume without causing severe damage to surrounding normal tissues. The goals are to achieve the highest probability of local and regional tumor control with the lowest achievable incidence of side effects (Figure 3.1) (1) and to prolong the life of the patient with the best possible quality of life (as few as possible anatomic defects or physiologic disturbances). This chapter reviews the principles and methodology of irradiation treatment planning.

Large tumors require higher doses than those used to control small lesions or subclinical/microscopic metastases (Figure 3.2) (2,3). Reports by Herring (4), Perez et al (5), Shukovsky and Fletcher (6), and Thames et al (7) indicate a close correlation between the dose of radiation given and the probability of tumor control at the primary site or in metastatic lymph nodes, which may be influenced by the initial number of clonogenic cells and tumor cell heterogeneity (8).

The first dose-response data were reported for skin cancer by Miescher (9) in 1934; 10 years later Strandqvist (10) published a dose-response curve for skin cancer. As Fletcher (11) pointed out, dose-response curves can be elicited only when a group of homogeneous tumors is given a range of radiation doses, indicating that tumor control is a probabilistic event. For every increment of radiation dose, a certain fraction of cells will be killed; therefore, the total number of surviving cells will be proportional to the initial number present and the fraction killed with each dose (11). Thus, various levels of irradiation will yield different probabilities of tumor control, depending on the extent of the lesion (number of clonogenic cells present) and cellular radiosensitivity. For subclinical disease in many malignant tumors, doses of 45 to 50 Gy will result in disease control in over 90% of patients (12,13). Subclinical disease has been referred to as deposits of tumor cells that are too small to be detected clinically and even microscopically but, if left untreated, may subsequently evolve to clinically apparent tumor (14). It must be emphasized that microscopic evidence of tumor, such as at the surgical margin, should not be regarded as subclinical disease; cell aggregates $10^6/cm^3$ or greater are required for the pathologist to detect them. Therefore, these volumes must receive higher doses of irradiation, in the range of 60 to 65 Gy in 6 to 7 weeks for epithelial or mesenchymal tumors.

For clinically palpable tumors, doses of 65 (for T1) to 80 Gy or higher (for T4 tumors) are required (2 Gy/day, five fractions weekly). The dose range and probability of tumor control have been documented for squamous cell carcinoma and adenocarcinoma (Table 3.1) (3,6,8, 11,15–24).

The effects of radiation on most normal tissues have been documented; an intricate interrelationship of total dose, fraction size, volume of organ irradiated, and mechanisms of injury repair (Figure 3.3) and lack of correlation between acute and late effects have been described (Figure 3.4) (25,26). The tolerance of normal tissues is related to the volume irradiated, the nature and function of organs within that volume, and the stage of cancer treated (3).

It has been postulated that for many normal tissues the dose to produce a particular sequela increases as the irradiated volume of the organ decreases (27,28). However, in a review of 268 patients with head and neck tumors treated with various total doses and fractions, Maciejewski et al. (29) observed no difference in acute or late effects

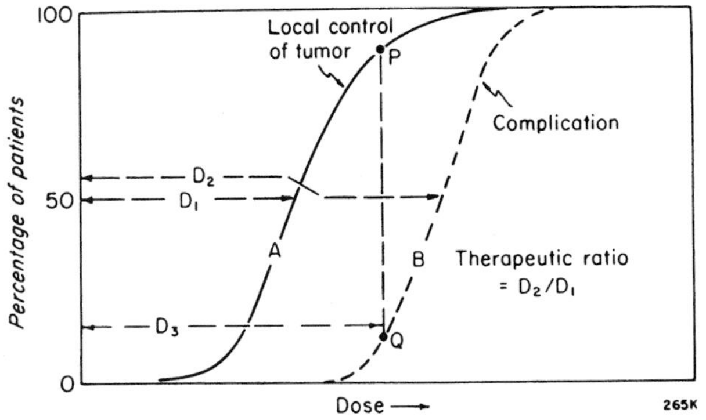

Figure 3.1. Response versus dose relationships for tumor and healthy tissue. (Reprinted with permission from Cunningham JR. Development of computer algorithms for radiation treatment planning. Int J Radiat Oncol Biol Phys 1989;16:1367-1376.) (1)

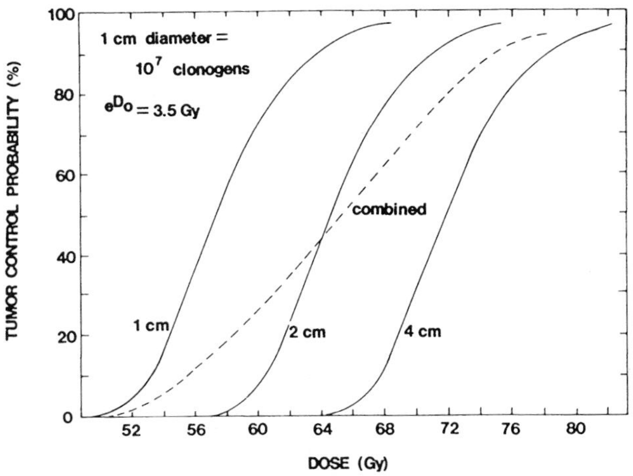

Figure 3.2. Theoretic tumor control probability (TCP) curves for three spherical tumors (solid lines) and one that would result from a study incorporating into the dose response analysis all three tumor sizes in equal proportions (broken line). They were calculated on the assumption that the dose was given in 2 Gy fractions, that the $_eD_0$ value for 2 Gy per fraction was 3.5 Gy, and that a 1 cm diameter spherical tumor contained 10^7 clonogens. (Reprinted with permission from Withers HR, McBride WH. Biologic basis of radiation therapy. In: Perez CA, Brady LW, eds. Principles and Practice of Radiation Oncology, 3rd ed. Philadelphia: Lippincott-Raven, 1998.)

in patients treated with small (50 to 80 cm^2) or large (100 to 140 cm^2) fields.

Several authors have reported higher tolerance doses than initially described for a variety of organs (30-34), which stresses the importance of updating this information in the light of more precise treatment planning and delivery of irradiation and more accurate evaluation and recording of sequelae. A compilation from the literature data of tolerance doses for whole or partial organ irradiation was published (35). These estimates were used by Burman et al (36) to develop a series of tolerance curves for multiple organs. However, it should be pointed out that this compilation of data was taken from the literature that predated three-dimensional (3-D) planning; thus the dose-volume data must be viewed cautiously.

Further, the combination of irradiation with chemotherapeutic agents usually results in greater effect on normal tissues, in some instances requiring adjustments in treatment planning and dose prescription.

Herring (4) discussed the theoretic consequences of lack of precision on dose-response curves for tumor control and normal tissue injury. The predicted consequences are based on the accuracy with which the dose and irradiated volume are defined. An imprecise treatment system could lead to a high incidence of necrosis with a low probability of tumor control (Figure 3.5) (37). Reducing irradiation doses in an effort to avoid complications further decreases the probability of achieving tumor control if such action is based on the wrong assumption that complications are only related to radiation dose levels. Cunningham (1) noted that the goal recommended by International Commission of Radiation Units and Measurements (ICRU) (38) of ±5% accuracy for dose delivery computations is difficult to achieve. Every effort should be made, however, to develop accurate dose calculation algorithms, including methods to correct for inhomogeneities in tissue density and the shape of the patient's body, and to develop practical treatment planning capabilities to obtain the highest possible dose optimization in the irradiated volume (tumor and normal tissues).

In addition to accurate treatment planning, optimal repositioning and immobilization techniques are needed to translate the dose optimization formulated in a plan to actual delivery in single or multiple fractions to the patient. Reproducible patient immobilization and repositioning involve the correct placement of the fields, to cover the entire planning target volume (PTV), with a margin to account for penumbra, and the proper setting of all treatment parameters, such as collimator jaw position, gantry, treatment table angles, monitor units, and time setting. Inaccuracies in field placement, as demonstrated by weekly localization films, have been reported (Table 3.2) (39).

Rabinowitz (40), in a comparison of simulator and portal films of 71 patients, noted some discrepancies between the simulator and the localization (treatment) portal films. With an average value of 3 mm standard deviation of the variations, the mean worst-case discrepancy averaged 3.5 mm in the head and neck region, 9.2 mm in the thorax, 5.1 mm in the abdomen, 8.4 mm in the pelvis, and 6.9 mm in the extremities. Other authors have documented similar localization errors on the basis of portal film review analysis (40,41).

Hendrickson (42) reported a 3.5% error frequency in multiple parameters (setting of field size, timer, gantry and collimator angles, and patient positioning) with one technologist working; the error rate declined to 0.82% when

Table 3.1. Tumor Control Probability Correlated with Irradiation Dose and Volume of Cancer

Dose	Squamous Cell Carcinoma of Upper Respiratory and Digestive Tracts	Adenocarcinoma of Breast
50 Gy*	>90% subclinical (3) 60% T1 lesions of nasopharynx (16) ≈50% 1–3 cm neck nodes (17)	>90% subclinical (15)
60 Gy*	≈90% T1 lesions of pharynx and larynx† ≈50% T3 and T4 lesions of tonsillar fossa (18,19) ≈90% 1–3 cm neck nodes (20) ≈70% 3–5 cm neck nodes (21)	90% clinically positive axillary nodes 2.5–3 cm‡ (15)
70 Gy*	≈90% T2 lesions of tonsillar fossa and supraglottic larynx (6,22) ≈80% T3 and T4 lesions of tonsillar fossa (6)	65% 2–3 cm primary (23)
70–80 Gy (8–9 weeks)	⟶	30% >5 cm primary (23)
80–90 Gy (8–10 weeks)	⟶	56% >5 cm primary (23)
80–100 Gy (10–12 weeks)	⟶	75% 5–15 cm primary (23)

* 10 Gy in five fractions each week.
† Universal experience.
‡ The control rate is corrected for the percentage of nodes that would be positive histologically had a dissection of the axilla been done.
(Reprinted with permission from Fletcher GH, Shukovsky LJ. The interplay of radiocurability and tolerance in the irradiation of human cancers. J Radiol Electrol 1975;56:383–400.)

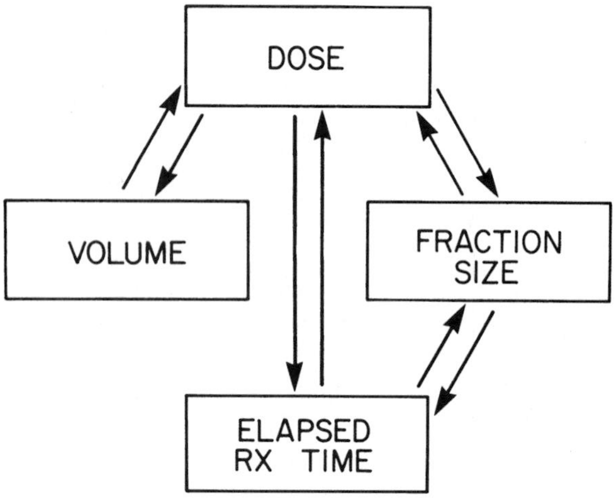

Figure 3.3. Basic dosimetric parameters determining normal tissue effects in radiation therapy. (Reprinted with permission from Perez CA, Brady LW, Roti Roti JL. Overview. In: Perez CA, Brady LW, eds. Principles and Practice of Radiation Oncology, 3rd ed. Philadelphia: Lippincott-Raven, 1998.)

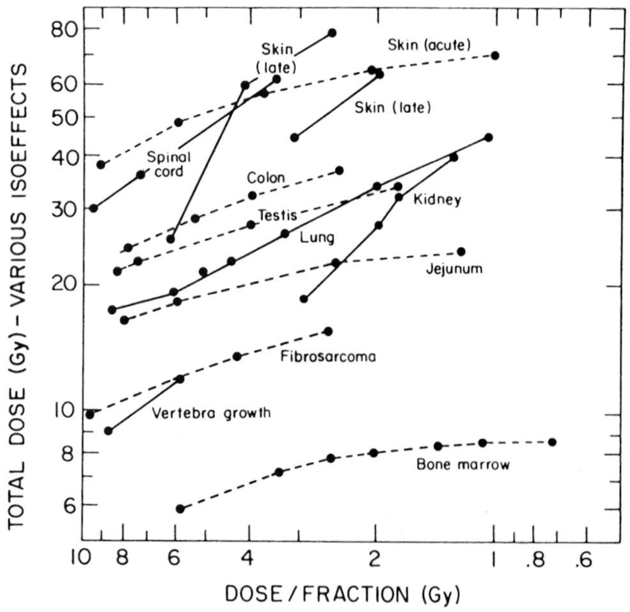

Figure 3.4. Isoeffect curves in which the total dose necessary for a certain effect in various tissues is plotted as a function of dose per fraction (late effects: solid lines; acute effects: broken lines). Data were selected to exclude an influence of regeneration on total dose during multifraction experiments. The isodoses for late effects increase more rapidly with decrease in dose per fraction than is the case for acute effects. (Reprinted with permission from Withers HR. Biologic basis for altered fractionation schemes. Cancer 1985;55:2086-2095.)

two technologists worked together. Marks et al (43,44) demonstrated, by systematic use of verification films, a high frequency of localization errors in patients irradiated for head and neck cancer or malignant lymphomas. These errors were corrected with improved immobilization of the patients; for instance, the use of a bite block in patients with head and neck tumors reduced localization errors from 16 to 1% (43). Extra care is taken in defining the volume to be irradiated because small inaccuracies may result in appreciable variations of dose in the critical volume (target volume).

Doss (45), in a study of patients with upper airway carcinoma, showed that in 21 of 28 patients (75%) with treatments in which 30% or more portals exhibited a blocking error, a recurrence developed, whereas tumor failure was noted in only 2 of 12 patients (17%) without such errors.

Perez et al (46) also reported a higher incidence of failures in patients with carcinoma of the nasopharynx on

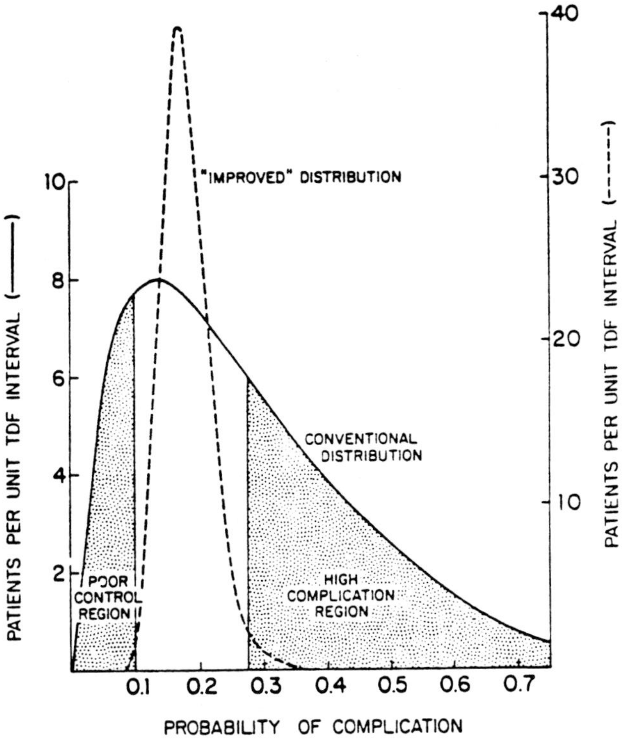

Figure 3.5. Frequency distribution of patients receiving treatment and different probabilities of complication. (Reprinted with permission from Orton CG. Other Considerations in Three-Dimensional Treatment Planning. In: Bagne F, ed. Computerized Treatment Planning Systems. HHS Publications FDA 84-8223;1984:136-141.)

whom shielding of the ear inadvertently caused some blocking of tumor volume (Table 3.3).

More recently, on-line electronic portal imaging verification studies have been reported (Table 3.4) (47). In a review of 48 patients on whom multiple digital portal verification images were obtained, Bissett et al (48) noted that displacements of the field were 2.9 mm in the transverse and 3.4 mm in the craniocaudal dimensions. Mean rotational displacement was 2 degrees. The mean treatment field coverage in this set of images was 95%. There were some variations in the assessment of the translational errors when observations of several radiation oncologists were analyzed.

Suit et al (49) reviewed various recent technologic developments that through more precise treatment planning and delivery techniques will reduce volume irradiated and improve dose distributions, which should enhance therapeutic outcome.

Although treatment planning is extremely helpful in determining the best form of therapy, the responsibility for critical judgment and execution rests with the radiation oncologist, who, to treat patients effectively, must: (1) have sufficient training (particularly in cross-sectional anatomy) to define the target volume and critical structures, to interpret treatment planning information, and to guide the physicist or dosimetrist in achieving the best dose distribution; (2) have sufficient knowledge to select the best possible combination of dose and fractionation for a given site and volume; (3) be competent to judge the quality of the dose distribution and the technical feasibility and accuracy of a proposed plan; and (4) understand the capabilities and limitations of the staff and computer systems involved in the radiation treatment planning process. No computer software can correct the radiation oncologist's errors of clinical judgment, misunderstanding of physical concepts, or inadequate treatment delivery.

LIMITATIONS OF RADIATION THERAPY

The failure of radiation therapy to eradicate a tumor can result not only from suboptimal dosimetry and treatment planning but also from a variety of factors.

Clinical factors include:

1. Inadequate appraisal of the full extent of the tumor in the surrounding tissues or regional lymph node metastases that are not irradiated.

Table 3.2. Type and Degree of Field Placement Errors Detected by Weekly Localization Films (Verification Film + Beam Film)

					Degree Misplaced	
Anatomic Region of Primary Tumor	Field Malposition (%)	Field Malrotation (%)	Patient Malposition (%)	Block Misplaced (%)	Range (cm)	Average (cm)
Ear-nose-throat	78	9.5	9.5	3	0.5–3.0	0.92
Cranial	75	17	0	17	0.5–3.0	0.85
Chest	68	12	17	2.4	0.5–2.0	1.0
Pelvis	72.5	25	0	2.5	0.5–4.0	1.5
Extrapelvic Abdomen	75	17	0	8.5	0.5–3.0	1.4
Bones	67	11	22	0	0.5–3.0	1.15
Total	74	14	8.5	4	0.5–4.0	1.1

(Reprinted with permission from Byhardt RW, Cox JD, Hornburg A, et al. Weekly localization films and detection of field placement errors. Int J Radiat Oncol Biol Phys 1978;4:881–887.)

Table 3.3. Carcinoma of Nasopharynx: Correlation of Quality of Portal Films with Primary Tumor Control

	Local Tumor Control			
	1956-1965 (n = 30)	1966-1975 (n = 54)	1976-1986 (n = 59)	Total (n = 143)
Simulation done	0	12/21 (57%)	43/57 (75%)	55/78 (71%)
Simulation not done	18/30 (60%)	16/31 (52%)	0	34/61 (56%)
				p = 0.1
>75% adequate portal films	8/11 (73%)	16/28 (57%)	42/56 (75%)	66/95 (69%)
<75% adequate portal films	10/19 (53%)	12/24 (50%)	1/1 (100%)	23/44 (52%)
				p = 0.07
Percent of films with ear block shielding nasopharynx				
≤25%	11/17 (65%)	22/36 (61%)	42/56 (75%)	75/109 (69%)
26% to 50%	7/12 (58%)	4/9 (44%)	1/1 (100%)	12/22 (55%)
≥51%	0/1	2/7 (29%)	0/0	2/8 (25%)
				p = 0.04

(Reprinted with permission from Perez CA, Devineni VR, Marcial-Vega V, et al. Carcinoma of the nasopharynx: Factors affecting prognosis. Int J Radiat Oncol Biol Phys 1992;23:271–280.)

Table 3.4. Mean Image Shift Parameter *d* at End of Treatment

	Visit 1			Visit 2			Visit 3			Visit 4			Overall		
	No.	*d*	(SD)	No.	*d*	(SD)	No.	*d*	(SD)	No.	*d*	(SD)	No.	*d*	(SD)
Anterior															
Conventional	5	2.5	(1.8)	5	5.4	(2.9)	6	4.6	(2.9)	5	4.1	(1.6)	21	4.1	(2.5)
Intervention	6	3.1	(1.4)	6	2.3	(1.6)	6	2.1	(1.3)	5	2.6	(2.3)	23	2.5	(1.6)
Posterior															
Conventional	6	5.3	(2.2)	4	6.9	(0.6)	5	6.2	(2.8)	5	6.5	(2.0)	20	6.1	(2.0)
Intervention	6	1.8	(1.6)	5	1.4	(1.7)	6	1.2	(1.4)	5	1.6	(1.1)	22	1.5	(1.4)
Right lateral															
Conventional	5	5.3	(2.3)	3	5.2	(1.7)	4	2.3	(2.3)	4	6.0	(3.1)	16	4.7	(2.6)
Intervention	4	2.8	(1.2)	3	2.0	(0.9)	5	2.2	(1.4)	4	2.1	(1.5)	16	2.3	(1.2)
Left lateral															
Conventional	5	4.9	(1.8)	3	7.0	(2.3)	4	4.6	(1.4)	4	7.2	(1.2)	16	5.8	(1.9)
Intervention	4	1.5	(0.0)	3	2.5	(0.9)	5	1.7	(1.2)	3	1.0	(0.9)	15	1.7	(0.9)

No. is the number of patients from which the associated average *d* is computed; *d* in the final column is the average over the four visits. (Reprinted with permission from Gildersleve J, Dearnaley DP, Evans PM, et al. A randomised trial of patient repositioning during radiotherapy using a megavoltage imaging system. Radiother Oncol 1994;31:161–168.)

2. Clinically unrecognized distant metastases at the time of initial treatment, which are a major cause of failure in some tumors, such as breast or lung primary tumors. Their management requires effective systemic therapy.
3. Inaccurate definition of gross tumor volume (GTV), clinical target volume (CTV), and PTV.
4. Inaccurate definition or difficulty in determining critical normal structures (e.g., optic chiasma, brachial plexus).

Physical and technical factors can also affect radiation therapy:

1. Inadequate treatment planning with inhomogeneous dose distributions in planning target volumes or dose exceeding tolerance of critical normal structures.
2. Unreliable patient repositioning and immobilization techniques, with faulty reproducibility in daily treatments resulting in inadequate doses or volumes treated.

3. Lack of adequate verification-dosimetry techniques, except in cases in which small in vivo dosimeters can be used.
4. Inadequate dose prescription (i.e., low dose).

Biologic factors affecting treatment outcome include:

1. Large initial cell burden; small tumors are more easily eradicated than large tumors.
2. Hypoxic cell subpopulations, which require greater doses of irradiation. This problem is resolved in part by the reoxygenation that occurs between fractionated doses of irradiation (50).
3. Repair of sublethal or potentially lethal damage between fractions (51).
4. Variation in radiosensitivity throughout cell proliferative cycle (52).
5. Lack of knowledge of human cell kinetics and biologic equivalents for various dose rate-fractionation regimens (53,54).
6. Limited tolerance of normal tissues to irradiation (55).

Less well-defined factors include the general condition, nutritional status, metabolism, and immune response of the individual patient. This subject was thoroughly discussed by Bush and Hill (56).

STEPS INVOLVED IN TREATMENT PLANNING

The procedures involved in effective planning and administration of radiation therapy comprise a complex, closely integrated process that should include the following:

1. Thorough knowledge of the natural history and pathologic characteristics of the tumor.
2. Adequate evaluation of the patient and staging procedures to determine the full extent of the tumor.
3. Definition of treatment strategy to select the best method or combinations of therapies to be applied, which may depend on the stage, type of tumor, and routes of spread.
4. Treatment planning volumetric imaging study, with accurate definition of the target volume, critical normal structures, and radiation beam portals.
5. Treatment isodose (volumetric) computations and plan evaluation to determine the optimum distribution of irradiation within the volume of interest.
6. Accurate and reproducible repositioning and immobilization techniques for daily treatment delivery.
7. Applicable in vivo dosimetry, portal localization, and verification procedures to ensure quality control throughout the therapeutic process.
8. Periodic evaluation of the patient during and after therapy, to assess the effects of treatment on the tumor and the tolerance of the patient.

The steps and personnel involved in the radiation therapy process are summarized in Figure 3.6 (57) and Table 3.5 (58).

The treatment strategy must include, in addition to clinical, physical, and radiobiologic concepts that provide a rational basis for the therapy, thoughtful consideration of the treatment's psychologic repercussions, acute side effects, and late sequelae, all of which may affect the quality of life of the patient. Supportive care during treatment is important. Although treatment guidelines may be established and dosimetry patterns compiled, the treatment plan may be individualized to suit the needs of each patient.

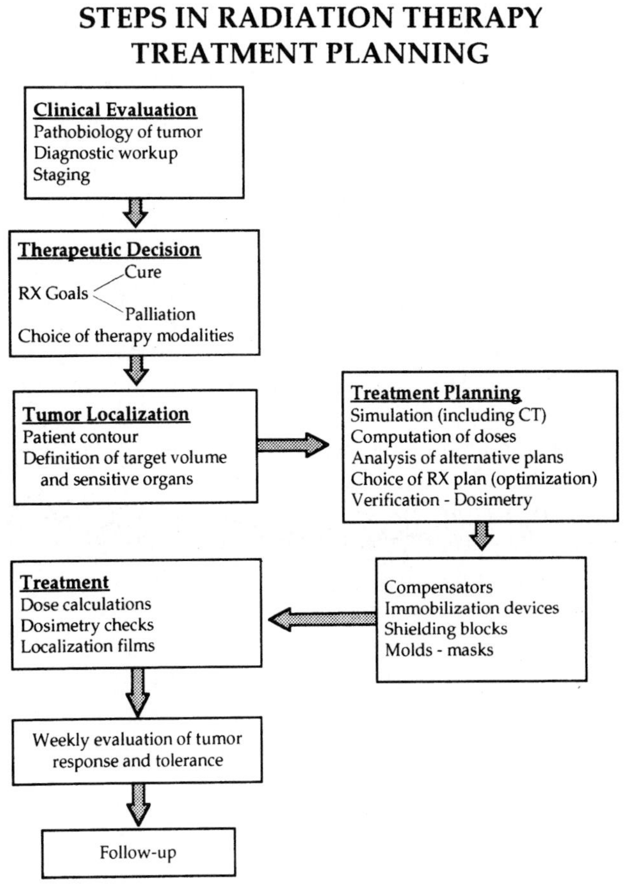

Figure 3.6. Steps in radiation therapy treatment planning. (Modified from Perez CA, Thomas PRM. Radiation Therapy: Basic Concepts and Clinical Implications. In: Sutow WW, Fernbach DJ, Vietti TJ, eds. Clinical Pediatric Oncology, 3rd ed. St. Louis: CV Mosby, 1984:167-209.)

Table 3.5. Process and Staff in Clinical Radiation Therapy

	Key Staff	Supportive Role
Clinical evaluation	Radiation oncologist	
Therapeutic decision	Radiation oncologist	
Target volume localization		
Tumor volume	Radiation oncologist	Simulation technologist/dosimetrist
Sensitive critical organs	Radiation oncologist	Simulation technologist/dosimetrist
Patient contour	Dosimetrist	Simulation technologist/dosimetrist
Treatment planning		
Beam data computerization	Physicist	
Computation of beams	Physicist	Dosimetrist
Shielding blocks, treatment aids, etc.	Dosimetrist/mold room technologist	Radiation oncologist/physicist
Analysis of alternate plans	Radiation oncologist/physicist	Dosimetrist
Selection of treatment plan	Radiation oncologist/physicist	
Dose calculation	Dosimetrist	Physicist
Simulation/verification of treatment plan	Radiation oncologist/simulation technologist	Dosimetrist/physicist
Treatment		
First day setup	Radiation oncologist/physicist/therapy technologist	Dosimetrist/physicist
Localization films	Radiation oncologist/therapy technologist	
Dosimetry checks/initial chart review	Physicist/radiation oncologist	Dosimetrist/chief technologist
Repositioning/retreatment	Therapy technologist	Dosimetrist/technologist
Periodic evaluation (during treatment)		
Tumor response/tolerance	Radiation oncologist	Nurse/radiation therapy technologist
Follow-up evaluation	Radiation oncologist	Nurse

(Reprinted with permission from Inter-Society Council for Radiation Oncology: Radiation Oncology in Integrated Cancer Management. November 1986.)

Definition of Tumor Volume

From a cell burden standpoint, a clinical tumor can be considered to encompass several compartments: macroscopic (visible or palpable) disease, microextensions into adjacent tissues, and subclinical disease, presumed to be present but not detectable even under the microscope. Treatment portals must adequately cover all three compartments in addition to margins to compensate for geometric inaccuracies and beam characteristics (penumbra) during irradiation exposure.

According to ICRU No. 50 (59), volumes of interest in treatment planning are defined as follows. The GTV is all known gross disease including abnormally enlarged regional lymph nodes. When GTV is being determined, it is important to use the appropriate computed tomography (CT) window and level settings that give the maximum dimension of what is considered potential gross disease. The CTV encompasses the GTV plus regions considered to harbor potential microscopic disease. The PTV provides a margin around the CTV to allow for variation in treatment setup and other anatomic motion during treatment such as respiration. Finally, an additional margin must be added beyond the PTV to account for treatment machine beam characteristics such as penumbra (Figure 3.7) (60). More detail on ICRU No. 50 nomenclature is presented in Chapter 9.

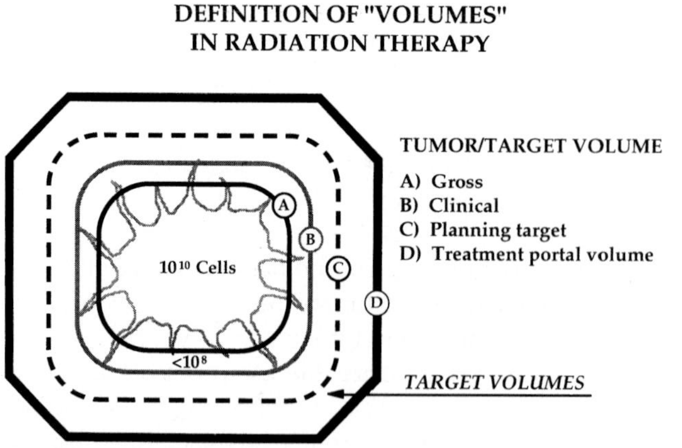

Figure 3.7. Definition of tumor volume and target volume. Target volume includes tumor volume, potential areas of local and regional microscopic disease around tumor, and margin of surrounding normal tissue. (Reprinted with permission from Perez CA, Brady LW, Roti Roti JL. Overview. In: Perez CA, Brady LW, eds. Principles and Practice of Radiation Oncology, 3rd ed. Philadelphia: Lippincott-Raven, 1998.)

Definition of Relevant Normal Structures

Sensitive structures (ICRU calls these "organs at risk") within the irradiated volume should be clearly identified, and the maximum doses and fractionation to be delivered to them must be specified.

When late radiation effects are studied, an organ can be considered to be made up of multiple functional subunits (FSUs) arranged in either series or parallel (61,62). For organs structured in a series, such as gastrointestinal tract or nervous tissue, damage to one portion of the organ may render the entire organ dysfunctional. In contrast, in a parallel-structured organ, FSU damage may not impair the entire organ function because the remaining FSUs operate independently from the damaged group, and clinical injury occurs only when a critical volume of the organ (or proportion of FSUs) is damaged and the surviving FSUs are unable to maintain organ function. Therefore, the sensitivity of an organ depends on the number of FSUs. Marks (63) discussed the importance of organ structure in determining late radiation effects and pointed out that conventional dose-volume histograms (DVHs) and normal tissue complication probability (NTCP) models are frequently inadequate because they ignore functional and structural heterogeneities. He suggested incorporation of functional heterogeneities with improved assessment of normal tissue effects in treatment planning.

Jackson et al (64) presented a thorough discussion of the subject, including its mathematical basis, and addressed the problem of calculating NTCP for inhomogeneously irradiated organs with parallel quantal architecture. They showed that variations in FSUs and functional reserve in a patient population may produce NTCP dose-response curves, the widths of which are comparable to those observed clinically.

Structural alterations without anatomic or functional impairment may be noted, whereas in other instances substantial injuries with tissue destruction, severe dysfunction, or even death may occur. Normal tissues have a substantial capacity to recover from sublethal or potentially lethal damage induced by radiation (at tolerable dose levels). Injury to normal tissues may be caused by the radiation effect on the microvasculature or the support tissues (stromal or parenchymal cells) (65).

Rubin et al (66) indicated the usefulness of assigning a certain percentage of risk of complication, depending on the dose of the radiation. The minimal tolerance dose is defined as $TD_{5/5}$, which represents the dose of radiation that would cause no more than a 5% severe complication rate within 5 years after treatment. An acceptable complication rate for severe injury is 5 to 10% in most curative clinical situations. Moderate sequelae are noted in varying proportions (10 to 25% of patients), depending on the dose of irradiation given and the organs at risk.

Chronologically, the effects of irradiation have been subdivided as *acute* (first 6 months), *subacute* (second 6 months), or *late* (depending on the time they are observed). The gross manifestations depend on the kinetic properties of the cells (slow or rapid renewal) and the dose of irradiation given (67).

Simulation

After appropriate evaluation of the patient and determination of therapeutic goals, the treatment planning process begins with the simulation, which in most instances accurately defines the tumor volume and sensitive structures and documents the configuration of the portals and volume to be irradiated (68). Conventional simulators and their use have been described previously (69-73).

Perez et al (60) described the conceptual structure and process for the use of a fully integrated 3-D CT simulator. The elements of an optimal device include: 1) volumetric definition of tumor volume and patient anatomy obtained with a CT scanner, 2) virtual simulation for beam setup and digitally reconstructed radiographs (DRRs), 3) 3-D treatment planning for volumetric dose computation and plan evaluation, and 4) patient-marking device to outline portal or fiducial marks on patient's skin.

The process of CT simulation and 3-D conformal radiation therapy (3-D CRT) will be explained in detail later.

Treatment Aids and Repositioning Devices

Treatment aids, such as shielding blocks, molds, masks, immobilization devices, and compensators, are extremely important in treatment planning and delivery to achieve optimal radiation dose distribution. The radiation oncologist should be familiar with the physical characteristics of these devices and use them to achieve optimal therapeutic results. Simpler treatment delivery techniques that yield an acceptable dose distribution are preferred over more costly and complex ones, in which a greater margin of error in a day-to-day treatment may be present. Repositioning and immobilization are critical because the only effective irradiation is that which strikes the clonogenic tumor cells. Therefore, in fractionated irradiation accurate setup should be such that the patient will maintain the desired position during every daily treatment. Repositioning and immobilization devices, such as the Alpha cradle, plaster casts, thermoplast molds, bite blocks, and arm boards, are invaluable in assisting radiation therapists in patient positioning.

Improved accuracy in treatment planning and delivery may give credence to a long-heralded goal of optimizing the dose of irradiation given to a patient through conformational dynamic therapy. New approaches to the delivery of irradiation, with multiple portals and dynamic beam modifiers (multileaf collimator, wedges, etc.) and beam-intensity modulation will optimize the clinical applications of 3-D radiation treatment planning (3-D RTP) and conformal irradiation (74). Computer interplay between the CT simulator/3-D planning system and the radiation therapy machines allows the highly complex treatment plan generated by computational techniques to be transferred to the treatment machine through a computer interface, which conforms the shape of the collimator as the therapy is delivered (75).

Computer-aided integration of the data generated by 3-D RTP with parameters used on the treatment machine, including gantry and couch position, may decrease localization errors and enhance the precision and efficiency with which irradiation is administered. Several authors have reported improved dose distribution with less-irradiated volume of normal lung (76), liver (77), bladder, or rectum using 3-D conformal techniques (78-82).

Accuracy is periodically assessed with portal (localization) films or on-line imaging verification (electronic portal imaging) devices (83-85). Portal films, used for geometric/anatomic verification, are generally of fair to poor quality, making accurate identification of internal landmarks difficult. Real-time on-line electronic portal imaging devices (EPIDs) allow monitoring of the position of the area to be treated during the radiation exposure (86). Geometric verification primarily ensures reproducibility. There is a paucity of noninvasive techniques to verify dosimetrically the implementation of an optimized treatment plan.

Portal localization errors may be systematic or occur at random; EPID images were used to document inter- or intratreatment portal displacement in patients treated with pelvic irradiation (84). In this study, intertreatment displacement exceeding 10 mm was seen in 3% of the patients in the mediolateral, 16% in the craniocaudal, and 23% in the anteroposterior directions. There was no intratreatment displacement exceeding 10 mm in 547 images.

TREATMENT PLANNING AND GOAL OF THERAPY

Treatment planning, because of its cost, should be reserved primarily for patients treated with a curative aim using high doses of irradiation or in selected patients receiving palliative therapy who require complex treatment techniques or higher irradiation doses (i.e., greater than 45 Gy).

Techniques of Irradiation

In patients treated with isocentric techniques or multiple fields or using special beam-modifying devices (e.g., wedges, multileaf collimator), treatment planning with CT is widely used to optimize the dose distribution. Isodose curves are displayed on CT scan images using two-dimensional (2-D) or 3-D techniques for better appreciation of the dose to tumor volume and normal tissue.

In patients treated with brachytherapy, treatment planning accurately documents the placement of the radioactive sources and the dose distributions in the treatment volume in several planes or in 3-D displays.

Beam Quality

Depending on whether photons, electrons, or protons will be used, it is critical to determine the dose distributions in the target volume related to the physical characteristics of the beams. Electrons have a sharp dose gradient in tissues, and the depth at which a certain dose is required must be determined to accurately select the electron beam energy. Also, the depth-dose curves for high linear energy transfer particles such as protons are characterized by the Bragg peak in which the maximum dose is delivered with no dose beyond that point, again requiring an extremely accurate definition of target volumes (87).

Therapeutic Ratio (Gain)

It is apparent that there is (or should be) an optimal dose that will produce the maximum probability of tumor control with a minimum (reasonably acceptable) frequency of complications (preferably called sequelae of therapy).

The farther the two curves diverge, the more favorable is the therapeutic ratio (88). The therapeutic ratio or therapeutic gain factor (TGF) of a given regimen could be expressed as follows:

$$\text{TGF} = \frac{\%\ \text{tumor control A versus B therapy}}{\%\ \text{major complications A versus B therapy}}$$

The higher the TGF, the more efficient a particular therapy. Such a quantitative expression could be used to compare different therapeutic strategies. Mendelsohn (89) expressed this concept in terms of "uncomplicated tumor ablation" (Figure 3.8). The selection of a dose must weigh the probability of major complications against any potential enhancement of tumor control. Models for decision-making, using Bayesian theory, incorporate values assigned to positive or negative outcomes: Positive outcome—uncomplicated cure, negative outcome—complicated cure, uncomplicated recurrence, or complicated recurrence (90).

Andrews (91,92) emphasized that in radiation therapy, even though there is a recognized correlation between total dose delivered to the tumor and probability of control, efforts to reduce the risk of failure cannot be made at the cost of increasing the risk of injury (beyond reasonable levels). This principle was illustrated by Herring (4) using clinical data from Shukovsky et al (93) for carcinoma of the glossopalatine sulcus.

Dose Optimization

In seeking maximum application of treatment planning, we should keep in mind several factors that will affect its impact on the outcome of radiation therapy.

1. Optimal dose distribution, which is typically achieved using multiple stationary or dynamic beams. In addition, the optimal dose distribution in many tumors requires more than one beam energy or beam modifiers such as wedges or compensating

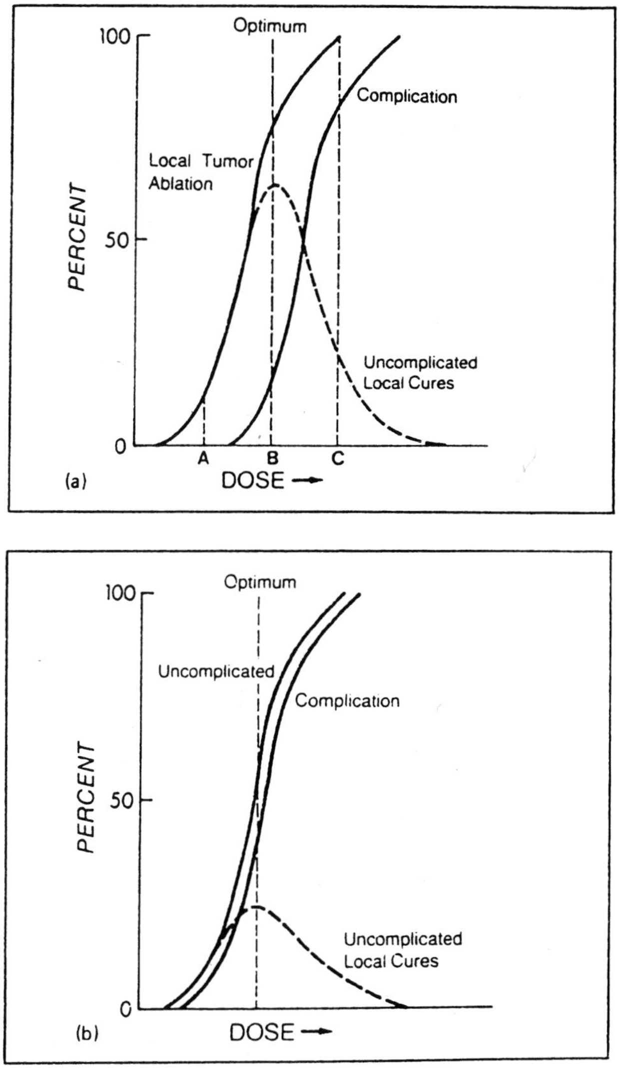

Figure 3.8. Treatment outcomes. Uncomplicated curves (dashed lines) are the desired results of treatment. This is illustrated as a function of the therapeutic ratio; that is, the greater the separation of the tumor control curve and the normal tissue complication curve, the greater number of uncomplicated cures will result. The letters A, B, and C represent three different dose levels, which, if chosen, would lead to three different outcomes: A would result in few tumor cures but no complications; C would lead to complete cure in many cases, but virtually all patients would suffer complications. The optimal choice in this group of dose levels is B, which would result in the greatest number of cured patients without complications. (Modified from Mendelsohn ML. The biology of dose-limiting tissues. In: Time and Dose Relationships in Radiation Biology as Applied to Radiotherapy, Brookhaven National Laboratory Report 5023. Upton, NY: Brookhaven National Laboratory, 1969:154-173. In: Rubin P, Siemann DW. Principles of Radiation Oncology and Cancer Radiotherapy. In: Rubin P, ed. Clinical Oncology: A Multidisciplinary Approach for Physicians and Students, 7th ed. Philadelphia: WB Saunders, 1993:71-90.)

filters. A combination of external beams and intracavitary or interstitial therapy also may be required, depending on the location of the tumor and the beam type and energies used. New techniques are being used such as intensity-modulated radiation therapy (IMRT) in which nonuniform beam fluences are used either in an arc-based approach or with multiple static fields.

2. Small integral dose. The ideal situation is represented by an optimal dose to the target volume with a minimum dose to the rest of the patient.

THREE-DIMENSIONAL TREATMENT PLANNING AND CONFORMAL RADIATION THERAPY

Three-dimensional treatment planning and conformal irradiation promise high-precision dose delivery to a specified target volume with better sparing of normal tissues than 2-D RTP (94,95). The rationale for using 3-D CRT for treatment of patients with cancer has been discussed in numerous publications (95,96). Although preliminary reports are very encouraging, it remains to be demonstrated that this new technology will result in more long-term cures of patients with cancer.

Dose escalation may be difficult or unfeasible in certain sites with organs having serial architecture, such as brain or spinal cord, due to the potential for higher complication rates. Caution should be used in considering other organs for dose escalation using 3-D CRT. For example, the esophagus, although not considered a tissue with serial architecture, may experience severe complications (stricture or possible perforation) with doses beyond tolerance of the organ.

Tumors arising from tissues with parallel architecture such as lung, prostate, head and neck (certain sites), and liver are being treated by 3-D CRT at an increasing number of institutions. The benefit of 3-D CRT hypothetically could be linked to improved local tumor control because of better coverage of the target volume with a specific dose of irradiation, less acute and late morbidity, possibility of carrying out dose-escalation studies if morbidity is held to acceptable levels, and improved survival. Several single institutions, the Radiation Therapy Oncology Group, and nine institutions under cooperative agreement with the National Cancer Institute are conducting phase I/II dose-escalation studies in carcinoma of the prostate and lung.

We identified cases that would benefit most from this technology, including patients with tumors in sites with complex anatomy, irregular-shaped tumors, tumors adjacent to radiation-sensitive normal structures, and small-volume or high-dose treatment. As our efficiency improves, we are able to treat more patients, and greater productivity is being achieved. We implemented 3-D CRT with current technology, but the use of innovative engineering, such as computer-controlled linear accelerators with improved planning and delivery techniques, and accessories such as multileaf collimation and dynamic wedges, has enhanced the efficiency of 3-D planning and delivery, decreasing its overall cost.

Process of 3-D Conformal Radiation Therapy

Three-dimensional CRT, which conforms the prescription dose to the target volumes while lowering dose to normal tissues, is considered an integrated process that involves constructing a patient repositioning/immobilization device, obtaining a volumetric image data set of the patient, defining image-based target volumes and organs at risk, designing beam shapes and beam orientations, calculating volumetric dose distributions, evaluating/optimizing the 3-D plan, delivering a conformal dose distribution, and verifying the treatment plan implementation. This topic is addressed fully in Chapter 9, and only a brief overview of the 3-D CRT treatment planning process is presented here.

Step 1: Evaluation of the patient, tumor (staging), and functional status of uninvolved organs.

Step 2: CT scanning of the patient (CT simulation). At our institution, we use the AcQsim (Varian-Picker International). Patients are scanned, and reference marks are placed on both the patient and the immobilization device to aid in repositioning. Generally, we obtain 3 mm thick CT slices throughout the target volume and 6 to 8 mm thick slices in other areas to further define normal patient anatomy in the treatment position.

Step 3: Outline of target volumes (GTV, CTV, and PTV) and relevant surrounding normal structures (Figure 3.9). The CT data are transferred to the Voxel-Q workstation (Varian-Picker International), and volumes are contoured slice by slice. For target volume definition, we have adopted the ICRU Report No. 50 recommendations (59). The contour data are transferred to the 3-D RTP system, and realistic reconstruction of all target volumes and normal tissue structures is carried out.

Step 4: Design appropriate portals using the beam's eye view (BEV) (Figure 3.10) tool and beam arrangements using room-view display tools. We have found room-view display to be useful for setting the isocenter position and evaluating multiple-beam arrangements.

Step 5: Dose calculation and plan evaluation using tools such as the room-view 3-D isodose-volume display (Figure 3.11), dose statistics, and DVH (Figure 3.12) (96). After trial and error and changes for improvement, the final plan (most appropriate) is selected.

Step 6: Obtain and review final set of DRRs. Geometric information obtained at this step is used either to make Cerrobend blocks or for multileaf collimation.

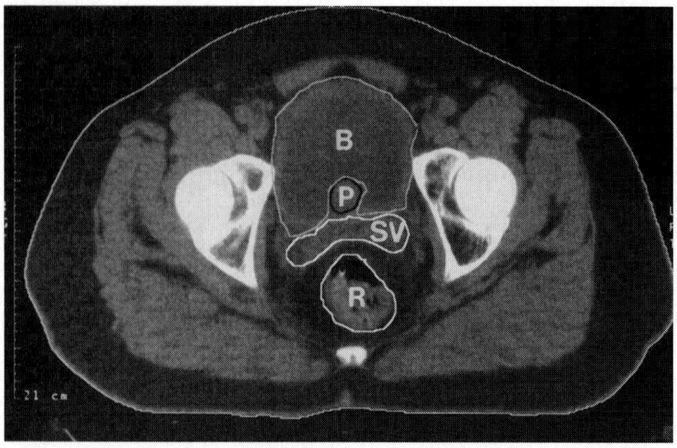

Figure 3.9. CT scan of the pelvis illustrating the outline of the prostate, seminal vesicles, bladder, and rectum, which must be carried out in all CT slices in order to proceed with 3-D volume reconstruction.

A radiographic verification simulation procedure is used in selected patients to confirm the accuracy and validity of 3-D plans; films of each portal are visually compared with the DRR generated from the 3-D system using multiple bony landmarks. Monitor unit calculations are performed, and all treatment parameters are transferred and recorded on the treatment record.

Several tumor sites have been treated with 3-D CRT (to various degrees of conformity) including prostate, lung, head and neck, brain, and hepatobiliary tract. In general, clinical research in 3-D CRT can arbitrarily be divided into three categories: technical innovations and improvements including target volume delineation, treatment planning, immobilization, and dose delivery; clinical trials aimed at the reduction of dose to normal structures to reduce complication rates; and dose-escalation studies aimed at increasing dose to the target volume to improve local tumor control and survival.

Readers interested in 3-D CRT will appreciate a complete treatise by Webb (97), many articles on the subject in a special issue of the *International Journal of Radiation Oncology Biology Physics* (98), and a monograph on 3-D treatment planning and conformal therapy edited by Purdy and Emami (94).

The actual initial cost of 3-D CRT is somewhat higher than standard irradiation techniques (99). Cost-benefit studies should be undertaken in which the actual cost of treating a patient who is cured is computed according to the long-term probability of tumor control, survival, and quality of life. This should be compared with the cost of a

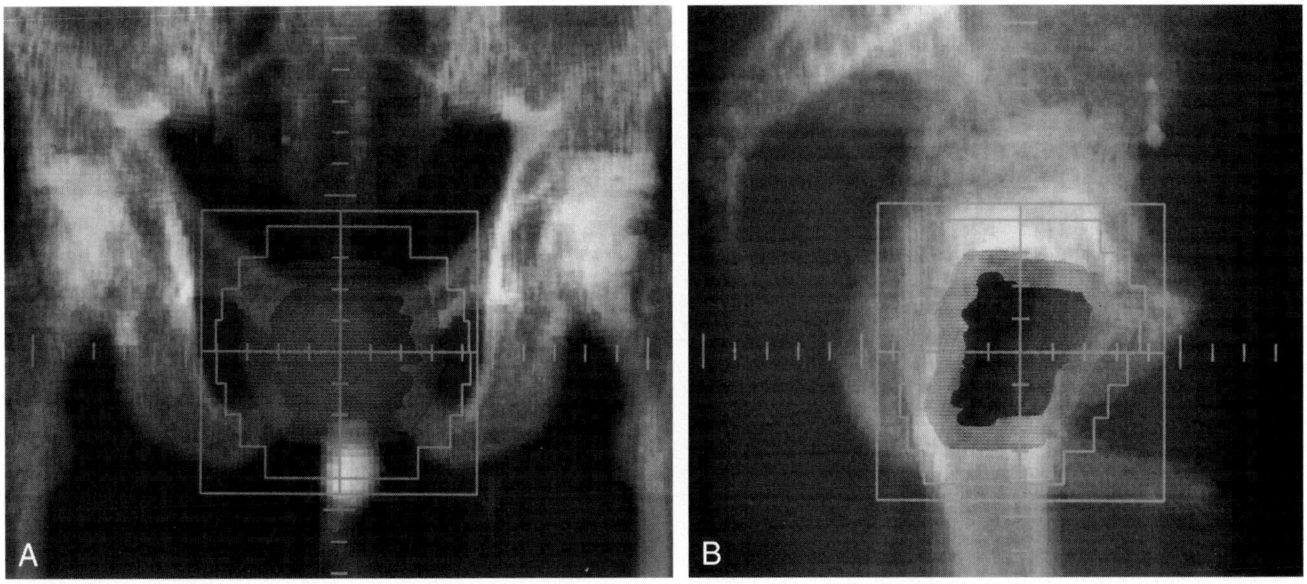

Figure 3.10. Anteroposterior (**A**) and lateral (**B**) digital reconstructed radiograph with outline of prostate (GTV) and planning target volume (PTV) as well as portal outline for 3-D conformal therapy.

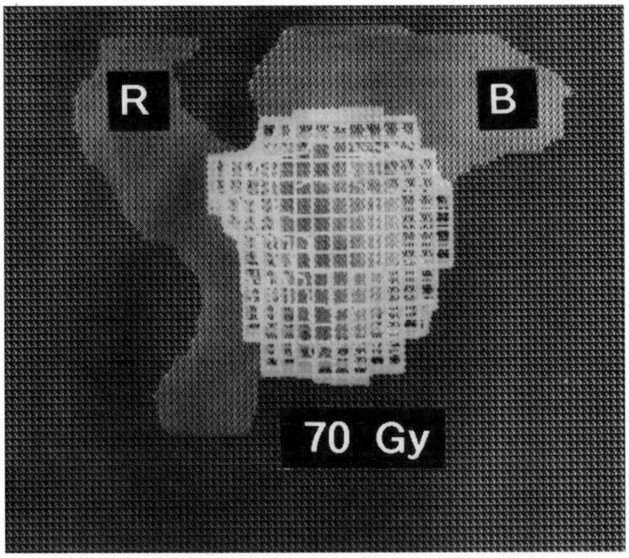

Figure 3.11. Example of room-view display of volumetric dose distribution (70 Gy) covering the entire prostatic volume. The bladder (B) and rectum (R) are identified.

patient similarly treated who develops locoregional tumor recurrence or distant metastases. The cost of treating clinically significant treatment sequelae must be included. If tumor control and survival are enhanced and morbidity decreased with optimal 3-D CRT, prospective cost-benefit analysis should document that this is a worthwhile investment (100).

IMPACT OF TREATMENT PLANNING ON OUTCOME OF THERAPY

Goitein (101) hypothesized that the impact of CT treatment planning on survival would be limited, because other factors can affect the overall prognosis of patients. Using theoretic assumptions, Goitein calculated that the improvement in survival was approximately 4%. Although this estimate is conservative, it represents a significant number of patients, considering that over 1.2 million new cancer patients were diagnosed in the United States in 1997, and approximately 650,000 were treated with radiation therapy, with more than 50% of patients receiving treatment with a curative aim.

Because of the emphasis on control of systemic disease, mostly by medical oncologists, assessment of the importance of locoregional tumor control in patients with malignant tumors has been relatively underemphasized (102). Table 3.6, compiled from data reported by the American Cancer Society (103), illustrates that in 1997 in the United States, 69% of patients died with locoregional disease, which is just as prevalent as distant metastases. A large proportion of patients (50%) have *both* locoregional recurrence and distant metastases.

As more effective systemic adjuvant therapies are designed, it becomes imperative to improve locoregional tumor control, the first step in the overall eradication of the tumor and prolongation of patient survival.

Suit and Westgate (104) noted that improvements in locoregional tumor control will result in a decreased incidence of distant metastases and better survival in patients

Target Volume Assessment for PTV1
Matched Tissue: TARGET_VOLUME1

Patient ID: B950773 | Total Organ Volume: 119 cc | Date: Fri Aug 25 13:56:18 1995
Patient Name: | | Disease Site: Prostate
Dose Bin: 0.10 Gy | Sample Resolution: 1.0 mm | Rank: 7

Plan	Plan ID	Plan Description	%Vol. >= Rx Dose	Maximum Dose (Gy)	Minimum Dose (Gy)	Mean Dose (Gy)	ICRU Ref Dose (Gy)
A ———	120ARCS	120 DEG ARCS	68.30	69.20	65.40	68.10	67.70
B ········	4FIELD	4 FIELD	37.70	69.00	64.80	67.90	67.70
C – – –	CONFORMAL3D	3D CONFORMAL	100.00	71.70	68.00	70.60	70.20

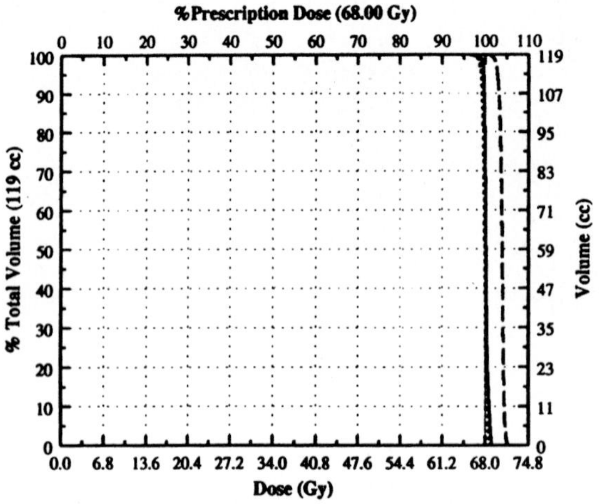

A

Normal Tissue Assessment for RECTUM
Matched Tissue: RECTUM

Patient ID: B950773 | Total Organ Volume: 84 cc | Date: Fri Aug 25 13:56:18 1995
Patient Name: | | Disease Site: Prostate
Dose Bin: 0.10 Gy | Sample Resolution: 1.0 mm | Rank: 7

Plan	Plan ID	Plan Description	%Vol. >= Ref. Dose	Maximum Dose (Gy)	Minimum Dose (Gy)	Mean Dose (Gy)
A ———	120ARCS	120 DEG ARCS	65.00	69.00	9.70	58.10
B ········	4FIELD	4 FIELD	14.80	68.40	1.90	40.20
C – – –	CONFORMAL3D	3D CONFORMAL	17.30	71.10	2.00	31.60

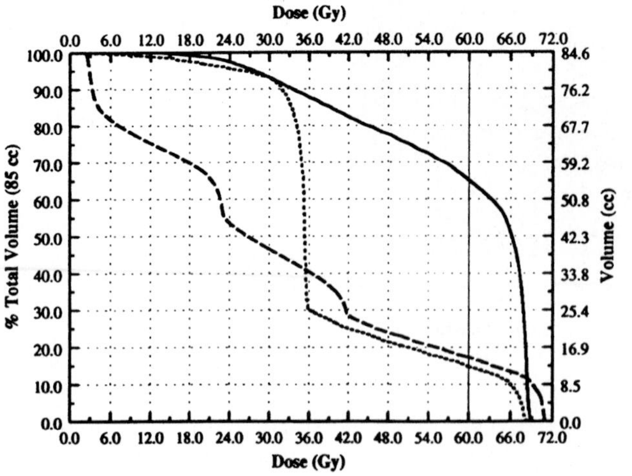

B

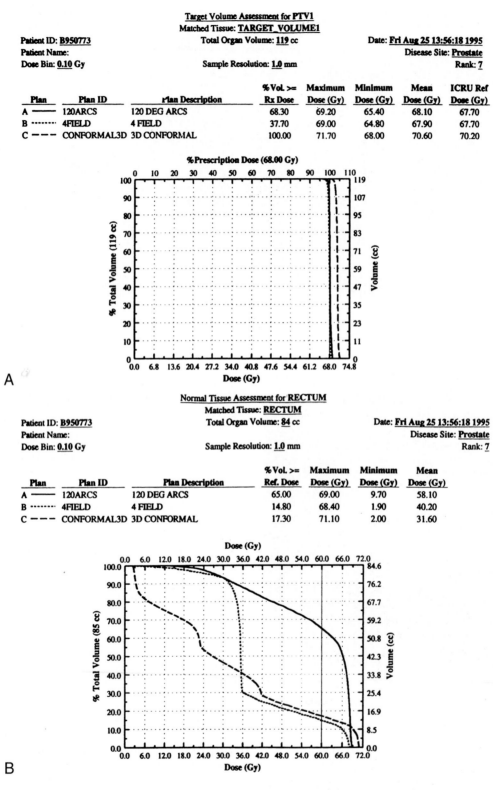

Figure 3.12. (A) Dose-volume histogram for PTV1 (planning target volume) indicating that 100% of the volume is receiving the prescribed tumor dose (58 Gy) with 120-degree bilateral arcs, four-field conformal, or seven-field 3-D conformal techniques. (B) Dose-volume histogram showing different volumes receiving given doses of irradiation with the three techniques described. (Reprinted with permission from Perez CA, Michalski J, Drzymala R, et al. 3D Conformal therapy and potential for IMRT in localized carcinoma of the prostate. In: Sternick ES, ed. The Theory and Practice of Intensity Modulated Radiation Therapy. Madison, WI: Advanced Medical Publishing, 1997.)

Table 3.6. Cancer in the United States–1997: Estimated Incidence, Mortality, and Sites of Failure in Most Common Types

			Distribution of Failures (Deaths)			
	New Cases/Year	Deaths/Year	Locoregional Only	Locoregional and Distant Metastases	Distant Metastases Only	Total Deaths Locoregional Tumor
Lung	178,100	160,400	56,140	56,140	48,120	112,280
Colon and rectum	99,000	47,740	4,740	11,935	31,031	16,675
Breast	181,600	44,190	6,629	26,514	11,048	33,143
Prostate	334,500	41,800	6,270	27,170	8,360	33,440
Uterus*	49,400	10,800	2,160	5,400	3,240	7,560
Oral, pharynx, larynx	41,650	12,670	6,335	3,801	2,534	10,136
Bladder	54,500	11,700	3,510	2,925	5,265	6,435
Lymphomas	61,100	25,280	5,056	5,056	15,168	10,112
Pancreas, biliary	48,100	44,000	8,800	26,400	8,800	35,200
Esophagus, stomach	34,900	25,500	7,650	12,750	5,100	20,400
Leukemia	38,300	21,310	8,524	8,524	4,262	17,048
Ovary	26,800	14,200	12,780	710	710	13,490
Brain, CNS	17,600	13,200	12,738	330	132	13,068
Total	1,165,550	472,790	141,332	187,655	143,770	328,987

* Cervix, invasive and endometrium.
(American Cancer Society: Cancer Facts and Figures–1997. Atlanta: American Cancer Society, 1997.)

with a variety of tumors. These observations were confirmed by Perez et al in carcinoma of the lung (105), uterine cervix (106), and prostate (Figure 3.13) (107). Suit et al (49) pointed out the benefits of reducing the treatment volume in an effort to deliver higher doses of irradiation, which may improve the quality of tumor control without excessively irradiating surrounding normal tissues, thereby decreasing treatment-related morbidity. Furthermore, with emphasis on organ preservation (which is being applied to patients with tumors in the head and neck, breast, and rectosigmoid and soft tissues sarcomas), treatment planning is critical to achieving these goals with maximum tumor control probability and satisfactory cosmetic results.

Many of the reports of the Patterns of Care Study demonstrate a definite correlation between the quality of the radiation therapy delivered at various types of institutions and the outcome of therapy (108).

Preliminary reports, most of them on localized carcinoma of the prostate, point out a greater probability of local tumor control (over 90%) in patients with stage T1c and T2 tumors treated with 3-D CRT. Also, the data suggest that biochemical disease-free survival is improved with this innovative technology (99,109,110).

Normal tissue effects can be viewed from two different viewpoints: potential of 3-D CRT to (1) decrease dose to normal tissue or organs, which results in reduction of radiation-induced short- and long-term sequelae, and (2) study volumetric relationships between dose of irradiation and normal tissue late sequelae.

Because of the procedures performed and the special treatment techniques sometimes required for quality assurance, greater time and effort are necessary. In the United States, the estimated overall cost per patient for a quality assurance review is approximately $300. This investment is small in that, on average, the cost to successfully treat a patient with cancer is about $15,000, whereas $45,000 (over three times as much) is needed to cover all treatment expenses of the patient who has an initial treatment failure (99).

TREATMENT PLANNING IN INTENSITY-MODULATED RADIATION THERAPY

This new approach to 3-D treatment planning and conformal therapy optimizes the delivery of irradiation to irregularly shaped volumes through a process of complex inverse treatment planning and dynamic delivery of irradiation that results in modulated fluence of photon beam profiles (111).

Carol et al (74) described a novel approach to external irradiation with modulated photon beams using dynamic multileaf collimators designed to deliver specific doses to irregularly shaped volumes. Scanning fields are subdivided into subfields of uniform intensity.

The intensity-modulated technique narrows radiation beams, each 2 cm wide, which are further divided into four small beams that can each be turned on or off by the multileaf collimator of the linear accelerator as the exposure proceeds. One rotation treats two slices, and the treatment table is indexed by a specially designed apparatus attached to the table to conform the irradiated volume. The collimating system includes a controller that implements computer-driven treatment instructions to drive the collimating system and the accelerator throughout the treatment (112).

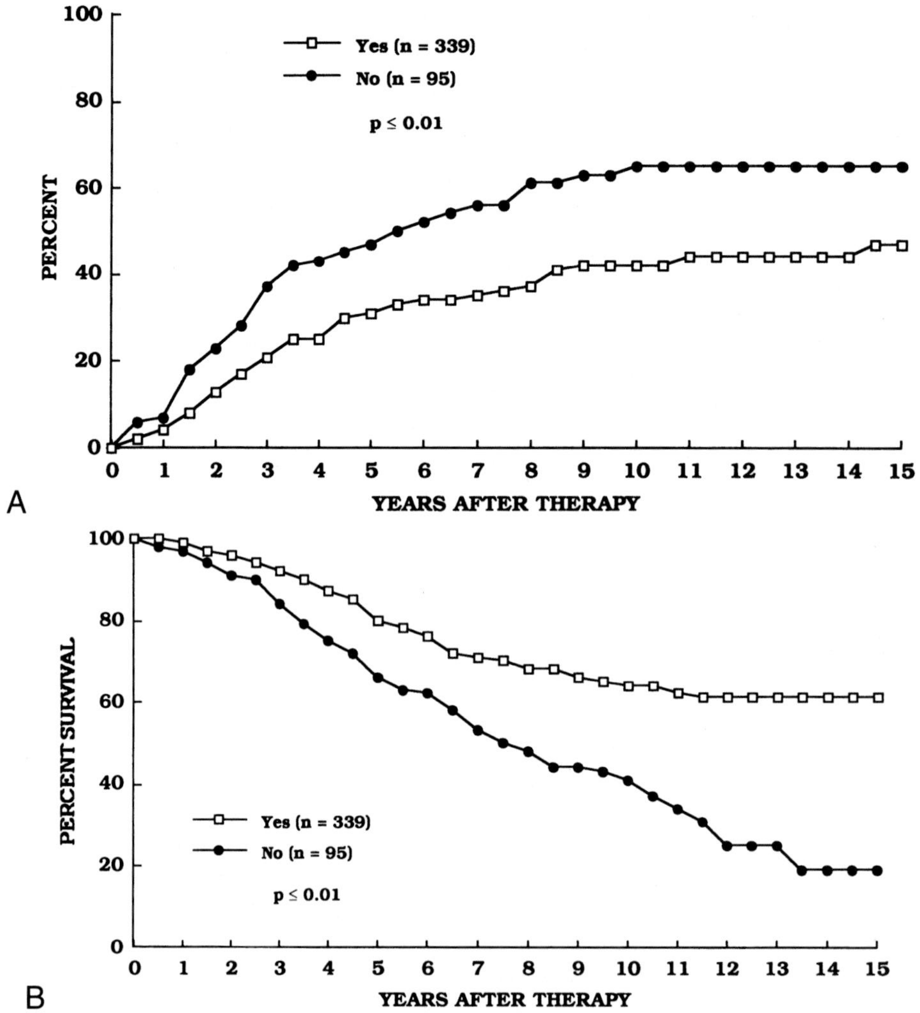

Figure 3.13. Distant metastasis rate (**A**) and cause-specific survival (**B**) correlated with pelvic tumor control (yes, no) in patients with stage **C** (T3) carcinoma of the prostate treated at Mallinckrodt Institute of Radiology.

The intensity of the beam across the field and the field shape are continuously varied by a special collimator called a multileaf intensity modulating collimator (MIMIC) throughout the rotation of accelerator. The collimator consists of 40 divergent tungsten vanes, each 8 cm thick, and it functionally narrows the beam coming from the accelerator down into two thin slices, further dividing these slices into four small beams, 20 for each slice. Each beam projects to 8.5 by 10 mm at 100 cm distance from the target, and all beams are divergent. As the gantry rotates around the patient, each of these 40 small beams can be turned on or off by movement of its vane for a variable period of time, thus creating intensity modulation required in the inverse solution. Because a rotation about the patient treats only the equivalent of two slices throughout the patient (e.g., 17 mm in length), the treatment couch must be successively indexed between rotations when longer targets are treated. A region of adjacent field mismatch between two successive rotations is created for each index of the treatment couch. To minimize the magnitude of mismatch and to allow the correct dose modeling of regions in which such mismatch exists, precise and predictable indexing of the treatment couch is required. This is accomplished with a special couch indexing device with a 0.1 mm resolution digital readout, which clamps to the rail supports on the side of the treatment couch.

For treatment planning, contouring of tumor/target volumes and normal anatomic structures is carried out on multiple CT scans obtained with the patient in the treatment position using appropriate immobilization devices.

The treatment planning system generates an optimal set of beam weights on a planar basis; dose simulation is volumetric. Dose is calculated using a modified path length algorithm and measured beam data. Validation studies showed that the nonuniformity introduced by correctly delivered segmental strip plans adds only 1 to 2%, regardless of target size, to the nonuniformity resulting from the intensity-modulation delivery paradigm (113,114).

The dose-distribution and field-shaping parameters are based on inverse 3-D planning using specially defined minimal dose to target and dose constraints for surrounding normal tissues (111,115-117). Inverse planning starts with an ideal dose distribution and finds the beam characteristics (fluence profiles), through trial and error or multiple iterations (simulated annealing), then produces the best approximation to the ideal dose defined in a 3-D array of dose voxels organized in a stack of 2-D arrays (96,118). A back-projection technique through careful choice of filters, beam placement, and shaping of the portals conforms the irradiation dose to the shape of the tumor, minimizing dose to critical adjacent structures. When this technique is used, it is critical to adhere to basic concepts of treatment planning and evaluation of the pathobiology of malignant disease. Well-designed treatment plans based on radiographic imaging (CT scanning or magnetic resonance imaging), which, in most instances, demonstrates gross disease, are necessary to minimize the risk of missing or underirradiating adjacent microscopic or subclinical tumor (112).

Further refinements are in progress to enhance the clinical applications of intensity-modulated radiation therapy. For additional details, see Chapters 9 and 10.

SPECIAL PARTICLES

Special particles, such as neutrons, protons, or heavy ions, provide better dose distributions and some biologic advantages, and in preliminary studies they have been reported to yield a high probability of tumor control with relative sparing of normal tissues (119-122). Treatment planning for these radiations is more specialized and beyond the scope of this chapter.

TREATMENT PLANNING SYSTEMS

Computers have been used in planning radiation therapy over a period approaching 40 years (123). The first dedicated 2-D RTP minicomputer system, the forerunner of today's dedicated 3-D RTP systems, grew out of efforts at Washington University's Biomedical Computer Laboratory in the 1960s (124).

Limitations of 2-D RTP systems include lack of software aids to define the clinical problem, deficiencies in the dose calculation algorithm, inability to handle treatments with noncoplanar beams, lack of efficient tools for assessing alternative plans, inadequate definition of geometric coverage of anatomic structures, and failure to provide tools for specifying and verifying the accuracy in treatment delivery.

For photon dose calculations, most commercial 2-D RTP systems still use methods that were developed before the advent of CT with inherent limitations (125).

More advanced algorithms that compute the dose from a first-principles approach rather than correcting parameterized dose distributions measured in a water phantom are now being implemented in commercial 3-D RTP systems. Examples of the more advanced algorithms include the superposition/convolution method developed by Mackie et al (126) and the differential pencil beam method developed by Mohan et al (127). These methods use convolution energy deposition kernels that describe the distribution of dose about a single primary photon interaction site. The convolution kernels are most often obtained by using the Monte Carlo method to interact monoenergetic primary photons at the origin in a phantom and to transport the charged particles and scattered and secondary photons that are set in motion. The energy that is deposited about the primary photon interaction site is tabulated and stored for use in the convolution method. In addition to describing how scattered photons contribute to dose absorbed at some distance away from the interaction site of primary photons, the convolution kernels take into account charged particle transport. This information can be used to compute dose in electronic disequilibrium situations such as occur in the buildup region and the beam penumbra.

Most methods used for electron dose calculation in commercial 2-D RTP systems also were developed before the advent of CT (128). Such algorithms are based on determining parameters of dose distributions in water phantoms under standard conditions and applying correction factors to the beam representations. For dose calculation for the patient, empiric absorption equivalent thickness corrections typically are used. These methods, however, are inadequate for inhomogeneity corrections, particularly in their inability to predict "hot" and "cold" spots in the electron beam dose distribution near boundaries.

The pencil beam method, based on a semiempiric adaptation of the Fermi-Eyges multiple scattering model, overcomes such difficulties and has been implemented in most commercial 3-D RTP systems (129,130).

There is no doubt that the correction for inhomogeneities in the medium and their effect on dose distribution, as well as computations with beam modifiers such as wedges or shielding blocks and the effect they may have on the dose distribution, have been greatly improved with the advent of 3-D RTP.

Imaged-based 3-D RTP will see a growing demand to incorporate the complementary information available from magnetic resonance (MR) and other imaging modalities such as single photon emission computed tomography (SPECT) and positron emission tomography (PET) into the planning process. In some sites, MR is already known to be a better imaging modality for defining the boundaries of the gross tumor, while SPECT and PET provide detailed functional information concerning tissue metabolism and radioisotope transport (131-133). Research to automate the image correlation task in 3-D RTP is an important area for advancing the use of multimodality imaging to more accurately define target volumes.

THREE-DIMENSIONAL TREATMENT PLANNING SYSTEMS

Three-dimensional RTP and conformal delivery techniques are increasingly used worldwide (94,95); 3-D techniques will continue to be refined and usher in changes in the way radiation oncology is practiced. One of the most important directions is the increased use of multimodality imaging to more accurately define the GTV and CTV. MR, SPECT, and PET are already used to supplement CT data. However, improved correlation software allowing these imaging studies to be effectively used is sorely needed. In addition, new imaging modalities such as magnetic resonance angiography and magnetic resonance spectroscopy imaging are also likely to have an impact in this area.

Determining target volumes and organs at risk by drawing contours on the CT image on a slice-by-slice basis as opposed to drawing portals on a radiograph is a major paradigm shift for the radiation oncologist and treatment planner. Software for contouring normal structures and target volumes and virtual simulation that previously required a significant investment of time and effort by the radiation oncology staff continue to be significantly improved. The treatment planner/radiation oncologist can now draw contours around the tumor, target, and normal tissues on a slice-by-slice basis, and, at the same time, view a cross-reference to planar images from both the anteroposterior and lateral projections. In addition, improved edit functions allow the user to move, scale, and rotate an entered contour in addition to providing tools for rapid corrections, changing the shape of a contour, automatic adjusting of a copied contour to fit a new organ boundary, and copying to inferior and superior slices. Three-dimensional RTP software provides improved capability over a conventional x-ray simulator by allowing rapid computation of DRRs, giving BEV displays showing the delineated contours and the projection of the beam aperture. However, continued refinement is necessary to increase the efficiency of 3-D RTP.

Quantitative data for specifying the boundary of the planning target volume for many sites are lacking. Considerable effort is being expended in conducting uncertainty studies aimed at determining patient setup errors and organ motion ranges and will likely continue for many more years.

Three-dimensional RTP BEV displays and room-view displays (134) help treatment planners better appreciate the 3-D geometry, but they can be confusing when there are large numbers of overlapping structures or beams. More refined software is needed in most planning systems to prevent use of beams that may lead to collision of the head of the accelerator with the patient or the support system.

An essential component of any advanced 3-D RTP system is an adequate method of dose calculation. Although a goal of about 3% accuracy in dose calculations has been suggested, in practice, calculation accuracy still does not meet this goal in many heterogeneous regions of the patient. As previously discussed, most photon dose calculation methods presently used in 3-D RTP provide explicit calculations of the primary photon transport component but, inevitably, approximate the effects due to scattered photons and the secondary electrons. However, the use of Monte Carlo calculations to account for these effects now appears promising, and it is likely that Monte Carlo-based algorithms (or at least full scatter ray-trace algorithms) will be available and will be practical for clinical 3-D RTP by the end of the decade (135).

Plan optimization is a difficult, if not impossible, task at this time. Current technology relies heavily on subjective evaluation by the physician using 2-D isodoses or color washes superimposed on multiple gray scale CT images. This task is made easier by tools such as volumetric displays (Figure 3.1) and DVHs (Figure 3.2) such as the real-time room-view of 3-D dose surfaces. In addition, biologic indices for evaluating 3-D plans, such as tumor control probability and NTCP models are being investigated; this is already a very active area of research.

Modern 3-D RTP systems are capable of generating extremely high quality DRRs that simulate portal films for comparison with the treatment portal film to verify treatment geometry. EPID, dose monitoring, verify and record, and computer control feedback systems are methods that play a role in verifying 3-D CRT treatments.

The link between RTP and treatment delivery systems will become vital. Computer-controlled 3-D CRT delivery systems (e.g., beam-intensity modulation) will require that the planning system generate the computer files needed to implement the 3-D CRT technique. Research and development are just starting in this field.

Integrating the management of diagnostic, planning, and treatment verification data in radiation therapy must be accomplished. A dedicated radiation oncologist's workstation networked to the 3-D RTP database will allow the physician to review organ and target volume delineation, plan parameters and dose statistics, and verify treatment images in the office or other work areas, thus saving considerable time and effort.

QUALITY ASSURANCE AND TREATMENT PLANNING

Treatment planning is a complex process that involves a complete evaluation of the patient's condition, knowledge of the extent and characteristics of the tumor, and selection of optimal therapy.

Each institution must establish standard treatment guidelines or investigational protocols that contain detailed information to guide the radiation oncologist on the indications for radiation therapy, depending on anatomic location, extent (stage) and histologic features of the tumor, and general condition of the patient. The description of radiation therapy must include details on the target volume, tumor dose, and fractionation schedule, all critical elements in treatment planning.

Inasmuch as higher doses of irradiation and adequacy of treatment portals (volume treated) appear to correlate with greater tumor control and sequelae, the need to optimize treatment planning and quality assurance in radiation therapy is critical (Table 3.7).

To verify the validity of treatment administration at the initiation of the radiation therapy, data concerning the planned treatment techniques, technical factors, and dose prescription should be reviewed by both the radiation oncologist directing the treatment and the physics/dosimetry staff. Simulation, localization films, Polaroid pictures, and the like are required to document the appropriateness of the irradiation portals. The dosimetry review includes a complete verification of the doses delivered at the periphery of the tumor, draining lymphatics, and critical normal structures.

Quality assurance procedures in radiation therapy vary, depending on whether a standard treatment or a clinical trial is carried out at single or multiple institutions. Particularly in multiinstitutional studies, the need is clear for instructions and standardized parameters in dosimetry procedures, treatment techniques, and treatment planning to be carried out by all participants.

Some of the essential components of a sound quality assurance program include:

1. Tumor registry that collects information useful in epidemiologic studies or in the planning of regional health care cancer programs.
2. Standardization of hospital and radiation therapy records to ensure the collection of reliable information.
3. Formulation of consensus guidelines of cancer management, such as those generated by the Patterns of Care Study in the United States to ensure uniformity of management and consistency of data that will allow better evaluation of therapy results.
4. Guidelines regarding patient services, staff needs, organization, and training, and criteria for equipment availability consistent with state-of-the-art development that provides the best possible patient care (within the limitations of the resources available).
5. Quality assurance procedure and assessment programs in radiation dosimetry and guidelines detailing specific minimal and optimal requirements to fulfill these programs should be formulated and individually tailored to the needs and resources of specific institutions.
6. Radiation safety and other types of measures (e.g., Occupational Safety and Health Administration) to ensure the welfare of personnel and patients.
7. Educational programs and training opportunities for physicians, physicists, dosimetrists, technologists, and allied health personnel to upgrade cancer management and radiation therapy practice.

Table 3.7. Quality Assurance: Treatment Planning

		Quality Assurance Action
Diagnostic patient data acquisition	Diagnostic x-ray, nuclear medicine, ultrasound	Image quality assurance procedures are established in diagnostic departments.
	CT	Special procedures relating to therapy.
	Simulator	Image quality and mechanical integrity.
Treatment decision, tumor localization	Data synthesis, contours, delineation of target volume and sensitive organs	Clinical quality assurance. Accuracy of contouring equipment. Simulator quality assurance.
Computation of dose and dose distribution	Tissue-air ratio and/or other dose concepts, algorithms, computer, field shaping	Data verification for individual machines. Accuracy of calculational methods. Input-output devices of computer. Documentation of dose distribution data and calculational procedures.
Immobilization blocks and wedges	Immobilization devices, mold materials, and block cutters	Frequent alignment and stability checks. Personnel safety in regard to material toxicity (lead, cadmium, tin, etc.) and shop procedures. Patient safety.
Treatment verification	Portal film verification	Field delineation and adequacy of tumor coverage (physicians should sign films). Image quality.
	Patient charts	Dose summations and treatment prescriptions.
	Equipment log books	Adequate calibration records. Machine problems and performance.
	On/in patient dosimetry	Dosimetry and equipment verification. Dosimeter placement. Analysis and reporting of results.

(Reprinted with permission from Inter-Society Council for Radiation Oncology: Radiation Oncology in Integrated Cancer Management. Philadelphia: American College of Radiology. November 1986.)

Quality Assurance in Three-Dimensional Treatment Planning

It is now recognized that the treatment flexibility that image-based, 3-D RTP systems facilitate is accompanied by significantly increased technical complexity and potential hazards (136-139). The attendant safety and quality assurance considerations, therefore, must be more elaborate. Today, computerized 3-D RTP systems integrated with dose delivery on computer-controlled treatment equipment are being implemented in clinics around the world. Exactly where the 3-D RTP system ends and where the treatment delivery system begins is becoming blurred. Simply checking that the 3-D RTP system is accurately reproducing the input data is no longer considered adequate quality assurance. While there are not yet formal recommendations on 3-D RTP quality assurance, several groups have published their initial experience (138,140). In addition, the American Association of Physicists will soon publish a report on this subject (141). Our 3-D RTP quality assurance program is divided into three main areas: dose algorithm verification test, systemic validation tests (including dosimetric and nondosimetric) of the 3-D RTP system hardware and software, and formal quality assurance procedures for the individual patient undergoing the 3-D planning process. Details are presented in Chapter 9. We emphasize that any 3-D quality assurance program requires the active involvement of physicists, dosimetrists, physicians, and the treating radiation therapists.

References

1. Cunningham JR. Development of computer algorithms for radiation treatment planning. Int J Radiat Oncol Biol Phys 1989;16:1367-1376.
2. Withers HR, McBride WH. Biologic Basis of Radiation Therapy. In: Perez CA, Brady LW, eds. Principles and Practice of Radiation Oncology, 3rd ed. Philadelphia: Lippincott-Raven, 1998.
3. Fletcher GH. Clinical dose-response curves of human malignant epithelial tumours. Br J Radiol 1973;46:1-12.
4. Herring DF. The consequences of dose response curves for tumor control and normal tissue injury on the precision necessary in patient management. Laryngoscope 1975;85:1112-1118.
5. Perez CA, Carmichael T, Devineni VR, et al. Carcinoma of the tonsillar fossa: A nonrandomized comparison of irradiation alone or combined with surgery: Long-term results. Head Neck 1991;13:282-290.
6. Shukovsky LJ, Fletcher GH. Time-dose and tumor volume relationships in irradiation of squamous cell carcinoma of tonsillar fossa. Radiology 1973;107:621-626.
7. Thames HD Jr, Peters LJ, Spanos W Jr, et al. Dose response of squamous cell carcinomas of the upper respiratory and digestive tracts. Br J Cancer 1980;41(Suppl 4):35-38.
8. Fletcher GH, Shukovsky LJ. The interplay of radiocurability and tolerance in the irradiation of human cancer. J Radiol Electrol 1975; 56:383-400.
9. Miescher G. Erfolge der karzinombehandlung an der Dermatologischen Klinik Zurich. Einzeitige Hochstdosis and Fraktionierte Behandlung. Strahlentherapie 1934;49:65-81.
10. Strandqvist M. Studien uber die kumulative wirkung der rontgenstrahlen bie frakionierung. Acta Radiol (Suppl) (Stockh) 1944;55:1-300.
11. Fletcher GH, ed. Textbook of Radiotherapy, 3rd ed. Philadelphia: Lea & Febiger, 1980.
12. Fletcher GH. Keynote address: The scientific basis of the present and future practice of clinical radiotherapy. Int J Radiat Oncol Biol Phys 1983;9:1073-1082.
13. Mendenhall WM, Million RR, Cassisi NJ. Elective neck irradiation in squamous cell carcinoma of the head and neck. Head Neck Surg 1980;3:15-20.
14. Parsons JT. Time-Dose-Volume Relationships in Radiation Therapy. In: Million RR, Cassisi NJ, eds. Management of Head and Neck Cancer: A Multidisciplinary Approach. Philadelphia: JB Lippincott, 1984: 137-172.
15. Fletcher GH. Local results of irradiation in the primary management of localized breast cancer. Cancer 1972;29:545-551.
16. Moench HC, Phillips TL. Carcinoma of the nasopharynx: Review of 146 patients with emphasis on radiation dose and time factors. Am J Surg 1972;124:515-518.
17. Northrop M, Fletcher GH, Jesse RH, et al. Evolution of neck disease in patients with primary squamous cell carcinoma of the oral tongue, floor of mouth, and palatine arch, and clinically positive neck nodes neither fixed nor bilateral. Cancer 1972;29:23-30.
18. Fayos JV, Lampe I. Radiation therapy of carcinoma of the tonsillar region. Am J Roentgenol Radium Ther Nucl Med 1971;111:85-94.
19. Perez CA, Ackerman LV, Mill WB, et al. Malignant tumors of the tonsil: Analysis of failures and factors affecting prognosis. Am J Roentgenol Radium Ther Nucl Med 1972;114:43-58.
20. Schneider JJ, Fletcher GH, Barkley HT Jr. Control by irradiation alone of nonfixed clinically positive lymph nodes from squamous cell carcinoma of the oral cavity, oropharynx, supraglottic larynx, and hypopharynx. Am J Roentgenol Radium Ther Med 1975;123: 42-48.
21. Votava C Jr, Fletcher GH, Jesse RH Jr, et al. Management of cervical nodes, either fixed or bilateral, from squamous cell carcinoma of the oral cavity and faucial arch. Radiology 1972;105:417-420.
22. Shukovsky LJ. Dose, time, volume relationships in squamous cell carcinoma of the supraglottic larynx. Am J Roentgenol 1970;108:27-29.
23. Calle R, Fletcher GH, Pierquin B. Le bases de la radiotherapie curative des eiptheliomas mammaires. J Radiol Electrol 1973;54:929-938.
24. Meoz-Mendez RT, Fletcher GH, Guillamondegui OM, et al. Analysis of the results of irradiation in the treatment of squamous cell carcinomas of the pharyngeal walls. Int J Radiat Oncol Biol Phys 1978;4: 579-585.
25. Perez CA, Brady LW, Roti Roti JL. Overview. In: Perez CA, Brady LW, eds. Principles and Practice of Radiation Oncology, 3rd ed. Philadelphia: Lippincott-Raven, 1998.
26. Withers HR. Biologic basis for altered fractionation schemes. Cancer 1985;55:2086-2095.
27. Paterson R. The Treatment of Malignant Disease by Radium and X-ray: Being a Practice of Radiotherapy. Baltimore: Williams & Wilkins, 1949.
28. Spanos WJ Jr, Shukovsky LJ, Fletcher GH. Time, dose, and tumor volume relationships in irradiation of squamous cell carcinomas of the base of the tongue. Cancer 1976;37:2591-2599.
29. Maciejewski B, Withers HR, Taylor JMG, et al. Dose fractionation and regeneration in radiotherapy for cancer of the oral cavity and oropharynx. II. Normal tissue responses: Acute and late effects. Int J Radiat Oncol Biol Phys 1990;18:101-111.
30. Marcus RB Jr, Million RR. The incidence of myelitis after irradiation of the cervical spinal cord. Int J Radiat Oncol Biol Phys 1990;19:3-8.
31. McCunniff AJ, Laing MJ. Radiation tolerance of the cervical spinal cord. Int J Radiat Oncol Biol Phys 1989;16:675-678.
32. Montana GS, Fowler WC, Varia MA, et al. Carcinoma of the cervix, stage III: Results of radiation therapy. Cancer 1986;57:148-154.
33. Pourquier H, Delard R, Achille E, et al. A quantified approach to the analysis and prevention of urinary complications in radiotherapeutic treatment of cancer of the cervix. Int J Radiat Oncol Biol Phys 1987; 13:1025-1033.
34. Pourquier H, Dubois JB, Delard R. Cancer of the uterine cervix: Dosimetric guidelines for prevention of late rectal and rectosigmoid complications as a result of radiotherapeutic treatment. Int J Radiat Oncol Biol Phys 1982;8:1887-1895.
35. Emami B, Lyman J, Brown A, et al. Tolerance of normal tissue to therapeutic irradiation. Int J Radiat Oncol Biol Phys 1991;21:109-122.

36. Burman C, Kutcher GJ, Emami B, et al. Fitting of normal tissue tolerance data to an analytic function. Int J Radiat Oncol Biol Phys 1991;21:123-135.
37. Orton CG. Other Considerations in Three-Dimensional Treatment Planning. In Bagne F, ed. Computerized Treatment Planning Systems. Washington, DC: HHS Publications FDA 84-8223, 1984.
38. International Commission of Radiation Units and Measurements. Determination of Absorbed Dose in a Patient Irradiated by Beams of X or Gamma Rays. In Radiotherapy Procedures, ICRU Report 24. Washington, DC: ICRU, 1976.
39. Byhardt RW, Cox JD, Hornburg A, et al. Weekly localization films and detection of field placement errors. Int J Radiat Oncol Biol Phys 1978;4:881-887.
40. Rabinowitz I, Broomberg J, Goitein M, et al. Accuracy of radiation field alignment in clinical practice. Int J Radiat Oncol Biol Phys 1985; 11:1857-1867.
41. Marks JE, Haus AG. The effect of immobilization on localization errors in the radiotherapy of head and neck cancer. Clin Radiol 1976;27:175-177.
42. Hendrickson FR. Four P's of human error in treatment delivery. Int J Radiat Oncol Biol Phys 1978;4:913-914.
43. Marks JE, Haus AG. The effect of immobilization on localization error in the radiotherapy of head and neck cancer. Clin Radiol 1976; 27:175-177.
44. Marks JE, Haus AG, Sutton HG, et al: Localization error in the radiotherapy of Hodgkin's disease and malignant lymphoma with extended mantle fields. Cancer 1974;34:83-90.
45. Doss LL. Localization error and local recurrence in upper airway carcinoma. Proceedings of the Workshop on Quality Control in the Radiotherapy Department of the Cancer and Leukemia Group B (CALGB), New York, May 31, 1979.
46. Perez CA, Devineni VR, Marcial-Vega V, et al. Carcinoma of the nasopharynx: Factors affecting prognosis. Int J Radiat Oncol Biol Phys 1992;23:271-280.
47. Gildersleve J, Dearnaley DP, Evans PM, et al. A randomised trial of patient repositioning during radiotherapy using a megavoltage imaging system. Radiother Oncol 1994;31:161-168.
48. Bissett R, Leszczynski K, Loose S, et al. Quantitative vs. subjective portal verification using digital portal images. Int J Radiat Oncol Biol Phys 1996;34:489-495.
49. Suit HD, Becht J, Leong J, et al. Potential for improvement in radiation therapy. Int J Radiat Oncol Biol Phys 1988;14:777-796.
50. Kallman RF. The phenomenon of reoxygenation and its implications for fractionated radiotherapy. Radiology 1972;105:135-142.
51. Elkind MM, Sutton H. Radiation response of mammalian cells grown in culture. I. Repair of x-ray damage in surviving Chinese hamster cells. Radiat Res 1960;13:556-593.
52. Terasima T, Tolmach LJ. Variations in several responses of HeLa cells to x-irradiation during the division cycle. Biophys J 1963;3:11-33.
53. Brown BW, Thompson JR, Barkley T, et al. Theoretical considerations of dose rate factors influencing radiation strategy. Radiology 1974;110:197-202.
54. Hethcote HW, Waltman P. Theoretical determination of optimal treatment schedules for radiation therapy. Radiat Res 1973;57:150-161.
55. Withers HR, Thomas HD, Peters LJ. Differences in Fractionation Response of Acutely and Late Responding Tissues. In Karcher KJ, ed. Progress in Radio Oncology II. New York: Raven, 1982.
56. Bush RS, Hill RP. Biologic discussions augmenting radiation effects and model systems. Laryngoscope 1975;85:1119-1133.
57. Perez CA, Thomas PRM. Radiation Therapy: Basic Concepts and Clinical Implications. In: Sutow WW, Fernbach DJ, Vietti TJ, eds. Clinical Pediatric Oncology, 3rd ed. St. Louis: CV Mosby, 1984:167-209.
58. Inter-Society Council for Radiation Oncology. Radiation Oncology in Integrated Cancer Management. Philadelphia: American College of Radiology, November, 1986.
59. International Commission on Radiation Units and Measurements. Prescribing, Recording, and Reporting Photon Beam Therapy: ICRU Report 50. Bethesda: International Commission of Radiation Units and Measurements, 1993.
60. Perez CA, Purdy JA, Harms W, et al. Design of a fully integrated three-dimensional computed tomography simulator and preliminary clinical evaluation. Int J Radiat Oncol Biol Phys 1994;30:887-897.
61. Schultheiss TE, Stephens LC, Ang KK, et al. Volume effects in rhesus monkey spinal cord. Int J Radiat Oncol Biol Phys 1994;29:67-72.
62. Withers HR, Taylor JM. Critical volume model. Int J Radiat Oncol Biol Phys 1992;25:151-152.
63. Marks LB. The impact of organ structure on radiation response. Int J Radiat Oncol Biol Phys 1996;34:1165-1171.
64. Jackson A, Kutcher GJ, Yorke ED. Probability of radiation-induced complications for normal tissues with parallel architecture subject to non-uniform irradiation. Med Phys 1993;20:613-625.
65. Travis EL. Primer of Medical Radiobiology, 2nd ed. Chicago: Year Book Publishers, 1989.
66. Rubin P, Cooper R, Phillips TL, eds. Radiation Biology and Radiation Pathology Syllabus (Set RT 1: Radiation Oncology). Chicago; American College of Radiology, 1975.
67. Rubin P, Casarett GW. Clinical Radiation Pathology, vols 1 and 2. Philadelphia: WB Saunders, 1968.
68. Dritschilo A, Sherman D, Emami B, et al. The cost effectiveness of a radiation therapy simulator: A model for the determination of need. Int J Radiat Oncol Biol Phys 1979;5:243-247.
69. Bentel GC, ed. Radiation Therapy Planning, 2nd ed. New York: McGraw-Hill, 1996.
70. Bomford CK, Craig LM, Hanna FA, et al. Treatment simulation. Br J Radiol 1981;Suppl 16:1-31.
71. Day MJ, Harrison RM. Cross sectional information and treatment simulation. In Bleehen NM, Glatstein E, Haybittle JL, eds. Radiation Therapy Planning. New York: Marcel Dekker, 1983.
72. Mizer S, Scheller RR, Deye JA. Radiation Therapy Simulation Workbook. New York: Pergamon Press, 1986.
73. Washington CM, Leaver DT, eds. Principles and Practice of Radiation Therapy: Physics, Simulation, and Treatment Planning, vol 1. St. Louis: Mosby, 1996.
74. Carol MP, Targovnik H, Smith D, et al. 3-D planning and delivery system for optimized conformal therapy. Int J Radiat Oncol Biol Phys 1992;24(suppl 1):158.
75. Lichter AS, Fraass BA, McShan DL. Recent advances in radiotherapy treatment planning. Oncology 1988;2:43-57.
76. Graham ML, Purdy JA, Emami B, et al. Preliminary results of a prospective trial using three-dimensional radiotherapy for lung cancer. Int J Radiat Oncol Biol Phys 1995;33:993-1000.
77. Lawrence TS, Tesser RJ, Ten Haken RK. An application of dose-volume histograms to treatment of intrahepatic malignancies with radiation therapy. Int J Radiat Oncol Biol Phys 1990;19:1041-1047.
78. Hanks GE. Conformal radiation in prostate cancer: Reduced morbidity with hope of increased local control. Int J Radiat Oncol Biol Phys 1993;25:377-378.
79. Perez CA, Purdy JA, Harms W, et al. Three-dimensional treatment planning and conformal radiation therapy: Preliminary evaluation. Radiother Oncol 1995;36:32-43.
80. Robertson JM, Kessler ML, Lawrence TS. Clinical results of three-dimensional conformal irradiation. J Natl Cancer Inst 1994;86:968-974.
81. Sandler HM, McLaughlin PW, Ten Haken RK, et al. Three dimensional conformal radiotherapy for the treatment of prostate cancer: Low risk of chronic rectal morbidity observed in a large series of patients. Int J Radiat Oncol Biol Phys 1995;33:797-801.
82. Soffen EM, Hanks GE, Hunt MA, et al. Conformal static field radiation therapy treatment of early prostate cancer versus non-conformal techniques: A reduction in acute morbidity. Int J Radiat Oncol Biol Phys 1992;24:485-488.
83. Michalski JM, Wong JW, Gerber RL, et al. The use of on-line image verification to estimate the variation in radiation therapy dose delivery. Int J Radiat Oncol Biol Phys 1993;27:707-716.
84. Tinger A, Michalski JM, Bosch WR, et al. An analysis of intratreatment and intertreatment displacements in pelvic radiotherapy using electronic portal imaging. Int J Radiat Oncol Biol Phys 1996;34:683-690.
85. Verhey LJ, Goitein M, McNulty P, et al. Precise positioning of patients for radiation therapy. Int J Radiat Oncol Biol Phys 1982;8:289-294.
86. Wong JW, Binns WR, Cheng AY, et al. On-line radiotherapy imaging with an array of fiber-optic imaging reducers. Int J Radiat Oncol Biol Phys 1990;18:1477-1484.

87. Chen GTY, Singh RP, Castro JR, et al. Treatment planning for heavy ion radiotherapy. Int J Radiat Oncol Biol Phys 1979;5:1809-1819.
88. Rubin P, Siemann DW. Principles of Radiation Oncology and Cancer Radiotherapy. In: Rubin P, ed. Clinical Oncology: A Multidisciplinary Approach for Physicians and Students, 7th ed. Philadelphia: WB Saunders, 1993;71-90.
89. Mendelsohn ML. The biology of dose-limiting tissues. In: Time and Dose Relationships in Radiation Biology as Applied to Radiotherapy, Brookhaven National Laboratory (BNL) Report 5023 (C-57). Upton: Brookhaven National Laboratory, 1969:154-173.
90. Mendelsohn ML. Radiotherapy and tolerance. In: Vaeth JM, ed. Frontiers of Radiation Therapy and Oncology. Baltimore: University Park Press, 1972:512-528.
91. Andrews JR. Optimization of radiotherapy: Some notes on the principles and practice of optimization of cancer treatment and implications for clinical research. Cancer Clin Trials 1981;4:483-495.
92. Andrews JR. Benefit, risk and optimization by ROC analysis in cancer radiotherapy. Int J Radiat Oncol Biol Phys 1985;11:1557-1562.
93. Shukovsky LJ, Baeza MR, Fletcher GH: Results of irradiation of squamous cell carcinomas of the glossopalatine sulcus. Radiology 1976; 120:405-408.
94. Purdy JA, Emami B, eds. 3D Radiation Treatment Planning and Conformal Therapy: Proceedings of an International Symposium. Madison: Medical Physics Publishing, 1995.
95. Meyer JL, Purdy JA, eds. 3-D Conformal Radiotherapy, vol 29, Frontiers in Radiation Therapy Oncology, Basel: Karger, 1996
96. Perez CA, Michalski J, Drzymala R, et al. 3D Conformal Therapy and Potential for IMRT in Localized Carcinoma of the Prostate. In: Sternick ES, ed. The Theory and Practice of Intensity Modulated Radiation Therapy. Madison, WI: Advanced Medical Publishing, 1997.
97. Webb S. The Physics of Three-Dimensional Radiation Therapy: Conformal Radiotherapy, Radiosurgery and Treatment Planning. Bristol, England: Institute of Physics Publishing, 1993.
98. International Journal of Radiation Oncology Biology Physics, volume 34, number 5, 1995.
99. Perez CA, Michalski J, Ballard S, et al. Cost benefit of emerging technology in localized carcinoma of the prostate. Int J Radiat Oncol Biol Phys (In press).
100. Perez CA. The critical need for accurate treatment planning and quality control in radiation therapy. Int J Radiat Oncol Biol Phys 1977;2:815-818.
101. Goitein M. Computed tomography in planning radiation therapy. Int J Radiat Oncol Biol Phys 1979;5:445-447.
102. DeVita VT, Lippman M, Hubbard SM, et al. The effect of combined modality therapy on local control and survival. Int J Radiat Oncol Biol Phys 1986;12:487-501.
103. American Cancer Society. Cancer Facts and Figures—1997. Atlanta: American Cancer Society, 1997.
104. Suit HD, Westgate SJ. Impact of improved local control on survival. Int J Radiat Oncol Biol Phys 1986;12:435-438.
105. Perez CA, Pajak TF, Rubin P, et al. Long-term observations of the patterns of failure in patients with unresectable non-oat cell carcinoma of the lung treated with definitive radiotherapy: Report by the Radiation Therapy Oncology Group. Cancer 1987;59:1874-1881.
106. Perez CA, Kuske RR, Camel HM, et al. Analysis of pelvic tumor control and impact on survival in carcinoma of the uterine cervix treated with radiation therapy alone. Int J Radiat Oncol Biol Phys 1988;14:613-621.
107. Perez C, Pilepich MV, Zivnuska F. Tumor control in definitive irradiation of localized carcinoma of the prostate. Int J Radiat Oncol Biol Phys 1986;12:523-531.
108. Hanks GE, Kinzie JJ, White RL, et al. Patterns of care outcome studies: Results of the National Practice in Hodgkin's disease. Cancer 1983;51:569-573.
109. Hanks GE, Lee WR, Schultheiss TE. Clinical and biochemical evidence of control of prostate cancer at 5 years after external beam radiation. J. Urol. 1995;154:456-459.
110. Leibel SA, Zelefsky MJ, Kutcher GJ, et al. Three-dimensional conformal radiation therapy in localized carcinoma of the prostate: Interim report of a phase I dose-escalation study. J Urol 1994;152:1792-1798.
111. Brahme A. Optimization of stationary and moving beam radiation therapy techniques. Radiother Oncol 1988;12:129-140.
112. Woo SY, Sanders M, Grant W, et al. Does the "Peacock" have anything to do with radiotherapy? Int J Radiat Oncol Biol Phys 1994; 29:213-214.
113. Carol MP. Integrated 3-D conformal planning/multivane intensity modulating delivery system for radiotherapy. In: Purdy JA, Emami B, eds. 3D Radiation Treatment Planning and Conformal Therapy. Madison: Medical Physics Publishing, 1993.
114. Shaw E, Kline R, Gilin M, et al. Radiation Therapy Oncology Group: Radiosurgery quality assurance guidelines. Int J Radiat Oncol Biol Phys 1993;27:1231-1239.
115. Bortfeld T, Schlegel W. Optimization of beam orientations in radiation therapy: Some theoretical considerations. Phys Med Biol 1993; 38:291-304.
116. Carol MP, Targovnik H. Importance of the user in creating optimized treatment plans with Peacock. Med Phys 1994;21:913.
117. Yorke ED, Kutcher GJ, Jackson A, et al. Probability of radiation-induced complications in normal tissues with parallel architecture under conditions of uniform whole or partial organ irradiation. Radiother Oncol 1993;26:226-237.
118. Rosen II: Treatment planning for intensity modulated radiation therapy. Presented at the Intensity Modulated Radiation Therapy Workshop, Durango, CO, May 17-18, 1996.
119. Fowler JF. Rationale for High Linear Energy Transfer Radiotherapy. In: Steel GG, Adams GE, Peckham JM, eds. The Biological Basis of Radiotherapy. Amsterdam: Elsevier Science, 1983:261-268.
120. Griffin TW, Pajak TF, Maor MH, et al. Mixed neutron/photon irradiation of unresectable squamous cell carcinomas of the head and neck: The final report of a randomized cooperative trial. Int J Radiat Oncol Biol Phys 1989;17:959-965.
121. Kelland LR, Steel GG. Inhibition of recovery from damage induced by ionizing radiation in mammalian cells. Radiother Oncol 1988;13: 285-299.
122. Suit HD, Urie M. Proton beams in radiation therapy. J Natl Cancer Inst 1992;84:155-164.
123. Tsien KC. The application of automatic computing machines to radiation treatment planning. Br J Radiol 1955;28:432-439.
124. Holmes WF. External beam treatment-planning with the programmed console. Radiology 1970;94:391-400.
125. Wong JW, Purdy JA. On methods of inhomogeneity corrections for photon transport. Med Phys 1990;17:807-814.
126. Mackie TR, Ahnesjö A, Dickof P, et al. Development of a convolution/superposition method for photon beams. In: Bruinvis IAD, van Kleffens HJ, Wittkamper FW, eds. Proceedings of the 9th International Conference on the Use of Computers in Radiation Therapy. Scheveningen, The Netherlands: Elsevier Science Publishers, 1987: 107-110
127. Mohan R, Chui C, Lidofsky L. Differential pencil beam dose computation model for photons. Med Phys 1986;13:64-73.
128. Hogstrom K, Steadham R. Electron Beam Dose Computation. In: Palta J, Mackie TR, eds. Teletherapy: Present and Future. College Park, MD: Advanced Medical Publishing, 1996:137-174.
129. Hogstrom KR, Mills MD, Almond PR. Electron beam dose calculations. Phys Med Biol 1981;26:445-459.
130. Hogstrom KR. 3-D Electron Beam Dose Algorithms. In: Purdy JA, Emami B, eds. 3D Radiation Treatment Planning and Conformal Therapy. Madison, WI: Medical Physics Publishing, 1995:245-263.
131. Austin-Seymour M, Chen GTY, Rosenman J, et al. Tumor and target delineation: Current research and future challenges. Int J Radiat Oncol Biol Phys 1995;33:1041-1052.
132. Kuszyk BS, Ney DR, Fishman EK. The current state of the art in three dimensional oncologic imaging: An overview. Int J Radiat Oncol Biol Phys 1995;33:1029-1039.
133. Hamilton RJ, Sweeney PJ, Pelizzari CA, et al. Functional imaging in treatment planning of brain lesions. Int J Radiat Oncol Biol Phys 1997;37:181-188.
134. Purdy JA, Harms WB, Matthews JW, et al. Advances in 3-dimensional radiation treatment planning systems: Room-view display with real time interactivity. Int J Radiat Oncol Biol Phys 1993;27:933-944.
135. Hartmann Siantar CL, Chandler WP, Weaver KA, et al. Validation and performance assessment of the peregrine all-particle Monte Carlo code for photon beam therapy (abstract). Med Phys 1996;23: 1128-1129.

136. Curran BH. A Program for Quality Assurance of Dose Planning Computers. In: Starkschall G, Horton JL, eds. Quality Assurance in Radiotherapy Physics. Madison, WI: Medical Physics Publishing, 1991; 207-228.
137. Fraass B. Quality Assurance for 3D Treatment Planning. In: Palta J, Mackie TR, eds. Teletherapy: Present and Future. College Park, MD: Advanced Medical Publishing, 1996:253-318.
138. Harms WB, Purdy JA, Emami B, et al. Quality Assurance for Three-Dimensional Treatment Planning: In: Purdy JA, Fraass BA, eds. Syllabus: A Categorical Course in Physics: Three-Dimensional Radiation Therapy Treatment Planning. Oak Brook, IL: Radiological Society of North America, 1994:161-167.
139. Jacky J, White CP. Testing a 3-D radiation therapy planning program. Int J Radiat Oncol Biol Phys 1990;18:253-261.
140. Ten Haken RK, Fraass BA. Quality Assurance in 3-D Treatment Planning. In: Meyer JL, Purdy JA, eds. Frontiers in Radiation Therapy and Oncology, Vol 29,3-D Conformal Radiotherapy. Basel: Karger, 1996:104-114.
141. Fraass BA, Doppke KP, Hunt MA, et al. AAPM TG 53 Report: Quality Assurance of Radiotherapy Treatment Planning Systems. In press.

Chapter 4

The Simulation Process in the Determination and Definition of the Treatment Volume and Treatment Planning

Bruce J. Gerbi

The goal of radiation therapy is to deliver a homogeneous tumoricidal dose to a well-defined region while minimizing the dose to the surrounding normal tissue. To achieve this goal, a high degree of accuracy in dose delivery is required along with a systematic and logical approach to the treatment of the particular disease. Essential to this is accurate determination of the volume of tissue to be treated.

Over the past several decades, the process of simulation and the method by which treatment fields are set up in radiation oncology have changed dramatically. Initially, treatment fields were demarcated by the physician based on indications of pain determined by palpation or on the knowledge of patient anatomy and external bony landmarks. Port films on the treatment unit were later taken in some cases to document the treatment area and to determine if the proper areas were being covered by the treatment field.

In the 1970s, simulators became more prevalent in the positioning of radiation treatment fields. These modified diagnostic units capable of duplicating the mechanical movements of the treatment machine have offered several advantages to treatment planning:

1. More accurate, high-contrast radiographs are possible compared to those obtained from a megavoltage beam;
2. Diagnostic x-ray beams are much less destructive of tissue than beams in the megavoltage range, and therefore more beam time over volumes larger than the treatment area can be used without excessive damage to normal tissue;
3. The availability of fluoroscopic imaging on simulators allows the beam to be placed and adjusted in real time and permits the evaluation of tissue motion during treatment.

Further developments in imaging technology with computed tomography (CT) in the 1970s and magnetic resonance imaging (MRI) in the 1980s now permit full three-dimensional (3D) visualization of the treatment region and the surrounding sensitive normal structures. The ability of these imaging devices to enhance anatomical visualization and improve identification of the true target led to additional developments in simulation. In recent years, importance has been placed on the use of CT or MRI scans to digitally represent the patient, do all planning of field or portal definition on the digital representation of the patient, and verify the planned fields using the simulator (1). The development of commercially available CT simulators has fused the processes of patient scanning, tumor and target localization, treatment planning, and treatment field verification into a single integrated operation. In all, the new simulation process has streamlined the way radiation treatment portals can be accurately positioned, verified, documented, and treated.

Successful treatment field placement, however, is not simply a technical process demanding advanced equipment and technology. Rather, it requires the expertise of several specialists in the radiation oncology department. The medical aspects, clinical progress, and overall responsibility for proper patient treatment ultimately lie with radiation oncologists. Their role is to decide the actual target to be treated and the dose to be delivered to the region of interest, as well as to ensure that the normal tissue tolerances of the adjacent sensitive structures are not exceeded. The technical aspects of radiation therapy such as patient positioning, immobilization, computerized treatment planning, and actual dose delivery are largely the domain of the clinical physics and radiation therapy staff. In meeting these technical challenges and achieving treatment success, the process of simulation is critical.

SIMULATION PROCESS

Several steps are involved in the simulation process, depending on the complexity of the case:

1. Presimulation planning
2. Patient positioning
3. Treatment field localization
4. Beam orientation
5. Documentation of treatment field location
6. External patient contours
7. Compensating filters
8. Custom field blocking
9. Treatment planning: CT and MRI scans
10. Target volume localization
11. Computerized treatment planning
12. Verification simulation.

The actual order in which these steps are performed depends on the type and location of the equipment available to the radiation oncology staff. Each of these steps is discussed in greater detail below in the following sections. The final step of the simulation process and the first step of implementing the treatment plan is the accurate transfer of information from the simulator to the treatment unit, which is described later in this chapter.

Presimulation Planning

For the treatment of any patient, the crucial step that should be undertaken well before the patient is brought into the simulator room is the accurate determination of the volume to be irradiated. Description of the volumes to be treated has been aided by standard nomenclature developed by the International Commission on Radiation Units and Measurements (ICRU) to define target structures (2). Five different target structures are defined:

1. Gross tumor volume (GTV) is the "gross palpable or visible/demonstrable extent and location of malignant growth;
2. Clinical target volume (CTV) is "a tissue volume that contains a demonstrable GTV and/or subclinical microscopic malignant disease, which has to be eliminated";
3. Planning target volume (PTV) is "a geometric concept . . . to select appropriate beam sizes and beam arrangements, taking into consideration the net effect of all the possible geometrical variations, in order to ensure that the prescribe dose is actually absorbed in the CTV";
4. Treated volume is the volume enclosed by an isodose surface, selected and specified by the radiation oncologist as being appropriate to achieve the purpose of treatment (e.g., tumor eradication, palliation);
5. Irradiated volume is the tissue volume that receives a dose considered significant in relation to normal tissue tolerance. Organs at risk are specified as normal tissues whose radiation sensitivity may significantly influence treatment planning and/or prescribed dose (2). The GTV and CTV are anatomic and biologic concepts whereas the PTV is a geometric concept (see Figure 4.1).

Determination of the GTV is the first step in presimulation planning, followed by determination of the CTV and finally the PTV. Both CTV and PTV determination depend on the staging of the disease and on all available diagnostic information including diagnostic radiographs, CT and MRI images, nuclear medicine scans, operating room reports, the pathology report, patient and organ motion, and uncertainties in beam placement. The presumed microscopic invasion of the disease is also taken into account in the determination of the CTV. The PTV does not include any margin for beam characteristics such as beam penumbra.

For difficult cases, possible treatment approaches are discussed between the staff physician and the clinical

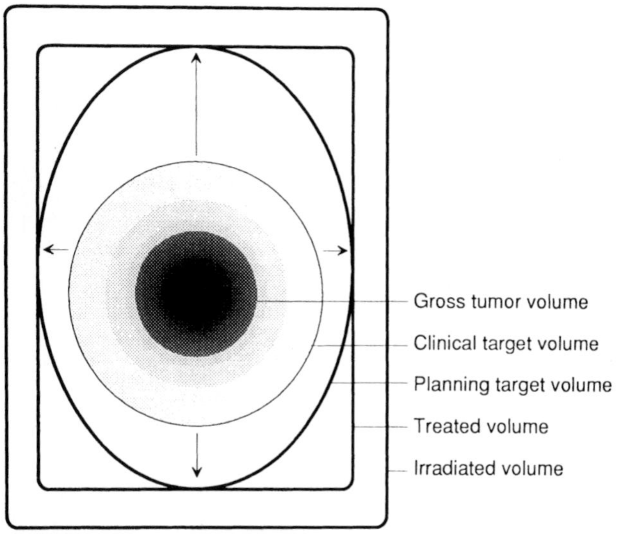

Figure 4.1. Diagram illustrating the ICRU 50 definitions of gross tumor volume (GTV), clinical target volume (CTV), planning target volume (PTV), and other planning related nomenclature.

physicist several days before the simulation. Preliminary plans may be performed before the patient has been seen in the department. For all cases, if a clear treatment approach is known at the beginning of the simulation process, the procedure will be done more efficiently and accurately. This will enhance the patient's confidence in the entire process, reduce the time needed to complete the simulation, and reduce the likelihood of a repeat simulation.

Patient Positioning

Establishing a stable and reproducible patient position is the first function performed at the start of simulation. This step is paramount and has been emphasized by several investigators (3–10). The accurate and reproducible positioning of the patient is increasingly important as 3D conformal therapy and intensity modulated radiation therapy (IMRT) become more common. The general consensus among authors is that if a stable position cannot be maintained and reproduced on a day-to-day basis, either geometric miss of the PTV will result or greater amounts of uninvolved normal tissue will be irradiated. The treatment position should be suitable for both the initial treatment fields and any boost fields that are to be treated at a later time. This eliminates the uncertainty in the position of the internal structures from one treatment position to another and reduces the amount of time required for an additional setup. Establishing a reproducible treatment position essentially defines a patient-based frame of reference to which all other patient specific data is referenced.

The supine position with the arms at the side is the preferred treatment position we use in the Department of Therapeutic Radiology—Radiation Oncology at the University of Minnesota, because the patient rests firmly on the couch with little tendency toward movement or rotation. It is also an easy position to document and reproduce throughout the course of treatment. We use a bare treatment couch surface since this tends to reduce patient setup discrepancies in moving from the simulator couch to the treatment machine couch, and reduces the inaccuracy in measuring the height of the isocenter above the tabletop (11). A sagittal or midline laser is used to align the patient along the longitudinal axis of the beam while a parallel opposed pair of lateral lasers indicate the location of the isocenter above the tabletop (See Figure 4.2). Treatment positions with the arms placed above the head are avoided unless absolutely necessary. This position tends to promote patient movement, especially rotation, and is less comfortable for the patient. It is also more difficult to accurately describe and is more difficult for the treatment therapists to accurately reproduce on the treatment machines. If the treatment must be done with the arms above the head, additional measures are taken to ensure an accurate treatment position.

Improved immobilization and patient repositioning are possible using one of the many devices that are commercially available. Polyurethane foam casts are commonly used in our clinic and are easily made by mixing two chemical components together and then pouring the material into a plastic bag. The patient is positioned for simulation on top of the bag and the foam resulting from the chemical reaction between the two components expands to surround the patient. The material hardens in about 15 minutes and forms an exact copy of the external surface of the patient. If a treatment field intersects the cast, that part can easily be cut away to preserve skin sparing. However, little skin sparing is lost at megavoltage energies even if the field does impinge on the foam at some point (12). Vacuum bags are another immobilization device proven to be useful in the clinic. They offer the added advantages of being reusable and easy to make. Thermoplastics are

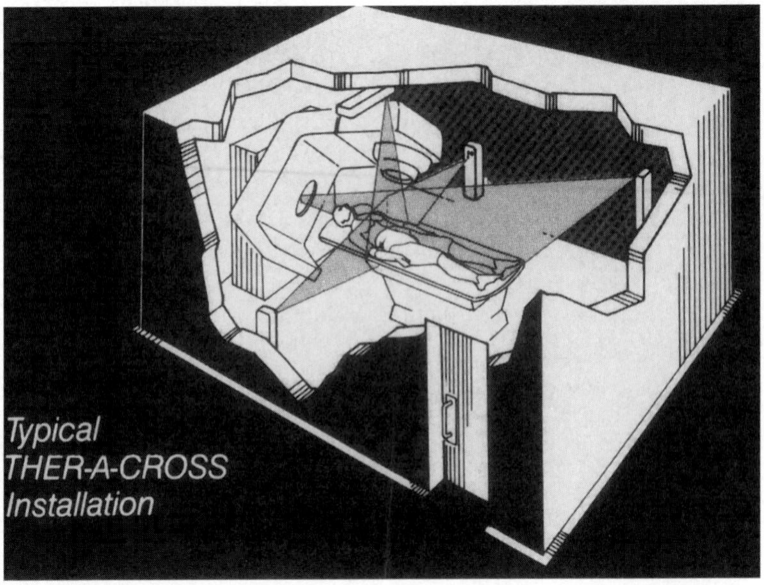

Figure 4.2. Use of sagittal and midline lasers to accurately define the location of the isocenter of the machine during patient treatment.

also convenient for patient positioning and immobilization and are our primary method of immobilization for head and neck treatments (13). However, when using casts, changes in the external shape of the patient during treatment that reduce the effectiveness of the cast must be constantly monitored.

Treatment Field Localization

The primary goal of the simulation process is to localize the isocenter, the central axis of the beam, and the edges of the treatment field to optimize coverage of the PTV and minimize irradiation of normal tissue. The location of the central axis of the beam and the field edges are specified in terms of fixed anatomical bony landmarks or with respect to surface anatomy. Depending on the complexity of the case, adequate field localization may be accomplished in one simulation session. More complicated cases may require two or more simulations before the treatment course can be started.

Simple cases are those where the location of the PTV can be easily determined with respect to either bony anatomy that is visible on the radiograph or by surface anatomy. In these cases, there is little doubt about the location of the PTV, and the treatment position determined at the start of simulation has little influence on the applicability of previous diagnostic information in locating the proper region to be irradiated. As such, the margins of the treatment field can be easily localized and accurately delineated with only one simulation. Whole brain or pelvic fields are examples of these types of cases.

The simulation process becomes more complicated when the PTV cannot be easily or accurately localized either before or during the course of the simulation. This difficulty occurs either because the PTV is not visible on routine radiographs or because previous diagnostic studies identifying the location of the PTV were performed with the patient in a position different from that of the simulation. In these cases, the primary purpose of the first simulation is to establish a reproducible treatment position. This stable treatment position forms the frame of reference that is used to coordinate data from the simulation, previously obtained diagnostic information, and future treatment planning CT or MRI scans. This is important so that the location of the PTV can be accurately drawn on the contour taken in simulation or on the treatment planning CT scan if one is performed. This task can be quite difficult considering the fact that previous studies often are done with the patient in a variety of positions, all of which can differ considerably from the treatment position established in the simulator.

Beam Orientation

Isocentric treatment fields that take advantage of the mechanical accuracy of modern treatment units are preferred over fixed source-skin distance (SSD) fields. With an isocentric beam arrangement, the only motion necessary to treat multiple fields once the position of the isocenter is located within the patient is gantry rotation, table rotation, or collimator rotation (11). The mechanical accuracy of these motions on modern accelerators is within a sphere whose maximum diameter is less than 2 mm. When the margins of the field have been established, an orthogonal film pair is taken to provide 3D information concerning the region of interest (see Figure 4.3). The orthogonal film

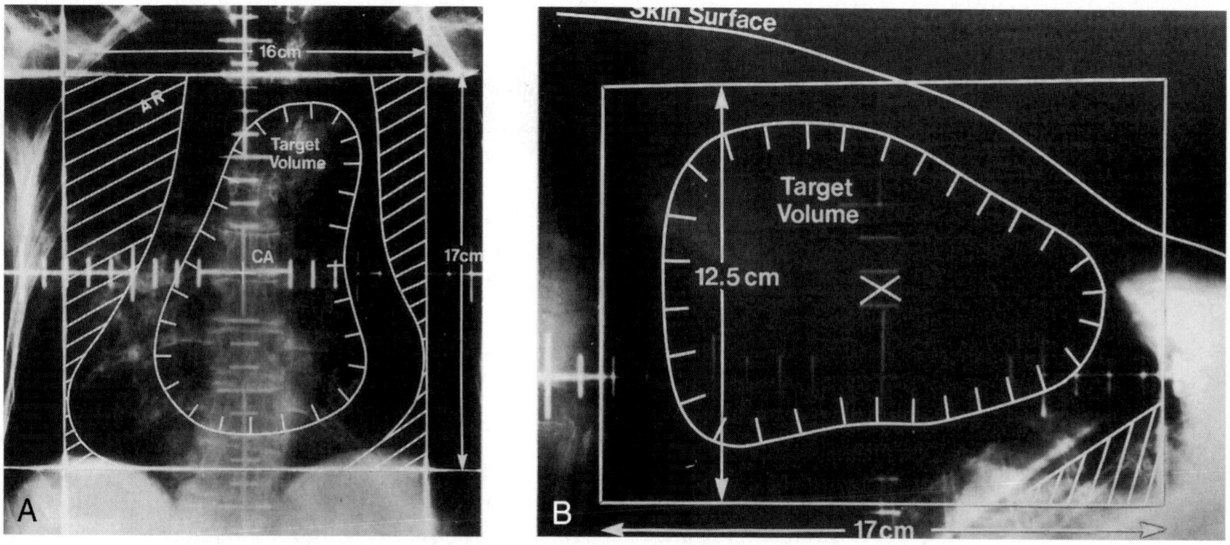

Figure 4.3. An orthogonal film pair used to document the location of the treatment fields in three dimensions. The anterior film **(A)** shows right-left and superior-inferior information while the lateral film **(B)** gives anterior-posterior and superior-inferior information. The location of the PTV is marked on both films.

pair provides a great deal of anatomic information that can be directly transferred to the patient contour. The anterior field of the orthogonal pair supplies right-left and superior-inferior information about the treatment region, while the lateral film of the pair orients structures in the anterior-posterior and the superior-inferior direction. Patient thicknesses measured at the central axis and at both the superior and inferior borders of the field are written on the anterior film. When taking the lateral film, a chain or some other radiopaque marker is placed along the midline of the patient to help visualize the location of the anterior skin surface. This procedure, by default, also yields a sagittal contour. The location of the tumor and the PTV is marked on each of these films of the orthogonal pair using previous diagnostic information and through consultation with a diagnostic radiologist.

Documentation of Treatment Field Location

After determining the location of the treatment portals, it is essential to properly document the location of the treatment field. This step requires measuring the distance from easily identified bony landmarks to the location of the central axis and the field edges. Describing the location of the treatment field versus bony landmarks has several advantages over the use of skin marks:

1. Skin marks are highly mobile, especially for obese patients, whereas the location of the PTV remains essentially constant with respect to bony structures.
2. A resimulation is not required if the skin marks are lost.
3. The treatment field can easily be reconstructed long after the current course of therapy has been delivered.

The treatment chart should allow for easy documentation of patient positioning information and immobilization devices used for the treatment. The parameters needed to set up and locate the isocenter in the patient should also be part of the treatment documentation, as well as field diagrams showing the body region treated along with the associated blocking. Treatment machine setup parameters for each field, such as the SSD, the field size, collimator, table and gantry rotation, and machine wedges, if used for treatment, are all necessary to document. Special treatment devices such as bolus, compensating filters, custom blocks, or multileaf collimation should also be indicated in the patient's chart, as well as photographs of the treatment position or any other pertinent data. Three-dimensional conformal treatment field arrangements often require additional amounts of space for adequate documentation since the beam, collimator, and wedge orientations are commonly complicated and difficult to visualize. Record and verify systems are a tremendous aid in ensuring that these complicated machine related treatment parameters are correctly transferred from the simulator to the treatment machines (14).

External Patient Contours

After the prospective fields have been radiographed, external patient contours are obtained. These contours are usually taken through the central axis of the primary simulated field and through the central axis of any cone-down boost field. If there is a large variation in patient thickness across the field, additional contours are taken so that planning can be done in these regions. In all cases, a contour is taken through the center of the region that is to receive the maximum prescribed dose.

A pantograph device (11) is used to obtain patient contours, although many other methods have been described (15–19). To provide accurate correlation of information between the simulation radiographs and the contours, the location of the central axis of the AP and lateral radiographs, the midline of the patient, and the field edges are all marked on the contour. Any other important anatomical features (e.g., surgical incisions, the eyes, external nodules) are also indicated on the contours. Even when treatment planning CT or MRI scans are performed, contours taken in the simulator provide a good check of the fidelity of the scanned data. It is essential that the patient-centered frame of reference is maintained from the simulator, through the treatment planning CT or MRI scans, to computerized treatment planning.

Compensating Filters

During simulation, the need for compensating filters is also evaluated. Many methods have been described in the literature to account for tissue deficits in the treatment field (20–25). Some methods can account for more than just missing tissue, and compensate for dose variations across the field (26) or include the effect of tissue inhomogeneities within the treatment field (27). At the University of Minnesota, we have found that a two-dimensional compensating filter may suffice for the chest where there is little variation in patient thickness in the transverse direction but large thickness variations in the sagittal dimension. By taking thickness measurements at the central axis and at the inferior and superior borders, or by using the lateral film of the orthogonal pair to determine tissue deficits, a simple compensating filter can be easily made from acrylic. If more than a 5% variation in dose exists without compensation in both the transverse and sagittal planes, a more elaborate three-dimensional compensating filter is made. The system that we currently use to make three-dimensional compensators is the commercially available Clinicomp-100 system (Varian Associates). This system uses a mechanical linkage between a stylus that is traced over the patient's surface and a dental drill bit that cuts a depression in a block of Styrofoam. For each centimeter of missing tissue, an appropriate amount of Styrofoam is routed from the foam block. The actual amount depends on the beam energy, field size, and depth of compensation for that particular treatment. The cavity in the foam is later filled with cerrobend™, which provides the proper amount of attenuation to the beam (28). Before any compensating filter is used for patient treatment, the amount of transmission through the device is checked at several points to ensure that the amount of compensation is correct. The compensator checking technique we use at the University of Minnesota is fully described elsewhere (29).

Custom Field Blocking

Field shaping is done using custom cerrobend™ blocks as described by Powers et al (30) or by multileaf collimation (see Figure 4.4). The necessary blocking is indicated on the approved simulator films and the custom blocks are fabricated using these films as the template for cutting. For parallel opposed treatments, both blocks of the pair are cut from the outline drawn on one of the simulator films. Doing this increases the likelihood that the blocks will be true mirror images of one another and that each field of the parallel opposed pair irradiates the same volume of tissue.

Custom blocking has many advantages:

1. It produces sharper beam edges since the shape of the block exactly matches the divergent edge of the beam;
2. The treatment time per patient is reduced since hand placement of individual blocks is eliminated;
3. The day-to-day reproducibility of field positioning is enhanced with rigidly mounted blocks;
4. It is possible to spare more normal tissue since more complicated blocking arrangements can be designed with this system.

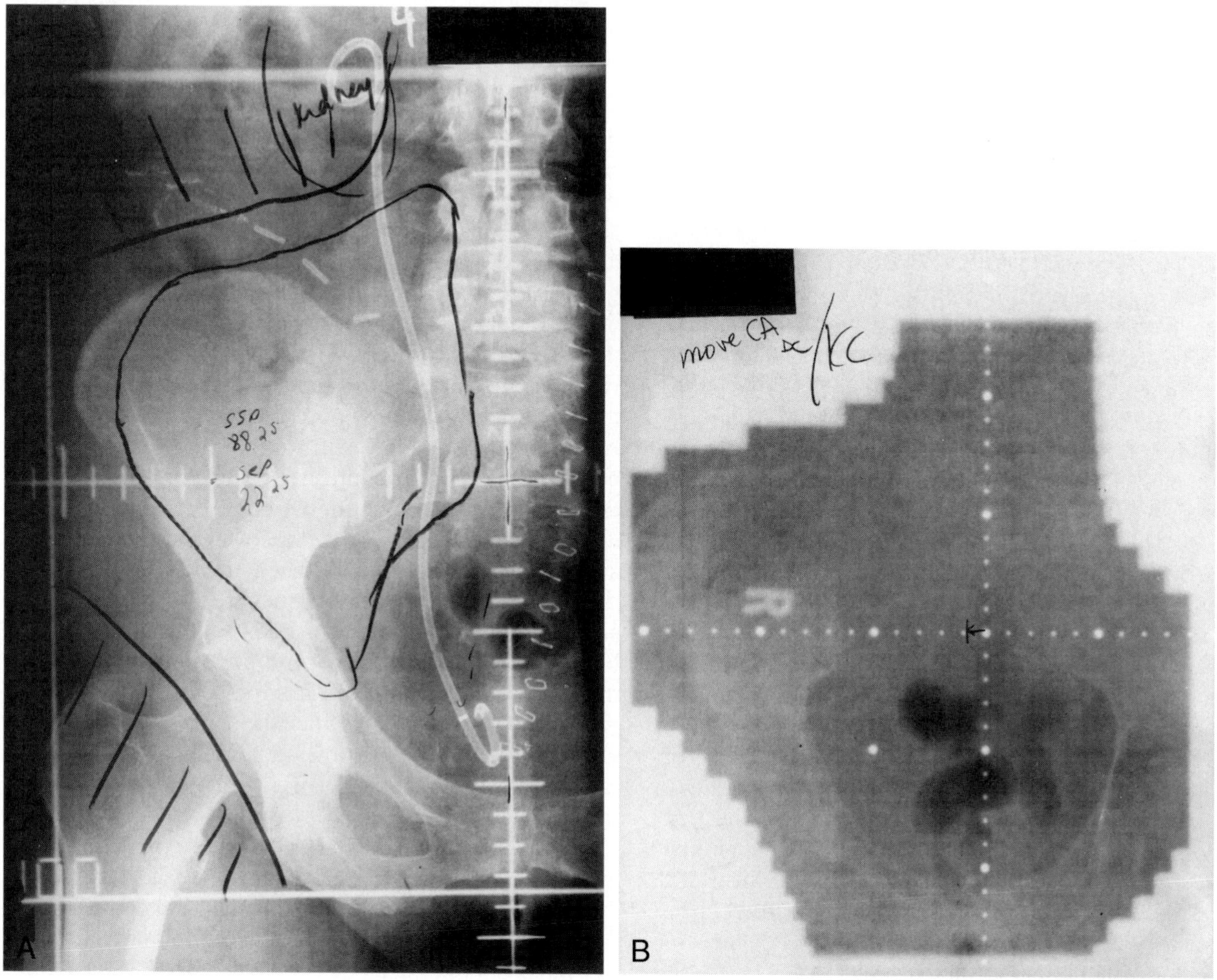

Figure 4.4. The desired treatment field indicated on simulator radiograph **(A)** and the corresponding multi-leaf collimated field port film **(B)** of the treated area.

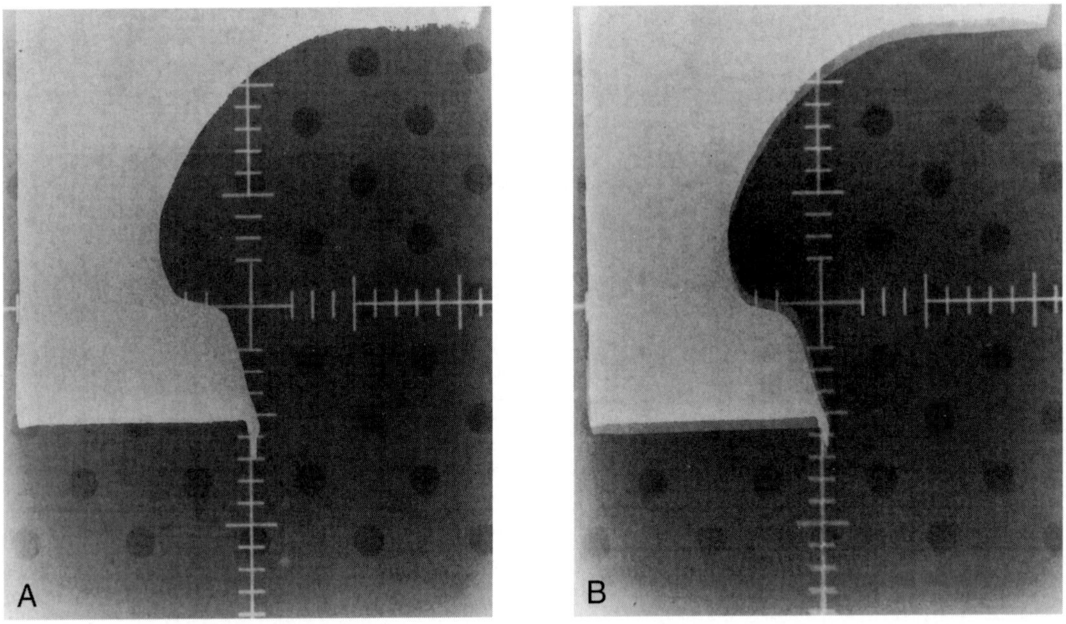

Figure 4.5. Block check film resulting from an exposure made with the right lateral block in place, then rotating the gantry 180° and making an exposure on the same film with the left lateral block in place. **A.** An example of a block pair with no mismatch between blocks. **B.** Right-left lateral block check film showing a mismatch between the two blocks of the pair.

Despite these many advantages, many sources of error are possible in both the fabrication and use of custom blocking. Incorrectly orienting the block on the tray or improperly setting the source-tray distance (STD) or source-film distance (SFD) before cutting the Styrofoam can lead to incorrect treatments. An error of approximately ±3 mm in the size of the finished blocks can result if either too little or too much tension is applied to the cutting wire during the cutting procedure. Any other inaccuracies or defects in the block cutter itself will result in blocks that are different from what was intended. To ensure that the custom blocks for each patient are accurately cut and mounted, we follow a three step block-checking procedure (31). These steps include a static light check, a parallel opposed film check, and a block check on the simulator involving the patient.

The static light check is performed in the simulator room and is done to confirm that the size and shape of the blocks is correct and are properly positioned on the block tray. The film from which the blocks were cut is placed at the proper SFD to ensure that the central axis of the film is aligned with the central axis of the light field. The blocks are inserted into the standard blocking tray slot, positioned to match the outline on the film, and then tightened to hold them in place. In performing this static block check, we have found that over 80% of the blocks need some type of adjustment before they meet our acceptance criteria of ±2 mm at 140 cm SFD.

The parallel opposed film check is performed on blocks that are made for a parallel opposed field arrangement. This check is done even though each individual block receives the static light check because of the possible misalignment of the blocks when compared to each other as a pair. Since the check film is placed at 100 cm source axis distance (SAD), all discrepancies visible on the radiograph reflect the magnitude of the misalignment occurring at the patient's treatment isocenter. The film obtained from this check visually illustrates the congruence between the two custom blocks in the actual treatment orientation. If they are truly a parallel opposed set, all blocked edges will match (see Figure 4.5A). Any mismatches due to irregular cutting, improper mounting, or collimator offset will appear as a light gray area on the film (see Figure 4.5B).

The final block check is done with the patient on the simulator. With the patient in the treatment position, a radiograph is taken of each treatment field using two exposures per film. The first exposure is done with the custom block in place while the second exposure is made with the custom block removed from the beam. The double exposure allows visualization of the surrounding anatomy, which aids in the evaluation of field adequacy. If the check radiographs are acceptable, the patient is ready to start treatment.

In performing the third check, we have found that even after successfully completing the first two checks, discrepancies are still present between the films taken during the first simulation and the check simulation. Since the first two block checks ruled out any block related inaccuracies, we know that the discrepancies found in the third block check are due to patient positioning. This block checking procedure has virtually eliminated most of the problems usually associated with the use of custom blocks, and, if a problem does arise, we are better aware of its source. Under this system, our patients are consistently treated with greater precision.

When multileaf collimation (MLC) is used to define the treatment field, a static light field check is done on the linac. The procedure exactly mimics the block field check for cerrobend blocks that is done on the simulator. This check of the MLC positions is done to ensure the accuracy of the treatment field and to facilitate the start of treatment on the first day.

Treatment Planning: CT and MRI Scans

Computed tomography and MRI scans offer the most useful information for treatment planning purposes because these scans can produce a 3D representation of the patient and the associated treatment region. Treatment planning CT scans are often performed after the initial simulation to obtain information about the location of the PTV and internal structures when the patient is in the treatment position. For the scans, radiopaque markers are placed on the skin surface to mark the location of the central axes from the anterior and lateral films of the orthogonal film pair. Other surface anatomical features are marked in a similar way so that they can also be seen on the CT scans.

Treatment planning CT scans can produce external contours that are more accurate than those obtained by other means such as pantographs, solder wire, or plaster casts. However, the patient position during the CT scan must be exactly the same as it was in the simulator (32,33). Failure to do this will produce scans of limited use for treatment planning except for their diagnostic value. If the CT scanner has a curved couch, an insert should be made to provide a flat surface for the patient to lie upon as in the simulator. The effect of a curved versus a flat couch on the location of internal organs is illustrated in Figure 4.6. In addition, the scans should be taken through the same anatomical locations as the simulator contours with radiopaque markers on the anterior and lateral central axes. This will produce both a cross-check with the simulator contour information and provide reference points that match those of the simulator radiographs.

The exact treatment position cannot always be produced on the CT scanner because of the small scan-ring size of some units. This is especially true for tangential breast treatments where the arm is usually positioned 90° to the sagittal axis of the patient. Also, for wide body sections such as the shoulders and pelvis, there can be some side cut-off of the scans resulting in an incomplete external contour. This is not a major problem unless lateral fields are required. However, relating the CT scan data to the data taken in the simulator is more difficult because of the loss of the lateral central axis markers.

Respiration during the scan can also lead to an inaccurate representation of the patient's external and internal contours. It was found that quiet respiration during the scan resulted in patient representation that was within one cm for all areas of the body (27,32). Holding a deep breath during the scan should be avoided since this tends to increase the thickness of the patient on the CT scan as compared to the contour obtained in the simulator. A sufficient number of scans must be taken to accurately represent the target in 3D space without introducing the problem of volume averaging over the scan slice thickness. Thin CT scans with no more than 5 mm spacing between scans is desirable to produce digitally reconstructive radiograph (DRRs) with acceptable contrast and bony detail. Figure 4.7 shows the effect of slice thickness and table indexing on the final quality of the DRR.

The CT scans are read directly into the treatment plan-

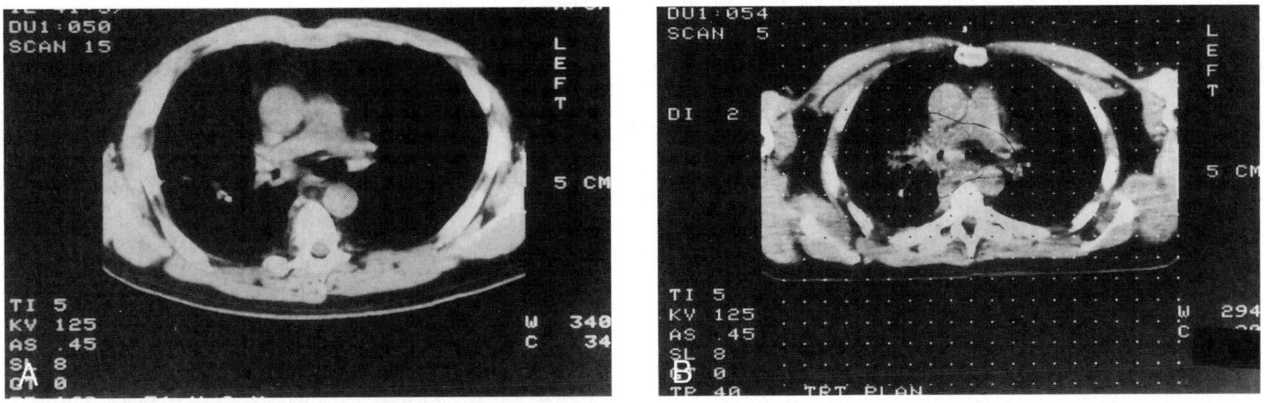

Figure 4.6. Effect of the shape of the CT scanner couch on the internal and external contours. The CT scans are for the same patient at the same anatomical location. **A.** Routine diagnostic scan performed with a curved couch in place. **B.** A treatment planning CT scan with a flat insert added to the curved couch to provide the same surface as in the treatment rooms. Lateral cutoff seen on both scans is due to the small scan ring size.

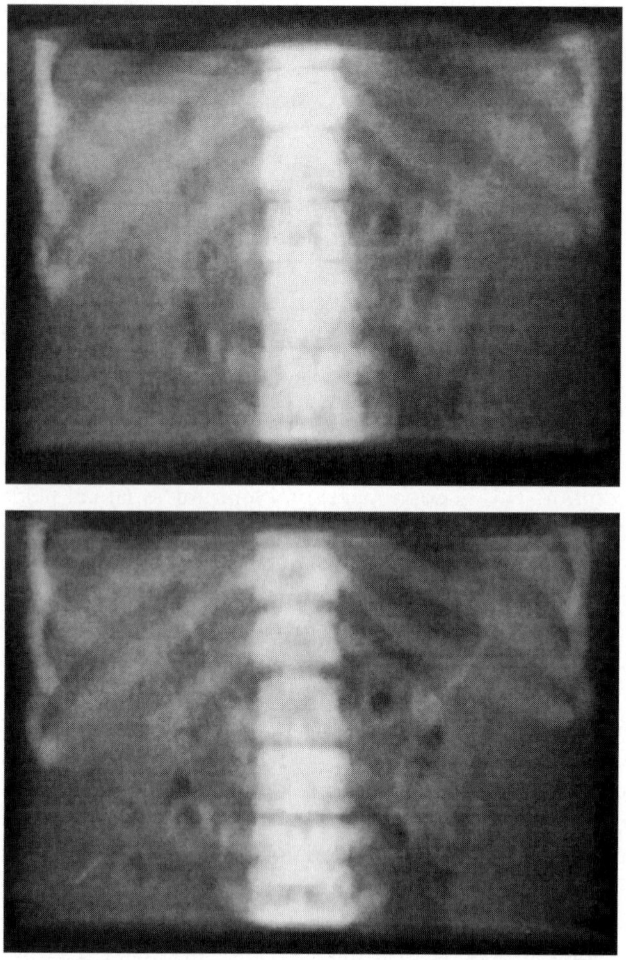

Figure 4.7. The effect of slice thickness and table indexing on the digitally reconstructed radiograph of the abdomen of a CT phantom. **A.** A 5 mm slice and 5 mm table increment image. **B.** A DRR reconstructed from 2 mm slices and 2 mm table increments. (Reprinted with permission from Advanced Medical Publishing: Madison, Wisconsin, 1995; Figure 5, p. 48.)

ning computer where field shaping is determined using beams eye view (BEV) representations of the treatment field. Computerized treatment planning is performed to determine the location of the isocenter, and the number, size, energy, and orientation of the beams to be used. Three-dimensional dose calculations are performed to optimize the dose uniformity throughout the PTV and to ensure that normal structures receive an acceptable dose. Commercially available computerized treatment planning systems that utilize CT data in their dose computation algorithms provide accurate dose representations in all regions except close to the interface between inhomogeneities (34–36).

Target Volume Localization

If the treatment planning CT scan is available and does not suffer from the problems mentioned above, the PTV can either be marked on the CT scan radiographs or directly on the video display image of the treatment planning computer. Care must be taken so that possible distortion of the radiographic image caused by the photographic process does not lead to unacceptable errors in the final computed isodose distribution (18,37). If the target is marked on all the CT scans along with the blocking needed to shield sensitive structures, DRRs are obtained along with 3-D calculations. In all instances where CT or MRI scans are used for target identification, it must be kept in mind that these studies represent a snapshot of the individual at the time of the study. Organ motion and scan related uncertainties are not easily quantified using only static data sources such as radiographs, CT, and MRI scans.

Computerized Treatment Planning

The goals of computerized treatment planning are 1) to maximize the dose in the PTV, 2) to minimize the dose to the surrounding uninvolved tissue, and 3) to provide a homogeneous dose with less than 5% variation through the PTV. The treatment plan should specify the field sizes that optimally cover the PTV, the energy of the radiation beams, and the orientation of the radiation fields. This topic is covered in previous chapters and is treated extensively in several published books on this topic (11,27,38–41).

Verification Simulation

After the completion of computerized treatment planning, a verification simulation is performed to evaluate the feasibility of the plan. This simulation is done to ensure that the beam arrangement shown on the computer plan is indeed what is desired or required for proper treatment. It is during this step that the orientation of the beams on the computer is compared to the bony anatomy on the radiographs to verify proper field position. This is also where the coverage of the beams with respect to surface anatomy is checked clinically so that the fields do not pass too close to sensitive structures (i.e., spinal cord, eyes). Once the position of the fields has been checked and radiographed, precise custom blocks can be designed to limit the dose to uninvolved regions. When 3D conformal planning has been performed, the custom blocks are cut prior to simulation using the BEV representation of the treatment field and generated using a digitally reconstructed radiograph. Figure 4.8 shows the BEV for a treatment of the brain. The PTV is clearly shown in the diagram. Because some combinations of gantry, table, and collimator orientation cannot be radiographed on the simulator due to the presence of the image intensifier, we also develop a DRR of the anterior setup field and the orthogonal lateral field to ensure that the location of the isocenter is correct. The final step of this simulation is to produce an

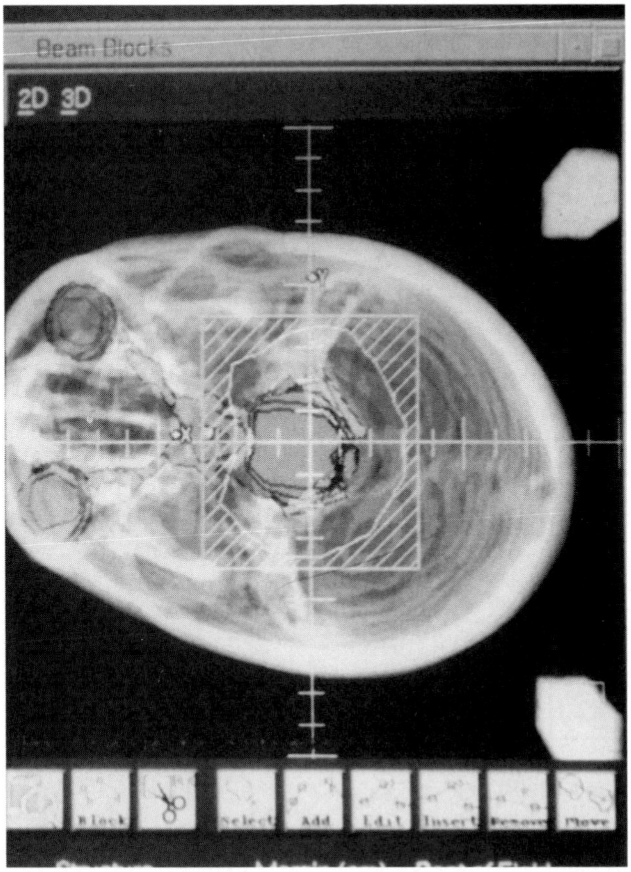

Figure 4.8. A digitally reconstructed radiograph of a brain field used to compare with a simulator field of the same port.

accurate setup diagram describing the exact anatomic location of the treatment fields. Machine orientation data is captured on the simulator using the record and verify system, and downloaded directly to the treatment accelerators.

IMPLEMENTATION OF THE TREATMENT PLAN

Accurate transfer of information from the simulator to the treatment unit is critical to the success of treatment. Even the most accurate simulation and treatment plan is of no use if that information is not properly transferred to the treatment machine. To ensure an accurate transfer of this information, the staff physician along with the involved physicist are always present for the first treatment. Before treatment, the setup diagrams, the calculations, the patient position, and the placement of custom blocks or special treatment devices are reviewed. The importance of initiating the treatment correctly can be put in perspective by reviewing published results (9). These results show considerably greater discrepancies between simulator films and portal films than from one portal film to the next. This indicates that setup errors and treatment inaccuracies are more likely to occur when going from the simulator to the treatment machine than after the patient is under treatment.

To ensure the long-term accuracy of treatment, port films are taken after the first treatment and on a weekly basis thereafter. These port films should always be checked versus the simulator films so that small variations from one port film to the next do not combine to produce large changes over the course of the patient's treatment. The importance of this continued surveillance is of major importance in ensuring that local failure does not occur purely because of geometric miss (42,43). In an unpublished retrospective review of upper airway carcinoma (44), a clear correlation between local recurrence and errors in blocking was shown. The author observed a 75% recurrence rate associated with treatments in which 30% or more of the portals exhibited a blocking error compared to a 17% recurrence rate for patients that had no such errors in blocking. This information highlights the importance of precision field placement in radiotherapy.

Technical improvements have been made in response to this need for greater accuracy. Two of these advances are record and verify systems (14,45) and on-line real-time portal imaging systems (46–49). Record and verify systems improve the accuracy of patient treatments and provide greater insight into the areas where treatment errors are most likely to occur (14). In comparison to non-verified treatments, these systems have all but eliminated treatment errors related to parameters set on the treatment unit.

On-line real-time imaging is a fairly new capability that is an improvement over taking port films for field verification. The poor contrast associated with port films has always been their main disadvantage even though much work has gone into improving techniques and overcoming the physical limitations imposed by megavoltage radiations (50,51). The advantage of on-line real-time digital imaging is the speed with which an image can be displayed (usually 3–4 seconds) as well as its ability to enhance images to improve the image contrast. Thus, bones and other detail are more easily discerned and the processed image is closer in contrast to what is seen on a typical simulator or diagnostic radiograph (52,53). To evaluate the correctness of the treated volume, the image of the treatment field that was approved in simulation is placed on a monitor and the acquired image from the treatment being delivered is shown on the same monitor. In this fashion, the two images can be immediately and directly compared for every field and evaluated for positional accuracy. Yet another capability of these systems is their ability to act as a dose verification system. Since the image detector is simply an array of radiation detectors, the signal from these detectors can be used to verify the transmitted dose through the treatment region (48). Thus, this one system has the ability to provide visual verification of the treatment field, to enhance the image to produce greater contrast, and to verify the dose that was delivered to the irradiated region.

Virtual Simulation

In recent years, CT simulation or virtual simulation has become more common in radiation oncology (54,55). The steps required to perform CT simulation are essentially the same as those required for conventional simulation. In conventional simulation the field locations are first set, the target is defined, and then the fields are shaped to treat the target. However, with virtual simulation, the target is first defined and then the fields are shaped to conform to the target. Virtual simulation represents the end result of an evolutionary process of simulation that applies advanced technology to the problem of setting fields more accurately and delivering a more homogeneous dose to the target region. In fact, a virtual simulator is simply a set of software routines that allows the physician to define and evaluate a treatment and then simulate the case using DRRs (54,55). Conventional simulators are still used in many cases to verify the CT simulation derived treatment fields, but the promise of virtual simulation is to eliminate conventional simulators altogether. Since virtual simulation must emulate conventional simulation, the virtual simulator must contain the same functionality as a conventional simulator. This means that the field size, gantry, collimator, and table rotations must all be correctly and accurately represented on the virtual simulator and must be accurately transferred to the patient to be treated.

The two main components of a CT simulation package are a target localization routine that allows for the target to be defined and transfers the appropriate marks to the patient skin surface, and the virtual simulation package that generates the DRRs that are used for treatment. Since the accuracy of this process depends entirely on the accuracy of the CT data, the patient position in the CT scanner and the accuracy of the CT data set itself are essential. The accuracy of the CT data set must be checked to ensure that the physical dimensions of the anatomical structures are accurately portrayed. This must be done for the images from the scanner and the images transferred to the treatment planning computer. Testing procedures using standard phantoms must be performed on a routine basis to verify the accuracy of the CT data (1). A host of other tests must also be performed to ensure the accuracy of the virtual simulator routines. A comprehensive list of these tests is documented in the literature (1).

Virtual simulation has not changed the goal of the simulation process but has made the attainment of those goals more accurate and efficient in cases where extreme accuracy is required. Large, irregularly shaped intracranial lesions that are not appropriate for stereotactic radiotherapy can be accurately simulated virtually while the utility of virtual simulations in prostate and lung cancer treatments are currently under investigation. For some cases, however, virtual simulation is not needed and may be less useful than conventional simulation, such as the placement of mantle fields for Hodgkin's disease.

CONCLUSION

The simulation process has changed significantly over the years. Initially simulators became popular because of their ability to improve the accuracy of treatment field placement and to increase the cost efficiency of preparing patients for treatment (56,57). As the need for increased accuracy became more important to treatment success, so did the demand for greater accuracy in treatment field localization.

In the near future, the accepted standard of practice may be to digitally record all aspects of the patient's treatment beginning with the original simulated and verified fields with the custom blocks or MLCs in place. The machine parameters including the beam angles, the field sizes, the collimator rotation, and table position parameters would all be included as part of the archived data. This information would be directly transferred to the treatment unit awaiting the arrival of the patient for their first day of treatment. The therapists on the treatment unit will then put the patient in the treatment position, have the machine automatically moved to the coordinates established in simulation, and then recall the DRR onto the monitor for visual verification of the treated region. While the treatment is delivered, the irradiated region will be shown on the monitor next to the approved simulation image and the portal imaging system will verify that the correct dose was delivered to the correct region. All these data for that field, and ultimately, all fields for all patients would be digitally stored to form the permanent treatment record.

References

1. Coia LR, Schultheiss TE, Hanks GE, eds. A practical guide to CT simulation. Madison, WI: Advanced Medical Publishing, 1995.
2. International Commission on Radiation Units and Measurements (ICRU): Report 50. Prescribing, recording, and reporting photon beam therapy. Bethesda, MD, 1993.
3. Bentel GC, Marks LB, Krishnamurthy R, Prosnitz LR. Comparison of two repositioning devices used during radiation therapy for Hodgkin's disease. Int J Radiat Oncol Biol Phys 1997;38:791-5.
4. Bentel GC, Marks LB, Krishnamurthy R. Impact of cradle immobilization on setup reproducibility during external beam radiation therapy for lung cancer. Int J Radiat Oncol Biol Phys 1997;38:527-31.
5. Bentel GC, Marks LB, Hendren K, Brizel DM. Comparison of two head and neck immobilization systems. Int J Radiat Oncol Biol Phys 1997;38:867-73.
6. Bentel GC, Marks LB, Sherouse GW, Spencer DP. A customized head and neck support system. Int J Radiat Oncol Biol Phys 1995;32:245-8.
7. Bentel GC, Marks LB, Sherouse GW, Spencer DP, Anscher MS. The effectiveness of immobilization during prostate irradiation. Int J Radiat Oncol Biol Phys 1995;31:143-8.
8. Carter DL, Marks LB, Bentel GC. Impact of setup variability on incidental lung irradiation during tangential breast treatment. Int J Radiat Oncol Biol Phys 1997;38:109-15.
9. Rabinowitz I, Broomberg J, Goitein M, McCarthy K, Leong J. Accuracy of radiation field alignment in clinical practice. Int J Radiat Oncol Biol Phys 1985;11:1857-1867.
10. Verhey LV, Goitein M, McNulty P, Munzenrider JE, Suit HD. Precise positioning of patients for radiation therapy. Int J Radiat Oncol Biol Phys 1982;8:289-294.

11. Khan FM. The physics of radiation therapy. Baltimore: Williams & Wilkins, 1984.
12. Mondalek, PM, Orton, CG. Transmission and build-up characteristics of polyurethane foam immobilization devices. J Amer Assoc Med Dos 1980; 7:510.
13. Gerber RL, Marks JE, Purdy JA. The use of thermal plastics for immobilization of patients during radiotherapy. Int J Radiat Oncol Biol Phys 1982;8:1461-1462.
14. Podmaniczky KC Mohan R, Kutcher GJ, Kestler C, Bhadrasain V. Clinical experience with a computerized record and verify system. Int J Radiat Oncol Biol Phys 1985;11:1529-1537.
15. Carson PL, Wenzel WW, Avery P, Hendee WR. Ultrasound imaging as an aid to cancer therapy—Part I. Int J Radiat Oncol Biol Phys 1975; 1:119. Part II, 1976;2:335.
16. Clark HC. A contouring device for use in radiation treatment planning. Brit J Radiol 1969;42:858.
17. Clayton C, Thompson D. An optical apparatus for reproducing surface outlines of body cross sections. Brit J Radiol 1970;43:489.
18. Hills JF, Ibbott GS, Hendee WR. Computerized patient contours using the scanning arm of a compound B-scanner. Med Phys 1979;6:309-311.
19. Kuisk H. "Contour maker" eliminating body casting in radiotherapy planning. Radiol 1971;101:203.
20. Boyer AL, Goitein M. Simulator mounted Moire topography camera for constructing compensating filters. Med Phys 1980; 7:19-26.
21. Ellis F, Hall EJ, Oliver R. A compensator for variations in tissue thickness for high energy beams. Brit J Radiol 1959;32:421-422.
22. Gerbi BJ. Compensating filter design using radiographic stereo shift information. Med Phys 1985;12:646-648.
23. Khan FM, Moore VC, Burns DJ. An apparatus for the construction of irregular surface compensators for use in radiotherapy. Radiol 1968; 90:593-594.
24. Purdy JA, Keys DJ, Zivnuska F. A compensation filter for chest portals. Int J Radiat Oncol Biol Phys 1977;2:1213-1215.
25. Van de Geijn J. The construction of individualized intensity modifying filters in cobalt 60 teletherapy. Brit J Radiol 1965;38:865-870.
26. Leung PMK, Van Dyk J, Robins J. A method of large irregular field compensation. Brit J Radiol 1974;47:805-810.
27. Bentel GC, Nelson CE, Noell KT. Treatment planning and dose calculation in radiation oncology, 4th ed. New York: Pergamon, 1989.
28. Henderson SD, Purdy JA, Gerber RL, Mestman SJ. Dosimetry considerations for a lipowitz metal tissue compensator system. Int J Radiat Oncol Biol Phys 1987;13:1107-1112.
29. Johnson JM, Ali MM, Khan FM. Quality control of custom-made compensators. Med Dosim 1988;13:109-111.
30. Powers WE, Kinzie JJ, Demidecki AJ, Bradford JS, Feldman A. A New System of Field Shaping for External-Beam Radiation Therapy. Radiol 1973;108:407.
31. Johnson JM, Gerbi BJ. Quality control of custom blockmaking in radiation therapy. Med Dosim 1989;14:199–202.
32. Goitein M. Computed tomography in planning radiation therapy. Int J Radiat Oncol Biol Phys 1979;5:445-447.
33. Hobday P, Hodson NJ, Husband J, Parker R, Macdonald JS. Computed tomography applied to radiotherapy treatment planning: techniques and results. Radiol 1979;133:477-482.
34. Cunningham JR. Tissue inhomogeneity corrections in photon-beam treatment planning. Prog Med Rad Phys 1982;1:103-131.
35. Sontag MR, Cunningham JR. The equivalent tissue-air-ratio method for making absorbed dose calculations in a heterogeneous medium. Radiol 1978;129:787-794.
36. Van Dyk J. Lung dose calculations using computerized tomography: Is there a need for pixel based procedures?.Int J Radiat Oncol Biol Phys 1983;9:1035-1041.
37. Ibbott GS. Radiation therapy treatment planning and the distortion of CT images. Med Phys 1980;7:261.
38. Dobbs J, Barrett A. Practical radiotherapy planning. London: Edward Arnold, 1985.
39. Mould RF. Radiotherapy treatment planning (Medical Physics Handbooks 7). Bristol: Adam Hilger Ltd., 1981.
40. Vaeth JM, Meyer J, eds. Frontiers of radiation therapy and oncology, Vol. 21: Treatment planning in the radiation therapy of cancer. Basel: Karger, 1987.
41. Wright AE, Boyer AL, eds. Advances in radiation therapy treatment planning. New York: American Institute of Physics, 1983.
42. Marks JE, Davis MK, Haus AG. Anatomic and geometric precision in radiotherapy. Radiol Clin Biol 1974;43:1-20.
43. Marks JE, Haus AG, Sutton HG, Griem ML. Localization error in the radiotherapy of Hodgkin's disease and malignant lymphoma with extended mantle field. Cancer 1974;34:83-90.
44. Doss LL. Localization error and local recurrence in upper airway carcinoma. Proceedings of the Workshop on Quality Control in the Radiotherapy Department of the Cancer and Leukemia Group B (CALGB), New York, 1979.
45. Mohan R, Podmaniczky KC, Caley R, Lapidus A, Laughlin JS. A computerized record and verify system for radiation treatments. Int J Radiat Oncol Biol Phys 1984;10:1975-1985.
46. Baily NA, Horn RA, Kampp TD. Fluoroscopic visualization of megavoltage therapeutic x-ray beams. Int J Radiat Oncol Biol Phys 1980; 6:935-939.
47. Lam KS, Partowmah M, Lam WC. An on-line electronic portal imaging system for external beam radiotherapy. Brit J Radiol 1986;59:1007-1013.
48. Leong J. Use of digital fluoroscopy as an on-line verification device in radiation therapy. Phys Med Biol 1986;31:985-992.
49. Meertens H. Digital processing of high-energy photon beam images. Med Phys 1985;12:111-113.
50. Droege RT, Bjärngard BE. Influence of metal screens on contrast in megavoltage x-ray imaging. Med Phys 1979;6:487-493.
51. Droege RT, Bjärngard BE. Metal screen-film detector MTF at megavoltage x-ray energies. Med Phys 1979; 6:515-518.
52. Lam WC, Partowmah M, Lee DJ, Wharam MD, Lam KS. On-line measurement of field placement errors in external beam radiotherapy. Br J Radiol 1987;60:361-367.
53. Meertens H, Bijhold J, Strackee J. A method for the measurement of field placement errors in digital portal images. Phys Med Biol 1990; 35:299-323.
54. Sherouse GW, Bourland JD, Reynolds K, McMurry HL, Mitchell TP, Chaney EL. Virtual simulation in the clinical setting: some practical considerations. Int J Radiat Oncol Biol Phys 1990;19:1059-65.
55. Sherouse GW, Chaney EL. The portable virtual simulator. Int J Radiat Oncol Biol Phys 1991;21:475-82.
56. Supplement 16: Treatment Simulators. Br J Radiol 1981;1-31.
57. Horton JL. Handbook of radiation therapy physics. Englewood Cliffs: Prentice Hall, 1987.

Chapter 5

Complex Field Arrangements: Field Shaping and Separation of Adjoining Fields

Faiz M. Khan

In the early days of radiotherapy, field blocking was seldom used. Rectangular fields defined by the collimating jaws were mostly used to encompass the tumor bearing areas, with no undue concern to shape the field to conform to the imagined target volume. Later in the 1960s and early 1970s, standard lead blocks of various shapes and dimensions were used, primarily to block off radiation to sensitive structures or to avoid unnecessary treatment of normal tissues. With the increasing use of linear accelerators which have small focal spots (2 to 3 mm), the need for divergent blocks became apparent and eventually gave way to individualized custom blocks, cut divergently with a block cutting machine. In the modern era of conformal radiotherapy, extensive field shaping is done using cerrobend lead custom blocks and/or multileaf collimators installed in the head of the machine.

This chapter describes various methods of field blocking, both for photons and electron beams, and discusses related problems especially of skin dose, electron backscatter, and separation of adjoining fields.

Standardized Lead Blocks

The construction of shielding blocks involves time and cost. For relatively simple cases of shielding, therefore, it is desirable to have a stock of precut lead blocks of various geometric shapes available. Some of the blocks may be contoured to block specific organs (e.g., kidneys, eyes, head of humerus, and skin edges).

Block Thickness

Shielding blocks are most commonly made of lead. The thickness of blocks depends on the beam energy and the allowed transmission through the block. A primary beam transmission of 5% through the block is acceptable—that means a thickness corresponding to a little more than four half-value layers (HVL). In the case of cobalt-60 (^{60}Co), 5-cm thick lead is considered adequate. The radiation quantity of interest is the dose received in the shielded volume, which may be 10 to 15% of the dose in the open beam, depending on energy and location, because of the added contribution of radiation scattered from the adjoining open areas of the field.

Dose at a given point in the shielded volume depends on the proximity of that point to the surrounding exposed volume. When lungs are shielded in a mantle field, the shielded apex areas may receive two to three times the dose received under the middle of the shield. There is also a gradient of dose across the block edges where the dose changes from a full value in the open area to a low value within the shielded area. Sharpness of this gradient depends on many factors, such as block divergence, position in the field, source size, block-to-surface distance (BSD), and beam energy.

Ordinarily, it is not advantageous to increase the thickness of the blocks beyond what is needed for 5% primary beam transmission. The blocks get heavier without much further diminution of the dose in the shielded volume.

Block Divergence

Because the treatment beam is divergent, the blocks may be tapered, with the sides conforming to the direction of rays. Straight (untapered) blocks, in general, produce a less sharp dose gradient at the edge than divergent blocks. The advantage is not significant in the case of beams emanating from a large source, such as ^{60}Co; the geometric penumbra dominates the effect on dose gradient. Divergent blocks are suitable for beams with small focal spots and especially when a large BSD is used. Another advantage is that, by employing divergent shields, the shields can be placed closer to the source, thus reducing the size of otherwise bulky and heavy blocks. The size of the block should be considered when the area to be shielded is large (e.g., lungs in a mantle field treatment).

Straight-cut blocks are easier to construct and are mostly prefabricated to various shapes and sizes. Because the sides of the blocks are not parallel to the rays (nondivergent), a partial transmission of beam results at the block edges. To minimize this effect, the blocks should be placed close to the patient surface, which calls for bigger blocks and introduces the problem of increased skin dose. A distance of 15 to 20 cm between the plastic block-supporting tray and the skin surface is a good compromise for most megavoltage beams.

The BSD is important from the point of view of setup accuracy. If the BSD is too large, a small displacement in the position of the shield in the beam is magnified at the position of the shielded area. It is desirable to use a minimum BSD, provided the surface dose is kept within acceptable limits.

Shadow Tray and Skin Sparing

The skin-sparing effect is one of the most desirable features of megavoltage beams. This effect may be reduced or lost if the photon beam is contaminated excessively with secondary electrons. An air gap of 15 to 20 cm between the tray and the skin surface is required to maintain the skin-sparing effect (i.e., surface dose of less than 50%) (1,2).

The surface dose also increases with field size and may become prohibitively excessive for extremely large fields. The range of surface-dose values and build-up characteristics of a beam may vary with energy and from machine to machine. The effect of field size on surface dose has been discussed in the literature (3–5).

The amount of electron contamination produced in the beam depends on the atomic number of the absorber or the electron scattering material. Low-atomic number absorbers, such as a Lucite shadow tray, produce more forward scatter of electrons than the high-atomic number materials and, therefore, give rise to a greater surface dose. It has been shown both theoretically and experimentally that the absorbers of an intermediate atomic number such as tin (Z = 50) produce minimum electron contamination (4–8). A sheet of this material, known as electron filter, may be placed under the shadow tray to minimize skin dose. The thickness of electron filter should approximately equal the range of the secondary electrons produced in that material. For ^{60}Co gamma rays, a tin sheet of approximately 1-mm thickness is adequate. Figure 5.1 shows the effect of tin in reducing surface dose. Qualitatively similar results are obtained using linac x-ray beams (4). Figure 5.2 shows data for a 10 MV x-ray beam.

In modern linear accelerators with 100-cm source-axis distance (SAD), the BSD is usually greater than 20 cm; therefore, the electron contamination produced by the blocking tray is considerably reduced by electron scatter in air before incidence on the skin surface. Thus, the use

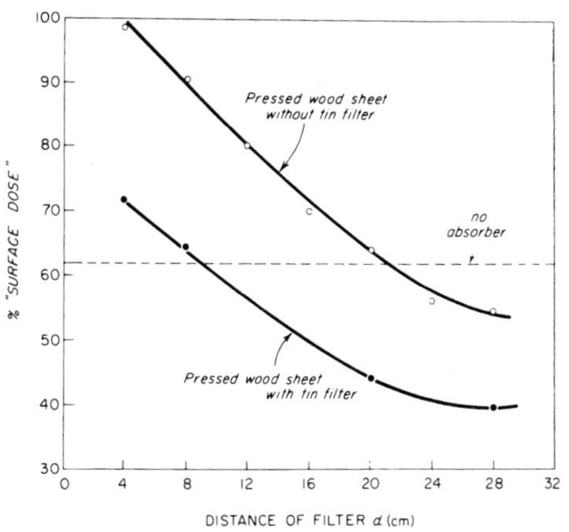

Figure 5.1. Percent surface dose versus absorber to surface distance *(d)* for pressed wood tray and tray plus tin filter.
^{60}Co beam; field size, 20 × 20 cm, source-surface distance, 80 cm; source-to-diaphragm distance, 45 cm. (Reprinted with permission from Khan FM. Use of electron filter to reduce skin dose in cobalt teletherapy. AJR 1971;111:180.)

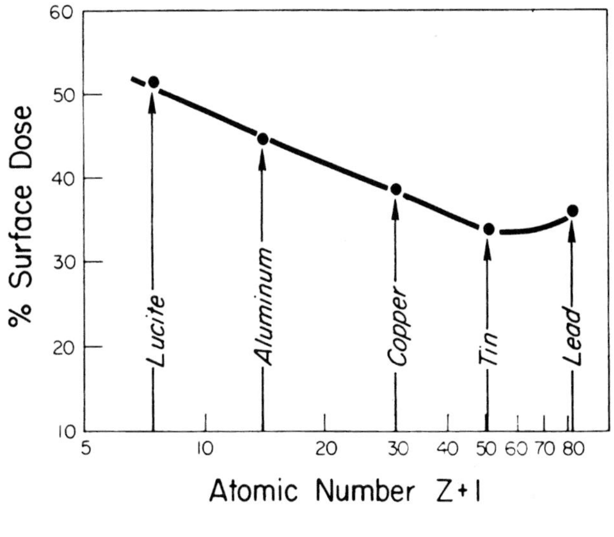

Figure 5.2. Variation of percent surface dose with atomic number of absorber inserted in the beam. Absorber thickness = 1.5 g/cm^2, mounted underneath an acrylic shadow tray of thickness = 6 mm; 10 MV x-ray beam; field size = 15x15 cm; absorber to surface distance = 15 cm. (Reprinted with permission from Khan FM, Moore VC, Levitt SH. Effect of various atomic number absorbers on skin dose for 10-MeV x-rays. Radiology 1973;109:209.)

of electron filters is usually unnecessary. However, situations of reduced tray-surface distance may arise, especially when treating large patients isocentrically, and in those cases the use of electron filter may be considered to reduce surface dose.

Construction of Custom Blocks

Various methods have been proposed for the construction of individualized blocks. The reader is referred to several sources (9–16). The method described here is similar to that described by Powers et al (15).

A device for cutting Styrofoam cavities divergently with an electrically heated wire is in common use today. Such a device is commercially available, as are Styrofoam and cerrobend lead. Outline of the treatment field is made on a simulator radiograph or a port film. The film, the Styrofoam block, and the wire apparatus are adjusted so that the treatment geometry is obtained. The lower end of the wire traces the outline on the film. For lung blocks, cavities are cut in the Styrofoam with the heated segment of the wire and subsequently filled with melted cerrobend (an alloy of lead, bismuth, and cadmium; melting point 70° C, density at 20° C = 9.4 g/cm^3). The required thickness of cerrobend block (for 5% narrow-beam transmission) is approximately 3 inches, depending on energy, from ^{60}Co energy to 22 MV x-rays (15). The material is poured slowly into the Styrofoam cavities to prevent formation of air bubbles. The Styrofoam block may be pressed tightly against a rubber pad at the bottom to avoid leakage of the liquid material. The inside of the cavities may be sprayed with silicone for easy release of the Styrofoam from the block.

Making a "negative" block, with central area open and blocking around the periphery, is a bit more cumbersome. First, the inner cut is made in the Styrofoam block to outline the given field. An outer rectangular cut is made corresponding to the overall field (defined by the collimator) with 1- to 2-cm margin. The two cuts give rise to three Styrofoam pieces. The intermediate piece, corresponding to the areas to be shielded, is removed, retaining only the outermost and the innermost pieces. Alignment of pieces is carefully maintained relative to central axis. Cerrobend is then poured into the cavity between the inner and the outer pieces.

The blocks are mounted on a 1/4-inch plexiglass plate with cross hairs drawn on the plate. One way of mounting blocks is to have fixed pegs on the plate. The plate is placed under the Styrofoam blocks when the cerrobend is poured, thus creating corresponding holes for the pegs in the lead block. These plates are individualized for each patient. Figure 5.3 shows blocks that were constructed for a mantle and a head and neck field.

Multileaf Collimators

An alternative to custom-designed cerrobend lead blocking is to use multileaf collimators (MLC) for shaping photon fields (Figure 5.4). Typical MLC systems consist of 80 leaves (40 pairs) with individual leaf width of 1 cm, projected at isocenter. The leaves are made up of tungsten alloy (ρ = 17.0–18.5 g/cm^3) with thickness ranging from 6 cm to 7.5 cm, depending on the type of accelerator. Primary x-ray transmission through the leaves is less than 2% and intra-leaf (leaf sides) transmission is less than 3%. These values are lower than the primary beam transmission for cerrobend blocks (~3.5%) and higher than that for the collimator jaws (~1%). As discussed earlier, the dose under the block, jaw, or the MLC is the sum of the primary transmission dose and the scattered dose contributed by photons scattered from the adjoining open areas of the field.

Advantages of MLC over cerrobend blocking are: 1) lifting of heavy blocks is eliminated; 2) field shaping by MLC, being computer-controlled, is reproducible and much faster than designing blocks; 3) MLC-shaped fields are ideal for treatments requiring large number of multiple fields because of automation of the field shaping procedure and significantly reduced setup time; 4) dynamic mo-

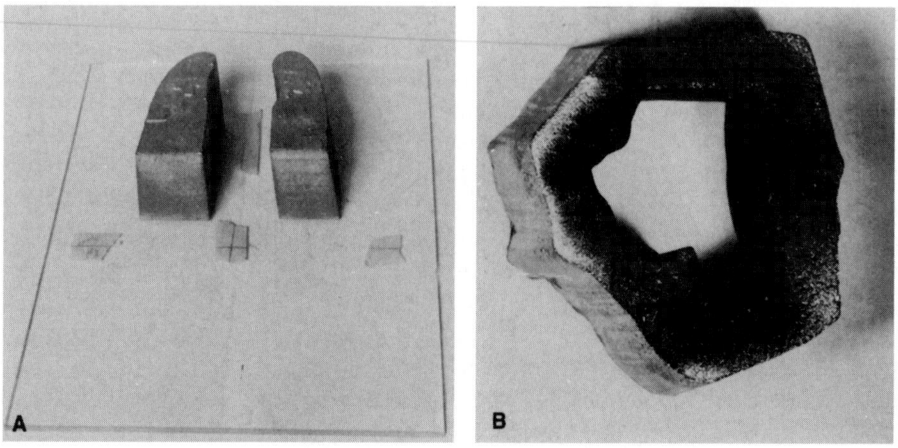

Figure 5.3. Cerrobend blocks. **A,** Lung blocks for a mantle field. **B,** Block for shaping a head and neck field.

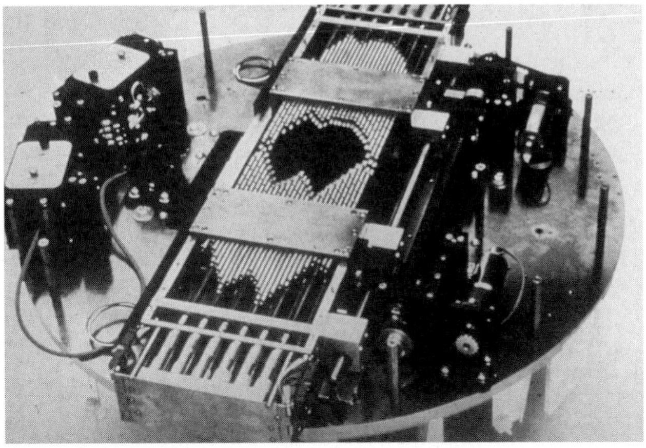

Figure 5.4. Varian multileaf collimator. (Courtesy of Varian Associates, Palo Alto, CA.)

tion of the leaves allows for new techniques such as generating enhanced dynamic wedges (wedge fields created by MLC motion in any part of the field), dynamic compensators and intensity modulated radiotherapy (IMRT).

The disadvantages of the MLC over cerrobend blocking include: 1) jaggedness of the field border because of the finite leaf width. This can be a serious drawback when field sizes are small and critical structures are located close to the target volume; 2) the physical penumbra, due to lateral dose distribution near the field edge, is larger for the MLC (because of the step size) compared to the physical penumbra associated with cerrobend blocks or the collimator jaws (Figure 5.5); 3) blocking a part of the field within the open field or "island" blocking is difficult if not impossible; and 4) matching of adjoining field is difficult if not impossible.

It should be emphasized that the importance of MLC in radiation therapy is not just the replacement of cerrobend blocking with multileaf collimation. The greatest impact of this technology is in the automation of field shaping and modulation of beam intensity. These capabilities allow complex field arrangements in conjunction with three-dimensional treatment planning, dynamic wedge and compensator design, and the intensity modulated radiotherapy (see chapter 9). As these techniques become more and more feasible, MLC will become a standard component of any modern linear accelerator. A detailed review of multileaf collimators is provided by Boyer (17).

Electron-Beam Shielding

Considerable beam shaping is required in treating superficial tumors with electron beams (6 to 20 MeV). Lead or cerrobend cutouts are often used to shape fields. The cutouts can be placed directly on the skin surface or in the applicator at a distance of not more than 5 cm from the surface.

Electron beams require thicker lead sheets for 5% transmission than do superficial x-rays and the orthovoltage. Figure 5.6 gives the thickness of lead for transmitted surface doses for electrons. A rule of thumb in electron shielding is to use thickness of lead in millimeter equal to one-half the incident energy of electrons in MeV. If the lead is too thin, the surface dose may be enhanced rather than reduced (because of more scattering than attenuation).

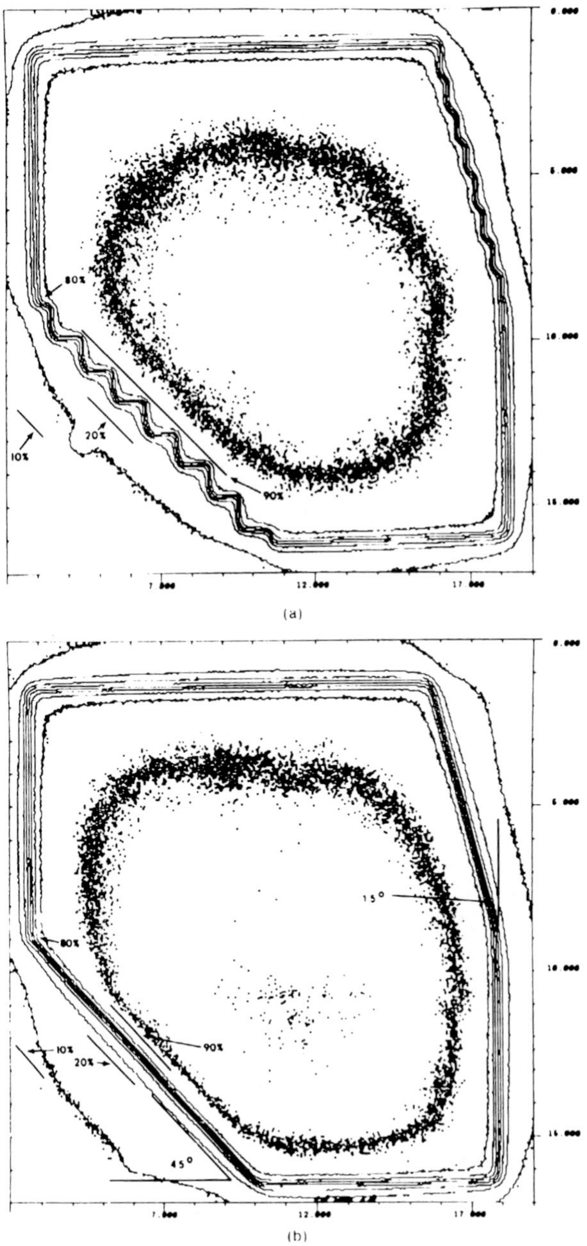

Figure 5.5. Comparison of dosimetric penumbra associated with MLC (a) and cerrobend blocks (b). Field size 15 × 15, depth 10 cm, and energy 6 MV. Dose distribution normalized to 100% at central axis. (Reproduced with permission from Galvin JM, Smith AR, Moeller RD, Goodman RL, Powlis WD, Rubenstein J, et al. Int J Radiat Oncol Biol Phys 1992;23:789-801.

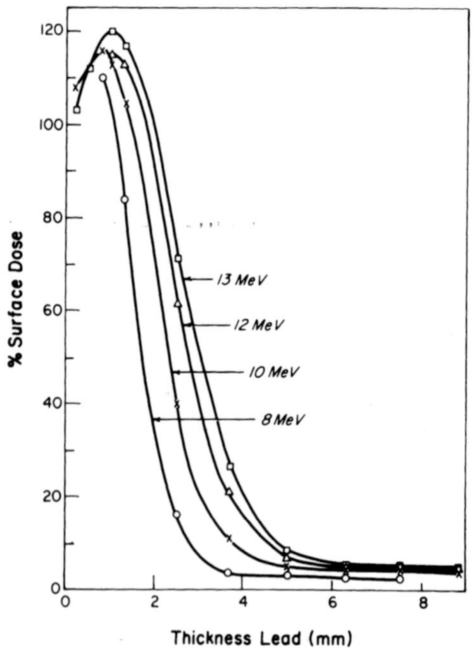

Figure 5.6. Shielding for electrons. Surface dose versus lead thickness as a percentage of maximum dose in phantom without lead. Shielding thickness may be determined for 5% transmission. (Reprinted with permission from Khan FM, Moore VC, Levitt SH. Field shaping in electron beam therapy. Br J Radiol 1976;49:883.)

X-ray contamination is slightly increased when lead shields are used because of the increased bremsstrahlung interactions with lead. In treating small volumes, however, the x-ray contamination associated with lead shielding is not of much concern.

In some situations, such as the treatment of lip and buccal mucosa lesions, internal shielding is useful to protect the internal structures. The problem with such shielding is the electron backscatter (EBS), resulting in an increase in dose at the lead-tissue interface of approximately 40 to 50% (Figure 5.7). This effect has been discussed by Okumura et al (18), Saunders and Peters (19), Nüsslin (20), Weatherburn et al (21), and Khan et al (22). It has been suggested to interpose 5 to 10 mm of tissue-equivalent bolus between the internal shield and the preceding tissue. The lead shield alternatively may be sheathed with 2 to 3 mm of aluminum to absorb the backscattered electrons of electron beams up to 15 MeV.

Separation of Adjacent Fields

Adjacent fields are commonly used in external-beam radiotherapy. Many treatment techniques involve the junction of fields with the adjoining margins abutted or separated, depending on various circumstances. The radiation distribution in the junction volume is profoundly changed as a result. These changes can be observed by placing isodose charts side by side and determining the sum of the doses in the junction area. Because of a rapid falloff of the dose near the boundary of the field, a small change in the relative spacing of the field margins produces a large change in dose distribution in the junction volume. Knowledge of the distribution of dose at the junction is important so that the fields are arranged to avoid a junctional dose that either exceeds normal tissue tolerance or is inadequate to sterilize the tumor.

If the adjacent fields abut on the surface, the fields overlap to an increasing degree with depth because of divergence. This overlapping causes a substantial increase in dose over a large area. In clinical practice, head and neck fields most often abut (provided the spinal cord dose does not exceed the tolerance dose) because of relative superficiality of tumor. The fields of the thorax, pelvis, or such a critical structure as the spinal cord, are usually separated.

In some cases of adjacent fields, the doses at the junction are delivered over about twice the time period as the central axis dose for the individual fields; an example is the mantle and the inverted-Y fields. From the time-dose effect perspective, a somewhat higher dose at the junction may be desirable (23), provided the tolerance of the normal tissue or a critical organ is not exceeded.

Methods of Field Separation

Geometric It is possible to achieve dose uniformity at the junction of two fields from geometric considerations, provided the geometric boundary of the field is defined by the 50% decrement line (i. e., the line joining the points at the depth where the dose is 50% of the central-axis dose at the same depth). The separation of the fields at the surface can then be calculated so that the adjacent field boundaries join at the chosen depth.

If two adjacent fields are incident from one side only,

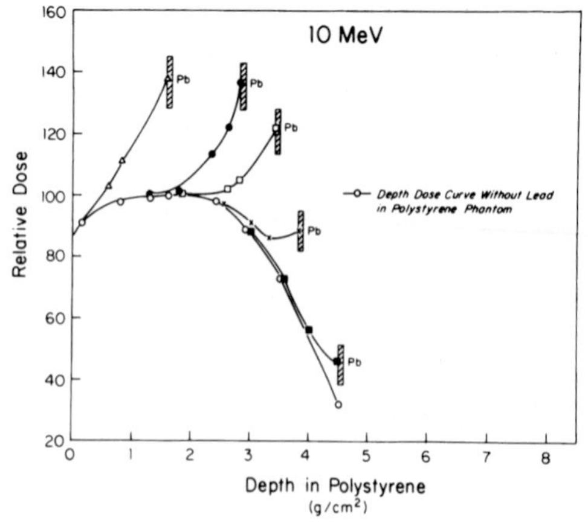

Figure 5.7. Modification of depth dose by electron backscattering from lead placed at various depths in phantom. Lead thickness = 1.7 mm. (Reprinted with permission from Khan FM, Moore VC, Levitt SH. Field shaping in electron beam therapy. Br J Radiol 1976;49:883.)

and if the fields are separated to junction at a given depth, the dose lateral to the junction is made uniform. The dose to the entrance side will be lower and the dose to the exit side will be higher than the junction dose.

In the equally weighted four-field technique, in which two adjacent fields are incident from one side and two are from the parallel opposed direction, the corresponding opposing fields are usually made to junction at the midline depth. The result is a uniform dose lateral to the junction and lower doses above and below the junction. Abutting and geometrically separated fields are compared in Figure 5.8. This example qualitatively applies to the mantle and inverted-Y fields.

Figure 5.9 illustrates the calculation of field separation. Let L_1 and L_2 be the field lengths, d be the depth of the junction point at which dose uniformity is desired, *SSD* be the source-surface distance; the field separation S on the surface is then given by: (23,24)

$$S = \frac{L_1}{2}\left(\frac{d}{SSD}\right) + \frac{L_2}{2}\left(\frac{d}{SSD}\right)$$

Dosimetric With the availability of computers for radiotherapy treatment planning, separation of fields to achieve uniform dose at a desired depth can be planned easily by optimizing the placement of fields on the contour and

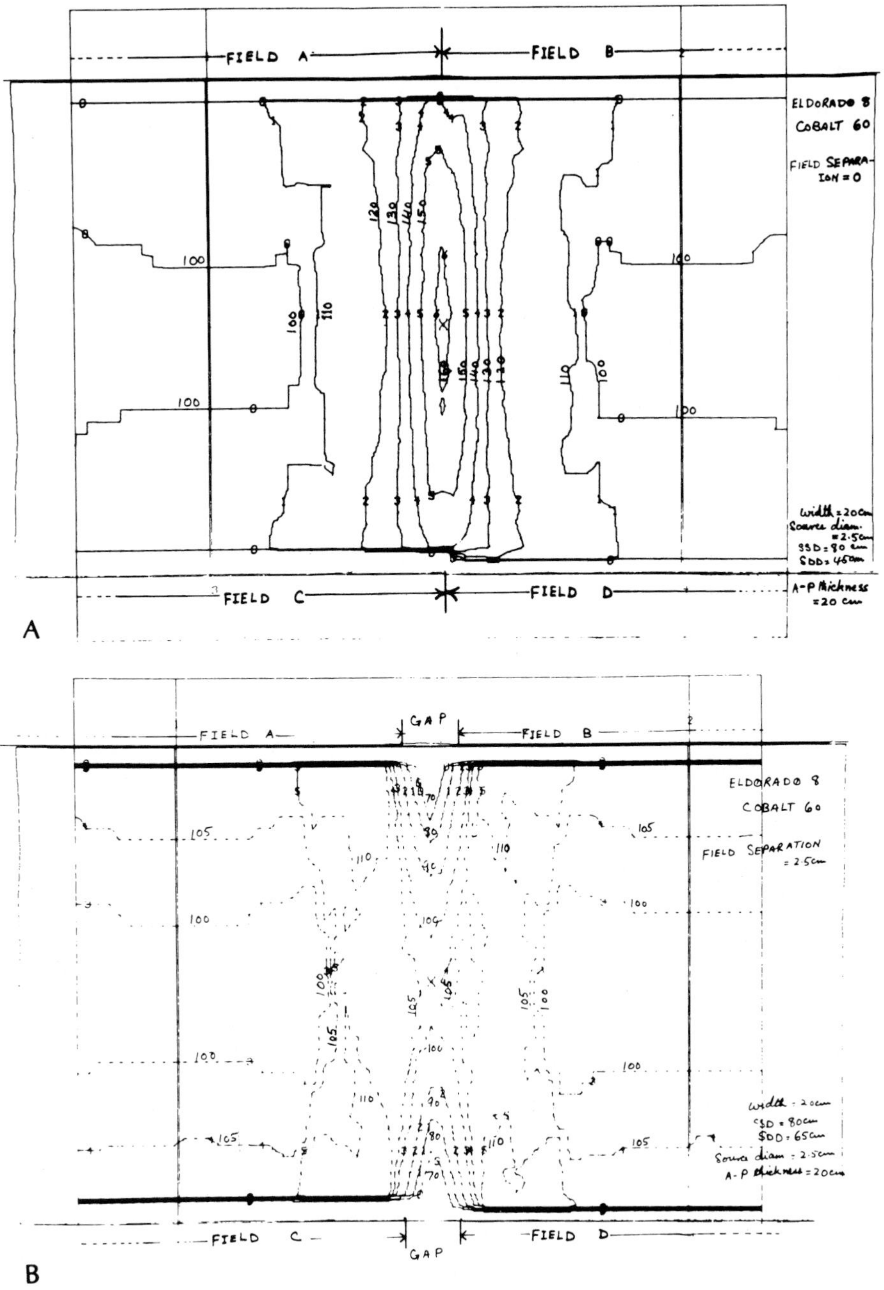

Figure 5.8. Dose distribution in junction volume of two anterior and two posterior fields. **A,** Abutting fields; **B,** Fields geometrically separated to junction at midline depth.

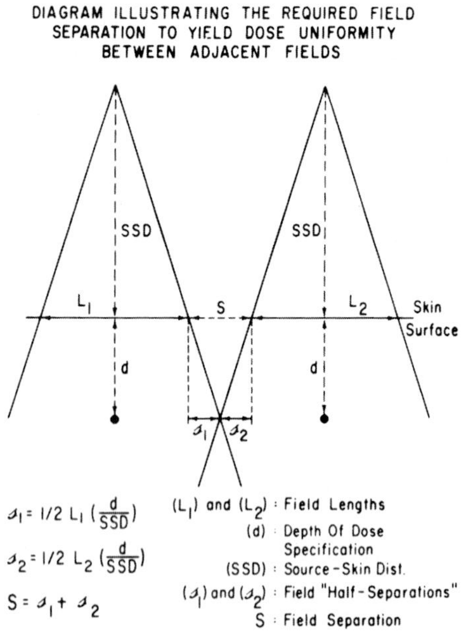

Figure 5.9. Geometric method for calculation of separation between adjoining fields. (Reprinted with permission from Cundiff JH, et al. The calculation of dose in the radiation treatment of Hodgkin's disease. In: Dosimetry Workshop. Hodgkin's Disease. Chicago: American Association of Physicists in Medicine, 1970).

obtaining isodose curves in the plane containing the central axes of all the beams. This method is more informative in the sense that uniformity as well as "hot" and "cold" spots can be visualized in an individual patient. The accuracy of this method depends on the accuracy of the individual field isodose curves.

Compensating Wedges It is possible to design compensating wedges so that an artificial dose falloff is created at the adjacent field borders that when summated at a given depth, gives a uniform dose distribution (25). A similar technique has been used by Griffin et al (26) for cranial-spinal irradiation.

Junction Shift In this method, the fields abut on the surface but the junction is moved to different positions on different days of treatment, so that the hot spot is spread over a distance. This method may also be applied to field separation to avoid hot and cold spots at one place.

Half-Beam Block or Independent Jaw Overlapping of adjacent fields at depth due to beam divergence can be avoided by blocking the adjoining fields along respective central axis. The blocking can be achieved by cerrobend "half-beam blocks" or by using independently movable collimator jaws ("independent jaws"). In either case, half the field is blocked along central axis and the fields are allowed to abut along a common junction line, the central axis.

The use of independent jaws has become quite common since the introduction in the early 1980s. Independently movable jaws allow asymmetric blocking as well as field matching by making the adjacent rays parallel. Although beam divergence of the abutting fields can be removed (by blocking half the field) or made equal by independent jaws, it may be prudent in some cases to move the junction line a few times during the course of treatment to smear out the lateral dose distribution across the junction line.

Guidelines for Adjacent-Field Irradiation

The decision whether the fields should abut or be separated is based on dosimetric data and clinical considerations (e.g., the presence of a critical organ and under- or overdosage of the tissues around the junction volume).

The site of field matching should be chosen carefully so that, as far as possible, it does not contain a tumor-involved area or a sensitive critical organ.

In field separations calculated by the geometric method, the margin of the field must coincide with the 50% decrement line. Also, the radiation beam must be aligned accurately with the beam-defining light.

References

1. Johns JE, Epp ER, Cormack DV, Fedoruk SO. Depth dose data and diaphragm design for Saskatchewan 1000 Curie cobalt unit. Br J Radiol 1952;25:302.
2. Richardson JE, Kerman HD, Brucer M. Skin dose from cobalt 60 teletherapy unit. Radiol 1954;63:25.
3. Dutreix J, Dutreix A, Tubiana M. Electronic equilibrium and transition stages. Phys Med Biol 1965;10:177.
4. Khan FM, Moore VC, Levitt SH. Effect of various atomic number absorbers on skin dose for 10 MeV x-rays. Radiol 1973;109:209.
5. Saylor WL, Quillin RM. Methods for the enhancement of skin sparing in cobalt 60 teletherapy. AJR 1971;111:174.
6. Hine GJ. Scattering of secondary electrons produced by gamma rays in materials of various atomic numbers. Phys Rev 1951;82:755.
7. Hine GJ. Secondary electron emission and effective atomic numbers. Nucleonics 1952;10:9.
8. Khan, FM. Use of electron filter to reduce skin dose in cobalt teletherapy. AJR 1971;111:180.
9. Earl JD, Bagshaw MA. A rapid optical method for preparation of complex field shapes. Radiol 1967;88:1162.
10. Edland RW, Hansen H. Irregular field-shaping for ^{60}Co teletherapy. Radiol 1969;92:1567.
11. Jones D. A method for the accurate manufacture of lead shields. Br J Radiol 1971;44:398.
12. Karzmark CJ, Huisman PA. Melting, casting and shaping lead shielding blocks: method and toxicity aspects. AJR 1972;114:636.
13. Maruyama Y, et al. Individualized lung shields constructed from lead shot embedded in plastic. Radiol 1969;92:634.
14. Parfitt R. Manufacture of lead shields. Br J Radiol 1971;44:895.
15. Powers WE, et al. A new system of field shaping for external-beam radiation therapy. Radiol 1973;108:407.
16. Khan FM. The physics of radiation therapy. Baltimore: Williams & Wilkins, 1994.
17. Boyer AL. Basic applications of a multileaf collimator. In: Mackie TR, Palta JR, eds. Teletherapy: present and future. College Park, MD: American Association of Physicists in Medicine, 1996.

18. Okumura U, Mori T, Kitagawa T. Modifications of dose distributions in high-energy electron beam treatment. Radiol 1971;99: 683.
19. Saunders JE, Peters VG. Backscattering from metals in superficial therapy with high energy electrons. Br J Radiol 1974;47:467.
20. Nüsslin F. Electron back-scattering from lead in a perspex phantom. Br J Radiol 1975;48:1041.
21. Weatherburn H, McMillan KTP, Stedeford B, Durrant KR. Physical measurements and clinical observations on back-scattering of 10 MeV electrons from lead shielding. Br J Radiol 1975;48:229.
22. Khan FM, Moore VC, Levitt SH. Field shaping in electron beam therapy. Br J Radiol 1976;49:883.
23. Faw FL, Glenn DW. Further investigations of physical aspects of multiple field radiation therapy. AJR 1970;108:184.
24. Cundiff JH, et al. Dosimetry workshop, Hodgkin's disease. Chicago: American Association of Physicists in Medicine, 1970.
25. Glenn DW, Faw FL, Kagan R, Johnson RE. Field separation in multiple portal radiation therapy. AJR 1968;102:199.
26. Griffin TW, Schumacher D, Berry HC. A technique for cranial-spinal irradiation. Br J Radiol 1976;49:887.

Chapter 6

Electron Beam Therapy

Faiz M. Khan and Marsha D. McNeese

Basic physics of electron beams has been discussed in several books and reports (1–6). Clinical applications are discussed in the classic book by Norah duV. Tapley (7). This chapter provides a review of the use of electrons in radiotherapy. Physical beam characteristics are discussed in relation to treatment planning, as are certain techniques that have been found useful in electron therapy.

BEAM ENERGY

Most modern high-energy linear accelerators provide a number of electron beam energies along with one or two x-ray beam energies. The most useful electron energy range for radiotherapy is 6 to 20 MeV, so the electron linear accelerator should be equipped with five or six different energy beams interspersed in this range.

The energy of a clinical electron beam is specified by what is called the most probable energy at the surface of a phantom at the standard source-surface distance (SSD) used for electron beam therapy. As illustrated in Figure 6.1, a small energy spread of the beam occurs at the phantom surface, and the most probable energy corresponds to the peak of the energy spectrum, i.e., the energy of most of the incident electrons. The energy indicated on the machine console is the nominal energy, which usually is set as a rounded number for the most probable energy at the surface.

An electron beam loses its energy at almost a constant rate as it penetrates the phantom or patient. This rate is approximately 2 MeV/cm of water. Thus, the maximum penetration or range of electrons is limited to approximately (E/2) cm of water, in which E is the incident energy (the most probable energy at the surface) in MeV. At the end of the range, the energy and dose approach zero, with a small fraction of dose persisting because of bremsstrahlung x-rays. The latter is seen as a tail of the depth dose curve in Figure 6.2.

The most useful range or the therapeutic range of electrons is given by the depth of the 90% depth dose. Although beam characteristics vary from machine to machine, the therapeutic range lies approximately between (E/4) and (E/3) cm. The depth of the 80% depth dose falls a little beyond (E/3) cm. The depth of maximum dose (D_{max}) represents a relatively broad region and varies between machines of different design. Also, it is not linearly dependent on energy, i.e., depth of D_{max} first increases with energy up to approximately 12 MeV and then decreases or broadens with energy. Figures 6.3 and 6.4 show these relationships for two different linear accelerators

Although the aforementioned relationships between energy, range, and depth doses are useful to keep in mind, it is absolutely essential to plan an electron beam treatment using the beam data that have been measured specifically for the given machine. Because the dose drops off precipitously beyond the therapeutic range, the target volume must be covered by the reference isodose curve (e.g., 90% isodose curve) with suitable margins (6). Selection of beam energy is more critical for electrons than for photons.

Depth Dose Distribution

The central axis depth dose distribution for several electron energies is illustrated in Figure 6.5. It is instructive to examine these curves in the context of treatment planning.

Surface Dose

The percent surface dose increases with an increase in electron energy, because electrons scatter into wider angles at lower energies than at higher energies. Therefore,

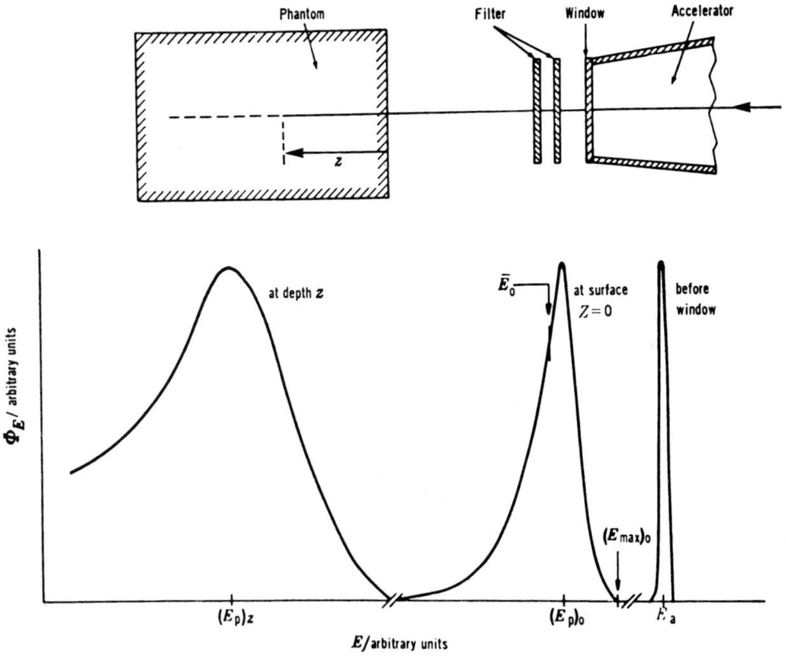

Figure 6.1. Energy spectrum of an electron beam. (Reprinted with permission from ICRU Reports No. 21: Radiation dosimetry: electrons with initial energies between 1 and 50 MeV. Washington, D.C.: International Commission on Radiation Units and Measurements, 1972.)

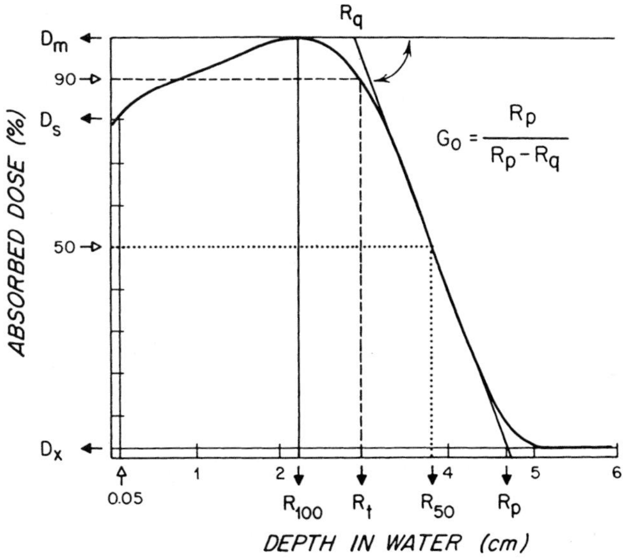

Figure 6.2. Parameters of electron beam depth dose curve. (Reprinted with permission from Brahme A, Svensson H. Specification of electron beam quality from the central-axis depth absorbed-dose distribution. Med Phys 1976;3:95.)

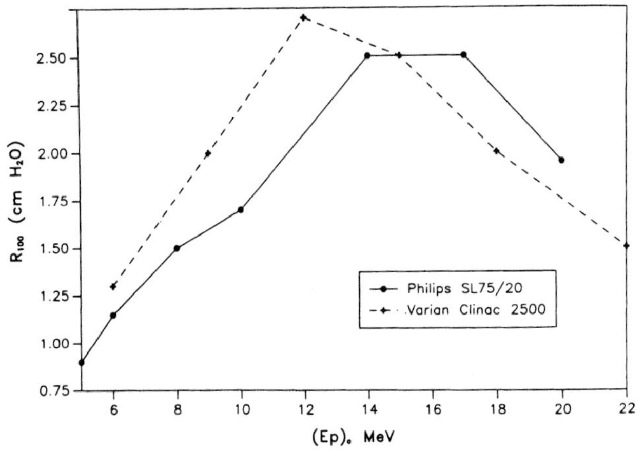

Figure 6.3. Depth of $(D_{max})(R_{100})$ plotted as a function of most probable energy at the surface, $(E_p)_6$. (Reprinted with permission from Khan FM. In American Association of Physicists in Medicine: Radiat Oncol Phys, Monograph No. 15. New York: American Institute of Physics, 1986.)

as the beam enters the patient, the lower energy electrons give rise to greater scatter at the depth of D_{max} than the higher energy electrons. The surface dose, as a percentage of D_{max}, is therefore lower for lower energy electrons.

In treatment planning, the radiotherapist needs to know the percent surface dose because dose to the skin is a major consideration in radiotherapy. Depending on the beam energy, the skin dose varies between 70 and 100%. In general, the scanning electron beams tend to give less skin dose than the beam scattered by scattering foils. Surface dose data for various accelerators (Figure 6.6) demonstrate that surface dose depends not only on energy but also on the type of accelerator.

Dose Gradient

The steepness of the depth dose falloff beyond the therapeutic range is a parameter of quality for an electron beam. Clinically, it is desirable to have the longest thera-

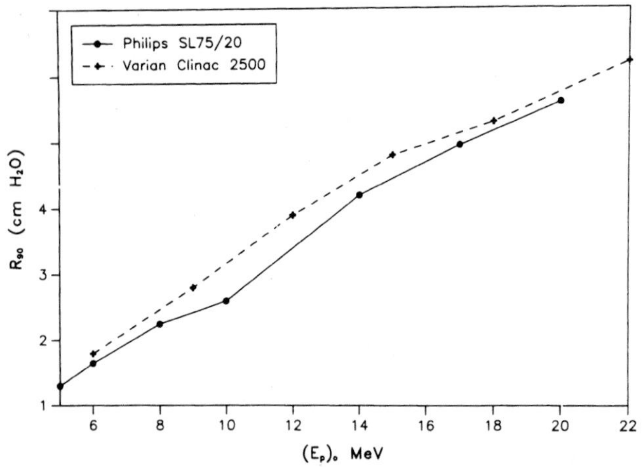

Figure 6.4. Depth of 90% dose (R_{90}) as a function of electron beam energy, $(E_p)_o$. (Reprinted with permission from Khan FM. Clinical Electron Beam Dosimetry. In American Association of Physicists in Medicine: Radiat Oncol Phys, Monograph No. 15. New York: American Institute of Physics, 1986.)

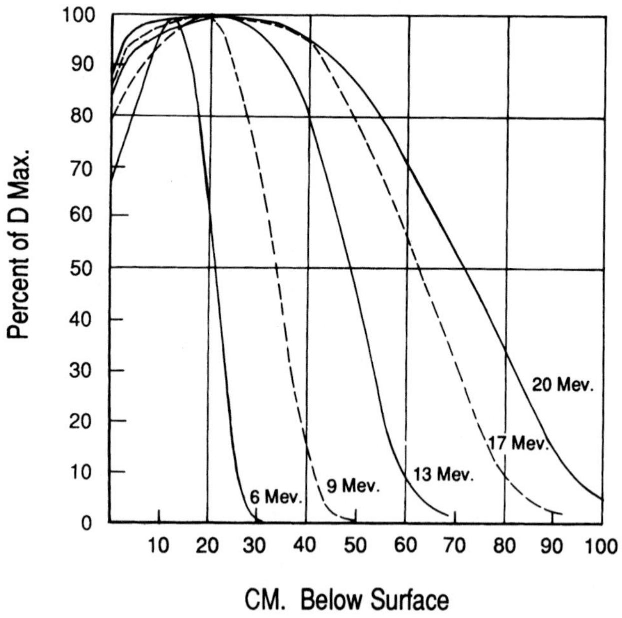

Figure 6.5. Central axis depth dose distribution of the AECL Therac 20 electron beams.

Figure 6.6. Surface dose, D_s, expressed as a fraction of maximum dose, D_m, plotted as a function of energy, $(E_p)_o$, for different accelerators and theoretic monoenergetic electron beams. (Reprinted with permission from ICRU Report No. 35: Radiation dosimetry: electron beams with energies between 1 and 50 MeV. Washington, DC: International Commission on Radiation Units and Measurements, 1984.)

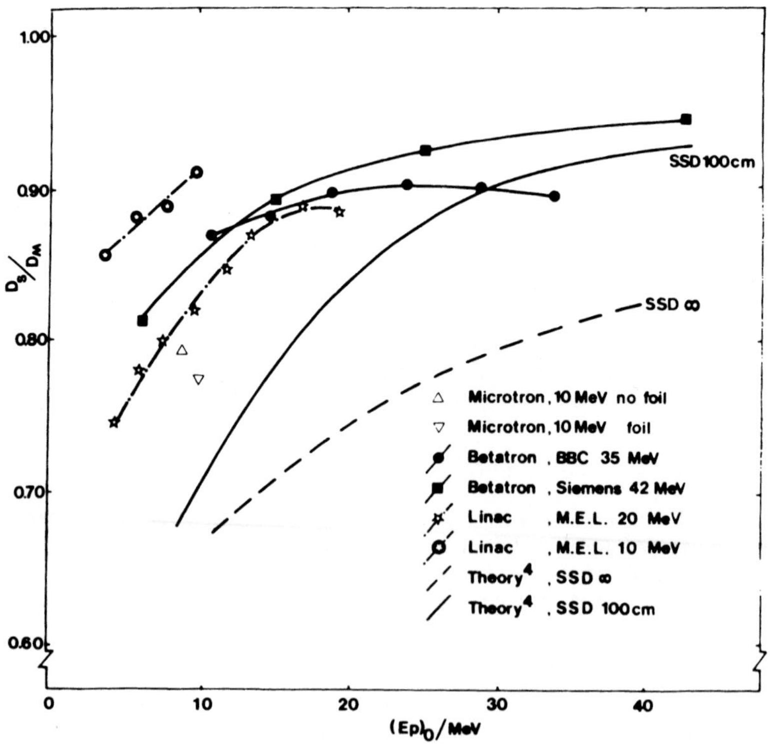

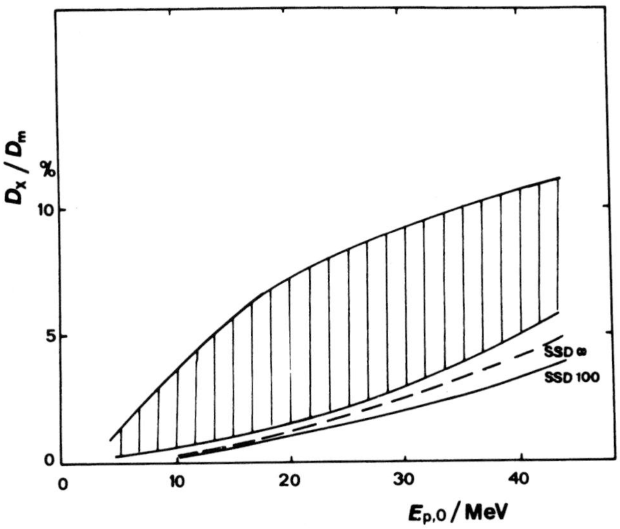

Figure 6.7. Photon background dose, D_x, expressed as a percentage of maximum dose D_m, plotted as a function of energy, $(E_p)_o$. Cross-hatched area shows large variation in photon background between various accelerators. Curves labeled with SSD give photon background dose produced in phantom. (Reprinted with permission from Brahme A, Svensson H. Specification of electron beam quality from the central-axis depth absorbed-dose distribution. Med Phys 1976;3: 95.)

peutic range for a given energy. Brahme and Svensson quantitated this parameter, the *reduced dose gradient,* G_o, given by

$$G_o = R_p/(R_p - R_q);$$

all the parameters are illustrated in Figure 6.2 (8). Rp is the practical or extrapolated range and R_q is the depth at which the tangent to the curve at the point of inflection meets the level of D_{max}. This equation may be used to compare quality of different accelerator beams in terms of their dose gradient beyond the therapeutic range.

X-Ray Background

Electron interactions with the exit window of the accelerator, scattering foils, monitoring ion chambers, collimator jaws, cones, trimmers, and air contribute to bremsstrahlung x-rays. Additional x-rays are produced within the body of the patient. The contribution of x-ray dose to the patient varies with energy and the type of accelerator. The percent of x-ray dose from various energy electron beams and accelerators is presented in Figure 6.7. Note that the x-ray dose increases with electron energy, and ranges from less than 1% for 4 MeV to approximately 5% for 20 MeV. The scanning beams that do not use scattering foils to spread the beam give the least x-ray contamination.

The x-ray contamination dose is acceptable for most electron beam applications. It becomes a critical factor in total skin electron irradiation, however, in which x-ray dose must be kept to a minimum, e.g., less than 1% of the surface dose.

ISODOSE DISTRIBUTION

Uniformity

Dose is never uniform in the entire field. Depending on the energy, field size, beam collimation, and depth, the lateral width of the isodose curves varies. Constriction of the therapeutic isodose curve (e.g., 90% isodose curve) with depth was first pointed out by Tapley (7). As seen in Figure 6.8, the width of the 90% isodose curve decreases with increasing depth. In treatment planning, however, allowance must be made for this constriction of the isodose curves. A larger field size may be required to adequately cover a target volume than would be called for in the case of photon beams. The isodose constriction effect is more dramatic for smaller fields and higher energy electron beams. Therefore, isodose planning for electron beam treatments is important to ensure adequate isodose coverage of the target volume.

Beam Obliquity

An obliquely incident beam creates an isodose distribution that may be significantly different from the beam incident perpendicularly on a flat surface (9,10). If the angle of obliquity (the angle between the beam ray and the perpendicular to the surface) is greater than 30°, the D_{max} dose is increased, the depth of D_{max} is decreased, and the therapeutic range (e.g., depth of 90%) is decreased. These effects are evident in Figure 6.9. The entire depth dose distribution is altered with extreme beam obliquity.

In chest wall irradiation, the obliquity of the beam relative to the surface tends to create the effects just described while the increasing air gap between the plane of the treat-

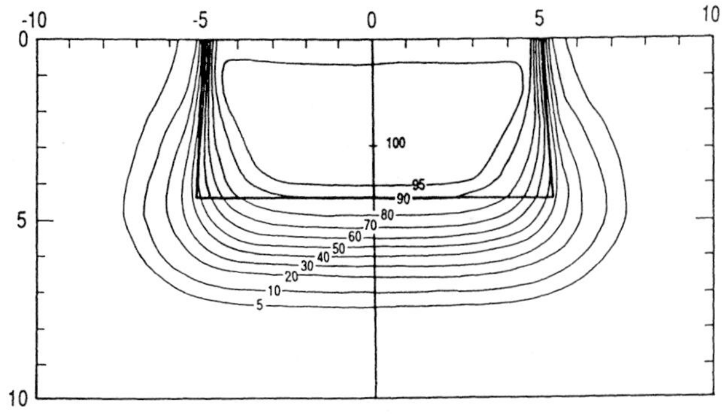

Figure 6.8. Isodose curves for a 10 × 10 cm field, 15-MeV electron beam on a Siemen's Mevatron 771. Note lateral constriction of 90% curve with depth. (Reprinted with permission from American Association of Physicists in Medicine: Task Group 25 Report: Clinical electron beam dosimetry. Med Phys, 1991;18:73-109.)

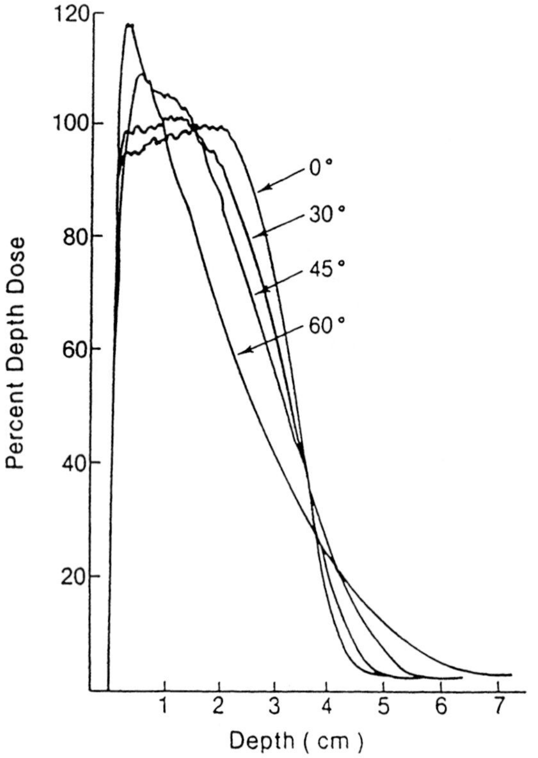

Figure 6.9. Variation of depth dose distribution with beam obliquity (angle between ray and a line perpendicular to surface) for a 9-MeV electron beam. (Reprinted with permission from Ekstrand KE, Dixon RL. The problem of obliquity incident beams in electron-beam treatment planning. Med Phys 1982;9:276.)

ment SSD and the skin decreases the dose because of beam divergence. The net effect is that the isodose curves do not exactly follow the curvature of the chest wall. As seen in Figure 6.10, the isodose curves at the lateral chest wall exhibit large penumbra and are shallower than the isodose curves at the medial chest wall. The chest wall treatment with electrons therefore requires meticulous treatment planning to ensure uniformity of dose distribution along the chest wall and adequate depth coverage of the target volume. Depending on the shape of the chest wall, multiple electron beams (see Figure 6.19A) or electron arc therapy (Figure 6.11) may be used to obtain acceptable uniformity of target dose distribution.

Tissue Heterogeneities

Depth dose distribution in a medium depends on its electron density (electrons/cm^3). Because the number of electrons per gram is almost the same for all materials (except hydrogen), the mass density primarily determines the depth of penetration of electrons. Thus, the depth dose distribution in a medium of mass density, ρ_{med}, may be obtained by scaling the depth by ρ_{med}: $Z_{water} = Z_{med}\,\rho_{med}$, in which Z is the depth. For example, 1 cm of bone (ρ = 1.8 g/cm^3) is equivalent to 1.8 cm of water or soft tissue and 1 cm of lung (ρ = .25 g/cm^3) is equivalent to 0.25 cm of water. This relationship is only approximate because it does not take into account the scattering power of the medium. In addition, it is valid only for large slabs (larger than the range of the laterally scattered electrons) of heterogeneities.

For small inhomogeneities (small air cavities, small bony structures, etc.), the local scattering of electrons at

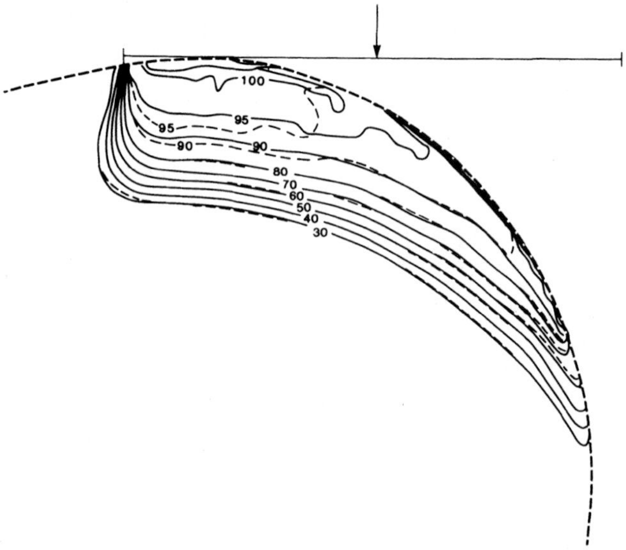

Figure 6.10. Measured *(solid lines)* and calculated *(dashed lines)* isodose distribution for an electron beam incident on cylindric polystyrene phantom. (Reprinted with permission from Khan FM. The physics of radiation therapy. Baltimore: Williams & Wilkins, 1984.)

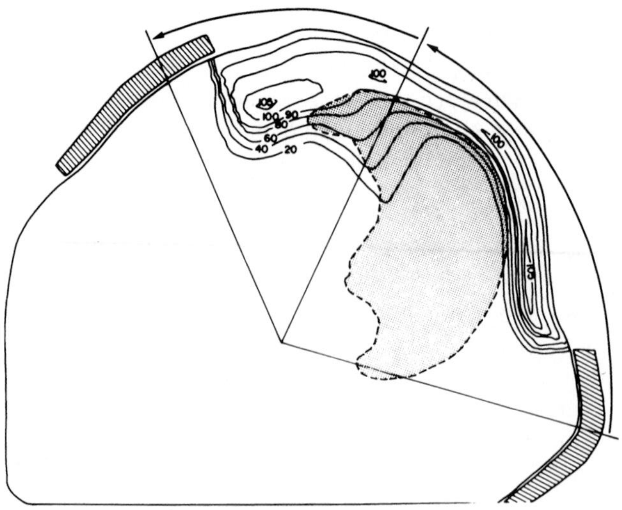

Figure 6.11. Isodose distribution for chest wall irradiation using electron arc therapy. (Reprinted with permission from Leavitt DD, Peacock LM, Gibbs FA, Stewart JR. Electron arc therapy: physical measurement and treatment planning techniques. Int J Radiat Oncol Biol Phys 1985;11:987.)

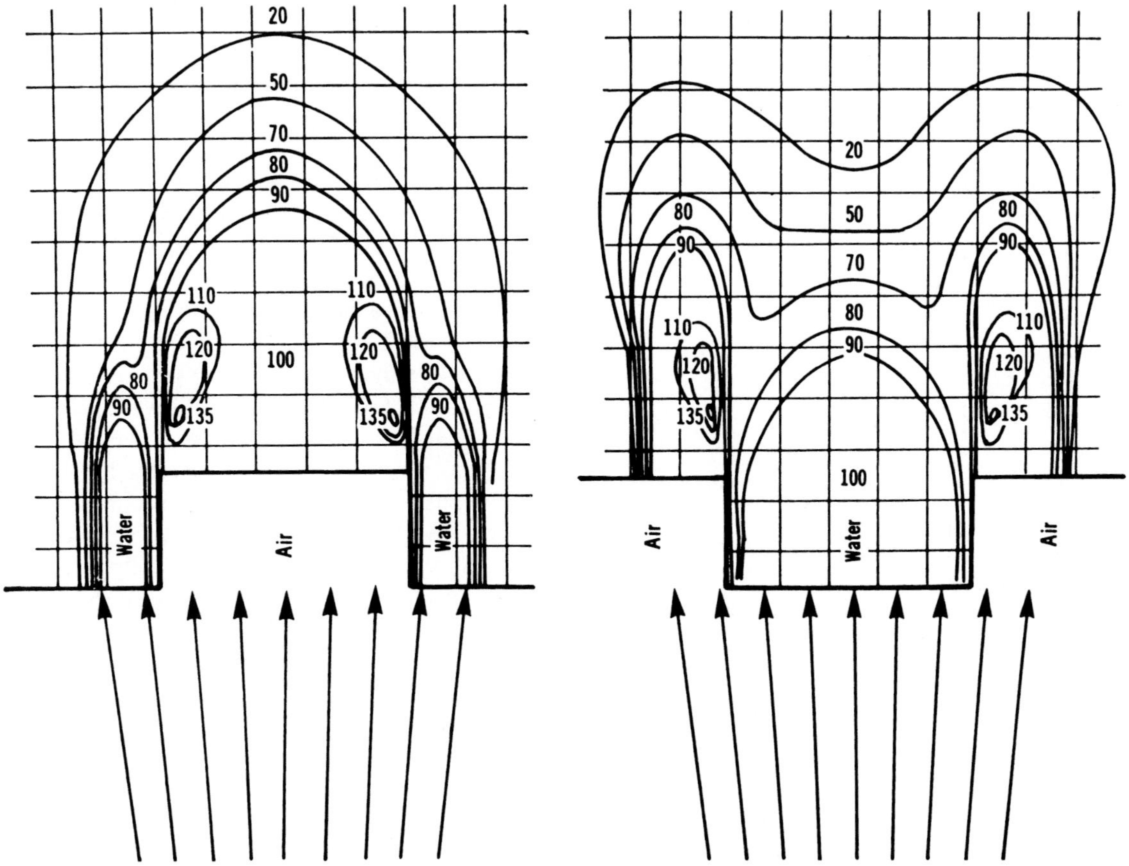

Figure 6.12. Hot spots created by electron beam incident on water phantom with sharp irregularities in surface contour. (Reprinted with permission from Dutreix J. Dosimetry. In: Gil G, Gayarre G, eds. Symposium on high-energy electrons. Madrid: General Directorate of Health, 1970.)

the edge is the predominant effect. At a straight edge of a material, the scattering of electrons gives rise to a hot spot on one side and a cold spot on the other side (Figure 6.12).

The effect of electron scattering creating a hot spot at the edges of materials or surface contour can be minimized by making the edge smoother with a bolus or tapering the edge to give a gradual slope to the contour. The effect of small internal heterogeneities on dose distribution is difficult to assess quantitatively. Sophisticated computer algorithms have been developed to take these effects into account.

Field Shaping

Lead or Cerrobend apertures are often used to shape electron fields. The thickness of lead must be sufficient to absorb the electron beam so that the transmitted dose is only from bremsstrahlung x-rays. Lead causes an increase in the x-ray contamination by a small percentage depending on energy, but for most treatments, this increase is not of much concern.

A rule of thumb developed to determine the thickness of lead required for blocking is $t_{\text{lead}} = c \cdot E$, in which t_{lead} is the lead thickness in millimeters, c is 0.5 mm/MeV, and E is energy in MeV incident on lead.

Electron blocking is mostly external when using custom-made Cerrobend inserts or lead sheets placed at the end of the cone or directly on the skin. Occasionally, it is possible to use lead blocking internally, such as in the treatment of eyelid lesions or tumors in the buccal mucosa. In such cases, one must be aware of electron backscatter that occurs at the lead-tissue interface on the entrance side of the beam, which increases the dose at and within a few millimeters of the interface (Figure 6.13). The enhancement in dose from backscatter can be substantial (e.g., about 50% for 6 MeV at the interface).

Internal shielding with lead requires the use of shields coated with a low atomic number material such as plastic or a bolus material to absorb as much of the backscatter electrons as possible (4,5).

Air Gaps

Air gaps between the standard treatment SSD (defined at or a few centimeters away from the cone or trimmers) and the patient surface can give rise to several effects. The

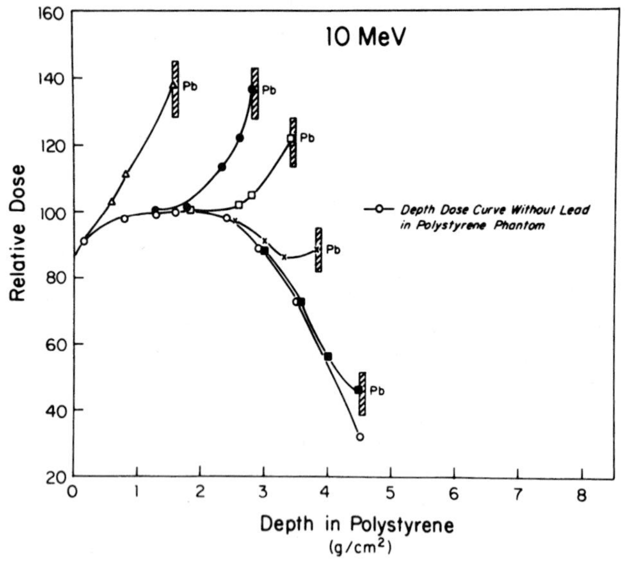

Figure 6.13. Plot showing increased dose at lead-polystyrene interface because of electron backscatter. (Reprinted with permission from Khan FM, Moore VC, Levitt SH. Field shaping in electron beam therapy. Br J Radiol 1976;49:883.)

dose decreases with increasing air gap, and electron scattering in air tends to offset flatness. Large air gaps produce rounded or gaussian dose profiles, and penumbra at the beam edges is broadened. The problem becomes more complex when the air gaps are not uniform across the field or if the beam is incident obliquely.

If bolus is used, it must be placed directly on the skin surface. Large air gaps between the bolus and the skin surface result in a significant decrease in dose, because electrons are scattered by bolus into larger angles than by air, resulting in a greater loss of electrons reaching a point at the center of the field and greater spread laterally. Because of these effects, air gaps should be minimized between bolus and surface and extended SSD treatments should be avoided.

With a small unavoidable gap between applicator and surface (less than 10 cm or so), air gap correction in output for an open beam may be used by using inverse square law. A virtual or effective SSD is used in the inverse square law expression. For small field sizes and lower energies, the effective SSD may be field size and energy dependent. A table of effective SSD as a function of field size and energy is required as a reference to make air gap corrections. (For further discussion of air gap corrections, see references 2, 4, 6, and 11.)

Bolusing

Bolus in electron beam therapy may be needed to:

1. Build up skin dose, if skin is involved with tumor;
2. Moderate electron beam energy to achieve a desired isodose surface at the maximum depth of the target; and
3. Even out sharp edges (depressions and elevations) in the surface contours.

The use of bolus requires recalculation of depth dose distribution, because electrons traversing the bolus lose energy as they do in the tissues and, therefore, the therapeutic range is altered by bolus placement. With photon beams, skin dose can be increased by placing a thin sheet of bolus without significantly altering the depth dose distribution.

Several kinds of bolus materials are available: "Superstuff," "Superflab," paraffin wax, polystyrene, and Lucite. The usefulness of these materials for electron bolusing has been discussed previously (12). In most situations, bolus is placed directly on the skin surface. Flexible bolus, such as Superflab, has the advantage of conforming to the skin contours. A Lucite or polystyrene plate can also be used, provided it can be placed stably on the skin surface. Minimizing the air gaps between the skin surface and the bolus is important because large air gaps result in reduction in dose as well as lateral electron scatter, which may not be predictable unless special dosimetry is performed.

Adjacent Fields

Electron beams usually are used for superficial tumors. When the need arises for abutting two electron fields or an electron field with a photon field, one cannot separate the fields at the surface by a gap unless the region between the two fields is at no risk for tumor. When the target volume is contiguous with the surface, the adjacent fields should be abutted with no separation. This positioning will create a hot spot at the junction regions. The hot spot may be acceptable or not depending on its extent and location. A composite isodose plan is needed to evaluate the acceptability of a given beam arrangement. If needed, the extent of hot spots is minimized by angling each beam away from the other by a small angle $\theta = tan^{-1}(1/2w/SSD)$, in which w is the field width. Isodose curves are again needed to evaluate the dose distribution in the junction region. Even if the isodose distribution looks perfect on paper, it is probably a good idea to move the junction line two or three times, if feasible, during the treatment course.

When an electron field is placed abuttingly with a photon field (e.g., anterior neck field treated with photons and posterior neck nodes treated with electrons), a hot spot is created in the photon field near the junction line and a corresponding cold spot develops in the electron field. This is caused by greater side scatter of electrons into the photon field than the side scatter of photons into the electron field. The extent of hot and cold spot is modified when electron field is treated with an unavoidable air gap of 10 to 20 cm between the electron applicator and the

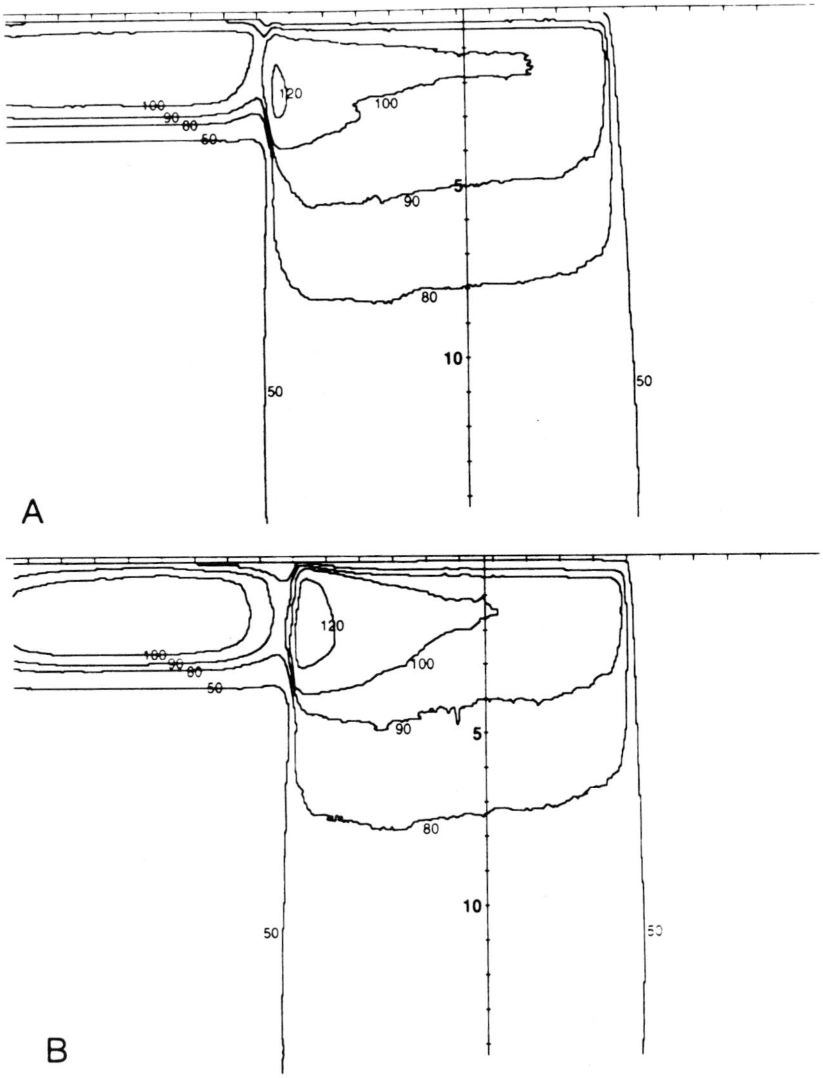

Figure 6.14. Composite isodose distribution in abutting photon and electron beam fields. 9 MeV electron beam; field size = 10x10; 6 MV photon beam; SSD = 100 cm. **A.** Electron beam at standard SSD of 100 cm. **B.** Electron beam at extended SSD of 120 cm. (Reprinted with permission from Johnson JM, Khan FM. Dosimetric effects of abutting extended SSD electron fields with photons in the treatment of head and neck cancers. Int J Radiat Oncol Bio Physics 1992;24:202.

surface (e.g., when shoulders are in the way). The effect on dose distribution in such cases is shown in Figure 6.14 as an example (13).

COMPUTER TREATMENT PLANNING

Computer algorithms have been developed to calculate dose distributions using computed tomographic (CT) scan data (14–16). Some commercial treatment planning computers provide treatment planning programs, but these must be tested carefully for the user's beam data. When planning complex electron beam treatments (e.g., field shaping, mixing electron and photon beams, and multiple electron fields), it is as essential to have a computer treatment planning system for electrons as it is for photons. Without such a system, we advise staying with simple field arrangements for which dosimetry has been established experimentally in suitable phantoms.

CLINICAL APPLICATIONS

In many instances, electron beam is a superior method of treatment, such as in lateral lesions of the oral cavity or parotid tumors, in treating the posterior cervical chain nodes and avoiding the underlying spinal cord, in treating scar extensions, and also in treating the radically dissected neck. In some cases, no alternative treatment is effective, such as in massive lesions of the skin of the face and scalp. In other cases, the use of electrons makes certain treatments easier than when photons are used, such as when boosting lymph nodes or treating the chest wall after mastectomy. Usual applications are listed in Table 6.1

Skin Cancers Involving the Eyelid(s)

The best cosmetic results are obtained by protracting the treatment over several weeks and treating daily with 5 fractions/week. Lesions that measure 1 to 4 cm can be treated with doses in the range of 55 Gy over 4 to 4 ½ weeks, although smaller lesions (<1 cm) can be treated effectively with 45 Gy in 3 weeks. In the elderly, for whom cosmesis may not be as important, effective tumor control can be done with several large dose fractions such as 11 Gy × 3 or 4.0 Gy × 10. Large lesions (>5 cm) require higher doses, in the range of 60 to 75 Gy over 6 to 7 weeks, with a field reduction at 50 Gy. Postoperative recurrences also generally receive 60 to 65 Gy in 5 ½ to 6 weeks. Figure 6.15A depicts a patient with carcinoma of the lower eyelid. Although the main lesion is visible centrally, biopsy showed that most of the lower lid exhibited some evidence of basal cell carcinoma. In the treatment setup (Figure 6.15B), a gold-plated eyeshield is inserted beneath the lid to protect the lens and eye, and a custom-made lead mask is used to outline the treatment field. The light field should protect onto the eyeshield approximately 1 cm around the treatment field to avoid cold edges. The patient received 60 Gy in 5 ½ weeks. One year later (Figure 6.15C), the atrophy of the treated left eyelid is no worse than the untreated right eyelid.

In one of our favorite examples of how effective electron beam therapy can be, a patient had a squamous cell carcinoma (Figure 6.16A and B) that had been neglected: any attempt at resection with plastic reconstruction would have resulted in resection of a large amount of the face.

Table 6.1. Applications of 7- to 18-MeV Electrons

Skin and lip cancers
Chest wall and regional lymphatics
Lateral head and neck tumors
Electron beam alone or combined with photons or interstitial
As boost treatment to primary
Boost to nodes, scars, posterior cervical strip

The patient received 70 Gy with the electron beam, beginning with an energy of 15 MeV; the energy was reduced as the lesion regressed. Follow-up 2 years after radiation (Figure 6.16C) revealed the patient remained free of disease in that area.

The Nasal Vestibule

A patient received treatment through a boost field after initial treatment of the entire nose and mustache area. He did well from the standpoint of tumor control, but approximately 2 years after treatment, he developed maxillary necrosis (Figure 6.17A). This treatment was done before the availability of CT planning and computer algorithms to account for tissue inhomogeneities. A two-dimensional calculation (Figure 6.17B) shows the significant amount of side scatter into the premaxilla, as well as the cold spot along the nasal septum. A review of 32 patients treated with electrons to the nasal vestibule for squamous cell carcinomas showed that local control was gained in 31 of 32 patients, and only this one patient developed maxillary necrosis. One other patient had persistent epistaxis, but this individual also had hypertension.

Our cosmetic results improved remarkably when we changed our technique to account for tissue inhomogeneities. One of our patients treated in 1982 had involvement of the nasal septum as well as the nasal vestibule. Figure 6.18A and B shows the dosimetry with and without heterogeneity correction, and demonstrates the importance of using the heterogeneity correction with the electron beam. Figure 6.18C shows the heterogeneity correction with external wax bolus as well as internal bolus placed in the nostrils. An intraoral stent is used to depress the tongue, protect the mouth, and provide an airway. The nose is treated with high energy electrons and with photons, usu-

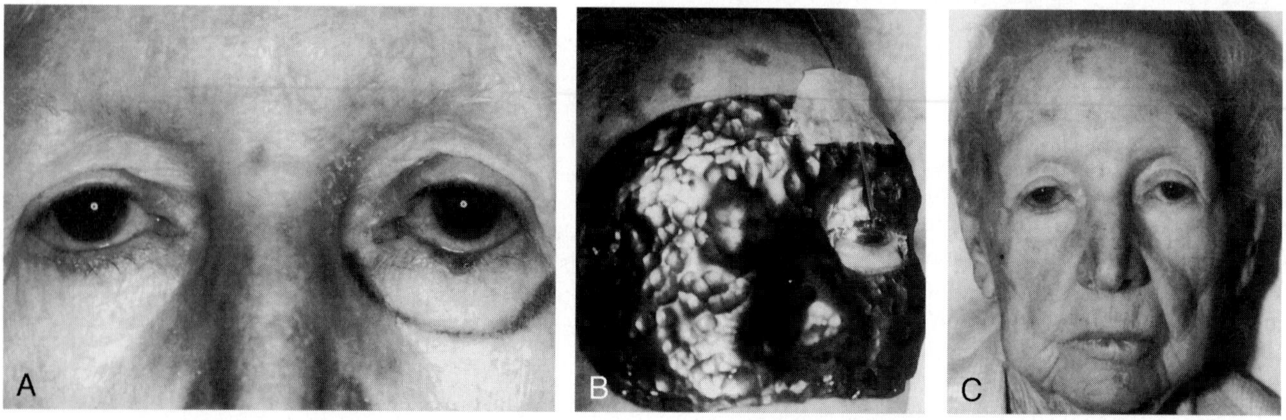

Figure 6.15. A. Basal cell carcinoma of lower eyelid. Although main lesion is visible centrally, biopsy results showed almost entire lower lid was involved. **B.** Treatment setup, using gold-plated eyeshield and custom-made lead mask. **C.** 1 year after receiving 60 Gy in 5-1/2 weeks. (**A–C** reprinted with permission from McNeese MD, Sinesi C. Radiotherapy for eyelid carcinomas. Cancer Bull 1986;38:91.)

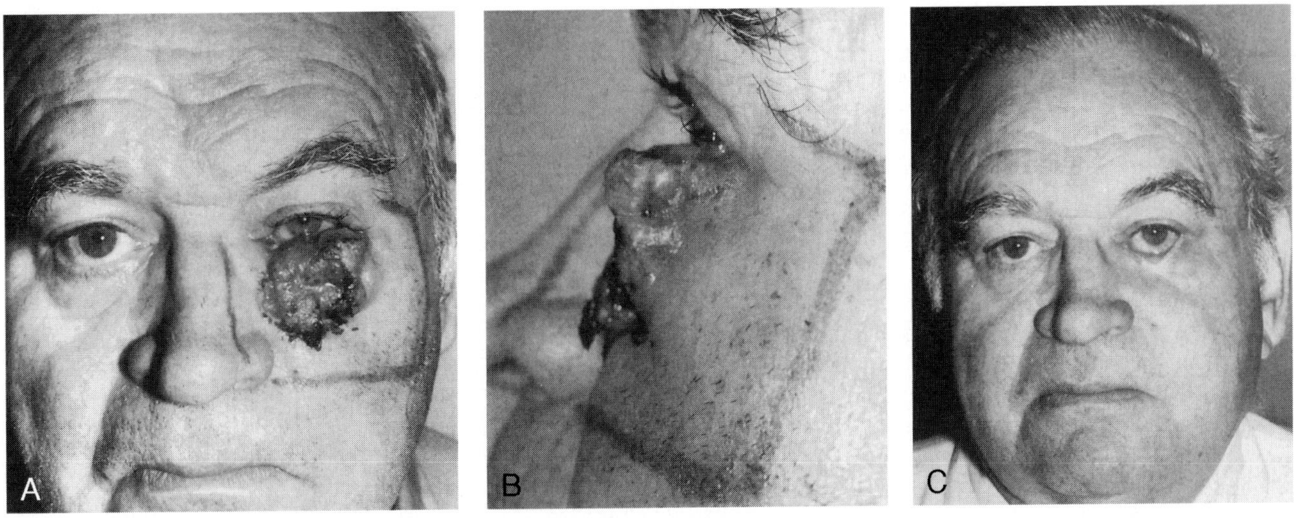

Figure 6.16. **A** and **B.** Large squamous cell carcinomas destroying lower eyelid was treated to 70 Gy in 6-1/2 weeks with electrons. **C.** 2 years after irradiation. (**A–C** reprinted with permission from Sinesi C, et al. Electron beam therapy for eyelid carcinomas. Head Neck 1987; 10:31.)

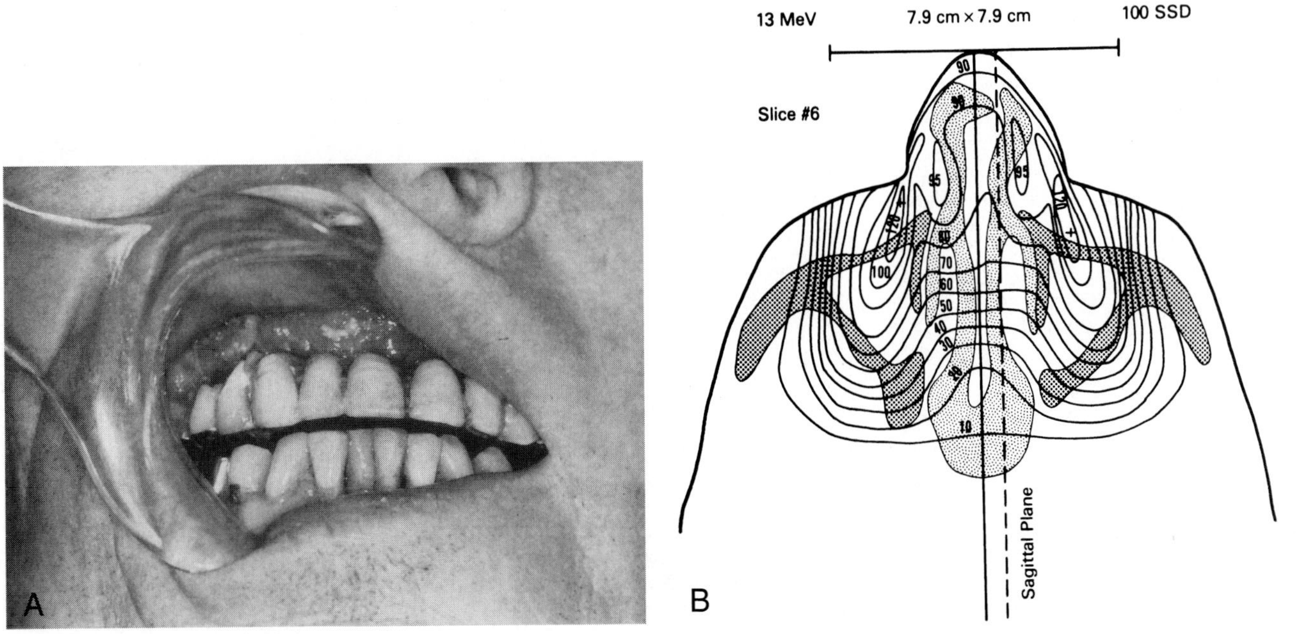

Figure 6.17. **A.** Maxillary necrosis 2 years after electron beam therapy for squamous cell carcinoma of nasal vestibule. **B.** Two-dimensional calculation showing effect of tissue inhomogeneity. Note increased dose in maxilla because of side scatter. (Reprinted with permission from Chobe R, McNeese MD, Weber RS, et al. Radiation therapy for carcinoma of the nasal vestibule. Otolaryngol Head Neck Surg 1988;98:67.)

ally in a ratio of 4:1. Facial nodes and lymphatics are treated with 6- or 7-MeV electrons to the mustache distribution (Figure 6.18D and E). Figure 6.18E illustrates the placement of the wax bolus before treatment. The bolus was removed during photon therapy for skin sparing. Two years after treatment, the cosmetic result was excellent (Figure 6.18F).

Lateral Head and Neck Tumors

Patients with parotid gland carcinomas or lesions involving the buccal mucosa or retromolar trigone are well treated by the use of electron beam therapy. An example of the treatment fields in a patient with a high grade parotid lesion is provided in Figure 6.19A. Low energy electrons

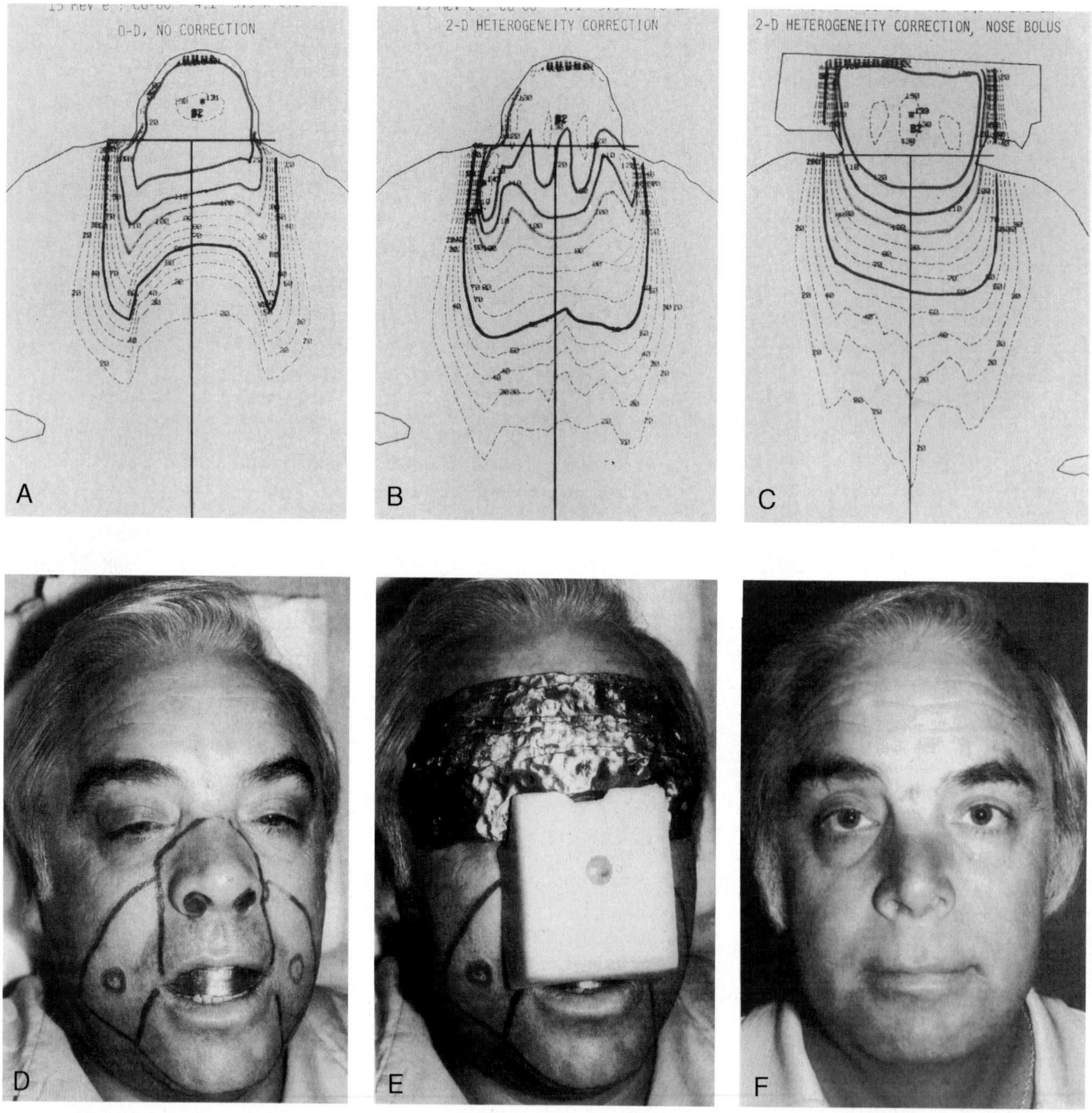

Figure 6.18. A. Dosimetry without heterogeneity correction gives false impression of isodose distribution. **B.** Dosimetry with heterogeneity correction shows more accurate isodose distribution. **C.** Improved isodose distribution with use of internal and external bolus. **D.** Actual treatment fields, with bolus placed in nostrils and intraoral stent in place. (Reprinted with permission from McNeese MD. Cancer Bull 1989;41:88.) **E.** Completion of treatment setup with external wax bolus and lead eyeshield in place. **F.** 2 years after completion of therapy. (Reprinted with permission from McNeese MD, Cancer Bull 1989;41: 88. Chobe R, et al. Radiation therapy for carcinoma of the nasal vestibule. Otolaryngol Head Neck Surg 1988;98:67.)

are used to treat the scar extension above the zygoma, high energy electrons are used to treat the parotid bed, and intermediate energy electrons are used to treat the undissected neck. Of 116 patients treated postoperatively at this institution, local control has been achieved in 90%. For these patients, intraoral stents are used to protect the opposite mucosa as well as the opposite salivary gland tissue, and computer planning is done to evaluate the homogeneity caused by surface irregularity as well as mandibular absorption. The usual treatment involves a mixture of high energy electrons and photons in a 4:1 ratio to achieve some skin sparing (Figure 6.19B). Ipsilateral neck

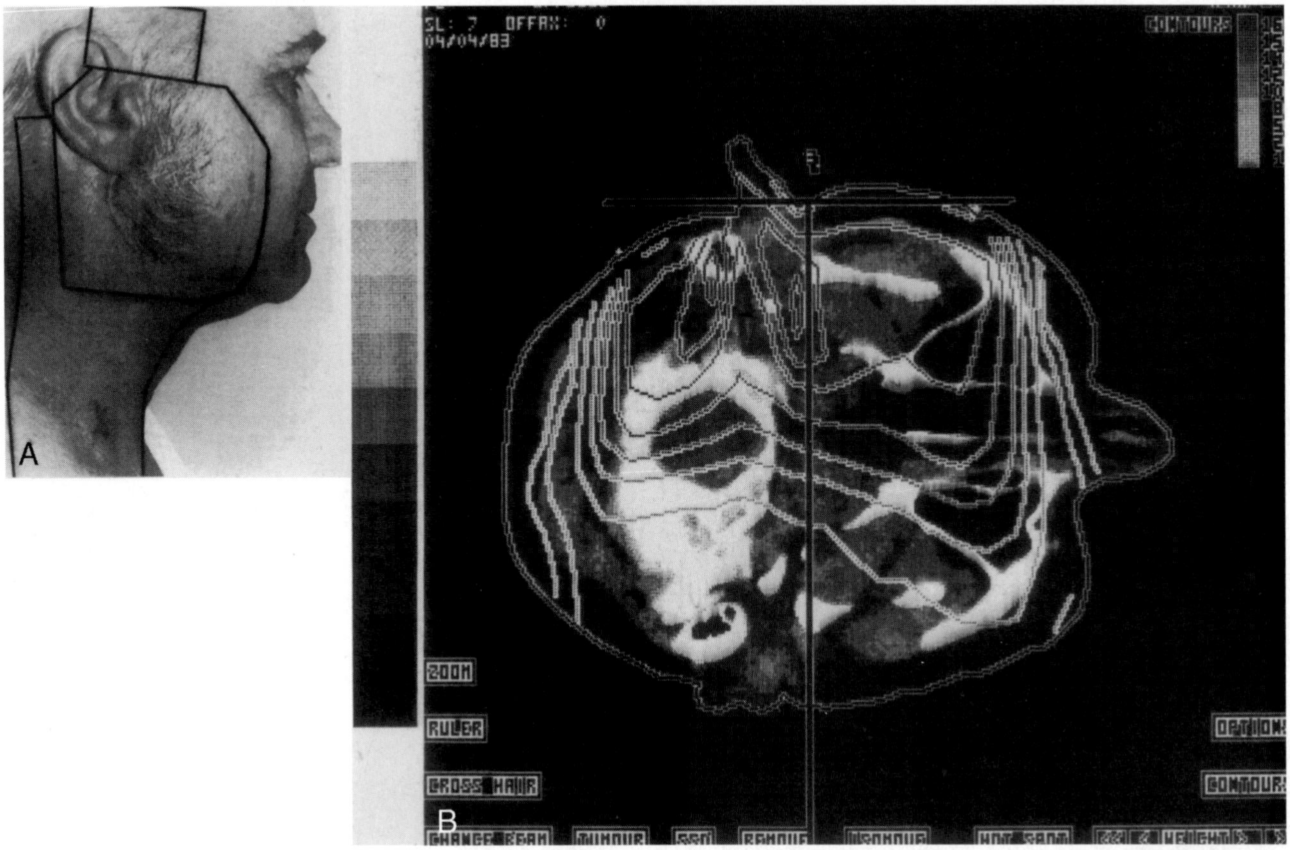

Figure 6.19. A. Treatment fields for high-grade parotid malignancy (see text). (Reprinted with permission from McNaney D, et al. Postoperative irradiation in malignant epithelial tumors of the parotid gland. Int J Radiol Oncol Biol Phys 1983;9:1289.) **B.** Computed tomographic dosimetry, with 4:1 ratio of high-energy electrons and photons.

irradiation with electrons is appropriate in certain situations, as listed in Table 6.2. The ear is taped flat to improve tissue homogeneity.

Postoperative Chest Wall and Peripheral Lymphatics

Electron beam therapy is extremely useful in patients who have undergone modified radical mastectomy because the use of photon tangentials would result in significant lung irradiation. One of the problems with electron beam dosimetry relates to the curvature of the chest wall. Figure 6.20 demonstrates the treatment fields commonly used (A) and the "hot spot" seen at the point at which the medial and lateral tangential fields overlap (B and C). One way to improve the dosimetry is to move the junction between the two fields weekly. Again, meticulous dosimetry is an absolute necessity, because too high an energy can also result in an increased dose to lung tissue. Another useful technique is arc electron therapy, although the planning and execution of treatment is more time consuming and requires sophisticated computer dosimetry. An equally important application of electron beam therapy for patients with locally advanced carcinomas is the coverage of the nodes of the internal mammary chain with electrons, because of the significantly decreased danger of any cardiotoxicity. Many of these patients will also receive Adriamycin chemotherapy at some time, and the avoidance of cardiac problems becomes even more important.

Table 6.2. Ipsilateral Neck Irradiation

Clinical situations
- Contralateral neck at negligible risk of developing metastatic disease
- Well-lateralized cancers of:
  - Gingiva
  - Buccal mucosa
  - Lateral floor of mouth
  - Retromolar trigone-anterior tonsillar pillar
- Maxillary antrum carcinoma
- Major salivary gland tumors
- Skin cancers (excluding midline area)

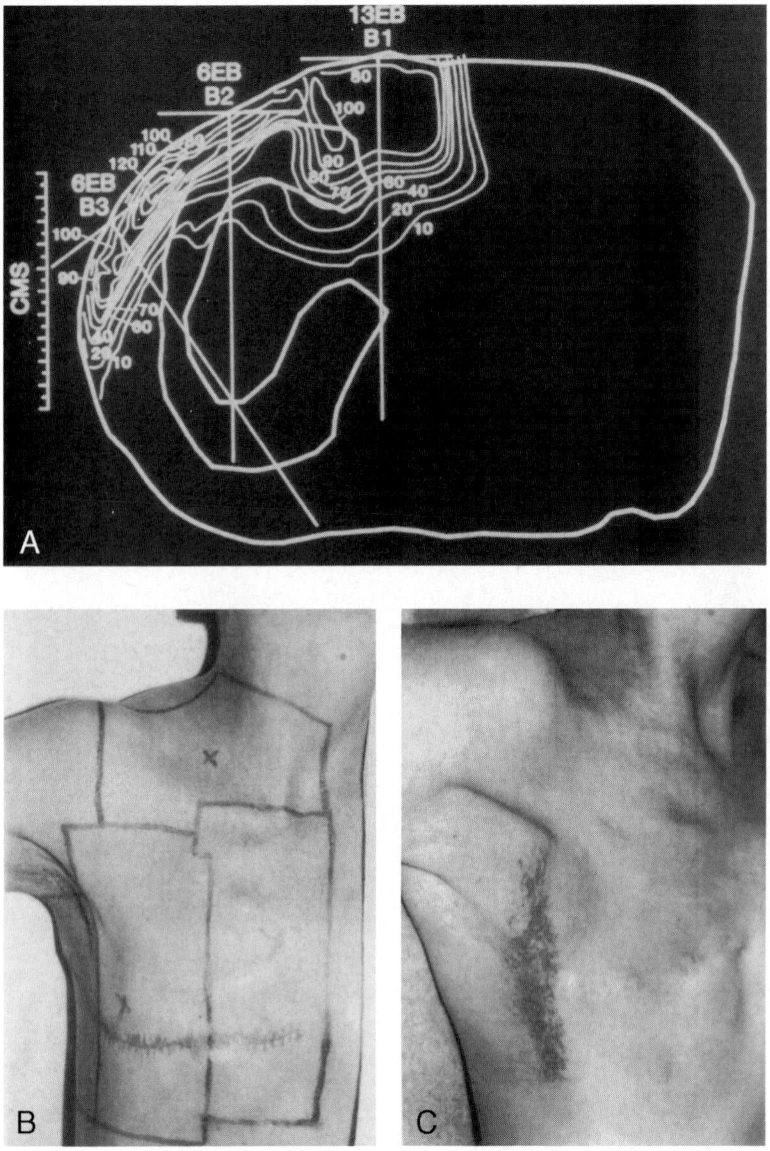

Figure 6.20. A. Electron treatment fields for post-mastectomy patient. Chest wall usually is treated with 6 or 7 MeV electrons, internal mammary chain with 12 or 13 MeV, and supraclavicular area with 9 or 10 MeV electrons. **B.** Overlap of 6-MeV electron fields and resultant hot spot. **C.** Area of overlap, with telangiectasis.

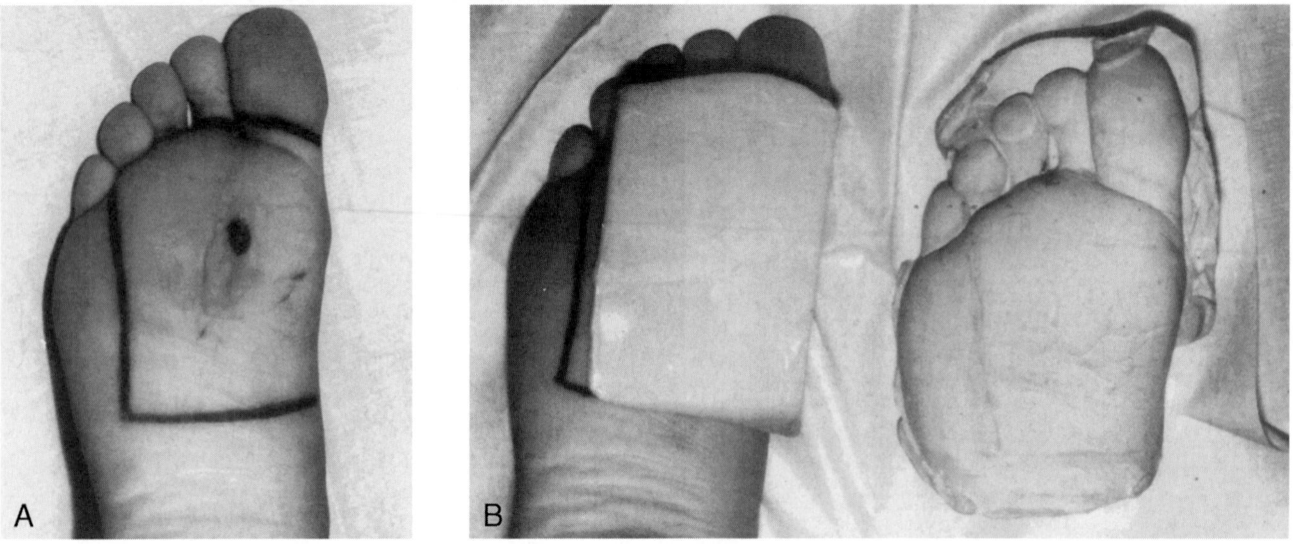

Figure 6.21. A and **B.** Electron beam therapy for Ewing's sarcoma of foot, using wax bolus to improve homogeneity.

Miscellaneous Uses

Tumors of the hands and feet frequently are treated with electron beam. A Ewing's sarcoma of the foot (Figure 6.21) was treated with chemotherapy and electron beam radiotherapy, using a wax bolus to help make the dose distribution more homogeneous.

Multiple boost fields, as in patients with head and neck carcinoma (Figure 6.22), can also be done easily with electron beam. Areas in the breast tissue can be boosted with photons after completion of external treatment to the entire breast, but electron beam frequently is easier to use because an energy can be chosen that will not enter the lungs.

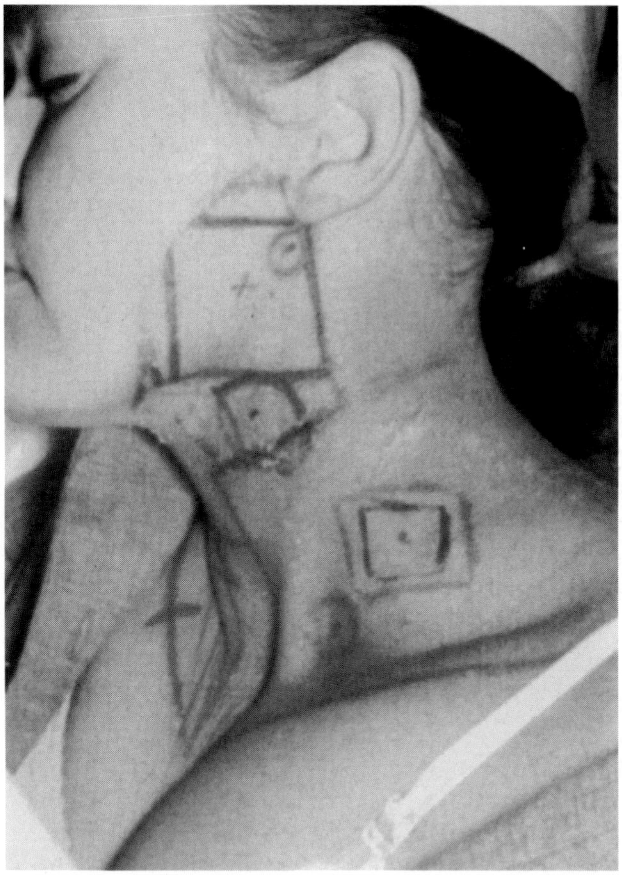

Figure 6.22. Multiple boost areas, where lymphadenopathy was detected, receive electron beam therapy. (Reprinted with permission from Fletcher GH. Textbook of radiotherapy. 3rd ed. Philadelphia: Lea & Febiger, 1980.)

Total Skin Electron Beam Treatment

Patients such as those with mycosis fungoides or Kaposi's sarcoma may benefit from this technique. The actual treatment requires only a few minutes, but significant physics time and machine time are needed to achieve this technique. The output of the machine is increased to 10,000 monitor units/minute at the isocenter, therefore the machine must be recalibrated before and after treatment. Because these tumors are rare, our recommendation is to refer such patients to a major institution. (For details regarding dosimetry and technique of total skin irradiation, see reference 3.)

References

1. American Association of Physicists in Medicine: Radiat Oncol Phys, Monograph No. 15. New York: American Institute of Physics, 1986.
2. American Association of Physicists in Medicine: Task Group 25 Report: Clinical electron beam dosimetry. Med Phys 1991;18: 73–109.
3. ICRU Report No. 35: Radiation dosimetry: electron beams with energies between 1 and 50 MeV. Washington, D.C.: International Commission on Radiation Units and Measurements, 1984.
4. Khan FM. The physics of radiation therapy. Baltimore: Williams & Wilkins, 1994.
5. Klevenhagen SC. Physics of electron beam therapy. Bristol: Adam Hilger, Ltd., 1985.
6. AAPM, Task Group 25: Clinical electron beam dosimetry. Med Phys 199;18:73.
7. Tapley N duV. Clinical applications of the electron beam. New York: John Wiley & Sons, 1976.
8. Brahme A, Svensson H. Specification of electron beam quality from the central-axis depth absorbed-dose distribution. Med Phys 1976;3: 95–102.
9. Ekstrand KE, Dixon RL. The problem of obliquity incident beams in electron-beam treatment planning. Med Phys 1982;9:276.
10. Khan FM, Deibel FC, Soleimani-Meigooni A. Obliquity correction for electron beams. Med Phys 1985;12:749.
11. Roback DM, Khan FM, Gibbons JP, Sethi A. Effective SSD for electron beams as a function of energy and beam collimation. Med Phys 1995; 22:2093–2095.
12. Sharma SC, Deibel FC, Khan FM. Tissue equivalence of bolus materials for electron beams. Radiology 1983;146:854.
13. Johnson JM, Khan FM. Dosimetric effects of abutting extended SSD electron fields with photons in the treatment of head and neck cancers. Int J Radiat Oncol Biol Phys 1992;24:202.
14. Hogstrom KR. Evaluation of electron pencil beam dose calculation. In AAPM Monograph No. 15, Radiat Oncol Phys. NY: American Institute of Physics, 1986.
15. Hogstrom KR, Fields RS. Use of CT in electron beam treatment planning: current and future development. In: Ling CC, Rogers CC, Morton RJ, eds. Computed Tomography in Radiation Therapy. NY: Raven, 1983.
16. Werner BL, Khan FM, Deibel FC. Model for calculating electron beam scattering in treatment planning. Med Phys 1982;9:180.

Chapter 7

Treatment Aids for External Beam Radiotherapy

Donald M. Roback and Faiz M. Khan[a]

Positioning a patient relative to the treatment beam has always been important in radiation therapy, but recently, as conformal therapy has become more popular, the need to accurately reposition the patient has become crucial. According to the International Commission on Radiation Units and Measurements (ICRU) Report 24, the treatment target must be irradiated uniformly to ±5% for adequate tumor control (1). At the same time, many treatment courses are limited by dose delivered to normal tissue. These two factors result in the necessity for accurate reproduction of anatomy relative to treatment beam for every dose fraction.

In this chapter, we survey devices that can be used to attain excellent accuracy and reproducibility. Other previously published material on these devices may be useful as supplemental reading (2–4). In the first section, we review patient data acquisition and registration aids used to attain accurate patient anatomy and the position of various anatomical landmarks relative to the treatment beam. In the second section, we review tools used to modify treatment beams so that the desired dose distributions can be achieved. In the third section, we categorize patient immobilization devices by the general anatomical area being treated. This section also includes devices that are especially useful to certain special treatment procedures such as total body photon irradiation, total skin electron irradiation, stereotactic radiosurgery and radiotherapy, and craniospinal irradiation. The last section covers several miscellaneous devices that can also be used to aid in accurate patient setup.

PATIENT DATA ACQUISITION AND REGISTRATION

It is necessary to know the position of internal and external patient anatomy relative to the treatment beam in order to accurately calculate and deliver dose. In this section, several devices used to measure patient anatomy are reviewed (Figures 7.1–7.7). Several simple devices exist to measure external contours and patient thicknesses, but in a modern radiation oncology clinic, computed tomography (CT) and magnetic resonance imaging (MRI) scanning are the preferred methods of obtaining data on internal anatomy.

Beam Modifiers

Several devices exist to alter the dose distribution as delivered by the treatment beam (Figures 7.8–7.17). This dose alteration is necessary to protect normal structures, deliver an even dose across an uneven patient surface, or to treat superficial disease by increasing the skin dose.

HEAD AND NECK

This and the following two sections review patient immobilization devices specific to anatomical regions. In this section, we consider immobilization devices useful for brain and head and neck treatments (Figures 7.18–7.27). Because of the number and location of critical dose limiting structures in the head and neck, patient setups must be accurate and reproducible. This task is aided, however, by the bony head and neck anatomy.

PELVIS

In this section, we consider immobilization devices useful for pelvis treatments (Figures 7.28–7.34). Maintaining accuracy and reproducibility in this region is hindered by the relative lack of bony anatomy and by any excess tissue in the stomach or hips that can change the patient

Text continued on page 97

[a] The authors acknowledge the contributions of previous authors of this chapter: Luis Delclos and Vincent A. Sampiere.

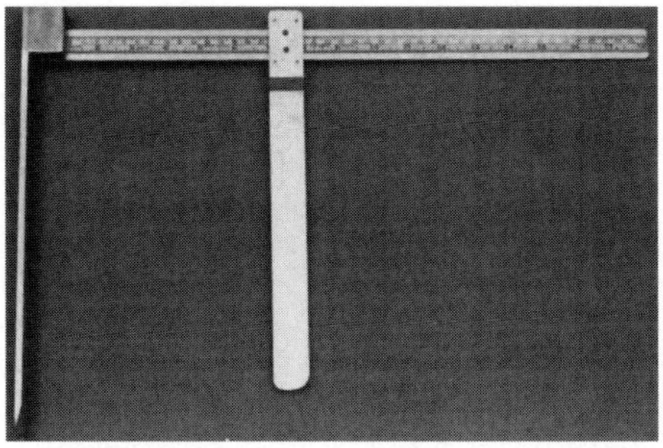

Figure 7.1. Caliper. This device is used to measure thicknesses parallel to the beam axis at a point in the treatment field. The moveable arm is parallel to the base arm and moves smoothly along the vertical bar by means of a nylon sleeve. The instrument has either an analog or digital scale.

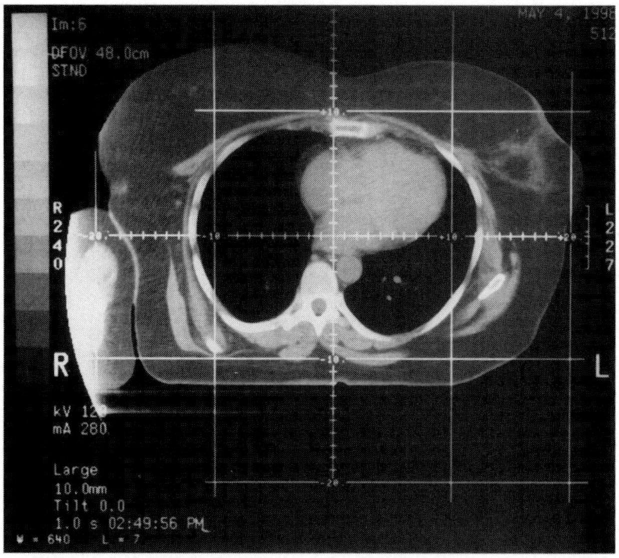

Figure 7.3. CT/MRI Scans. The most accurate method to acquire internal patient anatomy is to use either a CT or MRI scan. The films generated by these units are commonly used for treatment planning but the digital data can also be fed directly into most modern treatment planning computers. Because CTs are so commonly used for treatment planning, many radiation therapy departments have installed a dedicated CT scanner. But even without a dedicated unit, most departments have easy access to CT and MRI scanners.

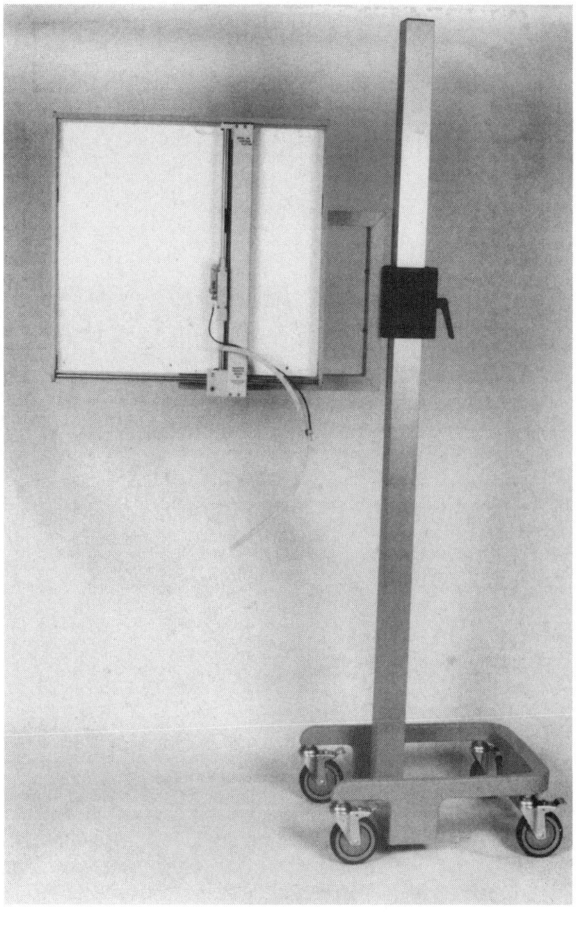

Figure 7.2. Pantograph. This device consists of a mechanical arm that links an ink pen to a stylus arm mounted on a drawing plane. When moved over a patient's contour, the stylus motion is directly translated to the pen which draws a scale contour on the drawing plane. (Courtesy of Radiation Products Design, Albertville, MN.)

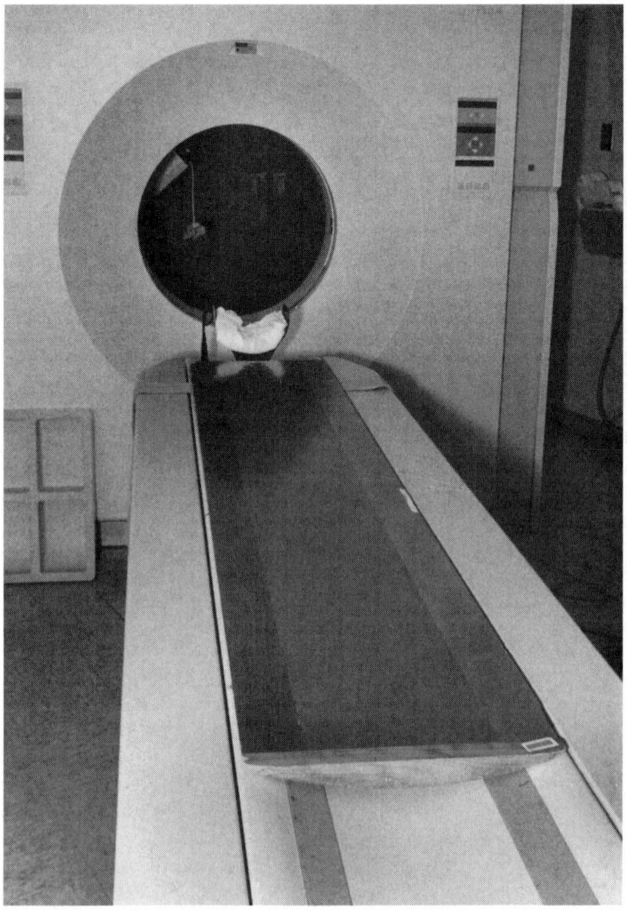

Figure 7.4. CT/MRI Table Inserts. To align a patient's anatomy to the treatment beam, the patient must be imaged in the same position as he or she will be treated. Because patients are imaged on a curved profile couch but treated on a flat profile couch, errors can occur if the imaging setup is not modified. Computed tomography and MRI table inserts fit inside the curved CT or MRI couches and make them flat. They are constructed of wood covered by felt or rubber so that they do not cause image artifacts or slip during patient positioning. (Manufactured by Scientific Apparatus, University of Minnesota.)

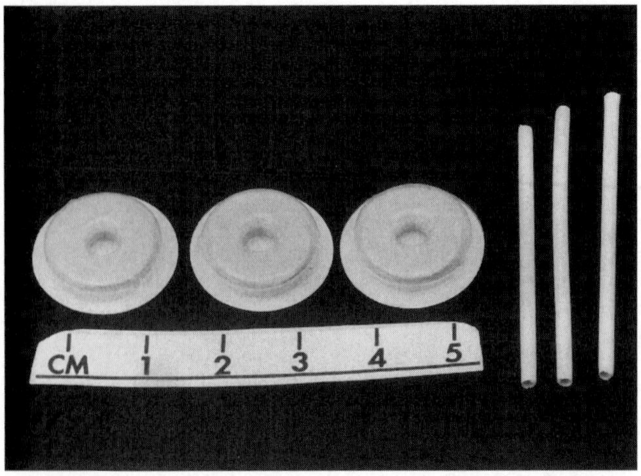

Figure 7.5. CT/MRI Markers. Markers can be used to identify simulator skin marks on a CT or MRI scan. As long as the markers don't create any imaging artifact, they are useful to correlate the simulator setup with the CT or MRI images. Hollow plastic catheters make excellent CT markers and Vitamin E capsules make excellent MRI markers.

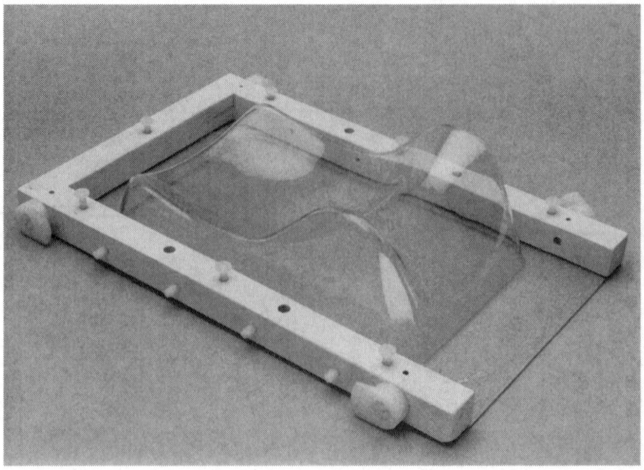

Figure 7.6. Aquaplast Frame. The device pictured is useful as an aquaplast face mask holder because it can be used for simulation, imaging, and treatment. It is made smaller than the standard aquaplast mask holder to fit into an MRI scanner and it is made of mostly radio-paque material to minimize treatment beam attenuation. (Manufactured by Scientific Apparatus, University of Minnesota.)

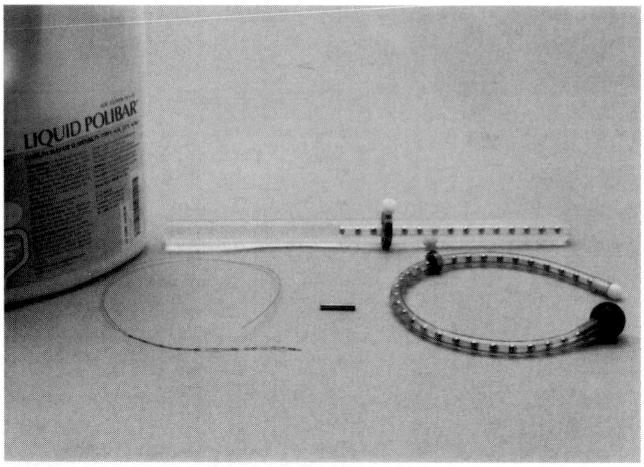

Figure 7.7. Contrast Materials. This figure shows several items that aid in localizing patient anatomy during simulation. The contrast material $BaSO_4$ can be used to image small bowel and large bowel. The various markers shown are used to image the genitourinary or gastrointestinal systems during simulation. The dummy seeds are the same size and shape of radioactive seeds used for brachytherapy applications. They are used to image where the radioactive seeds will be placed relative to the pre-implanted brachytherapy loading devices.

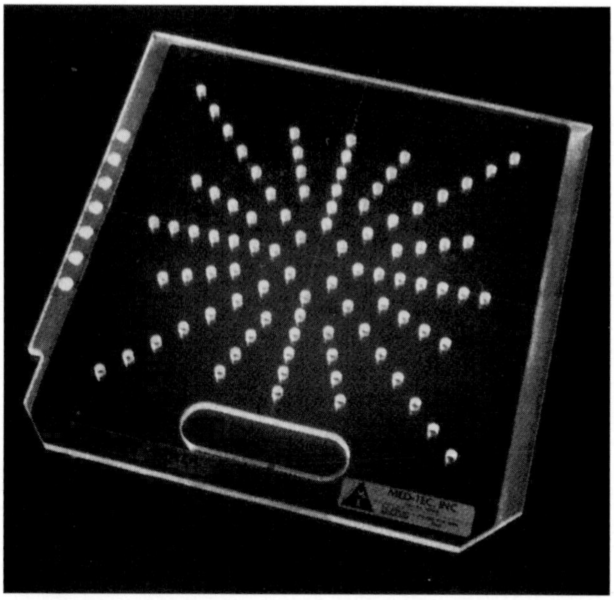

Figure 7.8. Blocking and Compensator Trays. These acrylic trays are used to support cerrobend field-shaping blocks and missing tissue compensators. The trays are mounted in the collimator head of a linear accelerator or cobalt teletherapy unit. The trays usually have several holes drilled in them to allow for block mounting but they can also be slotted to allow for adjustment of the blocks during patient setup. (Courtesy of Med-Tec, Inc. Orange City, IA.)

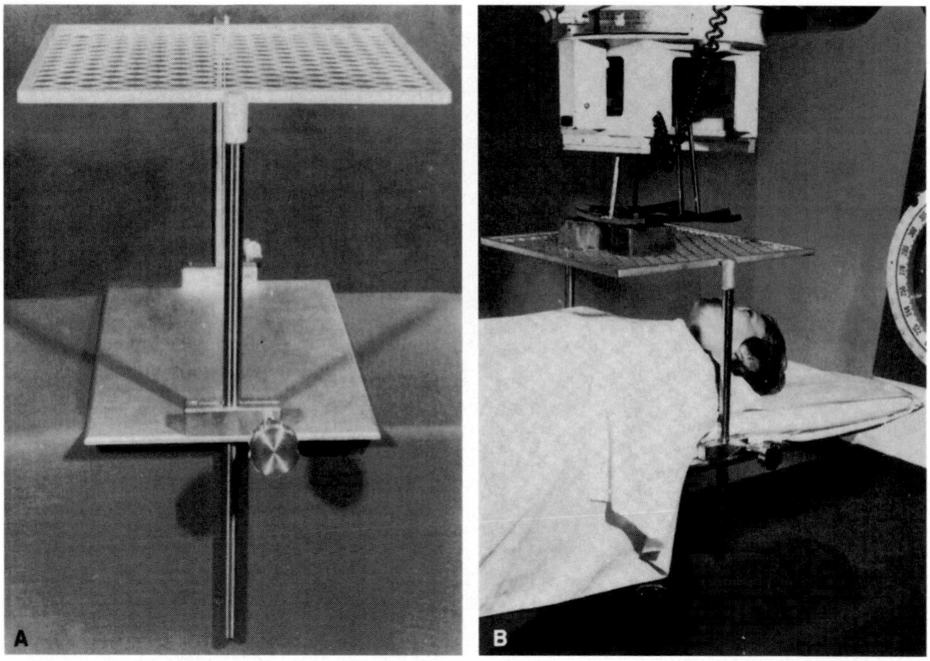

Figure 7.9. Table-Mounted Blocking Tray. This blocking tray is constructed to cover a larger area and support more weight than the trays mounted in the linear accelerator collimator head. Tray height is adjustable so that it can be used for many treatment techniques. The base that locks the supporting columns (A) at the proper height lies beneath the patient on top of the treatment table (B).

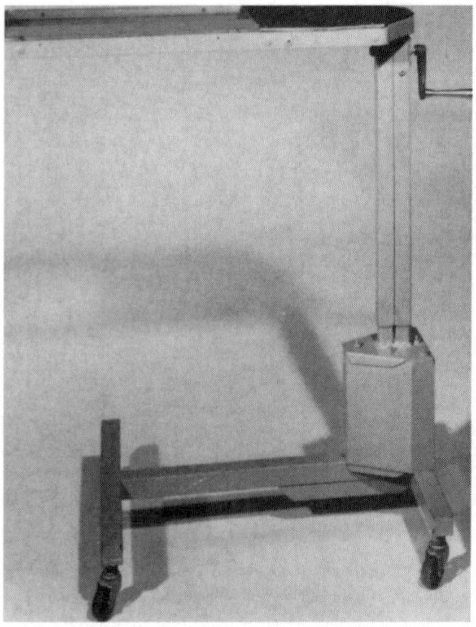

Figure 7.10. Floor-Mounted Blocking Tray. This blocking tray can be used to treat patients in stretchers or patients treated on the floor. The tray height is adjustable so that it can be used for many treatment techniques.

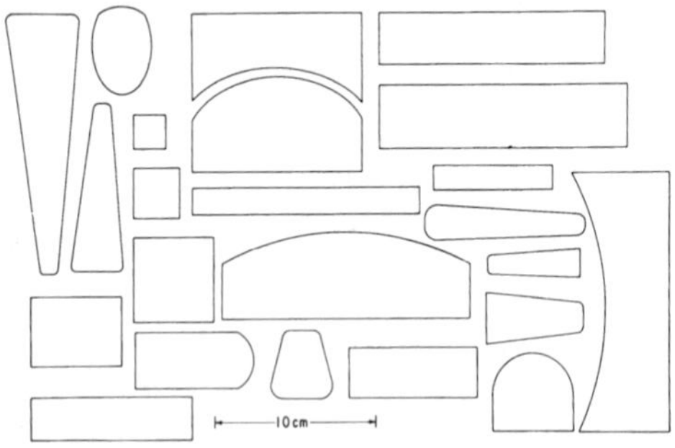

Figure 7.11. Standard Cerrobend Blocks. Each machine has an assortment of secondary cerrobend or lead blocks to reduce a rectangularly collimated field to the desired irregularly shaped field. Also, for some blocking configurations, such as whole brain and pelvis fields, standard cerrobend blocks can be used instead of making custom blocks.

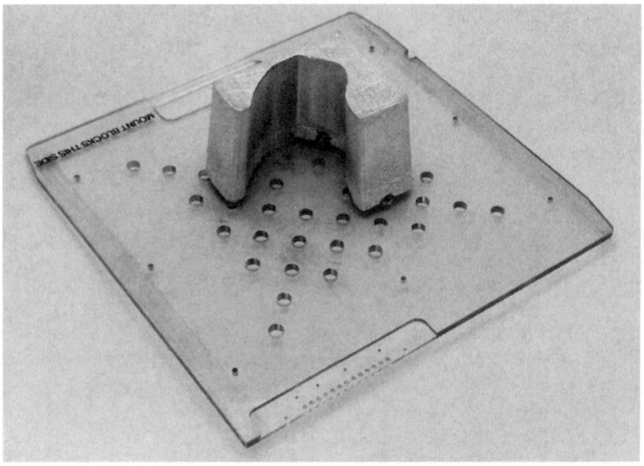

Figure 7.12. Custom Cerrobend Blocks. For most patients, custom cerrobend blocking is necessary. The blocking shape is cut out of a Styrofoam block on a hot-wire apparatus and filled with cerrobend. For x-ray radiation, these blocks are approximately 7 cm thick. If made thinner, these blocks can also be used to transmit partial dose. As an example, partial transmission lung blocks can be made to reduce the lung dose to 50% of the prescription point dose.

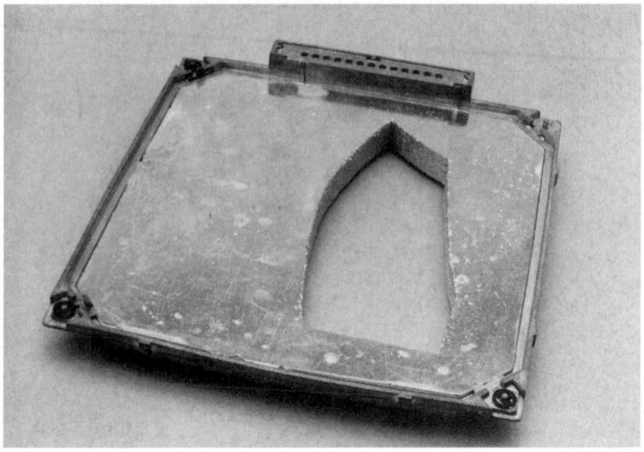

Figure 7.13. Cerrobend Electron Cutouts. Custom blocking can also be performed when treating with electrons. These cutouts are made approximately 1.5 cm thick. The custom insert is placed at the end of the electron collimating device on the linear accelerator. This cutout performs the final collimation of the electron beam either at or within about 5 cm of the patient's surface.

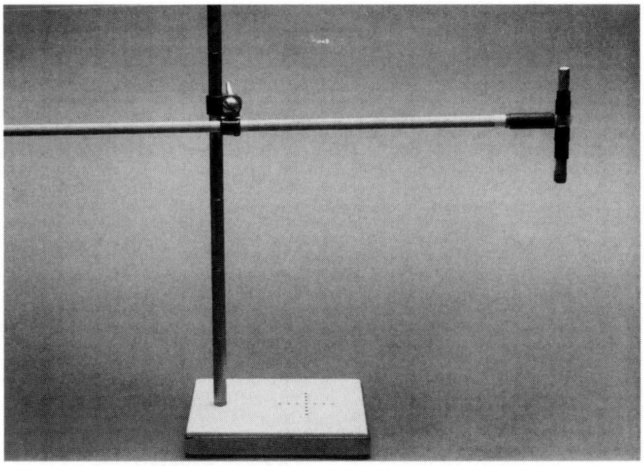

Figure 7.14. Eye Block. A small diameter cerrobend or lead block can be used to shield the lens of the eye when treating the cornea or orbit. This block is made the same thickness as an x-ray block and is mounted to a wooden rod or other similar device. The block should be aligned according to the patient's anatomy every day instead of permanently mounting it to a block tray.

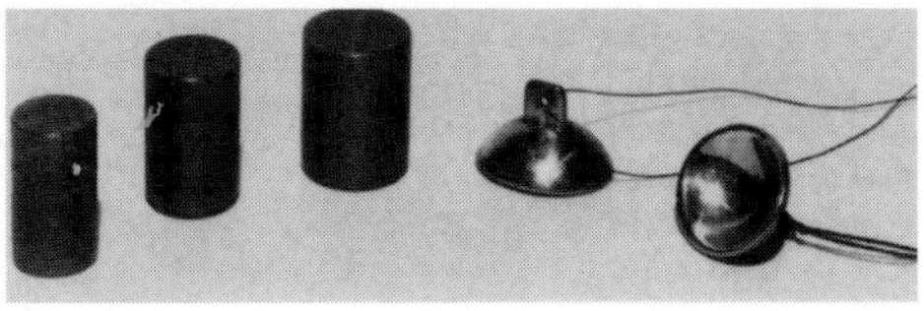

Figure 7.15. Eye Shields. Two types of eye shields. Shields at right, inserted beneath the eye lids, provide protection from superficial and orthovoltage x-rays and low-energy electrons (7 MeV or less). Shields at left are lead cylinders in three different diameters (1.0, 1.5 and 2.0 cm) that can be suspended above the patient on a Mylar tray. Appropriate thickness is specified by the radiation oncologist. Tungsten eye shields have been recently recommended. (From Shiu AS, et al. Int J Radiat Oncol Biol Phys 1996;35(3):599.)

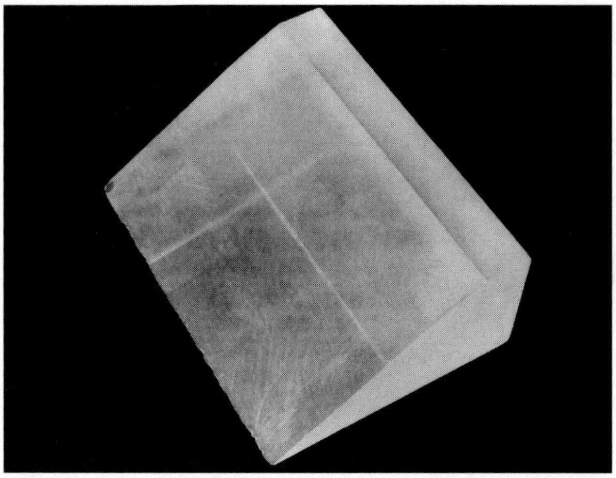

Figure 7.16. Compensators. To deliver a uniform dose to a volume beneath a nonuniform surface, missing tissue compensators can be placed in front of the beam. Several types of missing tissue compensators exist. The simplest, which only compensates in one direction, is an acrylic slab placed on a blocking tray between the accelerator and the patient. More complicated compensators account for thickness changes in both the length and width directions and require special machinery to generate. (Manufactured by Scientific Apparatus, University of Minnesota.)

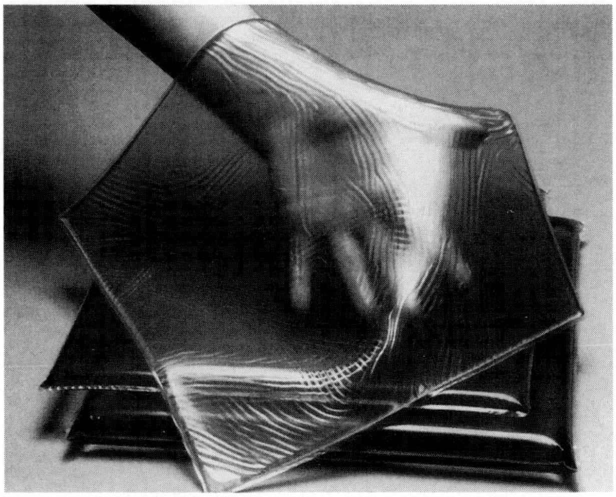

Figure 7.17. Bolus. Bolus is a tissue substitute useful for increasing surface dose or filling in small amounts of missing tissue. Slabs of 0.5 cm or 1.0 cm thick material are placed on the skin surface to increase skin dose. Custom thickness bolus can be created using wax to equalize the amount of tissue seen by the treatment beam. Computed tomography or MRI studies can be used to determine the amount of bolus necessary throughout the field. (Courtesy of Med-Tec, Inc., Orange City, IA.)

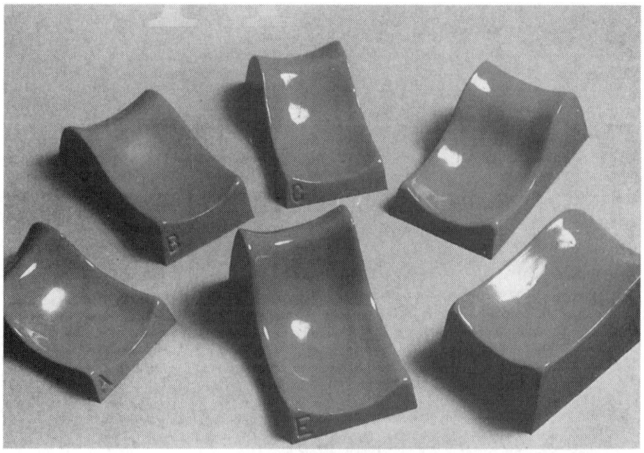

Figure 7.18. Head and Neck Supports. These devices provide head stability for supine patients. They are available in various height and contour combinations so that a patient's head angulation is adjustable. The same set of head and neck supports is available in clear plastic which only minimally attenuates the treatment beam. (Courtesy of Med-Tec, Inc., Orange City, IA.)

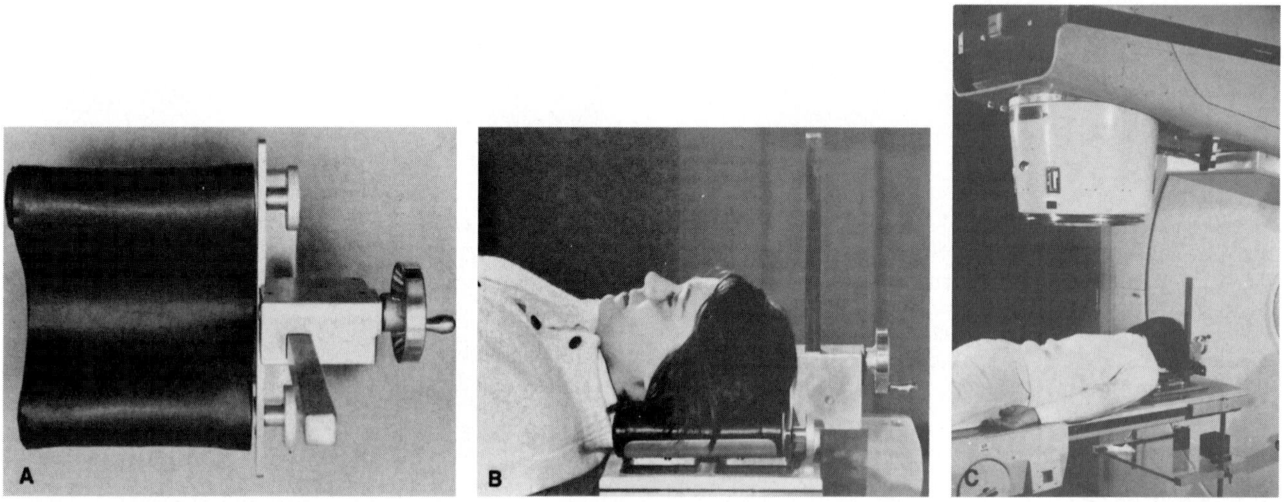

Figure 7.19. Head and Face Holder. This apparatus is designed for the proper positioning of the head or face (**A**). When the patient is in the supine position, the head rests on a vinyl sheet suspended between two bars (**B**). Vertical height is adjustable to provide proper tilt or leveling of the head. For a patient in the prone position, the same device is used as a face rest (**C**). The bars are covered with Styrofoam and vinyl, and can be moved laterally to provide a comfortable and secure face rest without hindering breathing. The adjustments are made by a gear crank arrangement. This device can also be used for lateral positioning of the head.

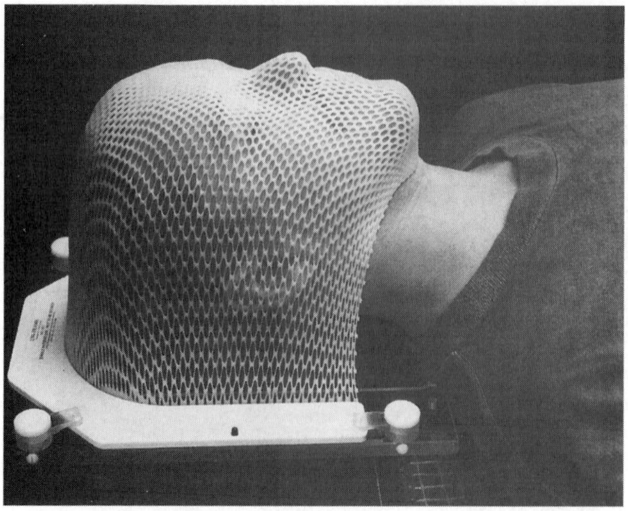

Figure 7.20. Aquaplast Mask. This plastic mask and frame combination provide excellent head immobilization. The mask derives its accuracy from the chin, nose, and brow. Small areas can also be cut out for treatment or comfort without compromising the integrity of the mask. The frames also come in tilting and prone configurations. (Courtesy of Med-Tec, Inc., Orange City, IA.)

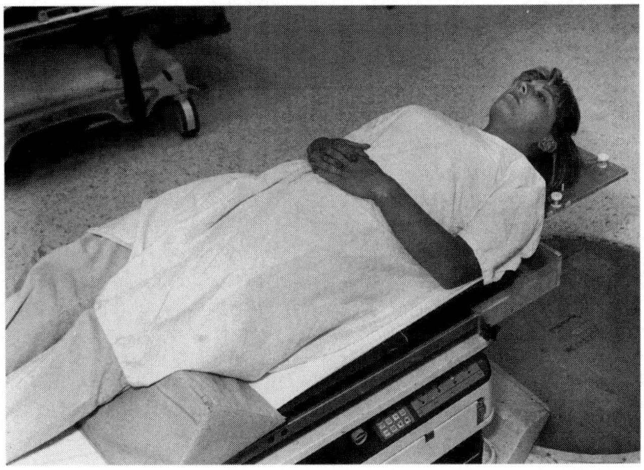

Figure 7.21. Off Treatment Table Head Holder. A head rest can be mounted at the end of the treatment table to allow more gantry and couch angle combinations to be treated for conformal noncoplanar brain treatments. The holder is made of a honeycomb fiberglass laminate composite and is radiopaque. It attaches to the couch side rails and includes the hardware necessary to accept an aquaplast face mask. (Manufactured by Scientific Apparatus, University of Minnesota.)

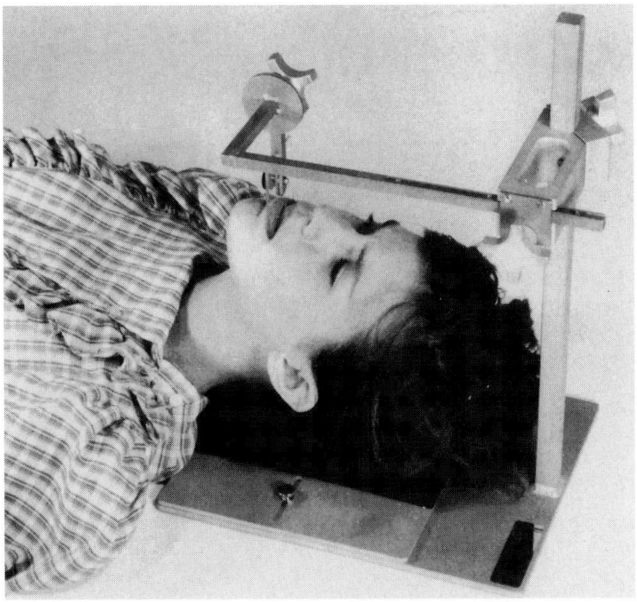

Figure 7.22. Bite Block. This device consists of a head and neck support and a formed mouthpiece attached to a rigid stand. The mouthpiece and stand ensure that the extension of the chin is constant and the patient head is immobilized for every treatment. The rigid stand can also be made in a "C" shape to allow anterior fields to be treated. (Courtesy of Radiation Products Design, Albertville, MN.)

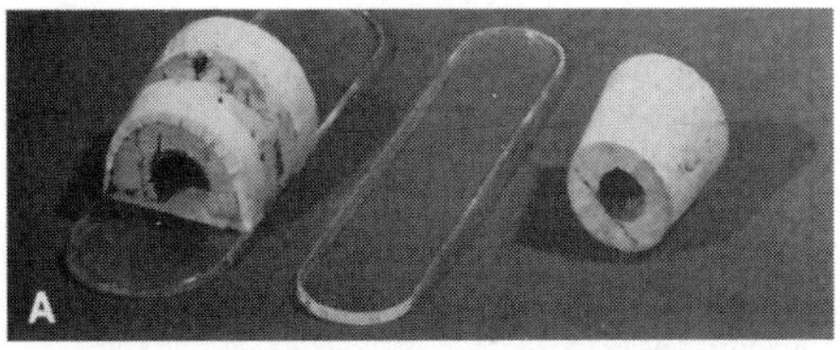

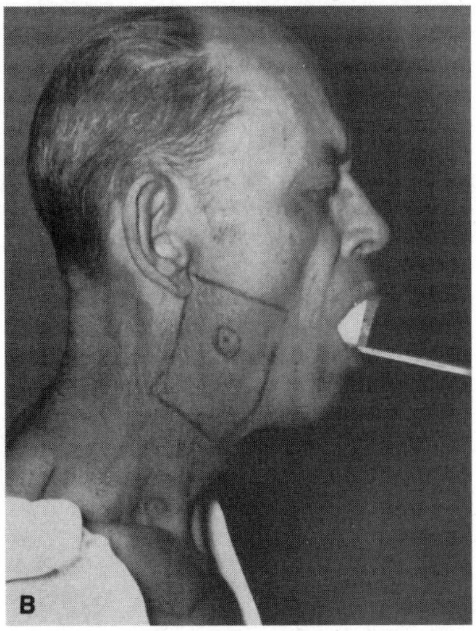

Figure 7.23. Cork and Tongue Blade. A cork is mounted on a wooden or plastic tongue blade (**A**) to move the tongue out of the radiation field or to ensure that the tongue is included in the radiation field. A gum or tooth groove is cut in the top of the cork to stabilize the cork in the mouth (**B**). An air hole is drilled through the center of the cork for breathing. (Reprinted with permission from Fletcher GH. Neck nodes. In: Fletcher GH, ed. Textbook of radiology. 3rd ed. Philadelphia: Lea and Febiger, 1980.)

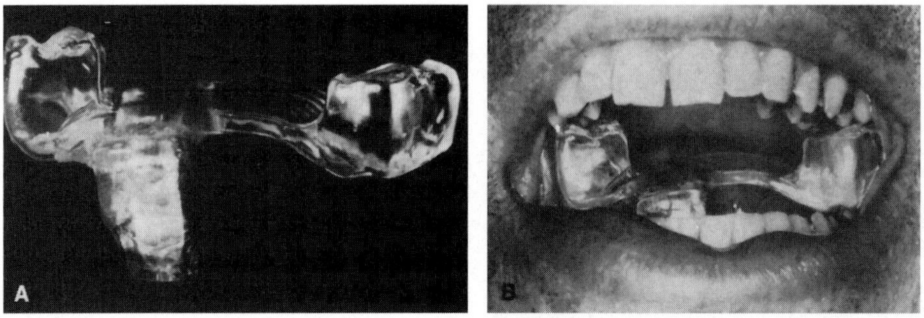

Figure 7.24. Intraoral Stent. A dentist can make a stent to a radiation oncologist's specifications that provides heavy-metal protection for the tongue and gingiva when the cheek and lip are treated with electrons (**A**). Stents are made of a dental acrylic that encompasses the heavy metal. These devices can also be made to displace the tongue to a desired position (**B**). (Reprinted with permission from Tapley NduV. Skin and lips. In: Tapley NduV. Clinical applications of the electron beam. New York: John Wiley, 1976.)

Figure 7.25. Intraoral Cone Holder and Periscope. The intraoral cone holder accepts the desired intraoral cone and interlocks the linear accelerator to fix the collimator field size. The periscope is used to visualize the area at which the intraoral cone is aimed. (Courtesy of Radiation Products Design, Albertville, MN.)

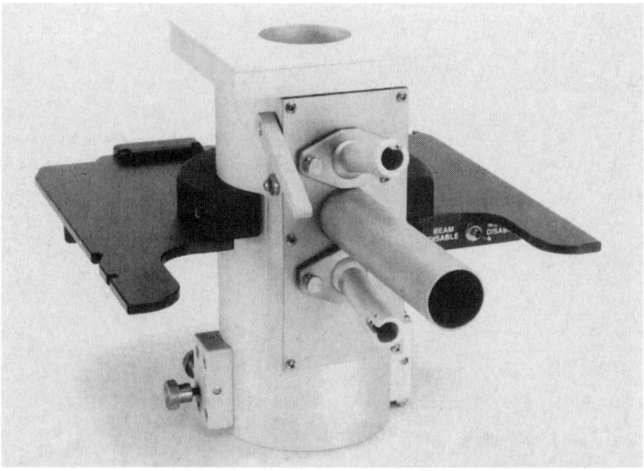

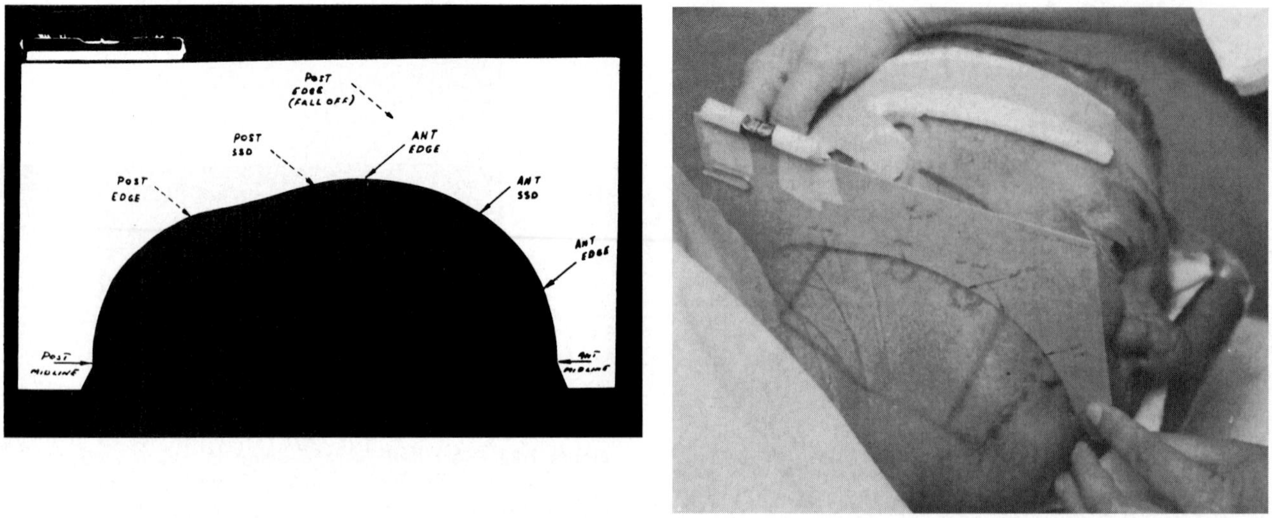

Figure 7.26. Cardboard Cutout. A cardboard cutout is made by transferring a patient's contour outline and beam parameters on a treatment plan to a sheet of cardboard. This template can then be used to transfer field edges, source to skin distance (SSD) positions, and anatomic landmarks from the treatment plan to the patient. A pocket bubble level attached to the upper surface of the cardboard ensures that the cutout is level every time the position is checked. This device is especially useful for lateral head and neck and tangential breast treatments. (Reprinted with permission from Sampiere VA. Radiation measurement and dosimetric practices. In: Fletcher GH, ed. Textbook of radiology. 3rd ed. Philadelphia: Lea & Febiger, 1980.)

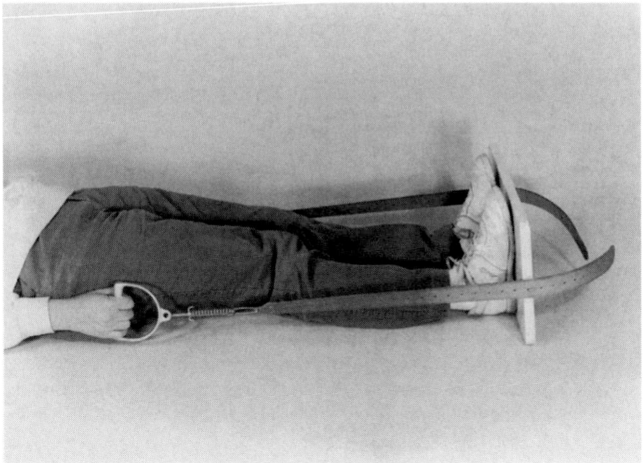

Figure 7.27. Shoulder Swing. The rope handles on this device are held by the patient to aid in pulling down the shoulders. Lower shoulders lead to lower inferior borders of lateral head and neck fields. The rope lengths are adjustable for patient height and arm length. (Courtesy of Radiation Products Design, Albertville, MN.)

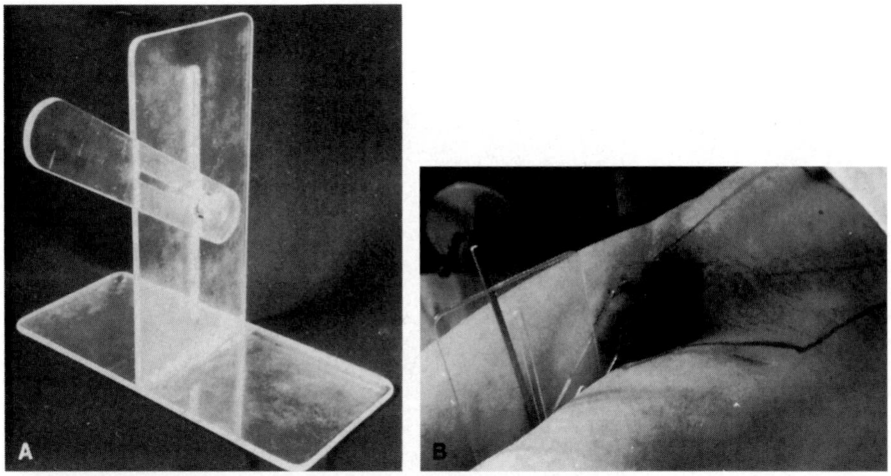

Figure 7.28. Testicular Retractor. This device moves the untreated testicle and part of the scrotum from the direct treatment beam path. The T-shaped device has a groove along the vertical support that allows positioning of the narrower blade, also with a groove (**A**), in any vertical or angled orientation to the patient. It is fixed in position by means of a locking screw (**B**). (Reprinted with permission from Delclos L. Radiologia 1971; 13:283.)

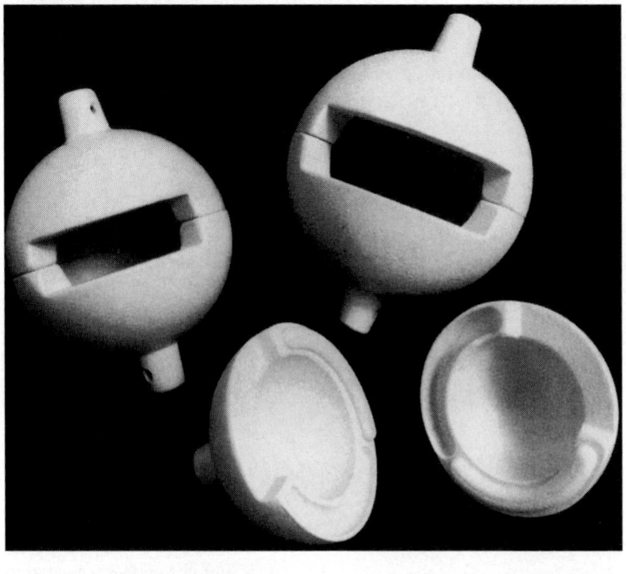

Figure 7.29. Testicular Shield. This lead device is designed to reduce scatter radiation to the testicles. The device is oriented to minimize the amount of scatter radiation reaching the testicles through the entrance slit. (Courtesy of Med-Tec, Inc., Orange City, IA.)

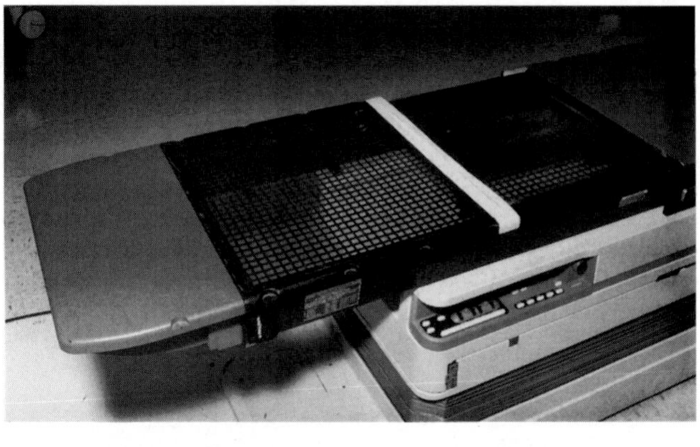

Figure 7.30. Mylar Window. This couch insert allows posterior fields to be visualized and treated with minimal additional buildup material in the beam path. The window is designed to provide rigid support to patients and sag minimally under their weight.

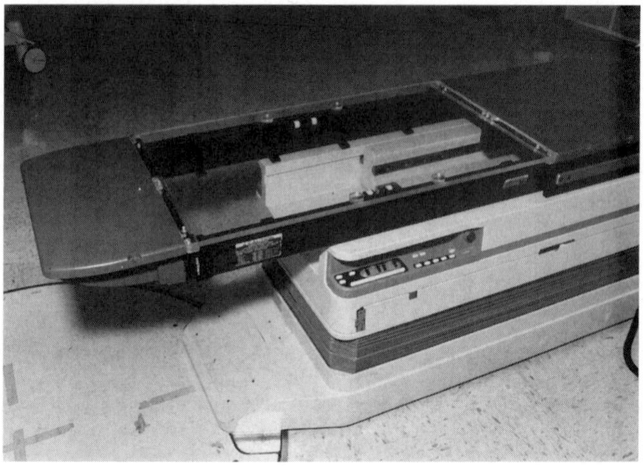

Figure 7.31. **Acrylic Insert.** This couch insert allows anterior/posterior and lateral fields to be treated during the same session without changing the couch configuration. For anterior and posterior beams, the acrylic acts as extra tissue. For lateral beams, the acrylic is a solid table which does not allow any sag. The insert corresponds to 1.4 cm of tissue equivalence which must be considered in the dose calculation for the posterior field. (Manufactured by Scientific Apparatus, University of Minnesota.)

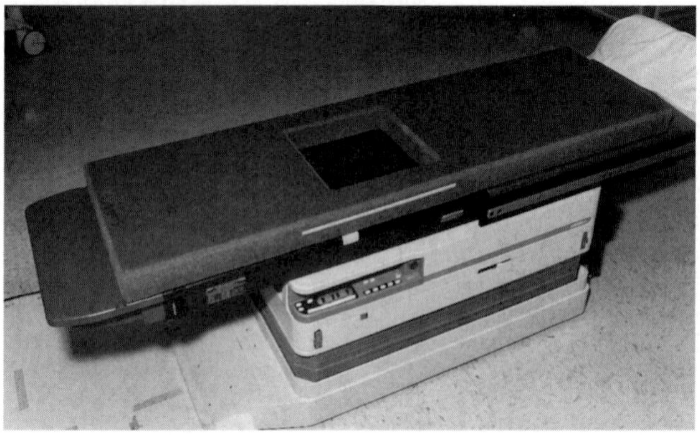

Figure 7.32. **Window Board.** This board is used to move small bowel out of a treatment field. Patients are laid prone on the board with their pelvis over the opening. Either by letting the belly hang into the opening or allowing the opening to push the belly superiorly, the bowels can be moved from the area to be treated.

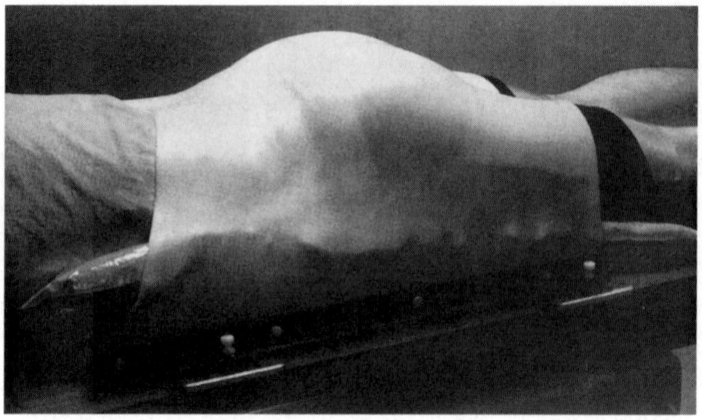

Figure 7.33. **Aquaplast Immobilizer.** Aquaplast can be used to immobilize the pelvis with this device. A large perforated or solid sheet of aquaplast material can be attached to the sides of the board and to a point between the legs. The patient can be treated in either the prone or supine position. (Courtesy of Med-Tec, Inc., Orange City, IA.)

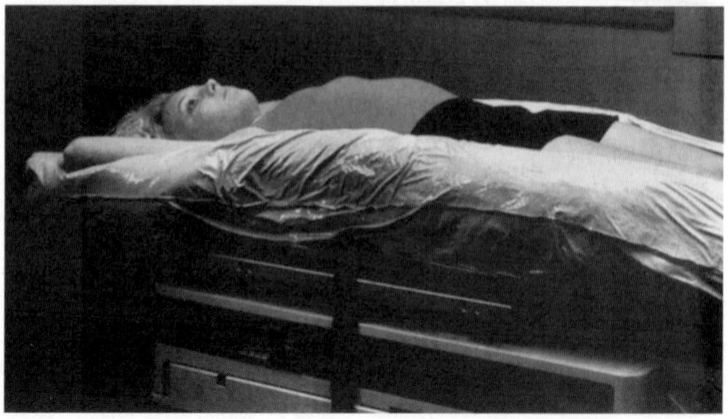

Figure 7.34. **Vacuum Bag.** This radiopaque vacuum bag is filled with tiny polystyrene beads. The bag is deflated and formed around a patient previously set up in the desired treatment position. Next, a vacuum is drawn and the bag becomes rigid. These vacuum bags can be used to immobilize nearly any body part. (Courtesy of Med-Tec, Inc., Orange City, IA.)

contour for each treatment. For pelvic treatments, ink marks on the skin cannot be relied on because of extensive skin movement. Since organs such as the bladder, rectum, and kidneys are all dose limiting structures, delivering dose accurately in the pelvis is critical. It is important, therefore, to have either rigid immobilization or to move critical structures out of the treatment beam path.

THORAX

In this section, we consider immobilization devices useful for thorax treatments such as lung, mantle, and breast irradiation (Figures 7.35–7.40). There is significant bony anatomy in the thoracic region to aid daily setup, but anatomy such as the breast, for example, can hinder reproducibility. The spinal cord, heart, lungs, and liver are all dose limiting structures in the thoracic region, so accuracy needs to be maintained.

SPECIAL PROCEDURES

The next four sections show devices that can be used for total body irradiation, total skin irradiation, stereotactic radiotherapy, and craniospinal irradiation. These special procedures require unique equipment to ensure a uniform dose over a large area, a high dose over a small area, or a nonuniform dose over a small area.

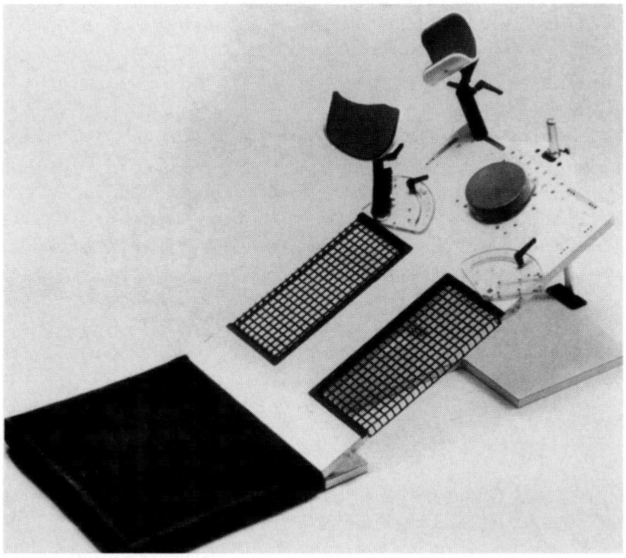

Figure 7.35. Breast Board. This device is useful for treating breast cancer with tangential x-ray beams. The tilt is adjustable to make the angle of the patient's chest wall parallel to the treatment couch. The board also has cups for the patient's elbow and wrist for comfort. Carbon fiber panels allow lateral tangent fields to be treated with negligible attenuation. Aquaplast sheets can also be attached to the board to provide more rigid immobilization. (Courtesy of Med-Tec, Inc., Orange City, IA.)

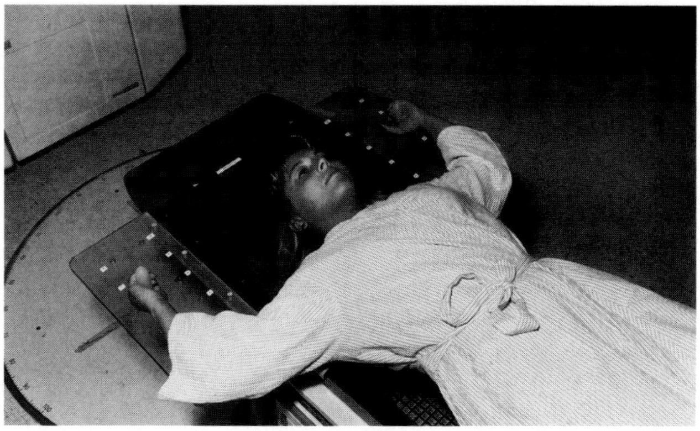

Figure 7.36. Mantle Board. This device has several holes for positioning pegs. Once the patient's treatment position is determined, pegs are placed in the appropriate holes for reproducibility. The mantle board is made of acrylic and can be treated through with minimal attenuation. (Manufactured by Scientific Apparatus, University of Minnesota.)

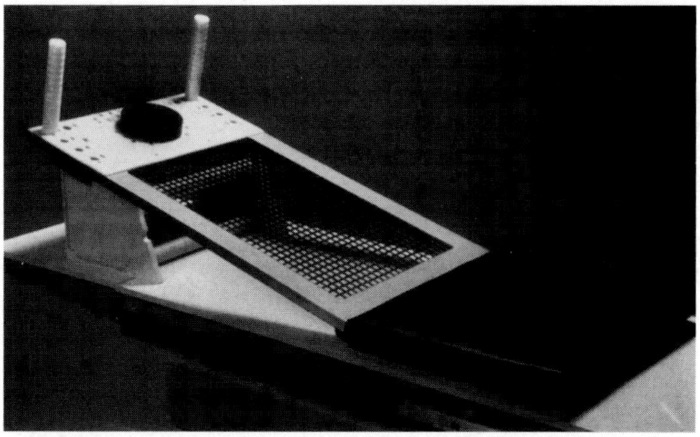

Figure 7.37. Angle Board. The angle board is a device similar to the breast board that can be used to treat tangential breast patients, but it is also useful for patients that cannot lay horizontally. The angle of the board is adjustable and can be treated through if necessary. (Courtesy of Med-Tec, Inc., Orange City, IA.)

Total Body Irradiation

The goal of total body irradiation is to deliver a uniform dose to a patient's bone marrow. This therapy is often given as preparation for bone marrow transplantation. The two most popular beam arrangements for total body irradiation are bilateral and anterior/posterior opposing beams. With compensation, dose uniformity of ±10% can be achieved with either technique (Figures 7.41–7.43).

Total Skin Irradiation

The goal of total skin irradiation is to deliver a uniform dose to the entire skin surface. The treatment generally is

Text continued on page 100

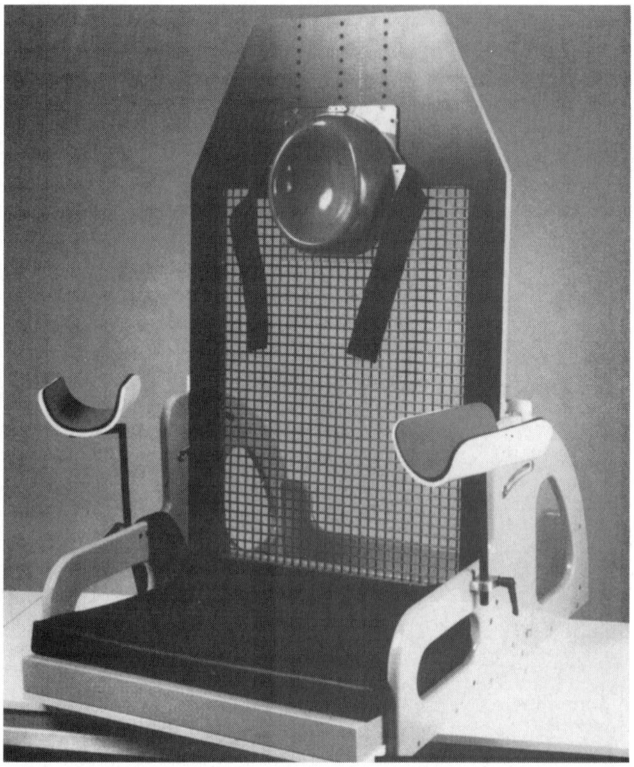

Figure 7.38. Treatment Seat. The treatment seat is a device that allows a patient to be accurately repositioned daily in a seated position. There are several means of stabilizing the patient including hand grips, elbow holders, and a seatbelt. The back of the seat is carbon fiber and can be treated through. The angle of the seat back is adjustable. (Courtesy of Med-Tec, Inc., Orange City, IA.)

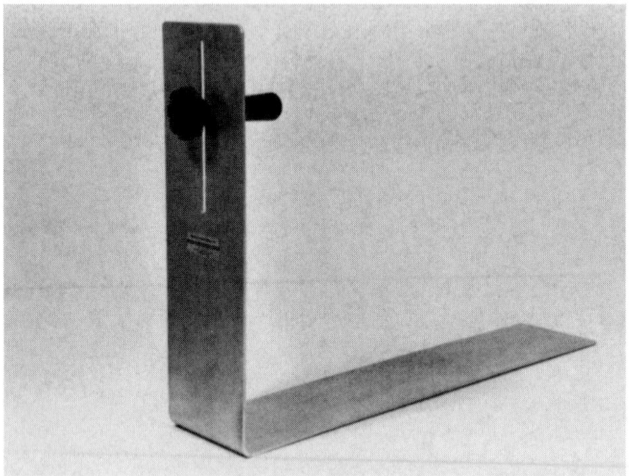

Figure 7.39. Arm Board. The arm board is an L-shaped device placed under the patient before lying down which provides vertical support for the hand and arm. It can be used for tangential breast treatments and other treatment that require the arm to be pulled away from the body including treatment of the arm itself. (Courtesy of Radiation Products Design, Albertville, MN.)

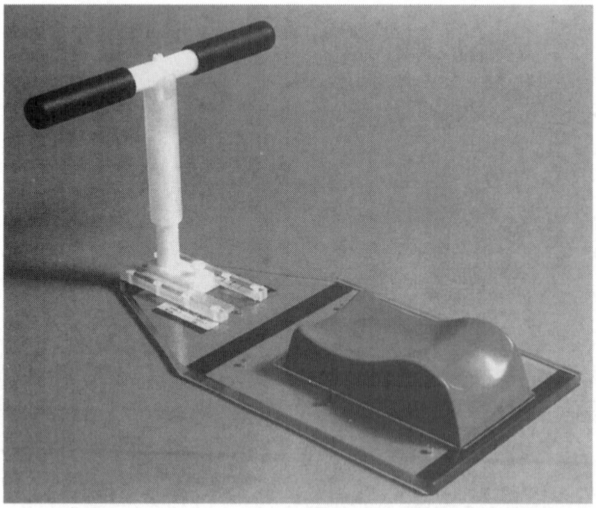

Figure 7.40. Overhead Arm Positioner. This device is used to move both arms from the patient's sides. The patient holds onto the adjustable hand rests pulling the arms overhead. This position allows lateral lung and mediastinal fields to be treated without treating the arms. (Courtesy of Med-Tec, Inc., Orange City, IA.)

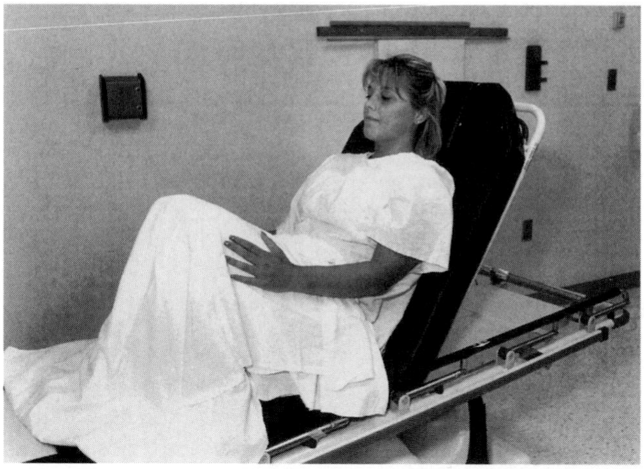

Figure 7.41. Treatment Chair for Lateral Fields. A patient treated with bilateral fields is placed on a treatment couch in a relaxed position with the torso reclined and the knees bent. The upper arms provide compensation for the lungs and custom designed aluminum compensators are added to make the doses to the head, neck, lower legs, and feet match the prescription dose.

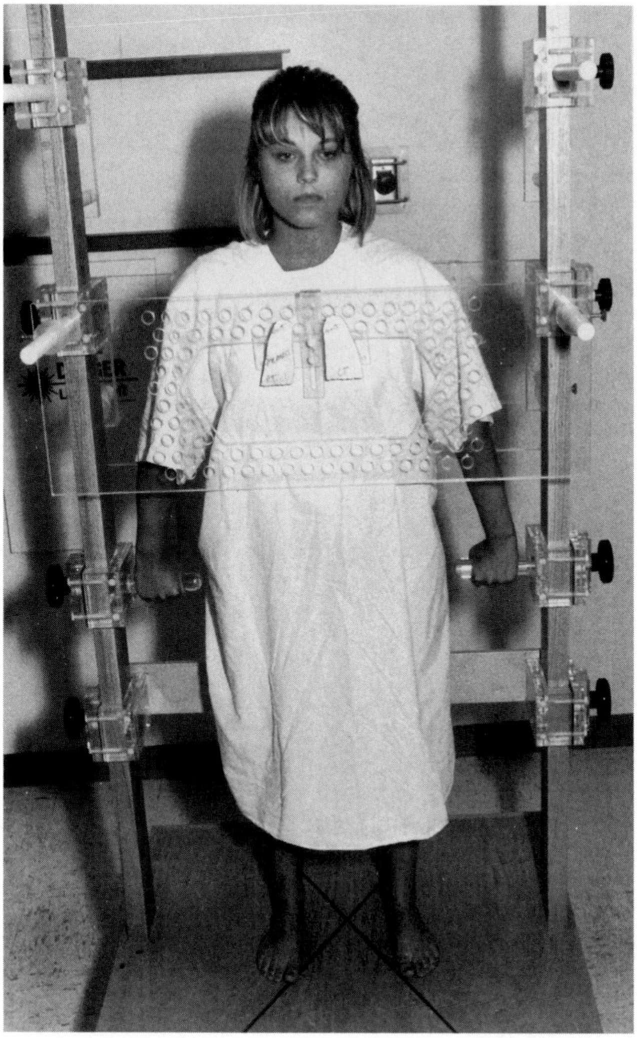

Figure 7.42. Treatment Stand for Anterior and Posterior Fields. When treating a patient with the anterior and posterior total body irradiation technique, a stand is provided for patient positioning and for holding equipment such as lung blocks or port films. This same stand can be used for total skin irradiation. (Manufactured by Scientific Apparatus, University of Minnesota.)

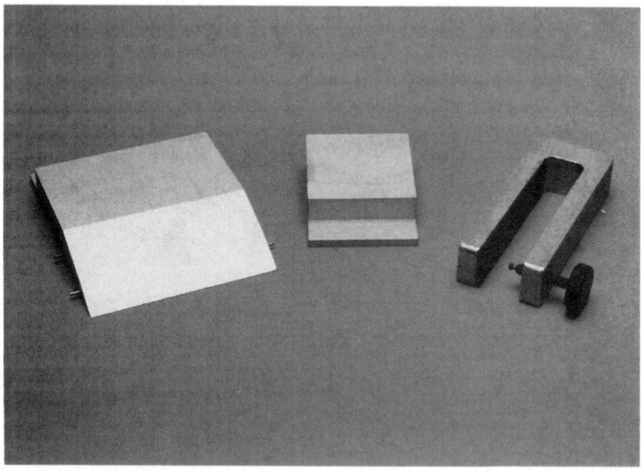

Figure 7.43. Compensators. Aluminum compensators are used to equalize the dose to all anatomical locations. For the bilateral technique, the compensators are attached to a standard blocking ray by special clamps. The leg and foot compensator is outfitted with small alignment pins which cast a shadow on the wall behind the patient. The compensators are adjusted until the shadows match the patient's knee and ankle positions. The head and neck compensator is clamped to the blocking tray such that the thickest edge (for the neck) aligns inferior to the patient's neck along the shoulder. For the anterior/posterior technique, the compensators for lungs are usually mounted on the treatment stand. Other compensators such as those for arms, legs, head, and neck can be mounted either on the treatment stand or on the blocking tray. (Manufactured by Scientific Apparatus, University of Minnesota.)

delivered with 9 MeV electrons at an extended source to patient distance. Often, due to patient contours, small boost fields are added to increase shielded anatomical areas to the prescription dose. Note that the same stand used to treat anterior and posterior total body irradiation patients can be used to treat total skin irradiation patients (Figures 7.44–7.45).

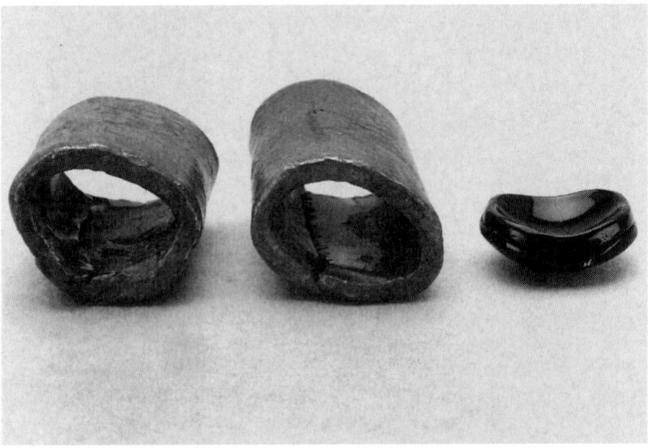

Figure 7.44. Eye and Nail Shields. Since the dose tolerance of the eyes is low, eye shields are used throughout the treatment. In addition, fingernails and toenails generally cannot tolerate the prescription dose so small pieces of lead are placed over the finger and toe tips during the course of treatment.

Stereotactic Radiosurgery and Radiotherapy

Stereotactic radiosurgery and radiotherapy require accurate setups due to the small field sizes used and the critical structures near the treatment area. In radiosurgery, accuracy is achieved by both imaging and treating a patient with a head frame attached to his or her skull (Figures 7.46 and 7.47). Four small screws are used to affix the head ring to the patient on the treatment day.

Craniospinal Irradiation

Several techniques have been developed to treat the entire craniospinal axis at one time. At the University of Minnesota, we treat the brain with right and left lateral x-ray fields and we treat the spine with either posterior x-ray or electron fields (for pediatric patients). The junction of these three fields along the craniospinal axis must be carefully set up to avoid any overdoses or severe underdoses (Figure 7.48).

MISCELLANEOUS

The following devices do not fit into any general category above, but are useful for general patient positioning (Figures 7.49–7.51) or patient setup verification (Figures 7.52 and 7.53).

Text continued on page 103

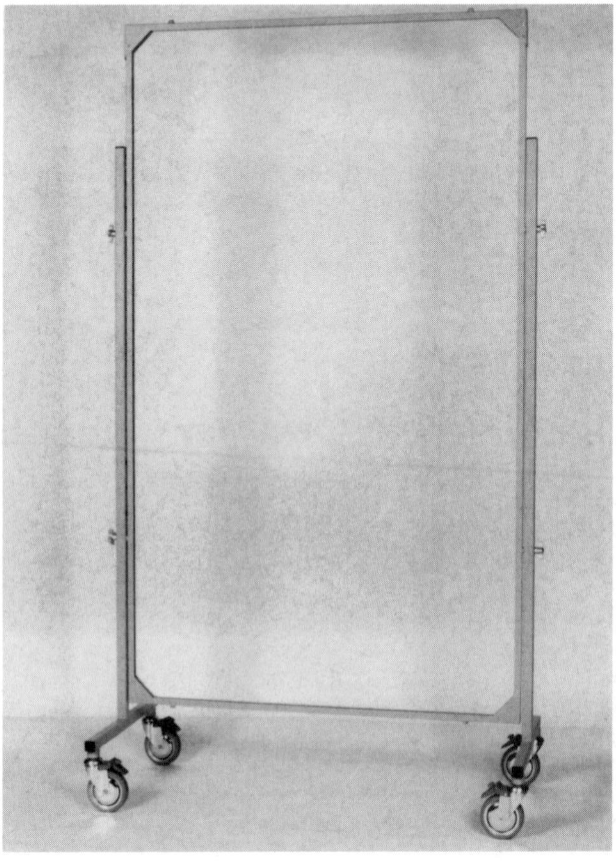

Figure 7.45. Beam Spoiler. An acrylic beam spoiler (3/8" or 1/2" thick) can be placed near the patient during treatment to further scatter the electron beam over the patient's skin surface. (Courtesy of Radiation Products Design, Albertville, MN.)

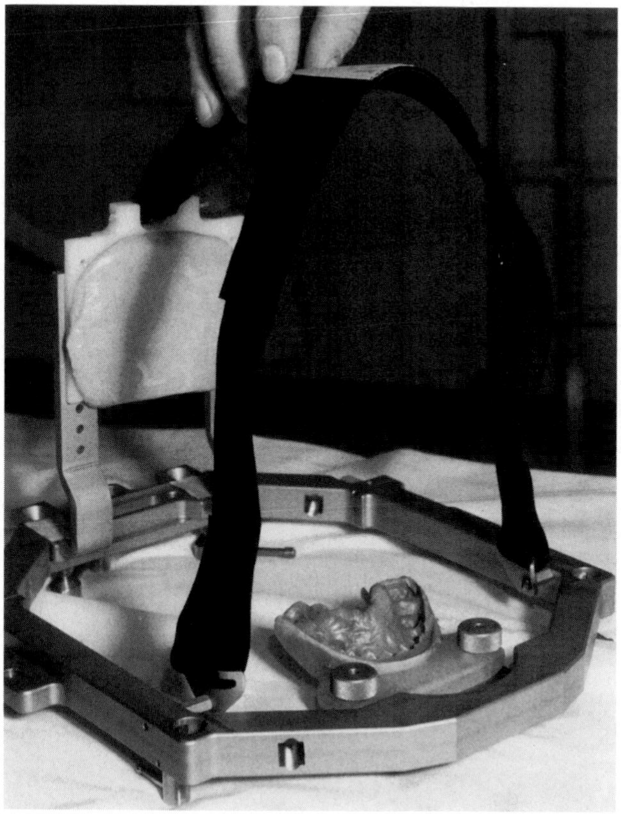

Figure 7.46. BRW and CRW Head Immobilizers. For fractionated stereotactic radiotherapy treatments, a mold of the patient's dentition and a cast of the occiput are used to reproduce the position of the skull every treatment. (Manufactured by Radionics, Burlington, Massachusetts.)

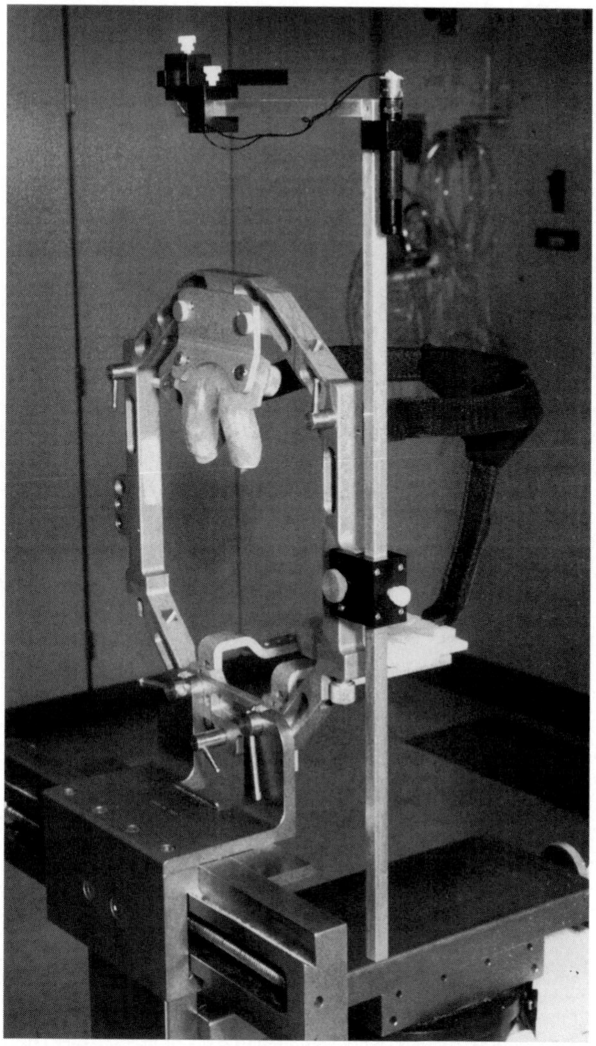

Figure 7.47. Head Ring Mounted Light. The treatment of certain diseases with stereotactic radiotherapy calls for the patient's eye to maintain a certain position. This task is made simpler if the patient can stare at an object. Shown in this figure is an adjustable head-ring mounted light. (Manufactured by Scientific Apparatus, University of Minnesota.)

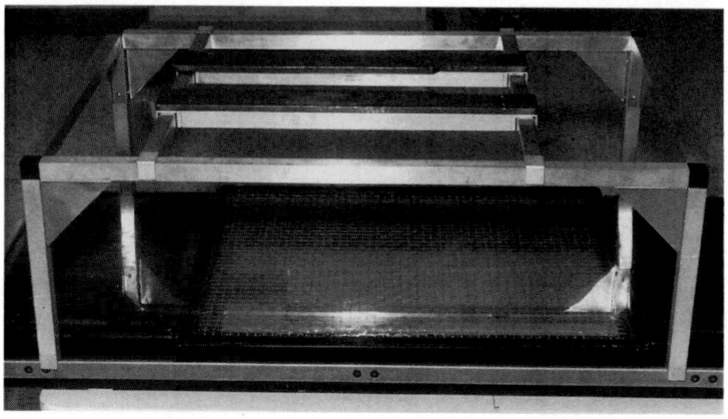

Figure 7.48. Tertiary Collimator Stand. The mediastinum and lungs can receive a high dose when treated with a posterior x-ray field. If the spinal cord is shallow enough (as is the case in many pediatric patients) then exit dose is minimal. To treat a long electron field, however, an extended source to surface distance is necessary. A tertiary collimation system is used in these cases to collimate the beam near the patient's surface which minimizes penumbra and widens the higher percent isodose curves. The stand shown in this figure has an adjustable length and width and mounts to the treatment couch. Lead pieces are then placed on the stand to collimate the beam based on the patient's anatomy. (Manufactured by Scientific Apparatus, University of Minnesota.)

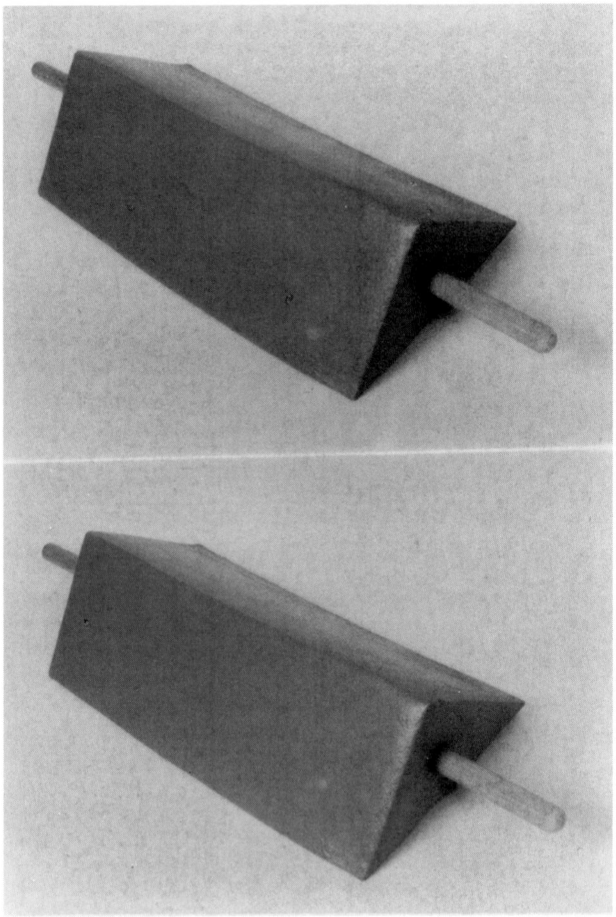

Figure 7.49. Sponges. Various foam shapes can be used to support a patient's body during treatment. For example, triangular sponges hold the knees bent to relieve strain on the low back. Also, sponges can be wedged under a patient's hips and back to stabilize him or her in a lateral setup position. (Courtesy of Radiation Products Design, Albertville, MN.)

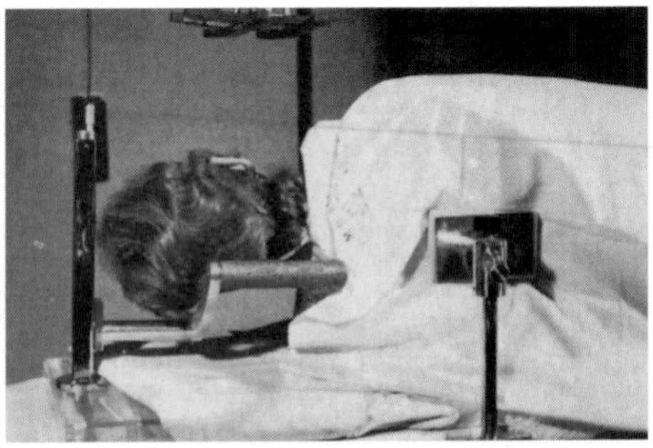

Figure 7.50. Body Brace. This device is used to support patients in a lateral setup position. It is mounted on a base that rests on the table top beneath the patient. Foam rubber pads are mounted on the arms that can be moved vertically or horizontally and placed against the patient. Two braces usually are used, one anteriorly and one posteriorly.

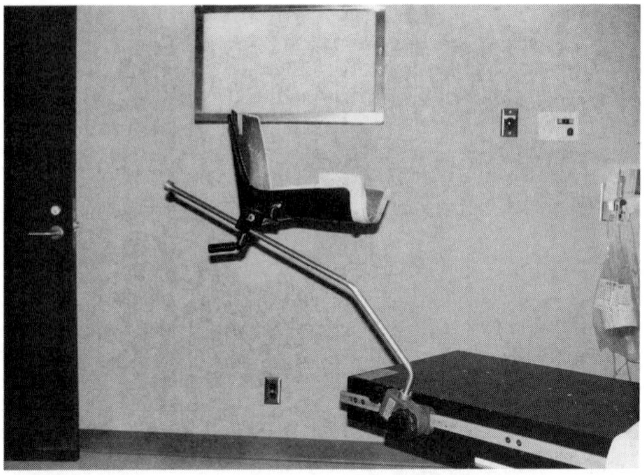

Figure 7.51. Stirrups. To treat a leg with lateral or oblique fields, it is often necessary to move the untreated leg out of the way. Stirrups mounted to the treatment couch can be adjusted to provide a stable and comfortable holder for the untreated leg.

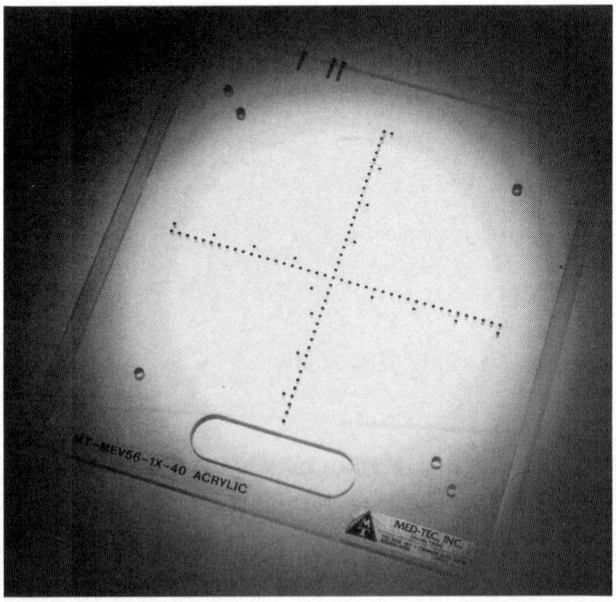

Figure 7.52. Graticule. A graticule will project a series of small dots onto port films. The spacing between the dots is usually chosen to be 1 cm at the machine isocenter. The graticule is made of acrylic or other radiopaque material outfitted with small tungsten dots. The graticule fits into either the wedge slot or block tray slot in he head of the accelerator. (Courtesy of Med-Tec, Inc., Orange City, IA.)

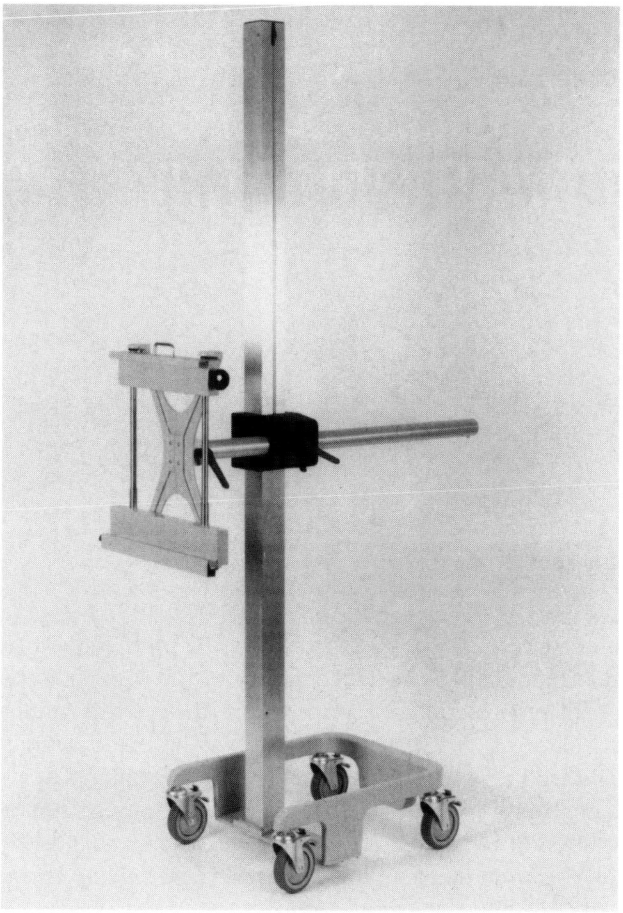

Figure 7.53. Port Film Holders. This device is used to position port films behind the patient. The freestanding holder is especially useful for oblique treatment angles where the films cannot be supported by the treatment couch. The holder is mounted on wheels so it is easy to roll to the necessary position. The holder may also have a inclinometer mounted on it to set accurate angles of port film to match the oblique treatment angles. (Courtesy of Radiation Products Design, Albertville, MN.)

References

1. ICRU report 24. Determination of absorbed dose in a patient irradiated by beams of X or gamma rays in radiotherapy procedures. International Commission on Radiation Units and Measurements, 1976.
2. Balter JM, Ten Haken RK, Larn KL. Immobilization and treatment setup verification. In: Mackie TR, Palta JR, eds. Teletherapy: present and future. Madison, WI: Advanced Medical Publishing, 1996.
3. Purdy JA, Gerber R, Harms W. Patient positioning, immobilization, and treatment verification. In: Purdy JA, ed. Advances in radiation oncology physics. Woodbury, NY: American Institute of Physics, Inc., 1992.
4. Reinstein LE. Patient positioning and immobilization. In: Khan FM, Potish RA, eds. Treatment planning in radiation oncology. Baltimore, MD: Williams & Wilkins, 1998.

Chapter 8

Three-Dimensional Treatment Planning and Conformal Therapy

James A. Purdy, Bahman Emami, Mary V. Graham, Jeff Michalski, Carlos A. Perez, and Joseph Simpson

In the treatment of cancer with radiation, the radiation oncologist is faced with the dilemma of prescribing a treatment that either cures or controls the disease but is not associated with an unacceptable incidence of serious complications. The difficulty of this task is best illustrated by the dose-response relationships between tumor/normal tissues and the radiation dose delivered. Published clinical and experimental results show tumor control or normal tissue effect response as a steep function of radiation dose, e.g., a small change in the dose delivered (±5%) can result in a dramatic change in the local response of the tissue (±20%) (1–3). Moreover, the prescribed curative doses are often, by necessity, close to the dose tolerated by the normal tissue. For optimum treatment, the radiation dose must be delivered with a high degree of accuracy.

It has been argued that when the treatment involves multiple dose fractions, the requirement for accurate dose delivery can be relaxed (4). This statement may be true when all the errors involved in dose delivery are random and independent and tend to cancel each other, e.g., patient's breathing motion and daily misalignment of radiation fields; although in radiation therapy, systematic errors also occur, e.g., inaccurate localization of the target volumes and/or critical structures, inaccurate dose calculation, and erroneous machine calibration. Presumably, if all patients were identical in their responses to the dose administered, any systematic error would be corrected when the radiation oncologist readjusted the treatment regimens (e.g., by enlarging field sizes or increasing the time of irradiation). Unfortunately, because of biologic variations, the systematic errors for individual patients are different and are not detected easily. Inappropriate dose calculations in patients with different anatomic characteristics fall into this category. Furthermore, these errors cannot be reduced by increasing the numbers of dose fractions so that some patients consistently receive suboptimal treatment. Therefore, careful treatment planning (e.g., tumor localization and dose calculation) is needed on an individual basis to minimize the occurrence of systematic errors in the treatment of each patient.

The degree of accuracy required in dose delivery is difficult to determine, but the International Commission on Radiation Units and Measurements (ICRU) recommended a value of ±5%, a standard representing the best that can be achieved at present (5). Loevinger and Loftus reported that even the straightforward procedure of delivering the dose to a water phantom has an uncertainty of 2.5% under optimum conditions (6). Considering the many steps involved in the clinical dosimetric procedure in which the dose is delivered to a target volume in a heterogeneous patient rather than to a uniform phantom, each step must be performed with accuracy of better than ±5% to achieve the ICRU recommendation. If, for example, only three steps were involved (e.g. tumor localization, dose calculation, and machine calibration) and the uncertainties presumably add in quadrature, a ±3% accuracy would be required for each step. Therefore, to improve outcome in radiation therapy, more accurate treatment planning is required.

The treatment planning process comprises several steps, including: a) accurate spatial and density determination of the target volume and critical structures; b) prescription of dose to the target volume(s) and assignment of normal tissue tolerance doses; c) initial plan setup; d) dose calculation; e) plan evaluation and optimization; and f) plan implementation and verification. Imaging technologies such as x-ray computed tomography (CT) and magnetic resonance (MR) have impacted greatly on the planning process and have set the stage for three-dimensional radiation therapy treatment planning (3DRTTP) as a standard of practice.

In addition to advances in medical imaging, a virtual revolution in computer capability for radiation oncology occurred in the 1980s and continues in the 1990s, based largely on rapidly decreasing costs and increasing computer processor power and mass storage capability. Powerful CT simulation and 3DRTTP systems are now commercially available and are likely to replace the conventional radiation therapy x-ray simulator and two-dimensional (2-D) dose planning systems as the standard of practice early in the next century (7). These advances in treatment planning have prompted medical accelerator manufacturers to use advanced electronics and computer technology to produce sophisticated treatment delivery systems capable of precise shaping of dose distributions via computer-controlled multileaf collimators (MLC) and beam-intensity modulation (8,9).

TECHNICAL ASPECTS OF COMPUTED TOMOGRAPHY

Computed tomography consists of the reconstruction by computer of a tomographic plane of a patient's anatomy developed from multiple x-ray attenuation measurements made around the patient. The CT image is formed by using a mathematics technique known as reconstruction from projections. The data for the reconstruction process are obtained by rotating an x-ray source about the patient's body within a stationary circular array of detectors which provide x-ray transmission data in many different directions (10).

Once the data have been measured and stored in the computer, the processing of this information and image reconstruction begin. Simply stated, the reconstruction algorithm consists of calculating the linear attenuation coefficient for each pixel element and assigning a corresponding CT number to it. The CT scan is composed of individual volume elements, each with its own characteristic attenuation properties. These volume elements are reduced to a 2-D array of picture elements or pixels. The computer displays this array on a display monitor using varying shades of gray to represent the CT numbers. The CT numbers associated with the various tissues are related to the linear attenuation coefficient, μ, by the following equation:

$$\text{CT number} = \frac{K(\mu_{\text{tissue}} - \mu_{\text{water}})}{\mu_{\text{water}}}$$

in which K is a constant typically chosen to be 1000 (Hounsfield unit). Thus, it is the linear attenuation coefficient that is actually measured by a CT scan.

The CT numbers may be correlated with the electron density of the corresponding tissues, as shown in Figure 8.1. This correlation is important because for the types of photon beam used primarily in radiation therapy (cobalt 60 through 25 MV x-rays), Compton scattering is the dominant mode of interaction. In Compton scattering, the absorption and scattering of photons in tissue depend primarily on the electron density of the tissue, which is the pertinent parameter for photon beam inhomogeneity corrections used in current dose calculation algorithms.

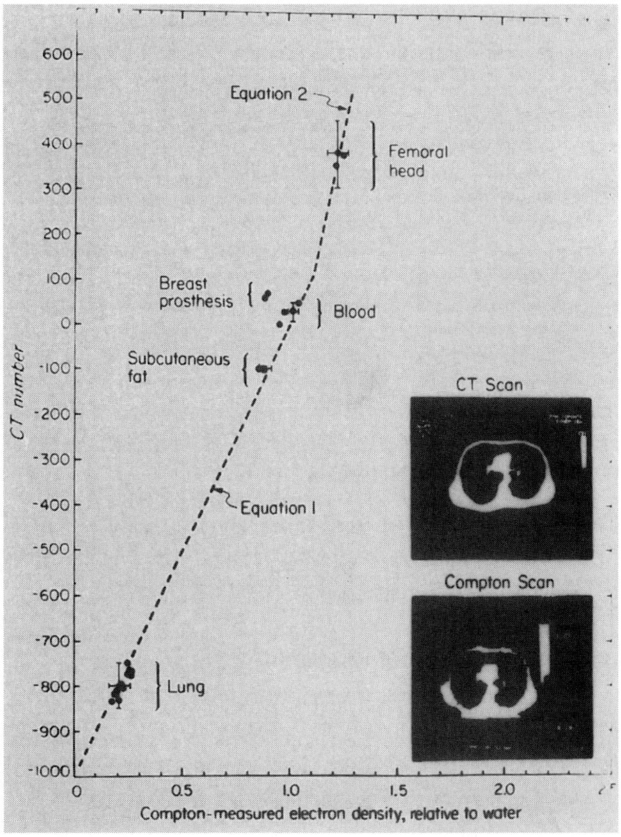

Figure 8.1. Relation of tissue computed tomography (CT) numbers to electron density (electrons per cm^3) in vivo. Patients were imaged by both CT and Compton scanning, and corresponding tissue regions in same patient were compared. For such regions, average CT number is plotted against average electron density, obtained by Compton scanning. Uncertainty bars correspond to standard deviations of individual tissue elements sampled and reflect heterogeneity of tissue in vivo. CT number scale used ranges from −1000 (air) to +1000 (twice attenuation of water). CT scanner was operated at 135 kVp, with 3 mm of added aluminum filtration (half-value thickness of 7.2 mm aluminum). (Reprinted with permission from Battista JJ, Rider WD, Van Dyk J. Computed tomography for radiation therapy planning. Int J Radiat Oncol Biol Phys 1980;6:99.)

Efforts continue in industry toward obtaining CT images for treatment planning using a conventional radiation therapy simulator (11). In these systems, referred to as *simulator-CT* systems, the image intensifier output at various angles about the patient is taken in the form of television raster scan lines, which are used to reconstruct a tomographic image in a manner that is similar to that used in conventional CT scanners. Although this approach appears useful for 2-D treatment planning, this system cannot be used for real 3DRTTP because scan times are on the order of 1 minute and resolution is well below that needed for good critical structure and target volume delineation.

This has led manufacturers to integrate a diagnostic CT scanner with features designed for radiation therapy with an advanced 3DRTTP computer. Such a system is referred to as a *CT-simulator* and provides many advanced image manipulation and viewing advantages including *beam's eye view* (BEV) display, which allows the anatomy to be viewed from the perspective of the radiation beams and allows field shaping electronically at the graphics display station. A CT-simulator introduces the concept of virtual simulation whereby the generation and comparison of BEV digitally reconstructed radiographs (DRRs) can be done in the absence of the patient. While some development work still remains (e.g., larger scan tunnel, improved image segmentation and correlation software), CT-simulators will likely render conventional simulators obsolete by the year 2000.

Table 8.1. 3-D Treatment Planning and Delivery Process

1. Pre-planning and Localization:	• Position patient in proposed treatment position • Fabricate immobilization devices • Mark repositioning lines on patient and immobilization devices • Obtain orthogonal localization images
2. CT Imaging Study:	• Perform volumetric CT scan of patient in treatment position
3. Dose-Volume Prescription:	• Transfer CT images to 3DRTTP system • Contour target and normal anatomy • Specify prescription dose and tolerance doses to critical structures
4. Treatment Planning:	• Setup initial beam geometry and portal shapes • Compute 3D dose matrix • Evaluate/optimize/approve treatment plan • Calculate treatment machine monitor unit setting • Physicist check
5. Plan Verification on Simulator: (optional)	• Verify patient position and isocenter placement using orthogonal DRR's and sim films • Compare treatment field DRR's with sim films
6. Treatment Verification:	• Initial verification of plan on treatment machine (orthogonal DRR's/films, treatment field DRR's/port films, diode measurement, record & verify • Periodic verification checks during treatment (orthogonal DRR's/films or DRR's/port films, record & verify)

THREE-DIMENSIONAL RADIATION THERAPY TREATMENT PLANNING

The routine use of three-dimensional treatment planning typically involves a series of procedures that are listed in Table 8.1 and are discussed in subsequent paragraphs.

Localization and Immobilization

An important part of the 3-D planning process is ensuring that the patient is in a treatment position consistent with the potential geometric beam arrangements that can be applied to the site being treated. This requires some discussion with the physician and other personnel involved in the planning process to ensure that treatment unit limitations are not encountered during the planning or implementation phase. After the treatment position has been established the patient must be immobilized in a reproducible manner such that the geometric parameters defined during the data acquisition can be accurately transferred from the CT-simulator to the virtual simulation or 3DRTTP system and ultimately reproduced on the treatment unit on the first day setup.

We have implemented an immobilization device registration system for indexing repositioning devices to the couch during each phase of our treatment planning process (Figure 8.2A–D). The registration of the immobilization device begins at the CT-simulation procedure where the patient's custom immobilization device is constructed and fitted to a registration device attached to the couch. The registration device consists of a plastic base plate with two nylon pins, 10 inches apart, and protruding upward from the couch top approximately 2 inches. The base plate attaches to all of the tables (CT scanner, x-ray simulator, and the treatment machines), providing a mounting mechanism for thermoplastic repositioning masks and custom foam Alpha Cradles. Once the immobilization device is constructed, table coordinates relative to a designated point on the registration device are established. These coordinates are the same on the CT simulator, the conventional simulator, and the linear accelerator tables. Because the immobilization device is securely attached and referenced to these tables, the daily setup is facilitated by driving the couch to a set of coordinates established at the time of 3-D planning. Provided the patient is securely immobilized, he or she will be accurately positioned for each treatment. This system has proven to be an easy method

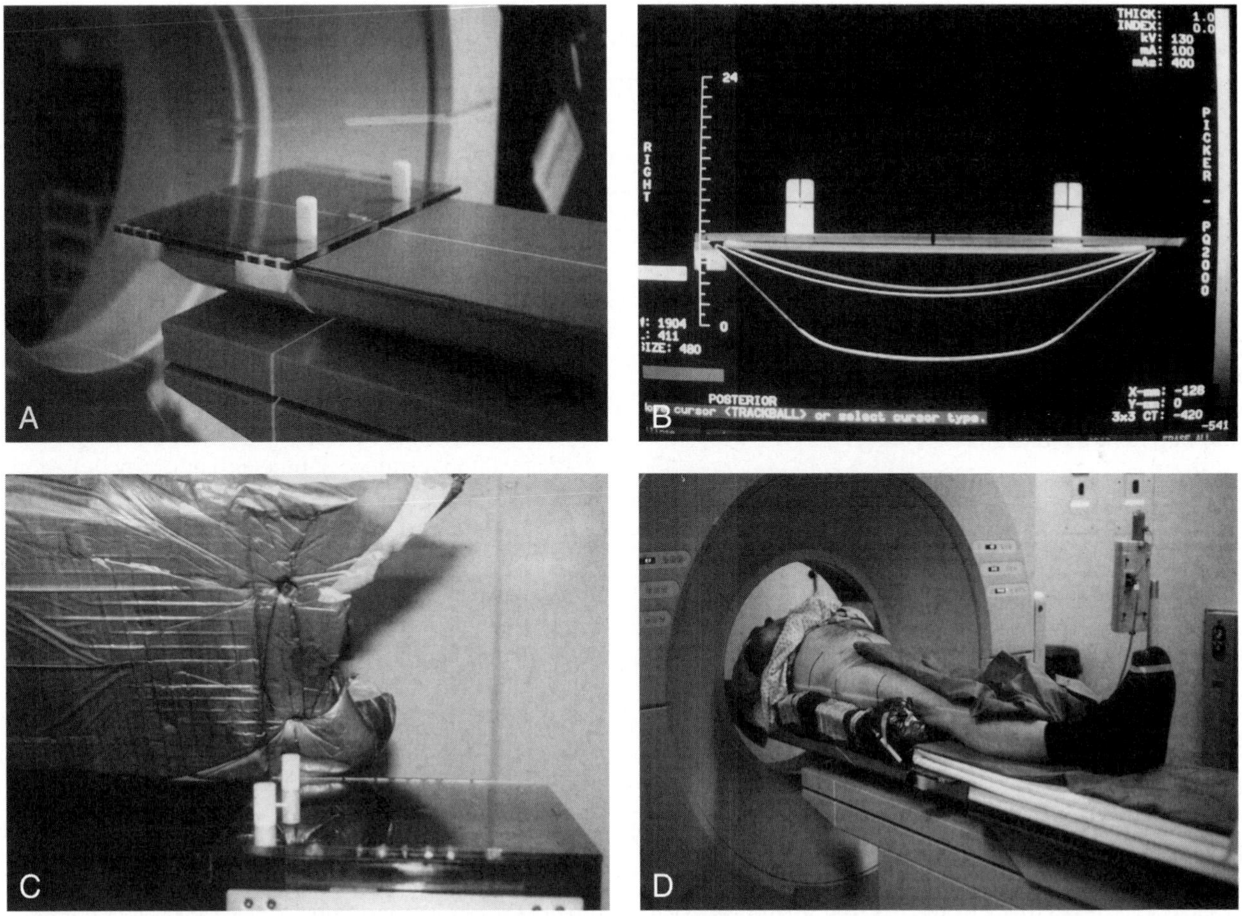

Figure 8.2. **A.** Plastic pegs attached to CT couch used to register (and fix) the immobilization device to the patient support couch (similar device on simulator and treatment machine) and aid in the establishment of a coordinate system for the planning and implementation of 3-DCRT; **B.** CT scan slice showing center of plastic pegs used to calibrate CT-simulator coordinate system; **C.** Alpha Cradle immobilization form being put in place utilizing plastic peg registration system; **D.** Prostate cancer patient in Alpha Cradle immobilization form held in place with plastic pegs in preparation for CT planning scan. Note multiple laser set-up points on the patient and positioning device to assist in coordinate transformation for 3D planning and eventual plan implementation.

for reconciling coordinate systems from data acquisition (CT scan) to treatment planning (virtual simulation/3-D planning system) to treatment delivery (linac) and aids in evaluating gantry-couch clearance issues for plan implementation.

While a variety of immobilizing casts and molds are currently in use for 3-D treatment, the majority of centers that have implemented 3-D therapy on a large scale are using combinations of thermoplastic masks and alpha cradles (12). At Mallinckrodt Institute of Radiology (MIR), thermoplastic masks are used for head and neck treatments, and alpha cradles are often used to build up and support the neck and shoulder areas. It is critical that the mask have a good fit around the chin, nose, and intercanthal areas to properly immobilize the patient. For chest and prostate treatments, our institution has employed alpha cradles that are larger than traditionally used. For chest treatments the alpha cradle is fabricated from the hips, up around the chest and shoulders, neck and head. The patients are immobilized with their arms above their head to keep the arms away from oblique beams. However, this may create an inherently unstable position, so the mold must be built up around the shoulders, neck, and arms to adequately support the arms in this position. For prostate patients the alpha cradle is made from the level of the waist to the knees. It is also important for the prostate patients to have their feet immobilized (at our institution the patient's feet are taped or banded together). Because alpha cradles are less immobilizing than masks or casts that fit over the patient, multiple laser light setup points are designated and marked on the patient and on the immobilizing device. These marks are used to properly position the patient in the alpha cradle each day for treatment. A reference line near the center of the volume also needs to be marked to serve as a reference for any required isocenter coordinate shifts after the planning is completed.

If the localization process begins in a conventional simulator, orthogonal radiographs are needed for confirming patient position and relative isocenter placement for comparison with the DRRs generated from the virtual simulation software. If the initial localization process begins in a CT-simulator, the scout or pilot films provide the initial orthogonal beam information and are used to check patient alignment. However, scout/pilot films from the scanner do not represent the patient data with divergence in the scanning axis but are representative of the patient in the other axis. Orthogonal DRRs generated from the volumetric data set provide the necessary image data for isocenter localization setup comparisons on the simulator or treatment machine.

CT Imaging Procedure

The next step is to obtain a volumetric CT scan of the patient. The CT data are the basis for 3DRTTP because they provide an accurate geometric model of the patient along with the electron density information needed for the calculation of inhomogeneity-corrected dose distributions. The CT study is performed with the patient in the treatment position determined in the pre-planning step, using any immobilization devices deemed necessary in the previous step. The skin marks are made visible on the CT images by the use of radio-opaque markers. The CT scan protocols used for 3-D planning are tumor site dependent and typically slice thickness ranges from 2 to 10 mm and the total number of slices from 50 to 120 slices. However, the introduction of spiral CT in the planning process has resulted in data sets as large as 200 slices, which greatly improve the quality of the DRR.

Tumor, Target Volume, and Critical Structure Delineation

In the next phase of the process, the CT scans are transferred to the 3DRTTP or virtual simulation system, typically via a local area computer network. The CT data are used to define the critical structures and tumor and target volumes. The CT data are displayed and contours are drawn around the tumor, target, and normal tissues on a slice-by-slice basis. In a 3DRTTP system, these contours can be used to generate realistic solid-shaded surface graphic representations of structures. 3-D displays of the patient data can be confusing when large numbers of structures overlap, but color, depth perception, and interactive manipulation of the image help to clarify the display.

Currently, automatic contouring of the CT data can be done only for those structures with distinct boundaries. For medium and low contrast structures, this task must be accomplished manually by trained professionals. This process can take as long as 1 hour for a complete 3-D CT series because typically many structures are of interest, depending on the site of the disease. Several different approaches have been investigated in an attempt to minimize the time spent in this step of the planning process. McShan et al developed a large screen digitizer system that they claim has accelerated contour entry considerably, contributing significantly to the clinical utility of 3-D planning in their clinic (13). Other groups are working on automated structure recognition algorithms (14).

Determining target volumes and organs at risk by drawing contours on the CT image on a slice-by-slice basis as opposed to drawing portals on a radiograph is a major paradigm shift for the radiation oncologist and treatment planner. Software for contouring normal structures and target volumes and virtual simulation that previously required a significant investment of time and effort by radiation oncology staff continue to be significantly improved as shown in Figure 8.3. The treatment planner/radiation oncologist can now draw contours around the tumor, target, and normal tissues on a slice-by-slice basis, and, at the same time, view a cross-reference to planar images from both AP and lateral projections. In addition, improved edit functions allow the user to move, scale, and rotate an entered contour in addition to providing tools for rapid corrections, changing the shape of a contour, automatic adjusting of a copied contour to fit a new organ boundary, and copying to inferior and superior slices. However, while software for the contouring task continues to improve, additional improvement is necessary to increase the efficiency of 3-D planning.

The recommendations for specifying volumes proposed in ICRU Report 50 are gaining widespread acceptance for 3-D radiation therapy (15). The ICRU Report 50 definition of target volume is now separated into the three distinct boundaries as illustrated in Figure 8.4. The *gross tumor volume* (GTV) is defined as the gross extent of the malignant growth as determined by palpation or imaging study. The terms $GTV_{Primary}$ and GTV_{Nodal} can be used to distinguish between primary disease and other areas of macroscopic tumor involvement such as involved lymph nodes. The *clinical target volume* (CTV) is defined as the tissue volume that contains a GTV and/or subclinical microscopic malignant disease. In specifying the CTV, the physician must consider microextensions of the disease in the vicinity of the GTV and the natural avenues of spread for the particular disease and site including lymph node, perivascular, and perineural extensions. The GTV and CTV are anatomic-clinical concepts that must be defined before a choice of treatment modality and technique is made. The *planning target volume* (PTV) is defined by specifying the margins that must be added around the CTV to compensate for the effects of organ, tumor, and patient movements and inaccuracies in beam and patient setup. The PTV is a static, geometric concept used for treatment planning and specification of dose. Its size and shape depend primarily on the GTV and CTV and the effects caused by internal motions of

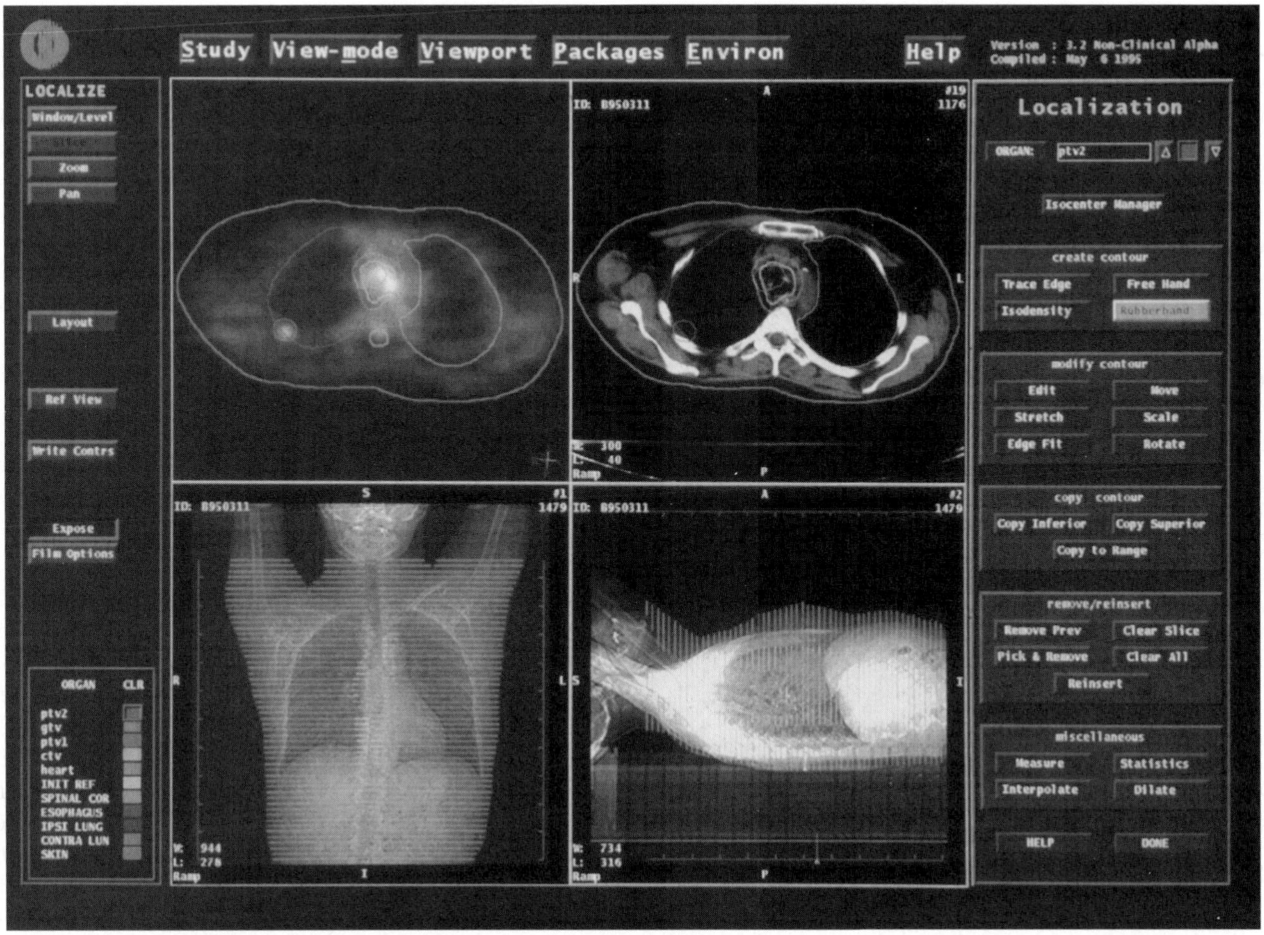

Figure 8.3. Image segmentation software provides tools for radiation oncologists and treatment planner to determine critical structures, tumor, and target volumes for 3-D planning. CT data are displayed and contours are drawn by the treatment planner/radiation oncologist around the tumor, target, and normal tissues on a slice-by-slice basis as seen in upper right panel. At the same time, planar images from both AP and lateral projections are displayed in bottom right and left panels. Upper left panel shows PET scan data with overlying contours after image registration with the CT data.

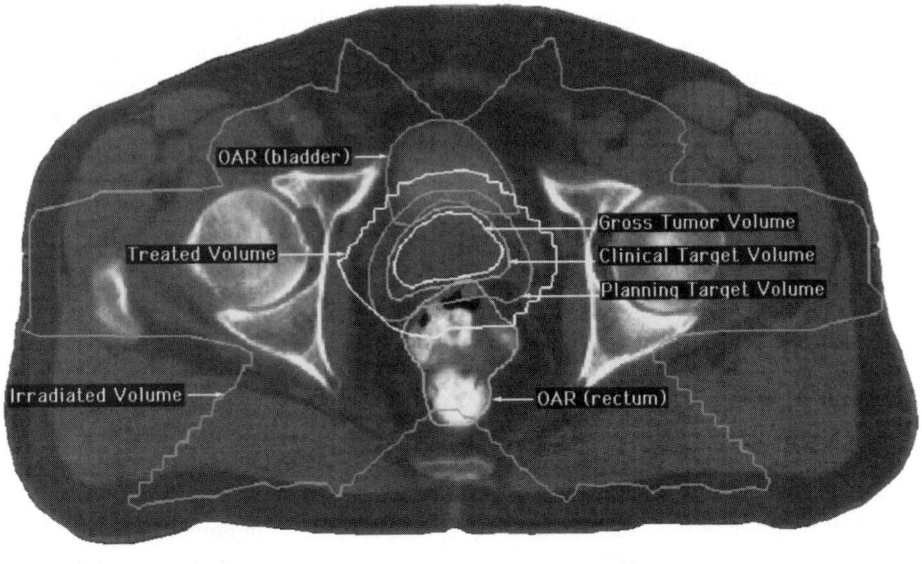

Figure 8.4. CT slice for prostate cancer patient showing the different contours of the volumes defined for 3DCRT by ICRU Report No. 50. *Gross Tumor Volume* (GTV), the demonstrated tumor; *Clinical Target Volume* (CTV), the demonstrated tumor (when present) and also volumes with suspected (subclinical) tumor (e.g., margin around the GTV); *Planning Target Volume* (PTV), consists of the CTV(s) and a margin to account for variations in size, shape, and position relative to the treatment beams(s); *Treated Volume,* the volume that receives a dose that is considered important for local cure or palliation; *Irradiated Volume,* the volume that receives a dose that is considered important for normal tissue tolerance (other than those specifically defined for organs at risk).

organs and the tumor as well as the treatment technique (beam orientation and patient fixation) used. The PTV can be considered a 3-D envelope fixed in space in which the tumor and any microscopic extensions reside. The GTV and CTV can move within this envelope, but not through it.

Once the PTV is defined, the beam geometry is determined. Beam apertures having appropriate margins are drawn around the PTV to provide the prescribed dose coverage. The definitions of two dose volumes have been retained from ICRU Report 29 pertaining to this task of the treatment planning process (16). They are the *treated volume,* which is the volume enclosed by an isodose surface that is selected and specified by the radiation oncologist as being appropriate to achieve the purpose of treatment (e.g., prescription isodose surface), and the *irradiated volume,* which is the volume that receives a dose considered significant in relation to normal tissue tolerance (e.g., 50% isodose surface).

Organs at risk are defined as normal tissues whose radiation sensitivity may significantly influence treatment planning or prescribed dose.

ICRU Report No. 50 recommends that dose to the PTV be reported for the *ICRU Reference Point,* along with the minimum, maximum, and mean dose. Information should be included about how the mean dose was computed to ensure consistency among reported mean dose values. In addition, dose volume histograms (DVHs), which will be discussed later, for PTVs and for all organs at risk should be reported to facilitate interpretation of treatment outcome and comparison of the relative merits of different techniques. Note that the prescription can be specified by the radiation oncologist at any one of the reported doses.

The ICRU Reference Point must be: a) defined in an unambiguous way and be clinically relevant; b) located where the dose can be accurately determined; and c) in a region in which there are no steep dose gradients. In general, this point is in the central part of the PTV. In cases where multiple beams intersect at a given point, the intersection point is recommended to be the ICRU reference point.

Using The ICRU Report 50 Recommendations

Purdy has reported on the use of the ICRU 50 recommendations in 3DRTTP which is summarized in this section (17,18). The physical treatment planning process is dependent on the delineation of the three volumes (GTV, CTV, and PTV) and the prescription of the target dose. These factors constitute the medical decision that must precede the determination of the dose distribution in the patient. The GTV, CTV, and PTV must be specified independent of the dose distribution: the GTV in terms of the patient's anatomy, the CTV in terms of the patient's anatomy or as a quantitative margin to be added to the GTV, and the PTV in terms of a quantitative margin to be added to the CTV to account for positional uncertainties.

When the GTV is delineated, it is important to use the appropriate CT window and level settings to determine the maximum dimension of what is considered to be potential gross disease. Defining the CTV is even more difficult than defining the GTV or any normal organs at risk and must be defined by the radiation oncologist based on clinical experience since current imaging techniques are not capable of detecting subclinical tumor involvement directly. Because most radiation oncologists are unfamiliar with defining target volumes and normal tissue on axial CT slices, assistance from a diagnostic radiologist is often needed in these early years of 3DRTTP. Image-based cross-sectional anatomy training is now needed in radiation oncology residency training programs as the radiation oncologist of the future will need to become much more expert in image recognition of normal tissue anatomy and gross tumor changes for accurate CTVs to be defined.

The PTV margin is specified by the radiation oncologist, in consultation with the radiation oncology physicist, based on clinical experience. Unfortunately, data for internal organ motion and setup error for most sites are lacking, although uncertainty studies addressing these issues for some sites (e.g., prostate) are increasingly being reported. When defining the PTV, the radiation oncologist must account for the asymmetric nature of positional uncertainties. For example, it is now recognized that prostate organ motion and daily setup errors may be anisotropic (side-to-side or rotational shifts of patients are likely to be different from movement in the anteroposterior direction). Thus, the PTV margin around a CTV should not, in general, be uniform.

Some limitations and practical issues must be clearly understood when the ICRU Report 50 methodology is used (17,18). Perhaps the most criticized limitation of this methodology is that positional uncertainties for normal structures are not accounted for. While this is a weakness, the practical utility of the PTV concept for planning and reporting 3DCRT (3-D conformal radiation therapy) results clearly overshadows this limitation. Another point of clarification is that ICRU Report 50 does not address directly how to combine the different positional uncertainties (e.g., setup and internal organ motion) that make up the PTV margin. Simple addition of the margins to account for each of their independent effects could make the PTV inappropriately large. A software model has been developed that creates the PTV based on a defined CTV using a biostatistical technique (the square root of the sum of the squares) (19). At Washington University, the radiation oncologist specifies the PTV margin as an estimate based on clinical experience, taking into account published literature and intramural uncertainty studies, and not treating it as a simple summation.

When a PTV overlaps with a contoured normal structure, a quandary is created as to which volume the overlapping voxels should be assigned to for DVH calculations. At Washington University, the overlapping voxels are assigned to both volumes. This ensures that the clinician is aware of the potential for this high-dose region to include the normal structure as well as the CTV/GTV when reviewing the DVHs.

Many 3DRTTP systems cannot account for a PTV contour that goes outside the skin surface. In those cases, one must accept the limitation that the PTV margin coincides with the skin surface.

In addition, one must understand that the PTV concept treats all points within the PTV as equally likely for the CTV to occupy all of the time, and this obviously does not occur in practice. A probabilistic approach in which the positional uncertainties are convolved mathematically with the dose calculation will likely evolve over the next several years. However, until such time, the ICRU Report 50 PTV methodology provides the most practical way to account for positional uncertainties to ensure coverage of the CTV.

Finally, the authors wish to emphasize that one of the most effective QA measures regarding 3DCRT plans is a weekly 3-D Case Review Conference where physicians, physicists, dosimetrists, and therapists review the plans using a high-resolution large screen video projector connected to the 3DRTTP network (Figure 8.5). GTV, CTV and PTV contours, DRRs and dose distributions can all be reviewed efficiently. This type of QA conference helps the staff to develop a consistent approach in implementing ICRU 50 methodology for specifying volumes and provides an effective peer review mechanism for a 3DCRT clinical program.

Designing Beams and Field Shaping

Design of the beam arrangement requires that the 3DRTTP system have the capability to simulate each of the treatment machine motion functions, including collimator length, width, and angle; gantry angle; couch angle; and couch latitude, longitude, and height position. This ability to orient beams in three dimensions allows the development of treatment plans that involve non-coplanar sets of fields. However, the effectiveness of this advanced capability is greatly improved if the 3DRTTP software truly models any beam setup limitations of the treatment machine in order to prevent wasted and inefficient time in the planning process.

An essential feature in a three-dimensional 3DRTTP system is the BEV display (Figure 8.6), in which the observer's viewing point is at the source of radiation looking out along the axis of the radiation beam (20–22). This type of display of the patient model is analogous to the simulator and port film. The BEV display is an extremely effective way to view the target volume(s) and normal structures, in that it quickly points out the regions that require shielding from the beam and clearly demonstrates the coverage of the target volume by the beam. Shielding blocks are designed on a 3-D system by drawing the block aperture on a BEV display with a light pen or joystick. In addition, modern 3DRTTP systems now have features that take advantage of the three-dimensional data to design the beam aperture automatically to encompass the planning target volume based on a prescribed margin.

The increased computational power of today's workstations permits real-time interactivity in many of the tasks of treatment planning and led to the development of the real-time Room-View display (23–24). Whereas the

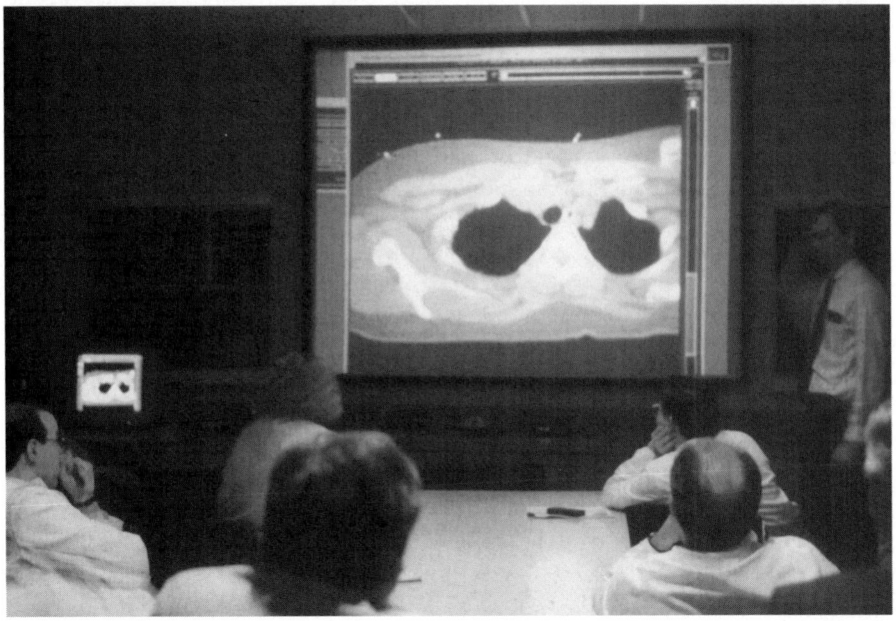

Figure 8.5. 3D Case Review Conference at MIR where physicians, physicists, dosimetrists, and therapists review the plans including GTV, CTV and PTV contours, DRRs and dose distributions, using a high resolution large screen video projector connected to the 3DRTTP network.

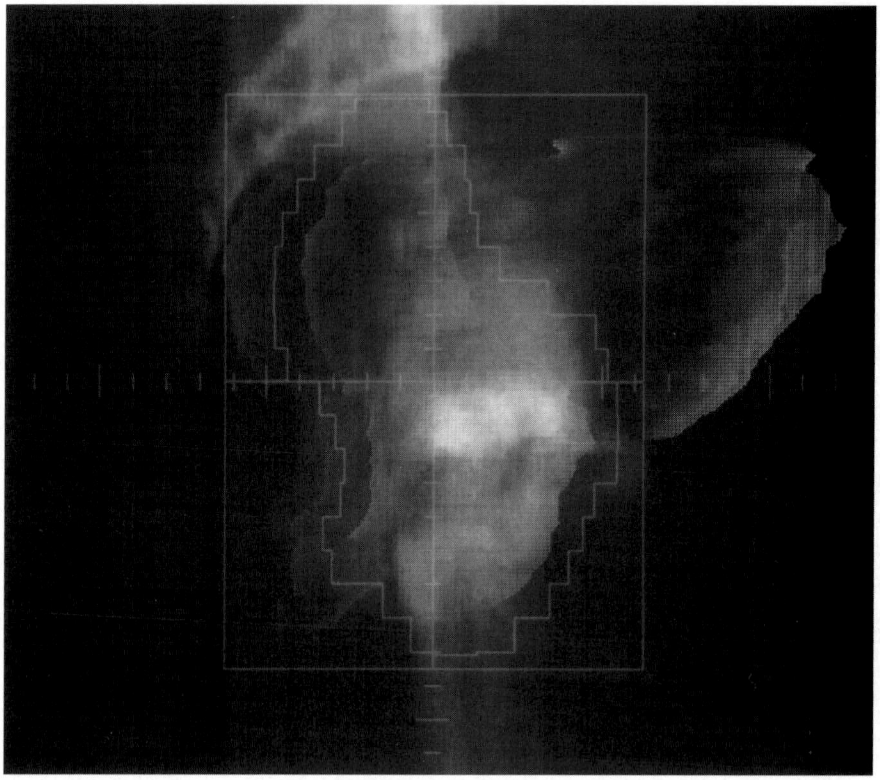

Figure 8.6. Beam's eye view (BEV) display is useful in identifying best gantry, collimator, and couch angles at which to irradiate target and avoid irradiating adjacent normal structures by interactively moving patient and treatment beam. Critical structures and target volumes are outlined on patient's serial CT sections. Contours are seen in perspective, as though observer's eye is at radiation source looking out along axis of the radiation beam. Outline of beam-shaping blocks are displayed.

BEV display provides the treatment planner a viewing point simulated at the source of radiation looking out along the axis of the radiation beam, the Room-View display illustrated in Figure 8.7 simulates any arbitrary viewing location within the treatment room. The real-time Room-View display significantly complements the BEV in the beam design phase of treatment planning, particularly in the positioning of the beam isocenter depth and in allowing for the display of all, or selected, beams to better appreciate the treatment technique geometry. The Room-View's display is even more valuable in the plan evaluation phase of 3DRTTP by providing a real-time capability for viewing 3-D isodose volumes.

Dose Calculation

After the initial plan(s) are designed, dose calculations are performed. In most 2-D planning, the dose calculations are done assuming all densities are that of water. The change in dose due to the presence of tissue inhomogeneities such as the lungs, bony structures, air cavities, and metal prostheses is related to the perturbation of the transport of primary and scattered photons and that of the secondary electrons set in motion from photon interactions. Depending on the energy of the photon beam, the shape, the size, and the constituents of the inhomogeneity, the resultant change in dose can be substantial.

Perturbation of photon transport is more noticeable for the lower energy beams, as appreciated by their larger mass attenuation coefficients. Usually, an increase in transmission, and therefore dose, occurs when the beam traverses a low-density inhomogeneity. The reverse applies when the inhomogeneity has a density higher than that of water. The change in dose usually is lessened, however, because of the concomitant decrease or increase in the scatter dose. For a modest lung thickness of 10 cm, the increase in the dose to the lung for the cobalt 60 and the 6 MV x-ray beams would be about 15%, reducing to about 5% for the 18 MV x-ray beams (25).

When there is a net imbalance of electrons leaving and entering the region near an inhomogeneity, a condition of electron disequilibrium is created. The effects are similar to those in the buildup region, near a beam edge, or in a small beam. Because electrons have finite travel, the resultant change in dose usually is local to the vicinity of the inhomogeneity and may be large. The effects are more noticeable for the higher photon energy beams because of their increased energy and range. Near the edge of the lungs and air cavities, the reduction in dose can be greater than 15% (26). For inhomogeneities with density greater than water, an increase in dose occurs locally simply because of the generation of more electrons. Most dense inhomogeneities, however, have atomic numbers higher than that of water such that the resultant dose perturbation

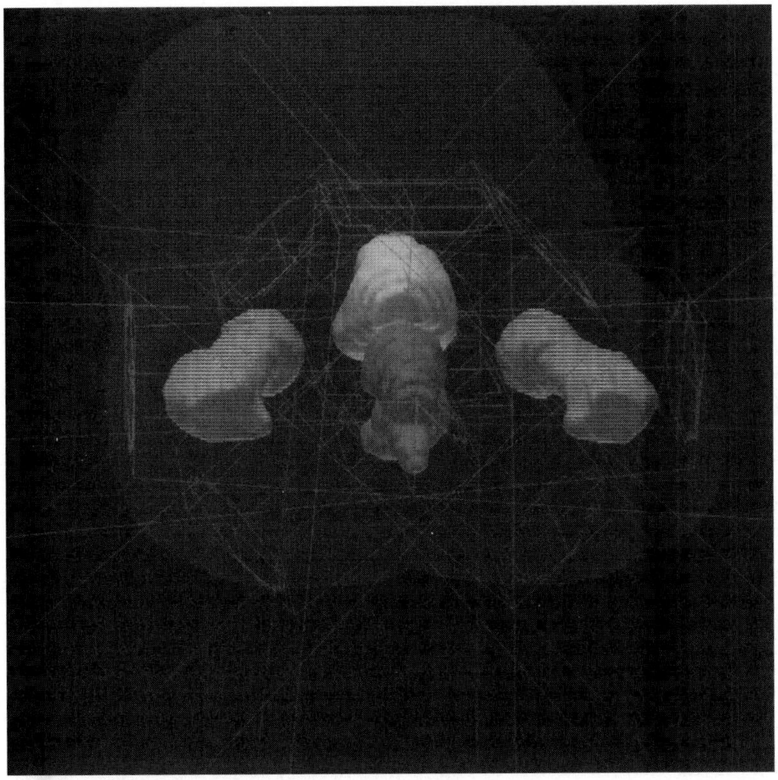

Figure 8.7. Real-time interactive Room-View display showing simulated patient and radiation beams is ideal for visualizing multi-beam arrangements and setting isocenter position during virtual simulation process.

is compounded further by the perturbation of the multiple coulomb scattering of the electrons. Near the interface between a bony structure and water-like tissue, large hot and cold dose spots can be present.

In the past, dose calculation methods have traditionally been based on parameterizing dose distributions measured in water phantoms under standard conditions and applying correction factors to the beam representations for the nonuniform surface contour of the patient or the obliquity of the beam, tissue heterogeneities, and beam modifiers such as blocks, wedges, and compensator. However, in the past decade, several, more advanced models have been developed for 3DRTTP that compute the dose more from first principles and only use a limited set of measurements to obtain a better fit of the model. Examples of the more advanced type algorithms include the superposition/convolution method developed by Mackie and associates (27) and the differential pencil beam method developed by Mohan and colleagues (28). The reader is referred to published reviews for the rigorous mathematical formalism of dose calculation algorithms as only a brief review is presented here (25,29).

These 3DRTTP methods utilize convolution energy deposition kernels that describe the distribution of dose about a single primary photon interaction site. The convolution kernels are most often obtained by using the Monte Carlo method to interact monoenergetic primary photons at the origin in a phantom and to transport the charged particles and scattered and secondary photons that are set in motion. The energy that gets deposited about the primary photon interaction site is tabulated and stored for use in the convolution method. In addition to describing how scattered photons contribute to dose absorbed at some distance away from the interaction site of primary photons, the convolution kernels take into account charged particle transport. This information can be used to compute dose in electronic disequilibrium situations such as occurs in the buildup region and in the beam penumbra.

Eventually, the direct use of Monte Carlo simulations will likely be the preferred method for 3DRTTP dose computation. It is the only method capable of computing the dose accurately near interfaces of materials with dissimilar atomic numbers, as, for example, near metal prostheses. Researchers are actively working on reducing the computation time to make this approach practical (30,31). As the price/performance ratio of computer workstations continues to decrease by almost a factor of two each year, Monte Carlo simulation should be practical for 3DRTTP dose computation sometime early in the next century.

Plan Optimization and Evaluation

Conventional 3DCRT plan optimization relies on iterative, interactive geometric plan optimization, which is more accurately described as plan improvement as opposed to automated computer optimization. Typically, the initial beam arrangement is selected based primarily on clinical experience using BEV and Room-View displays. The 3-D display of the dose distribution is a critical part of the evaluation methodology, as the dosimetrist and radiation oncologist must be able to decipher a huge amount of data in a relatively short time. Planning tools that can spotlight the areas of particular concern for a certain plan are essential. Numerous types of presentations of the anatomic and dosimetric information are useful in 3DRTTP, including DVH (32); multilevel 2-D displays showing isodose lines superimposed on CT images or as a spectrum of colors superimposed on the anatomic information (color wash); and 3-D dose surfaces (24). In addition, biologic models of normal tissue complication probability (NTCP) and tumor control probability (TCP) are now being used by some research groups in evaluating treatment plans.

The review of 3-D dose distributions using only multiple 2-D transverse sections is difficult, but displays that present multiple views of reconstructed sections, such as sagittal and coronal sections, on a single screen are helpful. Arbitrary plane sections may yet prove to be of some use, but they are difficult to interpret. No doubt, the DVH as shown in Figure 8.8 is one of the most useful 3-D plan evaluation tools. A set of DVHs provides a complete summary of the entire 3-D dose matrix showing the amount of target volume or critical structure receiving more or less than a specified dose level. They do not, however, give the spatial information and thus must complement, not replace, spatial dose distribution displays. The DVH display effectively points out the critical structures that are overdosed as well as any target volume(s) that may be underdosed.

In addition to DVHs, Room-View 3-D isodose surface displays with real-time interactivity (Figure 8.9) are invaluable for the efficient evaluation of the dose distribution and complement the DVH in providing spatial dose information. This type of display enables the treatment planner to view the target volume or normal tissue volume(s) with superimposed isodose surfaces from any arbitrary viewing angle, and thus it is extremely useful for evaluating adequate coverage of the target volumes and sparing of critical structures.

Three-dimensional radiation therapy treatment planning has renewed the interest in automatic computer optimization in an effort to improve efficiency as the planner has to deal with so much more information. Automatic computer optimization can be better understood by considering it as made up of two components: 1) an objective (score) function which describes a figure of merit of a par-

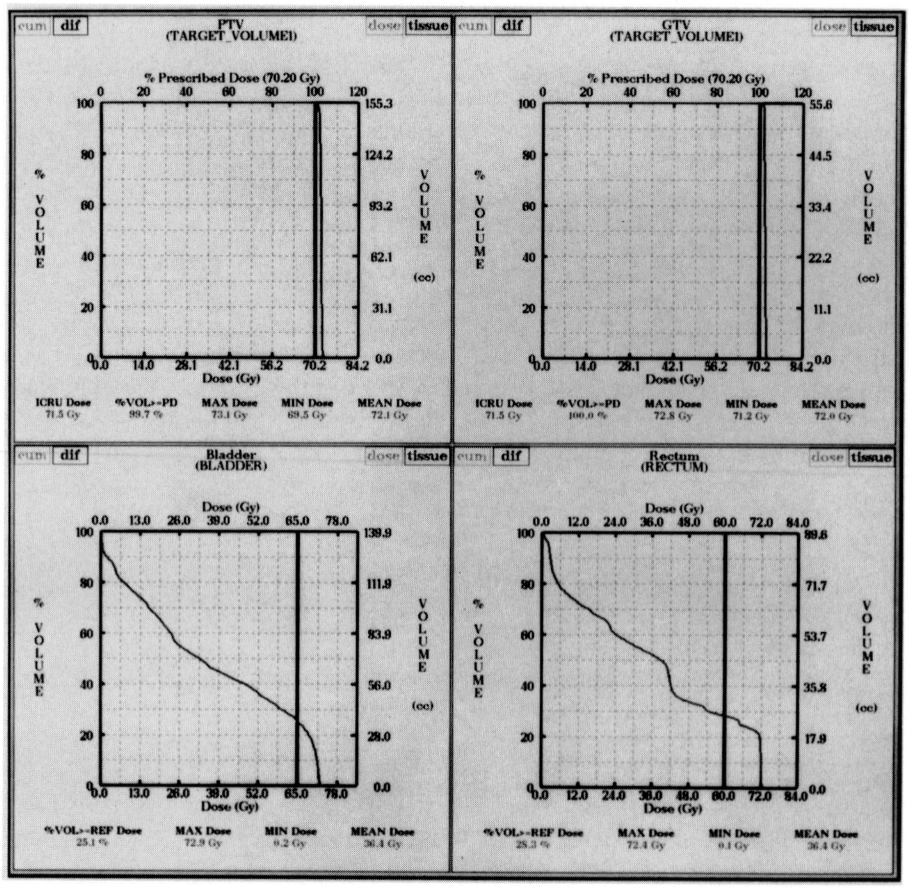

Figure 8.8. Dose-volume histograms (DVH) provide complete summary of entire dose-volume data, showing amount of target volume or critical structure receiving more or less than a specified dose level. Shown is the cumulative DVH's for prostate cancer patient treated with 3DCRT for the planning target volume (PTV); gross target volume (GTV); bladder; and rectum.

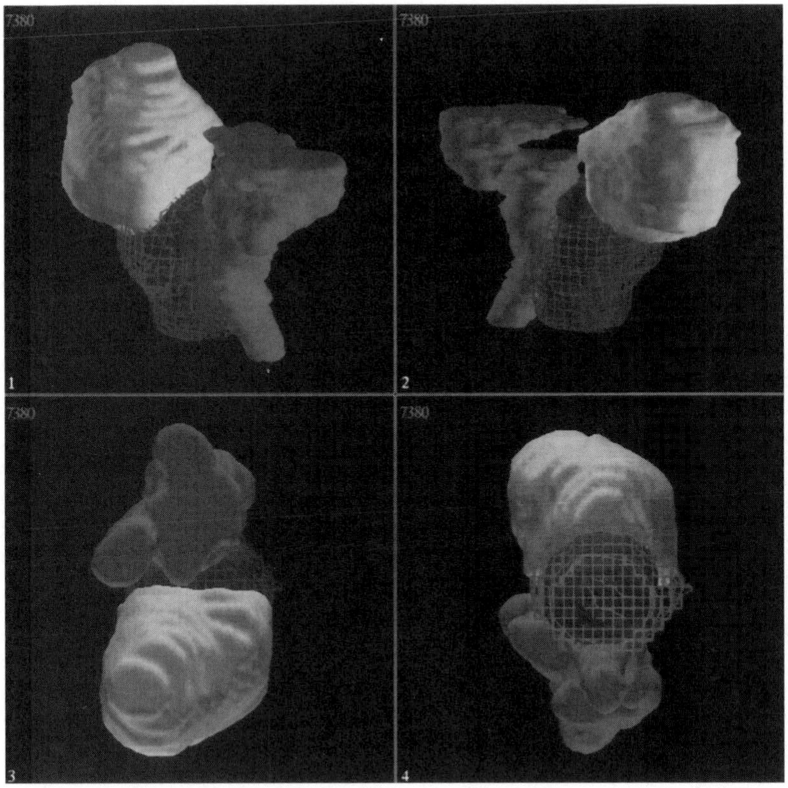

Figure 8.9. Room-View 3D isodose surface display with real-time interactivity is a valuable tool for evaluation of 3D dose distributions in terms of adequate coverage of target volumes and sparing of critical structures. The Room-View display enables radiation oncologists to view target volume or normal tissue volume with superimposed isodose surfaces or "dose clouds" from any arbitrary viewing angle. Shown is a four window Room-View display of the 73.8 Gy isodose volume, the prostate PTV, bladder, and rectum of a prostate cancer patient treated with a 7-field technique. The location of the PTV region not covered by the specified dose are easily discernible using this type display.

ticular plan that is to be maximized or minimized; and 2) an optimization (search) algorithm that searches the domain of plan variables to find the optimal plan; i.e., the set of plan parameters that maximize/minimize the chosen objective function subject to specified constraints. A recent review of the various computer optimization methods being investigated for 3DRTTP is provided by Niemierko (33).

Objective functions that have been utilized include those based on dose-volume criteria such as minimum dose to the target volume and/or some dose-volume constraint on critical normal structure volumes. More recently, objective functions have been expressed in terms of biological indices such as some weighted combination of TCP and NTCPs. The development of robust TCP and NTCP models that accurately predict clinical outcome will emerge from the 3DCRT era as dose-volume outcome data is gathered and analyzed, but to date these models should be viewed with some skepticism.

One of the most promising search algorithms for 3DRTTP is simulated annealing which was first applied to radiation therapy plan optimization in 1989 (34). This algorithm is derived from statistical mechanics and attempts to mimic the behavior of a system of interacting particles that are progressively cooled and allowed to maintain thermal equilibrium while reaching the ground state. With this approach, there is no restriction on the order (e.g., quadratic) of the objective functions or on the number of constraints. In addition, it has the ability to escape from local minimum of the objective function, and thus find the global minimum, i.e., the best plan. However, simulated annealing is generally slower than the deterministic optimization algorithms that have been used in the past for computer optimization, and thus, from a practical standpoint, may limit the search domain (e.g. table and couch positions).

Today, the term "inverse method" is being used to describe most forms of automated computer optimization. That is, in this method, a physician prescribes the dose distribution (objective function constraints) as input into the computer planning system and the computer then determines the beam geometries, including the nonuniform beam intensities for intensity modulated radiation therapy (IMRT), required to generate the dose distribution. Strictly speaking, Brahme and associates are generally credited as the first to state the radiation therapy optimization problem in terms of an inverse-method of treatment design (35). Their method was similar to the problem of reconstructing a tomographic image from projections at many angles.

Plan objective function and optimization search algorithms are an important research area for 3DCRT with no clear winner established as yet. As computer power increases, the optimization search algorithm will likely not pose the real problem for practical widespread implementation of computer optimization. Rather, the more difficult problem is likely to be the development of robust optimi-

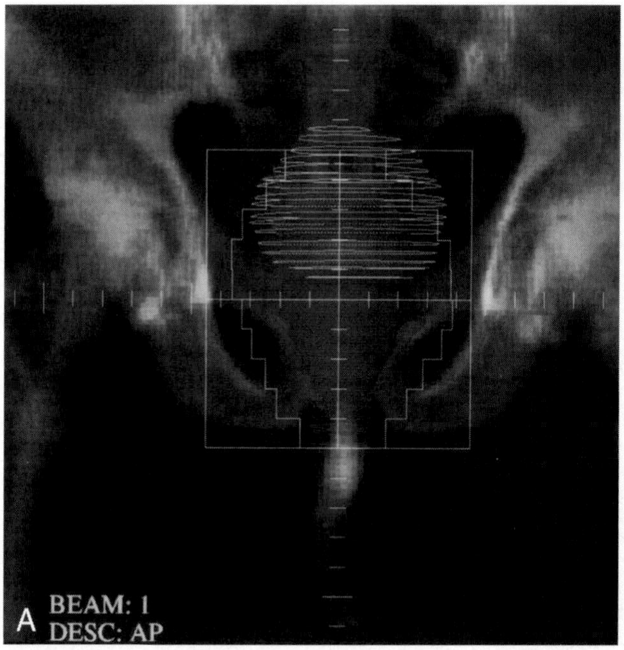

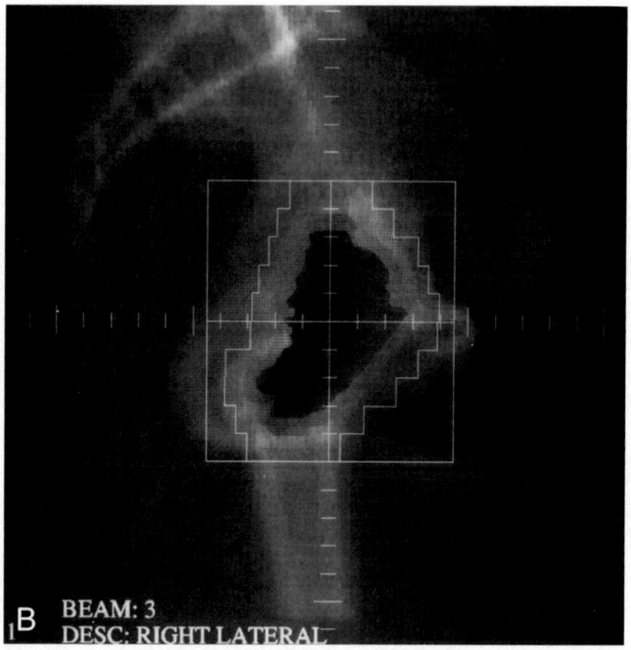

Figure 8.10. **A.** Anterior/posterior digitally reconstructed radiograph (DRR) for prostate cancer patient illustrating target volume, bladder, and outline of treatment portal. **B.** Lateral digitally reconstructed radiograph with structures and treatment portal outline. Similar orthogonal simulator or portal films can be taken with the patient in treatment position and compared to the orthogonal DRRs.

zation objective functions that will be applicable to the diverse population of cancer patients and also satisfy individual physician preferences. Until such objective functions are developed, inverse planning will more resemble the iterative forward approach in which a physician will be forced to review the dose distribution and make changes to the objective function input until an acceptable plan is obtained.

Plan Implementation and Treatment Verification

A verification simulation procedure is sometimes used to confirm the validity and accuracy of a 3-D CT-based treatment plan. To be effective, the 3DRTTP system must have the capability of generating DRRs from the CT data for comparison with verification simulation radiographs (22,36) as shown in Figure 8.10A and 8.10B. The DRR provides a plane film representation with the same perspective as a simulator or portal film. The target volume and critical structure contour ring stacks as well as the beam-defining apertures can be superimposed on the DRR to aid the radiation oncologists in their understanding of 3-D volumetrics.

For the verification simulation procedure, the patient is placed on the simulator table in the treatment position, using the immobilization device employed in the initial plan localization. Orthogonal radiographs are taken and then compared to the original simulator radiographs if obtained in the plan localization simulation or orthogonal DRRs. After verification of the treatment isocenter, the treatment fields are filmed and compared to the DRRs prepared from the plan. This tedious verification check is extremely important, because with many 3-D plans utilizing noncoplanar fields, one cannot identify reliably the normal anatomy on portal films taken from unusual oblique angles.

Finally, beam arrangements developed using 3DRTTP systems must be verified for accurate implementation on the treatment machine. The customary first day isocenter verification and treatment port film and subsequent weekly check procedure is typically used. Any extreme or unusual beam orientation may require more frequent verification. Online electronic portal imaging systems are just now coming into use and may allow more frequent verification of each treatment. Several systems, such as the matrix ionization device and TV camera-based units, are now commercially available but more development work is needed before the systems can replace film totally (37).

COMPUTER-CONTROLLED CONFORMAL RADIATION THERAPY TREATMENT MACHINES

One of the major driving forces behind the implementation of 3DCRT has been the development of the MLC (Figure 8.11) (38–40). To perform any kind of conformal field shaping, it was necessary to develop an individualized beam aperture out of a lead-based shielding material. To treat the patient with more than one field, the therapist was forced to enter the treatment room and change the field aperture manually. The MLC replaces the simple rectangular jaw system on the treatment machine with a set of thin blades that can be individually positioned, under computer control. The MLC, which typically has between 26 and 40 pairs of leaves that are 1.0 to 1.25 cm wide (projected to 100 cm), can therefore create an individually shaped beam aperture under computer control and without a therapist having to enter the treatment room. The ability to change the field shape without a manual action by a treatment therapist makes computer control of other functions of the treatment machine take on new importance. One can easily consider using the computer control system to automatically move the machine between field positions, since the field shaping can now be accomplished by the MLC.

The new computer-controlled treatment machines are much more sophisticated than the previous generation of medical linear accelerators (linacs). The new generation of linacs are now capable of performing what is called computer-controlled conformal radiation therapy (CCRT) (41,42). Currently, two different kinds of CCRT have been defined. *Segmental CCRT* uses fixed beam portals ("segments"), where multiple segments of the treatment are delivered automatically under computer control. *Dynamic CCRT* involves motion of the linac and MLC while the beam is on.

Most CCRT development work currently is based on computer-controlled but otherwise somewhat standard medical accelerators equipped with MLCs (42,43). However, other approaches are also possible, as illustrated by the use of fully computer-controlled industrial robots, equipped with a small linear accelerator at the end of the robot arms (44). This device, based on relatively standard industrial robot technology, can be used for treating small tumors in a highly conformal way. However, this type of treatment is just beginning its testing, and much work remains to be done before it is in routine clinical use.

The latest development in dynamic CCRT exploits techniques in which beam intensity is varied across the field. This has been referred to as intensity-modulated radiation therapy (IMRT). This approach is capable of generating concave dose distributions and providing specific sparing of sensitive normal structures within complex treatment geometries. The beam intensity is made to be proportional to the target thickness as assessed from a BEV as the beam rotates around the patient. Where the target is "thickest," the beam intensity is at its greatest; where it is at its thinnest, the intensity is at its lowest. IMRT is discussed in detail in Chapter 10.

These new technologies change the kinds of treatments that are possible, and this changes the process with which treatment planning and treatment delivery are performed. It is clear that 3-D radiation therapy shows significant potential for improving the quality of radiation therapy and will, in the long run, improve the efficiency with which it can be delivered once the systems are integrated and networked.

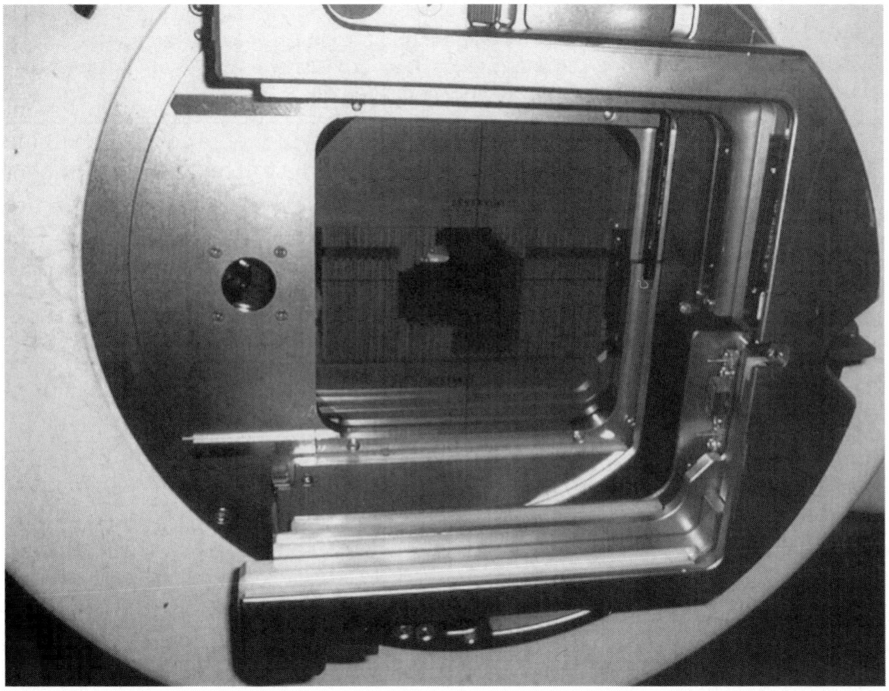

Figure 8.11. Medical linac equipped with multileaf collimator (MLC) system. The development of the MLC has been a major driving force behind the implementation of 3DCRT. The ability to change the field shape without a manual action by a treatment therapist makes computer control of other functions of the treatment machine take on new importance.

3DCRT CLINICAL STUDIES

Prostate Cancer

Between January 1992 and December 1995, a total of 119 patients were treated at our institution with 3DCRT and 138 with standard radiation therapy (SRT) for clinical stage A2 (T1c) or B (T2) histologically confirmed carcinoma of the prostate. The pelvic lymph nodes were electively irradiated (45 Gy in 5 weeks) in 11 patients in the 3DCRT and 32 in the SRT groups. Mean follow-up for all patients is 1.4 years (1 to 4 years).

Standard irradiation consisted of bilateral 120-degree rotational arcs, with portals approximately 10 × 12 cm (2 cm margins around the prostate) to deliver 68 to 70 Gy to the prostate.

For 3DCRT following ICRU 50 guidelines, GTV for stages A2 and B (T1c, T2) was the prostate. The CTV was arbitrarily set as 0.5 cm around the prostate for stage A2 and B1 tumors and 0.8 to 1 cm around the prostate and seminal vesicles for stage B2 (0.5 cm in the rectal area). The PTV was 0.8 to 1 cm in all patients. Four anterior and posterior oblique fields, one anterior, and two lateral fields were used (Cerrobend blocks or MLC) (Figure 8.7) to deliver 68 to 73.8 Gy to the prostate (the latter as participants in Radiation Therapy Oncology Group [RTOG] protocol 94-06). Patients with B2 lesions were treated to the whole pelvis with four fields (45 Gy) and additional dose to complete 67 to 70 Gy with SRT or 3DCRT techniques. Treatment planning was carried out in all patients; isodose curves were generated, and percent of target volume receiving maximum, mean, and minimum tumor dose was determined. In all 3-D planned and in 87 bilateral arc patients, DVHs were calculated for GTV, PTV, bladder, rectum, and femora (Fig. 8.8).

Tumor control was assessed by periodic rectal examination and serial prostate-specific antigen (PSA) determinations; when indicated, radiographic or radionuclide scan studies were obtained. The criterion for chemical disease-free survival was postirradiation PSA value of 1.5 or 2 ng/ml or less at all follow-up evaluations.

Acute morbidity of therapy was assessed on a weekly basis in specially designed forms (graded from 0 to 4), and late morbidity was evaluated at periodic follow-up.

Time and Effort for Three-Dimensional Conformal or Standard Irradiation

Average time and effort for contouring of the target volume and sensitive structures were 66 minutes. In the virtual simulation and plan evaluation, both the physics/dosimetry staff and the radiation oncologist closely interacted to subjectively identify the plan most appropriate for the individual patient; the average time was 55 minutes.

Average time for plan preparation and documentation was 39 minutes, and for physical simulation, 65 minutes. The radiation oncologist is responsible for final approval of the plan and verification radiographs, which take approximately 20 minutes.

Greater familiarity of the staff and simplification of 3DCRT techniques have already resulted in significant savings in time and effort. Furthermore, having several VOXEL-Q devices (Picker Corp., St. Davids, PA.) for contouring and networking to transfer information throughout the radiation oncology facility has resulted in greater ability and efficiency to define target and normal tissue volumes, which has facilitated the optimization of dose distributions.

The maximum and mean average patient daily treatment times with 3DCRT and SRT were calculated (16 minutes with seven-field MLC 3DCRT, 19 minutes with Cerrobend blocking 3DCRT, and 10 minutes with SRT) (45).

Dosimetric Analysis

On 3-D isodose curves or DVHs, either bilateral-arc rotation or 3DCRT provided similar coverage of the target volume. However, significantly less volume (about 50%) of bladder and rectum received doses greater than 65 or 70 Gy with 3DCRT (Table 8.2).

Chemical Disease–Free Survival

In both the 3DCRT and SRT groups chemical disease-free survival was equivalent for patients with clinical stage A2 (T1c) or B (T2) tumors. Comparison of treatment outcome is made merging both clinical stage groups.

Mean follow-up is 1.4 years; preliminary analysis shows no difference in chemical disease-free survival using a postirradiation PSA level of 1.5 ng/ml as an arbitrary end point (Figure 8.12A). If a postirradiation level of

Table 8.2. Comparison of Mean Dosimetric Parameters for 3-D Conformal or Standard Bilateral Arc Rotation Radiation Therapy in Carcinoma of Prostate

	Prostate Irradiation Only	
Parameter	3-D Conformal Therapy	Standard Therapy
Number of observations	87	87
Percent PTV receiving ≥ prescribed dose	92.9 ± 13.9	92.9 ± 10.8
ICRU dose (Gy)	69.1 ± 2.6	69.2 ± 2.6
Minimum tumor dose (Gy)	66.3 ± 5.3	63.5 ± 8.6
Mean tumor dose (Gy)	69.8 ± 2.6	69.7 ± 2.8
Maximum dose (Gy)	71.7 ± 2.4	71.3 ± 2.8
Percent volume rectum ≥65 Gy	33.7 ± 15	62.7 ± 21
Percent volume rectum ≥70 Gy	8.5 ± 11.8	28.8 ± 28.9
Percent volume bladder ≥65 Gy	22.3 ± 12.5	50.5 ± 22.8
Percent volume bladder ≥70 Gy	6.3 ± 8.4	19.4 ± 24.4

Reprinted with permission from Perez CA, Michalski J, Ballard S, et al. Cost benefit of emerging technology in localized carcinoma of the prostate. Int J Radiat Oncol Biol Phys, 1997;39(4):875–883.

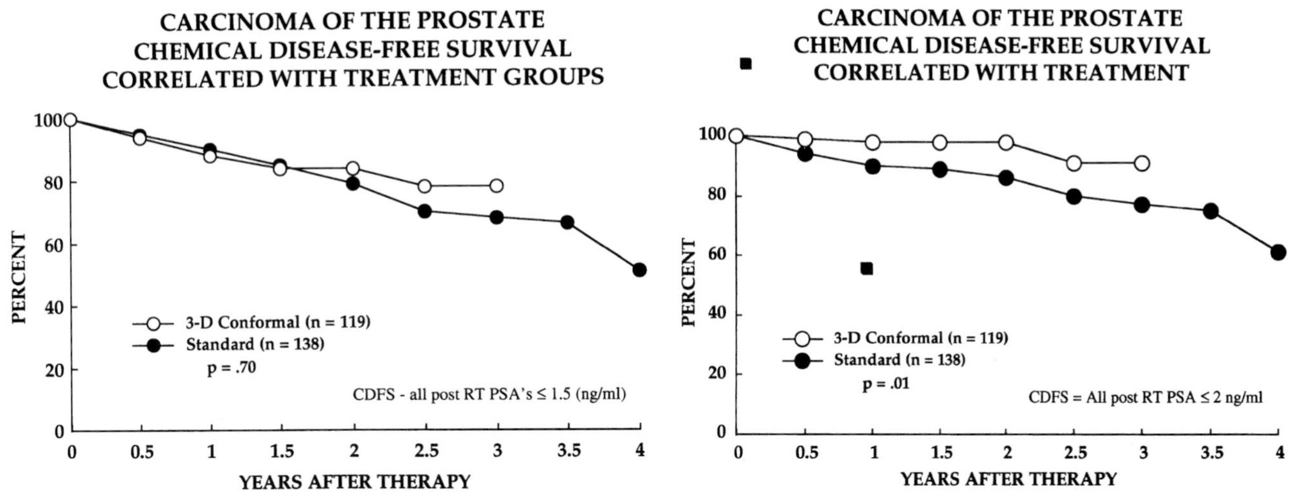

Figure 8.12. Chemical disease-free survival for stage T1b,c and T2 patients with postirradiation PSA of ≤1.5 ng/ml **(A)** or postirradiation PSA of 2 ng/ml **(B)** correlated with treatment technique (84).

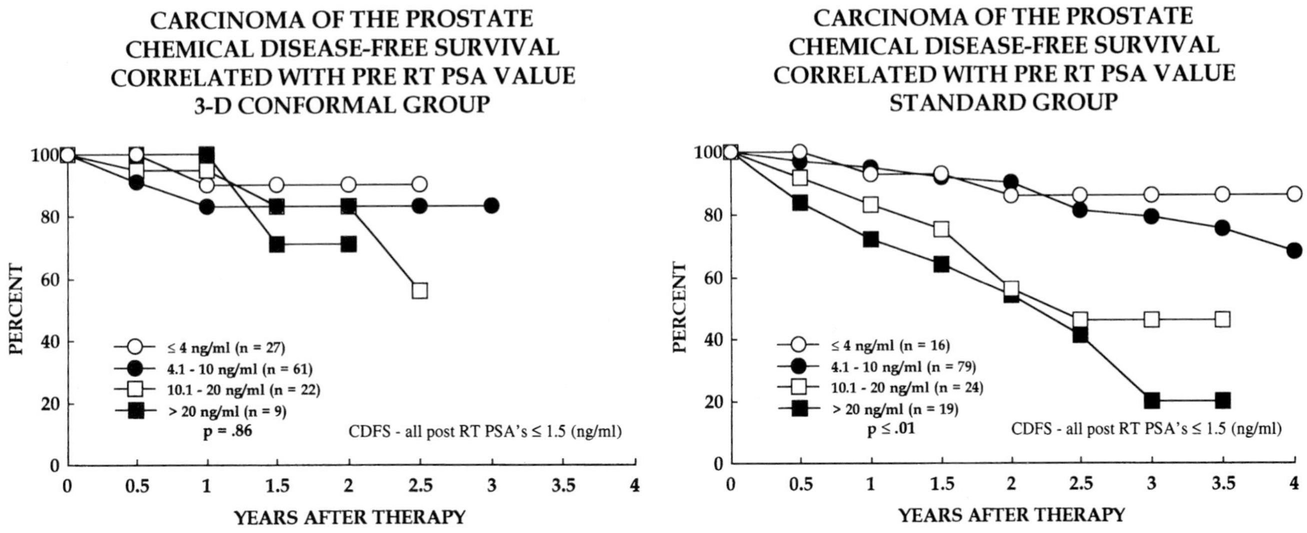

Figure 8.13. Chemical disease-free survival correlated with pretreatment PSA values for patients treated with **(A)** 3-D conformal radiation therapy or **(B)** standard irradiation.

2 ng/ml is used, the 3-year survival rates are 90% with 3DCRT and 80% with standard bilateral-arc rotation (P = .01) (Figure 8.12B).

There is no statistically significant difference (P = .15) in chemical disease-free survival in either treatment group when correlated with histologic tumor differentiation (Gleason score). However, in both treatment groups chemical disease-free survival is higher (80% at 3 to 4 years) in patients with pretreatment PSA levels below 10 ng/ml (Tandem-R, Hybritech). In contrast, in patients with PSA higher than 10 ng/ml, chemical disease-free survival is better in the 3-D CRT group (70 to 90%) than in the SRT group (20 to 45%) (P = .01) (Figure 8.13A and 8.13B).

At this time, there is no significant difference in survival in the 3DCRT patients treated with irradiation doses higher than 67 Gy; this may be a reflection of more adequate coverage of the target volume. However, in the SRT group there is a strong trend toward improved survival with higher doses (difference not statistically significant, P = .10).

Acute Toxicity

Moderate difficulty in urinating was reported by 6 to 9% of patients treated with SRT in contrast to 2 to 5% of patients treated with 3DCRT. Moderate dysuria and noctu-

Table 8.3. Carcinoma of the Prostate: Late Sequelae Correlated with Treatment Group

	3-D Conformal Therapy (n = 119)		Standard Radiation Therapy (n = 138)	
	Grade 2	Grade 3	Grade 2	Grade 3
Proctitis	4 (3%)		16 (12%)	
Perianal abscess				1 (.7%)
Small bowel obstruction				1 (.7%)
Cystitis			4 (3%)	
Urethral stricture	2 (2%)		1 (.7%)	

Note: The statistical significance of the incidence of proctitis in the two treatment groups is P = 0.01.
Reprinted with permission from Perez CA, Michalski J, Ballard S, et al. Cost benefit of emerging technology in localized carcinoma of the prostate. Int J Radiat Oncol Biol Phys, 1997;39(4):875–883.

ria were reported by 25 to 36% of patients in the SRT group and 27 to 33% treated with 3DCRT. Differences are not statistically significant.

The incidence of moderate (grade 2) diarrhea, usually after the fourth week of treatment, was 9 to 21% in the SRT group and 3 to 6% in the 3DCRT patients. Grade 2 rectal morbidity (proctitis, rectal bleeding) was low (3%) in the 3DCRT group in contrast to 12% in the SRT patients (Table 8.3) (P = .01).

As in our experience, decreased toxicity has been observed by others with 3DCRT, even when higher-than-standard irradiation doses are administered. Hanks et al (46) reported 34% grade 2 toxicity in 247 patients treated with conformal irradiation in comparison with 57% in 162 patients receiving standard radiation therapy. Sandler et al (47), in an update of their experience in 721 patients treated with 3DCRT, noted only 3% incidence of grade 3 and 4 rectal morbidity, similar to our experience.

Improved tumor control and disease-free survival with 3DCRT, in comparison with SRT, have been reported. Leibel et al (48), in an update of preliminary results on 324 patients with carcinoma of the prostate (48 with stage T1c, 39 with stage T2a, 135 with stage T2b,c, and 102 with stage C), irradiated a PTV defined as 1 cm margin around the identifiable prostate gland, except at the interface with the rectum where a 0.6 cm margin was used, on a dose-escalation protocol (64.8 to 66.6 Gy in 70 patients, 70.2 Gy in 102, 75.6 Gy in 57, and 81 Gy in 25 patients). The overall 3-year actuarial PSA normalization rate was 97% in patients with stage T1c-T2a, 86% with T2b, 60% with stage T2c, and 43% with stage C tumors. Only 15% of patients had grade 2 or 3 acute morbidity, and 34% exhibited urinary sequelae requiring short-term medication; only one patient (0.4%) has developed a severe late complication. Hanks et al (49) observed a 50% 4-year actuarial survival in 373 patients treated with conformal irradiation and 39% in 129 patients receiving conventional radiation therapy. Median follow-up was short (14 months for 3DCRT patients and 50 months for the SRT group).

The benefit of 3DCRT is hypothetically linked to improved local tumor control because of better coverage of the target volume with a specific dose of irradiation, less acute and late morbidity, possibility of carrying out dose-escalation studies if morbidity is held to acceptable levels, and improved survival. Several institutions, RTOG, and 10 institutions under cooperative agreement with the National Cancer Institute are conducting phase I/II dose-escalation studies in carcinoma of the prostate and carcinoma of the lung. Depending on the results, the cost benefit of 3DCRT must be further evaluated in dose-escalation and in larger multiinstitutional phase III studies comparing it with standard techniques to justify its somewhat higher initial cost.

3D Therapy for Lung Cancer

Clinical studies utilizing 3DCRT for lung cancer can be arbitrarily divided into two groups, those relating and testing the technical feasibility of 3DCRT for lung cancer and those reporting clinical results of patients treated with 3DCRT.

Technical Innovations-Lung 3DCRT

The technical complexities of treating intrathoracic malignancies to high doses of radiation therapy are great. Early work utilizing 3DCRT delineated several issues (Table 8.4).

Application of the ICRU 50 target delineation recommendations to the treatment of lung cancer were described by Graham et al (50). Definition of GTV depends on CT window and level settings and is often obscured by post-obstructive pneumonitis or partial lung collapse. The authors suggested that target delineation was often inadequate on hard copy film (i.e., simulator films) and that CT designation of tumor was considered more accurate. Vijayakumar et al also noted that real or dosimetric geographic misses in treating lung cancer could be reduced with the BEV tool(s) (51). Further BEV has been used as an interactive tool to exclude critical structures such as lung(s) and/

Table 8.4. Technical Issues for 3D CRT of Lung Cancers

- Physiological movement, i.e. tumors, lungs, heart
- Target delineation-where are involved cancerous lymph nodes?
  -where is nodal irradiation?
  -where is the cancer relative to the lung pathology?
- Dose calculation-accounting for density heterogeneity
- Understanding of partial organ radiation dose tolerances

or heart (51,52). Ross et al measured tumor movement using ultrafast computerized tomography (53). The greatest tumor movements averaging 9.2 mm were in lesions near the heart or diaphragm. They also noted major geographic misses secondary to tumor movement in 15% of patients. These papers gave guidelines for margins of the PTV necessary when treating lung primaries. For upper lobe lesions, approximately 7 mm (GTV-PTV) are the minimum margins necessary. For lower lobe tumors, or those near the heart, 10 mm or greater may be necessary.

Numerous authors have reported planning studies utilizing 3DCRT for lung cancer (50,51,54-56). Each of these authors reported improvement in either tumor target prescription dose coverage and/or reduction in dose to surrounding normal organs by utilizing 3DCRT compared to conventional treatment planning. Ha et al (56) and Graham et al (50) independently reported from their dosimetric studies that dose to lung cancers could be safely increased up to 80 Gy for most patients.

Computer-assisted decision making and DVH analysis were evaluated using lung cancer patients by Viggars et al (57) and Graham et al (58). The authors concluded that rapid, reliable, and consistent choices between alternative plans could be achieved using objective score fractions and quantitative analysis of DVHs of intrathoracic organs (and tumor targets). These score functions are expected to have increasing significance and utility as more data is obtained that correlate clinical outcomes with biologic models and physical dose distributions (and DVHs).

Martel et al published results of a retrospective analysis of 3-D radiation dose distributions (DVHs) and the incidence of pneumonitis (59). The authors concluded that NTCPs: (a) would allow clinicians to assess the risk of pneumonitis (low-risk versus high-risk) and (b) establish a framework for a dose escalation protocol for the treatment of non-small cell lung cancer based on risk of development of pneumonitis. Similar reports have corroborated these results and a realistic assessment for the prediction of pneumonitis seems possible (60,61). Stratifying patients by their risk of development of pneumonitis can be done by utilizing NTCPs, percent volume of the total lung volume that exceeds 20 Gy (threshold dose for lung injury), or total lung mean dose. Additional work may delineate further if any of these parameters (or possible newer models) are the most predictive.

Tissue inhomogeneity in the thorax poses significant dose calculation challenges. It has been stated that "a protocol designed to give equal doses to the center of lung tumors under the assumption of completely water equivalent patients, will lead to a spread in delivered dose and patients will not get equivalent treatments" (62). Unfortunately, the reproducibility between 3-D treatment planning systems and the predictability of current algorithms that "correct" for inhomogeneities are certainly less tumor perfect. Other than Monte Carlo calculations (which have not been implemented in 3-D treatment planning systems) all correction calculations are estimates and approximations of how radiation interacts in complicated anatomic heterogeneous matter. Human phantom measurements compared with two different 3-D heterogeneity corrected algorithms were performed by Klein et al (63). Their results indicated that the heterogeneity corrected algorithms overestimate the dose delivery when tumors are surrounded by lung. Essers et al, in contrast, reported good agreement between transmission dose profiles (from Electronic Portal Imaging Devices) (EPID) and CT-based dose calculations (64). One criticism of their results is that they only tested rather simple beam shapes and arrangements (AP/PA only) and did not test the complex and often unique beam arrangement that might be necessary to treat lung cancers. The Photon Treatment Planning Collaborative Working Group concluded that full quantitative evaluation of the role of inhomogeneity corrections in treatment planning requires a yet unavailable all-encompassing accurate method of dose calculation (65).

Further dose optimization studies for lung cancer have proposed that the tumor/target dose uniformity should be relaxed (greater tumor target prescription *inhomogeneity* accepted) and that this would allow for improved ability to optimize dose delivery (66). This has great implications to the application of inverse radiation therapy technique and dose optimization for intrathoracic malignancies. Mohan et al reported the inverse technique *not* suitable for situations where dose-volume considerations and biologic indices are important (67). While adequate dose distributions were achieved for prostate cancers with the inverse solution, the performance of this technique was considerably inferior for lung tumors. Specifically, the inverse techniques appear to fail because the objectives are specified in terms of desired dose or dose ranges—but cannot be stated in terms of the dose limits, fractional volumes, or biological indices (as discussed above).

Further attempts to optimize the intensity distributions employing an objective function based on biological indices still proved inferior (68). Thus, further work in the area of dose optimization for lung cancer is needed.

Clinical Investigations—Lung 3DCRT

Four institutions have reported clinical results of 3DCRT for patients with non-small cell lung cancer (Table 8.5). These results are notable for two reasons. First, the doses delivered were modest and have not reflected any significant dose escalation. This would imply that simply improving the accuracy of subtumoricidal dose delivery will not improve the results of lung cancer. Second, the survival statistics are remarkably similar to the "best" results reported with chemoradiotherapy trials. This may suggest that improving the radiation therapy delivery may mitigate the need for chemotherapy. It could also mean

Table 8.5. Clinical Results of 3D CRT for Patients with Non-Small Cell Lung Cancer

Survival Author/Institution	No. Pts (by Stage)	Dose (median cGy)	Median (mo.)	1 yr (%)	2 yr (%)
Leibel et al (MSKCC)	45	(70.2)	16.5	—	33
Graham (MIR)	70	(70)	—	56	44
Hazuka (UM)	88	(7.60)	14–26	—	36
Sibley (U of Chicago)	37	(66)	19.5	75	37

the patients were "better selected" in the 3-D trials. At least four radiation therapy dose escalation trials have been initiated. The University of Michigan has initiated a dose escalation trial stratifying patient dose upon the risk of pneumonitis as assessed by NTCPs. Patients have been dose escalated to ≥90 Gy without complications (69). Similarly, the Memorial Sloan-Kettering Cancer Center has implemented a dose escalation trial also based on NTCPs for pneumonitis (70). The RTOG dose escalation trial stratifies patients for risk of pneumonitis based on the percent volume of the total lung greater than 20 Gy. The Dutch Cancer Group is stratifying patients by total lung mean dose. The results of these trials are highly anticipated. It appears that the safety of delivering high radiation dose for lung cancer can be improved (if one modifies or optimizes the treatment based on DVH analysis of lungs). It remains to be proven whether higher radiation doses will improve survival for lung cancer.

Central Nervous System Tumors

Many brain tumors, especially glial and neoplasms, have a high local failure rate despite radiation doses that approach or exceed the tolerance of the adjacent normal brain tissues. Nearly 80% of all glioblastomas fail within 2 cm of the contrast enhancing lesion seen on enhanced CT or magnetic resonance imaging (MRI) images following radiotherapy (71,72). Again, 3DCRT offers an opportunity to treat the primary glial neoplasms more aggressively while sparing the adjacent critical structures and allowing dose escalation to the primary target volume. In an analysis of the brain tumor study group protocols, an improvement in the median survival time was demonstrated with increasing radiation therapy doses from 18 weeks without radiation to 28 weeks with 50 Gy, 36 weeks with 55 Gy, and 42 weeks with 60 Gy (73). In another randomized dose escalation study conducted by the RTOG and Eastern Cooperative Oncology Group (ECOG), no benefit was demonstrated in patients receiving 70 Gy compared to patients receiving only 60 Gy. This lack of benefit may be related to increased toxicity associated with conventionally fractionated and standardly planned radiation therapy (74). Indeed, Marks, et al have reported an 18% incidence of brain necrosis with doses higher than 64.8 Gy compared to 0% with radiation doses <57 Gy (75).

Data from the University of Michigan have demonstrated that there is a significant saving of dose to normal brain with the use of conformal radiation therapy when compared to conventional treatment plan with parallel opposed lateral beams (76). In the University of Michigan studies, a 3-D treatment plan reduced the volume encompassed by the 95% isodose by over 50% when compared with conventional opposed partial brain fields. A small series of patients with conformally planned fields treated to doses of >70 Gy demonstrated no significant increase in morbidity (77). An added benefit of 3-D conformal radiation therapy is that the adjacent normal brain is irradiated at a lower dose per daily fraction when all fields are treated than in patients who are treated with conventional radiation therapy. Late central nervous system radiation effects are clearly related to dose per fraction and as a result it is expected that 3-D planned patients will tolerate higher doses to essential tumor and target volume because of the lower dose per fraction to which the adjacent normal tissues are exposed (78).

Other nonglial neoplasms also may benefit from the use of conformal radiation therapy. Tumors of the pineal gland, posterior fossa, or suprasellar region are often diagnosed in children and they may benefit tremendously from the use of conformal radiation therapy even with conventional radiation therapy doses. With the use of conformal radiation therapy it is possible to minimize the radiation dose delivered to the developing cerebral hemispheres, middle ear, optic nerves and chiasm with the use of well-designed conformal radiation therapy plans. Although some patients may require whole neuroaxis or craniospinal irradiation, the high dose that is necessary for local tumor control can be conformed to exclude some of the normal critical structures in the young child.

Patients are generally positioned supine and immobilization masks are used to facilitate a reproducible setup and minimize patient movement during treatment. Occasionally a prone position is used if the tumor is located posterior, to simplify field placement. Generally the planning CT scan extends from the vertex through the base of the skull, often to the level of the chin or midcervical spine in order to insure complete acquisition of anatomies that will be irradiated. In the head and neck or central nervous system region, 3 to 5 mm CT scan thickness and spacing is used. Intravenous contrast may assist in the delineation of the GTV if the patient is known to have a contrast enhancing tumor.

Target volumes and normal tissues are defined as they are for other clinical sites. In the head and neck the critical structures to be defined should include the eyes, lenses, optic nerves, optic chiasm, brain stem, and spinal cord.

Gross tumor volume can often be contoured on the planning CT scan if the tumor enhances and intravenous contrast was employed. T1 enhanced MRI scans may provide better tumor visualization and if available will complement the definition of the GTV. Image fusion or merge protocols linking an MRI to the planning CT may simplify the definition of the GTV and the CTV. A T2 weighted MRI scan can clearly show signal changes consistent with peritumoral edema. This edema has been shown to contain microscopic tumor deposits and may be included as a separate clinical target volume in order to allow treatment of subclinical disease.

In the postoperative setting, contrast enhancement at the time of CT planning may show postoperative effects and therefore a preoperative scan should be used to define the GTV and CTV. Again, image fusion or merging may help. Occasionally, following large tumor resections, normal brain tissue may migrate into the resection cavity. Care should be taken to avoid treating excessive normal brain tissue that has migrated into an area that was previously occupied by a mass occupying lesion.

A CTV is generally added to treat microscopic disease surrounding the GTV. The magnitude of such a margin is controversial. Because clinical data has demonstrated that most recurrences are found within 2 cm of the GTV, most clinicians add at least that much of a margin to the GTV. This, however, results in treating a large volume of normal brain tissue in some circumstances. Clinical discretion should be used when defining large CTV, especially if the clinician desires to escalate the radiation therapy doses above 60 Gy.

Noninfiltrative or nonglial neoplasms may be treated with a smaller CTV margin. Noninvasive pituitary tumors, some pineal tumors, or craniopharyngiomas can be treated with CTV of 10 mm or less. Barriers to tumor infiltration should be considered when defining the CTV. The cranial bones or meninges are infrequently invaded by central nervous system tumors and hence the CTV can often be reduced when abutting these tissues.

A PTV needs to be added because of the presence of daily setup errors and patient movement during radiation therapy. With well-constructed immobilization masks, a PTV of 3 to 5 mm is often adequate. Relocatable stereotactic radiotherapy frames may allow for even smaller PTV margins.

Treatment planning should capitalize on BEV displays to select beam orientation that minimizes incidental irradiation of normal tissues. Vertex or other noncoplanar fields often minimize the radiation therapy dose to uninvolved central nervous system structures. When using these noncoplanar fields, exit dose to the whole body and its detrimental consequences should be considered.

Field shaping generally can be conducted using an MLC. In some regions of the brain, MLC step size may be inadequate to properly shield some of the small critical structures such as the optic nerves or chiasm. In this setting, low melting alloy blocking for more carefully tailored beam shaping may be appropriate.

Clinical experience and use of 3-D conformal radiation therapy for central nervous system tumors has demonstrated that there is a significant saving of dose to normal brain when conformal radiation therapy is used compared to conventional treatment with parallel opposed lateral beams. At the University of Michigan, a small series of patients treated with conformally planned beams to doses of >70 Gy has not been associated with any increase in morbidity. The RTOG is currently conducting a trial of 3-D conformal radiation therapy in the management of patients with glioblastoma multiforme. In that study patients will receive 46 Gy to a CTV that encompasses the postoperative gross tumor residuum plus 15 mm followed by a boost to the postoperative residuum to an additional dose of 20 to 38 Gy.

Upper Abdominal Malignancies

The relatively modest radiation tolerance of the upper abdominal organs has made the radiation therapy of upper gastrointestinal malignancies a disappointing challenge. Three-dimensional radiation therapy planning offers a new approach to managing these aggressive cancers of the stomach, pancreas, and hepatobiliary system. The liver, small bowel, stomach, kidneys, and spinal cord are the critical normal structures that have historically limited the curative role of high-dose radiation therapy. Local tumor recurrence remains a significant problem leading to premature death and morbidity from these cancers.

Generally, patients are placed in the supine position for treatment, unless the target is posterior, in which case a prone position may be more appropriate. Arms should be positioned above the trunk to allow for the use of lateral or similarly oriented fields. Immobilization devices should be used as appropriate. The upper abdominal organs can move as much as 2 cm (average) with normal respiration (79). This organ motion needs to be considered when defining the appropriate PTV. This motion is predominantly in the inferior to superior direction. Some institutions have suggested that the PTV can be reduced by either gating the treatment delivery with respiration or by the use of controlled breath holds or active breathing control devices (80-82).

The planning CT scan volume must include all tissues that will be irradiated by the incident radiation therapy fields. It is better to err on scanning too large a volume than insufficient volume, which may require repeat scanning. Superior or inferior directed radiotherapy beams may be required including the mid- to upper-chest superiorly or the pelvic region inferiorly in the planning scan.

Normal tissue and target volume contours are defined as they are for other clinical sites. The use of intravenous and gastrointestinal contrast may help define both the normal tissues and the gross tumor. Margins for subclinical extensions of disease are often necessary, especially for tumors that have an infiltrative nature such as hepatobiliary cancers and pancreatic tumors.

Defining tumors of the biliary tree can be assisted by the use of intraluminal stents placed at the time of endoscopic retrograde cholangiopancreatography or transhepatic cholangiography. In the absence of such helpful markers, the diagnostic images from these procedures may provide some assistance in the placement of contours defining the CTV. The regional lymph nodes of the porta hepatis or celiac axis need to be included in the treatment of many biliary and pancreatic tumors. The PTV margin should be added around the CTV to account for the daily setup errors and the internal organ motion from respiration.

Radiation beam arrangements should be chosen to minimize the critical structures receiving significant doses of incidental radiation. It is often helpful to start with a standard beam arrangement (the common four field "box") and then adjust table gantry and collimator angles to avoid unnecessarily including large volumes of liver, bowel, or kidney. Noncoplanar fields may help decrease the liver volume irradiated. Anterior placed inferior to superior fields can often spare significant volumes of liver. Again, the advantage from such noncoplanar field arrangements should be determined by comparing the dose volume histograms of these complex field arrangements to those of a conventional beam arrangement until adequate experience is gained with these techniques.

The University of Michigan has reported their results of treatment of nondiffuse hepatobiliary malignancies with combined intra-arterial fluorodeoxyuridine and conformal radiation therapy. Patients received 48 to 66 Gy in 1.5 to 1.65 Gy twice daily fractions. The final prescription dose was selected by the fractional volume of liver excluded from the high-dose treatment volume. This allowed patients to receive a higher PTV radiation dose as more liver could be spared. With a median follow-up of 54 months, the overall freedom from primary hepatic tumor progression was 50% with a 20% 4-year survival. No late hepatotoxicity was observed in this series (83).

CONCLUSION

Three-dimensional radiation therapy treatment planning is a major paradigm shift for the radiation oncologist and treatment planner. The major change for these individuals is the task of determining target volumes and organs at risk in 3-D by drawing contours on CT or MR images on a slice-by-slice basis as opposed to drawing beam portals on a simulator radiograph. IMRT planning will again be a major paradigm shift for the radiation oncologist and treatment planner, the major change this time being the use of the inverse method of treatment design. (Note this second paradigm shift will occur even before classical 3DRTTP is practiced in a majority of radiation therapy clinics world wide). Using the inverse method, the physician will be required to quantitatively prescribe the optimal dose distribution apriori to viewing a dose distribution. While this sounds rather straightforward, this is likely to prove problematic to many physicians trained in the traditional iterative forward planning approach.

The 3-D planning and delivery process will cause changes in the roles and responsibilities of the radiation oncology team. As seen, the radiation oncologist is responsible for the delineation of tumor and target volumes using ICRU 50 methodology. They review and approve critical normal structure input by the dosimetrist, add critical structure contours, develop the plan with the dosimetrist, and review and approve the final treatment plan, verification sim films, and port films. Thus, one clearly sees that in this 3-D era, the radiation oncologist needs a great deal of expertise in interpreting CT imaging studies and in the future must know other imaging modalities (MR SPECT, PET). In addition, they will have to be much more computer literate. A workstation will become an indispensable tool of the radiation oncologist in this new era. Fear of the keyboard and mouse must be overcome as we move to virtual simulation, electronic chart, and on-line electronic plan and portal imaging review.

The radiation oncology physicist will also need much more training in imaging physics as spiral CT and multimodality imaging become the foundation of the planning process. Also, just as accelerator physicists in the 1970s were indispensable, physicists with good computer backgrounds, particularly with regards to networking issues and integrating peripheral devices. Data accessibility and networking issues will be crucial to the radiation oncology clinics of the future.

Treatment plan optimization while still labor intensive will likely become more automated in the future requiring less of a dosimetrist's time. Instead, the dosimetrist will spend considerably more time contouring critical structures. Thus, the dosimetrist in the 3-D era will also need considerably more training in normal tissue anatomy and imaging. Already, the dosimetrists at MIR have become well versed in contouring critical structures.

The radiation therapist in the 3-D era is going to be dealing with much more complex treatment delivery systems. For example, on our multimodality linac, the radiation therapist has to deal with four or five monitors and keyboards. That's probably going to continue for a while until the various systems become integrated. When that occurs, once the patient is repositioned, the treatment will be highly automated using computer controlled and beam intensity modulation techniques. The therapist of the future will play a key role in monitoring patient position and treatment delivery system operation. Thus, the emphasis in training for radiation therapists is likely to be on patient positioning, image based anatomy, and complex systems operation.

The ability for 3DCRT (particularly IMRT) to delivery more conformal dose distributions and spare normal tissues more effectively shows significant potential for improving the quality of radiation therapy. However, its use widespread is just in the initial stages. The equipment and techniques used for the 3-D treatment planning and treatment delivery process are still in rapidly evolving states. Significant research and developmental work still remains to make systems efficient and capable to reach their full potential.

The instrumentation used for implementation and the methods used for quality assurance procedures and testing of traditional planning and delivery systems must be revised and/or redesigned for 3DRTTP to allow efficient clinical use of these new kinds of treatment techniques. Considerable dosimetric verification is typically required and until efficient routine quality assurance check procedures are fully developed and well-documented, full acceptance of this new process will be delayed.

Even though much work still lies ahead, there is no doubt that the era of 3-D radiation therapy has begun in earnest. The number of patient treatments planned using 3DRTTP will increase dramatically over the next few years. As planning and delivery systems mature and become more integrated, 3-D technology will likely lead to lower cost treatment machines and improved efficiency of planning, delivery, and verification, and thus lower the overall costs of radiation therapy (84).

References

1. Herring DF. The consequences of dose response curves for tumor control and normal tissue injury on the precision necessary in patient management. Laryngoscope 1975;85:119-125.
2. Shukovsky LJ. Dose, time, volume relationships in squamous cell carcinoma of the supraglottic larynx. Am J Roentgenol 1970;108:27-29.
3. Stewart JG, Jackson AW. The steepness of the dose response curve for both tumor cure and normal tissue Injury. Laryngoscope 1975; 85:1107.
4. Fischer JJ, Moulder JE. The steepness of the dose-response curve in radiation therapy. Radiology 1975;117:179-184.
5. ICRU. Washington, DC: International Commission on Radiation Units and Measurements, 1976.
6. Loevinger R, Loftus TP. Uncertainty in the delivery of absorbed dose. In Casnati E, ed. Ionizing Radiation Metrology, International Course, Varenna, Italy, 1974. Bologna: Editrice Compositore, 1977:459-473.
7. Purdy JA. 3-D radiation treatment planning: a new era. In Meyer JL, Purdy JA, eds. 3-D Conformal Radiotherapy. Basel: Karger, 1996:1-16.
8. Purdy JA, Emami B, eds. 3-D Radiation Treatment Planning and Conformal Therapy. Madison, WI: Medical Physics Publishing, 1995.
9. Meyer JL, Purdy JA, eds. 3-D conformal radiotherapy: a new era in the irradiation of cancer. Front Radiat Ther Oncol. Basel: Karger, 1996.
10. Seibert JA, Barnes GT, Gould RG, eds. Specification, acceptance testing and quality control of diagnostic x-ray imaging equipment. Woodbury, NY: American Institute of Physics, 1994.
11. Mallik R, Hunt P, Seppi E, Pavkovich J, Shapiro E, Henderson S. Simulator based CT: 4 years experience at the Royal North Shore Hospital, Sydney, Australia. In: Purdy JA, Emami B, eds. 3D radiation treatment planning and conformal therapy. Madison, WI: Medical Physics Publishing, 1995:177-185.
12. Graham MV, Gerber R, Purdy JA. Patient positioning devices: innovations for set-up precision, speed, and patient comfort. In: Meyer JL, Purdy JA, eds. 3-D conformal radiotherapy. Basel: Karger, 1996:115-122.
13. McShan DL, Matrone G, Fraass BA, Lichter AS. A large screen digitizer system for radiation therapy planning. Med Phys 1987;14.
14. Chaney EL, Pizer SM. Defining anatomical structures from medical images. Semin Radiat Oncol 1992;2:215-225.
15. ICRU. Report No. 50, Prescribing, recording, and reporting photon beam therapy. Washington, DC: International Commission on Radiation Units and Measurements, 1993.
16. ICRU. Report No. 29, Dose Specification for Reporting External Beam Therapy with Photons and Electrons. Washington, DC: International Commission on Radiation Units and Measurements, 1978.
17. Purdy JA. Defining our goals: volume and dose specification for 3-D conformal radiation therapy. In: Meyer JL, Purdy JA, eds. 3-D conformal radiotherapy. Basel: Karger, 1996:24-30.
18. Purdy JA. Volume and dose specification, treatment evaluation, and reporting for 3D conformal radiation therapy. In: Palta J, Mackie TR, eds. Teletherapy: present and future. College Park, MD: Advanced Medical Publishing, 1996:235-251.
19. Austin-Seymour M, Kalet I, McDonald J, et al. Three dimensional planning target volumes: a model and a software tool. Int J Radiat Oncol Biol Phys 1995;33:1073-1080.
20. Reinstein LE, McShan D, Webber BM, Glicksman AS. A computer-assisted three-dimensional treatment planning system. Radiology 1978;127:259-264.
21. McShan DL, Silverman A, Lanza D, Reinstein LE, Glicksman AS. A computerized three-dimensional treatment planning system utilizing interactive color graphics. Br J Radiol 1979;52:478-481.
22. Goitein M, Abrams M, Rowell D, Pollari H, Wiles J. Multi-dimensional treatment planning: II. Beam's eye view, back projection, and projection through CT sections. Int J Radiat Oncol Biol Phys 1983;9:789-797.
23. Purdy JA, Wong JW, Harms WB, Drzymala RE, Emami B, Matthews JW, Krippner K, Ramchander PK. Three dimensional radiation treatment planning system. In Bruinvis IAD, van der Giessen PH, van Kleffens HJ, Wittkamper FW, eds. Proceedings of the 9th International Conference on the Use of Computers in Radiation Therapy. Scheveningen, The Netherlands: Elsevier Science Publishers, 1987: 227-279.
24. Purdy JA, Harms WB, Matthews JW, Drzymala RE, Emami B, Simpson JR, Manolis J, Rosenberger FU. Advances in 3-dimensional radiation treatment planning systems: room-iew display with real time interactivity. Int J Radiat Oncol Biol Phys 1993;27:933-944.
25. Wong JW, Purdy JA. On methods of inhomogeneity corrections for photon transport. Med Phys 1990;17:807-814.
26. Kornelsen RO, Young MEJ. Changes in the dose-profile of a 10 MV x-ray beam within and beyond low density material. Med Phys 1982; 9:114-116.
27. Mackie TR, Ahnesjö A, Dickof P, Snider A. Development of a convolution/superposition method for photon beams. In Bruinvis IAD, van der Giessen PH, van Kleffens HJ, Wittkamper FW, eds. Proceedings of the 9th International Conference on the Use of Computers in Radiation Therapy. Scheveningen, The Netherlands: Elsevier Science Publishers, 1987:107-110.
28. Mohan R, Chui C, Lidofsky L. Differential pencil beam dose computation model for photons. Med Phys 1986;13:64-73.
29. Mackie TR, Reckwerdt P, McNutt T, Gehring M, Sanders C. Photon beam dose computations. In Palta J, Mackie TR, eds. Teletherapy: present and future. College Park, MD: Advanced Medical Publishing, 1996:103-136.
30. Mackie TR. Applications of the Monte Carlo method in radiotherapy. In Kase KR, Bjarngard BE, Attix FH, eds. The Dosimetry of Ionizing Radiation, Vol. III. San Diego: Academic Press, 1990.
31. Hartmann Siantar CL, Chandler WP, Weaver KA, Albright NW, Verhey LJ, Hornstein SM, Cox LJ, Rathkopf JA, Svatos MM. Validation and performance assessment of the peregrine all-particle monte carlo code for photon beam therapy (abstract). 1996;23:1128-1129.

32. Drzymala RE, Mohan R, Brewster L, Chu J, Goitein M, Harms W, Urie M. Dose volume histograms. Int J Radiat Oncol Biol Phys 1991;21: 71-78.
33. Niemierko A. Treatment plan optimization. In Purdy JA, Emami B, eds. 3D radiation treatment planning and conformal therapy. Madison, WI: Medical Physics Publishing, 1995:49-55.
34. Webb S. Optimization of conformal radiotherapy dose distributions by simulated annealing. Phys Med Biol 1989;34:1349-1370.
35. Brahme A. Inverse radiation therapy planning as a tool for 3D dose optimization. Physica Medica 1990;6:53-63.
36. Sherouse GW, Novins K, Chaney EL. Computation of digitally reconstructed radiographs for use in radiotherapy treatment design. Int J Radiat Oncol Biol Phys 1990;18:651-658.
37. Munro P. Portal imaging technology: past, present, and future. Semin Rad Oncol 1995;5:115-133.
38. Boyer AL, Ochran TG, Nyerick CE, Waldron TJ, Huntzinger CJ. Clinical dosimetry for implementation of a multileaf collimator. Med Phys 1992;19:1255-1261.
39. Boyer A. Basic applications of a multileaf collimator. In Palta J, Mackie TR, eds. Teletherapy: present and future. College Park, MD: Advanced Medical Publishing, 1996:403-444.
40. Klein EE, Harms WB, Low DA, Willcut V, Purdy JA. Clinical implementation of a commercial multileaf collimator: dosimetry, networking, simulation, and quality assurance. Int J Radiat Oncol Biol Phys 1995;33:1195-1208.
41. Fraass BA, McShan CL, Kessler ML. Computer-controlled treatment delivery. Sem Rad Oncol 1995;5:77-85.
42. Fraass BA, McShan DL, Kessler ML, Matrone GM, Lewis JD, Weaver TA. A computer-controlled conformal radiotherapy system: I. Overview. Int J Radiat Oncol Biol Phys 1995;33:1139-1157.
43. Mageras GS, Podmaniczky K, Mohan R. A model for computer controlled delivery of 3D conformal treatments. Med Phys 1992;19:945-954.
44. Boyer AL. Present and future developments in radiotherapy treatment units. Semin Rad Oncol 1995;5:146-155.
45. Perez CA, Purdy JA, Harms WB, Gerber RL, Graham JV, Matthews JW, Bosch WR, Drzymala RE, Emami B, Fox S, Klein EE, Lee HI, et al. Three-dimensional treatment planning and conformal radiation therapy: preliminary evaluation. Radiother Oncol 1995;36:32-43.
46. Hanks GE, Schultheiss TE, Hunt MA, Epstein B. Factors influencing incidence of acute grade 2 morbidity in conformal and standard radiation treatment of prostate cancer. Int J Radiat Oncol Biol Phys 1995; 31:25-29.
47. Sandler HM, McLaughlin PW, Ten Haken RK, et al. Three dimensional conformal radiotherapy for the treatment of prostate cancer: low risk of chronic rectal morbidity observed in a large series of patients. Int J Radiat Oncol Biol Phys 1995;33:797-801.
48. Leibel SA, Zelefsky MJ, Kutcher GJ, et al. Three-dimensional conformal radiation therapy in localized carcinoma of the prostate: interim report of a phase I dose-escalation study. J Urol 1994;152:1792-1798.
49. Hanks GE, Lee WR, Schultheiss TE. Clinical and biochemical evidence of control of prostate cancer at 5 years after external beam radiation. U Urol 1995;154:456-459.
50. Graham MV, Matthews JW, Harms WB, et al. Three-dimensional radiation treatment planning study for patients with carcinoma of the lung. Int J Radiat Oncol Biol Phys 1994;29:1105-1117.
51. Vijayakumar S, Myrianthopoulos LC, Rosenberg I, Halpern HJ, Low N, Chen GTY. Optimization of radical radiotherapy with beam's eye view techniques for non-small cell lung cancer. Int J Radiat Oncol Biol Phys 1991;21:779-788.
52. Chen GTY, Spelbring DR, Pelizzari CA. Use of beam's eye view volumetrics in the selection of non-coplanar radiation portals. Int J Radiat Oncol Biol Phys 1992;23:153-163.
53. Ross CS, Hussey DH, Pennington EC, et al. Analysis of movement of intrathoracic neoplasms using ultrafast computerized tomography. Int J Radiat Oncol Biol Phys 1990;18:671-677.
54. Hodapp N, Boesecke R, Schlegel W, et al. Three-dimensional treatment planning for conformation therapy of a bronchial carcinoma. Radiother Oncol 1991;20:245-249.
55. Emami B, Purdy JA, Manolis J, Barest G, Cheng E, Coia L, Doppke K, Galvin J, LoSasso T, Matthews J, Munzenrider J, Shank B. Three-dimensional treatment planning for lung cancer. Int J Radiat Oncol Biol Phys 1991;21:217-227.
56. Ha CS, Kijewski PK, Langer M. Gain in target dose from using computer controlled radiation therapy (CCRT) in the treatment of non-small cell lung cancer. Int J Radiat Oncol Biol Phys 1993;26:335-339.
57. Viggars DA, Shalev S, Stewart M, Hahn P. The objective evaluation of alternative treatment plans III: the quantitative analysis of dose volume histograms. Int J Radiat Oncol Biol Phys 1992;23:419-427.
58. Graham MV, Jain NL, Kahn MG, Drzymala RE, Purdy, JA. Evaluation of an objective plan-evaluation model in the three dimensional treatment of non-small cell lung cancer. Int J Radiat Oncol Biol Phys 1996; 34:469-474.
59. Martel MK, Ten Haken RK, Hazuka MB, Turrisi AT, Fraass BA, Lichter AS. Dose-volume histogram and 3-D treatment planning evaluation of patients with pneumonitis. Int J Radiat Oncol Biol Phys 1994;28: 575-581.
60. Graham MV, Drzymala RE, Jain NL, et al. Confirmation of dose-volume histograms and normal tissue complication probability calculations to predict pulmonary complications after radiotherapy for lung cancer. Int J Radiat Oncol Biol Phys 1994;30:198.
61. Oetzel D, Schraube P, Hensley F, et al. Estimation of pneumonitis risk in three-dimensional treatment planning using dose-volume histogram analysis. Int J Radiat Oncol Biol Phys 1995;33:455-460.
62. Ten Haken RK, Balter JM, Martel MK, Fraass BA. Tissue inhomogeneity in the thorax: implications for 3-D treatment planning. In Meyer J, Purdy JA, eds. Front Radiat Ther Oncol 1996:180-187.
63. Klein EE, Morrison A, Purdy JA, Graham MV, Matthews JW. A volumetric study of measurements and calculations of lung density corrections for 6 and 18 MV photons. Int J Radiat Oncol Biol Phys 1997; 37:1163-1170.
64. Essers M, Lanson JH, Leunens G, et al. The accuracy of CT-based inhomogeneity corrections and in vivo dosimetry for the treatment of lung cancer. Radiother Oncol 1995;37:199-208.
65. Photon Treatment Planning Collaborative Working Group: Role of inhomogeneity corrections in three-dimensional photon treatment planning. Int J Radiat Oncol Biol Phys 1991;21:59-69.
66. Langer M, Kijewski P, Brown R, Ha C. The effect on minimum tumor dose of restricting target-dose inhomogeneity in optimized three-dimensional treatment of lung cancer. Radiother Oncol 1991;21:245-256.
67. Mohan R, Wang X, Jackson A, Bortfeld T, Boyer AL, Kutcher GJ, Leibel SA, Fuks Z, Ling CC. The potential and limitations of the inverse radiotherapy technique. Radiother Oncol 1994;32:232-248.
68. Wang XH, Mohan R, Jackson A, et al. Optimization of intensity-modulated 3D conformal treatment plans based on biological indices. Radiother Oncol 1995;37:140-152.
69. Martel M. Personal communication. 1997.
70. Leibel SA, Kutcher GJ, Zelefsky MJ, Burman CM, Mohan R, Ling CC, Fuks Z. 3-D conformal radiation therapy for non-small cell lung carcinoma. Clinical experience at the Memorial Sloan-Kettering Cancer Center. In Meyer J, Purdy JA, eds. Front Radiat Ther Oncol 1996;199-206.
71. Wallner KE, Galicich JH, Krol G, Arbit E, Malkin MG. Patterns of failure following treatment for glioblatoma multiforme and anaplastic astorcytoma. Int J Radiat Oncol Biol Phys 1989;16:1405-1409.
72. Hockberg FH. Assumptions in radiotherapy of glioblastoma. Neuro. 1980;30:907-911.
73. Walker MD, Strike TA, Sheline GE. An analysis of dose-effect relationship in the radiotherapy of malignant gliomas. Int J Radiat Oncol Biol Phys 1979;5:1725-1731.
74. Chang CH, Horton J, Schoenfeld SO, Perez-Tamayo R, Kramer S, Weinstein A, Nelson JS, Tsukada Y. Comparison of post operative radiotherapy in combined post operative radiotherapy and chemotherapy in the multidisciplinary management of malignant gliomas. The Joint Radiation Therapy Oncology Group and The Eastern Cooperative Oncology Group Study. Cancer 1983;32:997-1007.
75. Marks JE, Wong J. The risk of cerebral radionecrosis in relation to dose, time and fractionation. Prog Exp Tumor Res 1985;29:210-218.
76. Thornton AF, Hegarty TJ, Ten Haken RK, Yanke BR, LaVigne ML, Fraass BA, McShan DL, Greenberg HS. Three-dimensional treatment planning of astrocytomas, a dosimetric study of cerebral irradiation. Int J Radiat Oncol Biol Phys 1991;20:1309-1315.
77. Lichter AS, Sandler HM, Robertson JM, Lawrence TS, Ten Haken RK, McShan DL, Fraass BA. Clinical experience with three-dimensional treatment planning. Semin Radia Oncol 1992;2:257-266.

78. Sheline GE, Wara WM, Smith V. Therapeutic irradiation in brain injury. Int J Radiat Oncol Biol Phys 1980;6:1215-1228.
79. Balter J, Ten Haken R, Lam K. Immobilization and setup verification. In Palta J, Mackie TR, eds. Teletherapy: present and future. College Park, MD: Advanced Medical Publishing, 1996:471-494.
80. Ten Haken RK, Balter JM, Lam KL, Mcginn CJ, Lawrence TS. Improvement of CT-based treatment planning models of abdominal targets using static exhale imaging. Int J Radiat Oncol Biol Phys 1996;36:187.
81. Wong J, Sharpe M, Jaffray D. The use of active breathing control (ABC) to minimize breathing motion in conformal therapy. In Leavitt DD, Starkschall G, eds. Proceedings of the XIIth International Conference on the Use of Computers in Radiation Therapy. Madison, WI: Medical Physics Publishing, 1997:220-222.
82. Hanley J, Debois MM, Roben A, Mageras GS, Lutz WR, Mychalczak B, Schwartz LH, Gloeggler PJ, Leibel SA, Fuks Z, Kutcher GJ. Deep inspiration breath-hold technique for lung tumors: the potential value of target immobilization and reduced lung density in dose excalation. Int J Radiat Oncol Biol Phys 1996;36:188.
83. Robertson JM, Lawrence TS, Andrews JC, Walker S, Kessler ML, Ensminger WD. Long-term results of hepatic artery fluorodeoxyuridine and conformal radiation therapy for primary hepatobiliary cancers. Int J Radiat Oncol Biol Phys 1997;37:325-330.
84. Perez CA, Michalski J, Ballard S, Drzymala RE, Kobeissi B, Lockett M, Wasserman TH. Cost benefit of emerging technology in localized carcinoma of the prostate. Int J Radiat Oncol Biol Phys 1997;39:875-883.

Chapter 9

Intensity Modulated Radiation Therapy

Daniel A. Low, James A. Purdy, Carlos A. Perez, K. S. Clifford Chao, and Russell L. Gerber

The next decade will bring dramatic changes in radiation therapy treatment planning and treatment delivery, driven largely by advances in computer hardware and software. These advances have inspired the development of sophisticated three-dimensional (3-D) radiation therapy treatment planning (3DRTTP) and delivery systems, making practical the implementation of three-dimensional conformal radiation therapy (3DCRT). The purpose of 3DCRT is to conform the prescribed dose distribution to the 3-D target volume (cancerous cells) shape while simultaneously minimizing the dose to neighboring normal patient structures (1,2). Modern 3DCRT delivery is implemented by conforming the incident beam portal outlines to the target volume projections for a specified set of beam directions or during rotational beam delivery. Typically, the radiation beams exhibit either uniform intensity or, where appropriate, the intensity is varied by beam modifiers such as compensating filters or wedges. This treatment method will be referred to as traditional 3DCRT.

A more general definition of 3DCRT is being rapidly developed and implemented, even before the widespread implementation of traditional 3DCRT. It is described by several different labels, including generalized 3DCRT, unconstrained 3DCRT, computer-controlled conformal radiation therapy (CCRT), or intensity modulated radiation therapy (IMRT) (3–5). These approaches use radiation fields with incident radiation fluence distributions that may vary dramatically across the portals. The planning and delivery of IMRT are significantly more complex than traditional 3DCRT, but have the potential of achieving a much higher degree of target conformity, especially for target volumes with complex 3-D geometries, including those with concave features.

Beam modifiers such as wedges and compensators have been used in radiation oncology for many years to account for missing tissue and in some cases to tailor dose distributions (6,7). To consider this type of beam-intensity modulation as IMRT is too restrictive, as IMRT is capable of generating complex 3-D dose distributions with concave features and can also provide sparing of selected nearby sensitive normal structures. With IMRT, as the beam is oriented around the patient, the beam intensity (fluence) is optimized using computer algorithms that consider the target and normal tissue dimensions and user-defined constraints such as dose limits. This process is sometimes referred to as the "inverse problem" or "inverse method" of treatment planning (Figure 9.1).

Experience with IMRT techniques is limited, and there is significant research and development work to be done to assist in the worldwide introduction and use of this new technology. One commercial IMRT system (Peacock, Nomos Corporation) is available and has been implemented in more than 19 clinics worldwide with more than 800 patients treated (8,9). The system is provided with an inverse treatment planning computer and computer-controlled beam modulating multileaf collimator (MLC). The treatment plan is generated and the computer-controlled MLC instructions are relayed using a floppy disk. The treatment planning system does not allow changes in the treatment plan once the floppy disk is produced, reducing the chance of a discrepancy between the plan and delivery. Several university-developed prototype IMRT systems are also being brought into clinical use (10).

Although dosimetric advantages of the inverse method of IMRT treatment design are easily demonstrated in planning exercises, clinical trials are required to determine if the use of IMRT leads to improved outcome. In addition, IMRT and inverse treatment planning offer practical advan-

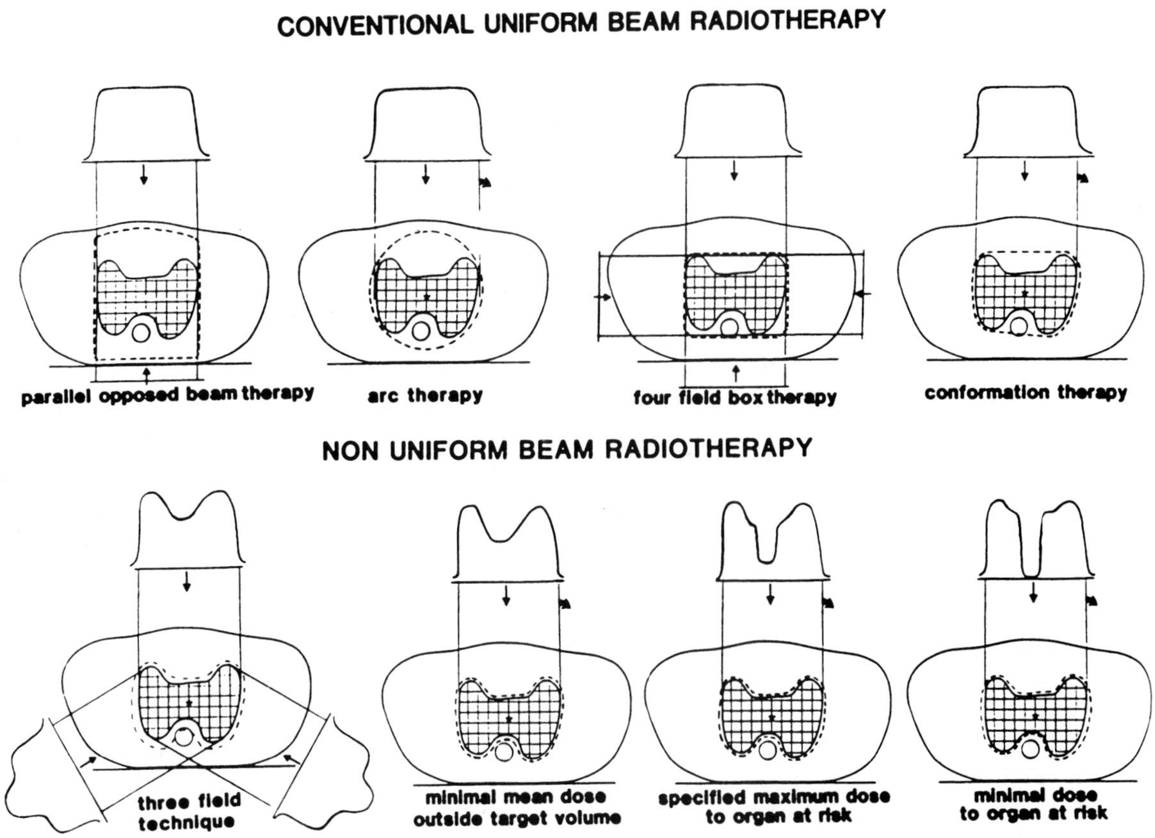

Figure 9.1. Conventional and IMRT dose distributions to a complex target volume (hatched) and critical structure geometry. The upper four figures indicate the dose distribution using conventional planning and delivery. The lower four figures indicate fixed-beam and arc-based IMRT with different optimization criteria. (Figure courtesy of Brahme [36].)

tages that may not yet be appreciated by the radiation oncology community. When fully developed, this integrated 3-D planning and delivery technology will likely lead to lower-cost treatment machines and improved efficiency of planning, delivery, and verification and will thus make a valuable contribution to reducing the overall costs of radiation therapy (2).

BASIC PHYSICAL PRINCIPLES OF IMRT

IMRT generates dose distributions that conform to complex target volume geometries in all three dimensions. The dose distributions can be considered to be produced by a series of individual beamlets, each consisting of a narrow incident photon beam (Figure 9.2). Ideally, all beam entry angles and positions would be available for use, but limitations of the dose delivery devices constrain the incident radiation beam fluence distributions to two types.

For IMRT delivery, the fluence is to be modulated as a function of entry angle for each point within the target volume. The dose at any point within the patient will be generated by a series of beamlets incident on that point,

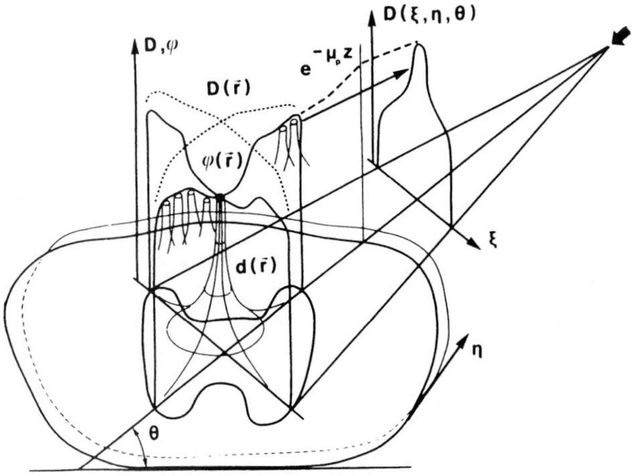

Figure 9.2. Sketch of beamlet-generated dose distribution. (Figure courtesy of Brahme [36].)

each with a unique entry angle. Currently, treatment accelerators are capable of simultaneously delivering fluence across a broad surface area of the patient in the form of a cone beam, with a unique patient entry angle for each position within the cone beam. The radiation fluence can be modulated within the cone beam using a physical modulator, a scanning dynamic MLC, a scanning bremsstrahlung photon beam, or a combination of these techniques (8,11–25). For each of these, significant time is required to deliver the incident fluence distribution. To limit the treatment to practical delivery times, the number of incident cone beams will be limited to a dozen at most. The beamlet distribution at each point within the patient when cone-beam IMRT is used is therefore limited principally in number, rather than in direction.

Alternatively, the accelerator can be operated using dynamic motion of one or more of the angular degrees of freedom (couch, collimator, and gantry). Of these, only dynamic gantry motion is currently being investigated (21,23,26). When dynamic motion of the gantry is used, there is insufficient time to arbitrarily adjust the fluence at each gantry angle using standard multileaf collimation. However, the fluence can be arbitrarily modulated along a one-dimensional array of beamlets using a rapidly actuating MLC (9,26–28). The collimator modulates the fluence by alternately opening and closing each leaf as the gantry rotates. This technique is termed fan-beam IMRT delivery. The fluence is modulated in time by opening and closing each of the multileaves over the course of a narrow gantry angle range. In this manner, modulated beams of 50 or more gantry angles are delivered to a roughly cylindrical volume with the cylinder thickness corresponding to the leaf opening size. A commercial MLC is designed using two adjacent independently actuated leaf banks, so two adjacent cylindrical volumes are simultaneously irradiated (29–31). After the dose is delivered to the first volumes, the patient is precisely moved and the next two cylindrical volumes treated. The couch angle can also be adjusted to allow a broad range of entry angles. The beamlet distribution for each point within the patient is limited principally by incident angular distribution (the beamlets are coplanar) rather than by number.

Standard MLCs can also be employed when using dynamic gantry motion (21). The MLC is moved during arc rotation such that an open field of predetermined shape is delivered for each gantry angle. To modulate the beam intensity for each beamlet, multiple arcs are delivered, each with a different portal shape such that the modulated final fluence is delivered. The beamlet distribution is similar to that of the fan-beam geometry.

In traditional radiation therapy, the photon beam energy selection is used to modify shallow doses and to limit dose heterogeneities along the beam path. In megavoltage therapy, shallow and deep tumors are treated with low- and high-beam energies, respectively. However, when beam-intensity modulation is used, much of the dose heterogeneity due to the depth dose can be removed by modulating nearly orthogonal beams (similar to the concept of a wedged pair). Therefore, the need for higher energy beams (greater than 10 MV), with potential neutron contamination, may be limited. In addition, the conformation of dose within the patient relies on each beamlet independently depositing dose within the patient, which requires that the secondary electron range be small with respect to the beamlet size. Studies have so far concluded that the ideal beam energy for intensity modulation lies between 4 and 10 MV.

INVERSE TREATMENT OPTIMIZATION (COST FUNCTION AND SEARCH ALGORITHM)

As previously indicated, IMRT requires a computer optimization method of determining the nonuniform beam fluence profiles. Early attempts at automated plan optimization methods were conducted by several groups, including Hope and Orr (32), Redpath et al (33), and McDonald and Rubin (34), but with limited acceptance. With the development of 3DCRT and the corresponding increase in image and graphic data, interest in computer optimization and automation has been renewed. Investigation of computer optimization has intensified because of the requirement for determining optimal nonuniform beam fluences for IMRT (35–37).

In 1982, Brahme et al (38) developed the concept of determining the modulated radiation field fluence distribution necessary to produce a desired dose distribution. An analytic solution of the beam fluence profile required to treat a circularly symmetric target with a critical structure at its center was developed. In 1987, Cormack (39,40) furthered this approach by extending it to targets with an axis of symmetry. In 1990, Barth (41) further developed this approach by describing a mathematical solution for a target of arbitrary shape by circular component target decomposition. For general solutions, the optimized incident fluence profiles contain negative fluence beamlets, an unphysically realizable result (42). Application of the nonnegativity constraint has been included in recent efforts to develop numerical solutions to calculate the incident fluence profiles. Reported methods include: 1) exhaustive search (41); 2) image reconstruction approaches (43,44); 3) quadratic programming (45); and 4) simulated annealing (46,47).

The task of generating an optimal plan can be separated into two parts: 1) specification of an optimization criterion and 2) the optimization algorithm used. The optimization criterion is expressed as a mathematical entity in the form of an objective or cost function. The objective function defines a plan's quality and is to be maximized or minimized, as appropriate, to satisfy a set of mathematical constraints. The objective function yields a single numerical value (sometimes referred to as a score) for the plan that is used for evaluating a set of competing treatment plans. Often an iterative computer search is made of the fluence distributions, with guidance by the objective function. Several types of objective functions have been investigated and have shown to be useful in some, but not all, clinical situations (47–57). Historically, plan optimization criteria have been based on dose parameters, but recent efforts are examining the use of biologically based indices (e.g., tumor control probability and normal tissue complication probability) (58,59).

Once the optimization criteria have been selected, an algorithm is used to automatically determine a set of plan parameters that optimizes the chosen objective function. There are a number of IMRT treatment planning optimization algorithms under investigation. If the objective function and constraints can be described by linear or quadratic functions of the plan parameters, efficient mathematical optimization techniques can be used that are guaranteed to find the best score (45,55,57,60). If the objective function is not linear or quadratic as a function of the optimization parameters, non-linear optimization techniques must be used (61). Other optimization approaches being used for IMRT are adopted from computed tomography (CT) image reconstruction techniques, with filtered back projection being the principal technique (44,62,63). If these techniques are used in an unmodified form, the optimized fluence distribution will have negative fluences. Nonnegativity constraints impact on the quality of the resulting distribution, so iterative techniques are often also required. One iteration method is a stochastic technique termed "simulated annealing," originally developed from statistical mechanics for finding the global minima of nonlinear objective functions (64,65). Webb (46) applied this approach to radiation therapy plan optimization; since then, several other researchers, as well as a commercial system, have used this method (47,66–73).

Optimization criteria and mathematical search algorithms are being vigorously investigated. As the capabilities of computers continue to improve, the time required to conduct an optimization search may become short, allowing the widespread implementation and practical use of IMRT. The biggest challenge may be the development of optimization criteria that will be appropriate for a wide variety of cancer sites and histologies and be able to account for individual physician preferences.

IMRT TREATMENT DELIVERY SYSTEMS

Historical Review

Early IMRT concepts were pioneered several decades ago. Seminal contributions were made by Dr. Shinji Takahashi and colleagues, from Nagoya, Japan (74). Their work illustrated some of the important concepts in both 3DCRT and IMRT treatment delivery. Dynamic treatments were planned and delivered by Takahashi's group using what may have been the first MLC system. The MLC used a mechanical control system to conform the beam aperture to the projected target shape as the machine was rotated around the patient.

In the late 1950s, another pioneering effort in IMRT was conducted by the group at the Massachusetts Institute of Technology Lahy Clinic (primarily Drs. Proimos, Wright, and Trump), who independently developed an asynchronous portal-defining device similar to that of Takahashi (75–78).

The Royal Northern Hospital in England also pioneered a 3DCRT effort (primarily Green, Jennings, and Christie) (79). The group developed a series of cobalt-60 teletherapy machines in which the patient was automatically positioned during rotational therapy by moving the treatment couch and gantry during the radiation delivery using electromechanical systems. This was called the "Tracking Cobalt Project" because the planning and delivery system attempted to track around the path of disease spread and subsequently conform the dose distribution. The work was extended in the 1970s and 1980s by Davy and Brace at the Royal Free Hospital in London (80–86).

The 1970s saw important advances in IMRT from the Harvard Medical School by Bjarngard, Kijewski, and others (87–91). Unfortunately, computer technology had not yet advanced to the capacity required for practical implementation of traditional 3DCRT and IMRT. This work and that of the previous researchers led the way for modern IMRT.

The recent introduction of commercially available MLCs (92–95) and the simultaneous development of medical accelerator computer control systems (92,96–99) assisted the rapid and widespread development of practical IMRT. Until recently, medical accelerators were produced with relatively primitive beam collimation systems consisting of opposed jaw pairs that were constrained to move symmetrically to provide square or rectangular beam apertures. A low melting point lead alloy was used to fabricate a customized beam block for each radiation portal to provide static conformal field shaping (100). This system was relatively inefficient, in that the radiation therapist was required to enter the treatment room and manually change the aperture block for each treatment portal. A limited improvement came when the collimator jaws were allowed to move independently, allowing the fabrication of lighter blocks. A rudimentary form of dynamic intensity modulation, the dynamic wedge was developed using independent jaws (91,101). The MLC replaced (or supplemented, depending on the accelerator manufacturer) the rectangular jaw system with a set of independently adjustable, relatively narrow, tungsten leaves (typically projecting to 1 or 1.25 cm wide at isocenter). The leaves were placed under computer control and were therefore able to create custom-shaped beam apertures and allow the change of portal shapes without the requirement of room entry by the radiation therapist. The computer control system was often used to automatically rotate the gantry (and collimator), position the treatment table, and control dose rate.

IMRT delivery is made practical by using a MLC in a dynamic mode similar to dynamic wedge (i.e., moving each pair of MLC leaves with the beam on while at a fixed gantry angle or during a gantry rotation). This method, and three others, for delivering IMRT are discussed in the following sections.

Arc-Based Fan-Beam Dynamic MLC IMRT

A commercial implementation of a fan-beam approach to IMRT uses a mini-MLC system that is mounted to an unmodified linear accelerator, and treatment is delivered to a narrow slice of the patient during arc rotation (8,26,27,30,102). The beam is collimated to a narrow slit and beamlets are turned on and off by driving the mini-MLC leaves out and in the beam path, respectively, as the gantry rotates around the patient. A complete treatment is accomplished by sequential delivery to adjoining slices. As previously indicated, this type of IMRT system (Peacock; Nomos Corp., Pittsburgh, PA) has been implemented in more than 19 clinics worldwide, and over 800 patients have been treated using this approach (9).

A variation of this approach, termed tomotherapy, has been suggested by Mackie et al (23). The dose is delivered using a narrow MLC and small linear accelerator mounted in a modified CT scanner gantry. The radiation will be delivered while the patient is moved through the gantry in the same way as a spiral CT study is conducted. The proposal includes a CT system mounted on the same gantry to allow the simultaneous acquisition of a CT verification scan study. This approach may provide a practical large-scale solution for the implementation of IMRT, and a prototype system is under development at the University of Wisconsin (103,104).

Fixed Portal Cone-Beam Dynamic MLC IMRT

Other IMRT researchers have concentrated on using the MLC to provide a full-field or cone-beam modulation technique (12,18–20,105–107). For IMRT, the MLC is operated in a dynamic mode where the gap formed by each opposing leaf sweeps under computer control across the target volume to produce the desired fluence profile. The technique for setting the gap opening and its speed for each MLC leaf pair was first determined by a technique introduced by Convery and Rosenbloom (12) and extended by Bortfeld et al (107) and Spirou and Chui (16). The Memorial Sloan Kettering Cancer Center has adopted a variation of this technique and is currently treating patients (10).

Fixed-Portal X-ray Compensating Filter IMRT

The original and common use of compensating filters is to account for missing tissue deficits while maintaining the skin-sparing benefit of megavoltage photon beams. Filters designed using 3DRTTP are capable of compensating for not only the missing tissue deficit, but also for internal tissue heterogeneities. Filters can be designed by calculating a thickness along a ray line using an effective attenuation coefficient for the filter material and dose-ratio parameters for effective depths may consider scattered radiation from the filter. The filter construction process can be automated using numerically controlled milling machines, and can be extended for use when inverse treatment planning is employed, fabricating the compensation filter that generates the desired IMRT fluence profile when the filter is placed in the radiation beam. A carousel or stack device could be supplied to hold multiple filters that would be automatically moved into the beam under computer control. Being relatively simple, this method of delivering IMRT may prove to be the easiest to clinically implement. Comparisons of IMRT dose distributions delivered using physical modulators and MLC-based approaches are under investigation, with indications that the dose distributions provided by these modalities are similar (25). Stein et al have developed a method for producing physical modulators by stacking layered filters up to 1.6 cm thick. The filters are fabricated using low melting-point alloy poured into foam molds, which are cut using a computer-controlled cutter. Others have also investigated the use of physical filters for IMRT (108,109).

IMRT QUALITY ASSURANCE (COMMISSIONING AND CLINICAL)

As for all treatment modalities, verification and characterization measurements are required before clinical implementation of IMRT. Dosimetric verification traditionally includes a comparison of measured and calculated dose distributions for selected test treatment plans. Acquisition of benchmark quality dose distributions for static beam therapy rely on ionization chambers, which measure doses at individual points. Acquisition of isodose distributions relies on the assumption that the dose distribution being delivered during the measurements is constant in time (at least to within an overall constant dose rate, monitored by a reference ionization chamber), and that the chamber can be scanned throughout the dose distribution during the measurement. Dynamic IMRT dose distributions are delivered using a temporal sequence of incident fluences, so this assumption does not hold. As a consequence, the measurement of dose at a single point using an ionization chamber requires that the entire fluence delivery sequence be delivered, requiring measurement times as long as 20 minutes. Similar difficulties are seen with all electronic point dosimeters (e.g., diodes). Stand-alone integrating point dosimeters, such as thermoluminescent dosimeters (TLDs), allow the simultaneous measurement of dose at numerous locations, but with the additional workload required for off-line readout. Practical application of real-time point dosimeters will provide, at most, dozens of measurement points within the treatment volume.

Characteristics of IMRT dose distributions include complex 3-D treatment volume geometries and high spatial dose gradients. The precise characterization of these distributions using only point dosimeters is not practical. To obtain the large quantity of dose measurements necessary for the description of the dose distributions, at least planar dosimeters are necessary. Currently, the only practical planar dosimeter is radiographic film, but benchmark quality dose distributions for megavoltage beams cannot be acquired using radiographic film due to its energy response and relative dosimetric characteristics (110–113). However, even with these dosimetric limitations, radiographic film is capable of accurately localizing regions of high spatial dose gradient. For example, in a region of a 5% mm^{-1} dose gradient, an error of 5% in the relative dose measurement results in a spatial error in the localization of that gradient region of only 1 mm. Radiographic film therefore provides an opportunity for accurately localizing a complex dose distribution within the two-dimensional measured area.

To determine the spatial accuracy of the treatment planning and delivery system, the spatial location of the measured and calculated doses must be accurately and independently determined. Most treatment planning systems use a Cartesian coordinate system to localize the calculated dose distribution. For example, the Peacock system ties the coordinate system directly to treatment delivery. Before acquisition of the volumetric CT scan of noninvasively immobilized patients, radiopaque markers are placed on the immobilization system (e.g., thermoplastic masks), corresponding to the lateral and anterior (for supine patients) projection of a selected point, termed the origin. During treatment planning, the origin location is identified on the CT scan data set and becomes the origin of the internal coordinate system. For the Peacock system, the X-axis corresponds to the horizontal transverse direction (lateral for a supine patient), while the Y and Z axes correspond to the anteroposterior and craniocaudal directions, respectively. For a supine patient, the positive directions correspond to the left, posterior, and superior directions for the X, Y, and Z directions, respectively.

During patient setup, the locations of the origin projections are aligned with the accelerator positioning lasers, placing the origin at isocenter. The treatment planning system provides instructions to offset the patient position a specified direction and distance to place the accelerator isocenter at the optimal location for treatment. Verification measurements should be made in the same way. Localization wires are placed on the dosimetry phantom identifying the projected origin. The wires are visualized on the CT scan data set to determine the origin location within the phantom. The dosimeter position locations are determined relative to the origin using physical measurements or machine drawings of the phantom.

Dosimetry System

A practical system has been developed to acquire quantitative dosimetry measurements for the verification of IMRT dose distributions (114). The optimal characteristics of TLD, film, and ionization chambers are exploited. Radiographic film is used to measure the spatial position of the dose distribution, while ionization chambers and/or TLDs are used to measure the absolute dose in relatively low dose gradient regions.

Careful dosimetry phantom design is important to the commissioning and quality assurance (QA) procedures. Anthropomorphic phantoms offer the advantage that they are shaped and sized similar to the patients to be treated. However, if the treatment planning system does not consider internal heterogeneities, determination of the cause of discrepancies between measured and calculated doses may be difficult, especially within and nearby bony anatomy. The spacing between locations for TLD chips may also be larger than desired. Film preparation is also made more difficult with anthropomorphic phantoms due to the irregular external contours. Preparation of the film may require careful cutting in the darkroom to conform to the phantom outline. Cuboid phantoms do not share these limitations.

Figure 9.3 shows the film phantom provided by the NOMOS Corporation for verification of IMRT dose distributions. The phantom is capable of holding up to 20 sheets of 12.7 × 14.0 cm^2 radiographic film, spaced 0.617 cm apart by polystyrene sheets. A standard paper cutter is used in the darkroom to cut the rectangular film pieces, and each piece is uniquely identified by trimming the corners. Thin brass shims are attached to the paper cutter board to assist in accurately placing and cutting the film.

The film phantom is irradiated using the entire IMRT delivery sequence. For patient QA, films are irradiated using the same treatment plan as the patient, but with the monitor units (MUs) scaled to yield doses within an optical density range of 0 to 2.0. This translates to a maximum dose of 100 cGy to the phantom for Kodak XV film. For optimal accuracy, a set of films from the same batch is irradiated to predetermined doses using fixed open fields. The films are placed in a water-equivalent phantom at a depth that corresponds to the average depth within the phantom and irradiated using an open field size similar to the tumor dimensions (e.g., 10 cm depth and a 6 × 6 cm^2 field). This irradiates the film under similar radiation conditions as for the arc treatments. For fixed-field IMRT, the depth can be the same as for the test films.

An automated film scanner is used to measure the optical density distribution of the film. The films are placed in a reproducible orientation such that the transverse treatment planning coordinate system axes are parallel to the scan axes. One corner of the film is designated as the scanning system origin, and the film is scanned using a 2 × 2 mm^2

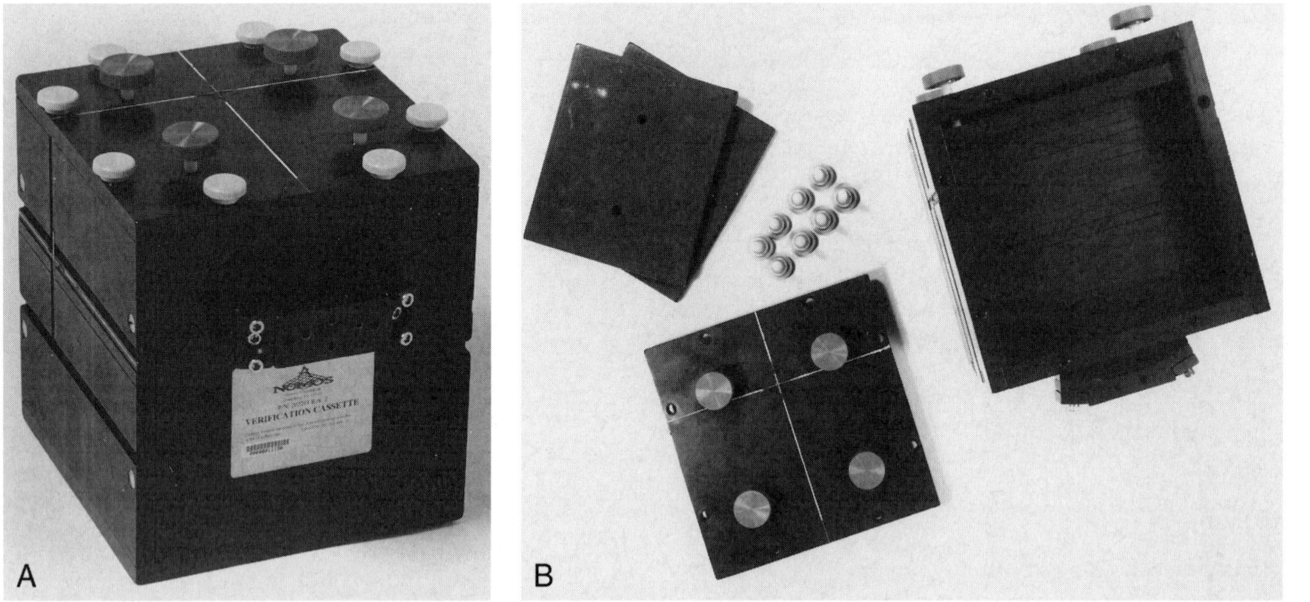

Figure 9.3. Film phantom provided by the NOMOS Corporation for intensity modulated radiation therapy treatment verification. (**A**) The phantom fully assembled. (**B**) The phantom from above with the lid and film compression sheets removed. The assembly screws are also shown.

grid spacing to include the entire film. The calibration films are also scanned, but only near the center of the irradiated field, and in a limited array of points. The calibration film scan provides a permanent record of the densitometer reading as a function of film optical density and absorbed dose.

The location of each film is determined relative to the treatment planning system coordinate system to enable comparison against a planar treatment plan dose distribution extraction. This can be done by direct measurement of the phantom relative to spatial alignment features (e.g., radiopaque localization wires), or by the use of machine drawings of the phantom. In theory, once the spatial location of the measured dose distribution is determined, direct comparison can be made against the calculated distributions. However, treatment planning companies have not provided the software to enable the necessary planar dose extractions and subsequent comparisons against measurement. Manual methods are still employed using scale printouts of measured and calculated distributions overlaid on a light box. Software is needed that will enable direct quantitative comparison of these distributions.

The comparison of single or limited multiple point dose measurements against calculated doses is simpler. If the treatment planning system allows a direct query of the dose distribution, the calculated doses can be recorded and compared against measurements. Point-dose measurements in high-dose gradient regions are of dubious value as a dose discrepancy because spatial misalignment cannot easily be distinguished from a calculation or delivery error. Therefore, point dose measurements are generally restricted to low-dose gradient regions ($<1\%$ mm^{-1}).

To enable measurements using TLDs and ionization chambers, Low et al (115) designed a phantom built using the NOMOS film phantom design. The phantom (shown in Figure 9.4) has the same external cross-section as the film phantom, to enable direct comparisons of measurements made using either phantom, but is filled with water-equivalent plastic. The water-equivalent plastic is fabricated such that the ionization chamber can be placed anywhere within the phantom in a $0.5 \times 0.5 \times 0.5$ cm^3 grid. TLD measurements are made using trays that have holes drilled in a 1×1 cm^2 spaced rectilinear array to hold $3 \times 3 \times 1$ mm^3 TLD chips. Some of the water-equivalent plastic sheets are replaced by the TLD trays for irradiation in the phantom.

An ideal dosimeter would be capable of providing dose measurements in a 3-D volume, with an energy response similar to that of water or muscle. A relatively new dosimeter, BANG^{TM} (bis, acrylamide, nitrogen, and gelatin) gel is being investigated for use in dynamic IMRT dose distribution measurements (116–120). The dosimeter is a gelatinous medium that relies on the polymerization and cross-linking produced by ionizing radiation and subsequent increases in the solvent proton relaxation in the presence of the polymer. The increased proton relaxation rate ($R_2 = 1/T_2$) can be imaged using magnetic resonance imaging (MRI). The gel is irradiated using IMRT delivery and subsequently imaged using a clinical MRI unit. T1 and T2-weighted scans are obtained for each gel and the volumetric distribution of R_2 is determined using these scans. A monotonic relationship exists between R_2 and absorbed dose, but because the gel radiation sensitivity is batch de-

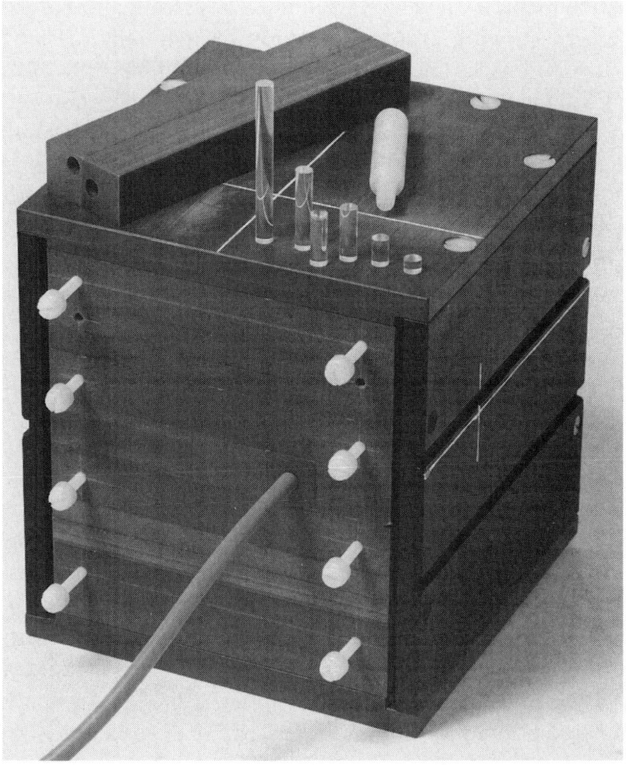

Figure 9.4. Ionization chamber and thermoluminescent dosimetry phantom. Shown are the three chamber holders, the longitudinal spacers, and a tool for removing the chamber holders. The ionization chamber cable is seen exiting from the phantom.

pendent, some gels are irradiated to known doses and scanned to obtain a dose calibration curve. A measurement of the full 3-D dose distribution is provided when this medium is used, with measurement voxels as small as $1 \times 1 \times 2$ mm^3. Currently, cost, thermal sensitivity, and the requirement of MRI for readout will limit the use of this detector medium to a few dosimetry studies. In addition to its MRI properties, the gel is normally transparent and becomes opaque on irradiation. Optical absorption imaging is also being investigated as a method for extracting the dose (118,119).

Commissioning

The core of a treatment planning system commissioning procedure is the comparison of calculated and measured dose distributions. Traditional commissioning procedures investigate beams incident on a water phantom for a variety of field sizes, blocking geometries, beam modulators (wedges), and incident angles. However, IMRT dose distributions are generated using a superposition of complex fluence distributions. Therefore, commissioning of these systems relies on developing dose distributions and fluence delivery sequences for a series of selected target and critical structure volume geometries. The volumes are selected based on expected sizes and shapes of clinical target volumes. Neighboring critical structures can also be defined to provide complex target geometries.

Treatment plans used for commissioning should include a variety of target sizes, shapes, and locations within the test phantom, as well as at least one test using phantoms of different sizes. The target can be cylindrical to simplify preparation and subsequent description of the target geometry. Both diameter and length of the targets should span the range of sizes used for clinical cases. Experiments should also include a broad range of optimization parameters.

Each commissioning experiment will include both film and absolute dose measurements (ionization chamber and/or TLDs). The results should be tabulated to show the dosimetric and spatial accuracy of the system.

System Quality Assurance

The accurate delivery of IMRT dose distributions will depend on thorough accelerator and delivery system QA programs. A description of all accelerator QA procedures is beyond the scope of this chapter. A thorough review was published by the American Association of Physicists in Medicine (121). Some of the specialized procedures specific to IMRT will be mentioned in this chapter.

The accurate localization of the accelerator isocenter relative to the patient alignment fiducial markers is important for noninvasively immobilized patients. The origin within the patient is aligned to the accelerator using the positioning lasers. As in all external beam therapy, if the lasers are not correctly aligned, the localization of the dose distribution within the patient will suffer. For IMRT treatment planning and delivery, dose distributions are generated using fluence distributions incident on the patient from a series of directions. The superposition of the fluence distributions generates the planned dose distribution, and the planning system assumes the orientation and position of each beam angle is accurate. Dose delivery errors can occur due to excessive gantry sag, especially for sequential arc-based therapy (e.g., the Peacock system). QA tests have been developed that check beam and isocenter alignment.

For indexed sequential arc therapy, accurate patient positioning between arcs is extremely important. Carol et al (26) determined that an incorrect placement of the patient between successive arc treatments will cause a 10% mm^{-1} dose heterogeneity in the abutment region. Consequently, the accuracy of the patient immobilization and placement system is critical to accurate dose delivery. Periodic testing of patient indexing system accuracy should be conducted. One method is to place a film at the plane of isocenter and irradiate it using the open collimated portal.

The film is then moved using the same apparatus as used in patient treatments, and the process is repeated six to ten times. Ideally, the film will have a homogeneous rectangular irradiated region, with no evidence of high- or low-dose regions. Overlaps or underlaps can serve to identify problems with either the positioning system or the treatment couch support structure or bearings. Tests are also being developed for the QA of dynamic MLC delivery (122).

The implications of incorrect treatment setup are being investigated. Studies by Low et al (123) and Convery and Rosenbloom (124) have shown that variations in the delivered dose distribution can arise when the gantry, collimator, or couch angle are incorrectly set.

Clinical Quality Assurance

The delivery of IMRT is similar in most respects to the delivery of standard conformal radiation therapy. The principal difference lies in the requirement to keep the patient stationary during the entire course of treatment. For traditional conformal therapy, the motion of the patient during treatment will result in minor dose variations within the portal outlines and a major dose variation near the portal boundaries. However, margins are typically applied to the tumor volumes to account for an expected amount of motion so that the targets will generally remain within the portal boundary. The exception to this rule is when compensating filters or wedges are used. In these cases, patient motion during treatment will alter the doses within the beams an amount proportional to the lateral fluence gradient. For example, the dose gradient for a 45 degree wedge is typically 4 to 5% cm^{-1}, so movement within the portal boundary of 5 mm will result in a dose delivery error of only 2 to 3%, respectively.

In IMRT, the dose distribution is due to a delivery sequence of incident fluences, each with a potentially large lateral fluence gradient. Patient motion between sequential arc deliveries in arc-based IMRT will yield dose heterogeneities similar to those encountered when incorrectly moving the patient (10% mm^{-1}). Patient immobilization is therefore extremely important when IMRT is used. The dose perturbations resulting from patient motion during dynamic MLC delivery are complex, being a function of the dose delivery sequence and patient motion. They can be of significant magnitude, especially for thorax irradiation (125).

One consequence of IMRT is the lack of a convenient open portal for image-based patient position and treatment verification. In IMRT, the two concepts must be separated; the patient position is verified separately from the treatment delivery. Patient positioning verification can be conducted using orthogonal portal films using fixed open fields and comparing against digitally reconstructed radiographs (DRRs) or simulator films. Figure 9.5 shows examples of the DRRs and portal films for a head and neck patient treated using arc-based IMRT. Determination of patient positioning accuracy is made by manually marking bony landmarks and overlaying the portal films and DRRs on a light box. Treatment verification can be conducted using measurement phantoms. The use of in vivo dosimetry may be limited to intracavitary dosimetry. Engler et al (126) used in vivo TLD dosimetry placed beneath bolus on the patient's skin to verify the delivered dose to arc-based fan-beam treatments. However, the acceptable dose tolerances were by necessity large due to the high spatial dose gradient near the patient surface.

SUMMARY OF CLINICAL EXPERIENCE WITH IMRT

Because this is new technology, reports on clinical applications are sparse. It is estimated that 500 patients have been treated with this modality. The academic institutions with the most experience are Methodist Hospital, Baylor University in Houston, Texas; Tufts Medical Center, Boston, Massachusetts; and Mallinckrodt Institute of Radiology, Washington University Medical Center, St. Louis, Missouri. As noted by Woo et al (9), because the concepts of treatment planning and delivery in IMRT break longstanding traditions, it is important that clinical procedures be followed, including:

1. Radiation oncologists, physicists, and dosimetrists must understand the accuracy of treatment planning information and become familiar with radiographic anatomy to more precisely outline target volumes and normal structures.
2. Immobilization of the patient on the treatment table is a high priority.
3. The dose inhomogeneity in the treated volume must be recognized, appropriate priority and various constraints incorporated into the system to achieve the highest dose homogeneity possible within the planning target volume (PTV), and dose contributions to adjacent normal structures be defined to minimize the dose. Because current imaging technology allows only definition of gross tumor, it is important to define clinical volume (microscopic disease) to which adequate minimal tumor doses must be delivered. Patient setup error and internal organ motion must be evaluated to determine the PTV. IMRT treatment planning systems should provide software tools to facilitate the generation of the PTV from the gross and clinical target volumes.

Engler et al (126) reported on 44 patients with advanced or recurrent malignant tumors treated with the NOMOS Peacock system using a 6 MV linear accelerator. The cost function embodied idealized dose-volume parameter sets of up to 21 regions of interest per patient.

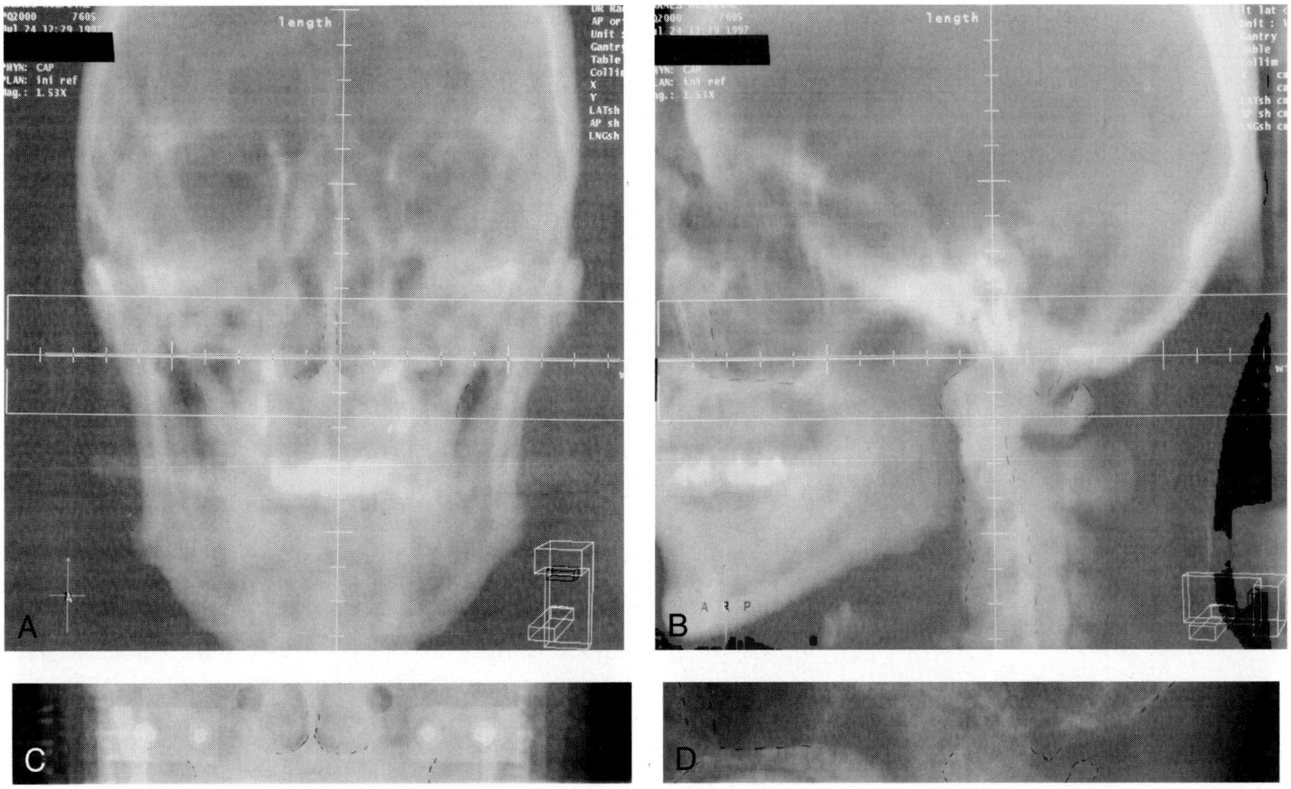

Figure 9.5. Patient with carcinoma of the nasopharynx and a 4 cm lymph node in left upper neck. (**A**) Anteroposterior and (**B**) lateral digitally reconstructed radiographs depicting one arc for intensity modulated radiation therapy through the midportion of the nasopharynx. (**C**) Anteroposterior and (**D**) lateral portal films on the linear accelerator corresponding to the same geometry as (a) and (b), respectively.

Relative importance and spatial preeminence of each region of interest were quantified into the constraint set, together with an instrument data file built from fixed-beam depth dose and crossplot of 8×8 to $40 \times 200\ mm^2$ field sizes. These radiation patterns were measured with a scanning diode in a water tank beam analyzing system. The instrument data file enforced constraints of gantry table angle and patient table geometry.

Treatment plans using the inverse planning system were generated, as well as two-dimensional coronal, sagittal, and cross-section dose distributions. Plans were approved after refining the simulated annealing parameters to provide dose distributions that closely reflected the clinical constraints. After the plan was approved by the radiation oncologist, it was copied onto a disk that was inserted into the MLC controller for treatment delivery.

These authors followed a similar system to the one we use for dose verification, which consisted of measurements with diodes or TLDs embedded in polystyrene calibration and anthropomorphic phantoms. Film dosimetry in the central axis of the anthropomorphic phantom, with optical density distributions of verification and film dose calibration curves, was obtained with a 300 point per inch scanner operated with Photoshop software.

Patients were monitored in vivo with film and thermoluminescent dosimeters under bolus on the patient surface, at a location expected to receive the maximum dose.

Alignment of immobilization devices was based on lasers projected laterally and in the midline over the patient's head. Alignment of face mask immobilization was based on lines and barium sulfate dots placed on the central axis of the face masks. Marker alignment was repeated before each treatment to verify the patient's repeated immobilization, and position was radiographically verified by portal films compared against simulation films.

Engler et al (126), in a study conducted using 550 treatment fractions, noticed position reproducibility within ± 1 mm and dose distribution verification delivered within 2 mm of the planned dose surface and within $\pm 5\%$ of the absolute dose in most cases with patients immobilized with head screws or face masks. Verification in three patients showed large dose discrepancies that were related to errors in image registration, dose calculation, and verification procedures. After correction of these errors, acceptable verification doses were obtained. Using a high dose rate linear accelerator with the capability of delivering up to 600 MUs per minute resulted in an average treatment time of 15 minutes (considering the time from the initial patient

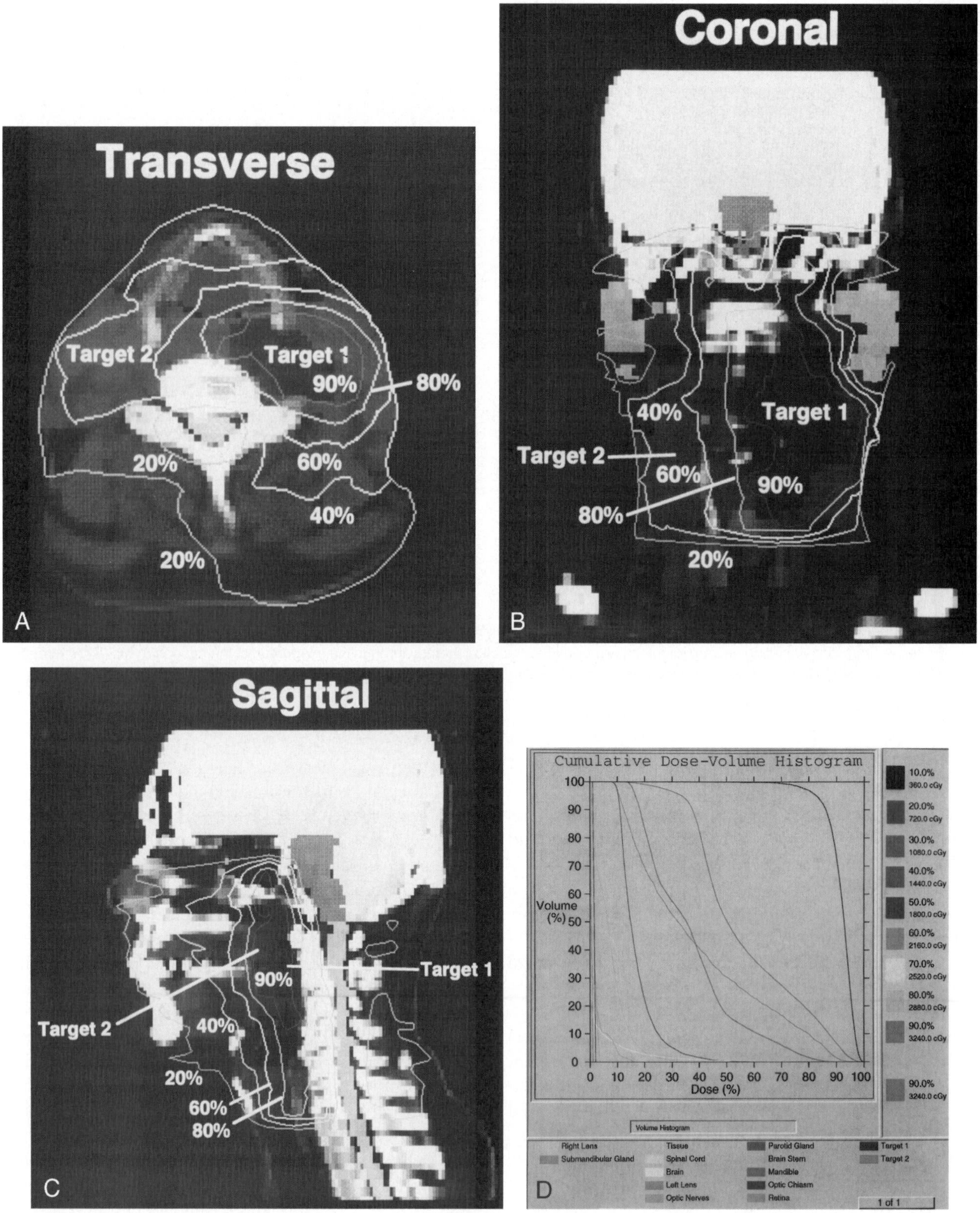

Figure 9.6. Isodose distributions for a patient with carcinoma of the nasopharynx. Isodose lines are shown as percents of the maximum dose within the patient plan. The 90% isodose line was used for the gross disease prescription. Also shown are the nodal disease, the spinal cord, the parotid glands, the mandible, and the brain. (**A**) Transverse isodose distribution. (**B**) Coronal isodose distribution. (**C**) Sagittal isodose distribution. (**D**) Cumulative dose-volume histogram.

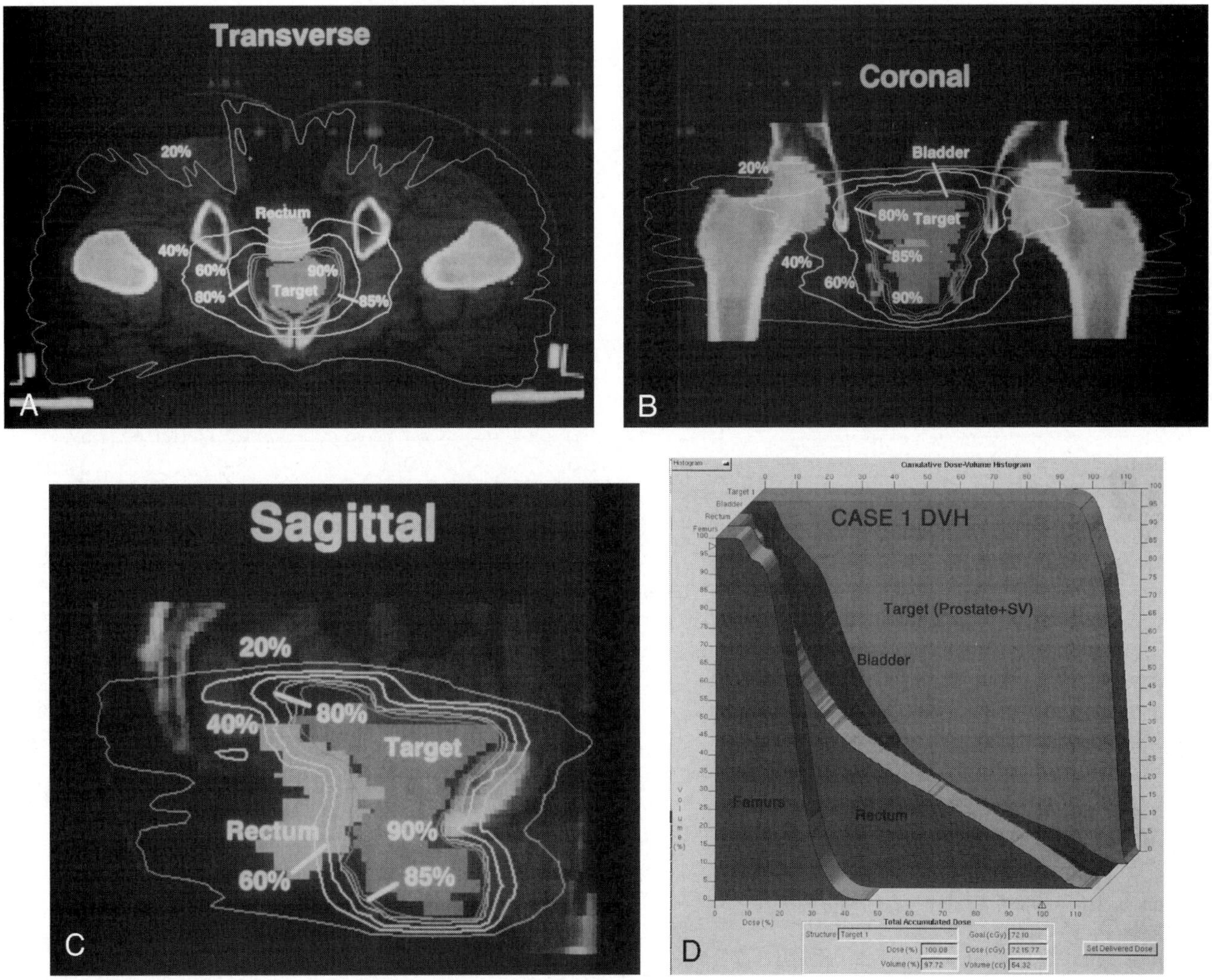

Figure 9.7. Isodose distributions for a patient with carcinoma of the prostate and seminal vesicles. Isodose lines are shown as percents of the maximum dose within the patient plan. The 85% isodose line was used for the target prescription. Also shown are the femurs, the rectum, and the bladder. (**A**) Transverse isodose distribution. (**B**) Coronal isodose distribution. (**C**) Sagittal isodose distribution. (**D**) Dose-volume histogram.

setup until the final arc was completed), which is shorter than what we have observed at our institution (20 to 45 minutes) with an older Varian Clinac 6 (Varian Associates, Palo Alto, CA) delivering up to 240 MU per minute.

As with static 3DCRT techniques, we believe that IMRT should be reserved for patients with significantly irregular tumor volumes, usually with a concave surface, in close proximity to a sensitive structure and when high irradiation doses are to be administered. These criteria are based mostly on the time and effort involved in the administration of these innovative modalities and the availability of scheduling for a significant number of patients. At the present time we use this modality to treat patients with head and neck (Figure 9.6) and intracranial lesions. Treatment planning and delivery exercises have also been conducted for carcinoma of the prostate (Figure 9.7), but potential patient motion may make this site unsuitable for tomotherapy. QA measurement results are shown for these treatments in Figures 9.8 and 9.9, respectively. Plans are underway to implement dynamic MLC-based IMRT for the treatment of prostate cancer. We have also treated one patient with a recurrent tumor in the vertebral column on whom lower doses to the spinal cord were desired. As our proficiency improves and dynamic MLC becomes available, we will expand patient eligibility for treatment with IMRT.

De Neve et al (127) used static beam-intensity modulation executed by beam segmentation to treat patients with head and neck or thyroid cancer. Doses of 70 to 80 Gy could be delivered to the primary tumor volume without exceeding tolerance of the spinal cord (50 Gy at highest voxel). In-target 3-D dose inhomogeneity was approximately 25%. The shortest time of execution of treatment (22 segments) on a patient was 25 minutes.

Verellen et al published a detailed description of the

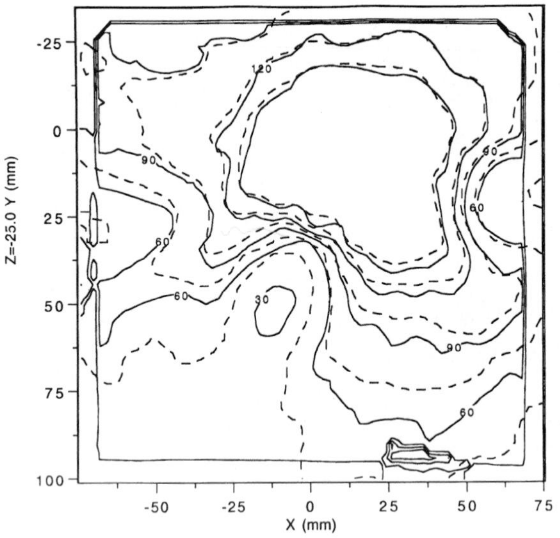

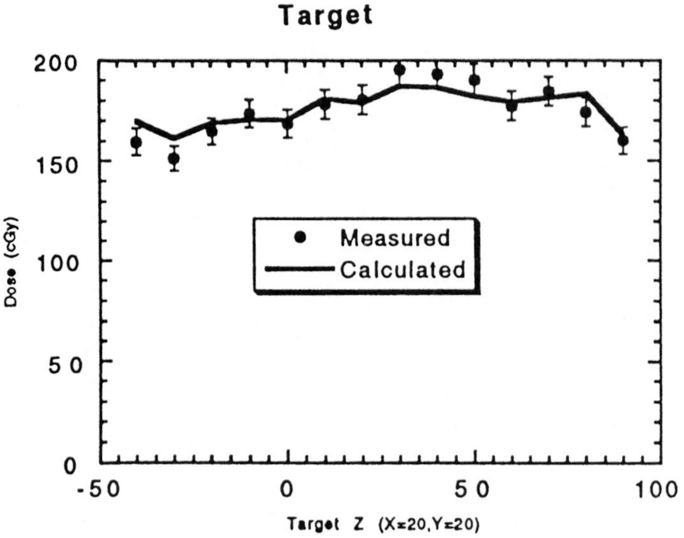

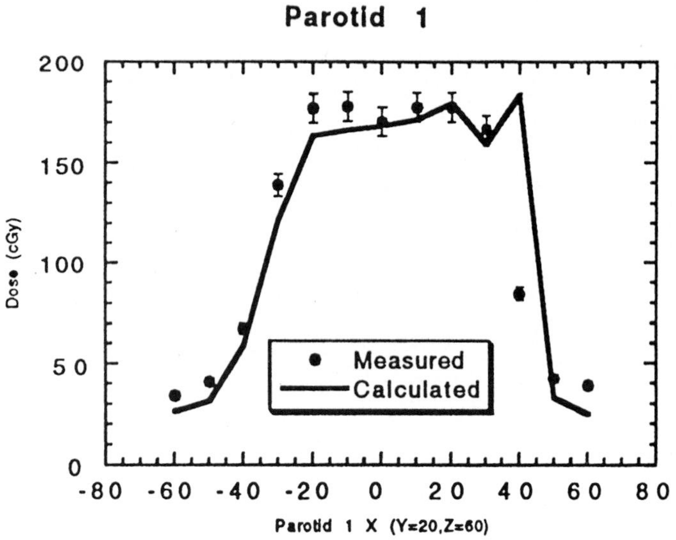

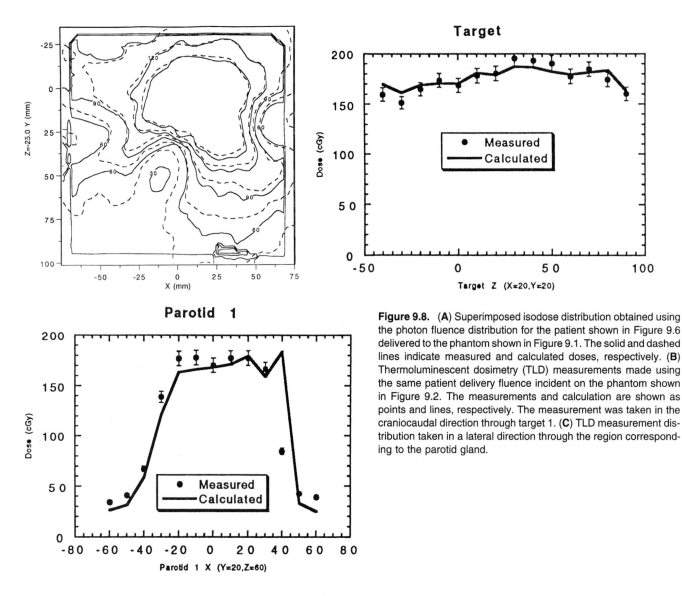

Figure 9.8. (**A**) Superimposed isodose distribution obtained using the photon fluence distribution for the patient shown in Figure 9.6 delivered to the phantom shown in Figure 9.1. The solid and dashed lines indicate measured and calculated doses, respectively. (**B**) Thermoluminescent dosimetry (TLD) measurements made using the same patient delivery fluence incident on the phantom shown in Figure 9.2. The measurements and calculation are shown as points and lines, respectively. The measurement was taken in the craniocaudal direction through target 1. (**C**) TLD measurement distribution taken in a lateral direction through the region corresponding to the parotid gland.

procedures used for the treatment of patients with head and neck tumors used in intensity-modulated conformal irradiation. Dose verification with alanine detectors, thermoluminescent dosimetry, and film dosimetry were conducted. Accuracy of patient positioning was within 0.3 cm and 2.0 degrees except in two cases. The authors concluded that noninvasive fixation techniques were acceptable for treatment of these patients. However, daily monitoring becomes mandatory if an accuracy better than 0.1 cm and 1 degree is required for patient setup.

Optimization

In traditional 3DCRT treatment planning, targets and critical structure geometries are used to determine beam orientations and weights and to prescribe the use of beam modulators such as wedges and compensating filters. IMRT dose planning also uses the geometry of targets and critical structures. However, instead of defining beams, the isodose distribution constraints are defined. These can include minimum target and maximum critical structure doses, requirements that often conflict, requiring the definition of a factor describing the relative importance of each dosimetric constraint. The treatment planning system will also be required to account for target setup uncertainty by allowing the specification of a planning target volume. The selection of these parameters may not be straightforward, and gaining experience of their effect on the resulting dose distribution will be necessary.

Chao et al (128) developed a method for assessing the optimization criteria for the NOMOS Peacock system. The input optimization parameters included the maximum target dose, minimum critical structure dose, and a weight factor ranging from 0 to 2 describing the importance of maintaining the requested dose limits for each structure. The treatment planning system described the patient structures in the CT voxel array, and each voxel was assigned at most a single structure. Spatial margins were considered

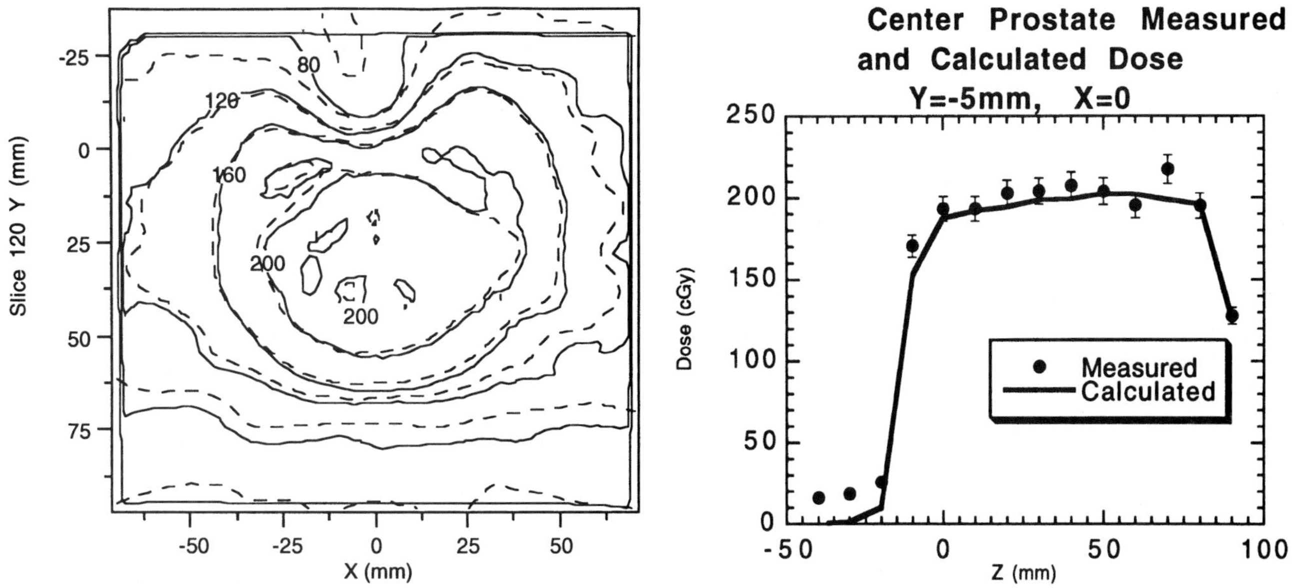

Figure 9.9. (**A**) Superimposed isodose distribution obtained using the photon fluence distribution for the patient shown in Figure 9.7 delivered to the phantom shown in Figure 9.1. The solid and dashed lines indicate measured and calculated doses, respectively. (**B**) Thermoluminescent dosimetry measurements made using the same patient delivery fluence incident on the phantom shown in Figure 9.2. The measurements and calculation are shown as points and lines, respectively. The measurement was taken in the craniocaudal direction through the target.

by "growing" a structure in three dimensions by the user-specified margin for that structure. The voxels enclosed in the enlarged margins became associated with that structure. If a voxel could be assigned to more than one structure, decision rules determined which structure was assigned. To provide user control in the determination of voxel assignments between targets and critical structures, a binary function, termed target priority, was assigned to each critical structure. If the target priority was selected, voxels with conflicting assignments were assigned to the target, and vice versa if target priority was deselected.

Because the effects of the structure weight and priority were unclear, Chao et al (128) conducted a study of the influence of these parameters on head and neck dose distributions in the region between the parotid gland and targets. Six plans were run, each with a common target weight of 1.0, but with variations in the parotid gland weight and target priority. The target coverage and parotid gland overdose were studied for a series of patients. Figure 9.10 shows an example of this evaluation. For this case, a comparison was made for parotid gland weights of 0.5, 1.0, and 2.0. The target margin was 0.5 cm, and no margin was placed on the parotid gland. Two sets of plans were run, one set with target volume superseding the parotid after the target volume margin was applied (target had priority) and one where the parotid was not (target did not have priority). Two quantities were evaluated, the percent of the target volume receiving less than 70 Gy (the prescription dose), and the percent parotid volume receiv-

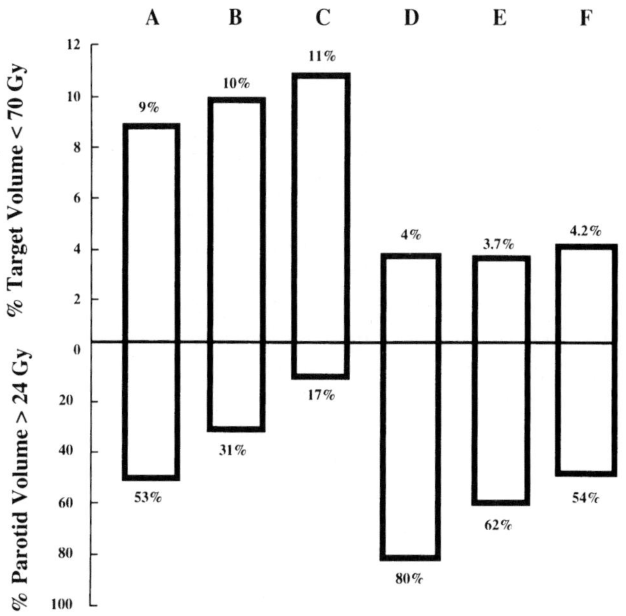

Figure 9.10. Analysis of treatment plan optimization parameters for a head and neck patient. The percent target volume receiving less than the prescription of 70 Gy is compared against the percent parotid gland volume receiving more than 24 Gy. This analysis was conducted for six treatment plan parameter sets to select the best plan and identify the sensitivity of the treatment plans to the optimization parameters.

ing more than 24 Gy. Plans A through C (target did not have priority, in increasing order of parotid weight) indicated slightly poorer coverage than did plans D through F (target had priority, in increasing order of parotid weight). This was due to the dose gradient at the edge of the target volume, a feature common with IMRT-generated dose distributions. A significant difference was seen in the volume of parotid gland exceeding the dose of 24 Gy. The plans with a higher parotid weighting consistently yielded a smaller overdosed parotid gland volume. However, the best plan with respect to parotid overdose yielded the poorest target coverage. The best compromise seemed to be with Plan F, yielding one of the lowest target underdose volumes (4.2%), with a relatively low parotid overdose volume (54%). Studies like these are important to understand the clinical implications of often obscure optimization parameters provided with an IMRT treatment planning system.

Under current 3DCRT clinical practice, patients are often treated using boost fields to deliver a variety of dose levels within the target volumes. Usually the main and boost treatments are delivered sequentially, often with the same daily dose to the planning target volumes. The Peacock (and Corvus) IMRT treatment planning systems do not enable the user to change the treatment volume during the course of therapy. The daily dose distribution is the same throughout the treatment. In order to deliver different total doses to the planning target volumes, the daily dose per fraction is adjusted, and is therefore not the same as delivered using conventional 3DCRT. Studies to determine the optimal or equivalent dose per fraction will be required to enable patient outcome comparisons between IMRT and 3DCRT.

Doses of Irradiation Outside the Treatment Volume

Followill et al (129), based on the observation that with IMRT some form of x-ray attenuation to modulate intensity is required, suggested that the number of MUs used to deliver a given treatment is increased over that used for conventional radiation therapy, resulting in the likelihood of increased whole-body dose to the patient by leakage and scattering of x-rays and, for higher energies, leakage of neutrons through the collimation and treatment head assemblies of the linear accelerator. These authors made estimates of the leakage neutron dose equivalent or photon dose at isocenter in the patient plane at a point 5 cm away from the central axis of a pelvic field and estimated the whole-body x-ray dose equivalent contribution for 50 cm from the center of a 20 × 20 cm treatment field based on previously measured data (3). They also calculated the MUs required to deliver a treatment with conventional x-rays (wedged or unwedged) and with beam-intensity modulated irradiation from two different systems (Varian MLC or NOMOS Peacock MLC). Average total MUs derived from treatment plans for six patients are shown in Table 9.1. The unwedged 6 MV beam required 20% more MUs than the 18 MV beam. With wedges, the 6 MV beam MUs increased by 60% over that for 18 MV. With the NOMOS Peacock system the total number of MUs per fraction increased with the number of arcs used. The total whole-body dose equivalent to a point 50 cm from the center of the pelvic field, when 70 Gy was delivered, was significantly higher with the intensity modulated plans (Table 9.2). The authors also calculated the estimated risk of any fatal secondary cancer associated with scattered dose from the prescribed treatment as a percentage increase in likelihood in nonirradiated populations. The smallest increased risk was 0.4% for the 6 MV unwedged conventional technique, and the highest risk was 24.4% with the tomotherapy technique using 25 MV x-rays. The authors caution against the use of 25 MV x-rays with intensity-modulated techniques, which may carry a serious high risk of second-

Table 9.1. MU/cGy and Total MU to Deliver Conventional and Modulated Beam Intensity Ratiotherapy

	Beam Energy	Conventional		Beam Intensity Modulated	
		Unwedged	Wedged	Varian MLC Modulated	NOMOS MLC Tomotherapy
		(MU/cGy)	(MU/cGy)	(MU/cGy)	(MU/cGy)
MU per dose*	6 MV	1.2	2.4	3.4	9.7
	18 MV	1.0	1.5	2.8	8.1
	25 MV	1.0	1.5	2.8	8.1
		(MU)	(MU)	(MU)	(MU)
Total MU†	6 MV	8,400	16,800	23,800	67,900
	18 MV	7.000	10,500	19,600	56,700
	25 MV	7,000	10,500	19,600	56,700

* The number of MU needed for the indicated technique to deliver 1 cGy to isocenter.
† The total MU needed, using the indicated technique and energy, to delivery 70 Gy to isocenter.
Reprinted with permission from Followill et al (129).

Table 9.2. The Estimated Whole-Body Dose Equivalent (mSv) From a Total Delivered Dose of 70.0 Gy at Isocenter

	6 MV		18 MV		25 MV	
	No Wedges	Wedges	No Wedges	Wedges	No Wedges	Wedges
Conventional	67	134	326	488	602	903
MLC modulated	190	—	911	—	1686	—
Tomotherapy	543	—	2637	—	4876	—

Reprinted with permission from Followill et al (129).

ary cancers, and recommend that the use of x-ray energies greater than 10 MV for beam-intensity modulated conformal therapy should not be attempted until the x-ray and neutron leakage dose and risks associated with the treatment have been carefully evaluated in long-term studies.

At our institution Mutic and Low (130) also measured whole-body irradiation doses from arc-based IMRT to the head and neck region using a water-equivalent plastic block whole-body phantom and a polystyrene phantom, placing TLDs in multiple locations arranged into orthogonal linear arrays. To assess the leakage dose component, the MLC leaves remained closed during treatment delivery. The total midplane whole-body dose from internal scatter and leakage was approximately 2.5% of the total target dose, decreasing to 0.5% at 30 cm from the target. The whole-body dose was entirely due to head irradiation leakage. The internal scatter dose was significant near the target but became negligible beyond 15 cm from the target in relation to the leakage dose. Therefore, the total-body dose was proportional to the total MUs used to deliver a given treatment.

DISCUSSION AND SUMMARY

The process of 3DCRT planning is significantly different from traditional two dimensional treatment planning and requires the retraining of the radiation oncologist and treatment planner. Most of the difference lies in the additional tasks of identifying target volumes and critical structures in three dimensions. The introduction of IMRT will again significantly change the roles of the radiation oncologist and treatment planner, principally because of the inverse planning method. With inverse planning, the physician prescribes the optimal dose distribution using tools provided by the software manufacturer. These may be simple text descriptions of minimum target doses and maximum critical structure doses, or they may include the specification of ideal dose-volume histograms (DVHs). The algorithms may have additional input parameters that specify the relative importance of sparing critical structures versus providing the requested target doses. While the process of inverse planning ideally removes the need for multiple plan development and evaluations, the lack of robust objective functions will continue to necessitate the execution of multiple plans, at least for the foreseeable future.

IMRT has the potential for delivering more conformal dose distributions, treating complex 3-D target volumes while sparing critical structures, and therefore improving the quality of radiation therapy. However, there are numerous clinical issues that remain unanswered in IMRT. Most important are the radiobiologic consequences of non-standard dose fractionation caused by having multiple dose prescription levels simultaneously delivered. With IMRT, there is significantly greater dose heterogeneity within the target than for conventional conformal therapy. The premise that the ideal dose distribution includes a homogeneous dose within the target will require reevaluation.

The dosimetry instrumentation used for both treatment delivery and QA needs to undergo reevaluation for IMRT. IMRT delivery places significant constraints on the design and operational characteristics of dosimetry equipment. The dynamic dose delivery and deficiencies of traditional QA techniques will leave many potential users cynical of this exciting development. Significant evidence of the clinical advantages and safeguards will be required before IMRT becomes routine clinical practice.

While significant efforts remain, the introduction of IMRT has been successful. The number of patients treated using commercial and developmental implementations of this modality will continue to increase. The introduction of multiinstitutional trials using IMRT is essential to document any clinical advantages. In the future, the further development of CT-based simulation, inverse planning systems, and linear accelerator systems designed to deliver IMRT-based dose distributions will likely reduce the overall cost of radiation therapy.

References

1. Meyer JL, Purdy JA, eds. 3-D Conformal Radiotherapy, Vol. 29, Frontiers in Radiation Therapy and Oncology, Basel: Switzerland, Karger AG, 1996.
2. Purdy JA. Intensity Modulated Radiation Therapy. Int J Radiat Oncol Biol Phys 1996;35:845–846.
3. Stovall M, Blackwell CR, Cundiff J, Novack DH, Palta JR, Wagner LK, Webster EW, Shalek RJ. Fetal dose from radiotherapy with photon beams: Report of AAPM Radiation Therapy Committee Task Group No. 36. Med Phys 1995;22:63-82.
4. Fraass BA. The development of conformal radiation therapy. Med Phys 1995;22:1911–1921.
5. Brahme A. Optimization of radiation therapy. Int J Radiat Oncol Biol Phys 1994;28:785–787.
6. Ellis F, Miller H. The use of wedge filters in deep x-ray therapy. Br J Radiol 1944;17:90.
7. Ellis F, Hall EJ, Oliver R. A compensator for variations in tissue thickness for high energy beams. Br J Radiol 1959;32:421–422.
8. Carol MP. Integrated 3D Conformal Planning/Multivane Intensity Modulating Delivery System for Radiotherapy. In: Purdy JA, Emami B, eds. 3D Radiation Treatment Planning and Conformal Therapy. Madison, Wisconsin: Medical Physics Publishing, 1995:435–445.
9. Woo SY, Sanders M, Grant W, Butler EB. Does the "Peacock" have anything to do with radiotherapy? Int J Radiat Oncol Biol Phys 1994; 29:213–214.
10. Ling CC, Burman C, Chui CS, Kutcher GJ, Leibel SA, LoSasso T, Mohan R, Bortfeld T, Reinstein L, Spirou S, Wang XH, Wu Q, et al. Conformal radiation treatment of prostate cancer using inversely-planned intensity-modulated photon beams produced with dynamic multileaf collimation. Int J Radiat Oncol Biol Phys 1996;35: 721–730.
11. Chui CS, LoSasso T, Spirou S. Dose calculation for photon beams with intensity modulation generated by dynamic jaw or multileaf collimations. Med Phys 1994;21:1237–1244.
12. Convery DJ, Rosenbloom ME. The generation of intensity-modulated fields for conformal radiotherapy by dynamic collimation. Phys Med Biol 1992;37:1359–1374.

13. Geis P, Boyer AL. Use of a multileaf collimator as a dynamic missing-tissue compensator. Med Phys 1996;23:1199–1205.
14. Grant W, Bellezza D. Leakage considerations with a multi-leaf collimator designed for intensity-modulated conformal radiotherapy (Abstract). Med Phys 1994;21:921.
15. Hounsell AR, Wilkinson JM. Head scatter modelling for irregular field shaping and intensity modulation. Phys Med Biol 1997;42: 1737–1749.
16. Spirou SV, Chui CS. Generation of arbitrary intensity profiles by dynamic jaws or multileaf collimators. Med Phys 1994;21: 1031–1041.
17. Stein J, Bortfeld T, Dorschel B, Schlegel W. Dynamic x-ray compensation for conformal radiotherapy by means of multi-leaf collimation. Radiother Oncol 1994;32:163–173.
18. Svensson R, Kallman P, Brahme A. An analytical solution for the dynamic control of multileaf collimators. Phys Med Biol 1994;39: 37–61.
19. Webb S, Bortfeld T, Stein J, Convery D. The effect of stair-step leaf transmission on the 'tongue-and-groove problem' in dynamic radiotherapy with a multileaf collimator. Phys Med Biol 1997;42:595–602.
20. vanSantvoort JPC. Dynamic multileaf collimation without 'tongue-and-groove' underdosage effects. Phys Med Biol 1996;41: 2091–2105.
21. Yu CX. Intensity-modulated arc therapy with dynamic multileaf collimation: An alternative to tomotherapy. Phys Med Biol 1995;40: 1435–1449.
22. Yu C, Symons MJ, Du MN, Martinez AA, Wong JW. A method for implementing dynamic photon beam intensity modulation using independent jaws and a multileaf collimator. Phys Med Biol 1995; 40:769–787.
23. Mackie TR, Holmes T, Swerdloff S, Reckwerdt P, Deasy JO, Yang J. Tomotherapy: a new concept for the delivery of dynamic conformal radiotherapy. Med Phys 1993;20:1709–1719.
24. Richter J, Neumann M, Bortfeld T. Dynamic Multileaf Collimator Rotation Techniques Versus Intensity Modulated Fixed Fields. In: Leavitt DD, Starkschall G, eds. XII International Conference on the Use of Computers in Radiation Therapy. Salt Lake City, UT: Medical Physics Publishing, 1997:335–337.
25. Stein J, Hartwig K, Levegrün S, Zhang G, Preiser K, Rhein B, Debus J, Bortfeld T. Intensity-Modulated Treatments: Compensators vs. Multileaf Modulation. In: Leavitt DD, Starkschall G, eds. XII International Conference on the Use of Computers in Radiation Therapy. Salt Lake City, UT: Medical Physics Publishing, 1997:338–341.
26. Carol M, Grant WH, Blier AR, Kania AA, Targovnik HS, Butler EB, Woo SW. The field-matching problem as it applies to the Peacock three dimensional conformal system for intensity modulation. Int J Radiat Oncol Biol Phys 1996;34:183–187.
27. Verellen D, Linthout N, Berge DVD, Bel A, Storme G. Initial experience with intensity-modulated conformal radiation therapy for treatment of the head and neck region. Int J Radiat Oncol Biol Phys 1997;39:99–114.
28. Webb S, Oldham M. A method to study the characteristics of 3D dose distributions created by superposition of many intensity-modulated beams delivered via a slit aperture with multiple absorbing vanes. Phys Med Biol 1996;41:2135–2153.
29. Wu A, Johnson M, Chen ASJ, Kalnicki S. Evaluation of dose calculation algorithm of the Peacock system for multileaf intensity modulation collimator. Int J Radiat Oncol Biol Phys 1996;36:1225–1231.
30. Carol M. Peacock: A system for planning and rotational delivery of intensity-modulated fields. Int J Imaging Systems Technol 1995;6: 56–61.
31. Low DA, Mutic S. Abutment region dosimetry for sequential arc IMRT delivery. Phys Med Biol 1997;42:1465–1470.
32. Hope C, Orr JS. Computer optimization of 4 MeV treatment planning. Phys Med Biol 1965;10:365–370.
33. Redpath AT, Vickery BL, Wright DH. A new technique for radiotherapy planning using quadratic programming. Phys Med Biol 1976; 21:781–791.
34. McDonald SC, Rubin P. Optimization of external beam radiation therapy. Int J Radiat Oncol Biol Phys 1977;2:307–317.
35. Gustafsson A, Lind BK, Svensson R, Brahme A. Simultaneous optimization of dynamic multileaf collimation and scanning patterns or compensation filters using a generalized pencil beam algorithm. Med Phys 1995;22:1141–1156.
36. Brahme A. Optimization of stationary and moving beam radiation therapy techniques. Radiother Oncol 1988;12:129–140.
37. Lind BK. Properties of an algorithm for solving the inverse problem in radiation therapy. Inverse Prob 1990;6:415–426.
38. Brahme A, Roos JE, Lax I. Solution of an integral equation in rotation therapy. Phys Med Biol 1982;27:1221–1229.
39. Cormack AM, Cormack RA. A problem in rotation therapy with x-rays: Dose distributions with an axis of symmetry. Int J Radiat Oncol Biol Phys 1987;13:1921–1925.
40. Cormack AM. A problem in rotational therapy with x rays. Int J Radiat Oncol Biol Phys 1987;13:623–630.
41. Barth NH. An inverse problem in radiation therapy. Int J Radiat Oncol Biol Phys 1990;18:425–431.
42. Cormack AM, Quinto ET. On a problem in radiotherapy: Questions on non-negativity. Int J Imaging Systems Technol 1989;1:120–124.
43. Bortfeld T, Burkelbach J, Boesecke R, Schlegel W. Methods of image reconstruction from projections applied to conformation radiotherapy. Phys Med Biol 1990;35:1423–1434.
44. Holmes T, Mackie TR, Simpkin D, Reckwerdt P. A unified approach to the optimization of brachytherapy and external beam dosimetry. Int J Radiat Oncol Biol Phys 1991;20:859–873.
45. Djordjevich A, Bonham DJ, Hussein EMA. Optimal design of radiation compensators. Med Phys 1990;17:397–404.
46. Webb S. Optimization of conformal radiotherapy dose distributions by simulated annealing. Phys Med Biol 1989;34:1349–1370.
47. Mohan R, Mageras GS, Baldwin B, Brewster LJ, Kutcher GJ, Leibel S, Burman CM, Ling CC, Fuks Z. Clinically relevant optimization of 3-D conformal treatments. Med Phys 1992;19:933–944.
48. Jain NL, Kahn MG, Graham MV, Purdy JA. 3D Conformal Radiation Therapy. V. Decision-Theoretic Evaluation on Radiation Treatment Plans. In: Hounsel AR, Wilkinson JM, Williams PC, eds. Proceedings of the XIth International Conference on the Use of Computers in Radiation Therapy. Manchester, UK: 1994:8–9.
49. Niemierko A, Urie M, Goitein M. Optimization of 3D radiation therapy with both physical and biological end points and constraints. Int J Radiat Oncol Biol Phys 1992;23:99–108.
50. Niemierko A. Random search algorithm (RONSC) for optimization of radiation therapy with both physical and biological end points and constraints. Int J Radiat Oncol Biol Phys 1992;20:1067–1073.
51. Rosen II, Morrill SM, Lane RG. Optimized dynamic rotation with wedges. Med Phys 1992;19:971–977.
52. Schultheiss TE. Models in radiotherapy: Definition of decision criteria. Med Phys 1985;12:183–187.
53. Soderstrom S, Brahme A. Optimization of the dose delivery in a few field techniques using radiobiological objective functions. Med Phys 1993;20:1201–1210.
54. Starkschall G. A constrained least-squares optimization method for external beam radiation therapy treatment planning. Med Phys 1984; 11:659–665.
55. Langer M, Brown R, Urie M, Leong J, Stracher M, Shapiro J. Large scale optimization of beam weights under dose-volume restrictions. Int J Radiat Oncol Biol Phys 1990;18:887–893.
56. Langer M, Brown R, Kijewski P, Ha C. The reliability of optimization under dose-volume limits. Int J Radiat Oncol Biol Phys 1993;26: 529–538.
57. Langer M, Leong J. Optimization of beam weights under dose-volume restrictions. Int J Radiat Oncol Biol Phys 1987;13:1255–1259.
58. Graham MV, Jain ML, Kahn MG, Drzymala RE, Purdy JA. Evaluation of an objective plan-evaluation model in the three dimensional treatment of nonsmall cell lung cancer. Int J Radiat Oncol Biol Phys 1996;34:469–474.
59. Brahme A. Treatment Optimization Using Physical and Radiobiological Objective Functions. In: Smith AR, ed. Medical Radiology, Radiation Therapy Physics. Berlin: Springer-Verlag, 1995:209–246.
60. Rosen II, Lane RG, Morrill SM, Belli JA. Treatment plan optimization using linear programming. Med Phys 1991;18:141–152.
61. Cooper RE. A gradient method for optimizing external-beam radiotherapy treatment plans. Radiology 1978;128:235–243.
62. Holmes T, Mackie TR. A filtered backprojection dose calculation method for inverse treatment planning. Med Phys 1994;21:303–313.
63. Gustafsson A, Lind BK, Brahme A. A generalized pencil beam algo-

rithm for optimization of radiation therapy. Med Phys 1994;21: 343–356.
64. Metropolis N, Rosenbluth A, Rosenbluth M, Teller A, Teller E. Equation of state calculations by fast computing machines. J Chem Phys 1953;21:1087–1092.
65. Kirkpatrick S. Optimization by simulated annealing. Science 1985; 220:671–680.
66. Mohan R, Wang X, Jackson A. Optimization of 3-D conformal radiation treatment plans. Frontiers of Radiat Ther Oncol 1996;29:86–103.
67. Morrill SM, Lane RG, Rosen II. Constrained simulated annealing for optimized radiation therapy treatment planning. Comput Meth Prog Biomed 1990;33:135–144.
68. Morrill SM, Lane RG, Jacobson G, Rosen II. Treatment planning optimization using constrained simulated annealing. Phys Med Biol 1991;36:1341–1361.
69. Mageras GS, Mohan R. Application of fast simulated annealing to optimization of conformal radiation treatments. Med Phys 1993;20: 639–647.
70. Webb S. Optimization by simulated annealing of three-dimensional conformal treatment planning for radiation fields defined by a multileaf collimator. Phys Med Biol 1991;36:1201–1226.
71. Webb S. Optimization of conformal radiotherapy dose distributions by simulated annealing. II. Inclusion of scatter in the 2D technique. Phys Med Biol 1991;36:1227–1237.
72. Webb S. Optimization by simulated annealing of three-dimensional, conformal treatment planning for radiation fields defined by a multileaf collimator: II. Inclusion of two-dimensional modulation of the x-ray intensity. Phys Med Biol 1992;37:1689–1704.
73. Sauer OA, Shepard DM, Angelos L, Mackie TR. A Comparison of Objective Functions for Use in Radiotherapy Optimization. In: Leavitt DD, Starkschall G, eds. XII International Conference on the Use of Computers in Radiation Therapy. Salt Lake City, UT: Medical Physics Publishing, 1997:313–316.
74. Takahashi S. Conformation radiotherapy: Rotation techniques as applied to radiography and radiotherapy of cancer. Acta Radiol Suppl 1965;242:1–42.
75. Proimos BS. Synchronous field shaping in rotational megavoltage therapy. Radiology 1960;74:753–757.
76. Proimos BS. Beam-shapers oriented by gravity in rotational therapy. Radiology 1966;87:928–932.
77. Trump JG, Wright KA, Smedal MI, Saltzman FA. Synchronous field shaping and protection in 2-million-volt rotational therapy. Radiology 1961;76:275.
78. Wright KA, Proimos BS, Trump JG, Smedal MI, Johnson DO, Salzman FA. Field shaping and selective protection in megavoltage therapy. Radiology 1959;72:101.
79. Green A. Tracking cobalt project. Nature 1965;207:1311.
80. Davy TJ, Johnson PH, Redford R, Williams JR. Conformation therapy using the tracking cobalt unit. Br J Radiol 1975;48:122–130.
81. Davy TJ, Brace JA. Dynamic 3-D treatment using a computer-controlled cobalt unit. Br J Radiol 1979;53:612–616.
82. Davy TJ. Physical Aspects of Conformation Therapy Using Computer-Controlled Tracking Units. In: Orton CG, ed. Progress in Medical Radiation Physics. 2nd ed. New York: Plenum, 1985:
83. Brace JA. A computer-controlled tele-cobalt unit. Int J Radiat Oncol Biol Phys 1982;8:2011–2013.
84. Brace JA, Davy TJ, Skeggs DBL, Williams HS. Conformation therapy at the Royal Free Hospital. A progress report on the tracking Cobalt project. Br J Radiol 1981;54:1068–1074.
85. Brace JA. Computer Systems for the Control of Teletherapy Units. In: Orton CG, ed. Progress in Medical Radiation Physics. 2nd ed. New York: Plenum, 1985.
86. Brace JA, Davy TJ, Skeggs DBL. A computer-controlled Cobalt unit for radiotherapy. Med Biol Eng Computing 1981;19:612–616.
87. Bjarngard BE, Kijewski PK. The Potential of Computer Control to Improve Dose Distributions in Radiation Therapy. In: Sternick ES, ed. Computer Applications in Radiation Oncology. Hanover: University Press, 1976.
88. Bjarngard B, Kijewski P, Pashby C. Description of a computer-controlled machine. Int J Radiat Oncol Biol Phys 1977;2:142.
89. Chin LM, Kijewski PK, Svensson GK, Chaffey JT, Levene MB, Bjarngard BE. A computer-controlled radiation therapy machine for pelvic and para-aortic nodal areas. Int J Radiat Oncol Biol Phys 1981;7: 61–70.
90. Chin LM, Kijewski PK, Svensson GK, Bjarngard BE. Dose optimization with computer-controlled gantry rotation, collimator motion and dose-rate variation. Int J Radiat Oncol Biol Phys 1983;9:723–729.
91. Kijewski PK, Chin LM, Bjarngard BE. Wedge-shaped dose distributions by computer-controlled collimator motion. Med Phys 1978;5: 426–429.
92. Mohan R, Lovelock M, Mageras G, LoSasso T, Chui C. Computer-Controlled Radiation Therapy and Multileaf Collimation. In: Meyer JL, Purdy JA, eds. 3-D Conformal Radiotherapy: A New Era in the Irradiation of Cancer. New York, NY: Karger, 1996:123–138.
93. Klein EE. Implementation and clinical use of multileaf collimation. In: Purdy JA, Fraass BA, eds. Syllabus: A Categorical Course in Physics, Three-Dimensional Radiation Therapy Treatment Planning. Oak Brook, IL: Radiological Society of North America, 1994.
94. Boyer AL, Ochran TG, Nyerick CE, Waldron TJ, Huntzinger CJ. Clinical dosimetry for implementation of a multileaf collimator. Med Phys 1992;19:1255–1261.
95. Webb S. The Physics of Three-Dimensional Radiation Therapy. Bristol: Institute of Physics Publishing, 1993:373.
96. Brahme A. Design principles and clinical possibilities with a new generation of radiation therapy equipment: A review. Acta Oncol 1987;26:403–412.
97. Fraass BA, McShan CL, Kessler ML. Computer-controlled treatment delivery. Sem Rad Oncol 1995;5:77–85.
98. Fraass BA. Computer-Controlled Three-Dimensional Conformal Therapy Delivery Systems. In: Purdy JA, Fraass BA, eds. Syllabus: A Categorical Course in Physics, Three-dimensional Radiation Therapy Treatment Planning. Oak Brook, IL: Radiological Society of North America, 1994:93–100.
99. Boyer AL. Present and future developments in radiotherapy treatment units. Semin Radiat Oncol 1995;5:146–155.
100. Powers WE, Kinzie JK, Demidecki AJ. A new system of field shaping for external-beam radiation therapy. Radiology 1973;108:407.
101. Leavitt DD, Martin M, Moeller JH, Lee WL. Dynamic wedge field techniques through computer-controlled collimator motion and dose delivery. Med Phys 1990;17:87–91.
102. Carol MP. 3-D planning and delivery system for optimized conformal therapy (abst.). Int J Radiat Oncol Biol Phys 1992;24:150.
103. Mackie TR, Aldridge S, Angelos L, Balog J, Coon S, Fang G, Fitchard E, Geiser B, Glass M, Iosevich S, Kapatoes J, McNutt T, et al. Tomotherapy: Rethinking the Process of Radiotherapy. In: Leavitt DD, Starkschall G, eds. XII International Conference on the Use of Computers in Radiation Therapy. Salt Lake City: Medical Physics Publishing, 1997:329–331.
104. Fang GY, Geiser B, Mackie RT. Software System for the UW/GE Tomotherapy Prototype. In: Leavitt DD, Starkschall G, eds. XII International Conference on the Use of Computers in Radiation Therapy. Salt Lake City: Medical Physics Publishing, 1997:332–334.
105. Källman P, Lind B, Eklof A, Brahme A. Shaping of arbitrary dose distributions by dynamic multileaf collimation. Phys Med Biol 1988; 33:1291–1300.
106. Galvin JM, Chen X-G, Smith RM. Combining multileaf fields to modulate fluence distributions. Int J Radiat Oncol Biol Phys 1993;27: 697–705.
107. Bortfeld TR, Kahler DL, Waldron TJ, Boyer AL. X-ray field compensation with multileaf collimators. Int J Radiat Oncol Biol Phys 1994; 28:723–730.
108. Low DA, Li Z, Klein EE. Verification of milled two-dimensional photon compensating filters using an electronic portal imaging device. Med Phys 1996;23:929–938.
109. Low DA, Zhu XR, Harms WB, Purdy JA. Beam-intensity modulation using physical modulators (abstract). Med Phys 1996;23:1001.
110. vanBattum LJ, Heijmen BJ. Film dosimetry in water in a 23 MV therapeutic photon beam. Radiother Oncol 1995;34:152–159.
111. Williamson JF, Kahn FM, Sharma SC. Film dosimetry of megavoltage photon beams: a practical method of isodensity-to-isodose curve conversion. Med Phys 1981;8:94–98.
112. Hale JI, Kerr AT, Shragge PC. Calibration of film for accurate megavoltage photon dosimetry. Med Dosim 1994;19:43–46.
113. Mayer R, Williams A, Frankel T, Cong Y, Simons S, Yang N, Timmerman R. Two-dimensional film dosimetry application in heterogeneous materials exposed to megavoltage photon beams. Med Phys 1997;24:455–460.

114. Low DA, Mutic S, Gerber RL, Bosch WR, Perez CA, Purdy JA. Quantitative dosimetric verification of an IMRT planning and delivery system (submitted). Radiother and Oncol 1997.
115. Low DA, Gerber RL, Mutic S, Purdy JA. Phantoms for IMRT dose distribution measurement and treatment verification. Int J Radiat Oncol Biol Phys 1997;40:1231-1235.
116. Maryanski MJ, Audet C, Gore JC. Effects of crosslinking and temperature on the dose response of a BANG polymer gel dosimeter. Phys Med Biol 1997;42:303–311.
117. Maryanski MJ, Schulz RJ, Ibbott GS, Gatenby JC, Xie J, Horton D, Gore JC. Magnetic resonance imaging of radiation dose distributions using a polymer gel dosimeter. Phys Med Biol 1994;39:1437–1455.
118. Maryanski MJ, Ibbott GS, Eastman P, Schulz RJ, Gore JC. Radiation therapy dosimetry using magnetic resonance imaging of polymer gels. Med Phys 1996;23:699–705.
119. Maryanski MJ, Zastavker YZ, Gore JC. Radiation dose distributions in three dimensions from tomographic optical density scanning of polymer gels: II. Optical properties of the BANG polymer gel. Phys Med Biol 1996;41:2705–2717.
120. Gore JC, Ranade M, Maryanski MJ, Schulz RJ. Radiation dose distributions in three dimensions from tomographic optical density scanning of polymer gels: I. Development of an optical scanner. Phys Med Biol 1996;41:2695–2704.
121. Kutcher GJ, Coia L, Gillin M, Hanson WF, Leibel S, Morton RJ, Palta JR, Reinstein LE, Svensson GK. Comprehensive QA for radiation oncology: Report of AAPM Radiation Therapy Committee Task Group 40. Med Phys 1994;21:581–618.
122. Chui CS, Spirou S, LoSasso T. Testing of dynamic multileaf collimation. Med Phys 1996;23:635–641.
123. Low DA, Zhu XR, Purdy JA, Söderström S. The influence of angular misalignment on fixed-portal intensity modulated radiation therapy. Med Phys 1997;24:1123–1139.
124. Convery D, Rosenbloom M. Treatment delivery accuracy in intensity-modulated conformal radiotherapy. Phys Med Biol 1995;40: 979–999.
125. Yu CX, Jaffray DA, Wong JW. Calculating the Effects of Intra-Treatment Organ Motion on Dynamic Intensity Modulation. In: Leavitt DD, Starkschall G, eds. XII International Conference on the Use of Computers in Radiation Therapy. Salt Lake City, UT: Medical Physics Publishing, 1997:231–233.
126. Engler MJ, Tsai J-S, Ling MN, Wu JK, Palano J, Koistinen M, Kramer B, Fagundes M, Dipetrillo T, Wazer DE. Physical and clinical aspects of the dynamic intensity modulated radiotherapy of 44 patients. In: 38th Annual Meeting of the American Society for Therapeutic Radiology and Oncology. Los Angeles, CA: 1996.
127. De Neve W, De Wagter C, De Jaeger I, Thienpont M, Colle C, Derycke S, Schelfhout J. Planning and delivering high doses to targets surrounding the spinal cord at the lower neck and upper mediastinal levels: Static beam-segmentation technique executed with a multileaf collimator. Radiother Oncol 1996;40:271–279.
128. Chao KC, Low DA, Gerber RL, Perez CA, Purdy JA. Clinical and technical considerations for head and neck cancers treated by IMRT: Initial experience (abstract). Int J Radiat Oncol Biol Phys 1997;39 (suppl):238.
129. Followill D, Geis P, Boyer A. Estimates of whole-body dose equivalent produced by beam intensity modulated conformal therapy. Int J Radiat Oncol Biol Phys 1997;38:667–672 (reprinted with permission from Elsevier Science).
130. Mutic S, Low DA. Whole body dose from arc-based IMRT treatments (abstract). Int J Radiat Oncol Biol Phys 1997;24:1368.

Chapter 10

Stereotactic Radiosurgery and Radiotherapy

Kwan H. Cho, Bruce J. Gerbi, and Walter A. Hall

Stereotactic radiosurgery (SRS) is a term coined by Lars Leksell in 1951 to describe any method of focusing small radiation beams on a small intra-cranial lesion (1). Incorporating technological developments that have occurred over the past several decades, such as the Gamma Knife unit in the 1950s, advanced imaging techniques in the 1970s and 1980s, and Linac-based stereotactic systems in the 1980s, the use of SRS has expanded from its original use to treat benign conditions (i.e., arteriovenous malformations (AVM), meningiomas, acoustic neuromas) to its current use to treat many malignant tumors (i.e., gliomas, brain metastases) and functional disorders (i.e., trigeminal neuralgia, movement disorders). Further developments permit fractionated treatments (referred to as stereotactic radiotherapy (SRT) as opposed to SRS for single fractional treatment), which are radiobiologically more advantageous in treating malignant tumors and lesions close to eloquent structures (i.e., optic pathway, brain stem).

This chapter provides a comprehensive description of the radiobiological, clinical, and technical aspects of SRS and SRT.

RADIOBIOLOGIC ASPECTS

The general practice in radiosurgery is to deliver a large dose of radiation in a single fraction to a relatively small circumscribed lesion (usually ≤4 cm) in the brain. This is contrary to the practice of conventional (fractionated) radiotherapy in which small doses are delivered in a number of fractions to the target, based on teachings over the past several decades on the four basic radiobiological principles of repair, reoxygenation, redistribution, and repopulation (referred to as the "4 Rs"). The potential benefits of the "4 Rs" are not considered with radiosurgery. The biological effects of a single large radiosurgical dose is a consequence of vascular effects (thrombosis in the case of AVM) and/or antiproliferative effects (reproductive cell death in the case of tumor).

The impact of ionizing radiation varies depending on the nature of the tissue, late-responding (slow proliferating) tissues or early-responding (rapidly proliferating) tissues. A single large fraction produces substantially greater damage in late-responding tissues (or tumors) and less damage in early-responding tissues (or tumors), whereas the opposite is true for fractionated radiotherapy if the linear quadratic equation is assumed to best represent the mammalian cell survival curve (Figure 10.1) (see also Chapter 1). Examples of late-responding tissue are the AVMs and possibly the slow growing benign tumors, such as meningioma, acoustic neuroma, pituitary adenoma, and chemodectoma. From a radiobiological standpoint, these lesions are suitable for a single large fractional treatment. Contrary to this, malignant tumors (rapidly proliferating) are more suitable for fractionated radiotherapy (see Fractionated Stereotactic Radiotherapy later in this section).

The process of radiation effect in the brain is highly complex and dependent on a number of factors including dose, volume, and the underlying cellular composition of the target.

Dose-Volume Relationship

The risks of radiation-induced brain necrosis are primarily dependent on total dose, the volume of tissue irradiated, and the fractionation scheme. For whole brain irradiation using conventional fractionation (1.8-2 Gy per fraction, daily at 5 days a week), $TD_{5/5}$ (tissue tolerance dose associated with a 5% rate of complications occurring

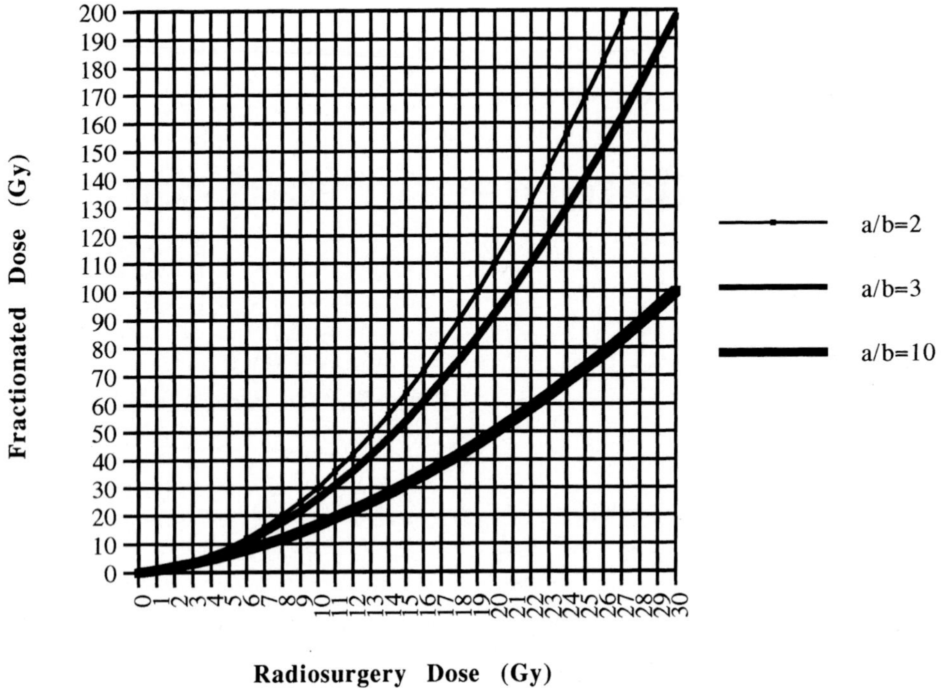

Figure 10.1. Radiosurgery dose (horizontal axis) versus total fractionated radiotherapy dose at 2 Gy per fraction to produce the same radiobiologic effect (vertical axis), both for late- (a/b = 2 or 3) and for early-responding (a/b = 10) tissue.

within 5 years of radiation treatment) is 45-60 Gy (2,3). With partial brain irradiation (25 to 67% of volume), the corresponding value is 50-70 Gy, implying that late injury is clearly volume-dependent. The use of just one fraction decreases the total numeric dose that can be delivered safely. In a series of experiments in monkeys (4), no histologic abnormalities were noted following whole brain irradiation with a single fraction of 10 Gy. With a single fraction of 15 Gy, discrete microfoci of white matter necrosis were identified. A single fraction of 20 Gy was uniformly fatal with scattered necrotic foci most dramatically affecting the brain stem. In humans, single fractional treatment to the whole brain has seldom been used. Although based on limited clinical data, 10 Gy in a single fraction can be delivered safely to the whole brain based on an RTOG (Radiation Therapy Oncology Group) study in which a single fraction of 10 Gy was used in patients with brain metastases with no serious toxicity. Long-term follow-up of these patients, however, was impossible because the majority of patients died of progressive disease within a few months before radiation-induced long-term toxicity became evident (5).

Radiosurgery is based on observations that when small volumes of brain tissues are irradiated, higher doses are necessary to cause brain injury compared to when large volumes of brain tissue are irradiated. Using a combination of animal and clinical experience, Kjellberg et al. (6) described dose-volume (or specifically, dose-diameter) isoeffect lines for brain necrosis at 1% or 99% risk levels. Their 1% dose-diameter isoeffect line is widely used as a guide for dose prescription for radiosurgery. It has been criticized, however, because the risk of necrosis observed was much higher than was represented by the 1% line (7). Another potential problem with using the proton 1% dose-volume isoeffect line as a guide for photon beam radiosurgery (Gamma Knife or LINAC radiosurgery) is the differences between the dose distributions in proton beam and those in photon beam. In addition, the 1% isoeffect line cannot account for the use of different isodoses, multiple isocenters, or combinations of fractionated whole brain irradiation with a radiosurgical boost.

Flickinger (8) proposed an integrated logistic formula that estimates the probability of necrosis within the entire volume-receiving radiation. Dose-volume isoeffect curves for a 3% risk of radionecrosis was predicted by the integrated logistic formula for treatment using the Gamma Knife or a 6-MV Linac (9). The current formula attempts to predict permanent complications (brain necrosis), but does not predict temporary complications or asymptomatic radiation-induced changes on MRI. It does not assign different risks for different portions of the brain depending on sensitivity, particularly for the cranial nerves. The integrated logistic formula will most likely be modified as more dose-volume data become available from clinical experience. The RTOG has completed a Phase I dose escalation study to establish maximum tolerable doses (MTDs) for

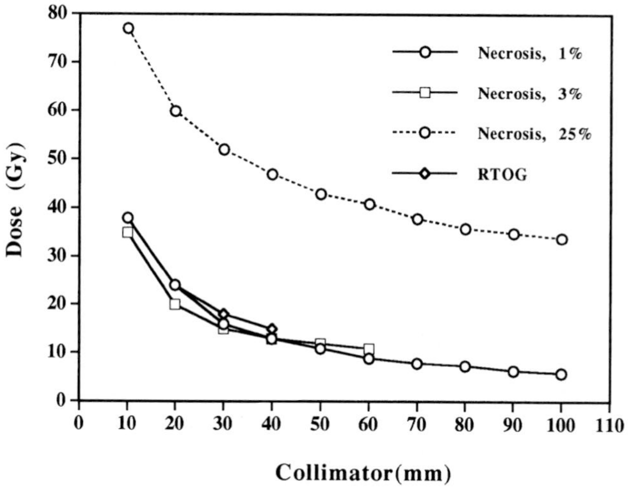

Figure 10.2. Dose-volume isoeffect curves in the literature. The curves for 1% and 25% risks of necrosis were adopted from the data of proton beam therapy (6). The curve for a 3% risk of radionecrosis was published as predicted by the integrated logistic formula for treatment using the Gamma Knife or a 6-MV Linac (9). The RTOG study used unacceptable neurotoxicities within 3 months as an endpoint (Grade 3, 4, or 5 using the RTOG central nervous system toxicity criteria, which is different from brain necrosis) to establish MTDs for various tumor diameters in patients with previously irradiated recurrent malignant gliomas and brain metastases. The MTD for <20, 21-30, and 31-40 mm tumor diameter was 24, 18, and 15 Gy, respectively (116).

various tumor diameters in patients with previously irradiated recurrent malignant gliomas and brain metastases. The MTD for <20, 21 to 30, and 31 to 40 mm tumor diameter was 24, 18, and 15 Gy, respectively (116). Three of 125 patients (2.4%) developed unacceptable toxicity within the range of doses used in this study. Unacceptable neurotoxicities within 3 months were used as an endpoint (Grade 3, 4, or 5 using the RTOG central nervous system toxicity criteria) instead of brain necrosis, which has been used as an endpoint in previous studies. Figure 10.2 depicts dose-volume isoeffect curves published in the literature.

Stereotactic Target Composition

To understand the radiobiologic basis for the efficacy and toxicity of single large fractional radiosurgery, it is necessary to know the radiosurgical target composition. The radiosurgical target may be an early- or late-responding tissue, whereas the surrounding normal tissues are always late-responding. All radiosurgery targets may be placed in one of four categories according to whether the target tissue is early- or late-responding and whether or not the target volume contains only abnormal tissue (Table 10.1) (11):

Category 1. These targets experience a large biologic effect both in normal and abnormal tissue within the target volume because abnormal tissue (AVM) is embedded within normal brain tissue in the diseased area.

Category 2. Abnormal tissue (meningioma) experience a large radiobiologic effect mainly because there is no brain tissue within the target.

Category 3. Normal tissue (late responding) experience a larger effect than abnormal tissue (early responding), and single fractional radiosurgery is not usually recommended. A fractionated regimen would be preferable to single fraction treatments particularly in this category.

Category 4. Abnormal tissue, in which the radiographically apparent target volume contains mainly malignant cells, experience a moderately large effect within the target when the target is limited to the enhancing region on CT/MRI. For targets in this category, the abnormal tissue is early-responding tissue, which may appear to indicate that a fractionated regimen would be preferable since tumor cells become more radiosensitive by reoxygenation and redistribution between fractions. However, this does not appear to be a substantial clinical problem for metastases as reported control rates range from 80 to 90% with acceptable complications (usually <5% of brain necrosis). The therapeutic ratio in the literature appears to be even better with radiosurgery than with conventional fractionated treatment. For glioblastomas, the therapeutic ratio with a brachytherapy boost is similar to that of a radiosurgery boost. This clinical consequence may have to do with a smaller target volume used in radiosurgery. Usually for smaller targets, not enough normal tissue is damaged with a single fraction to have clinical consequences.

Targets in category 1 or 2 appear to be ideal for a single high dose treatment because they are late-responding tissues in which no therapeutic gain is expected by fractionation. However, the toxicity from radiation could be different from one to the other because of differences in target composition. Arteriovenous malformations (category 1) are usually intermingled with normal brain tissue, but meningioma (category 2) are usually extra-axial expansile lesions with no normal brain tissue within the tumor. Conceptually, those in category 1 are at higher risk of de-

Table 10.1. Simplified Categorization of Radiosurgery Targets

Category	Example	Abnormal Tissue in Target Volume	Normal Tissue in Target Volume
1	AVM	Late responding	Late responding
2	Meningioma	Late responding	None
3	Low grade Astrocytoma	Early responding	Late responding
4	Metastases or Glioblastoma	Early responding	None

(Reprinted with permission from: Larson DA, Flickingger JC, Loeffler JS. The radiobiology of radiosurgery. Int J Radiat Oncol Biol Phys 1993;25:557, with permission from Elsevier Science.)

veloping radiation necrosis than those in category 2, since more normal tissue will be treated when the same dose is delivered to the same volume, although this has not been proved in the clinical setting.

Conceptually, targets in category 3 are at greater risk of radiation-induced toxicity than those in category 4, since normal tissue density within the target in category 3 will be greater than in category 4 (most of cells within the target will be tumorous in the latter). This, however, has not been proven mainly because limited data is available on patients with low-grade astrocytoma treated with single fraction radiosurgery.

Cranial Nerve Tolerance

Radiation tolerance of cranial nerves should be considered separately from the tolerance of brain parenchyma to irradiation. Experimental animal models that assessed the effects of radiation on peripheral nerves demonstrated that axonal degeneration, demyelination, and ischemia are important determinants of radiation injury (10). Tolerance of cranial nerves to single large fractional dose has been difficult to establish. Clinically useful dose-response information reported in the literature may serve as a guide to cranial nerve tolerance for single fraction radiosurgery (Table 10.2). Radiation tolerance may depend on the type or function of cranial nerve involved. Clinical experience suggests that special sensory nerves (optic or vestibulocochlear) are more sensitive to single stereotactic radiation than are motor nerves (12). It is unclear whether this is due to the difference in de novo sensitivity among nerves or due to the nerves carrying critical sensation (vision or hearing), which are more noticeable when impaired.

The optic pathway (optic nerves, optic chiasm, and optic radiation) is of special concern because of the impor-

Table 10.2. Cranial Nerve Tolerance to Single Fractional Radiosurgery

Cranial Nerve	Dose[a] (Gy)	Prevalence of Deficit[b] (%)	Common Temporal Pattern of Deficit[c]	Machine	IDS[d] (%) or Dmax (Gy)	Follow-Up Duration in Month[e] (range)	Comments[f]	References
II	*<8*	0/35 (0)	—	gamma, Linac	—	19 (3–49)		13
	>8	4/17 (24)	P	gamma, Linac	—	19 (3–49)		13
	10–20	2/34 (6)	P	gamma	≥50%	24 (6–54)	10.5 and 12 Gy delivered to optic chiasm	14
	7.5–1.5	0/13 (0)	—	gamma	—	(6–24)		15
	6–16.6	4/13 (31)	—	gamma	—	(6–24)	*visual deficit prior to radiosurgery*	15
III, IV, VI	*10–40*	3/62 (5)	P	gamma, Linac	10–40 Gy	19 (3–49)		13
	10–20	1/34 (3)	P	gamma	≥50%	24 (6–54)		14
	4.5–30	0/22 (0)	—	gamma		(6–24)		15
V	12–20	0/6 (0)	—	gamma	30–55%	21 (7–35)		16
	12–20	21/73 (29)	T	gamma	24–50 Gy	20.5 (3–36)	*nerve length*	18
	12–20	49/273 **(23)**	T	gamma	40–80%	30 (6–91)	*target diameter, MPD*	17
	10–40	5/62 (8)	T	gamma, Linac	10–40 Gy	19 (3–49)	*no correlation with Dmax*	13
	18–25	21/116 (18)	T	gamma	22–50 Gy	56 (8–154)		19
	10–20	1/34 (3)	T	gamma	≥50%	24 (6–54)		14
	10–22.5	6/32 (19)	T	Linac	68–90%	(4–59)	*target diameter*	20
	16–20	21/35 **(59)**	—	gamma	45–80%	16 (2.5–36)	*age, dose, target diameter*	21
	5–20	0/19 (0)	—	gamma		(6–24)		15
VII	12–20	22/70 (31)	T	gamma	24–50 Gy	20.5 (3–36)	*nerve length*	18
	12–20	36/260 **(17)**	T	gamma	40–80%	30 (6–91)	*target diameter, MPD*	17
	18–25	17/116 (15)	T	gamma	22–50 Gy	56 (8–154)		19
	10–22.5	5/32 (16)	T	Linac	68–90%	(4–59)	*target diameter*	20
	16–20	19/35 **(67)**	—	gamma	45–80%	16 (2.5–36)	*age, dose, target diameter*	21
VIII	12–20	53/146 **(45)**	P	gamma	40–80%	30 (6–91)	*target diameter, MPD*	17
	18–25	48/65 (74)	P	gamma	22–50 Gy	56 (8–154)		19
IX, X, XI	12–20	0/5 (0)	—	gamma	30–55%	21 (7–35)	—	16

[a] Dose delivered to the target (not to the nerves because it is difficult to delineate the individual nerve in most patients); it will be minimum peripheral dose of the target unless otherwise specified (it will be in *italic* when the maximum dose within the treatment volume is quoted).
[b] Number of patients developed deficit / number of patients treated, the **bold** number in parentheses is actuarial incidence of deficit at 2–3 years.
[c] Temporal pattern of deficit, P represents permanent and T represents temporary deficit, which recovers in most patients.
[d] Iso dose surface (expressed as a percent of the dose of maximum), which encompasses the target.
[e] This can be average, mean, or median.
[f] Important prognostic factors predicting nerve damage are *italic*. MPD, minimum peripheral dose.

tance of vision. For optic nerves and chiasm using conventional fractionation (180–200 cGy per fraction), $TD_{5/5}$ is 50–60 Gy (2,3). For SRS, the tolerance of the optic pathway may be much lower (probably ≤10 Gy) and a maximum of 8 Gy to the optic chiasm or optic nerves is generally recommended to avoid potential injury (13). Oculomotor nerves (III, IV, and VI) seem to tolerate higher doses and the risks of nerve damage appear to be acceptable within the range of doses (10–20 Gy) used in clinical practice (13–15). Trigeminal nerve damages have been reported primarily in patients with acoustic schwannomas or skull base meningiomas following radiosurgery. Wide ranges of trigeminal neuropathy (0 to 59%) have been reported after single fractional doses ranging from 5–40 Gy, which were prescribed to the margin of the target in most cases (not to the nerve) (13–21). However, the actual doses to the nerve have seldom been reported because it is hard to delineate nerves on stereotactic planning CT or MRI. The actual doses could have been much higher or lower than the marginal doses to the target. Subsequently, it appears to be difficult to determine dose-response relationship for nerve damage based on unreliable dosimetric data delivered to the nerves. However, the potential factors predicting nerve deficits following radiosurgery have been reported and include nerve length (18), target diameter (17,20,21), minimum peripheral dose (marginal dose) (17,21), and age younger than 65 (21). Trigeminal neuropathies are usually temporary and the majority of patients seem to recover with conservative measures (usually steroid therapy).

Facial neuropathies are also common adverse effects after radiosurgery for acoustic schwannomas and have been observed in 15 to 67% of patients following single fractional treatment of 10–25 Gy (17–21). The deficits are usually transient and the prognostic factors predicting the facial neuropathies are very similar to those of trigeminal neuropathies. Preservation of hearing is one of the potential advantages of radiosurgery over microsurgery in patients with acoustic schwannomas. However, 45 to 76% of patients with acoustic schwannomas had deterioration of their baseline hearing after single doses of 12–25 Gy (17,19). Preservation of baseline hearing was possible only in 26 to 55% of the patients, which is less than the optimum we would like to achieve. The prognostic factors predicting hearing deficits include target diameter and marginal dose (17). One of the approaches to preserve hearing could be lowering the marginal doses close to 12 Gy. The tumor control with lower doses has been so far comparable to that of higher doses, although longer follow-up is required. The information of cranial nerve damages with respect to nerves IX, X, and XI is scarce. One study demonstrated that none of five patients treated for jugular foramen schwannomas developed nerve deficit after single fractional doses of 12–20 Gy (16), although more information is required to determine nerve tolerance of this region.

Fractionated Stereotactic Radiotherapy

To ensure treatment accuracy, most current techniques use pins to attach a stereotactic head frame to the patient's skull, usually under local anesthesia. Fractionation, in general, has not been attempted because it would require doing this procedure for each fraction. Therefore, radiosurgery has been administered in a single high dose fraction, even though a fractionated regimen is known to be radiobiologically advantageous in certain circumstances. No attempt has been made in radiosurgery to spare normal tissue within the irradiated volume by dividing the total dose into a number of fractions. The rationale for this is based on the belief that the need for fractionation may not apply when the treatment volume is small and contains little functioning brain tissue.

A fractionated regimen, however, could be more beneficial to minimize potential toxicity in certain circumstances, such as treatments of a large volume of normal brain (target category 3 or large target), of lesions close to eloquent structures (such as brain stem or optic pathways), and of recurrent tumors after previous radiation. In addition, the use of a fractionated regimen may be radiobiologically more advantageous in malignant tumors because of the presence of hypoxic and/or noncycling tumor cells. A fractionated regimen results in more damage to the tumor cell population because the process of reoxygenation and redistribution of the cell cycle to a more sensitive phase is operative between the fractions. It has been demonstrated clearly over the years that a fractionated regimen is more effective than a single dose regimen in eradicating malignant tumors with minimum damage to normal tissue. Thus, fractionation can be used to exploit differences in the response to radiation between tumor and normal tissue, particularly in the treatment of malignant tumors.

Recently, relocatable stereotactic head frames have been developed that can reproduce patient position without attaching the head frame to the skull with pins. Instead, noninvasive techniques are used to fit the head frame on the patient's head (e.g., dental plates and an occipital mold are fitted to the patient), which facilitates the use of fractionation schemes.

Summary

The radiobiological consequence of a single large fractional treatment used in radiosurgery is different from that of multifractional treatment used in conventional radiotherapy. The response of the target and the toxicity of normal brain appear to depend on the total dose, the volume of normal tissue within the irradiated volume, the fractionation scheme, and the target composition (early- or late-responding). Currently available information of dose-volume relationship for the risk of toxicity was described in this section as a guide for dose prescription of single fraction radiosurgery. Because no attempt has been made in radiosurgery to spare normal tissue within the irradiated volume, conformity of isodose distribution is essential to minimize the volume of normal brain irradiated. Further investigation is required to determine the lowest possible control dose for individual targets to minimize toxicity without compromising tumor control. Target composition appears to be a useful piece of information for treatment decision. Cranial nerve tolerance should be considered separately from the tolerance of brain parenchyma. Caution should be given to the cranial nerves (particularly, the optic nerve pathways and vestibulocochlear nerves) when planning if the target is close to them. Fractionated SRT should be considered when treating large volumes of normal brain (target category 3 or large target, usually >4 cm in diameter), targets close to eloquent structures (such as brain stem or optic pathways), and recurrent tumors after previous radiation.

CLINICAL ASPECTS

Functional Stereotactic Radiosurgery

Intractable Pain

The first Gamma Knife was used for the treatment of intractable cancer pain by producing a ventromedial thalamotomy (22). Using 170–180 Gy, the gammathalamotomy achieved inconsistent pain relief in the upper part of the body, without loss of sensation (23). Of the 52 patients treated for intractable pain with gammathalamotomy, 24 had minimal relief, 18 moderate relief, and 8 had good relief.

Trigeminal Neuralgia

Using the first Gamma Knife, 46 patients with trigeminal neuralgia were treated. Of the 22 patients that had the trigeminal nerve localized by cisternography, 13 were pain-free at 6 months and 4 remained pain-free after 30 months (22,24). In a more recently reported multiinstitutional study using the gamma unit for trigeminal neuralgia, 50 patients were treated at 5 centers. The nerve root entry zone was targeted with a 4 mm isocenter using a radiation dose ranging from 60 to 90 Gy (25). After a median follow-up of 18 months, 29 patients (58%) were pain-free, 18 (36%) had good pain control, and 3 (6%) had no relief. The median time to pain relief was 1 month. In the three patients who experienced return of their facial pain, the time to relapse was 5, 7, and 10 months. A maximum radiosurgical dose of more than 70 Gy was associated with a significantly higher rate of pain relief (25). Linear accelerator radiosurgery for trigeminal neuralgia had a 70% therapeutic response rate that was either partial or complete (26).

Psychiatric Disease

Bilateral capsulotomies have been used with encouraging results for the treatment of obsessive-compulsive behavior and anxiety using the gamma unit. Five of seven patients treated with 160 Gy had benefit for more than 7 years (22).

Parkinson's Disease and Epilepsy

The tremor of Parkinson's disease has been treated with ventrolateral thalamotomy using the Gamma Knife and stereotactic coordinates obtained from MR imaging (22). A dose of 180–200 Gy was used to generate a lesion with a 4 mm collimator (24). Initial treatment results were poor and few patients have been treated with MR imaging. Patients with epilepsy related to an AVM usually have improvement after radiosurgery. One series reported 41 of 59 (69%) patients were significantly improved or seizure-free after treatment (27).

Nonfunctional Stereotactic Radiosurgery

Acoustic Tumors

The first acoustic tumor was treated with the gamma unit in Stockholm in 1969. Patients with acoustic tumors treated with SRS (Figure 10.3) are usually elderly, have medical problems that increase the risk of surgery, have type 2 neurofibromatosis and bilateral lesions, have a tumor in the only ear with preserved hearing, or refuse conventional neurosurgery (28). Histologically, acoustic tumors treated with SRS are acellular and have few blood vessels, abundant collagen, and central necrosis (29).

The largest number of acoustic tumors has been treated in Sweden with the Gamma Knife where the minimum dose to the lesion periphery was 18–25 Gy with a maximum central dose of 22–25 Gy (28). Patients with unilateral tumors followed for 12 to 206 months (mean, 54 months) after treatment demonstrated that 44 to 56% of tumors decreased in size, 32 to 42% were stable in size, and 9 to 15% grew (28,30–32). Overall tumor growth control rate was 86%. In patients with bilateral acoustic tumors and neurofibromatosis treated with the Gamma Knife, 25 to 32% of tumors decreased in size, 43% stabilized, and 25 to 33% progressed (31,32). Facial weakness occurred 4 to 15 months after treatment in 15% of people and usually resolved within 6 to 12 months (32). Hearing preservation was present in 56% at 1 year, 54% at 2 years, and 28% at 6 years (30). Transient facial numbness or weakness has decreased to 5% or less by decreasing the dose to the tumor periphery from 25–35 Gy to 10–15 Gy, without an increase in tumor growth rates (31).

When 20 Gy was administered to the tumor periphery, 60% decreased in size and 40% stabilized at a follow-up of more than 20 months (28,33). Tumor volumes ranged

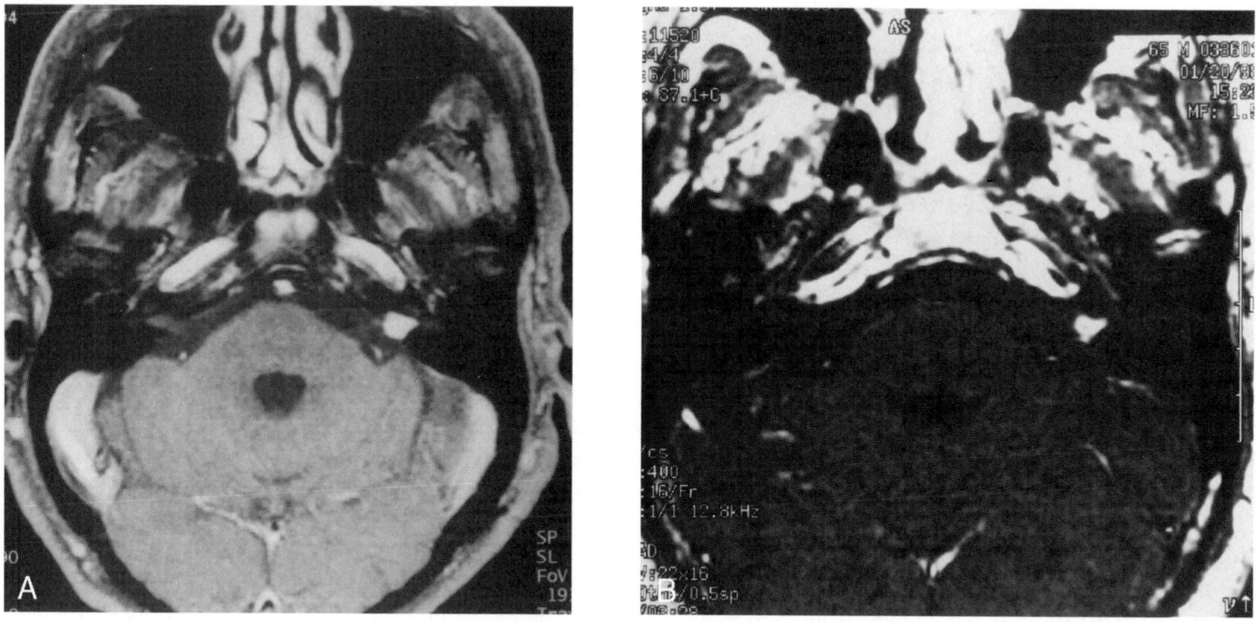

Figure 10.3. Acoustic tumor. (A) Left acoustic tumor prior to stereotactic radiosurgery. (B) Tumor appearance 3 years after radiosurgical treatment.

from 0.12 to 17 cm^3 (median, 2.75 cm^3) and the 4-year actuarial tumor growth control rate (reduced tumor size or absence of growth) was 89.2 ± 6% for 136 tumors (33). An absence of central contrast enhancement was seen in 78% of tumors at a median of 6 months after therapy (33). At a median duration of 5 months after radiosurgery, hearing deteriorated in 60% and 24% had transient facial weakness (28). In 92 patients treated with 16–18 Gy to the tumor margin, 21 (23%) tumors decreased in size, 68 (74%) stabilized, and 3 (3%) enlarged after an average period of 12 months (34,35). The 4-year actuarial incidence of postradiosurgical facial and trigeminal neuropathies was 29.0 ± 4.4% and 32.9 ± 4.5%, respectively (29,33).

An update of the series from Pittsburgh in 402 patients showed that 30% of acoustic tumors decreased in size, 63% stabilized, and 7% increased at a mean follow-up of 36 months (36). Loss of central contrast enhancement was seen in 41% of tumors. Using magnetic resonance (MR) imaging-based treatment planning, facial nerve function was preserved in 92%, trigeminal nerve function in 92%, and auditory nerve function in 68%. The decline in cranial nerve function is most likely to occur in the first 2 years after treatment. When comparing microsurgery to SRS for the treatment of acoustic neuromas less than 3 cm in diameter, radiosurgery was more effective in preserving normal postoperative facial function ($P < .05$) and hearing preservation ($P < .03$) with less treatment related morbidity ($P < .01$) (37). Hospital length of stay and total management charges were less in the radiosurgical group ($P < .001$). Other series have reported similar morbidity, mortality, and cranial nerve function preservation rates for SRS compared to microsurgery for tumors 3 cm or less in diameter with a 6.6 year median follow-up (38).

For larger acoustic tumors, fractionated SRT has been used with excellent results. In 33 patients with tumors having a mean volume of 7.8 cm^3, 25 tumors (74%) decreased in size and 9 (26%) remained stable at a median MR imaging follow-up of 18 months (39). Patients with tumors smaller than 3 cm in diameter received 500 cGy in 4 daily fractions or 400 cGy in 5 daily fractions for larger tumors. Of the 28 patients with measurable hearing, 4 (15%) improved, 21 (75%) had stable hearing, and 3 (10%) worsened. Two patients with facial weakness experienced improvement and no patient developed a new trigeminal or facial nerve neuropathy after treatment (39). In 26 patients with 27 acoustic tumors that were treated with fractionated SRT, none experienced a treatment-related facial neuropathy and 13% developed a trigeminal neuropathy (40).

Nonacoustic schwannomas have been successfully treated with SRS (41). At a mean follow-up of 21 months, all six patients with trigeminal nerve tumors had tumor stabilization whereas one of seven patients with a jugular foramen tumor experienced tumor growth at 7 months after radiosurgery. No patient sustained either a cranial nerve or brain stem injury after treatment.

Arteriovenous Malformations

Stereotactic radiosurgery is usually reserved for inoperable arteriovenous malformations (AVMs) of the brain. Arteriovenous malformations smaller than 2 cm in diameter are extremely sensitive to SRS (42). The 2-year obliteration rate for AVMs of this size treated with the Gamma Knife was 80 to 87%, 12% obliterated partially and 2% did not respond (29). The 1-year angiographically confirmed obliteration rate was 65% (43). At 2 years, there was a 66% complete obliteration rate in 66 AVMs treated with the linear accelerator (44). Friedman and Bova reported a higher 2-year obliteration rate of 81% for linac radiosurgery (45). Sources of error found in determining the nidus of the AVM on angiography compared to CT have included overlapping vessels, bony structures, fine filamentous arterioles, and irregular shapes for linac radiosurgery (46).

In 300 AVM patients treated with helium beam radiosurgery, the rate of complete obliteration was 65% at 2 years with 25% decreasing in size by more than 50% (47). The 2-year obliteration rate for 86 AVMs treated with stereotactic helium ion Bragg peak radiation was 94% for lesions <4 cm^3, 75% for those 4 to 25 cm^3, and 39% for those >25 cm^3 (28,48). The 3-year obliteration rates were 100%, 95%, and 70%, respectively. Lesion volumes measured 0.3 to 70 cm^3 and treatment doses ranged from 8.8–34.6 Gy. Ten (12%) patients experienced severe permanent neurological deficits prior to reducing the maximum dose to 19.2 Gy. Seizure frequency was improved in 63% and headaches were less intense in 68% of patients (48).

It is unknown whether the risk of hemorrhage for AVMs decreases after radiosurgical treatment, before obliteration is complete. Some investigators feel that the risk remains constant until obliteration occurs, while others think that radiosurgery affords a protective effect (49). In 153 patients, where the entire AVM nidus was irradiated with linac radiosurgery, the bleeding risk decreased after treatment from 4.8% in the first 6 months to 0% after 12 months (49). The risk of hemorrhage was 4% in the first 6 months, 10 to 12% from 6 to 18 months, before decreasing to 5.5% from 18 to 24 months for those 27 patients with incomplete irradiation of the nidus (49). No hemorrhage occurred after 24 months. After Gamma Knife radiosurgery, the risk of hemorrhage is approximately 5% and 3% will experience delayed radiation necrosis (29). Hemorrhage occurred in 10 (12%) patients at 4 to 34 months after helium ion radiosurgery. In 75 AVM patients treated with proton beam radiosurgery followed for 2 to 16 years, no protection from hemorrhage was noted in the first year (50).

The treatment of angiographically occult vascular malformations (AOVMs) with SRS remains controversial. These malformations are usually identified incidentally and their natural history is unknown. Treating these lesions is difficult because no imaging study can detect their obliteration. Indications for treatment of AOVMs with radiosurgery are multiple bleeding episodes that have caused repeated or progressive neurological deficits and surgical inaccessibility (51). In a series of 22 patients with cavernous malformations treated with the gamma unit, nine suffered posttreatment hemorrhage and six developed radiation injury (52). The annual posttreatment risk of hemorrhage was determined to be 8%. The incidence of radiation-induced complications with cavernous malformations was seven times higher than that for patients with AVMs who were treated with the same dose distributions (52). Based on these results, it was concluded that the high incidence of complications did not justify the limited protection afforded by the treatment except in exceptional cases. Another study reported an 8.8% annual hemorrhage rate for the first 2 years after radiosurgery, which decreased to 1.1% from years 2 to 6 (53).

In a series of 13 venous angiomas treated with radiosurgery, complete obliteration occurred in one case, three cases responded partially, and five cases did not respond (54). After treatment, one case developed cerebral edema and three cases had frank radionecrosis, one requiring surgical resection. Radiosurgery was not recommended for these lesions that have a benign natural history because of the risks associated with treatment (54).

The most common reasons for incomplete obliteration of the AVM after radiosurgery were incomplete angiographic definition of the nidus (57%) or "radiobiological resistance" (38%) (55,56). Retreatment for incompletely obliterated AVMs was associated with a 62% obliteration rate and a 14% complication rate (57). The complication rate was proportional to the previously administered dose of radiation. The incidence of hemorrhage after the second treatment was 1.8% in the first 2 years.

Meningiomas

Radiosurgery has been used to treat recurrent or inoperable meningiomas of the intracranial compartment. Small meningiomas have been treated with radiosurgery alone with large tumors requiring a combination of surgical resection and radiosurgery. Radiation doses administered to the periphery have ranged from 12–25 Gy. After treatment, most lesions are stable in size with central hypodensity suggesting necrosis developing at 6 to 12 months.

An early study with long-term follow-up in 30 patients showed a decrease in size in approximately half, 12 had growth stabilization, and 4 continued to grow (32,58). Seven of 20 (35%) had improvement in cranial nerve function and 5 (25%) had partial improvement. Eighteen (60%) patients did not improve after treatment and none had complications (32,58). Of 59 patients followed for 1 to 3 years, 31 (53%) had a decrease in tumor size, 23 had stabilization (39%), and 5 enlarged (8%) (32,59). Clinical improvement was seen in 9 (15%), 44 (75%) remained clinically stable, and 6 (10%) worsened (29,32). Decreased central contrast enhancement suggesting intratumoral necrosis was seen in 22 (37%) patients (32). The actuarial 2-year tumor control rate was 96% (59).

In one series of 28 meningiomas treated with linac radiosurgery and followed for 2 to 86 months (mean, 27 months), 4 (14%) decreased in size, 19 (68%) were unchanged, and 2 (7%) enlarged (32). Six (21%) patients improved clinically, 17 (61%) were unchanged, and 2 (7%) worsened (32). Another linac-based series of 55 patients with meningiomas reported tumor stabilization in 38 (69%), a decrease in 16 (29%), and progression in 1 (2%) (60). The length of follow-up for this series was 48.4 months. Magnetic resonance imaging demonstrated a decrease in the central enhancement in 20% of patients suggesting central necrosis. Fifteen patients (27%) improved neurologically and 34 were unchanged (63%). The 2-year actuarial control rate was 98% (60).

Lunsford has recently advocated SRS as an alternative treatment to microsurgery for meningiomas (61). Meningiomas are ideal for radiosurgery because they are well-circumscribed, are rarely invasive, are easily visualized by current imaging techniques, can be encompassed within the radiosurgical field even when irregular in shape, are identified when small, and their dural blood supply can be included in the treatment field (62). The 4-year actuarial control rate was 92% in 94 tumors treated with radiosurgery (61). Recurrent cavernous sinus meningiomas followed for a median of 26 months in 34 patients had 100% tumor control rate and permanent cranial nerve complications were seen in only 2 patients (63). In 72 middle fossa meningiomas treated with radiosurgery, 50 patients (69%) had tumor shrinkage, 18 (25%) had tumor stabilization, 2 (3%) initially had shrinkage followed by regrowth, and 2 (3%) had progression (64). Petroclival meningiomas treated with radiosurgery were associated with a low complication rate despite their proximity to critical structures (65). Volumes decreased in 14 patients (23%), remained stable in 42 (68%), and increased in 5 (8%) of 62 petroclival tumors after radiosurgery (65). Only 5 patients (8%) developed new cranial nerve deficits within 24 months of treatment, which resolved completely in 2 patients within 6 months of onset.

Pituitary Tumors and Craniopharyngiomas

Among the first tumors to be treated with SRS were pituitary adenomas. To date, nearly 3000 adenomas have been treated with charged-particle beam generators in Boston, Berkley, Moscow, and Leningrad of which 1149 had growth hormone-secreting tumors, 535 had ACTH-secreting tumors, 264 had prolactin-secreting tumors, and 220 had non-secreting tumors (66). Kjellberg from Harvard has treated the largest number of pituitary tumors using Bragg peak proton radiosurgery. Those conditions treated by Kjellberg included acromegaly, Cushing's disease, Nelson's syndrome, prolactinoma, and non-secreting adenoma. Panhypopituitarism following radiosurgery for acromegaly and Cushing's disease occurred in 10 to 15% and 2% of patients had temporary oculomotor disturbances (27). Visual field deficits and visual loss can occur because of the proximity of the pituitary gland to the optic chiasm and nerves.

Patients with acromegaly that were treated with 30 to 50 Gy of helium ion radiosurgery in four fractions over 5 days improved clinically and had decreased hormone levels within 3 to 6 months (66). Within 1 year, mean growth hormone levels decreased by 70% and some patients had normal levels for more than 10 years (32,66). Bragg peak proton irradiation demonstrated similar results with clinical improvement in 90% of patients within 2 years and growth hormone levels decreasing to <10 ng/ml in 60% (32,67). More than 50% Cushing's disease patients treated with 50 to 150 Gy in 3 or 4 fractions had normal cortisol levels within 1 year which were present at 10 years (32,66). After Bragg peak radiosurgery, complete clinical and endocrinological remission were seen in 65% of 175 patients with Cushing's disease, 20% had improvement, and 15% had no response (32,67).

Up to 3 treatments were necessary with the Gamma Knife to treat 21 acromegalic patients, using 40-70 Gy for each treatment or 30–50 Gy if prior radiation therapy was received (68). At follow-up of 1 to 21 years, 2 patients (10%) had near normal hormone levels with complete clinical remission, 8 (38%) improved clinically or endocrinologically, and 11 (52%) had little or no improvement (68). Two patients that had prior radiotherapy developed pituitary insufficiency (68).

In 35 adults and 8 children with ACTH-producing microadenomas treated with Gamma Knife radiosurgery, 1 to 4 small lesions were generated within the pituitary gland at 5 to 55 months (27,69). If the first lesion in the center of the adenohypophysis did not produce improvement, anterior and lateral lesions were created using 70 to 100 Gy in adults or 50 to 70 Gy in children (27,69). At follow-up of 3 to 9 years, 14 patients responded completely after one treatment with normal urinary cortisol levels and 8 patients had clinical remission and near normal urinary cortisol levels after 2 to 3 treatments (69). Five patients did not respond and 12 of 22 patients (55%) in remission developed panhypopituitarism (69). Seven of eight children (88%) had normal urinary cortisol levels and complete clinical remission and the child that did not respond was retreated, required bilateral adrenalectomy, and later lost pituitary function (32).

Pittsburgh has treated 18 pituitary tumors with the gamma unit with follow-up to 32 months (70). Four patients had acromegaly, six had Cushing's disease, and eight had non-secreting pituitary tumors. Nine (50%) patients had macroadenomas, 9 had microadenomas, normal vision (acuity and fields) was present in 12 (67%), and 6 (33%) had slight impairment (70). Eleven tumors were recurrent and five patients had received prior radiotherapy. After treatment with 28–60 Gy, eight (44%) tumors decreased in size, nine (50%) were unchanged, and one (6%) macroadenoma in the cavernous sinus progressed. Within 3 to 5 months, 3 of 10 patients had normal hormone levels and 3 had improved hormone levels. Those patients with normal vision remained stable and 2 of 6 patients with visual impairment improved. One patient that had prior radiotherapy experienced sudden, severe visual loss (70).

Craniopharyngiomas have been treated with a combination of SRS for the solid portion and intracavitary radionuclide for the cyst wall. Craniopharyngiomas in the sella turcica or that recur after microsurgery, which are at least 3 to 5 mm away from the optic chiasm or nerves, can be safely treated with SRS. Nearly 80 craniopharyngiomas have been treated with 20–50 Gy using the Gamma Knife (32). All patients had arrested tumor growth, none lost endocrine function, and two sustained visual impairment.

Metastatic Tumors

Stereotactic radiosurgery is an important treatment option for patients with brain metastases (Figure 10.4). Whether SRS alone without conventional radiation is satisfactory treatment for brain metastases is unknown. Radiosurgery has been used for lesions that are located in deep, inoperable areas or are recurrent/persistent after external beam radiation therapy. Although many metastases are considered radioresistant to fractionated radiation therapy based on their histology, these tumor types generally respond dramatically to radiosurgery. Brain metastases are considered ideal lesions for SRS because most are less than 3 cm at presentation and are not locally invasive, they are spherical and radiographically distinct from surrounding brain parenchyma on CT and MR imaging, and most displace normal brain tissue outside the radiosurgery treatment volume decreasing the potential for radiation injury (71–74). Lesions that have been treated with radiosurgery that infiltrate outside the enhancing tumor margin will ultimately recur at the edge of the treatment field (74,75).

In a large review of more than 20 independent reports where SRS was used to treat brain metastases, the results in >1250 patients with >2100 lesions were analyzed (71). The composite data revealed an average local control rate of 83% and a median survival of 9.6 months. This length of survival is comparable to that reported for patients with solitary brain metastases that have surgical excision followed by whole brain radiation therapy (73). Prognostic factors that were identified which were associated with prolonged survival were the presence of fewer than three lesions, Karnofsky performance status, and controlled systemic disease (71). There appeared to be a dose-response relationship when ≥18 Gy was the treatment dose administered. Whole-brain radiation therapy may enhance the rate of local control but does not seem to prolong survival. Most patients can be withdrawn from their corticosteroids within 1 to 3 months of radiosurgery and will have improved quality of life (75).

Astrocytomas

The infiltrative nature of astrocytomas with tumor cell extension into the area of increased signal on T2-weighted

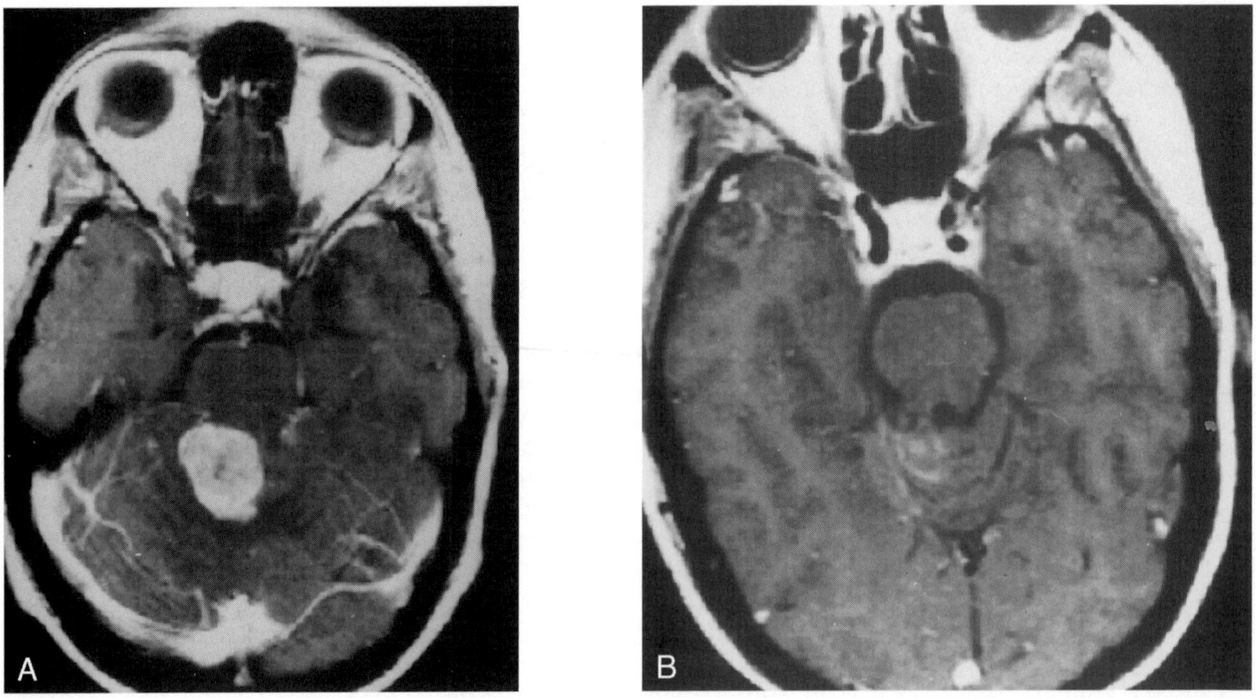

Figure 10.4. Brain metastasis. (A) Single colon carcinoma metastasis to the vermis of the cerebellum before stereotactic radiosurgery. (B) Metastatic lesion 3 months after radiosurgery.

MR images or the hypodense region on CT by stereotactic biopsy suggests that radiosurgery should not be beneficial for these tumors (76). For this reason, radiosurgery has been used primarily to "boost" a site of tumor recurrence in patients that have already received external beam radiation therapy. Stereotactic radiosurgery has been compared to brachytherapy using high-activity iodine-125 sources for the treatment of recurrent glioblastoma multiforme (77). For those patients having radiosurgery, the median actuarial survival was 10.2 months with 12- and 24-month survivals of 45 and 19%, respectively. The median actuarial survival was 11.5 months with 12- and 24-month survivals of 44 and 17%, respectively, for those receiving brachytherapy. The reoperation rate for radiosurgery was 22% in contrast to 44% for the brachytherapy group (77).

Whether radiosurgery for gliomas should be given immediately after the completion of conventional radiation therapy (up front) or at the time of tumor recurrence is not known. In 37 patients that received an up front linac radiosurgical dose of 13 Gy to the enhancing margin, the median actuarial survival was 26 months for 23 patients with glioblastoma multiforme and has not been reached for anaplastic astrocytoma (78,79). In 30 patients with malignant gliomas that received a radiosurgery boost immediately after the completion of external beam radiation therapy, the 1- and 2-year disease specific survivals from diagnosis were 57 and 25%, respectively, with a median survival of 13.9 months (80).

For 58 patients treated at the time of recurrence with radiosurgery as above and then followed for a median of 12 months, the median survival was 10 months for patients with glioblastoma multiforme and the median survival has not been attained for anaplastic astrocytoma. Of the 27 patients that have died, 4 failed locally at a median of 6 months, 12 had marginal failure at a median of 9 months, and 9 developed distant disease in the central nervous system at a median of 6 months (78). Twelve (21%) patients required reoperation at a median interval of 7 months after radiosurgery for mass effect with neurological deterioration (79). In another series of 35 patients with recurrent malignant gliomas that were treated with SRS, the actuarial survival from treatment to death was 8 months (81). Seven patients required reoperation for increasing mass effect at a mean of 4 months after radiosurgery for an actuarial rate of 31%.

At 3- to 24-month follow-up after Gamma Knife radiosurgery, 3 of 11 (27%) tumors decreased in size, 2 of 11 (18%) were stable, and 6 of 11 (55%) progressed (79). Five of 11 (45%) patients remained clinically stable and 6 of 11 (55%) died between 1 and 24 months after treatment due to progression at the tumor margin in 4 and distantly in 2 (79). The mean survival after radiosurgery was 7.3 months or 22 months from diagnosis.

Other Tumors

Recurrent chordomas and chondrosarcomas have been treated with Gamma Knife radiosurgery. A dose of 20 Gy delivered to the tumor periphery resulted in local tumor control (82). Neurologic improvement was seen in half of the treated patients and the others remained clinically stable.

Linac radiosurgery has been used to treat recurrent head and neck tumors that had been previously treated with external beam radiation therapy. Three patients with squamous cell carcinoma, one with mucoepidermoid carcinoma, and one with adenoid cystic carcinoma received 17.5 to 35 Gy to the tumor periphery (32). Within 5.5 to 7 months, all patients improved clinically, three tumors were smaller, and two were stable in size (32).

Pineal region tumors that included pineocytomas, pineoblastomas, metastases, gliomas, germinomas, ependymomas, craniopharyngiomas, and meningiomas have been treated with SRS. In a group of nine patients with pineal region tumors (four meningiomas, one ependymoma, one craniopharyngioma, one pineocytoma, and two anaplastic astrocytomas) who were followed for up to 32 months after Gamma Knife radiosurgery, three tumors were stable and six decreased in size (83). Seven patients with small germinomas treated with external beam radiation therapy (25–30 Gy) and linac radiosurgery (10–12 Gy) had tumor shrinkage at a follow-up of 26 to 86 months (84).

Glomus jugulare tumors, ocular melanomas, and hemangioblastomas have all been treated with SRS. A recent case report demonstrated no growth at 2 years for cerebellar hemangioblastomas that received 14-16 Gy to the tumor margin (85). A multiinstitutional series of 38 hemangioblastomas treated with SRS reported an actuarial freedom from tumor progression of 86 ± 12% (86). Better tumor control rates were seen with smaller treatment volumes and higher radiation doses.

In a report evaluating the efficacy of SRS in children, 11 recurrent brain tumors and 1 arteriovenous malformation were treated (87). Three of four children with malignant brain tumors died 6 to 9 months after treatment. Six of eight (75%) children with low-grade tumors had a substantial radiographic reduction in the size of their tumors. There was a relationship between lesion size and/or location and therapeutic response.

Complications

The development of radiation necrosis after SRS is related to the treatment volume and dose. Increased intracranial pressure, increased seizure frequency, and focal neurological deficits, most notably motor weakness, can be associated with radiation necrosis. Symptoms related to radiation injury develop between 3 to 18 months after treatment and usually resolve within 6 to 12 months in 50% of patients (29).

In 72 arteriovenous malformations treated with the Gamma Knife, areas of increased T2-weighted signal on MR imaging were seen 5 to 18 months after treatment in 20 (28%) patients, which were symptomatic in 9 (45%) (88). These imaging changes were symptomatic in six of seven patients where they were present in the brainstem. Radiographic resolution was seen between 4 and 19 months in 10 patients. The integrated logistic formula demonstrated that treatment volume was the only risk factor for predicting postradiosurgical imaging changes (88). Seventeen of 86 (20%) AVM patients treated with helium ion Bragg peak irradiation developed clinical symptoms between 4 and 26 months. Radiation doses associated with complications ranged from 18.5–34.6 Gy and treatment volumes were 0.85 to 40 mL (88). Complications that occur after AVM radiosurgery can be predicted with a statistical model that relates the risks of developing symptomatic postradiosurgical MR imaging changes to the 12 Gy treatment volume and location (89).

Symptomatic radiation necrosis will develop in ~5 to ~10% of patients with brain metastases that are followed for up to 18 months after radiosurgery (71,75). Clinical complications occurred in 14 of 40 (35%) patients with primary brain tumors after SRS (90). Five complications were characterized as moderate and 9 were severe (88,90). These complications were significantly related to tumor-dose inhomogeneity, maximum tumor dose, number of isocenters, maximum normal tissue dose, and tumor volume but not to the administration of prior radiotherapy (29,88).

The single fraction radiation tolerance of the optic nerves and chiasm is 8–10 Gy with a 3 to 5 mm clearance being necessary to treat lesions near these structures. Other cranial nerves have a greater tolerance to SRS but are vulnerable if they have received prior conventional radiation. Prescribing the radiation dose to a higher percentage isodose line does not decrease the incidence of trigeminal or facial nerve complications (88).

TECHNICAL ASPECTS

Precise dose delivery treatments required by SRS have been made possible by the unique mechanical devices and precise dosimetric evaluation of the small radiation fields used for stereotactic treatments in the intracranial region. Specialized hardware to immobilize and reposition the patient has been developed for this particular technique, which ensures that the patient is in the exact same position for the imaging studies, treatment planning, and treatment of this particular procedure. Image localizing devices have been developed that can accurately relate angiographic, CT, and MRI image information to the stereotactic frame of reference. Computerized treatment planning software has also been developed that can calculate and display this diagnostic information in the stereotactic reference frame and display the computed dose on the associated CT or MRI scans. Finally, treatment positioning devices have also been developed that ensure that the treatment parameters obtained from computerized treatment planning are accurately transferred back to the patient. Because of the numerous steps involved in delivering such precise treatments, the accuracy at all stages in the stereotactic process has to be ensured for these treatments to be successful.

The Stereotactic Process

Stereotactic treatments can be viewed as a two-step process: 1) accurate delineation of the shape and location of the target in addition to the surrounding neuroanatomy in the stereotactic reference frame using CT, MRI, or angiography, and 2) development and delivery of the planned treatment (91).

The basic sequence of treatment is to first attach the headring to the patient and then perform the imaging studies. The MR headring is attached if MR scans are required, otherwise the BRW headrings are used. At the University of Minnesota, a CT is always required since it is considered the most accurate scan sequence. MR scans or stereotactic angiography is performed next. Before each of these scan sequences, the location of the headring is checked using the depth helmet (Figure 10.5) to ensure that the position of the headring has not changed or shifted. The image

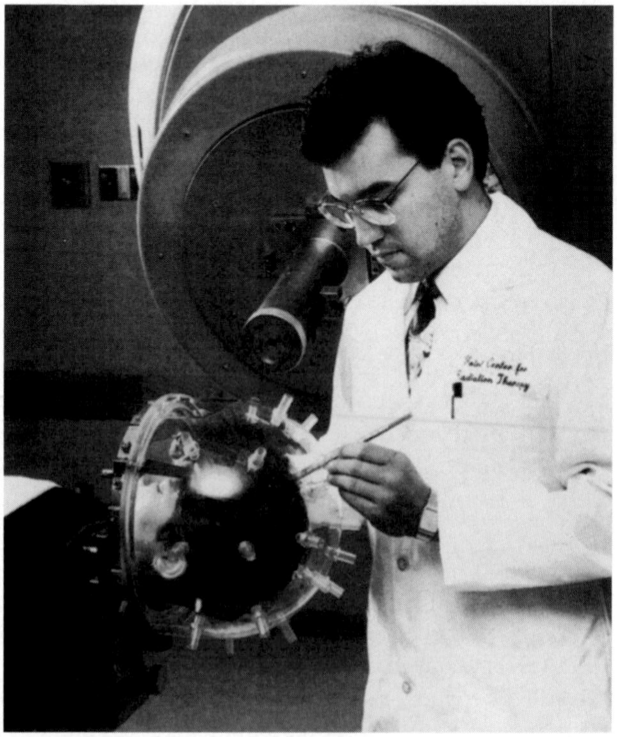

Figure 10.5. The depth helmet, shown in place on a patient, is used to verify that the position of the headring has not changed between the time of imaging and that of treatment.

sequence data is transferred to the treatment planning computer, and the stereotactic fiducial points are entered into the system. This imposes the stereotactic frame of reference onto the scan sequence and properly represents the imaging data in stereotactic space. External contours are entered from the CT scans, and other appropriate anatomic data, including the target to be treated, are digitized from the most useful data set. The beam arrangement and size of the collimators to use are optimized on the planning computer and the prescription dose is entered into the computer. Hard copy documentation is printed to provide a historical record of the plan and calculations of the number of monitor units to be delivered and the number of monitor units per degree are calculated. The accuracy of the treatment hardware is checked, the treatment parameters such as cone size, and vernier scale locations of the isocenter are triple checked, and the headring position is checked using the depth helmet to ensure it has not moved from the time of the imaging studies.

To deliver treatment, the patient is positioned on the treatment couch with all the couch motions locked and double immobilized using both the manufacturer provided couch locks as well as couch motion locks developed in the department. Ensuring that the height of the couch will not change is critical. For the actual treatments, each of the couch angles, and the start and stop angles of each arc, are double checked. The monitor units specified and the monitor units per degree settings are each double checked before treatment is delivered. If more than one isocenter is to be treated, the same checks described above are repeated in full.

This stereotactic process is the same for both SRS and SRT, except that fitting the headring is more involved for SRT because the bite block assembly, the back plate, and the velcro strap assembly all have to be custom fit to the patient.

Necessary Equipment

To adequately perform SRS and SRT, several pieces of equipment are required. The phantom base is the most important component in the entire stereotactic process and defines stereotactic space itself (Figure 10.6). It is the device to which all other steps in the stereotactic process are

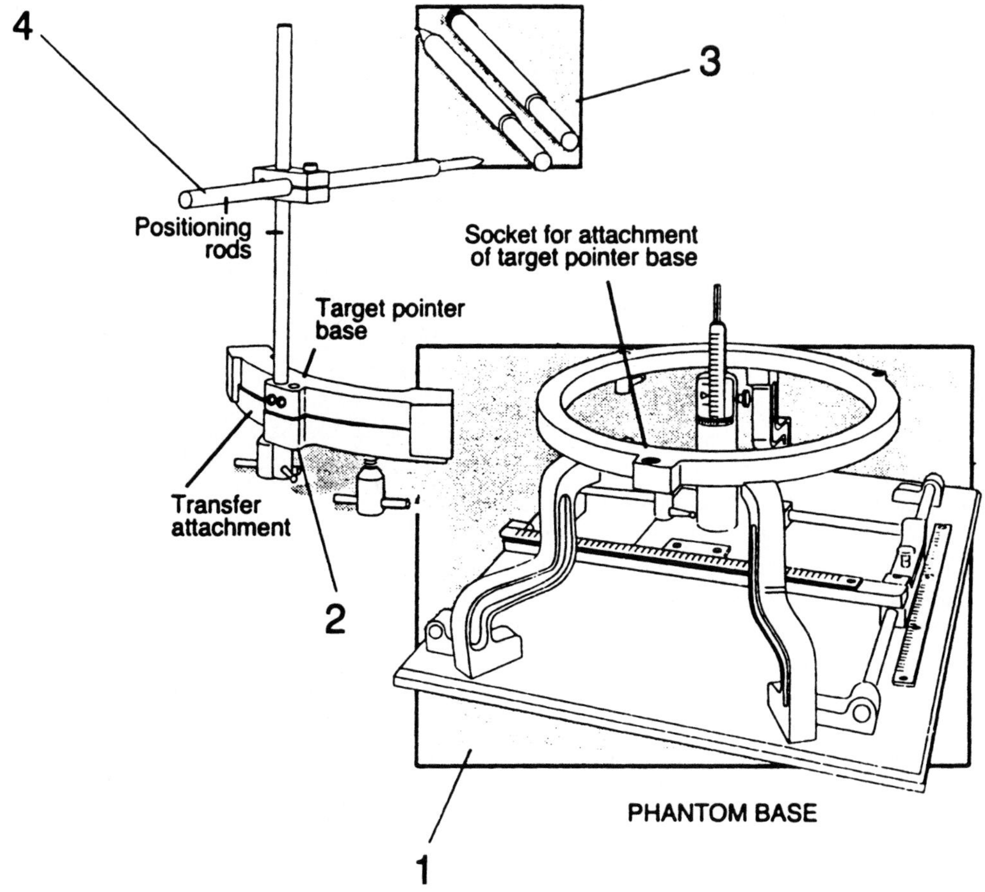

Figure 10.6. Phantom base (1) which is the basis of the BRW stereotactic coordinate system and is the source of accuracy for the stereotactic process. Also shown are the transfer pointer assembly (4), the interchangeable pointer, and target ball devices (3), and the transfer attachment (2) to fix the assembly to the ISS.

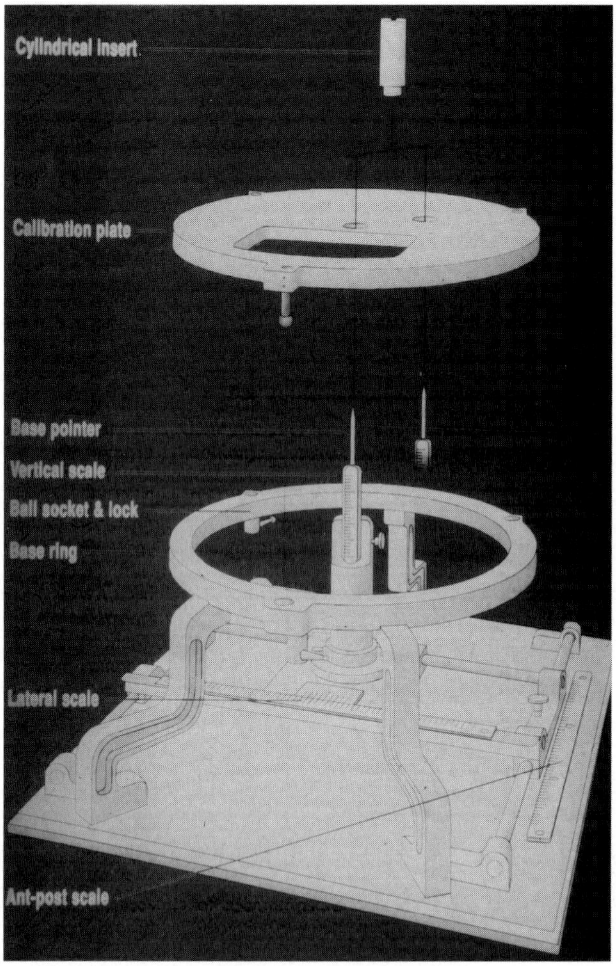

Figure 10.7. A simple and mechanically rugged device used to test routinely the accuracy of the phantom base.

referenced. It defines the AP, lateral, and vertical coordinates in stereotactic space for the independent support stand (ISS), the head immobilization system, and the imaging systems of CT, MRI, and angiography. This reference system must be consistent throughout all the mechanical devices and in the treatment planning computer. Because it is the key component of the system, its accuracy must be absolute and easily verified. At the University of Minnesota, we have designed a test jig to test the phantom base (Figure 10.7). It consists of a solid metal plate that fits snugly into the three holes in the ring of the phantom base. With the device in place, the AP, lateral, and vertical (0,0,0) position on the vernier scales can be quickly checked as well as the (5,5,0) position. This device is capable of ensuring the accuracy of the phantom base to within 0.1 mm. The construction and operation of this device have been described in more detail (92) and its use is highly recommended.

The three headrings used at the University of Minnesota are shown in Figures 10.8 to 10.10. Figure 10.8 shows the Brown-Roberts-Wells (BRW) CT headring and associated ancillary equipment. The extension posts that suspend the ring from the patient's head and the screws that attach the assembly to the patient are also required although they are not shown in the figure. The Gill-Thomas-Cosman (GTC) repeat fixation headring is shown in Figure 10.9A with the bite block assembly, the back headrest, and the velcro strap in place. Figure 10.9B shows the GTC headring in place. The MR headring is shown in Figure 10.10 and is required whenever MR scanning is used for the patient's treatment. The BRW headring attaches to the outside of this ring when the CT scan of the patient is performed and serves to support the CT localizer and is the means by which the patient is supported on the independent support stand (ISS) The purpose of these headrings is to directly, accurately, and rigidly transfer the stereotactic frame of reference from the phantom base to the head of the patient.

The angiographic and CT localizing frames are shown in Figure 10.11A and the MR localizer is shown in Figure 10.11B. These devices are required so that the position of the intracranial structures can be reconstructed from the information visible on the scan radiographs. The angiographic localizer attaches to the BRW headring in one specific orientation and consists of four plates. On each plate are four small lead markers positioned at the corners of a square. Since the precise location of each of these lead beads is known, the location in stereotactic space of any point can be reconstructed from projected radiographs (Figure 10.12). The CT localizer is another fiducial jig that allows the location of structures on each CT scan to be mapped into stereotactic treatment space. By knowing precisely the expected locations of the nine fiducial rods, the AP, lateral, and vertical stereotactic coordinates of any point in a CT scan sequence can be determined. Figure 10.13 shows a CT scan of the head with the nine fiducial points of the CT localizer visible on the scan.

The MR localizer (universal compact localizer frame, UCLF) can be used for both CT and MRI scans but is used primarily for MR scanning. Again, since the locations of the fiducial rods are known precisely, the location of points within the localizing cage can be reconstructed accurately from the fiducial points located on the particular MR or CT scans.

The mechanical equipment associated with the linear accelerator is illustrated in Figure 10.14. The commercially available (SRS 200 system; Elekta Oncology Systems, Inc., Norcross, GA) independent support stand and the subgantry assembly is the commercialized version of the unit designed at the University of Florida (93). The design goal of the system was that it provide the greatest possible mechanical accuracy on a scale comparable to the Gamma Knife unit (94). The secondary collimators are a series of circular cones made of 15-cm high stainless steel and cerro-

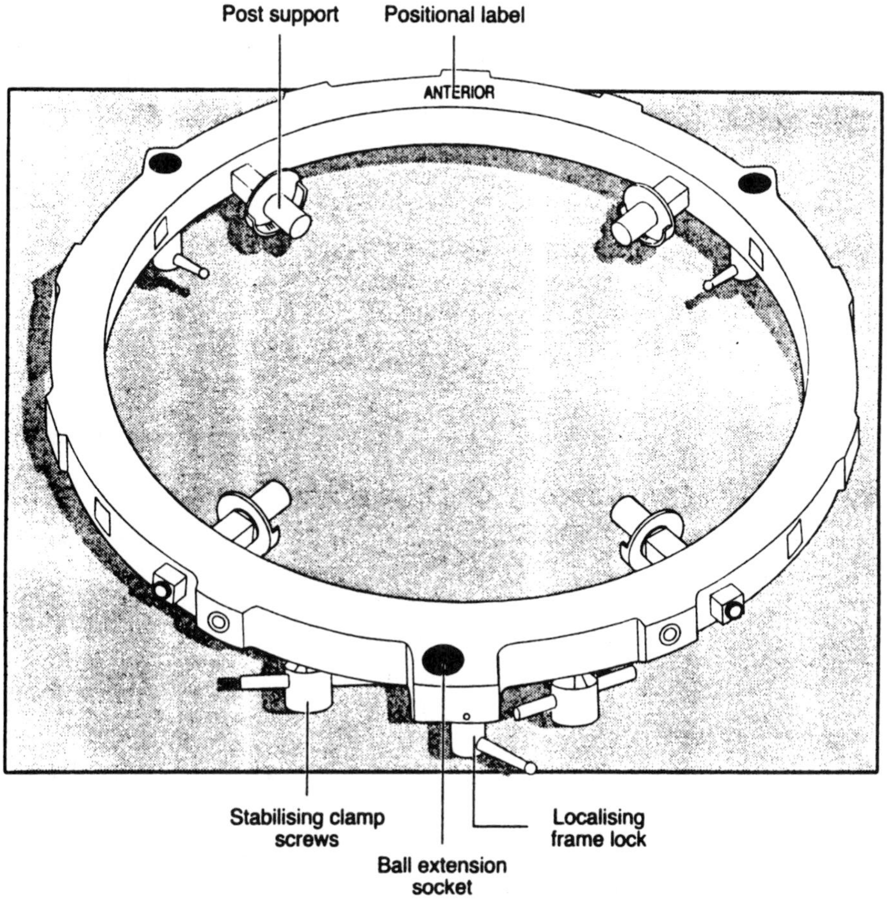

Figure 10.8. The Brown-Roberts-Wells (BRW) headring showing the post supports and the stabilizing clamp screws used to attach the frame to the ISS. The extension posts and head screws required for fixation of the ring to the patient are not shown.

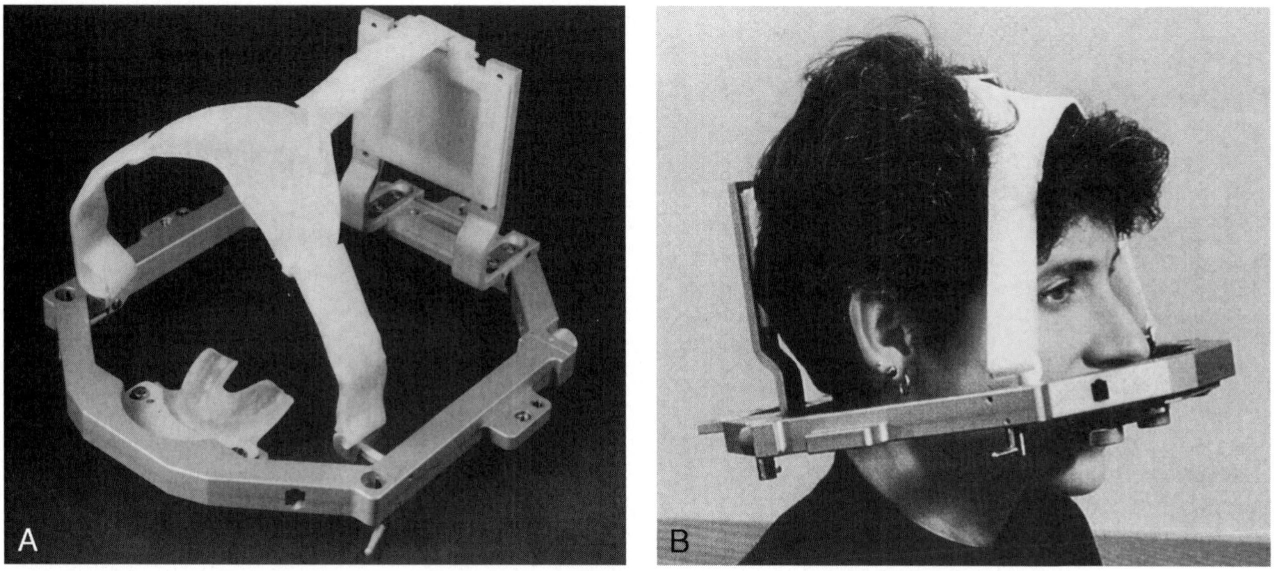

Figure 10.9. (A) The Gill-Thomas-Cosman (GTC) relocatable headring with the bite block, vertical bracket headrest, and velcro strap in place. (B) The GTC headring in place on a patient.

bend. A range of collimator opening from 5 mm diameter plus 10 mm diameter through 30 mm diameter in steps of 2 mm is supplied with the unit. Additional cones from 35 mm diameter through 75 mm diameter in steps of 5 mm were designed, tested, and put into use at our institution. These large collimator sizes became necessary as SRT became a more common application of the stereotactic process. The gimbal bearing with a sliding mount transfers the rotational force of the linac gantry to the ISS subgantry via the secondary collimators. This device allows the subgantry to determine gantry rotational accuracy, rather than the linear accelerator, and provides free rotation even though a slight misalignment may exist between the accelerator gantry and the ISS.

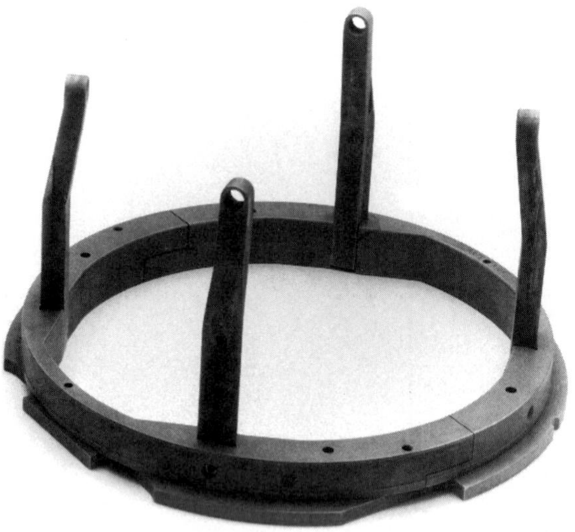

Figure 10.10. The headring supplied by RSA for use in MRI.

Tests of Mechanical Accuracy

The accuracy of all the mechanical components of the system must be verified before patient treatments can be initiated. The test of the phantom base using the phantom base test jig has already been described. Additional checks of the accuracy of the ISS and subgantry system, the angiographic, CT, and MRI localizers, and of the image transfer utilities must also be performed before stereotactic treatments can be initiated.

The ISS mechanical accuracy test very closely mimics that of Lutz et al. (95). It is performed by setting a particular point location on the phantom base then matching the tip of the transfer pointer to the phantom base pointer. The transfer pointer is then removed from the phantom base and the tapered pointer of the transfer pointer is replaced with a tungsten ball whose center is at the exact location of the tapered pointer. The same BRW coordinates that were set on the phantom base are set in the scales of the ISS. The transfer pointer is then attached to the ISS using the transfer attachment and a series of films is taken at eight different combinations of gantry and table angle settings (Table 10.3). Figure 10.15 illustrates the irradiation geome-

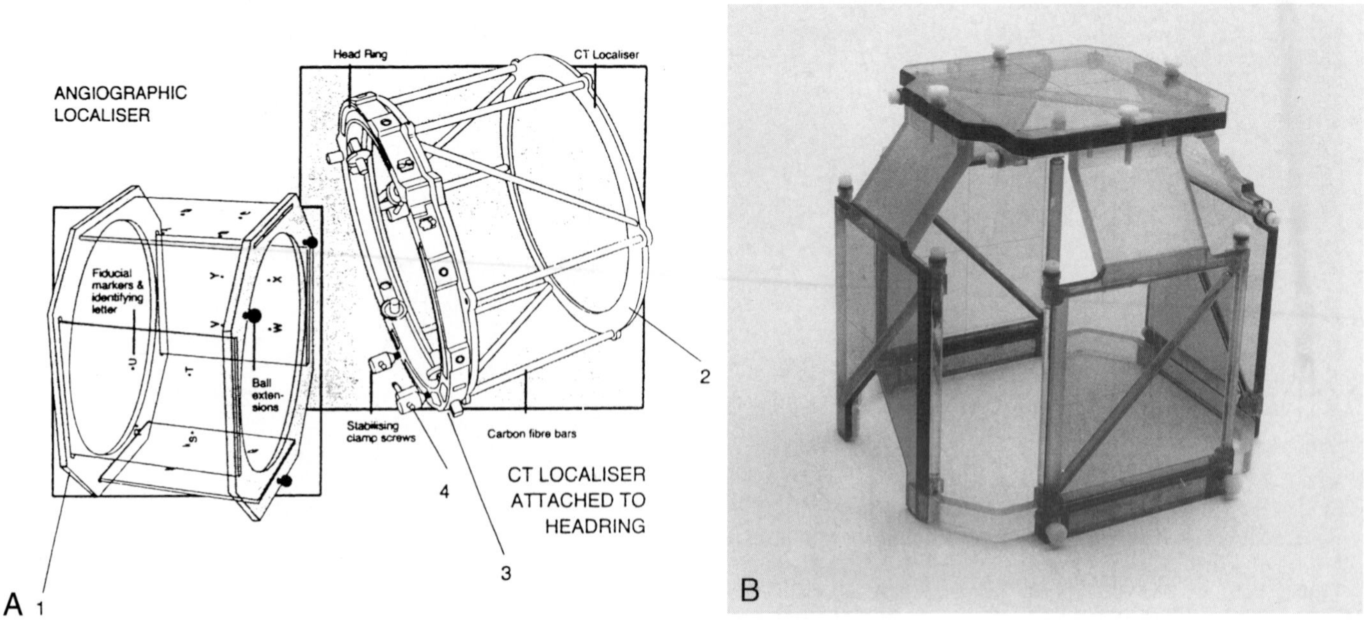

Figure 10.11. Localizing or fiducial devices used during angiography, CT scanning (A), and MRI scanning (B). The CT localizer is shown attached to the BRW headring.

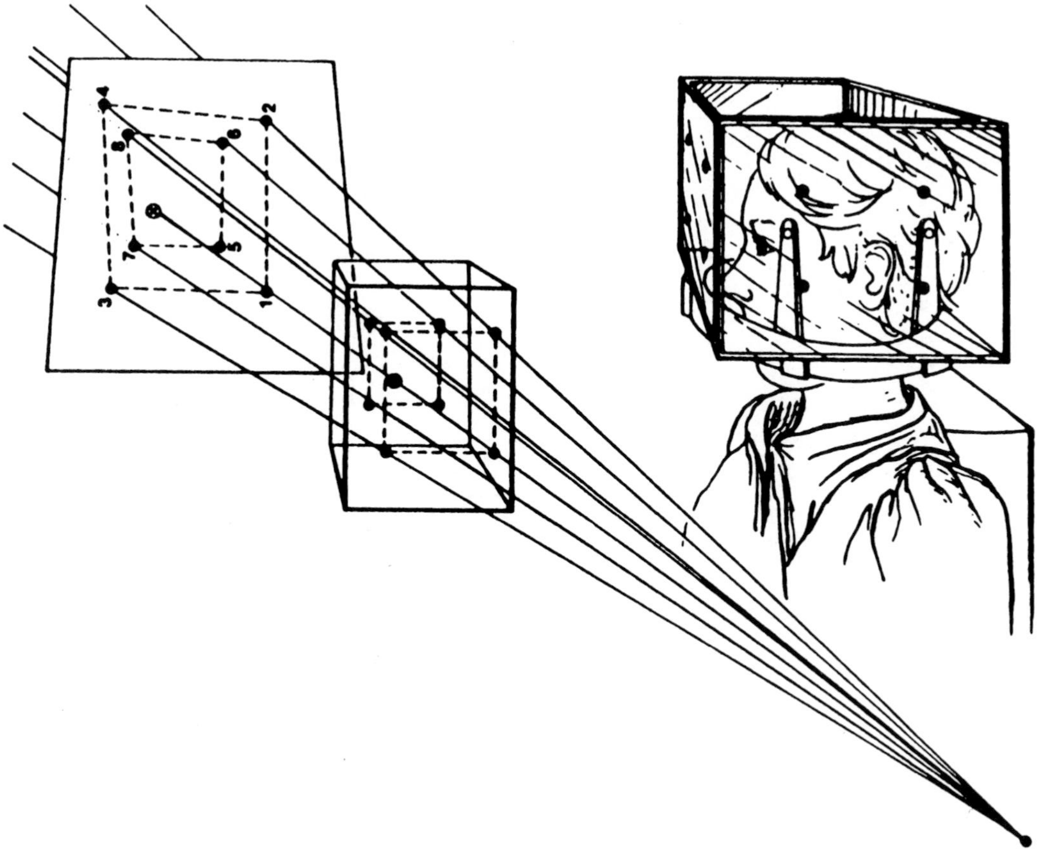

Figure 10.12. The angiographic localizer and a projected view showing how the location of an intracranial structure can be reconstructed from non-orthogonal projections. (Used with permission from Schell MC et al. AAPM Report 54. Stereotactic Radiosurgery. Report of Task Group 42. Radiation Therapy Committee. American Institute of Physics, 1995.)

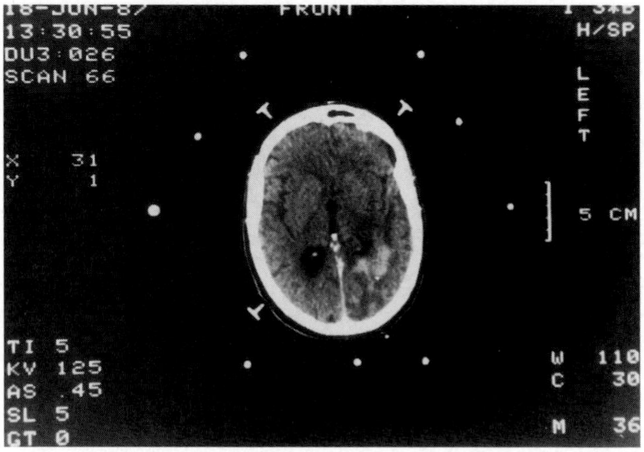

Figure 10.13. A CT scan showing the locations of the nine fiducial rods of the CT localizer.

try to perform the film test of the targeting accuracy. The test points are chosen to represent the center of stereotactic space (the 0,0,0 point) and the eight corners of a cube that exists in stereotactic space. Three of these points of the set are repeated to ensure reproducibility of the test series. Table 10.4 shows the BRW coordinates of the phantom base that were used for these tests. The unit was designed to be accurate to better than 0.3 mm with no single point deviating by more than 0.5 mm. Typical films from these types of tests are shown in Figure 10.16. When these films are checked using 8–10 × magnification, this test can accurately indicate the degree of alignment to within ±0.1 mm.

Tests of Imaging Accuracy

The test of imaging accuracy is done both on the CT and MRI scanners and on the images that are transferred from the scanners to the treatment planning computers. The most efficient means to accomplish this test is to have an accurate test phantom for comparison. One that is commercially available is illustrated in Figure 10.17 (Radionics Software Applications, Inc., Burlington, MA). The BRW coordinates of the top, center point of the internal test objects, a cube, sphere, cone, and cylinder, are known exactly. Using these values as the standard of comparison, the top, center point of each of these objects is identified on every CT and MRI scanner that is to be used for treat-

Figure 10.14. The mechanical components: (1) the secondary collimators for defining the treatment field diameter, (2) the independent support stand and sub gantry assembly, (3) the gimbal bearing assembly.

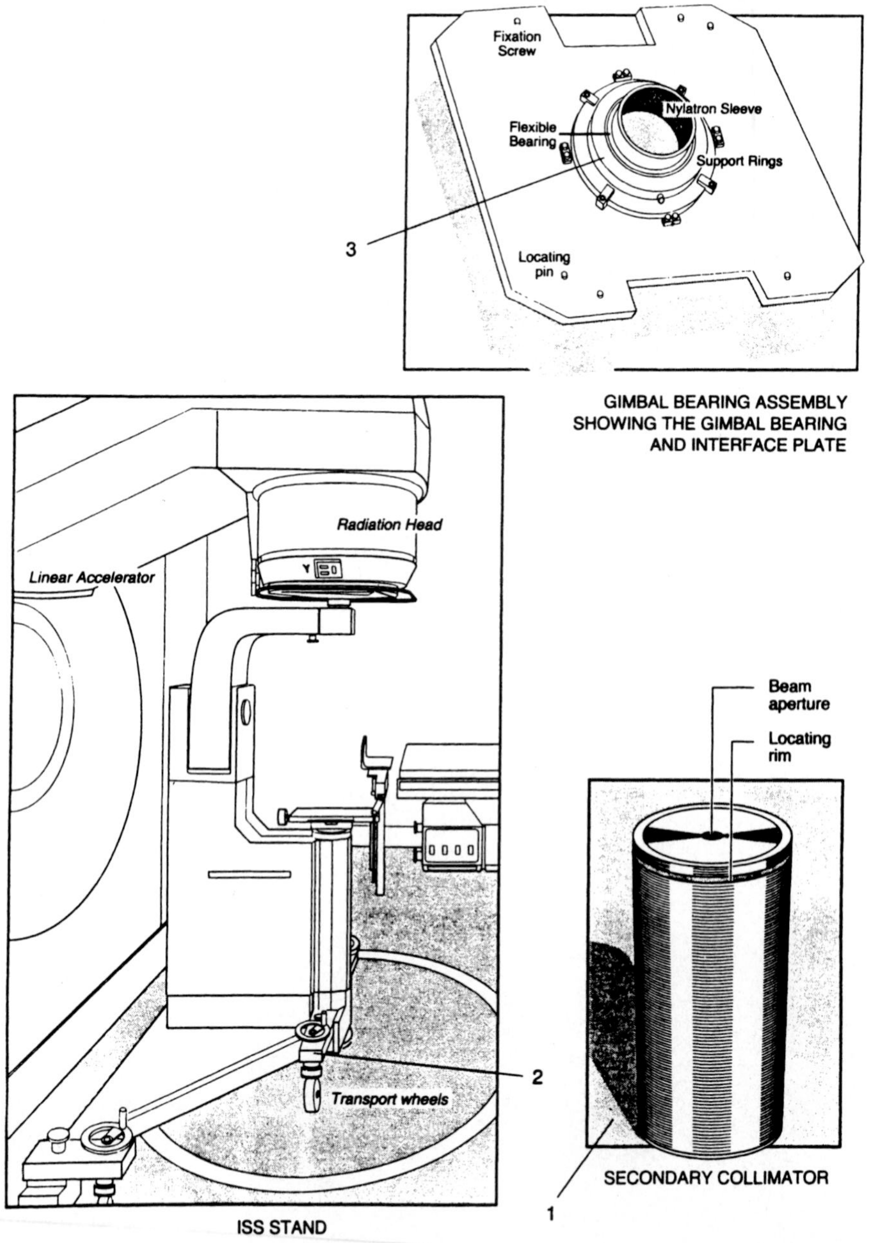

Table 10.3. The Combinations of Gantry and Couch Angle Used When Taking the Stereotactic Check Films

Gantry angle	240°	240°	315°	315°	45°	45°	120°	120°
Couch angle	270°	315°	315°	0°	0°	45°	45°	90°

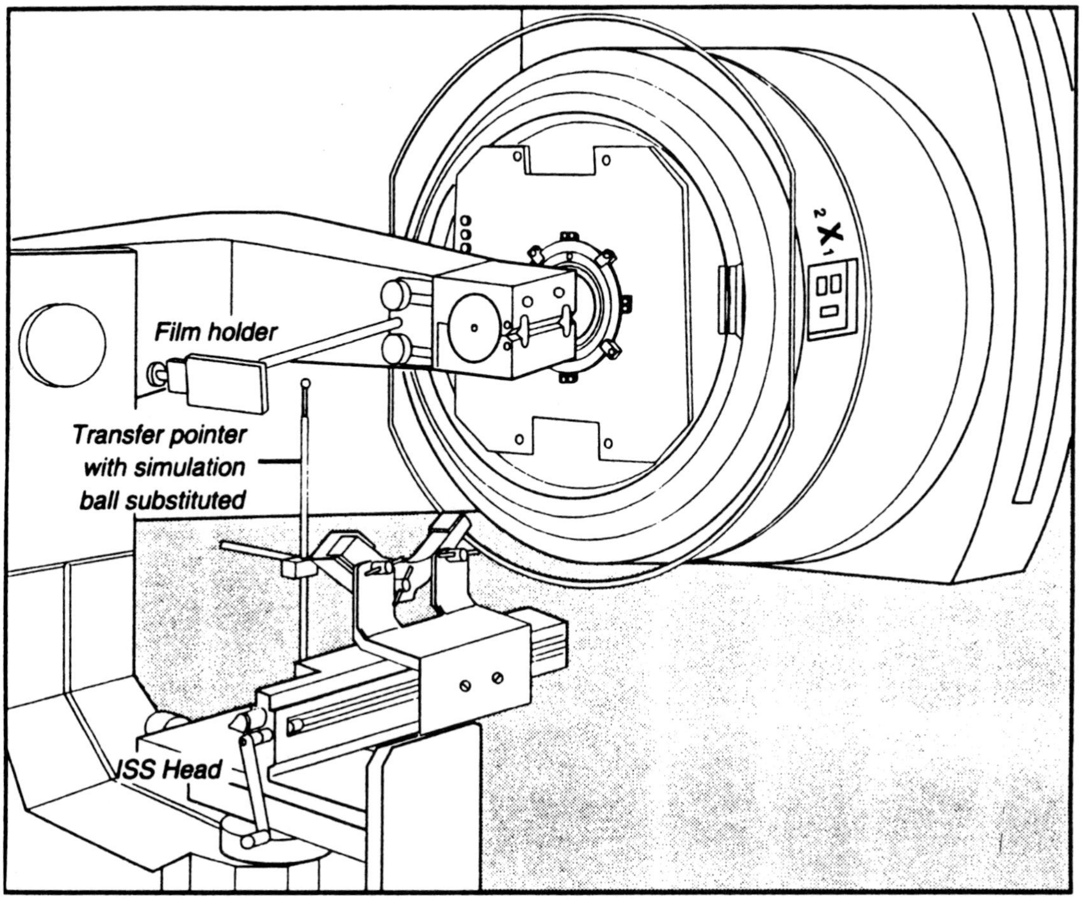

Figure 10.15. The transfer pointer with simulation ball in place. The film strip is attached to the film holder and a series of films are exposed at different table and gantry positions.

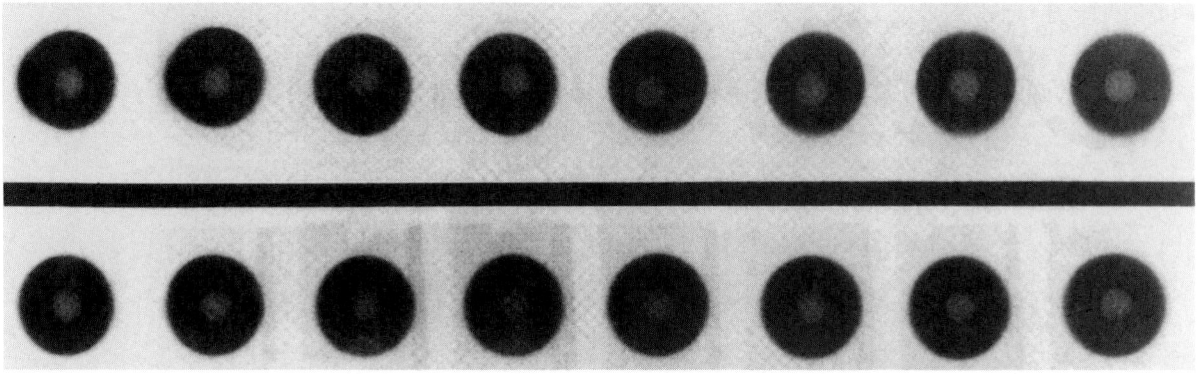

Figure 10.16. Two sets of test target films taken at the eight gantry-table angle combinations. The top film shows an average error of 1.5 mm with a minimum and maximum deviation of 0.2 and 2.4 mm, respectively. The bottom film has an average error of 0.2 mm with a minimum and maximum deviation of 0 and 0.3 mm, respectively. (Used with permission from Khan FM, Potish RA [eds]. Treatment Planning in Radiation Oncology. Baltimore: Williams & Wilkins, 1998.)

Table 10.4. The BRW Coordinates of the Test Points to Ensure the Accuracy of the Independent Support Stand Along with the Accuracy Obtained at Those Locations

Point Number	Vertical (mm)	Lateral (mm)	AP (mm)
1	0	0	0
2	0	0	50
3	0	0	−50
4	0	50	0
5	0	−50	0
6	50	0	0
7	−45	0	0
8	−45	−50	−50
9	50	50	50
3 repeat locations			
10	0	0	0
11	−45	−50	−50
12	50	50	50

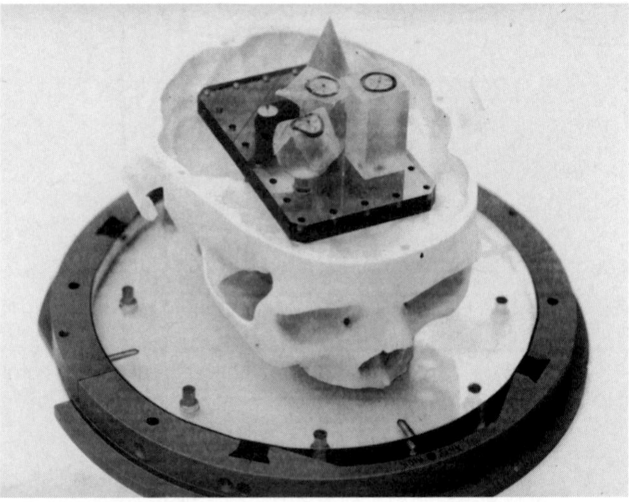

Figure 10.17. A commercially available head phantom used to verify the imaging accuracy of both CT and MRI scanners, in addition to the images transferred to the treatment planning computer. The BRW coordinate of the top, center point for the four internal test objects, the cube, sphere, cone, and cylinder, are all very accurately known.

ment planning, and the reconstructed BRW coordinate from the scanners is compared to the expected value.

The CT and MRI images on the scanners being commissioned are transferred to the treatment planning computer. The top, center points of the test phantom objects are identified on the reconstructed images in the treatment planning computer and the observed values are compared to the expected values for the test object. This ensures that the accuracy determined on the CT or MRI scanner is not degraded in being converted to a form usable by the treatment planning system. MRI units require more extensive commissioning since sagittal and coronal planes are reconstructed in addition to axial planes. Consequently, MRI image accuracy has to be quantified in each one of the reconstructed planes.

Dosimetry Data Required for Stereotactic Treatments

For most stereotactic treatment planning systems, the three primary dosimetric quantities required for dose computation are the cone output factors, TMR or %DD data, and off-axis ratio data. Because of the small field sizes common in SRS and SRT, simpler dose calculation algorithms can be employed than those required for routine radiation oncology (96). However, obtaining accurate dosimetry measurements for small field sizes is complicated by the relationship between detector size and field dimension and the lack of lateral charged particle equilibrium. Rice et al. (97) showed that the corrections to penumbra width ranged from 0.3 to 1.0 mm when beam profiles were measured with an ion chamber whose diameter was 3.5 mm. Investigations have also been done to deconvolve the effect of detector size from small field measurements (98,99).

Cone Output Factors

Detector size relative to the field size or cone aperture is also a major consideration in the determination of cone output factor. These field size dependent output factors are a key dosimetric parameter since they tie the treatment directly to the calibration of the accelerator (Figure 10.18). Since stereotactic treatments are delivered isocentrically, the cone output factor is defined as the dose delivered to

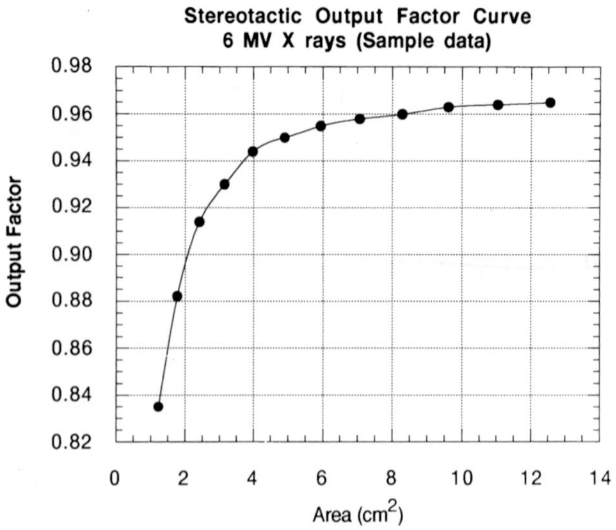

Figure 10.18. Typical cone output factors for 6 MV x-rays. (Used with permission from Schell et al. [91] AAPM Report #54. Stereotactic Radiosurgery. Report of Task Group 42, Radiation Therapy Committee. American Institute of Physics, 1995.)

the isocenter point divided by the dose delivered at the calibration point for the reference field size. For our treatment unit, the source-axis distance is 100 cm. The source-calibration distance is 101.6 cm because our accelerator calibration is done at 100 cm SSD with the chamber at the reference depth, t_o. A linac collimator setting of 5x5 cm^2 is used for cone diameters of 5 through 40 mm. For cone diameters of 45 through 75 mm, an $8 \times 8\ cm^2$ linac collimator setting is used. The cone output factors for stereotactic treatments were determined using multiple detectors: the Markus plane-parallel ionization chamber (PTW Freiberg, Freiberg, Germany), Kodak XV-2 film (Eastman Kodak Co., Rochester, NY), a Therados (Scanditronix AB, Radiotherapy Division, Uppsala, Sweden) electron diode with an active diameter of approximately 2.5 mm, and square, lithium fluoride thermoluminescent dosimeter (TLD) chips (Harshaw Filtrol Corp, Solon, Ohio). The field size dependence of cone output factors for cylindrical and plane-parallel ionization chambers has been discussed in the literature (97). These authors found that ionization chambers having inner diameters of 3.5 and 5.4 mm were capable of measuring output factors for cone diameters as small as 12.5 mm to within 0.5%. Our measurements showed that all detectors gave essentially the same cone output factors down to a cone diameter of 16 mm. However, for smaller cone diameters, we felt that the response of the Markus chamber (having a 5.4 cm diameter active volume) underestimated the true output. This could be due to the size of the active volume of the chamber, the criticality of accurate centering of the chamber in the radiation beam, or a combination of the two. We had higher confidence in the data obtained using diode and film for cone sizes from 10 to 14 mm in diameter. The 5-mm cone was particularly challenging to calibrate. Because of the small diameter, XV-2 film analyzed using the Wellhofer (Wellhofer Dosimetrie, Schwarzenbruck, Germany) scanner detector (0.8 mm effective aperture) was used for the cone output factor. The 5 mm output and the 10×10 field data were all taken on the accelerator at the same time (at the appropriate distances described above) and developed in the film processor at the same time.

Tissue Maximum Ratio Determination

Tissue maximum ratio (TMR) data was taken with Markus chamber, XV-2 film, and the Therados electron diode. Markus chamber measurements were performed in clear polystyrene for cone diameters down to 20 mm. The buildup data for the Markus Chamber was corrected for plate separation and guard width (100,101) and the depths in polystyrene were corrected to depths in water. These data were the standard of comparison for the cone data measured using other detectors. XV-2 film in clear polystyrene and the Therados electron diode in water were used for measurements of TMR for all cone sizes. A correction factor versus depth was determined from the 30 mm cone Markus chamber data and applied to the cone data measured for smaller cones using XV-2 film and the diode. The diode under responded by approximately 1% as a function of depth compared to the Markus chamber for the 30 mm cone. XV-2 film being energy dependent deviated progressively with depth as compared to the Markus chamber data. Depth dependent correction factors for the diode and XV-2 film were derived from the 30 mm cone data and applied to the raw data for the smaller cones. After correction the diode data and the film data agreed with Markus chamber data to within 2% or better at all depths.

Off-Axis Ratio Data

The off-axis ratio data was taken with XV-2 film and a Therados electron diode. The OAR profiles in the gun-target and right-left directions were averaged to yield one representative OAR for each of the cones. Film and diode data yielded essentially the same profile except for the extremely small cone diameters. We use film data for the off-axis ratios for all cone sizes as recommended by the AAPM task group (91). Typical data for the 10, 20, and 30 mm cones for three different detectors are illustrated in Figure 10.19.

Commissioning of the computerized treatment system is also an important facet of the technical aspects of SRS and radiotherapy. Commissioning of these systems follows the guidelines set by the AAPM (91,102) and of those published in the literature (103). The scope and magnitude of these checks are too lengthy to be covered here and the reader is encouraged to consult the literature. One check of the procedure that is of particular importance is to perform several dosimetric checks of the entire procedure and verify that the prescribed dose can be delivered correctly to the prescription point. This check should be a dry run of the entire procedure including imaging, computerized treatment planning, and final delivery of the dose to the prescription point. Our tests involved angiographic imag-

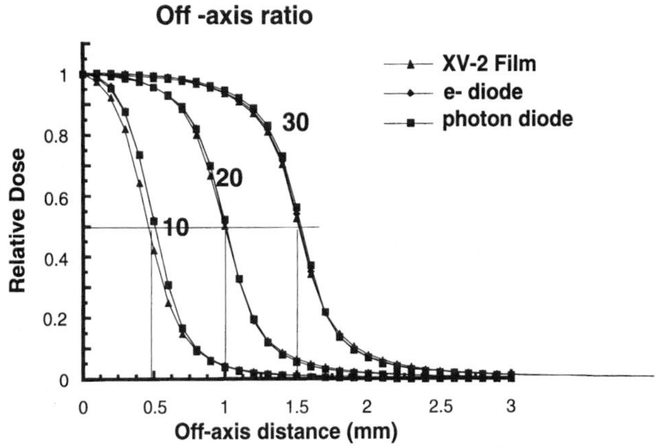

Figure 10.19. Typical off axis ratio data for 10 MV x-rays taken with different detectors.

ing, CT scanning, computerized treatment planning, and treating a solid water sphere measuring 15 cm in diameter. The 20 mm cone was used for the treatment so that the four TLD chips located at the treatment isocenter would be in the 99 to 100% dose region. For two independent checks, the dose measured at the location of the TLDs was within 1% of the expected dose. This gave us high confidence that the dose delivered and the accuracy of the system was within acceptable range.

Methods have been described in the literature to verify that the 3-D dose distribution generated by the computer is what is actually delivered. Arrays of TLDs have been used to make point dose samplings of the 3-D distribution but this method is time consuming and lacks sufficient detail to provide a comprehensive check (93). Fricke solution in an agarose gel medium has been shown to be a viable 3-D dosimeter (104–106) although original methods suffered from diffusion of the ion after irradiation and difficulty in preparing large samples of the material. Magnetic resonance scanning was taken of the irradiated gel and dose distributions determined from the resultant signal. Precision of the dosimeter compared to expected computerized dose distributions was within a few millimeters of the expected distribution (Figure 10.20A). Further advances along this line of 3-D dosimetry are the development of BANG polymers gels (MGS Research, Inc., PO Box 581, Guilford, CT 06437) using Fricke dosimetry solution imbedded in a plastic matrix (107). This technique has shown promise in developing 3-D dose distributions not only for SRS but in many other applications of radiation

A

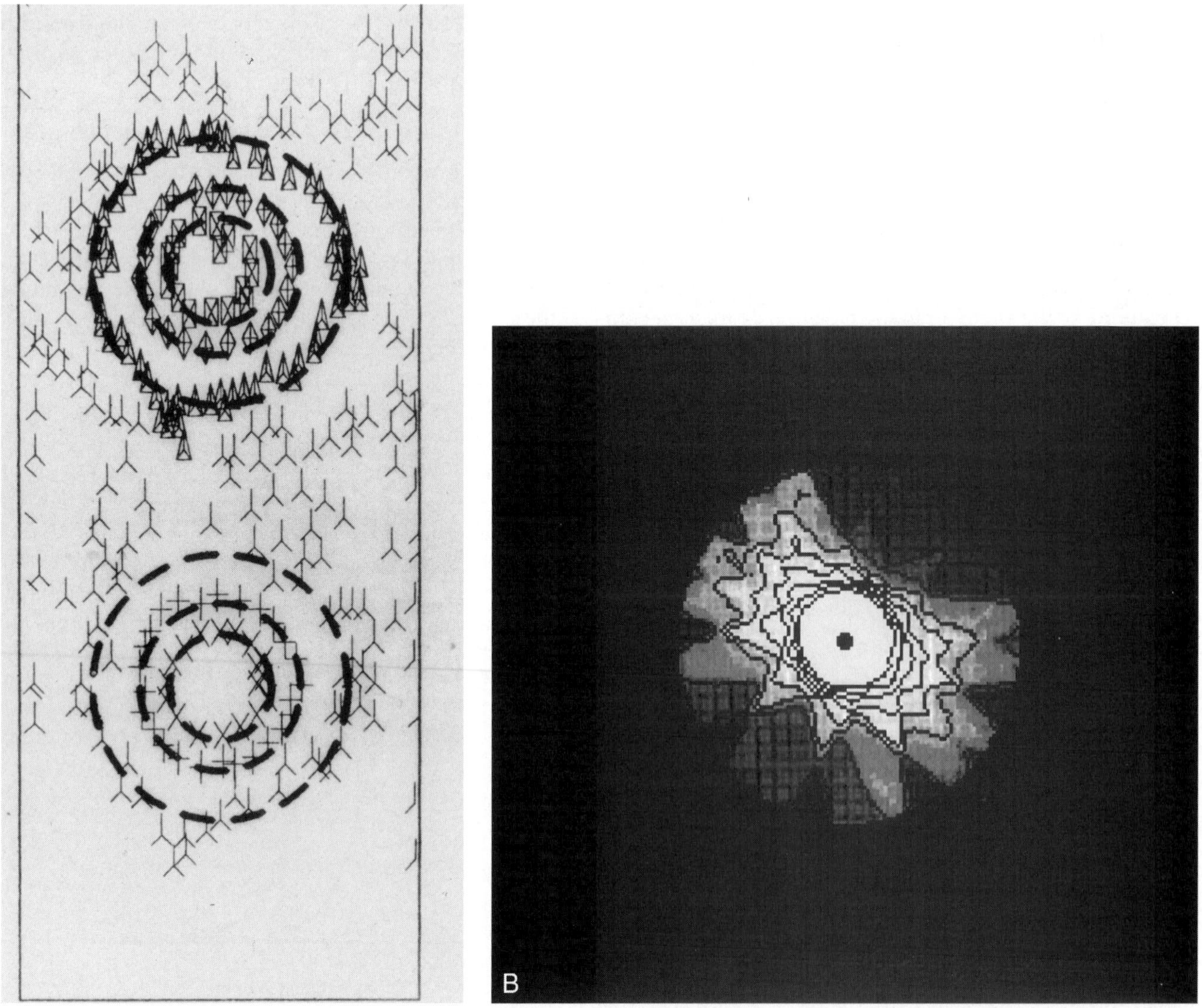

B

Figure 10.20. Dose distributions for (A) Fricke dosimeter solution in agarose gel material analyzed using magnetic resonance. (Used with permission from Maryanski et al. Magn Reson Imaging 1993;11:253–258.) (B) BANG polymer gel material for 3-D distribution verification.

therapy where 3-D integrated dose is necessary (Fig. 10.20b).

Quality Assurance

Quality assurance (QA) in stereotactic treatment is absolutely essential to maintain the accuracy of treatments. Published reports (91,95,108) give detailed explanations of the quality assurance that should be performed, how often the checks should be performed, and the rationale upon which these procedures is based. These publications and others dealing with various aspects of linac and stereotactic quality assurance should be consulted directly for details of these QA procedures.

Quality assurance for stereotactic treatments can be divided into treatment related quality assurance, and routine quality assurance. Treatment QA involves checks of the BRW reference system (the headring), the accuracy of the imaging and data transfer, confirmation of the target position, verification of the output factors, and patient setup verification. Checklists to document that these steps are all performed are highly recommended since inadequate performance at any step can easily degrade the accuracy of the final treatment. The checklist should follow the usual sequence of treatment and should be written in enough detail so as to minimize the chance of a treatment error. The checks should ensure the proper collimator setting, the proper collimator diameter, the couch immobilization locks are functional and set for treatment, the external target ball test is acceptable, the headring location check is acceptable, the target coordinates are properly set on the ISS, and that the safety straps are in place. Critical parameters should be double or even triple checked. Because of the difficulty in setting vernier scales accurately, we triple check these settings as well as the cone size and collimator settings.

Routine QA for stereotactic programs should include the inspection of both the hardware and the software to ensure that it meets the original specifications for the equipment. These checks should confirm the accuracy of the stereotactic frame system and its individual components. These should include the phantom base, transfer pointer assembly, and the CT, MR, and angiographic localizers. The accuracy of the head support system and gantry rotation should also be checked.

Quality assurance involving the therapy machine should verify the machine calibration along with the mechanical accuracy of the accelerator. This check should verify that the frame is aligned with both the gantry and couch rotations, and that the x-ray field is aligned with isocenter beam profiles.

Checks of the software should be done to ensure that the dose is properly calculated, that the stereotactic coordinate system is being accurately represented in the computer, and that the image display properly represents the dose.

Overall Accuracy in Stereotactic Treatments

Stereotactic radiosurgery and radiotherapy exist because of the need for extreme accuracy in the treatment of specific types of malignant and benign diseases. In light of this, it is essential to be aware of the true accuracies that can be achieved using a stereotactic treatment approach. The overall accuracy of the final treatment can be determined by quantifying the inaccuracy of each of the individual steps and components associated with the stereotactic process. The accuracy of various headframe systems has been investigated (109) and shown to be 0.6 mm in any orthogonal axis. Tumor definition with CT or MR scans depends on the resolution of the image and the spacing between the images. For CT, pixel dimensions are 0.7 × 0.7 mm and the slice spacing is not less than 1.0 mm. Therefore, in CT, the minimum accuracy for 1 mm slices is approximately 1.5 mm. For MR scans, the pixel size is on the order of 1.0 mm with slice spacing not less than 1.0 mm leading to a minimum accuracy of approximately 1.7 mm. Angiographic point identification accuracy has been shown to be on the order of 0.3–0.5 mm, while mechanical alignment of various systems range from 0.3 mm to 1.0 mm. Tissue motion also has to be taken into account and has been shown to be approximately 1.0 mm. Table 10.5 shows the achievable accuracies for stereotactic treatment for slice spacing of 1.0 mm and 3.0 mm. This 2 to 4 mm inaccuracy has to be kept in mind whenever a treatment plan is being evaluated for acceptability (91).

Future Directions

Stereotactic treatment of many diseases will continue to evolve to include a variety of treatment schemes. The treatment of large inoperable AVMs has combined endovascular neuroradiology and microsurgery with SRS. Volume staging which is defined as radiosurgery for portions of an AVM and dose staging or treatment of an AVM using multiple fractions have been advocated for large volume AVMs (110). For skull base meningiomas, a combination of cytoreductive surgery, conventional partial brain radiotherapy, and SRS may provide the best long-term control. Recurrent malignant glial tumors may be best treated with

Table 10.5. The Achievable Accuracies for Stereotactic Treatment for 1-mm and 3-mm CT Slice Thicknesses (2)

	1-mm CT slices	3-mm CT slices
Stereotactic Frame	1.0 mm	1.0 mm
Isocentric Alignment	1.0 mm	1.0 mm
CT Image Resolution	1.7 mm	3.2 mm
Tissue Motion	1.0 mm	1.0 mm
Angio (Point Identification)	0.3 mm	0.3 mm
St. Dev. of Point Uncertainty	2.4 mm	3.7 mm

fractionated SRS after conventional external beam radiotherapy to avoid the development of radiation necrosis. The benefit of SRS for three or more brain metastases is currently under investigation.

Techniques currently being developed, such as conformal and dynamic field shaping for linac-based SRS, will reduce the dose to normal tissue and dose inhomogeneity within the target. Frameless stereotaxy and the application of SRS to other parts of the body such as the spine and liver are also being developed (111).

Along with the increased efficacy to disease management, these developments in SRS and radiotherapy also are proving to be cost-effective. In an extensive analysis comparing the cost effectiveness of SRS to surgical resection for the treatment of solitary brain metastases, radiosurgery had a lower total cost per procedure, a lower uncomplicated procedure cost, and a lower average complication cost per case (73,112). Radiosurgery was more cost effective than surgical resection and had a better incremental cost effectiveness. Another study suggested that SRS and whole-brain radiation therapy had an equal or better local control rate than surgery and whole-brain radiation therapy and was 38% less expensive, based on average Medicare reimbursement rates (73,113). Further cost savings are seen in reduced hospitalization. Radiosurgery for meningiomas has reduced the length of hospitalization, the cost to patients, and allows for a rapid return to preoperative functional status (29,61). In an early publication evaluating SRS for acoustic tumors, AVMs, and meningiomas, the average length of hospitalization was 2.24 days for radiosurgery compared to 11.44 days for craniotomy, and hospital costs were reduced by 30 to 70% for patients who had radiosurgery instead of microsurgery (62,114).

As the number of new centers performing SRS continues to increase, the issue of quality assurance needs to be considered for this rapidly evolving field. Similarly, criteria for the appropriate training for all personnel involved with SRS need to be defined and established. A joint statement by the American Association of Neurological Surgeons and The American Society for Therapeutic Radiology and Oncology (115) recommends that training be received by both the radiation oncologists and physicists and that both groups should be board certified or board eligible.

References

1. Leksell L. The stereotactic method and radiosurgery of the brain. Acta Chir Scand 1951;102:316–319.
2. Rubin P, Cooper RA, Phillips TL, eds. Radiation biology and radiation pathology syllabus. Chicago: American College of Radiology, 1978.
3. Emami B, Lyman J, Brown A, et al. Tolerance of normal tissue to therapeutic irradiation. Int J Radiat Oncol Biol Phys 1992;21: 109–122.
4. Caveness WF. Experimental observations: delayed necrosis in normal monkey brain. In: Gilbert HA, Kagan AR, eds. Radiation damage to the nervous system. New York: Raven Press, 1980.
5. Borgelt B, Gelber R, Kramer S, et al. Ultra-rapid high dose irradiation schedules for the palliation of brain metastases: final results of the first two studies by the Radiation Therapy Oncology Group. Int J Radiat Oncol Biol Phys 1981;7:1633–1638.
6. Kjellberg RN, Koehler AN, Preston WM, et al. Intracranial lesions made by the Bragg-peak of a proton beam. In: Haley TJ, Sneider SR, eds. Response of the nervous system to ionizing radiation. Boston: Little, Brown and Company, 1974.
7. Wollin M, Kuruvilla A, Kagan AR, et al. Critique of "Stereotactic radiosurgery for intracranial arteriovenous malformations using a standard linear accelerator" [letter]. Int J Radiat Oncol Biol Phys 1990;18:1535–1536.
8. Flickinger JC. An integrated logistic formula for prediction of complications from radiosurgery. Int J Radiat Oncol Biol Phys 1989;17: 879–885.
9. Flickinger JC, Lunsford LD, Kondziolka D. Dose prescription and dose-volume effects in radiosurgery. Neurosurg Clin North Am 1992; 3:51–59.
10. LeCouteur RA, Gillette EL, Powers BE, Chowd G, McChesney SC, Ingram JT. Peripheral neuropathies following experimental intraoperative radiation therapy (IORT). Int J Radiat Oncol Biol Phys 1989; 17:583–590.
11. Larson DA, Flickinger JC, Loeffler JS. The radiobiology of radiosurgery. Int J Radiat Oncol Biol Phys 1993;25:557.
12. Kondziolka D, Lunsford LD, Coffey RJ, Flickinger JC. Stereotactic radiosurgery of meningiomas. J Neurosurg 1991;74:552–559.
13. Tishler RB, Loeffler JS, Lunsford LD, et al. Tolerance of cranial nerves of the cavernous sinus to radiosurgery. Int J Radiat Oncol Biol Phys 1993;27:215–221.
14. Duma CM, Lunsford LD, Kondziolka D, Harsh GR IV, Flickinger JC. Stereotactic radiosurgery of cavernous sinus meningiomas as an addition or alternative to microsurgery. Neurosurgery 1993;32: 699–705.
15. Leber KA, Bergloff J, Langmann G, Mokry M, Schrottner O, Pendl G. Radiation sensitivity of visual and oculomotor pathways. Stereotact Funct Neurosurg 1995;64(suppl 1):233–238.
16. Pollock BE, Kondziolka D, Flickinger JC, Maitz A, Lunsford LD. Preservation of cranial nerve function after radiosurgery for nonacoustic schwannomas. Neurosurgery 1993;33:597–601.
17. Flickinger JC, Kondziolka D, Lunsford LD. Dose and diameter relationships for facial, trigeminal, and acoustic neuropathies following acoustic neuroma radiosurgery. Radiother Oncol 1996;41(31): 215–219.
18. Linskey ME, Flickinger JC, Lunsford LD. Cranial nerve length predicts the risk of delayed facial and trigeminal neuropathies after acoustic tumor stereotactic radiosurgery. Int J Radiat Oncol Biol Phys 1993;25:227–233.
19. Hirsch A, Noren G. Audiologic findings after stereotactic radiosurgery in acoustic neurinomas. Acta Oto-Laryngologica 1988;106: 244–251.
20. Mendenhall WM, Friedman WA, Bova FJ. Linear accelerator-based stereotactic radiosurgery for acoustic schwannomas. Int J Radiat Oncol Biol Phys 1994;28:803–810.
21. Foote RL, Coffey RJ, Swanson JW, et al. Stereotactic radiosurgery using the Gamma Knife for acoustic neuroma. Int J Radiat Oncol Biol Phys 1995;32:1153–1160.
22. Alexander E III, Lindquist C. Special indications: radiosurgery for functional neurosurgery and epilepsy. In: Alexander E III, Loeffler JS, Lunsford LD, eds. Stereotactic radiosurgery. New York: McGraw-Hill, 1993.
23. Steiner L, Forster D, Leksell L, et al. Gammathalamotomy in intractable pain. Acta Neurochir 1980;52:173–184.
24. Lindquist C, Kihlström L, Hellstrand E. Functional neurosurgery—a future for the Gamma Knife? Stereotactic Func Neurosurg 1992;57: 72–81.
25. Kondziolka D, Lunsford LD, Flickinger JC, et al. Stereotactic radiosurgery for trigeminal neuralgia: a multiinstitutional study using the gamma unit. J Neurosurg 1996;84:940–945.
26. DeSalles AAF, Buxton W, Solberg T, et al. Linear accelerator radiosurgery for trigeminal neuralgia. In: Alexander E III, Kondziolka D, Lindquist C, Loeffler JS, eds. Radiosurgery 1997. Basel: Karger, 1998.
27. Steiner L, Lindquist C, Adler JR, et al. Clinical outcome of radiosurgery for cerebral arteriovenous malformations. J Neurosurg 1992; 77:1–8.
28. Loeffler JS, Alexander E III. The role of stereotactic radiosurgery in the management of intracranial tumors. Oncology 1990;4:21–31.

29. Hall WA. Stereotactic radiosurgery in perspective. In: Cohen AR, Haines SJ, eds. Concepts in neurosurgery: minimally invasive techniques in neurosurgery. Baltimore: Williams & Wilkins, 1995.
30. Norén G, Arndt J, Hindmarsh T. Stereotactic radiosurgical treatment of acoustic neuromas. In: Lunsford LD, ed. Modern stereotactic surgery. Boston: Martinus Nijhoff, 1988.
31. Norén G, Greitz D, Hirsch A, et al. Gamma knife radiosurgery in acoustic neuroma. In: Steiner L, Lindquist C, Forster D, Backlund EO, eds. Radiosurgery: baseline and trends. New York: Raven Press, 1992.
32. Walsh JW. Stereotactic radiosurgery. In: Morantz RA, Walsh JW, eds. Brain tumors. A comprehensive text. New York: Marcel Dekker, 1994.
33. Kondziolka D, Lunsford LD, Linskey ME, Flickinger JC. Skull base radiosurgery. In: Alexander E III, Loeffler JS, Lunsford LD, eds. Stereotactic radiosurgery. New York: McGraw-Hill, 1993.
34. Flickinger JC, Lunsford LD, Coffey RJ, et al. Radiosurgery of acoustic neurinomas. Cancer 1991;67:345–353.
35. Linskey ME, Lunsford LD, Flickinger JC, et al. Stereotactic radiosurgery for acoustic tumors. Neurosurg Clin North Am 1992;3:191–205.
36. Lunsford LD, Kondziolka D, Flickinger JC, et al. Acoustic neuroma management: evolution and revolution. In: Alexander E III, Kondziolka D, Lindquist C, Loeffler JS, eds. Radiosurgery 1997. Basel: Karger, 1998.
37. Pollock BE, Lunsford LD, Kondziolka D, et al. Outcome analysis of acoustic neuroma management: a comparison of microsurgery and stereotactic radiosurgery. Neurosurgery 1995;36:215–229.
38. Forster DMC, Kemeny AA, Pathak A, et al. Radiosurgery: a minimally interventional alternative to microsurgery in the management of acoustic neuroma. Br J Neurosurgery 1996;10:169–174.
39. Lederman GS, Wertheim S, Lowry J, et al. Acoustic neuromas treated by fractionated stereotactic radiotherapy. In: Alexander E III, Kondziolka D, Lindquist C, Loeffler JS, eds. Radiosurgery 1997. Basel: Karger, 1998.
40. Andrews DW, Silverman CL, Glass J, et al. Preservation of cranial nerve function after treatment of acoustic neurinomas with fractionated stereotactic radiotherapy. Preliminary observations in 26 patients. Stereotact Funct Neurosurg 1995;64:165–182.
41. Pollack BE, Kondziolka D, Flickinger JC, et al. Preservation of cranial nerve function after radiosurgery for nonacoustic schwannomas. Neurosurgery 1993;33:597–601.
42. Lunsford LD. The role of stereotactic radiosurgery in the management of brain vascular malformations. In: Alexander E III, Loeffler JS, Lunsford LD, eds. Stereotactic radiosurgery. New York: McGraw-Hill, 1993.
43. Steiner L, Lindquist C. Radiosurgery in cerebral arteriovenous malformations. Neurosurgery: state of the art reviews 1987;2:329–336.
44. Betti OO, Munari C, Rosler R. Stereotactic radiosurgery with the linear accelerator: treatment of arteriovenous malformations. Neurosurgery 1989;24:311–321.
45. Friedman WA, Bova FJ. Linear accelerator radiosurgery for arteriovenous malformations. J Neurosurg 1992;77:832–841.
46. Blatt DR, Friedman WA, Bova FJ. Modifications based on computed tomographic imaging in planning the radiosurgical treatment of arteriovenous malformations. Neurosurgery 1993;33:588–596.
47. Fabrikant JI, Lyman JT, Frankel KA. Heavy charged-particle Bragg peak radiosurgery for intracranial vascular disorders. Radiat Res 1985;104:S244–S258.
48. Steinberg GK, Fabrikant JI, Marks MP, et al. Stereotactic heavy-charged-particle Bragg-peak radiation for intracranial arteriovenous malformations. N Engl J Med 1990;323:96–101.
49. Colombo F, Pozza F, Chierego G, et al. Linear accelerator radiosurgery of cerebral arteriovenous malformations: an update. Neurosurgery 1994;34:14–21.
50. Kjellberg RN, Hanamura T, Davis KR, et al. Bragg-peak proton-beam therapy for arteriovenous malformations of the brain. N Engl J Med 1983;309:269–274.
51. Kondziolka D, Lunsford LD, Coffey RJ, et al. Stereotactic radiosurgery of angiographically occult vascular malformations: indications and preliminary experience. Neurosurgery 1990;27:892–900.
52. Karlsson B, Kihlström L, Lindquist C, et al. Radiosurgery for cavernous malformations. J Neurosurg 1998;88:293–297.
53. Kondziolka D, Lunsford LD, Flickinger JC, et al. Reduction of hemorrhage risk after stereotactic radiosurgery for cavernous malformations. J Neurosurg 1995;83:825–831.
54. Lindquist C, Guo WY, Karlsson B, et al. Radiosurgery for venous angiomas. J Neurosurg 1993;78:531–536.
55. Pollock BE, Kondziolka D, Lunsford LD, et al. Repeat stereotactic radiosurgery of arteriovenous malformations: factors associated with incomplete obliteration. Neurosurgery 1996;38:318–324.
56. Yamamoto Y, Coffey RJ, Nichols DA, et al. Interim report on the radiosurgical treatment of cerebral arteriovenous malformations. The influence of size, dose, time, and technical factors on obliteration rate. J Neurosurg 1995;83:832–837.
57. Karlsson B, Kihlström L, Lindquist C, et al. Gamma Knife surgery for previously irradiated arteriovenous malformations. Neurosurgery 1998;42:1–6.
58. Steiner L, Lindquist C, Steiner M. Meningiomas and Gamma Knife radiosurgery. In: Al-Mefty O, ed. Meningiomas. New York: Raven Press, 1991.
59. Kondziolka D, Lunsford LD, Coffey RD, et al. Stereotactic radiosurgery of meningiomas. J Neurosurg 1991;74:552–559.
60. Chang SD, Adler JR Jr. Treatment of cranial base meningiomas with linear accelerator radiosurgery. Neurosurgery 1997;41:1019–1027.
61. Lunsford LD. Contemporary management of meningiomas: radiation therapy as an adjuvant and radiosurgery as an alternative to surgical removal? J Neurosurg 1994;80:187–190.
62. Lunsford LD, Flickinger J, Linder G, Maitz A. Stereotactic radiosurgery of the brain using the first United States 201 cobalt-60 source Gamma Knife. Neurosurgery 1989;24:151–159.
63. Duma CM, Lunsford LD, Kondziolka D, et al. Stereotactic radiosurgery of cavernous sinus meningiomas as an alternative to microsurgery. Neurosurgery 1993;32:699–705.
64. Valentino V, Schinaia G, Raimondi AJ. The results of radiosurgical management of 72 middle fossa meningiomas. Acta Neurochir (Wien) 1993;122:60–70.
65. Subach BR, Lunsford LD, Kondziolka D, et al. Management of petroclival meningiomas by stereotactic radiosurgery. Neurosurgery 1998;42:437–445.
66. Levy RP, Fabrikant JI, Frankel KA, et al. Charged-particle radiosurgery of the brain. Neurosurg Clin North Am 1990;1:955–990.
67. Kjellberg RN, Kliman B. Lifetime effectiveness—a system of therapy for pituitary adenomas, emphasizing Bragg peak proton hypophysectomy. In: Linfoot JA, ed. Recent advances in the diagnosis and treatment of pituitary tumors. New York: Raven Press, 1979.
68. Thorén M, Rähn T, Guo W-Y, et al. Stereotactic radiosurgery with the cobalt-60 gamma unit in the treatment of growth hormone-producing pituitary tumors. Neurosurgery 1991;29:663–668.
69. Degerblad M, Rahn T, Bergstrand G, et al. Long-term results of stereotactic radiosurgery of the pituitary gland in Cushing's disease. Acta Endocrinol 1986;112:310–314.
70. Stephanian E, Lunsford LD, Coffey RJ, et al. Gamma Knife surgery for sellar and suprasellar tumors. Neurosurg Clin North Am 1992;3:207–218.
71. Mehta MP, Boyd TS, Sinha P. The status of stereotactic radiosurgery for cerebral metastases in 1998. J Radiosurgery 1998;1:17–30.
72. Hall WA. Stereotactic radiosurgery for brain metastases. Crit Rev Neurosurg 1996;6:257–262.
73. Hall WA. Solitary brain metastasis: surgery, stereotactic radiosurgery, and/or radiation therapy? In: Fischer III WS, ed. Perspectives in neurological surgery. New York: Thieme Medical Publishers, 1998.
74. Loeffler JS, Alexander E III. Radiosurgery for the treatment of intracranial metastases. In: Alexander E III, Loeffler JS, Lunsford LD, eds. Stereotactic radiosurgery. New York: McGraw-Hill, 1993.
75. Loeffler JS, Kooy HM, Wen PY, et al. The treatment of recurrent brain metastases with stereotactic radiosurgery. J Clin Oncol 1990;8:576–582.
76. Kelly PJ, Daumas-Duport C, Kispert DB, et al. Imaging-based stereotactic serial biopsies in untreated intracranial neoplasms. J Neurosurg 1987;66:865–874.
77. Shrieve DC, Alexander E III, Wen PY, et al. Comparison of stereotactic radiosurgery and brachytherapy in the treatment of recurrent glioblastoma multiforme. Neurosurgery 1995;36:275–284.
78. Loeffler JS, Alexander E III, Shea WM, et al. Radiosurgery as part of the initial management of patients with malignant gliomas. J Clin Oncol 1992;10:1379–1385.

79. Alexander E III, Coffey R, Loeffler JS. Radiosurgery for gliomas. In: Alexander E III, Loeffler JS, Lunsford LD, eds. Stereotactic radiosurgery. New York: McGraw-Hill, 1993.
80. Gannett D, Stea B, Lulu B, et al. Stereotactic radiosurgery as an adjunct to surgery and external beam radiotherapy in the treatment of patients with malignant gliomas. Int J Radiat Oncol Biol Phys 1995;33:461–468.
81. Hall WA, Djalilian HR, Sperduto PW, et al. Stereotactic radiosurgery for recurrent malignant gliomas. J Clin Oncol 1995;13:1642–1648.
82. Kondziolka D, Lunsford LD, Flickinger JC. The role of radiosurgery in the management of chordoma and chondrosarcoma of the cranial base. Neurosurgery 1991;29:38–46.
83. Dempsey PK, Lunsford LD. Stereotactic radiosurgery for pineal region tumors.Neurosurg Clin North Am 1992;3:245–253.
84. Casentini L, Colombo F, Pozza F, et al. Combined radiosurgery and external radiotherapy of intracranial germinomas. Surg Neurol 1990; 34:79–86.
85. Chandler HC Jr, Friedmen WA. Radiosurgical treatment of a hemangioblastoma: case report. Neurosurgery 1994;34:353–355.
86. Patrice SJ, Sneed PK, Flickinger JC, et al. Radiosurgery for hemangioblastoma: results of a multiinstitutional experience. Int J Radiat Oncol Biol Phys 1996;35:493–499.
87. Weprin BE, Hall WA, Cho KH, et al. Stereotactic radiosurgery in children. Pediatr Neurol 1996;15:193–199.
88. Flickinger JC. Dosimetry and dose-volume relationships in radiosurgery. In: Alexander E III, Loeffler JS, Lunsford LD, eds. Stereotactic radiosurgery. New York: McGraw Hill, 1993.
89. Flickinger JC, Kondziolka D, Pollack BE, et al. Complications from arteriovenous malformation radiosurgery: multivariate analysis and risk modeling. Int J Radiat Biol Phys 1997;38:485–490.
90. Nedzi LA, Kooy LI, Alexander E, et al. Variables associated with the development of complications from radiosurgery of intracranial tumors. Int J Radiat Oncol Biol Phys 1991;21:591–599.
91. Schell MC, Bova FJ, Larson DA, et al. AAPM report 54. Stereotactic radiosurgery. Report of Task Group 42, Radiation Therapy Committee. American Institute of Physics, 1995.
92. Gerbi BJ, Roback DM, Humphrey SD, Hall WA. Maintaining accuracy in stereotactic radiosurgery. Int J Radiat Oncol Biol Phys 1995; 32:1199–1203.
93. Friedman WA, Bova FJ. The University of Florida radiosurgery system. Surg Neurol 1989;32:334–342.
94. Wu A, Maitz AH, Kalend AM, Lunsford LD, Flickinger JC, Bloomer WD. Physics of Gamma Knife approach on convergent beams in stereotactic radiosurgery. Int J Radiat Oncol Biol Phys 1990;18: 941–949.
95. Lutz WA, Winston KR, Maleki N. A system for stereotactic radiosurgery with a linear accelerator. Int J Radiat Oncol Biol Phys 1988;14: 373.
96. Bova FJ, Meeks SL, Friedman WA. Linac radiosurgery: system requirements, procedures, and testing. In: Khan FM, Potish RA, eds. Treatment planning in radiation oncology. Baltimore: Williams & Wilkins, 1998.
97. Rice RK, Hansen JL, Svensson GK, Siddon RL. Measurements of dose distributions in small beams of 6-MV x rays. Phys Med Biol 1987; 32:1087–1099.
98. Higgins PD, Sibata CH, Siskind L, Sohn JW. Deconvolution of detector size effect for small field measurement. Med Phys 1995;22: 1663–1666.
99. Chang KS, Yin FF, Nie KW. The effect of detector size to the broadening of the penumbra—a computer simulated study. Med Phys 1996;23:1407–1411.
100. Gerbi BJ, Khan FM. Measurement of dose in the buildup region using fixed-separation plane-parallel ionization chambers. Med Phys 1990;17:17–26.
101. Sixel KE, Podgorsak EB. Buildup region of high-energy x-ray beams in radiosurgery. Med Phys 1993;20:761–764.
102. Kutcher GJ, Coia L, Gillin M, et al. Comprehensive QA for radiation oncology: report of AAPM Radiation Therapy Committee Task Group 40. Med Phys 1994;21:581–618.
103. Van Dyk J, Barnett RB, Cygler JE, Shragge PC. Commissioning and quality assurance of treatment planning computers. Int J Radiat Oncol Biol Phys 1993;26:261–273.
104. Schulz RJ, deGuzman AF, Nguyen DB, Gore JC. Dose-response curves for Fricke-infused agarose gels as obtained by nuclear magnetic resonance. Phys Med Biol 1990;35:1611–1622.
105. Olsson LE, Fransson A, Ericsson A, Mattsson S. MR imaging of absorbed dose distributions for radiotherapy using ferrous sulphate gels. Phys Med Biol 1990;35:1623–1631.
106. Maryanski MJ, Gore JC, Kennan RP, Schulz RJ. NMR relaxation enhancement in gels polymerized and cross-linked by ionizing radiation: a new approach to 3D dosimetry by MRI. Magn Reson Imaging 1993;11:253–258.
107. Ibbott GS, Maryanski MJ, Eastman P, et al. Three-dimensional visualization and measurement of conformal dose distributions using magnetic resonance imaging of BANG polymer gel dosimeters. Int J Radiat Oncol Biol Phys 1997;38:1097–1103.
108. Warrington AP, Laing RW, Brada M. Quality assurance in fractionated stereotactic radiotherapy. Radiother Oncol 1994;30:239–246.
109. Galloway RL Jr, Maciunas RJ, Latimer JW. The accuracies of four stereotactic frame systems: an independent assessment. Biomed Instr Tech 1991;25:457–460.
110. Lunsford LD. The future of gamma knife stereotactic radiosurgery. In: Alexander E III, Loeffler JS, Lunsford LD, eds. Stereotactic radiosurgery. New York: McGraw-Hill, 1993.
111. Blomgren H, Lax I, Göranson H, et al. Radiosurgery for tumors in the body: clinical experience using a new method. J Radiosurgery 1998;1:63–74.
112. Rutigliano MJ, Lunsford LD, Kondziolka D, et al. The cost effectiveness of stereotactic radiosurgery versus surgical resection in the treatment of solitary metastatic brain tumors. Neurosurgery 1995; 37:445–455.
113. Sperduto PW, Hall WA. The cost-effectiveness for alternative treatments for single brain metastases. In: Kondziolka D, ed. Radiosurgery 1995. Basel: Karger 1996.
114. Lunsford LD, Flickinger J, Coffey RJ. Stereotactic Gamma Knife radiosurgery: Initial North American experience in 207 patients. Arch Neurol 1990;47:169–175.
115. Lunsford LD, Larson DA. Consensus statement on stereotactic radiosurgery prepared by The American Association of Neurological Surgeons Task Force on Stereotactic Radiosurgery and The American Society for Therapeutic Radiology and Oncology Task Force on Stereotactic Radiosurgery. Neurosurgery 1994;34:193.
116. Shaw E, Farnan N, Souhami L, et al. Radiosurgical treatment of previously irradiated primary brain tumors and brain metastasis: final report of radiation therapy oncology group (RTOG) protocol 90-05. Int J Radiat Oncol Biol Phys 1995;32:145.

Chapter 11

Brachytherapy: Rules of Implantation and Dose Specification

Faiz M. Khan

GENERAL PRINCIPLES OF BRACHYTHERAPY

Inverse Square Law

One of the most important principles in brachytherapy is that the dose from a point source varies inversely as the square of the distance. The inverse square law is the dominant factor that influences the dose distribution around a source implanted in tissue, irrespective of the energy of the emitted radiation (see Figure 11.1). Another important feature of the inverse square law is that the dose varies more rapidly in the first 1 cm of distance than, say, between 1 and 2 cm or 2 and 3 cm and so on. The range of treatment from a single source is short indeed, and, if this range is to be increased, the source must be placed in a cylinder of appropriate diameter to achieve greater percent depth dose. This principle is followed in using ovoids or vaginal cylinders to expand the isodose distribution. The principle is violated (knowingly, I assume) when a few ^{125}I high intensity seeds are implanted to treat a brain tumor. To deliver a certain minimum dose in this case to the periphery of the tumor, a high dose or brain necrosing dose sometimes is received in the immediate vicinity (within 0.5 cm) of the sources.

Because of the inverse law effect, the traditional concept of dose uniformity does not hold in brachytherapy. The dose is not uniform, no matter what rules of implantation are followed. The dose gradients are so severe that the schemes of dose specification, so rigorously called for by various implant systems, seem academic or arbitrary. No matter what rules of implantation are followed, the resultant dose distribution has peaks and valleys, again because of the inverse square law.

Choice of Radioactive Sources

Because of the predominance of the inverse square law, the choice of a particular source for implantation is made on the basis of its half-life, radiation protection aspects, and mechanical properties rather than on its characteristics of dose distribution within the range of treatment distances. As shown in Figure 11.1, all sources except ^{125}I are indistinguishable from the inverse square law curve.

Table 11.1 is a summary of the physical properties of sources that are used most commonly in brachytherapy. The current trends are to use ^{137}Cs tube sources for intracavitary implants and ^{192}Ir for interstitial implants. ^{125}I and ^{103}Pd, because of their better radiation protection properties, are preferred for permanent implants. High intensity ^{192}Ir source is most commonly used in high dose rate remote afterloading units.

INTERSTITIAL BRACHYTHERAPY

Brachytherapy sources in the form of needles, wires, or seeds or seed-containing ribbons are inserted into the tumor-bearing tissue in a geometric pattern dictated by the distribution rules of a specific implant system. Several implant systems have been devised and each has its own rules of source distribution and a dose specification system. These systems are significantly different from each other and must not be mixed in any form. Shalek and Stovall caution that, "It is imperative that a radiotherapist use one radium system to the exclusion of the other" (1).

The availability of computers has simplified the problem of dosimetry. Instead of looking up tables for calculating or specifying doses, the planner can obtain isodose curves in any desired plane or view the entire dose distribution in three dimensions. In spite of all that capability, however, questions regarding dose specification remain. Is it the minimum dose or the maximum dose or 10% greater than the minimum dose or 85% of the "basal dose" that constitutes the prescribed dose in brachytherapy? The problem is complicated further by the lack of a clear definition of target volume and the severe dose gradients that characterize a brachytherapy application. The extent of the entire problem becomes evident when comparing the most commonly used systems and their seemingly idiosyncratic rules and dose specification schemes.

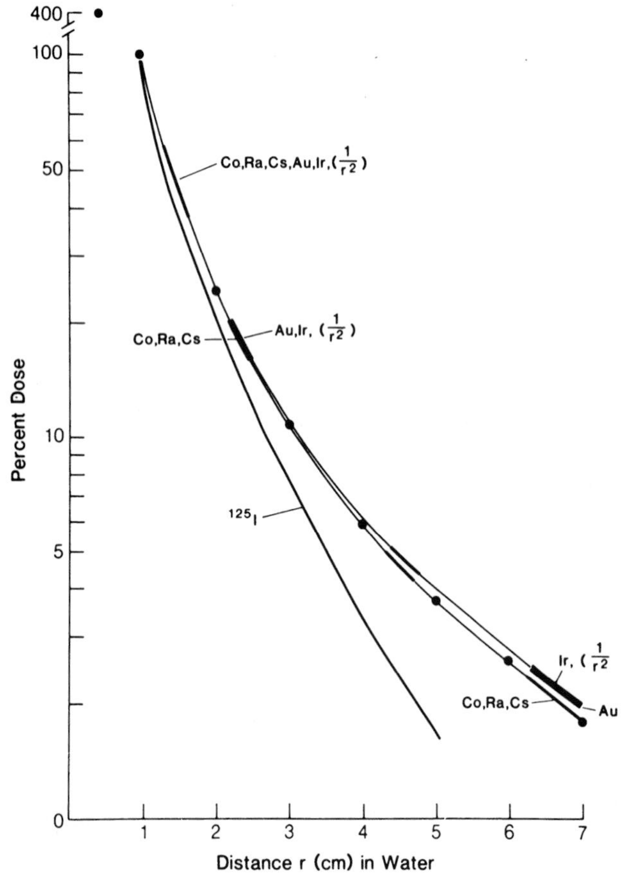

Figure 11.1. Percent depth dose as a function of distance from various point sources in water. Curves are compared with plot of inverse square law function ($1/r^2$). (Reprinted with permission from Khan FM. The physics of radiation therapy. Baltimore: Williams & Wilkins, 1984.)

Rules of Source Distribution

The principal characteristics of the most common implant systems are compared in Table 11.2. The Paterson-Parker and the Quimby rules were developed specifically for radium needles of limited active length (to about 5 cm). These may be adopted for cesium needles as well because the cesium sources are prepared with specifications similar to those of radium. Application of these systems to the iridium implants warrants caution, because the iridium sources come in any length and are flexible, giving rise to curvilinear implants or geometries that may differ from the simple planar or cylindric implants. Similarly, the dosage tables of Paterson-Parker or Quimby may not apply to iridium implants unless the rules of source distribution and the implant geometries are strictly in accordance with these systems.

Rules of Dose Specification

Considerable clinical experience with the use of various systems of interstitial implants has been accumulated. Broadly speaking, these systems can be divided into two schools: one advocating specific rules of source distribution to achieve as uniform a dose distribution as possible, and the other doing away with the uniformity of dose requirement in favor of simpler implantation rules, namely, uniform distribution of equal intensity sources. As noted previously, the dose distribution within the implant plane or volume is not uniform, regardless of the system of implantation followed. The uniform distribution of equal intensity sources, however, does give rise to a higher dose

Table 11.1. Physical Characteristics of Commonly Used Radionuclides in Brachytherapy

Radionuclide	Half-life	Photon Energy (MeV)	Half-Value Layer (mm lead)	Exposure Rate Constant (Rcm^2/mCi-hour)
^{226}Ra	1600 years	0.047–2.45 (0.83 avg)	8.0	8.25*,† Rcm^2/mg-hour
^{137}Cs	30.0 years	0.662	5.5	3.26‡
^{192}Ir	74.2 days	0.136–1.06 (0.38 avg)	2.5	4.69‡
^{192}Au	2.7 days	0.412	2.5	2.38‡
^{125}I	60.2 days	0.028 avg	0.025	1.46‡

* In equilibrium with daughter products.
† Filtered by 0.5 mm platinum.
‡ Unfiltered.
(Reprinted with permission from Khan FM. The physics of radiation therapy. Baltimore: Williams & Wilkins, 1984.)

Table 11.2. Rules of Interstitial Implant Systems

Characteristic	Paterson-Parker	Quimby	Paris	Computer
Linear strength	Variable (full intensity: 0.66 mg Ra/cm; half intensity: 0.33 mg Ra/cm)	Constant (full intensity: 1 mg Ra/cm; half intensity: 0.5 mg Ra/cm)	Constant (0.6 to 1.8 mg Ra eq./cm)	Constant (0.2 to 0.4 mg Ra eq./cm)
Source distribution	Planar implants: Area <25 cm^2: 2/3 Ra in periphery; area 25 to 100 cm^2: 1/2 Ra in periphery. Area > 100 cm^2: 1/3 Ra in periphery	Uniform	Uniform	Uniform
	Volume implants: Cylinder: belt, four parts; core, two parts; each end, one part. Sphere: shell, six parts; core, two parts. Cube: each side, one part; core, two parts.	Uniform distribution of sources throughout the volume	Line sources arranged in parallel planes	Line sources arranged in parallel planes or cylindric volumes
Line source spacing	Constant approximately 1 cm apart from each other or from crossing ends	Same as Paterson-Parker	Constant, but selected according to implant dimensions—larger spacing used in large volumes; 8 mm minimum to 15 mm maximum separation	Constant, 1 to 1.5 cm, depending on size of implant (larger spacing for larger size implants)
Crossing needles	Crossing needles required to enhance dose at implant ends	Same as Paterson-Parker	Crossing needles not used. Active length 30 to 40% longer than target length	Crossing needles not required. Active length of sources 30 to 40% longer than target length

centrally in an implant than in the case of a Paterson-Parker type distribution. Whether a centrally "hotter" implant is clinically acceptable or even desirable is a question that cannot be answered easily. Certain radiobiologic reasons favor having a higher dose in the central volume of the implant because the tumor in this area is believed to be thicker and more anoxic than that in the periphery. These ideas have been discussed by Pierquin et al (2) and Fletcher (3).

Paterson-Parker System

For planar implants, the dose is specified in a parallel plane at 0.5 cm from the plane of implant and within the area bounded by the projection of the peripheral sources on that plane. The prescribed or "stated" dose is 10% higher than the minimum dose in the specified plane. The maximum dose should not exceed 10% above the stated dose. For a volume implant, the prescribed dose is 10% higher than the minimum dose within the implanted volume.

The dose specification scheme just outlined applies only to the Paterson-Parker (P-P) rules of source distribution in which the amount of radium (or radium equivalent) is distributed between the peripheral and the central regions of the implant in a ratio that depends on the area (planar implants) or volume and shape (volume implants) (see Table 11.2). The philosophy of the P-P system is to achieve ± 10% dose uniformity in the specified plane for planar implants and to achieve as uniform a dose as possible for volume implants.

The ideals of P-P dose uniformity are achieved by following a relatively complex set of rules of source distribution. The system technically works well for small implants with Ra or Cs needles; considerable clinical experience has been obtained in hospitals all over the world. The P-P system, however, is not practical for ^{192}Ir sources because the linear activity (source strength/cm) cannot be varied as precisely or conveniently as with the traditional Ra or Cs inventory. Moreover, as mentioned previously, ^{192}Ir sources are flexible and can assume irregular shapes. Although the P-P system of dose specification can be applied to an ^{192}Ir implant, it should not be considered equivalent to the true P-P system unless its rules of source distribution have been followed.

Quimby System

The Quimby system is characterized by a uniform distribution of sources with intersource spacing of about 1 cm.

Such a distribution produces greater nonuniformity of dose distribution than is possible with the Manchester system. The dose in the central regions of the implant is higher than that in the periphery.

The Quimby system differs significantly from the P-P system with regard to dose specification. In the Quimby system, the stated dose is the maximum dose in the specified plane (e.g., parallel plane at 0.5 cm from the plane of implant). For volume implants, the stated dose is the minimum dose within the implanted volume. Thus, even if an implant satisfies both the P-P and the Quimby rules of source distribution, the stated dose will be different in the two systems because the dose specification systems are different.

Because ^{192}Ir implants use equal intensity sources with uniform spacing, a logical conclusion is that the Quimby rules are followed. Quimby tables should not be applied to these implants, however, without the realization that ^{192}Ir implants may not have the same geometric shape as assumed by Quimby, and that the Quimby system comes with its own dose specification system.

Memorial System

Laughlin et al introduced the Memorial System in 1963 (4). The system is an extension of the Quimby system and is characterized by implantation of point sources (e.g., ^{192}Ir seeds) of uniform strength spaced 1 cm apart. A volume implant is achieved with a cubic array of seeds. Tables have been constructed that give milligram-hours to deliver 1000 cGy at designated points, e.g., "minimum peripheral" and "reference maximum" dose points in the plane 0.5 cm from the source plane for the planar implants. For volume implants, "central line peripheral dose" points also are chosen for dose specification.

For permanent implants, a "dimension averaging" technique is used (5). The important feature of this method is the principle that dosages should be adjusted in accordance with the volume of the implant because the radiation tolerance of tissues depends on the size of the implant. The total activity for an implant is directly proportional to the average of the three dimensions of the implant. Mathematically, $A = K \cdot \bar{d}$, in which A is the total activity or strength and $\bar{d}$ is the average dimension ($\bar{d} = (a + b + c)/3$; a, b, and c are the three mutually perpendicular dimensions).

The proportionality constant K is based on clinical experience and is recommended to be equal to 5 for ^{125}I implants.

Paris System

The Paris System was developed for removable implants of long lines of sources, such as ^{192}Ir wires or ribbons containing seeds. The system recommends uniform spacing, determined by the size of the implant. Wider spacing is used for larger volumes or longer sources. As summarized in Table 11.2, the system uses uniform linear activity sources implanted in parallel lines. The details of the system were described previously by Pierquin et al (2).

The dose is specified by an isodose surface, called the *reference isodose*. The reference isodose surrounds the target volume within a few millimeters (6). In practice, the value of the reference isodose is fixed at 85% of the "basal

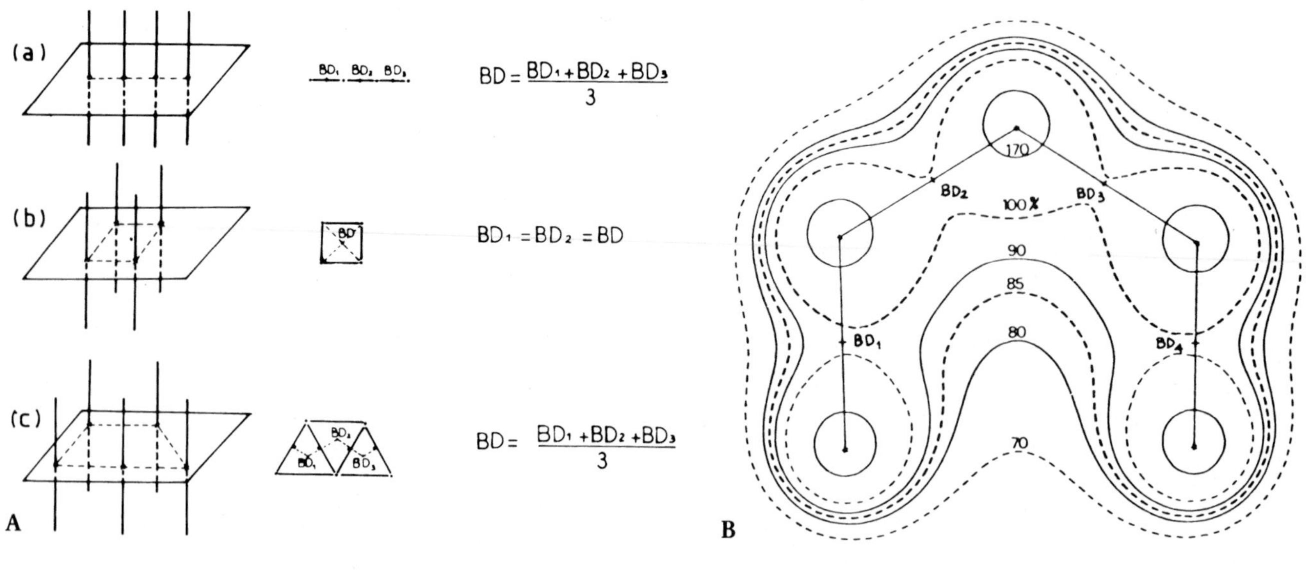

Figure 11.2. A. Calculation of average basal dose (BD) in implants using Paris system. Line sources implanted in patterns of (a) single plane; (b) squares; (c) triangles. **B.** Isodose curves in central plane (midplane perpendicular to line source) for a Paris-type implant. Isodose values are normalized relative to the average basal dose rate given by 1/4 (BD_1 + BD_2 + BD_3 + BD4). (Reprinted with permission from Pierquin B, Wilson JF, Chassagne D. Modern Brachytherapy. New York: Masson, 1987.)

dose," which is defined as the average of the minimum doses between sources. Figure 11.2A and 11.2B illustrate how the basal dose is calculated and the target dose is specified in different patterns of source implantation.

Computer System

A system that bears no formal name has been used in many institutions in the United States. We will call it the computer system. In this system, line sources of uniform linear activity are implanted, spaced uniformly (e.g., 1.0 to 1.5 cm) and cover the entire target volume. The dose prescription is based on the specification of an isodose surface that represents a minimum dose to the target volume. In practice, with the implant adequately covering the target volume, the isodose surface that just surrounds the implant (in the central plane perpendicular to the sources) is selected as the reference isodose for dose specification.

As discussed previously, the implantation of uniform activity sources gives rise to an implant that is "hotter" in the middle than in the periphery, as is the case with the Quimby and the Paris systems. The dose specification in these systems, however, is different (6–8). Overall, the computer system is more like the Paris system, with the exception that the reference isodose surface is not equated to the 85% value of the basal dose but rather to the actual isodose surface that just encloses the implanted volume.

As stated by Dutreix, the practice of specifying implant doses by subjectively selecting an isodose curve to represent a minimum target dose leads to uncertainty because of the high dose gradients that always exist around implants (6). The way to minimize this problem is to design the target volume before implanting with suitable margins around the tumor. The peripheral sources should be implanted on the outer surface of the target volume and the active length of the line sources should be suitably longer than the length of the target volume to compensate for uncrossed ends. The reference isodose curve is selected so that it just encloses the implant in the central-cross-sectional plane (see Figure 11.3A. Selecting a lower value isodose curve outside the implant for the purpose of providing greater (more generous) coverage of the target is avoided, because this could result in a substantially higher dose to the entire implant. To provide a bigger safety margin to the target volume, it is better to implant a larger volume than to select a lower value isodose curve.

Figure 11.3B shows the isodose distribution in the middle plane parallel to the implant planes. The dose distribution is viewed in this plane to ascertain that the selected isodose curve encompasses at least the target area. Coverage of the target in this plane usually indicates if the line sources used are long enough. Pre-implant planning may be helpful when deciding on appropriate length and spacing of the line sources.

For a single plane implant, the thickness of the treatment slab should first be decided. The reference isodose curve is selected in the central-cross-sectional plane such that it includes a slab thickness of 1 cm (0.5 cm on either side of the implant plane). If the target slab is thicker than 1 cm, more than one plane should be implanted (volume implant), with the peripheral sources placed on the outer surface of the target volume, as discussed previously.

INTRACAVITARY BRACHYTHERAPY

Numerous books and papers have been published on the use of radioactive sources for intracavitary implants.

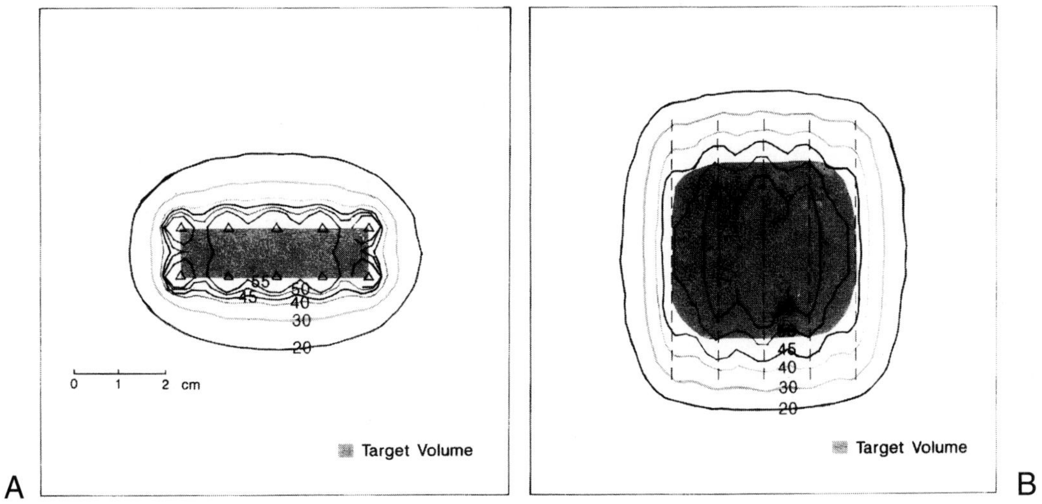

Figure 11.3. Computer-generated isodose curves for a volume implant using two parallel planes containing five ^{192}Ir wires per plane. Shaded area, target plus safety margin. **A.** Central plane perpendicular to line sources; **B.** Longitudinal plane through middle of implant. Reference isodose curve specified for this implant is 45 rad/hour, which just encloses implant in the central plane.

The subsequent discussion is confined to intracavitary therapy used for cancer of the uterine cervix.

The techniques of implantation vary only slightly, depending on the applicator used to hold the sources in a fixed configuration. Basically, the cervix applicator consists of a central tube, called the *tandem,* and lateral capsules, called the *ovoids* or *colpostats*. The tandem sources lie in the uterine cavity along its long axis and the ovoid sources are located on either side of the cervix.

Dose Specification

Pierquin et al. have reviewed various systems of intracavitary techniques and dose specification (2). The availability of computerized dosimetry has eliminated the need for prescribing dosages in terms of milligram-hours or milligram-hour equivalent. The latter is an elementary method of dose specification that is not only inadequate, but also is scientifically inaccurate in that it ignores differences between different source arrangements, applicator position, patient anatomy, etc. Several papers have been written to justify this system, but it is easy to demonstrate by actual dosimetry that a dose specification system based on milligram-hours alone is fraught with large uncertainties in the actual dose delivered.

From the never-ending debate regarding dose specification, two major contending systems have emerged: the Manchester System and the International Commission on Radiological Units and Measurements (ICRU) system.

The Manchester System

In this system, the application is characterized by doses to four points: point A, point B, a bladder point, and a rectum point. The duration of the implant is based on the dose rate calculated at point A.

Although points A and B have been defined in many different ways, according to the Manchester system, point A is located 2 cm superior to the external cervical os (or cervical end of tandem) and 2 cm lateral to the cervical canal, and point B is 3 cm lateral to point A (Figure 11.4) (9).

Historically, points A and B were defined to represent anatomic structures: point A was the point at which the uterine vessels cross the ureter (a critical structure) and point B signified the location of lateral structures in the pelvis, such as the obturator nodes. The anatomic significance of point A, however, has been questioned by several investigators (2,3,10). The critics pointed out the following limitations of point A: (1) it relates only to the position of the sources and not to the individual anatomy; (2) prescribing dose to point A does not take into account the size of the cervical cancer; and (3) dose to point A greatly depends on the position of the ovoid sources relative to the tandem sources (11). Thus, the implant times are dictated by the position of these sources relative to each other and not by the target dose rate.

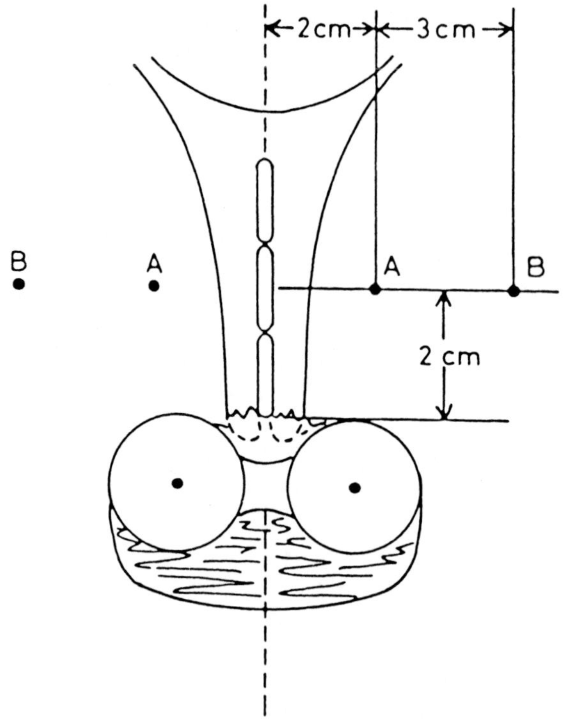

Figure 11.4. Definition of points A and B according to the Manchester system. (Reprinted with permission from Meredith WJ. Radium dosage: the Manchester system. Edinburgh: Livingstone, 1967.)

Although many investigators have considerable experience with using point A as the dosimetric reference, this system of dose specification has serious limitations and, in the final analysis, is not much better than the old system of milligram-hours.

ICRU System

In 1984, the ICRU recommended a system of dose specification that relates the dose distribution to the target volume, instead of the dose rate at a specific point (12). The duration of the implant is determined on the basis of isodose rate surface that surrounds the target volume.

The target volume is defined anatomically. It contains those tissues that are to be treated to a specified dose according to a specified time-dose pattern. In localizing the target volume, the demonstrated tumor, if present, and any presumed or microscopic disease are included. Figure 11.5 illustrates this concept when only intracavitary treatment is given and when intracavitary and external beam therapy are combined.

Table 11.3 is a summary of the ICRU system with regard to the various parameters needed to specify an intracavitary treatment in gynecology. These same parameters are discussed individually in subsequent sections.

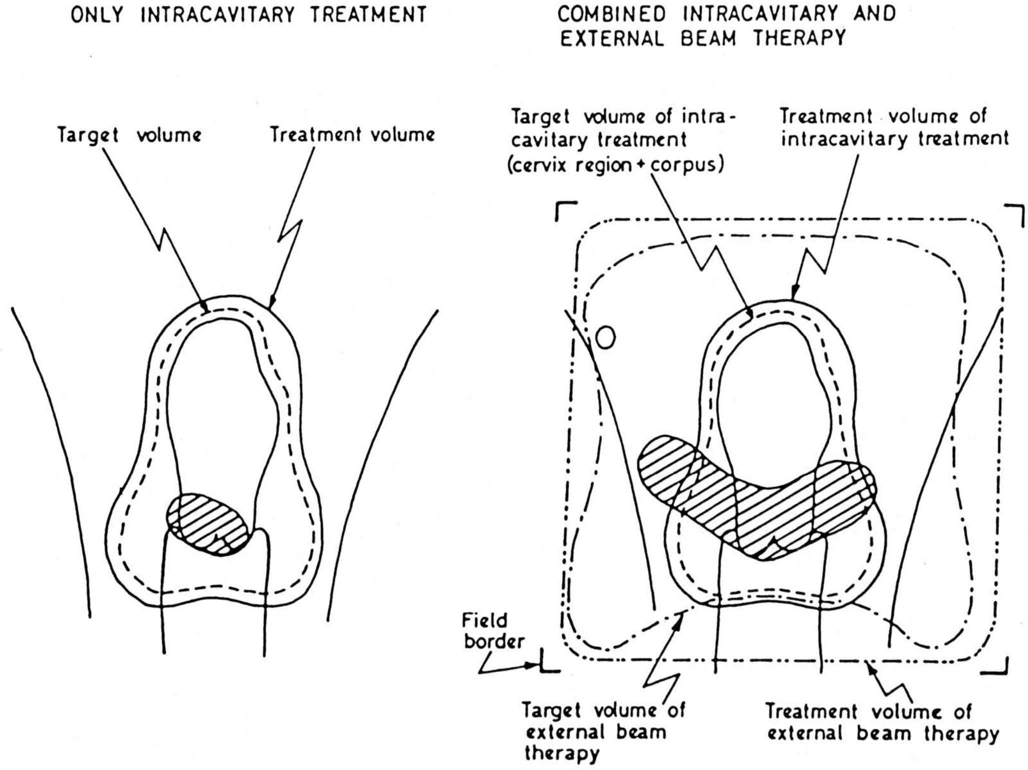

Figure 11.5. ICRU definition of treatment volume and other parameters for dose specification. (Reprinted with permission from ICRU Report 38. Dose and volume specification for reporting intracavitary therapy in gynecology. Radiological Units and Measurements, 1985.)

Table 11.3. Data Needed for Reporting Intracavitary Therapy in Gynecology (ICRU)

Description of the technique
Total reference air kerma
Description of the reference volume
Dose level if not 60 Gy
Dimensions of reference volume (height, width, thickness)
Absorbed dose at reference points
Bladder reference point
Rectal reference point
Lymphatic trapezoid
Pelvic wall reference point
Time-dose pattern

Description of the Technique The technique is described in terms of the radionuclide, source strength, shape and filtration, the applicator type, and the source arrangement. Orthogonal simulation radiographs are essential not only as a record but also for computer assisted dosimetry.

Total Source Strength Traditionally, this parameter has been recorded as total milligram-hours or total milligram radium equivalent-hours. The current ICRU recommendation is to express the total strength of sources in terms of total reference air kerma. This terminology is in keeping with the new specification of source strength that is in terms of air kerma strength, defined as the kerma rate to air in air, at a distance of 1 meter corrected for air attenuation and scattering. For example, a source containing 10 mg of radium, 1 mm platinum (Pt.) filtration, produces an air kerma rate of 67μ Gy $\cdot$ 1 hour^{-1} at 1 meter.

Reference Volume As mentioned previously, the ICRU system is characterized by the reference isodose surface that surrounds the target volume. Thus, an intracavitary application is specified in terms of the reference volume enclosed by the reference isodose surface. For example, the 60 Gy isodose surface is used in the Paris system to define the reference volume. This specification is similar to Fletcher's recommendation of specifying an isodose level of 31.5 Gy for each of the two intracavitary applications.

In Figure 11.6, a pear-shaped 60 Gy isodose surface defines the reference volume. The dimensions of this volume are recorded in terms of the height (d_h), width (d_w), and thickness (d_y) as determined from the oblique frontal and oblique sagittal planes. The reference volume is then approximated by ($d_h \times d_w \times d_t$) cm^3.

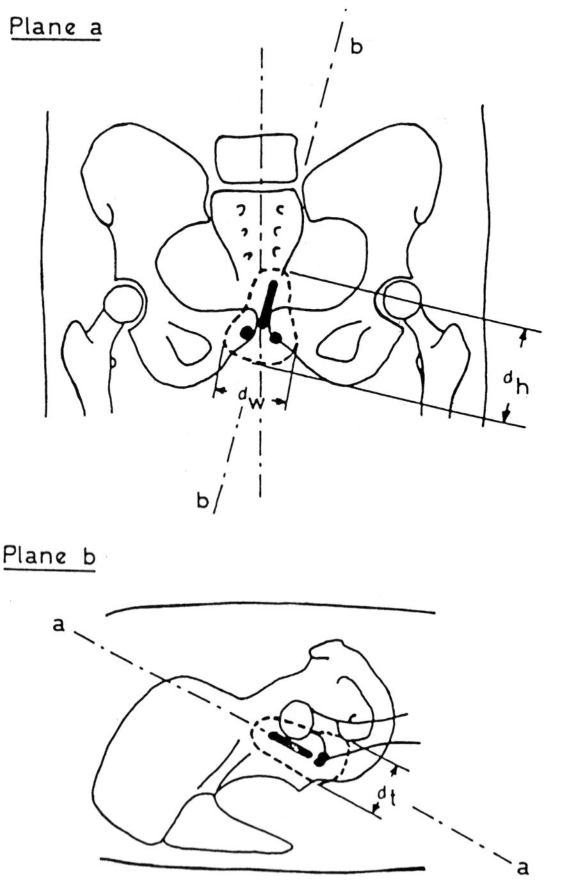

Figure 11.6. Dimensions (width d_w, height d_h, and thickness d_t) of the reference isodose surface in a typical treatment of carcinoma of cervix. (Reprinted with permission from ICRU Report 38. Dose and volume specification for reporting intracavitary therapy in gynecology. Bethesda: International Commission on Radiological Units and Measurements, 1985.)

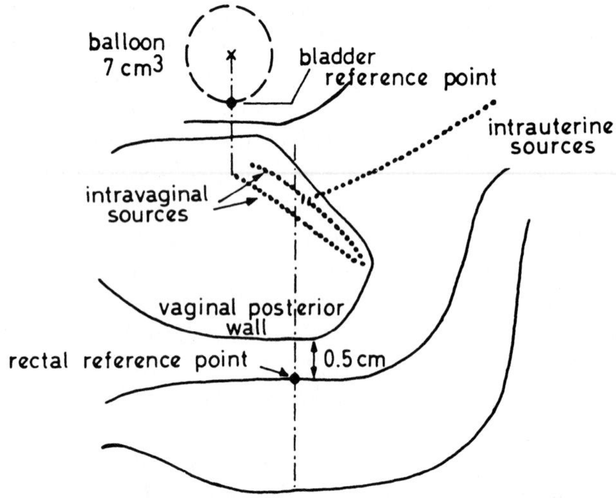

Figure 11.7. Localization of bladder and rectum points. (Reprinted with permission from ICRU Report 38. Dose and volume specification for reporting intracavitary therapy in gynecology. Bethesda, International Commission on Radiological Units and Measurements, 1985.)

Dose at Reference Points

Bladder Point This point is located by using a Foley catheter, with the balloon filled with contrast material. On the frontal radiograph, the reference point is taken at the center of the balloon; on the lateral radiograph, the reference point is obtained on an anteroposterior line drawn through the center of the balloon, at the posterior surface (Figure 11.7).

Rectal Point The rectal reference point is located on the anteroposterior radiograph at the midpoint of the ovoid sources (or at the lower end of the intrauterine source). On the lateral radiograph, the rectal reference point is located on an anteroposterior line drawn from the middle of the ovoid sources, 5 mm behind the posterior vaginal wall. The posterior vaginal wall may be visualized by using radio-opaque gauze for the vaginal packing.

Lymphatic Trapezoid of Fletcher These reference points are illustrated in Figure 11.8. The upper points, the middle points, and the lower points are used to calculate dose to the low para-aortic area, the common iliac nodes, and the mid-external iliac nodes, respectively.

Pelvic Wall Points The pelvic wall reference points (Figure 11.9) are determined as follows. On the anteroposterior radiograph, the points are located at the intersection

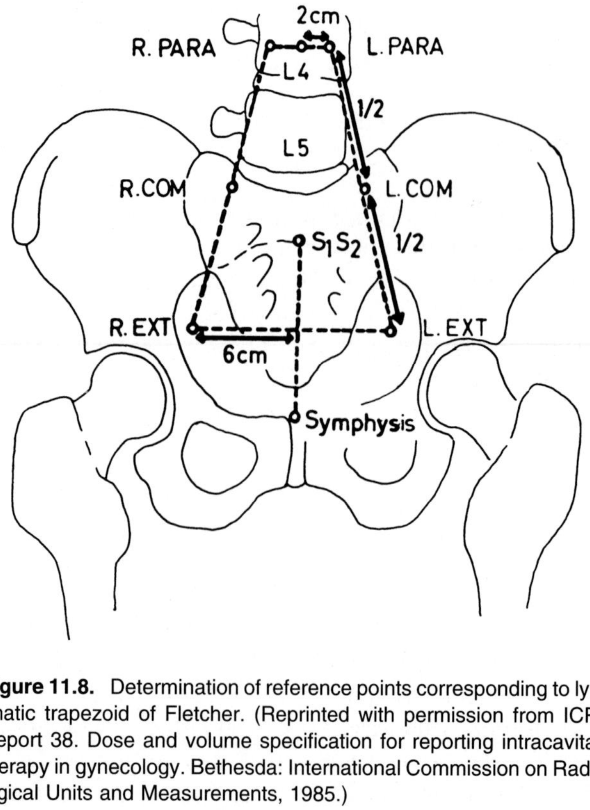

Figure 11.8. Determination of reference points corresponding to lymphatic trapezoid of Fletcher. (Reprinted with permission from ICRU Report 38. Dose and volume specification for reporting intracavitary therapy in gynecology. Bethesda: International Commission on Radiological Units and Measurements, 1985.)

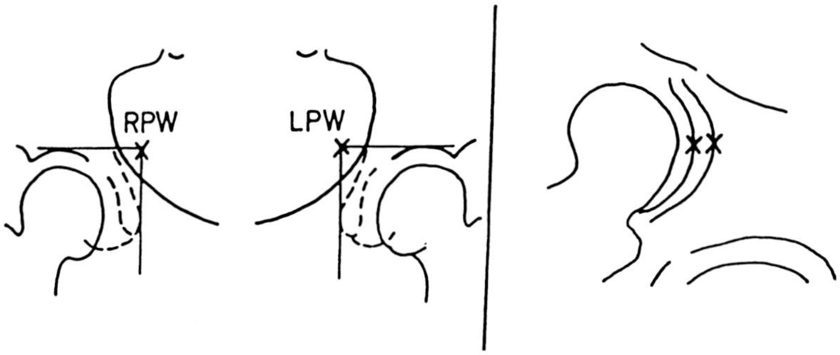

Figure 11.9. Definition of pelvic wall points. **A.** Anteroposterior view; **B.** Lateral view. (Reprinted with permission from ICRU Report 38. Dose and volume specification for reporting intracavitary therapy in gynecology. Bethesda: International Commission on Radiological Units and Measurements, 1985.)

of a horizontal line tangential to the superior aspects of the acetabulum and a vertical line to the medial aspect of the acetabulum. On the lateral view, the highest points of the right and left acetabulum are joined and the mid-distance points are marked to designate pelvic wall reference points. These points are selected to estimate dose to the distal parts of the parametrium and the obturator lymph nodes.

Time-Dose Pattern The duration of the implant should be reported so that the time-dose pattern is kept within the range of clinical experience. If more than one implant is applied, the duration of each as well as the time interval between applications should be reported.

Dose Rate and Implant Duration

The ICRU system of dose specification does not address the question of implant duration. It simply gives recommendations for reporting total absorbed doses and treatment volumes. The duration of an intracavitary implant, on the other hand, requires the knowledge of dose rate at a reference point or surface of a reference volume. To enclose the reference volume in the 60 Gy isodose surface requires selecting an appropriate combination of isodose rate surface and the implant duration.

The determination of reference volume and implant duration is linked to clinical experience or to a particular implant system. For example, Fletcher provided a complete set of guidelines for external beam irradiation and intracavitary therapy (3). The recommended techniques include loading of tandem and ovoids, implant duration, and reference isodose surfaces according to the size and extent of the cervical lesion. In his method, the dose rate is approximately 44 cGy/hour (31.5 Gy in 72 hours for each of two applications). According to the analysis by Pierquin et al., the Paris system uses a dose rate of approximately 40 cGy/hour (10 Gy/day for 6 days for a total dose of 60 Gy), the Stockholm method gives a dose rate of 100 to 120 cGy/hour in two applications of 24 to 36-hours duration, and the Manchester system employs a dose rate of 60 to 70 cGy/hour at point A in two 48-hour applications (13).

Table 11.4. Grading of Complications

Grade 3
Fatal
Fistulae
Requiring surgery
Grade 2
Continuous symptoms >6 months
Treatment >6 months
Hospitalization for treatment
Requiring transfusion
Radiologic stenosis (GI or GU)
Significant debility
Grade 1
Minor symptoms <6 months
Extremely intermittent minor symptoms
Responding rapidly to medical management

Reprinted with permission from Crook JM et al. Dose-volume analysis and the prevention of radiation sequelae in cervical cancer. Radiother Oncol 1987;8:321.

Crook et al analyzed the experience of the Centre Georges-Francois Lecterc with treatments given in accordance with the Fletcher guidelines (8). The data were analyzed using the ICRU system of dose specification (12) and correlated with radiation sequelae in cervical cancer. The authors present an interesting approach in which dosimetric parameters are determined by estimating risk of complications based on these data, allowing individual tailoring of treatment plans.

In Table 11.4, treatment complications are graded as mild (grade 1), moderate (grade 2), and severe (grade 3). Figure 11.10 illustrates scattergrams of rectal complications versus the reference volume (h × w × t) and mean rectal dose for intracavitary alone and intracavitary plus external beam treatment. Similar data for bladder complications are presented in Figure 11.11. These data may be used directly in conjunction with the treatment guidelines of Fletcher (3). The duration and loading of applicators can thus be individualized by analyzing the reference volume and its relationship with treatment complications. Such an approach is intended to fine-tune the dose specification system for individual patients.

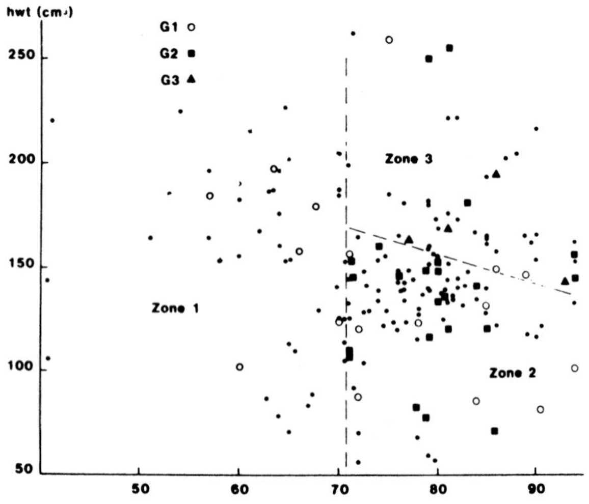

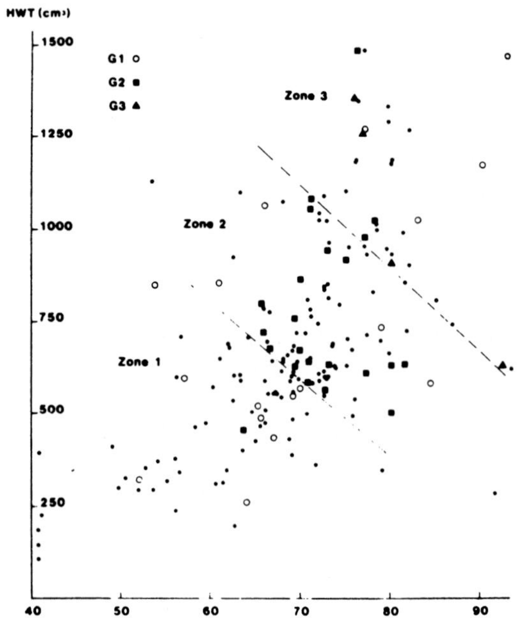

Figure 11.10. **A.** Scattergram of rectal complications in a plot of reference volume (h × w × t) of 60 Gy isodose surface as a function of rectal dose (CDR ref.) for intracavitary treatment alone. **B.** Scattergram of rectal complication in a plot (HWT) as a function of rectal dose (CDR ref.) for intracavitary plus external beam treatment. (Reprinted with permission from Crook JM et al. Dose-volume analysis and the prevention of radiation sequelae in cervical cancer. Radiother Oncol 1987;8: 321.

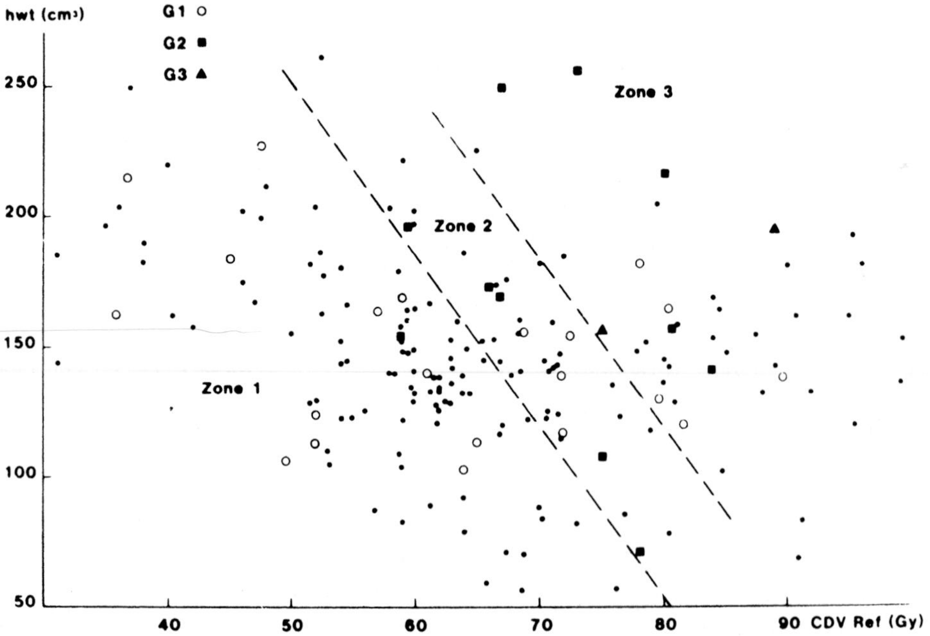

Figure 11.11. Scattergram of bladder complications in a plot of h × w × t as a function of reference vesical dose (CDV ref.) for intracavitary treatment alone. (Reprinted with permission from Crook JM et al. Dose-volume analysis and the prevention of radiation sequelae in cervical cancer. Radiother Oncol 1987;8:321.

References

1. Shalek RJ, Stovall M. Dosimetry in implant therapy. In: Attix FH, Tochilin E, eds. Radiation Dosimetry. Vol. III. New York: Academic Press, 1969.
2. Pierquin B, Wilson JF, Chassagne D. Modern brachytherapy. NY: Masson Publishing, 1987.
3. Fletcher GH. Squamous cell carcinoma of the uterine cervix. In: Fletcher GH, ed. Textbook of radiotherapy. 3rd ed. Philadelphia: Lea & Febiger, 1980.
4. Laughlin JS, Siler WM, Holodny EI, Ritter FW. A dose description system for interstitial radiation therapy. AJR 1963;89:470.
5. Anderson LL. Dosimetry in implant therapy. In: Hilaris BS, ed. Handbook of interstitial brachytherapy. Acton, MA: Publishing Sciences Group, 1975.
6. Dutreix A. Can we compare systems for interstitial therapy. Radiother Oncol 1988;13:127.
7. Gillin MT, Kline RW, Wilson F, Cox JD. Single and double plane implants: a comparison of the Manchester system with the Paris system. Int J Radiat Oncol Biol Phys 1984;10:921.
8. Olch AJ, et al. Multi-institutional survey of techniques in volume iridium implants. Endocuriether Hypertherm Oncol 1986;2:193.
9. Meredith WJ. Radium dosage: the Manchester system. Edinburgh: Livingstone, 1967.
10. Schwarz G. An evaluation of the Manchester system of treatment of carcinoma of the cervix. AJR 1969;105:579.
11. Potish TA, Deibel FC, Khan FM. The relationship between milligram-hours and dose to point A in carcinoma of the cervix. Radiology 1982;145:479.
12. ICRU Report 38. Dose and volume specification for reporting intracavitary therapy in gynecology. Bethesda: International Commission on Radiological Units and Measurements, 1985.
13. Crook JM, Esche BA, Chaplain G, et al. Dose-volume analysis and the prevention of radiation sequelae in cervical cancer. Radiother Oncol 1987;8:321.

Chapter 12

Radiobiology of Low and High Dose Rate Brachytherapy

Eric J. Hall

ABSORPTION OF RADIATION

When x- or γ-rays are absorbed in biological material, the first step is that part or all of the photon energy is converted into the kinetic energy of fast moving electrons.

A fast moving electron may interact directly with deoxyribonucleic acid (DNA) causing an excitation or ionization; this is called the direct action of radiation. It is the dominant process for high Linear Energy Transfer (LET) radiations such as α-particles illustrated in Figure 12.1. Alternatively, the electron may interact with other atoms or molecules in the cell, particularly water, to produce free radicals that can diffuse far enough to reach and damage DNA. This is referred to as the indirect action of radiation. A free radical is a free (not combined) atom or molecule which carries no electrical charge, but has an unpaired electron in the outer shell. This state is associated with a high degree of chemical reactivity. The most important radical produced from the interaction of radiation with water is the hydroxyl radical, OH·. There is evidence to support the notion that any OH· radicals produced within a cylinder of diameter about 4 nm around the DNA double helix is able to diffuse to the DNA and cause damage (see Figure 12.1). About two-thirds of the biological damage caused by x-rays is mediated via free radicals. This has been described in more detail by Hall (1).

DNA DAMAGE AND STRAND BREAKS

DNA consists of two strands that form a double helix. Each strand is composed of a series of deoxynucleotides, the sequence of which contains the genetic code. Sugar moieties and phosphate groups form the backbone of the double helix. The bases on opposite strands must be complementary; adenine pairs with thymine, while guanine pairs with cytosine. When cells are irradiated with x-rays, many breaks of a single strand occur. These can be observed and scored as a function of dose if the DNA is denatured and the supporting structure stripped away. In intact DNA, however, single-strand breaks are of little biological consequence as far as a cell killing is concerned because they are readily repaired using the opposite strand as a template (Figure 12.2). If the repair is incorrect (misrepair), it may result in a mutation. If both strands of the DNA are broken, and the breaks are well separated (see Figure 12.2), repair again occurs readily since the two breaks are handled separately.

By contrast, if the breaks in the two strands are opposite one another, or separated by only a few base pairs (see Figure 12.2), this may lead to a double-strand break (DSB); that is, the piece of chromatin snaps into two pieces. This picture of DNA damage has been described eloquently by Ward (2,3). A DSB is believed to be the most biologically important lesion produced in chromosomes by radiation; the interaction of two DSBs may result in cell killing, mutation, or carcinogenesis.

In practice, the situation is probably much more complicated than this, since both free radicals and direct ionizations may be involved. In particular, other base damage may be involved with the DSB to form a multiply damaged site (3).

CHROMOSOMAL ABERRATIONS

When cells are irradiated with x-rays, DSBs occur as described above. The broken ends appear to be "sticky" and can rejoin with any other sticky end. It would appear, however, that a broken end cannot join with a normal,

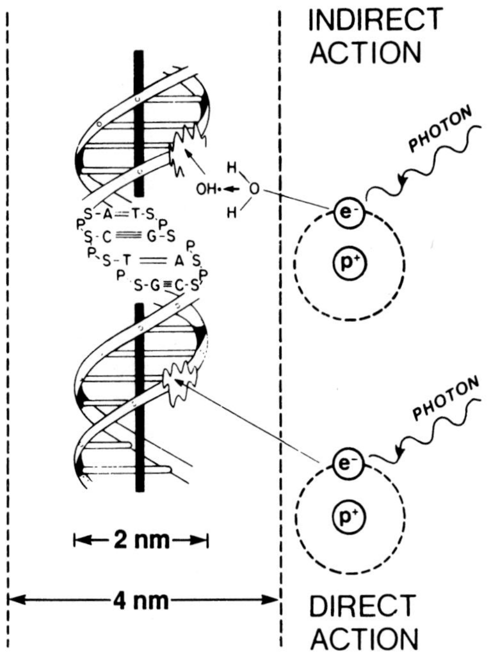

Figure 12.1. Direct and indirect actions of radiation. The structure of DNA is shown schematically; the letters S, P, A, T, G, and C represent sugar, phosphorus, adenine, thymine, guanine, and cytosine, respectively. In direct action a secondary electron resulting from absorption of an x-ray photon interacts with the DNA to produce an effect. In indirect action the secondary electron interacts with a water molecule to produce an OH•, which in turn diffused to the DNA to produce damage. The DNA helix has a diameter of about 2 nm. It is estimated that free radicals produced in a cylinder with a diameter double that of the DNA helix can affect the DNA. Indirect action is dominant for sparsely ionizing radiation, such as x-rays. (Redrawn from Hall EJ. Radiobiology for the Radiologist, 4th ed. JB Lippincott Company: Philadelphia, 1994.)

unbroken chromosome end (4). Once breaks are produced, different fragments may behave in a variety of ways:

1. The breaks may restitute, that is, rejoin in their original configuration. In this case, of course, nothing amiss will be visible at the next mitosis.
2. The breaks may fail to rejoin and give rise to an aberration, which will be scored as a deletion at the next mitosis.
3. Broken ends may reassort and rejoin other broken ends to give rise to chromosomes that appear to be grossly distorted when viewed at the following mitosis.

The aberrations seen at metaphase are of two classes: *chromosome* aberrations and *chromatid* aberrations. Chromosome aberrations result if a cell is irradiated early in interphase, before the chromosome material has been duplicated. In this case the radiation-induced break will be in a single strand of chromatin; during the DNA synthetic phase that follows, this strand of chromatin will lay down an identical strand next to itself and will replicate the break that had been produced by the radiation. If, on the other hand, the dose of radiation is given later in interphase, after the DNA material has doubled and the chromosomes consist of two strands of chromatin, then the aberrations produced are called chromatid aberrations.

Three types of aberrations are lethal to the cell, namely the dicentric and the ring which are chromosome aberrations, and an anaphase bridge, which is a chromatid aberration. For simplicity we will describe in detail the formation of a dicentric; similar considerations apply to rings and anaphase bridges.

The formation of a dicentric is illustrated in Figure 12.3. This aberration involves an interchange between two separate chromosomes. If a break is produced in each one early in interphase and the sticky ends are close to one another, they may rejoin in an illegitimate way as shown. This bizarre interchange will replicate during the DNA synthetic phase, and the result will be a grossly distorted chromo-

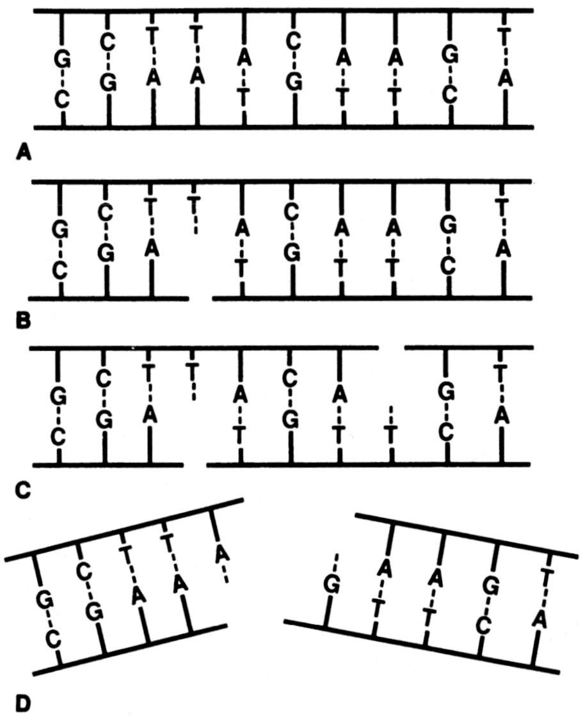

Figure 12.2. Diagrams of single- and double-strand DNA breaks caused by radiation. (**A**) Two-dimensional representation of the normal DNA double helix. The base pairs carrying the genetic code are complementary (i.e., adenine pairs with thymine, guanine pairs with cytosine). (**B**) A break in one strand is of little significance because it is readily repaired, using the opposite strand as a template. (**C**) Breaks in both strands, if well-separated, are repaired as independent breaks. (**D**) If breaks occur in both strands and are directly opposite or separated by only a few base pairs, this may lead to a DSB where the chromatin snaps into two pieces. (Drawn to illustrate concepts described by Ward JF. Radiat Res 1981;86:185–195; Ward JF. Progress in Nucleic Acids and Molecular Biology 1988;35:95–125.)

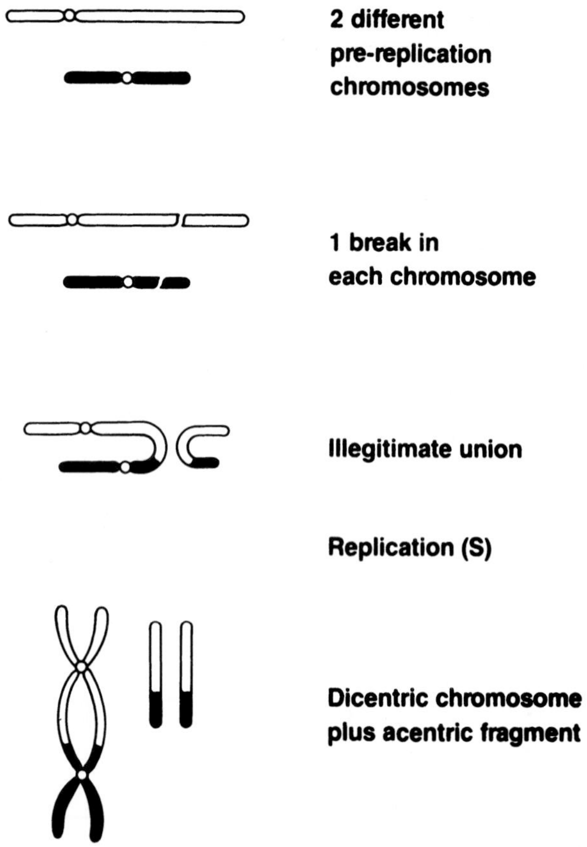

Figure 12.3. The steps in the formation of a dicentric by irradiation of prereplication (i.e., G_1) chromosomes. A break is produced in each of two separate chromosomes. The "sticky" ends may join incorrectly to form an interchange between the two chromosomes. Replication then occurs in the DNA synthetic period. One chromosome has two centromeres, a dicentric. The other is an acentric fragment, which will be lost at a subsequent mitosis, since, lacking a centromere, it will not go to either pole at anaphase. (Redrawn from Hall EJ. Radiobiology for the Radiologist, 4th ed. JB Lippincott Company: Philadelphia, 1994.)

some with two centromeres (hence, *dicentric*). There will also be a fragment that has no centromere (acentric fragment). The dose-response relationship for exchange type chromosomal aberrations, such as dicentrics, is a linear quadratic function of dose since they result from an interaction between breaks in two different chromosomes (5). The linear component is a consequence of the two breaks resulting from a single charged particle. If the two breaks result from different charged particles, the probability of an interaction will be a quadratic function of dose. The dose-response relationship for the formation of dicentrics is shown in Figure 12.4.

CELL SURVIVAL CURVES

A cell survival curve describes the relationship between the radiation dose and proportion of cells that survive. What is meant by "survival?" Survival is the opposite of death! For differentiated cells that do not proliferate, such as nerve, muscle, or secretory cells, death can be defined as the loss of a specific function. For proliferating cells, such as hematopoietic stem cells or cells grown in culture, loss of the capacity for sustained proliferation—that is, loss of reproductive integrity—is an appropriate definition. This is sometimes called *reproductive death* and a cell that survives by this definition is said to be clonogenic because it can form a clone or colony.

This definition is generally relevant to the radiobiology of whole animals and plants and their tissues. It has particular relevance to the radiotherapy of tumors. For a tumor to be eradicated, it is only necessary that cells be "killed" in the sense that they are rendered unable to divide and cause further growth and spread of the malignancy.

The classic mode of cell death following exposure to radiation is "mitotic death." Cells die in attempting to divide because of chromosomal damage, such as the formation of a ring or a dicentric that causes loss of genetic material and prevents the clean segregation of DNA into the two progeny. Death does not necessarily occur at the first mitosis following irradiation; cells can often manage to complete several divisions, but death is inevitable if chromosomal damage is severe.

The other form of cell death is programmed cell death or apoptosis first described by Kerr and colleagues (6).

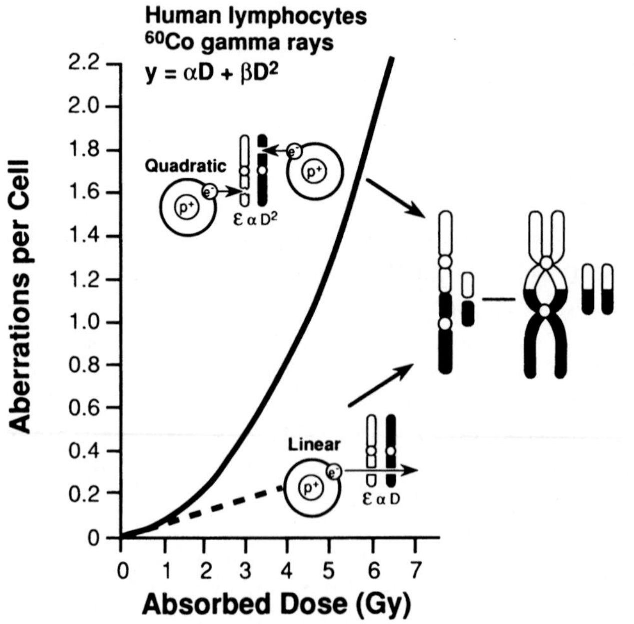

Figure 12.4. The frequency of interchange type chromosomal aberrations (dicentrics and rings) is a linear-quadratic function of dose because the aberrations are the consequence of the interaction of two separate breaks. At low doses, both breaks may be caused by the same electron; the probability of an exchange aberration is proportional to dose (D). At higher doses, the two breaks are more likely to be caused by separate electrons. The probability of an exchange aberration is then proportional to the square of the dose (D^2). (Redrawn from Hall EJ. Radiobiology for the Radiologist, 4th ed. JB Lippincott Company: Philadelphia, 1994.)

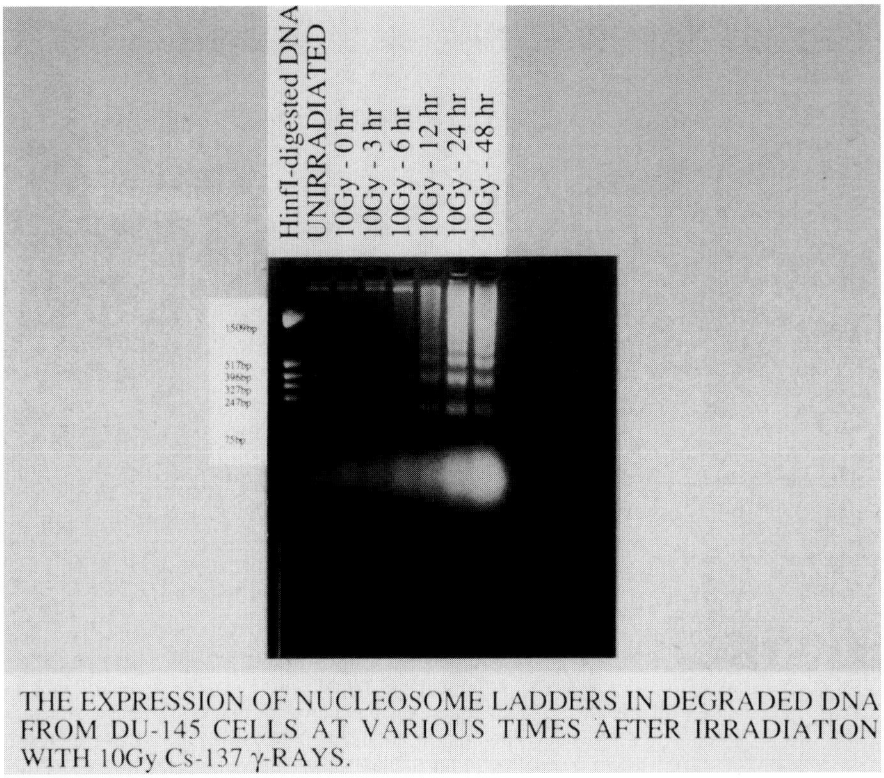

Figure 12.5. Illustrating the "laddering" of DNA as it breaks up into pieces of discreet sizes during the process of cell death by apoptosis. (Courtesy of Dr. Eileen Rakovitch).

This is an important form of cell death during the development of the embryo, and is implicated, for example, in the regression of the tadpole tail during metamorphosis. It is also important in many facets of biology including cell renewal systems and hormone related atrophy. Apoptosis is characterized by a sequence of morphological events; cells condense and the DNA breaks up into pieces of discreet size before the cells are phagocytosed and removed. The DNA "laddering" which is so characteristic of a cell undergoing apoptosis is shown in Figure 12.5. In radiation biology, apoptosis is a dominant mode of radiation-induced cell death in cells of lymphoid origin, but of variable importance in other cell types.

Most cell survival curves have been obtained by growing cells in vitro in petri dishes. Many cell lines have been established from malignant tumors and from normal tissues taken from humans or laboratory animals. If cells are seeded as single cells, allowed to attach to the surface of a petri dish, and provided with culture medium and appropriate conditions, each cell will grow into a macroscopic colony that is visible by eye in a period of a few weeks. If, in the other hand, the same number of cells are placed into a parallel dish and exposed to a dose of radiation just after they have attached to the surface of the dish, some cells will grow into colonies indistinguishable from those in the unirradiated dish—but others will form only tiny abortive colonies because the cells die after a few divisions. The surviving fraction is the number of macroscopic colonies counted in the irradiated dish divided by the number on the unirradiated dish. This process is repeated so that estimates of survival are obtained for a range of dishes; surviving fraction is plotted on a logarithmic scale against dose on a linear scale; the result is the solid line in Figure 12.6.

Qualitatively, the shape of the survival curve can be described in relatively simple terms. At low doses the survival curve starts out straight on the log-linear plot with a finite initial slope; that is, the surviving fraction is an exponential function of dose. At higher doses, the curve bends. This bending, or curving region, extends over a dose range of a few Gy. At very high doses the survival curve often tends to straighten again. In general, this does not occur until doses are in excess of 10 Gy.

The linear quadratic model is currently the model of choice for cell survival curves. This model assumes that there are two components to cell killing by radiation, one that is proportional to dose and one that is proportional to the square of the dose. The notion of a component of cell inactivation that varies with the square of the dose reflects the fact that cell death is due largely to complex chromosomal exchange-type aberrations that are the result of breaks in two separate chromosomes as previously described (see Figure 12.6).

By this model the expression for the cell survival curve is

$$s = e^{-} \alpha D - \beta D^2$$

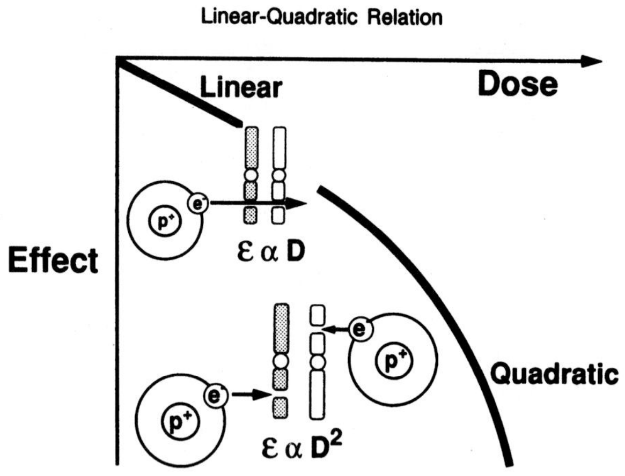

Figure 12.6. Relationship between chromosome aberrations and cell survival. Cells that suffer exchange-type chromosome aberrations (such as a dicentric) are unable to survive and continue to divide indefinitely. At low doses, the two chromosome breaks are the consequence of a single electron set in motion by the absorption of x- or γ-rays. The probability of an interaction between the breaks is proportional to dose; this is the linear portion of the survival curve. At higher doses, the two chromosome breaks may result also from two separate electrons. The probability of an interaction is then proportional to (dose)^2. The survival curve bends when the quadratic component dominates.

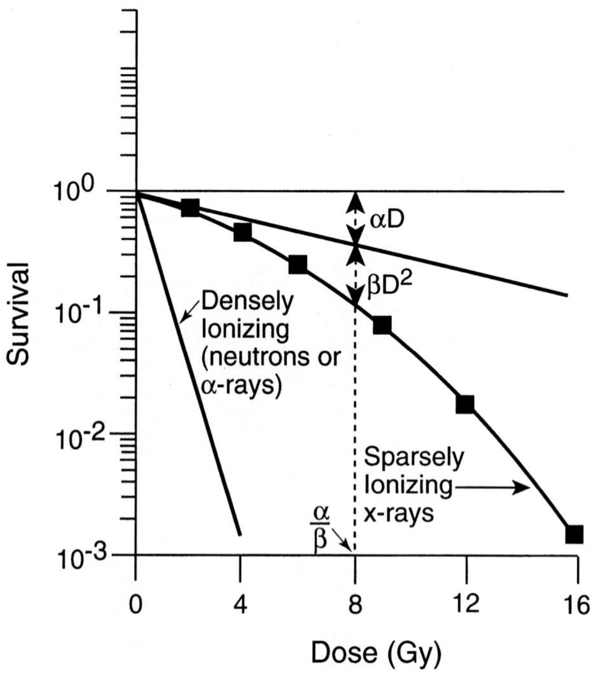

Figure 12.7. Shape of survival curve for mammalian cells exposed to radiation. The fraction of cells surviving is plotted on a logarithmic scale against dose on a linear scale. For α-particles or low-energy neutrons (said to be densely ionizing) the dose-response curve is a straight line from the origin (i.e., survival is an exponential function of dose). The survival curve can be described by just one parameter, the slope. For x- or γ-rays (said to be sparsely ionizing), the dose-response curve has an initial linear slope, followed by a region which curves. The experimental data are fitted to a linear-quadratic function. There are two components of cell killing: one is proportional to dose (αD), while the other is proportional to the square of the dose (βD^2). The dose at which the linear and quadratic components are equal is the ration α/β. The linear-quadratic curve bends continuously but is a good fit to experimental data for the first few decades of survival.

where S is the fraction of cells surviving a dose D, and α and β are constants. The components of cell killing that are proportional to dose and to the square of the dose are equal when:

$$\alpha D = BD^2$$

or

$$D = \alpha/\beta$$

This is an important point that bears repeating: the linear and quadratic contributions to cell killing are equal at a dose that is equal to the ratio of α/β (Figure 12.7). The ratio is a measure of the curviness of the survival curve. If α/β is small, the survival curve is very curvy; if α/β is large, the survival curve tends to be straighter and less curvy.

THE DOSE-RATE EFFECT

For x- or γ-rays, dose rate is one of the principal factors that determines the biological consequences of a given absorbed dose. As the dose rate is lowered and the exposure time extended, the biological effect of a given dose is generally reduced. Continuous low dose-rate irradiation may be considered to be an infinite number of infinitely small dose fractions; consequently the survival curve under these conditions would also be expected to have no shoulder and to be shallower than for single acute exposures at high dose rate, as illustrated by the dashed line in Figure 12.8. This is easy to understand in terms of the

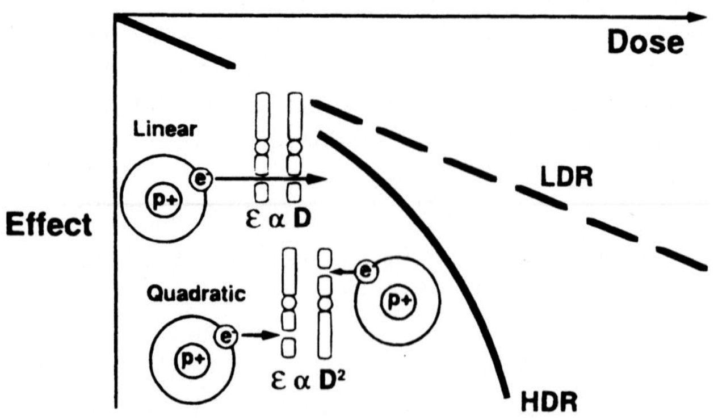

Figure 12.8. Cell killing by radiation is due largely to aberrations caused by breaks in two chromosomes. The dose response curve for high-dose rate irradiation (HDR) is linear-quadratic; the two breaks may be caused by the same electron (dominant at low doses) or by two different electrons (dominant at higher doses). For LDR irradiation, where radiation is delivered over a protracted period, the principal mechanism of cell killing is by the single electron. Consequently, the LDR survival curve is an extension of the low-dose region of the HDR survival curve.

repair of chromosome damage. The linear component of cell damage will be unaffected by dose-rate since the two chromosome breaks that interact to form a lethal lesion are caused by a single electron track. The quadratic component, however, is caused by two separate electron tracks; if there is a long time interval between the passage of the two electron tracks, then the damage caused by the first may be repaired before the second arrives. In this case an exchange type aberration would not be caused and the cell would survive. Under these circumstances the high dose component of the dose-response relationship is simply an extrapolation of the initial linear slope of the high dose-rate survival curve as illustrated in Figure 12.8. Sublethal damage repair, in this model, equates to repair of one double-strand chromosome break. This idea has its origins in a hypothesis of Gray, published in 1944, who wrote:

> It is postulated that in order to produce the biological effect under consideration, there must co-exist in a considerable proportion of the irradiated cells two separate injuries, each produced by a separate ionizing particle and each capable of restitution. In advancing this postulate we have of course type C chromosome aberrations particularly in mind.—Gray (7)

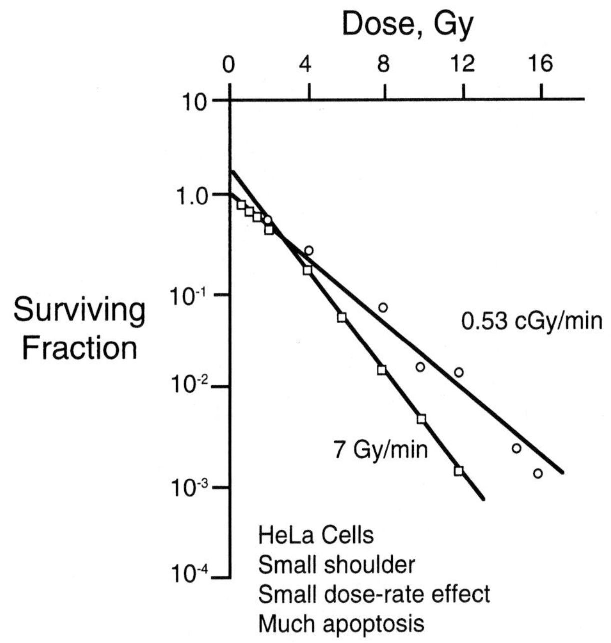

Figure 12.9. Survival curves for HeLa cells exposed to x-rays at high dose-rate and low dose-rate. (Redrawn from Hall EJ and Bedford JS. Dose-rate. Its effect on the survival of Hela cells irradiated with gamma-rays. Radiat Res 1964;22:305–315.)

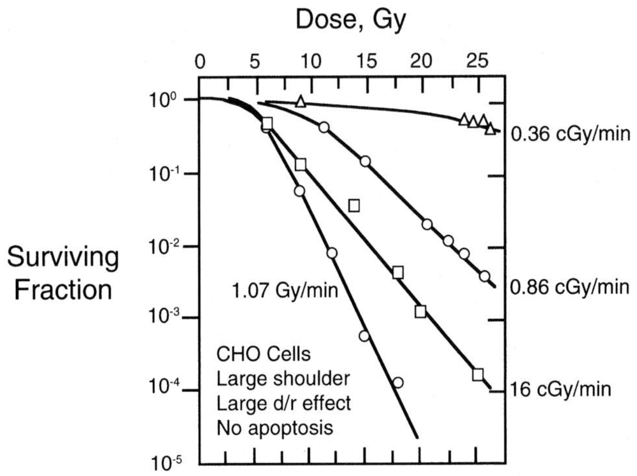

Figure 12.10. Survival curves for Chinese hamster (CHO) cells grown in vitro and exposed to x-rays at various dose-rates. (Redrawn from Bedford JS, Mitchell B. Dose-rate effects in synchronous mammalian cells in culture. Radiat Res 1973;54:316–327.)

The magnitude of the dose-rate effect from the repair of sublethal damage varies enormously between different types of cells. Cells characterized by a survival curve for acute exposures that have a small initial shoulder exhibit a modest dose-rate effect. This is to be expected, since both are expressions of the cell's capacity to accumulate and repair sublethal radiation damage. Cell lines characterized by a survival for acute exposures which have a broad initial shoulder exhibit a dramatic dose-rate effect. Survival curves for HeLa cells cultured in vitro over a wide range of dose rates, from 7.3 Gy minute to 0.535 cGy/minute are summarized in Figure 12.9, taken from the early work of Hall and Bedford (8). As the dose rate is reduced, the survival curve becomes shallower and the shoulder tends to disappear (i.e., the survival curve becomes an exponential function of dose). The dose-rate effect caused by repair of sublethal damage is most dramatic between 0.01 and 1 Gy/min. Above and below this dose-rate range, the survival curve changes little, if at all, with dose rate.

The magnitude of the dose-rate effect from the repair of sublethal damage varies enormously between different types of cells. HeLa cells are characterized by a survival curve for acute exposures that has a small initial shoulder, which goes hand in hand with a modest dose-rate effect. This is to be expected, since both are expressions of the cell's capacity to accumulate and repair sublethal radiation damage. By contrast, Chinese hamster cells have a broad shoulder to their acute x-ray survival curve and show a corresponding large dose-rate effect. As evidenced in Figure 12.10, (redrawn from the work of Bedford and Mitchell, [9]) there is a clear-cut difference in biological effect, at least at high doses, between dose rates of 1.07, 0.3 and 0.16 Gy min.

This difference in shoulder size and corresponding magnitude of the dose-rate effect correlates with the dominant mechanism of cell death. Chinese hamster ovary (CHO) cells (see Figure 12.5), like many cell lines selected to grow in culture, have an abrogated p53 status and do

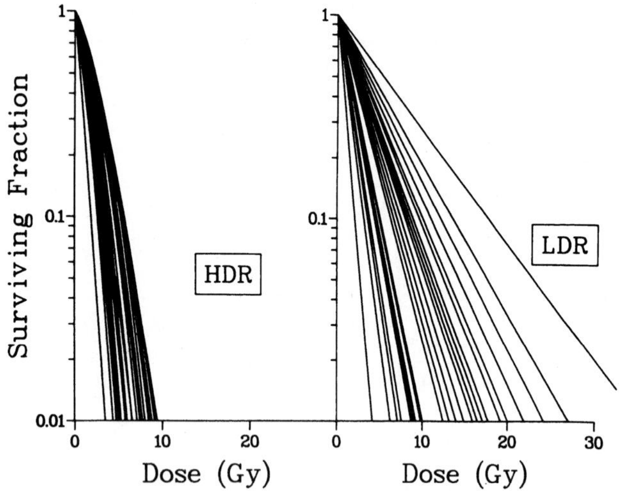

Figure 12.11. Dose survival curves at HDR and LDR for a large number of cells of human origin cultured in vitro. Note that the survival curves fan out at low dose rate because in addition to a range of inherent radiosensitivities (evident at HDR) there is also a range of repair times of sublethal damage. (Redrawn from Hall EA, Brenner DJ. The 1991 George Edelstyn Lecture. Needles, Wires and Chips—Advances in brachytherapy. Clin Oncol 1992;4:249–256.)

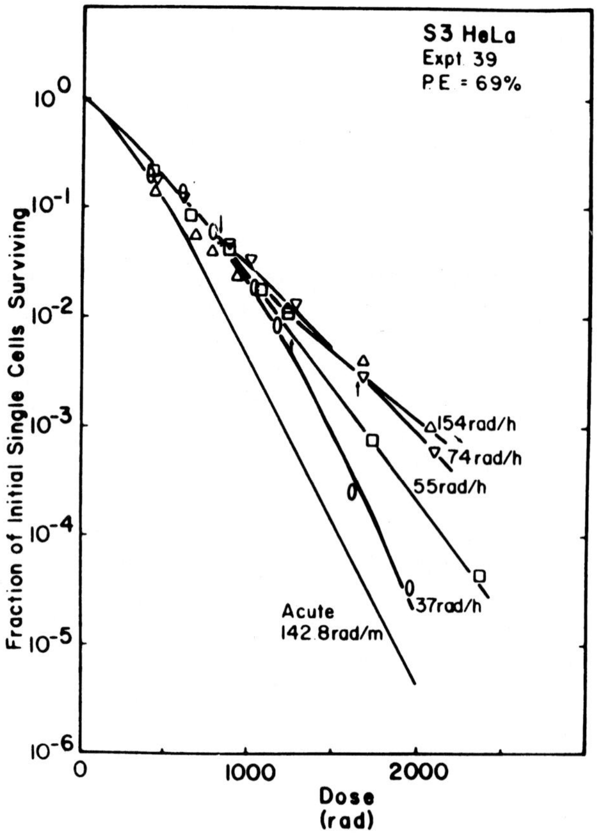

Figure 12.12. The inverse dose rate effect. A range of dose rates can be found for HeLa cells such that lowering the dose rate leads to *more* cell killing. At 1.54 Gy/h cells are "frozen" in the various phases of the cycle and do not progress. As the dose rate is dropped to 0.37 Gy/h, cells progress to a block in G_2, a radiosensitive phase of the cycle. (Redrawn from Mitchell B, Bedford JS, Bailey SM. Dose-rate effects in plateau-phase cultures of S3 Hela and V79 cells. Radiat Res 1979;79:520–536.)

not die an apoptotic death (Lowe et al [10]). On the other hand, apoptosis is an important (but not the only) form of radiation-induced lethality in HeLa cells. This accounts for the smaller shoulder to the survival curve and the less dramatic dose-rate effect.

Figure 12.11 shows survival curves for 40 different cell lines of human origin, cultured in vitro and irradiated at high dose rate (HDR) and low dose rate (LDR) (taken from Hall and Brenner [11]). At low dose rate, the survival curves fan out and show a greater variation in slope because in addition to the variation of inherent radiosensitivity evident at high dose rate, there is a range of repair times of sublethal damage. Some cell lines repair sublethal damage rapidly, some more slowly, and this is reflected in fanning out of the survival curves at low dose rate.

THE INVERSE DOSE-RATE EFFECT

In cells of human origin an inverse dose-rate effect is often seen over a narrow range of dose-rates, whereby decreasing the dose-rate actually increases the efficacy of cell killing. This was first reported by Mitchell, Bedford, and Bailey (12) for HeLa cells (see Figure 12.12. Decreasing the dose rate for this cell line from 1.53 to 0.37 Gy/h increases the efficiency of cell killing, so that this low dose rate is almost as effective as an acute exposure. The explanation of this phenomenon is illustrated in Figure 12.13, taken from Hall (13). At about 0.3 Gy/h, cells tend to progress through the cycle and become arrested in G2, a radiosensitive phase of the cycle. At higher dose rates they are frozen in the phase of the cycle they are in at the start

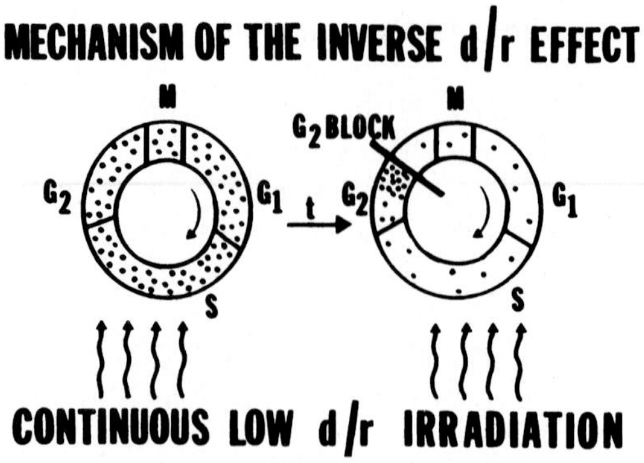

Figure 12.13. Explanation of the inverse dose-rate effect. A range of dose rates can be found, at least for many cells of human origin, that allows cells to progress through the mitotic cycle to a block in late G_2. Under continuous low dose rate irradiation, an asynchronous population becomes a population of radiosensitive G_2 cells. (Redrawn from Hall EJ. The biological basis of endocrine therapy. The Henschke Memorial Lecture 1984. Endocrine Hypertherm Oncology 1985;1: 141–151.)

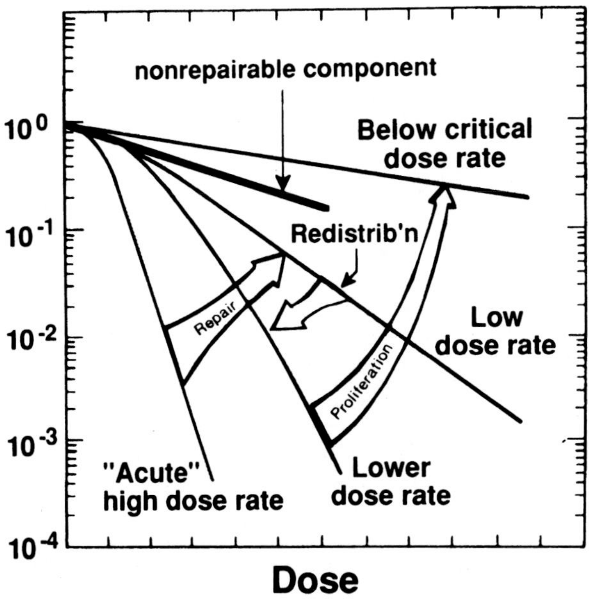

Figure 12.14. The dose rate effect due to repair of sublethal damage, redistribution in the cycle, and cell proliferation. The dose-response curve for acute exposures is characterized by a broad initial shoulder. As the dose rate is reduced, the survival curve becomes progressively shallower as more and more sublethal damage is repaired but cells are "frozen" in their positions in the cycle and do not progress. As the dose rate is lowered further and for a limited range of dose rates, the survival curve *steepens* again because cells can progress through the cycle to pile up at a block in G_2, a radiosensitive phase but still cannot divide. A further lowering of dose rate allows cells to escape the G_2 block and divide; cell proliferation may then occur during the protracted exposure, and survival curves become shallower as cell birth from mitosis offsets cell killing from the irradiation. (Based on the ideas of Dr. Joel Bedford).

of the irradiation; at lower dose rates they continue to cycle during irradiation.

The Dose-Rate Effect Summarized

Figure 12.14 summarizes the entire dose-rate effect. For acute exposures at high dose rate the survival curve has a significant initial shoulder. As the dose rate is lowered and the treatment time protracted, more and more sublethal damage can be repaired during the exposure. Consequently, the survival curve becomes progressively shallower, and the shoulder tends to disappear. A point is reached at which *all* sublethal damage is repaired, resulting in a limiting slope. In at least some cell lines, a further lowering of the dose rate allows cells to progress through the cycle and accumulate in G_2. This is a radiosensitive phase, and so the survival curve becomes steeper again. This is the inverse dose-rate effect. A further reduction in dose rate will allow cells to pass through the G_2 block and divide. Proliferation may then occur during the radiation exposure if the dose rate is low enough and the exposure time is long compared with the length of the mitotic cycle. This may lead to a further reduction in biological effect as the dose rate is progressively lowered, because cell birth will tend to balance cell death.

EARLY AND LATE RESPONDING TISSUES

Clinical and laboratory data suggest that there is a consistent difference between early and late responding tissues in their response to changes in the time course over which radiation is delivered.

The dose-response relationship for late-responding tissues is more curved than that for early-responding tissues as first described by Withers (14). In terms of the linear-quadratic relationship between effect and dose, this translates into a larger α/β-ratio for early than late effects. The difference in the shapes of the dose-response relationships is illustrated in Figure 12.15. The α/β ratio is the dose at which cell killing by the linear (α) and quadratic (β) components are equal. This difference in shape translates into a difference in response to changes in fractionation or dose-rate. Late effect tissues, characterized by a very curvy dose response relationship, show a much greater sparing in a multifraction or continuous low dose-rate regime than do early responding tissues, which include tumors.

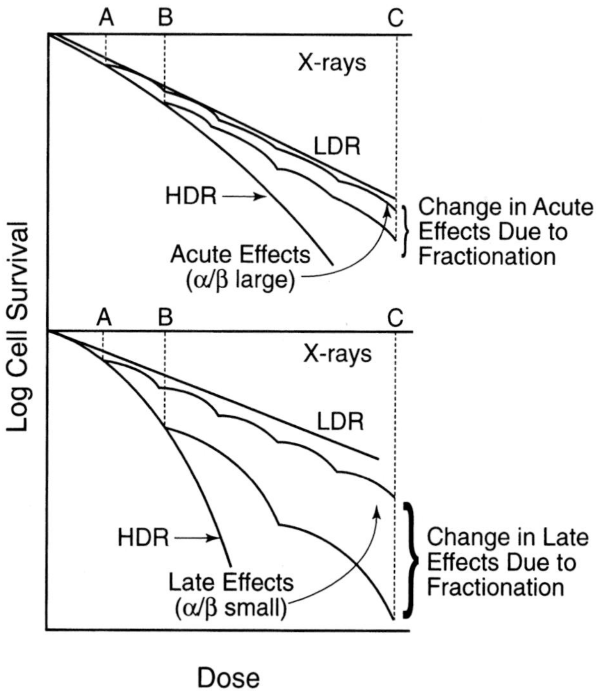

Figure 12.15. For x-rays late-responding tissues have a much more curved dose-response relationship and consequently show a much greater sparing in a multifraction regimen than early-responding tissues. Low dose-rate is, effectively, an infinite number of infinitely small doses. LDR therefore gives the maximum differential in sparing late responding normal tissues compared with early responding tissues, which includes tumors.

Consequently, it can be concluded that low dose-rate results in the maximal differential in response between late responding normal tissues and tumors. This is a significant biological advantage for brachytherapy, to be added to the physical advantage of good dose distribution resulting from the direct implantation of the tumor.

The Dose-Rate Effect and Clinical Data

Interstitial implants and intracavitary treatments typically involve the range of dose-rates where laboratory data would suggest that the biological effect should vary critically with dose rate. However, reports in the literature have been controversial. It was pointed out by Paterson in the 1960s that the dose-limiting factor in the case of interstitial implants is the tolerance of normal tissues (15). His philosophy was to push to the maximum dose tolerated by the normal tissues in order to maximize tumor control. Paterson published a curve relating total dose to overall time, with limiting normal tissue tolerance as the endpoint. Regarding 60 Gy in 7 days as the standard, he proposed that an implant of shorter duration should have a lower dose, and an implant of longer duration an augmented dose. The published curve represented his considerable clinical experience accumulated over many years and was unequivocally based on equalizing late effects in normal tissues. The experience was based on treatment with radium needles implanted according to the Manchester system. Ellis proposed an essentially identical scheme for use in clinical practice (16); the curve of Paterson and Ellis is reproduced in Figure 12.16, together with theoretical curves relating equivalent dose to overall time based on radiobiological data for early and late responding tissues, normalized to 60 Gy in 7 days. It is interesting to note that the calculated curve based on the radiobiological parameters for late responding tissues is virtually indistinguishable from the curves of Paterson and of Ellis who unequivocally based their judgment on obtaining equal late effects. The curve relating equivalent dose and overall time is steeper for late than for early responding tissues because of the smaller value of α/β.

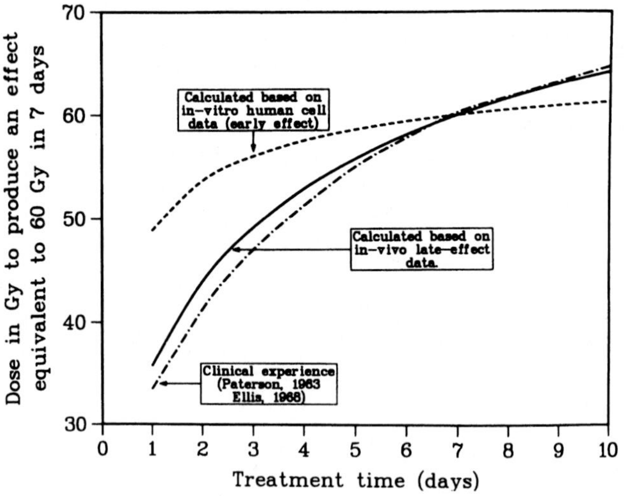

Figure 12.16. Dose equivalent to 60 Gy (6000 rads) in 7 days as proposed by Paterson (1963) and Ellis (1968) based on clinical observation of normal tissue tolerance, or calculated from radiobiological principles based on α/β ratios and T1/2 values characteristic of early and late responding tissues. (Redrawn from Hall EJ. Radiobiology for the Radiologist, 4th ed. JB Lippincott Company: Philadelphia, 1994.)

The introduction of iridium-192 as a substitute for radium needles in interstitial brachytherapy allowed greater flexibility and patient comfort, but also resulted in a much larger variation of dose-rate between individual implants. Two factors contribute to this:

1. As a consequence of the relatively short half-life of iridium-192 (74 days), the linear activity will vary significantly during the period of several months that the wires may be used or re-used.
2. The Paris system of dosimetry (17) developed for iridium-192 implants, where all sources have the same linear activity with varying separation between wires for different lengths (i.e. greater separation for larger wires) results in a wider range of dose-rates than was characteristic of radium implants using the Parker-Paterson dosimetry system, where internal needles had one-half or two-thirds of the linear activity of outer needles. Because all wires in an iridium-192 implant have the same linear activity, there is a correlation between implanted volume and dose-rate, with larger volumes being associated with higher dose-rates. The combination of those two factors results, in practice, in a three-fold variation in the overall irradiation time for the delivery of a given tumor dose. Nevertheless, Pierquin and his colleagues (18) came to the conclusion that in iridium-192 implants, the time factor, and therefore the dose rate, was unimportant. Consequently, the Paris school recommended the same prescribed dose irrespective of overall time within the range of 3 to 8 days. They were careful to point out that their conclusions were preliminary, but nevertheless concluded: "We can, however, say with certainty that the variation in overall treatment time for the same tumor dose from 3 days to 8 days does not appear to influence the frequency of recurrence of necrosis."

Based upon this conviction, many hundreds of patients were treated with iridium-192 implants using standard doses uncorrected for treatment time or dose-rate, despite the fact that this conflicts with the previously published clinical experience of Paterson and of Ellis, and does not agree with the experimental radiobiological data that would predict a substantial dose-rate effect over the dose-rate range in question.

Dose-Rate Effects from a Retrospective Analysis of the Iridium Implant Data

The large series of patients treated in Paris with iridium wire implants have been followed carefully over the years, and two important papers have appeared describing a retrospective analysis of these data. In the first, Mazeron and colleagues (19) studied the incidence of local tumor control and necrosis in T_1 and T_2 squamous cell carcinoma of the mobile tongue and floor of mouth treated with interstitial iridium-192. The data are shown in Figure 12.17 and compare tumor control and necrosis in patients treated at dose-rates above or below 0.5 Gy/hr. Two principal conclusions can be drawn from this analysis: 1) there is little or no difference in local control between the two dose-rate ranges provided a sufficiently high total dose is used (65 to 70 Gy), but there is a clear separation at lower doses (around 60 Gy) with the lower dose rate being significantly less effective; 2) over the entire range of doses used, there was a higher incidence of necrosis associated with the higher dose-rate range.

The clinical data are in line with the predictions that would be expected based on radiobiological considerations, particularly the more critical dependence on dose-rate of late responding tissues.

In a second study, Mazeron and colleagues (20) analyzed data from a large group of patients with carcinoma of the breast who received an iridium-192 implant as a boost to external beam radiotherapy. A fixed standard total dose was used, regardless of the dose rate, and there is a clear correlation between the proportion of recurrent tumors and the dose rate, as illustrated in Figure 12.18. For a given total dose, a clear difference in tumor control could be seen between 0.3 and 0.9 Gy/hr, as predicted from radiobiological experiments with cells in vitro.

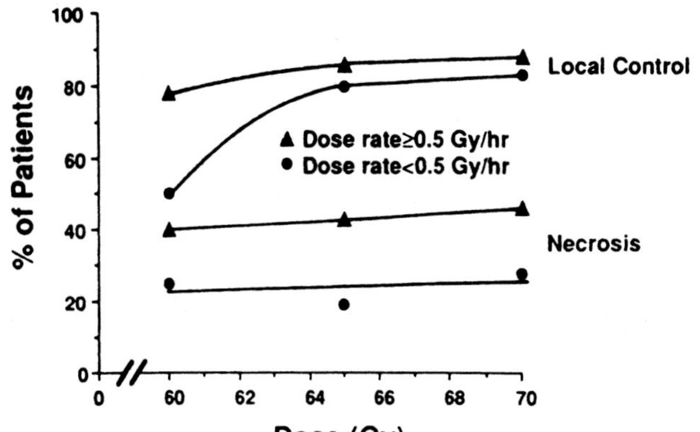

Figure 12.17. Local tumor control and necrosis rate at 5 years as a function of dose in patients treated for T1-2 squamous cell carcinomas of the mobile tongue and the floor of the mouth with interstitial iridium-192 implants. The patients were grouped according to whether the implant was characterized by a high dose rate (above 0.5 Gy/h) or low dose rate (below 0.5 Gy/h). The necrosis rate is higher for the higher dose rate at all dose levels. Local tumor control did not depend on dose rate provided the total dose was sufficiently large, but did vary with dose rate for lower total doses. (Redrawn from the data of Mazeron JJ, Simon JM, Le Pechoux C, et al). Effect of dose-rate on local control and complications in definitive irradiation of T_{1-2} squamous cell carcinomas of mobile tongue and floor of mouth with interstitial iridium-192. Radiother Oncol 1991;21:39–47.)

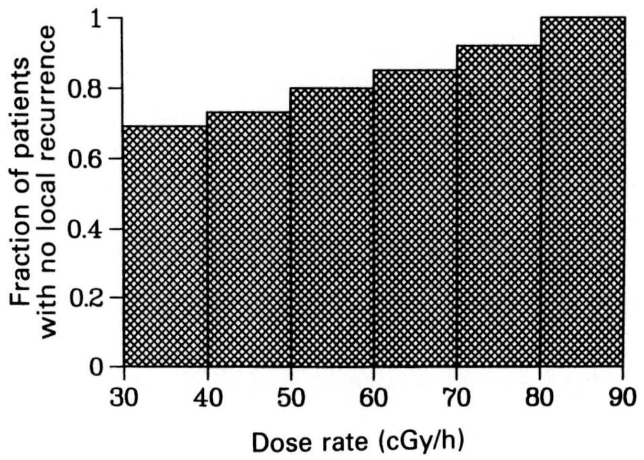

Figure 12.18. Percentage of patients who showed no local recurrence as a function of dose rate in patients treated for breast carcinoma by a combination of external-beam irradiation plus iridium-192 interstitial implant. The implant was used to deliver a constant dose of 37 Gy; the dose rate varied by a factor of 3 owing to different linear activities of the iridium-192 wire and to different size volumes implanted. (Drawn from the data of Mazeron JJ, Simon JM, Crook J, et al. Influence of dose-rate on local control of breast carcinoma treated by external beam irradiation plus iridium-192 Implant. Int J Radiat Oncol Biol Phys 1991; 21:1173–1177.)

The Bias of Tumor Size and Dose-Rate

A complication and confounding variable in the interpretation of these clinical data relating dose to produce an equivalent effect to implant time (and therefore to dose-rate) is the fact that, for interstitial implants, the dose-rate tends to increase as the size of the implant increases. This correlation is particularly true for implants using iridium-192 wires, as used in the Paris system, which are all of the same linear activity, but less so when there is a variation in linear activity, as in the Parker and Paterson system (21). The bias of larger tumors and larger volumes being associated with higher dose-rates, while smaller tumors and smaller treatment volumes are associated with lower dose-rates, was pointed out by Pierquin and his colleagues (18). Larger tumors of course require a larger dose for a given level of local control, while the maximum dose that can be tolerated by normal tissues decreases as the volume implanted increases. This will tend to flatten the isoeffect curve for tumor control and steepen the isoeffect curve for normal tissue tolerance.

Based on these considerations, then, it is clear why the Paris school and the Paterson/Ellis school differed so radically in their prescriptions for dealing with dose-rate changes. First, the Paterson/Ellis recommendations were based on equalizing only late effects where there is a clear change of equi-effect dose with dose-rate (solid curves in Figure 12.16). However, the Paris recommendations were based on an attempt to equalize late and early effects (with hindsight it is clear that when the dose-rate changes it is not possible to match both late and early effects). Second, the Paterson/Ellis recommendations date from the era of radium needles when there was less correlation between volume and dose rate. However, the Paris recommendations were based on iridium wire implants where there is strong correlation between tumor volume and dose-rate, which would tend to make the equi-effect curve for tumor control vary even less with dose-rate.

RATIONALE FOR LDR BRACHYTHERAPY

There are three factors that contribute to the efficacy of LDR brachytherapy.

1. The dose distribution is favorable because the radioactive sources are either implanted directly into the tumor, or contained in a body cavity close to the tumor. This allows a larger dose to be delivered to the tumor for a given dose to limiting normal tissues. It is interesting to note that this advantage for an implant was suggested by Alexander Graham Bell as early as 1903 in a letter to American Medicine (22). He wrote:
   Dear Dr. Sowers:
   I understand from you that the Röntgen rays and the rays emitted by radium have been found to have a marked curative effect upon external cancers, but that the effects upon deep-seated cancers have not thus far proved satisfactory.
   It has occurred to me that one reason for the unsatisfactory nature of these latter experiments arises from the fact that the rays have been applied externally, thus having to pass through healthy tissues of various depths in order to reach the cancerous matter.
   The Crookes' tube from which the Röntgen rays are emitted is of course too bulky to be admitted into the middle of a mass of cancer, but there is no reason why a tiny fragment of radium sealed up in a fine glass tube should not be inserted into the very heart of the cancer, thus acting directly upon the diseased material. Would it not be worth while making experiments along this line?
   (signed) Alexander Graham Bell
2. Low dose-rate is effectively an infinite number of infinitely small dose fractions; this exploits to the full the difference between tumors and late responding normal tissues that are a consequence of their different α/β ratios.
3. Brachytherapy is usually delivered over a shorter overall time period than conventional external beam radiotherapy; it constitutes accelerated treatment par excellence.

PULSED BRACHYTHERAPY PDR

A major innovation in brachytherapy during the past decade has been the introduction of pulsed brachytherapy (PDR), first described by Brenner and Hall (23). The principle of PDR is to replace the many individual wires ribbons or sources in a conventional implant or intracavitary treatment by a single iridium-192 source of about 37 Gbq. This source, under computer control from a remote afterloading device, steps through the implanted catheters with dwell times tailored to produce the dose distribution required. The principle is illustrated in Figure 12.19. Based on an analysis of a large body of data from cell lines of human origin, Brenner and Hall (23) came to the conclusion that a 10-minute pulse delivering 40 to 60 cGy and repeated every hour would adequately mimic continuous low dose rate (CLDR) irradiation at 40 to 60 cGy/hr. They concluded that, as long as the dose/pulse is kept low, a reasonable equivalence would be achieved in terms of both early and late effects. Between individual pulses, the source is returned to the safe.

This simple strategy leads to several important advantages.

1. Improved radiation safety because there is no individual source preparation beforehand, and during an implant the source can be returned to the safe while the patient is nursed, examined, or visited.
2. Only one source needs to be replaced instead of a whole inventory of sources, which leads to a substantial cost saving.

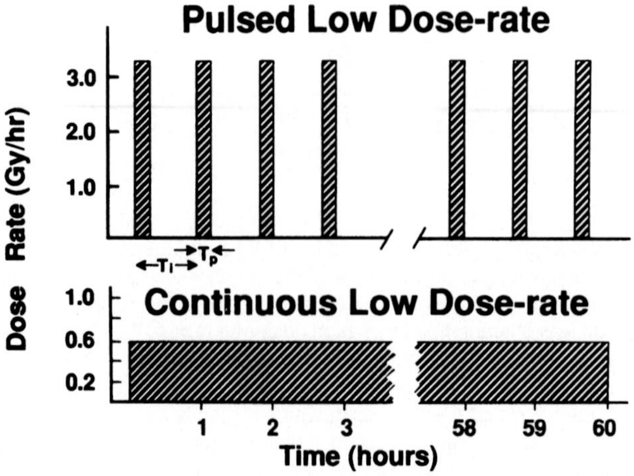

Figure 12.19. Illustrating the concept of replacing continuous low dose-rate irradiation by a series of short pulses, so-called PDR.

3. A stepping source under computer control, with variable dwell time in each position, allows improved optimization of the dose distribution.
4. The average dose rate can be kept constant for implants of different sizes and the iridium-192 source decays by the simple expedient of varying the pulse length. This is illustrated in Figure 12.20.

The pulsing schedule recommended by Brenner and Hall (23) was conservative and primarily designed to be safe for almost any conceivable set of biological response parameters characteristic of the relevant target tissues—whether early or late responding. For this reason, the proposed schedule maintained the same overall dose in the same overall time as the CLDR that the PDR replaced, and suggested frequent pulses with small doses per pulse. In this way the technical advantages offered by the new generation of computer controlled remote afterloaders could be combined with the true and trusted advantages of low dose-rate.

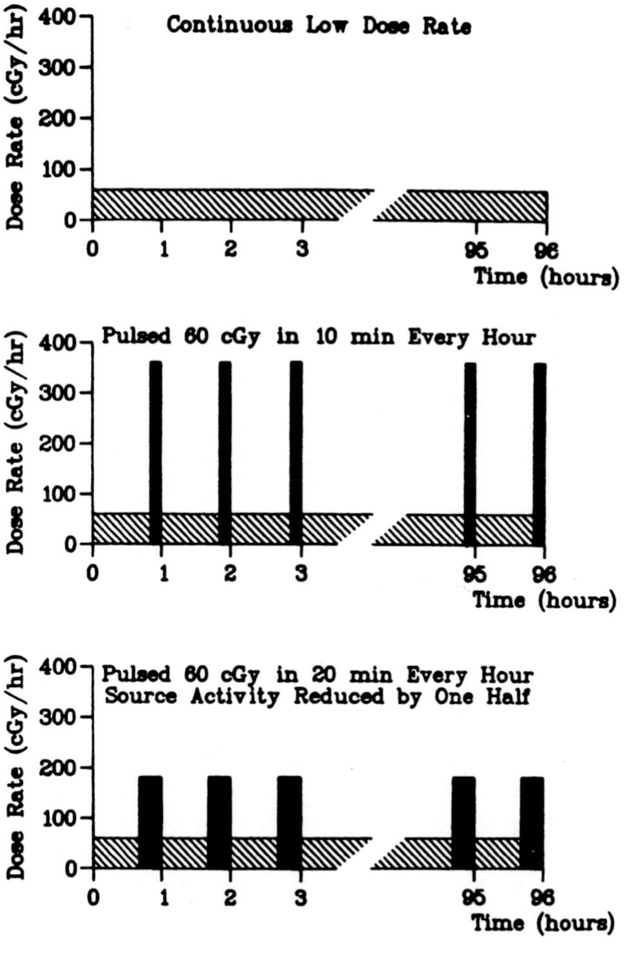

Figure 12.20. Illustrating the principle of pulsed brachytherapy. Continuous low dose rate irradiation at (for example) 60 cGy per hour is replaced by a relatively high-dose rate pulse of 60 cGy delivered once per hour. The pulse, during which the single iridium-192 source steps through the implant, would take about 12 minutes depending on the activity of the source and the size of the implant. Over a period of months as the activity of the iridium-192 source decays, the dose per pulse, and therefore the average dose rate per hour, can be maintained by simply increasing the pulse length. After one half-life of the radionuclide, which is 70 days, the pulse length would be doubled to 24 minutes in each hour. (Redrawn from Hall EJ, Brenner DJ. The 1991 George Edelstyn Lecture. Clin Oncol 1992;4:249–256.)

Experimental Validation of the PDR Concept

Conditions for the equivalence of pulsed and continuous low dose-rate irradiation have been investigated by a number of groups, always with a view to discover the limits of fraction number and dose per fraction where the equivalence breaks down, bearing in mind that fewer, more widely spaced fractions, would be logistically more convenient.

The first published experimental test of pulsed brachytherapy was by Armour and colleagues (24), using 9L rat gliosarcoma cells cultured in vitro. In this cell line, no difference in cell survival could be detected between CLDR at 0.5 Gy/h and pulsed schedules up to 3 Gy every 6 h. The equivalence broke down for a pulse schedule of 6 Gy every 12 h.

A later in vitro study by Chen and colleagues compared PDR and CLDR using three cell lines of human origin, one derived from a cervical carcinoma and two from breast carcinomas (25). There was no significant difference in cell survival between PDR and CLDR for any of the cell lines when a pulse interval of 1 hour (and a dose per pulse of about 0.6 Gy) was used, supporting the initial conservative recommendation of Brenner and Hall (23). As the pulse interval was increased, PDR became progressively more effective than CLDR for a given dose and there were significant differences for pulse intervals of 6 and 12 h. corresponding to large doses/pulse.

A comparison of CLDR and PDR was also published by Mason and colleagues from the MD Anderson Hospital (26) scoring regenerating crypts in the mouse jejunum-an in vivo early responding end point. They found an hourly PDR schedule to be indistinguishable from CLDR at 0.7 Gy/h, whether the pulse was delivered in 10 minutes or 1 minute. This is an important demonstration in vivo that agrees with the more extensive in vitro studies.

Brenner and colleagues (27) used a model late-effect system, namely cataract formation in the ocular lens of the rat, to compare PDR and CLDR. This is a true late effect, though not one that is generally dose limiting in radiation therapy. They found that, for the same total dose in the same overall time, there was no difference in overall time, cataractogenic potential between CLDR and hourly pulses (.62 Gy/pulse) or pulses repeated every 4 hours (2.48 Gy/pulse). The likely explanation of the fact that fewer larger pulses are still equivalent to CLDR in this system (whereas they were not in in vitro experiments) lies in a relatively slow rate of repair of sublethal damage in this late-responding tissue. There is good evidence from the clinic that sublethal damage responsible for late effects in the human also repairs relatively slowly. This has previously been discussed (28).

Armour and colleagues (29) later used late rectal stenosis in the rat as an endpoint to evaluate PDR. This is probably a consequential late effect, but highly relevant to intracavitary brachytherapy where late rectal damage can be dose limiting. They found that CLDR (0.75 Gy/hr) was indistinguishable from pulsed regimes consisting of 0.375 Gy every half-hour, 0.75 Gy every hour, or 1.5 Gy every 2 hours. However, a 3 Gy pulse every 4 hours was slightly more damaging while a 6 Gy pulse every 8 hours was much more damaging than CLDR to the same total dose in the same overall time.

In summary, these experimental studies confirm the conservative recommendations of Brenner and Hall (23), that small pulses repeated every 1 (or possibly 2) hours are indistinguishable from CLDR, but that bigger doses per pulse, with a longer separation between pulses, produce more severe biological damage. This is equally true for cells cultured in vitro and for tissues in vivo.

PRACTICAL CLINICAL SCHEDULES FOR PDR

While PDR has prospered in Europe and elsewhere, in the United States it has foundered on the Nuclear Regulatory Commission requirement that a physicist and/or radiotherapist (or some other suitably qualified person) be present throughout the treatment, that is, day and night, to deal with the possible, if unlikely, eventuality that the source becomes lodged inside the patient. An obvious way around this problem is to restrict treatment pulses to "office hours," when the need for the presence of a physicist and/or radiation oncologist is not a problem. This can only be done by dropping the constraint that was considered prudent in the original paper on this topic (that both the total dose and overall treatment time must be the same as the conventional CLDR brachytherapy treatment)—and instead allowing somewhat longer overall treatment times.

In addition, in order for the PDR to be equivalent to the CLDR, in terms of both early and late responding tissues, it must be assumed that the rate of repair of sublethal damage is slower in late than in early responding tissues. There is some evidence for this from animal experiments as well as from clinical data (30-33). The existing data summarizing repair half times in normal tissues are summarized in Tables 12.1 and 12.2. If these various assumptions are made, it is possible to design PDR schedules where pulses are given only during office hours. An extreme example of this is the protocol of Visser and colleagues (34) who proposed pulses at 3-hour intervals only during the working day. This is illustrated in Figure 12.21, which also shows how the overall pulsed schedule must be of longer duration than the CLDR protocol it replaces in order to achieve equivalence. Their early reports indicate no worse late effects in the patients treated with PDR, but since the implant was a boost, with the majority of the total dose being delivered in highly fractionated external beam radiotherapy, this is not really a critical test of the idea.

The total clinical experience with PDR to date is still limited. The first patient was treated in 1992 at the University of California at San Francisco. A survey conducted by Mazeron (35) concluded that by the end of 1995, over 1100 patients had been treated with PDR in 20 centers in North America, Europe, and Australia. Advantages of the new technology cited by the most frequent users included:

- better quality of treatment
- technical verification
- patient care during treatment
- radiation protection.

Table 12.1. Early and Late Responding Skin Damage (Turresson & Thames 1989)

	$T_{1/2}$ Slow min	$T_{1/2}$ Fast min
Early	75	25
Late	250	25

Table 12.2. Values of *α*, *β*, *α*/*β* and $T_{1/2}$ for Late Responding Normal Tissues Evaluated *In Vivo*

Endpoint	α Gy^{-1}	β Gy^{-2}	α/β Gy	$T_{1/2}$ min
Skin Telangiectasia				
fast repair	0.1	0.024	4.1	24
slow repair	0.1	0.024	4.1	210
Mouse lung (late damage)	0.31	0.072	4.3	39
Rat Spinal Cord (Paralysis)	**0.066**	**0.019**	**3.4**	**93**

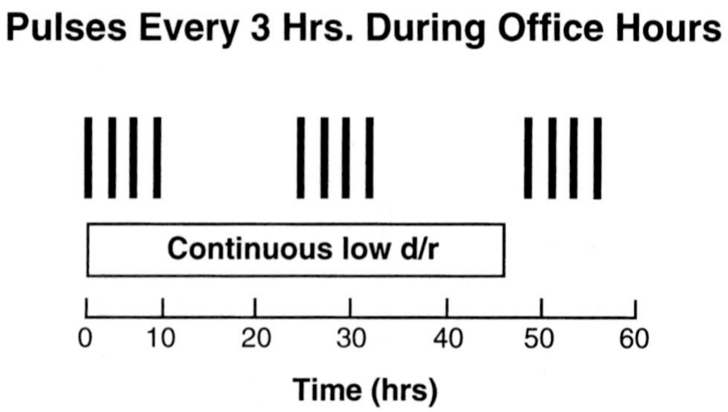

Figure 12.21. To illustrate the PDR Scheme proposed in Visser AG, et al. Pulsed dose rate and fractionated high dose rate brachytherapy. Int J Radiat Oncol Biol Phys 1996;34:497–505.

HIGH DOSE RATE VERSUS LOW DOSE RATE

The move towards high dose-rate brachytherapy has been fueled by a combination of many factors, including patient convenience, cost, radiation protection, and dose optimization made possible by the new generation of computer-controlled afterloading devices.

Since tumors are characterized in general by large α/β ratios (from 10 Gy to >) while late responding normal tissues have smaller α/β ratios (closer to 2 Gy) it is simply impossible to replace a continuous low dose-rate (CLDR) schedule with a high dose-rate (HDR) schedule consisting of a few fractions while preserving both local tumor control and normal tissue late effects. If doses are matched to produce the same tumor control, then late effects will inevitably be worse; if on the other hand doses are matched to result in equivalent normal tissue late effects, then tumor control will be jeopardized. This is an inevitable consequence of the biology involved. If the HDR is divided into a sufficient number of fractions (20 or more) to allow an approximate equivalence of both early and late effects, then all the advantages of patient convenience and cost would be lost. Fowler (36) summed it up well saying, "There is, therefore, a certain loss of therapeutic ratio when regimes of logistic convenience (that is, HDR) are used." What then is the place for HDR? There are two different situations where the convenience and cost savings associated with HDR can be exploited:

a) The implant as a boost

When the brachytherapy implant constitutes only one-third to one-half of the total radiation treatment, with the remainder of the treatment being delivered as highly fractionated external beam radiotherapy, then a few HDR fractions can be tolerated. This has been the approach, for example, of Levendag and his colleagues in the Netherlands (34). The HDR dose should be calculated to be equivalent to the CLDR regime it replaces for tumor control; the normal tissues are sufficiently "forgiving" that the slightly worse late effects will not be a problem because of all the other advantages of brachytherapy—limited volume, good dose distribution, etc.

b) Intracavitary brachytherapy for carcinoma of the uterine cervix

What makes this situation different from almost all others is that the radiation dose that produces unwanted late sequelae is significantly less than the treatment dose prescribed to the tumor. This is because the dose-limiting organs at risk (rectum and bladder) are some distance away from the brachytherapy sources, in contrast to the more usual situation in which the dose-limiting normal tissue is adjacent to the treatment volume. A further factor must be considered, namely that the short treatment time characteristic of HDR allows packing and retraction of the sensitive normal tissues estimated by Orton (37,38) to result in a further 20% reduction in dose to bladder/rectum compared with that associated with conventional LDR treatments.

Orton and colleagues (38) analyzed clinical data from a survey of 56 centers treating more than 17,000 cervical cancer patients with HDR. A wide range of doses and number of fractions were used. The average fractionation regime consisted of about 5 fractions of about 7.5 Gy each to Point A, regardless of the stage of the disease. Fractionation of the HDR treatments significantly influenced toxicity. Morbidity rates were significantly lower for Point A dose/fraction less than or equal to 7 Gy compared with greater than 7 Gy. This was true for both moderate and severe complications. The effect of dose/fraction on cure rates was equivocal. Some findings of the Orton survey are summarized in Table 12.3. Finally, the data showed that for conversion from LDR to HDR the total dose to Point A was reduced on average by a factor 0.54 + /-0.06. The overall conclusion of the survey was that HDR resulted in 5-year survival figure and complication rates that were at least as good as historical controls from the same centers treated with CLDR; however, none of these studies were prospective randomized trials.

Several critiques of the Orton study have been published, as well as a summary of the benefits of conventional LDR by Eifel (39). In summary, Eifel pointed out that HDR therapy can be expected to produce comparable results to LDR therapy only in situations where the dose to organ at risk for late complications is lower than the prescribed tumor dose. This leads to one of the clear guidelines as to when HDR is indicated as a good alternative to LDR.

The optimal number of fractions, and the dose per fraction for an HDR treatment is still a matter of debate. Using the linear quadratic formalism, and biological data from a battery of almost 40 cell lines of human origin, Brenner and Hall (40) calculated HDR schemes that were designed to be equivalent to many of the LDR protocols in common use. Distributions of HDR doses predicted to yield comparable acute effects to 60 Gy in two conventional LDR treatments are shown in Figure 12.22. The arithmetic mean of these dose distributions as a function of the number of fractions is plotted in Figure 12.23. The radiobiological predictions would suggest a dose per fraction of about 7.5 Gy if five fractions are used, which is in remarkable agreement with the average of the Orton survey.

A system has been described by Stitt and colleagues (41) and Thomadsen and colleagues (42), which provides

Table 12.3. Survey of HDR Schedules

	>7 Gy per fr	<7 Gy per fr
Mean # of fractions	3.8	5.6
Mean total dose (Gy)	35	30
Mean 5-year survival	66.2–2.2	56.8–2.1
Complication rate %	9.8	8.6
Severe complications %	3.4	1.4

a set of dose schedules and dose specification points for treatment of carcinoma of the cervix with HDR brachytherapy plus external beam radiotherapy. These various protocols, based on sound radiobiological principles, have been used to treat hundreds of patients. Local tumor control and complication rates are reported to be similar to LDR treatments, but these conclusions are based on historical controls.

The radiobiological principles summarized in this chapter lead to clear guidelines for the use of HDR brachytherapy for the uterine cervix.

1. When the dose to the dose limiting normal tissues is less than 75% of the prescribed tumor dose, for equal tumor control, HDR results in late effects that are comparable and no worse than for LDR.

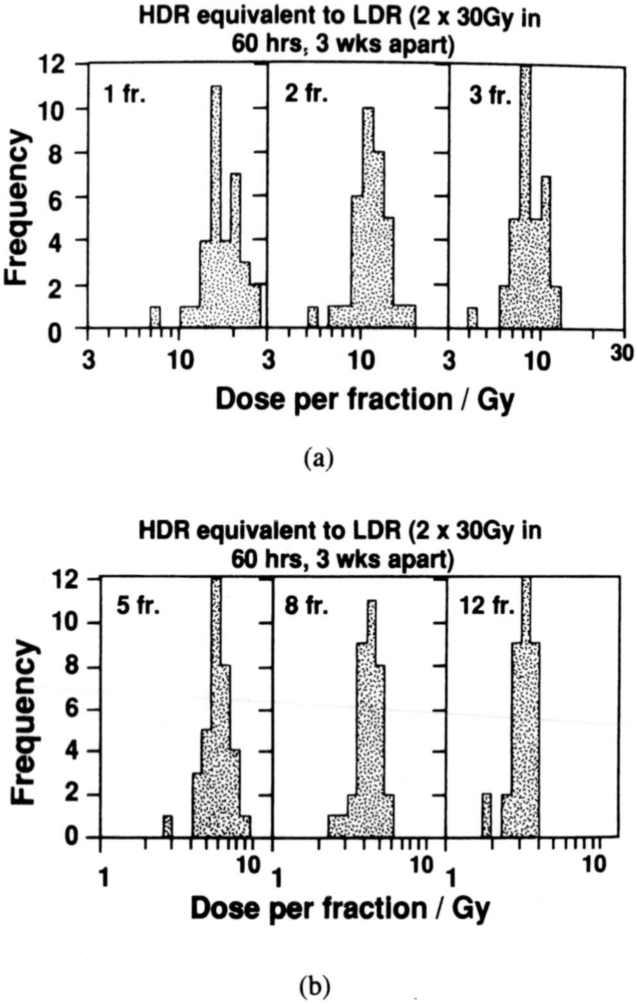

Figure 12.22. Distribution of doses delivered in one to twelve HDR fractions, equivalent to two LDR treatments of 30 Gy in 60 hours, based on data from cell lines of human origin as calculated in Brenner DJ, Hall EJ. Br J Radiol 1991;64:133.

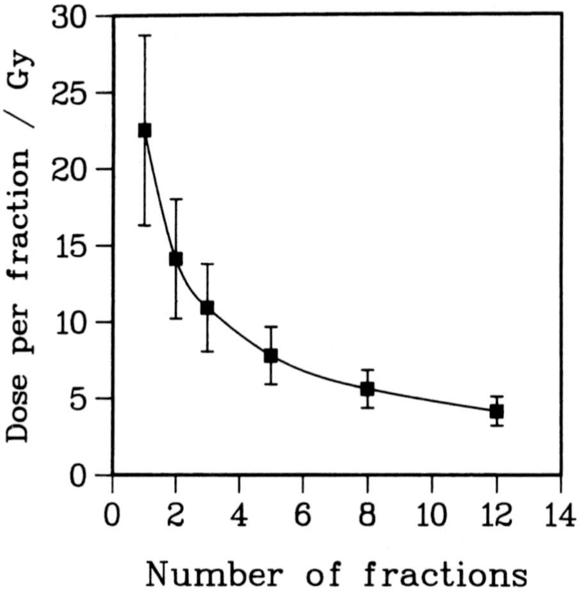

Figure 12.23. Dose/fraction as a function of the number of HDR treatments to achieve equal biological effect. The points plotted are the arithmetic means of the distributions shown in Figure 22 from Brenner DJ, Hall EJ. Br J Radiol 1991;64:133.

2. For patients in whom the dose to the bladder/rectum is comparable to the prescribed dose, HDR is contraindicated.
3. HDR protocols, comparable to LDR, should be designed based on matching early rather than late effects.

References

1. Hall EJ. Radiobiology for the Radiologist, 4th ed. JB Lippincott Company: Philadelphia, 1994.
2. Ward JF. Some biochemical consequences of the spatial distribution of ionizing radiation produced free radicals. Radiat Res 1981;86:185-195.
3. Ward JF. DNA damage produced by ionizing radiation in mammalian cells: Identities, mechanisms of formation and repairability. Progress in Nucleic Acids and Molecular Biology 1988;35:95-125.
4. Evans HJ. Chromosome aberrations induced by ionizing radiation. Int Rev Cytol 1962;13:22-321.
5. Lea DEA. Actions of radiations on living cells, 2nd ed. Cambridge, England: Cambridge University Press, 1956.
6. Kerr JFR, Wyllie AH, Currie AR. Apoptosis: A basic biological phenomenon with wide ranging implications in tissue kinetics. Brit J Cancer 1972;26: 239-257.
7. Gray LH. Dose-rate in radiotherapy. Brit J Radiol 1944;17:327-335
8. Hall EJ, Bedford JS. Dose-rate: Its effect on the survival of HeLa cells irradiated with gamma-rays. Radiat Res 1964;22:305-315.
9. Bedford JS, Mitchell B. Dose-rate effects in synchronous mammalian cells in culture. Radiat Res 1973;54:316-327.
10. Lowe SW, Schmitt EM, Smith SW, Osborne BA, Jacks T. P53 is required for radiation-induced apoptosis in mouse thymocytes. Nature 1993;362:847-849.
11. Hall EJ, Brenner DJ. The 1991 George Edelstyn Lecture: Needles, Wires and Chips—Advances in brachytherapy. Clin Oncol 1992;4: 249-256.
12. Mitchell B, Bedford JS, Bailey SM. Dose-rate effects in plateau-phase cultures of S3 HeLa and V79 cells. Radiat Res 1979;79:520-536.

13. Hall EJ. The biological basis of endocurie therapy. The Henschke Memorial Lecture 1984. Endocurie Hypertherm Oncology 1985;1: 141-151.
14. Withers HR, Thames HD, Peters LJ. Differences in the fractionation response of acutely and late-responding tissues. In: Karcher KH, Kolgelnik HD, Reinartz G, eds. Progress in radio-oncology. Vol II. New York: Raven Press, 1982:287-296.
15. Paterson R. Treatment of malignant disease by radiotherapy. Baltimore: Williams & Wilkins, 1963.
16. Ellis F. Dose time and fractionation in radiotherapy. In: Elbert M, Howard A (eds). Current Topics in Radiation Research. Amsterdam, North Holland, 1968;4:359-397.
17. Pierquin B. Dosimetry: The relational system. Proceedings of a Conference on Afterloading in Radiotherapy. Rockville, New York: US Department of Health, Education and Welfare. Publication number (FDA) 72-8024, 1971;204-227.
18. Pierquin B, Chassagne D, Baillet F, etal. Clinical observations on the time factor in interstitial radiotherapy using iridium-192. Clin Radiol 1973;24:506-509.
19. Mazeron JJ, Simon JM, Le Pechoux C, et al. Effect of dose-rate on local control and complications in definitive irradiation of T_{1-2} squamous cell carcinomas of mobile tongue and floor of mouth with interstitial iridium-192. Radiother Oncol 1991;21:39-47.
20. Mazeron JJ, Simon JM, Crook J, et al. Influence of dose-rate on local control of breast carcinoma treated by external beam irradiation plus iridium-192 implant. Int J Radiat Oncol Biol Phys 1991;21:1173-1177.
21. Meredith WJ, ed. Radium dosage: The Manchester system. 2nd ed. Edinburgh: Livingstone, 1967:42.
22. Bell AG. Correspondence. American Medicine, 1903.
23. Brenner DJ, Hall EJ. Conditions for the equivalence of continuous to pulsed low dose rate brachytherapy. Int J Radiat Oncol Biol Phys 1991bɔ:181-190.
24. Armour E, Wang Z, Corry P, Martinez A. Equivalence of continuous and pulse simulated low dose rate irradiation in 9L gliosarcoma cells at 37° and 41°C. Int J Radiat Oncol Biol Phys 1992;22:109-114.
25. Chen CZ, Huang Y, Hall EJ, Brenner DJ. Pulsed brachytherapy as a substitute for continuous low dose rate: An in vitro study with human carcinoma cells. Int J Radiat Oncol Biol Phys 1997;37:137-143.
26. Mason KA, Thames HD, Ochran TG, Ruifrok AC, Janjan N. Comparison of continuous and pulsed low dose rate brachytherapy: Biological equivalence in vivo. Int J Radiat Oncol Biol Phys 1994:28:667-671.
27. Brenner DJ, Hall EJ, Randers-Pehrson G, Huang YP, Johnson GW, Miller RW, Wu B, Vazquez ME, Medvedovsky C, Worgul BV. Quantitative comparisons of continuous and pulsed low dose-rate regimens in a model late-effect system. Int J Radiat Oncol Biol Phys 1996;34: 905-910.
28. Brenner DJ, Hall EJ, Huang Y, Sachs RK. Optimizing the time course of brachytherapy and other accelerated radiotherapeutic regimes. Int J Radiat Oncol Biol Phys 1994;29:893-901.
29. Armour E, White Jr A, Armin A, Lorry P, Coffey M, Dewitt C, Martinez A. Pulsed LDR brachytherapy in a rat model; dependence of late rectal injury on radiation pulse size. Int J Radiat Oncol Biol Phys 1997 (In press).
30. Moulder JE, Fish BL. Repair of sublethal damage in the rat kidney (abstract.). In: Chapman, Dewey JD, Dewey WC, Whitmore GF, eds. Radiation Research: A Twentieth-Century Perspective, Vol. 1. San Diego, CA: Academic Press, 1992:238.
31. Thames Jr HD, Withers HR, Peters LJ. Tissue repair capacity and repair kinetics deduced from multifractionated or continuous irradiation regimens with incomplete repair. Brit. J. Cancer 1984;49:263-269.
32. Turesson I, Thames HD. Repair capacity and kinetics of human skin during fractionated radiotherapy: erythenam desquamation, and telangiectasia after 3 and 5 years' follow-up. Radiother Oncol 1989;15: 169-188.
33. van Rongen E, Thames HD, Travis EL. Recovery from radiation damage in mouse lung: interpretations in terms of two rates of repair. Radiat. Res. 1993;133:225-233.
34. Visser AG, van den Aardweg JM, Levendag PC. Pulsed dose rate and fractionated high dose rate brachytherapy: Choice of brachytherapy schedules to replace low dose rate treatments. Int J Radiat Oncol Biol Phys 1996:34;497-505.
35. Mazeron JJ, Boisserie G, Baltas D. Pulsed dose rate brachytherapy: A survey. Curr Oncol 4: (suppl. 1) 1997ʧ-S6.
36. Fowler JF. Dose rate effects in normal tissues. In Mould RF, ed. Brachytherapy 2. The Netherlands, Nucletron p. 26, 1989.
37. Orton CG. Remote afterloading for cervix cancer: The physicist's point of view. In Brachytherapy HDR and LDR. Proceedings of brachytherapy meeting on remote afterloading: State of the Art, Dearborn, Michigan May 1989. Martinez AA, Orton, DG , Mould RF, eds. (Nucletron, The Netherlands).
38. Orton CG, Seyedsadr M, Somnay A. Comparison of high and low dose rate remote afterloading for cervix cancer and the importance of fractionation. Int J Radiat Oncol Biol Phys 1992;21:1425.
39. Eifel PJ. High-dose-rate brachytherapy for carcinoma of the cervix: High tech or high risk? Int J Radiat Oncol Biol Phys 1992;24:383.
40. Brenner DJ, Hall EJ. Fractionated high dose-rate versus low dose-rate brachytherapy of the cervix: I. General considerations based on radiobiology. Br J Radial 1991; 64:133
41. Stet JA, Fowler JF, Thomadsen BR, et al. High dose rate intracavitary brachytherapy for carcinoma of the cervix: The Madison system: I. Clinical and radiological considerations. Int J Radiat Oncol Biol Phys 1992;24:335
42. Thomadsen BR, Shahabi S, Stitt JA, et al. High dose rate intracavitary brachytherapy for carcinoma of the cervix: The Madison system: II. Procedural and physical considerations. Int J Radiat Oncol Biol Phys 1992;24:349.

Chapter 13

The Physics of High Dose Rate Brachytherapy

Gary A. Ezzell

SOURCES

The fundamental requirement for a treatment to be delivered at high dose rate is that the dose given to a cell must be received in a time shorter than compared with cellular repair processes. The International Commission on Radiation Units and Measurements (ICRU) Report 38 defines the high dose rate (HDR) regime as beginning at 0.2 gray/minute (1), but that value is arbitrary and not critical for this discussion. Few radioisotopes can be produced with specific activities and half-lives sufficient to make practical high dose rate sources. In the past decade, only cobalt 60 (Co-60) and iridium-192 (Ir-192) have been used commercially, and only with Ir-192 can sources which are small enough be achieved to permit interstitial treatments. Table 13.1 shows some of the pertinent characteristics of these two sources (2). Iridium-192 is superior with respect to source size and shielding requirements, but Co-60's longer half-life would make it the isotope of choice for a unit dedicated to intracavitary treatments.

The vast majority of installed HDR treatment units use Ir-192 sources because the small source size allows intracavitary, interstitial, and interluminal treatments to be performed. The strength of a new source is typically on the order of 4.0 cGy m^2 h^{-1} (370 MBq or 10 Ci). Such a source will produce an absorbed dose rate of about 7.7 gray/minute at 1 cm in tissue. Most centers replace their sources three or four times a year, after the source has decayed to 30 to 40% of its original strength.

Remote Afterloading Units

The intense radiation fields surrounding HDR sources dictate that the treatment delivery system be operated remotely, which in turn implies certain common elements in the design of the treatment unit. Although every commercial system differs in details, each contains (3,4):

1. A shielded storage safe in which the source resides when not actively treating the patient.
2. A mechanism for advancing the source(s) into and out of treatment applicators safely and with good precision.
3. An overall control system with which the user programs the treatment positions and times.
4. Associated safety systems that monitor system performance, prevent the source from advancing into potential hazards, and permit recovery from emergency conditions.

The storage safe must reduce radiation levels outside the remote afterloading unit to safe levels; in the United States these levels cannot exceed 0.25 mrem/h at one meter.

Source positioning systems have included pneumatic devices for HDR units having multiple Co-60 pellets and cable drive systems for those using single Ir-192 sources (5). Variants of this latter mechanism comprise the majority of installed HDR units today. In these systems, an encapsulated Ir-192 source is attached to the end of a cable, which can then be advanced and retracted in precise increments using stepper motors. This general scheme is often referred to as a "stepping source" method. The single source must sequentially advance to each programmed treatment position within the implanted applicators and remain at each position for a programmed "dwell time." The ability to control the locations and dwell times permits greater flexibility in modifying the dose distributions given the patient, as will be discussed in more detail below.

Table 13.1. Physical Characteristics for Common HDR Sources

Radioisotope	Half-life	Mean Energy	Energy Range	Half Value Layer-Lead	Typical Source Diameter
Co-60	5.26 y	1.25 MeV	1.17–1.33 MeV	1.1 cm	~2.5 mm
Ir-192	73.8 d	0.38 MeV	0.14–1.06 MeV	0.30 cm	~1 mm

The positioning accuracy of stepping source systems is generally ±1 mm. Stepping motors are capable of precise incremental motions, so the overall accuracy is to a large degree determined by how the afterloader establishes the reference position from which subsequent motions are measured. In some designs, the source is advanced to the end of the applicator and then retracted in precise increments. In others, the reference point is within the treatment head and the source is then advanced precisely from there. Either system works well, but each has its own ramifications for quality assurance (6).

Since patients often have more than one applicator in place (e.g. a tandem and two ovoids for an intracavitary cervix treatment, or multiple catheters for an interstitial implant), a treatment unit using one source must have a means of connecting these several applicators to the machine and then directing the source to each in turn. The terminology often applied refers to this selector unit as the "indexer," which directs the source to each "channel." Transfer tubes connect the applicator elements to the indexer, so that each element is associated with a particular channel. For example, channel one may be connected to the right ovoid, channel two to the left, and channel three to the tandem.

The safety systems for HDR remote afterloaders are all aimed at minimizing the chance that an unshielded source will inappropriately expose patients or personnel. For example, this could happen if the source is advanced at the wrong time, if the source cable becomes jammed and cannot retract, or if the source assembly detaches from the cable. Every HDR remote afterloading unit includes interlocks preventing initiation of treatment if the treatment door is open, if a programmed channel has no applicator attached, etc. In addition, each unit first tests each programmed treatment channel with a dummy source before advancing the real source. If the system detects blockages or excessive friction, then the treatment is aborted. Standard features also include emergency response capabilities, such as backup batteries to cope with power failure, and a manual source retraction mechanism.

Applicators

Virtually every type of brachytherapy applicator used for low dose rate temporary implants can be, or has been, adapted for HDR (7-15). There are some constraints; the applicator, transfer tube, and HDR unit must comprise a closed system, so there is no chance that a detached source could fall freely into a patient's body. Also, the safety mechanisms that detect potential blockages limit the radius of curvature that the source will negotiate. Another consideration is the mechanical flexing that might occur as the source advances rapidly through the applicator. Although not an issue for most situations, this could be a problem for some body sites. When internal shielding has been an important element in LDR applicator design (as for Fletcher-Suit colpostats), then changes in shielding patterns occasioned by changing to HDR applicators and sources should be evaluated (14).

One of the clear advantages that HDR brachytherapy has over LDR is the short treatment times. For intracavitary work, this means that the applicator is more likely to remain at the intended position over the course of treatment and also may permit more packing, retraction, or shielding than would be tolerated for an LDR treatment.

Facilities

An HDR brachytherapy program consists of several important elements which should be considered when developing a facility: implantation, imaging, planning, treatment, and applicator removal. It is perhaps obvious, but carefully thinking through the entire process for every type of anticipated implant is important for developing an efficient facility. What imaging will be needed: radiography, fluoroscopy, ultrasound? Will anesthesia be required? Are hospital gases and vacuum available? Can the imaging be done in the same room and on the same table as the implantation? A dedicated HDR suite which includes imaging equipment and an adjacent room for planning is preferable to sharing space with an existing simulator or external beam treatment unit. Sharing space means taking one machine out of service whenever the other is being used, which is often not cost effective. Keeping the planning area close to the treatment room is useful for efficiency and for dealing with unanticipated eventualities which require plans to be modified, but it is also important to have the planning team isolated enough to allow uninterrupted concentration.

The shielding requirements for each facility need to be evaluated, but 5 to 7 cm of lead or 35 to 50 cm of concrete are typically needed for Ir-192 (16,17).

Treatment Planning—General Concerns

The general principles for planning high dose rate brachytherapy treatments are the same as for any type of brachytherapy. One needs a dosimetric model of a single source giving the absorbed dose rate per unit source strength as a function of position around the source, and then the dose distribution for an array of sources is built by superimposing contributions from each source. The plan is then evaluated by analyzing the dose distribution within the target and normal structures, if explicitly identified, or with respect to the applicators, if not. What then is different for HDR planning? One aspect is the radiobiological consequence of operating at high dose rates, but that is beyond the scope of this chapter. A second concern is that the dose delivered while the source is in motion is not included in the planning calculations. The significance of this "transit dose" is discussed below. A third aspect is that stepping source systems provide the opportunity to improve dose distributions by varying the dwell time at each position. Methods for dwell time optimization of dose distributions are presented later in this review.

HDR Source Models

HDR sources using Ir-192 are small line sources attached to drive cables. Depending on the manufacturer, the source capsules range in size from 0.6 mm diameter × 10 mm long (Varisource) to 1.1 mm diameter by 6.5 mm long (GammaMed). These line sources produce dose rates in tissue that are best described in cylindrical coordinates where the dose rate at a point depends on the radial distance from the source center and the angle measured from the source axis.

A dose calculation formalism recommended by American Association of Physicists in Medicine (AAPM) Task Group 43 (18) includes terms that characterize the different phenomena that affect the dose rate at an arbitrary point in tissue. These phenomena include the source strength, the dose rate per unit source strength at a reference point (1 cm from the source along its transverse axis), the change in dose rate occasioned by the geometric extent of the source material, the change along the transverse axis caused by attenuation and scatter in tissue, and the change off the axis caused by attenuation within the source material and encapsulation. Data have been published for one HDR source in terms of the TG-43 formalism (19). More generally, data have been both measured and calculated using Monte Carlo techniques for HDR sources (20-22).

At the present time, most treatment planning systems use calculation methods less sophisticated than the TG-43 methodology. The simplest source models treat the radiation as coming from an isotropic point source, ignoring the physical extent of the source and its encapsulation, and reducing the dose rate dependency to a function of distance only. Such a model can speed the dose calculations but sacrifice accuracy, especially in regions relatively close to the source, i.e. at distances less than about three times the source length.

This simple model is improved in some planning systems by incorporating a one-dimensional anisotropy factor that depends on angle, but not distance, from the source (21,22). To illustrate the magnitude of the anisotropy effect, consider an endobronchial application using a common HDR device and associated planning system (Nucletron). For a 12 cm active length and constant dwell times, the dose rate at a prescription point 1 cm from the catheter axis at its midpoint is reduced by 6% when the anisotropy correction is turned on. The correction's effect diminishes at larger distances from the implant. This one-dimensional correction is an approximation to a two-dimensional phenomenon, but has been shown to be accurate to ±3% throughout most of the volume around the source and to ±8% for a small volume in line with the source cable (19).

The anisotropy correction itself does not account for the geometric extent of the source and its associated deviation from simple point source geometry. It has been shown, however, for the Nucletron HDR source (23) that this effect can be reduced to less than 0.5% if the prescription point is taken to be at least 1 cm from the source.

Transit Dose

The dose delivered while a stepping source is in motion is not accounted for in current planning calculations. The magnitude of the effect has been studied (24-26) and depends on the source speed, source strength, dwell times, and dwell positions. The dose delivered while the source moves within the implant may not be affected significantly if the afterloader subtracts the transit time from the destination's dwell time, as is done in at least one system. Nevertheless, the dose delivered while the source advances to the first position in a catheter and retracts from the last one is not accounted for and may be on the order of 0.1—0.15 Gy on the surface of a 2 mm catheter (24). Physicians and physicists should be aware of this deficiency in calculation models and be prepared to investigate the magnitude of the extra dose when the treatment involves a large number of source traversals.

Treatment Planning—Optimization

One of the attractions of HDR brachytherapy is the potential for tailoring the dose distributions by manipulating the dwell times. Planning systems which explicitly support HDR brachytherapy generally provide some tools for calculating dwell times in order to optimize the dose according to some explicit or implicit criteria. These useful methods improve dose distributions as a rule, but it is important that physicians and planners keep some caveats in mind.

One caveat is that spatial distribution of sources is more influential than temporal distribution, simply because the dose from one source element depends linearly on time but as the square of the distance. Correcting hot spots where applicators converge is easier than correcting cold spots where applicators are distant.

Another caveat is that any particular optimization tool has its individual range of applicability and may not work well in all cases. Just because the isodose plan is labeled "optimized" does not mean it is necessarily clinically best. For example, consider an endoesophageal treatment consisting of a single line of source positions with the dose prescribed to a distance of 1 cm from the sources. Every HDR planning system with optimization capability provides the tools to quickly and efficiently determine a pattern of dwell times that will maintain dose uniformity at the prescribed distance along the entire line. The dwell times at the ends of the line will be two to three times longer than those in the center. Closer to the sources, the highest doses will occur near these ends. (See Figure 13.1 for a similar example showing this effect.) If the obstructive disease is in the center with subclinical extensions toward the ends, one might question if the optimized distribution is clinically superior. Would it be better to keep all the dwell times uniform, leading to a naturally higher dose in the center? Or perhaps, following Jones et al (27), would it be better to specify higher doses in the center and conform the isodose surface to the presumed shape of the target? The point is that the optimization tools provided by the planning systems cannot be used uncritically. The physician must make clear to the planner what the clinical intent and concerns are, and the planner must then use the optimization tools to manipulate the dwell times to best advantage.

One should also keep in mind that optimized distributions are different than unoptimized and may cover more volume for a given set of dwell positions (28,29). A consequence is that clinical decisions about how to implant, active lengths to use, etc., may need reassessment if the change from LDR to HDR brachytherapy also includes a change in planning technique.

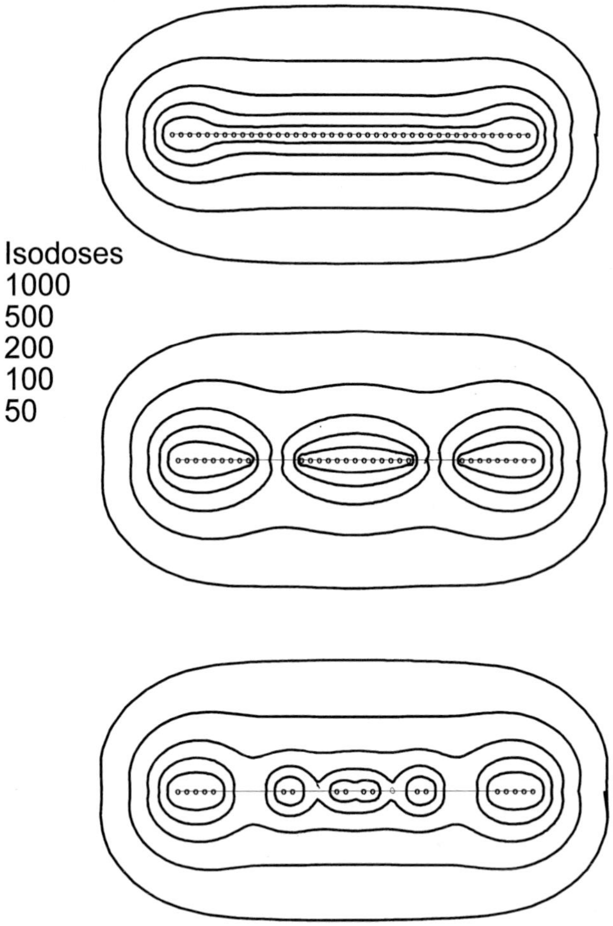

Figure 13.1. Isodose distributions for dwell time patterns optimized using three different algorithms. Each is for a 10 cm line of sources and is designed to produce a uniform dose of 1000 cGy at 2.0 cm from the sources. Top: Hill-climbing heuristic. Middle: Least squares minimization. Bottom: Linear programming.

Dose Point Optimization

Most optimization routines begin by having the planner designate a number of points in the volume and the desired dose for each point. For example, for a vaginal cylinder treatment one might locate a number of points parallel to the tandem at 0.5 cm outside the cylinder and continuing along the curved apex, and then indicate that the dose to each should equal the prescription dose. These dose points serve as constraints for the optimization code, which then searches for a pattern of dwell times that deliver the desired doses as closely as possible.

The possibilities for methods to define these dose points are many, and one way to judge a planning system is by the number of tools available for performing this task. Sometimes points are best placed relative to the applicator, such as for the vaginal cylinder example; sometimes the patient anatomy, as visualized on films or scans, is the better reference. The contour of a target volume can be sampled, for example, if that volume is visible on sequential scans. For practitioners familiar with the Paris system for interstitial implants, the basal dose points are key, and software which automatically locates them is valuable. In one system, one can essentially draw the desired isodose shape on the planning computer screen; dose points are then taken automatically from the desired isodose surface.

Once the dose points are defined, various mathematical algorithms can be used to achieve the desired doses. Among the techniques which have been used are least squares minimization (30,31), singular value decomposition (32-34), linear programming (35), simulated annealing (36), and an unnamed gradient search heuristic (37). Each technique is capable of meeting the dose constraints, but each may produce a different set of dwell times, leading to different doses at points away from the dose points. For example, Figure 13.1 displays three isodose distributions around a single treatment catheter. Each has been calculated using a different optimization algorithm but using the same dose points placed 2.0 cm from the source line. Note the similarity of the prescription isodose line and that each produces almost the same total air kerma, which is a measure of the total energy released in the implant. But notice also the difference close to the sources, which is a consequence of the different apportionment of dwell times between the available positions. The point here is that each optimization code succeeded in satisfying the problem as posed, but the different solutions have other consequences which may or may not be clinically significant. If doses nearer the sources need to be reasonably uniform, then some methods will accomplish that inherently and others will need to have additional constraints imposed, i.e. more dose points that define the problem more completely.

Geometric Optimization

An alternative to dose point optimization was developed by Edmundson (34,38). Termed "geometric optimization," this method uses the positions of the dwell positions themselves. The relative dwell time for each position depends on the sum of the inverse squares of the distances to all the other dwell positions. The more distant a dwell position is from the body of the implant, the larger its relative dwell time; the closer to the center it is, the smaller the dwell time. This algorithm uses the geometry of the implant itself to define the dwell time pattern and is most useful when the dwell positions fill the target volume fairly uniformly.

One system offers a combination of geometric and dose point optimization for multicatheter implants in which the geometric algorithm is used to apportion the total time between the catheters and then the dose point method determines the individual dwell times within each catheter (34,39).

Examples

Figure 13.2 shows isodose distributions for an idealized planar implant calculated with different optimization schemes. In each case, the prescription dose is delivered to a point 0.75 cm from the geometric center of the implant. Note the change in volume of the prescription isodose surface. Clearly, in order to cover a target of given volume, the implanted volume will decrease when optimization is employed. This observation has been made by others, at least for regular implants, with the concomitant finding that measures of dose uniformity improve with the use of optimization (28,40).

The utility of optimization has been studied for intracavitary treatment of gynecological cancers (8,10,11,41-44) using a variety of applicators. Jones et al (27,45) have shown the theoretical advantage of tailoring dose point optimization to the shape of the target structures for intraluminal treatments of the lung and esophagus, and Spratling and Speiser (46) have reviewed the role of opti-

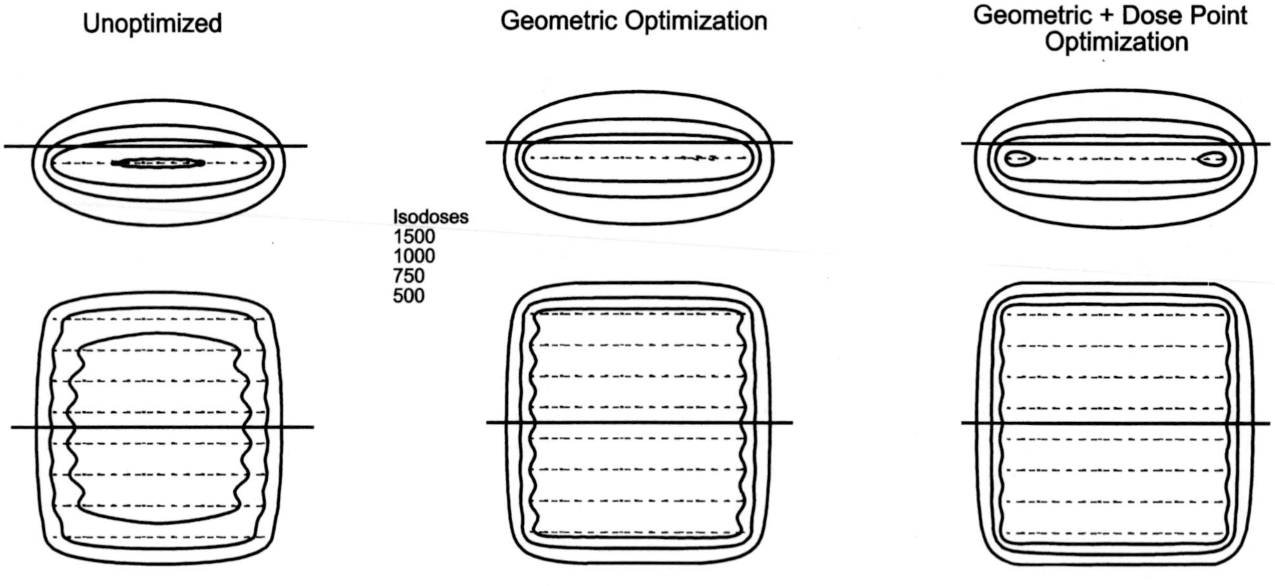

Figure 13.2. Isodose distributions for a 7×7 cm^2 planar source array for dwell times determined with different optimization algorithms. Each delivers 1000 cGy to a point 0.75 cm above the plane at its center.

mized intraluminal radiation of the bronchus in improving performance status and quality of life. Particularly elegant work has been done by Edmundson et al (47,48) on intraoperative optimization of HDR interstitial prostate implants.

In summary, optimization of dwell times has the potential for improving the physical dosimetry of brachytherapy applications. The clinician and planner must understand the new tools and communicate well together in order to maximize the benefit.

Quality Assurance

HDR brachytherapy is a complex process often performed quickly and with little opportunity for correction should errors occur. The very characteristics that make it attractive, such as fast treatment and sophisticated planning, also make the quality assurance problems more difficult. Various aspects of quality assurance for HDR brachytherapy have been addressed by a number of authors (16,49-54), and there are task group reports from the American Association of Physicists in Medicine (55-57) that are particularly relevant. It is useful to organize the discussion in terms of quality assurance of the devices on the one hand and of procedures on the other. Quality assurance of devices includes source calibration, afterloader performance, applicator characteristics, and planning system data and algorithms. Appropriate commissioning and ongoing quality control of these devices helps to prevent the kind of error that might affect a large number of patients. Procedures include the implantation, imaging and source localization, dose planning, and treatment delivery. Here the focus should be on developing methods for accurate documentation and double-checking so that the random human error that will inevitably occur has a high likelihood of being recognized and corrected.

Quality Assurance of Devices

The most fundamental requirement is that the source strength be accurately calibrated. This can be accomplished using in-air measurements with a Farmer-type chamber (58-62), in-phantom measurements (63), or most easily with a well-type ionization chamber (54,61,64,65). The manufacturer's source certificate provides a reasonability check on the local measurement, but it should not be regarded as more accurate. The source strength must be measured after each source change and should be checked periodically thereafter, at least monthly, in order to verify source decay and the ongoing operation of the remote afterloader.

It is recommended to express the source strength in units of air kerma rate at a reference distance (5,66-70), since this is the quantity that is actually measured for clinical sources and is most directly converted to absorbed dose. Use of quantities such as effective activity involves intermediate conversion factors (e.g. air kerma rate constant) that must be applied consistently in calibration and dose calculation. Inaccurate doses may be administered if this consistency is lost.

The positional and temporal accuracy of the source motion must also be assured. Positional accuracy has two components: the source positioning must be reproducible and must agree with expectation. Achieving the expected position means having correspondence between the radiographic markers used for localization and planning and the actual position of the source when extended to a programmed position. These two elements can be tested together or separately, and several techniques have been developed (4,6,16,51). For example, one can film the radiographic markers and then superimpose an autoradiograph of the source programmed to go to the same locations. Other techniques include using closed circuit television and a transparent source guide adjacent to a ruler, using a special shielded insert for a well chamber (50), using a diode imbedded next to a catheter (4), etc.

The accuracy of the dwell times should be determined. The linearity and reproducibility can be checked by integrating readings from a detector positioned close to the source for a variety of programmed dwell times. Since some charge will be accumulated during the advance and withdrawal of the source, the difference in readings obtained for two dwell times will provide a measure of the charge accumulated while the source is stationary. For example, subtracting a 5-second reading from a 6-second reading yields a net 1 second value unaffected by the transit exposure. The linearity of the timer can be assessed by finding the readings from a sequence of net times, and the absolute accuracy can be determined for a specific time using a stopwatch or the like.

Applicators should be put through a commissioning process that checks the source positioning, radiographic marker positioning, position and attenuation of any internal shields, interface to the remote afterloader, etc., and should be visually inspected before each use. It is especially critical that any applicator, commercial or otherwise, form a closed system with the remote afterloader so that a detached source cannot fall out and into the patient.

Basic safety interlocks, emergency off buttons, area radiation monitors, and indicator lights need to be checked initially and at regular intervals. Some should be checked on each day of use; others less frequently.

The treatment planning system is a key element of the treatment process. The accuracy of its input and output devices and dosimetry data, and the reliability of source localization and dose calculation routines need to be assessed initially during commissioning and also subjected to routine quality assurance tests (55,71).

A number of authors have discussed specific tests to be incorporated into a quality assurance program consisting of daily, monthly, quarterly, and/or annual procedures (6,16,51,72). Tables 13.2, 13.3, and 13.4 show some recommended checks.

A key point to be stressed is that the commissioning process for each of the devices involved in HDR brachytherapy includes understanding, documenting, testing, and training others in the intended use of the device. The output of the commissioning process should include written procedures for routine use as well as ongoing quality assurance. The next section addresses important concerns in the development of these procedures.

Table 13.2. Suggested Daily Quality Assurance Tests (Performed by Therapist)

Date, time, activity recorded by treatment unit.
Recall of standard program.
Positioning of source to within 1 mm of programmed locations.
Operation of interrupt key, door interlock, emergency off buttons.
Operation of door light.
Operation of area radiation monitor.
Operation of survey meter.
Operation of CCTV and intercom.
Operation of imaging devices.
Supply of printer paper.
Inspection of interconnect cables and applicators.
Supply of emergency response equipment.

Table 13.3. Suggested Monthly Quality Assurance Tests (Performed by Physicist)

Measure source strength.
Radiograph/autoradiograph of endobronchial, gynecologic, and interstitial applicators with localization markers.
Check operation of area radiation monitor with AC power off.
Check correct interlock function, e.g., indexer ring not latched, applicator not inserted, applicator obstructed.
Perform daily quality assurance test and review previous month's records.

Table 13.4. Suggested Quality Assurance Tests After Source Change (Performed by Physicist)

Review source change checks performed by the service engineer exchanging the sources.
Perform radiation survey of treatment unit with source retracted.
Perform radiation survey of treatment vault with source exposed.
Calibrate source strength.
Measure source strength with independent dosimetry system.
Prepare source strength decay table for new source.
Update source strength in treatment unit.
Update source strength in planning system.
Update treatment times for ongoing patients.
Perform monthly quality assurance tests.

Quality Assurance of Procedures

Unintended irradiation of patients or personnel can be the result of device malfunction, but it is more commonly caused by miscommunication, misunderstanding, or other mistakes by the humans involved. A recent study of misadministrations in HDR brachytherapy was done for the United States Nuclear Regulatory Commission (73). This analysis focused on the human factors involved in all aspects of the HDR brachytherapy process, identifying specific skills and tasks required and the accompanying opportunities for human error, and suggesting methods for reducing the likelihood of such errors. With this background information in hand, Task Group 59 (56) of the Radiation Therapy Committee of the American Association of Physicists in Medicine has prepared a report on HDR treatment delivery safety. The main points of their recommendations are to use written documentation, develop formal procedures, and double-check all key decision points. These recommendations overlap, of course. A formal procedure should be written and include pertinent checklists and forms; these forms should highlight key data points for double-checking.

The NRC and AAPM reports emphasize that some problems can make errors more likely, such as inadequate training, poor intrateam communication, confusing computer-human interfaces, difficult working conditions, and excessive time pressure. Alleviating these difficulties will reduce the chance of error. Nevertheless, even when conditions are optimal, random human error will sometimes occur. It is important to recognize the inevitability of such events and to design a program in which they are identified and corrected before the safety of patient or staff is compromised.

One should consider developing specific checklists for each type of application (endobronchial, vaginal cylinder, etc.) and include items for: pre-application inspection and testing of applicators and remote afterloading unit; documentation of the insertion and target definition; localization filming; completeness of prescription; documentation of optimization method and criteria; verification of data input for treatment planning; assessment of the reasonability of the dose calculations and plan; and verification of the programming of the remote afterloader. Such forms are valuable for ensuring that important items are not overlooked, that crucial data elements are documented and available for checking. The forms also become the framework for initial and ongoing training.

Checking the reasonability of the dose calculations with manual techniques is an important quality assurance tool. Several authors have published methods of quantitatively verifying HDR computer calculations to a precision of a few percent for different types of applications, such as single line (74,75), two-catheter endobronchial (76), planar (77), and volume (37,78). These techniques relate the total energy released, in terms of the product of source strength and total time, to the prescribed dose and some measure of implant size. Such a check is best performed by someone other than the primary planner using input data derived independently from the computer system. One group has also developed a means of using a diode-based dosimetry system to check the dose to a point on the patient's skin early in the progress of the treatment (79).

Emergency Procedures

High dose rate remote afterloaders have the potential for creating particularly hazardous emergency situations. Should the HDR source be lodged within the patient (either through failure of the drive mechanism, detachment of the source from the cable, or rupture of the source capsule), then the patient's tissues may be exposed to hundreds of cGy/minute while the operator entering the room to handle the emergency may be exposed to dose rates of about 1 cGy/minute. Since typical fractional doses to patients are a few hundred cGy and the annual exposure limit for personnel corresponds to 5 cGy, then the emergency response must be rapid and effective in order to prevent injury to the patient and personnel.

Every HDR facility must have written emergency procedures and a training program for all operators. The training should include how to recognize an emergency situation and how to deal with the potential variations for every type. Practice with a dummy source replacing the actual source is important.

Although specific emergency procedures depend on the remote afterloader involved, there are some common elements. The operator will: 1) recognize that an emergency exists, 2) press an emergency off button at or near the console, 3) enter the room with a survey meter and check the radiation levels using it and the area radiation monitor, 4) if high radiation levels persist, press an emergency off button on the remote afterloader, 5) if high radiation levels persist, retract the source manually, 6) if high radiation levels persist, remove the applicator from the patient and, if possible, place it in an emergency container, 7) remove the patient from the room and verify with a survey that the source is removed.

As mentioned above, it is critically important that the afterloader-transfer tubes-applicator remain a closed system so that the source elements cannot become lost within the patient's body. It is important to have procedures written and practiced so that each type of applicator can be quickly and safely removed. This may be particularly problematic in the case of interstitial catheters held in place with sutures and buttons. Each facility should have a dedicated emergency response kit containing long forceps, clamps, suture removal kit, betadine and swabs, suture kit, and flashlight. Outside the room, survey meters and emergency signs need to be available.

Personnel and Time Commitment

It is easy to underestimate the time required to set up a good HDR brachytherapy program. The afterloading devices themselves are simple machines compared to multimodality linear accelerators, but commissioning an afterloader itself is perhaps the smallest part of the task. Bringing the program on-line also requires licensing with regulatory agencies; commissioning a treatment planning system; developing detailed procedures that may be quite different from others already in place within the department; and training physicians, planners, and operators to capably handle routine and emergency situations. It is a task that should be measured in weeks, if not months, depending on the experience of the physicist undertaking the assignment.

References

1. International Commission of Radiation Units and Measurements. Dose and Volume Specification for Reporting Intracavitary Therapy in Gynecology, ICRU Report No. 38. Bethesda, MD: ICRU, 1985.
2. Meli JA. Dosimetry of some interstitial and intracavitary sources and their applicators. In: Williamson J, Thomadsen B, and Nath R, eds. Brachytherapy Physics. Madison, Wisconsin: Medical Physics Publishing Corporation, 1995.
3. Glasgow GP. Principles of remote afterloading devices. In: Williamson J, Thomadsen B, and Nath R eds. Brachytherapy Physics. Madison, WI: Medical Physics Publishing Corporation, 1995.
4. Glasgow GP, Bourland JD, Grigsby PW, et al. Remote afterloading technology: report of the American Association of Physicists in Medicine Task Group 41. New York: American Institute of Physics, 1993.
5. Chenery SGA, Pla M, Podgorsak EB. Physical characteristics of the Selectron high dose rate intracavitary afterloader. Brit J Radiol 1985; 58:735-740.
6. Williamson JF, Ezzell GA, Olch A, et al. Quality assurance for high dose rate brachytherapy. In: Nag S ed. High Dose Rate Brachytherapy: A Textbook. Armonk, NY: Futura Publishing Co, 1994.
7. Griffin PC, Amin PA, Hughes P, et al. Pelvic mass: CT-guided interstitial catheter implantation with high-dose-rate remote afterloader. Radiology 1994;191:581-583.
8. Maruyama Y, Ezzell GA, Porter AT. Afterloading high dose rate intracavitary vaginal cylinder. Int J Radiat Oncol Biol Phys 1994;30:473-476.
9. Meigooni AS, Zhu Y, Williamson JF, et al. Design and dosimetric characteristics of a high dose rate remote afterloaded endocavitary applicator system. Int J Radiat Oncol Biol Phys 1996;34:1153-1163.
10. Nair MT, Cheng MC, Barker A, et al. High dose rate (HDR) brachytherapy technique: for carcinoma of uterine cervix using Nucletron applicators. Medical Dosimetry 1995;20:201-207.
11. Noyes WR, Peters NE, Thomadsen BR, et al: Impact of "optimized" treatment planning for tandem and ring, and tandem and ovoids, using high dose rate brachytherapy for cervical cancer. Int J Radiat Oncol Biol Phys 1995;31:79-86.
12. Perera F, Chisela F, Engel J, et al. Method of localization and implantation of the lumpectomy site for high dose rate brachytherapy after conservative surgery for T1 and T2 breast cancer. Int J Radiat Oncol Biol Phys 1995;31:959-965.
13. Pla C, Evans MDC, Podgorsak EB. Dose distributions around Selectron applicators. Int J Radiat Oncol Biol Phys 1987;13:1761-1766.
14. Verellen D, DeNeve W. Van den Heuvel F, et al. On the determination of the effective transmission factor for stainless steel ovoid shielding

segments and estimation of their shielding efficacy for the clinical situation. Med Physics 1994;21:1677-1684.

15. Waterman FM, Holcomb DE. Dose distributions produced by a shielded vaginal cylinder using a high-activity iridium-192 source. Med Physics 1994;21:101-106.
16. Ezzell GA. Commissioning of single stepping-source remote afterloaders. In: Williamson J, Thomadsen B, and Nath R eds. Brachytherapy Physics. Madison, Wisconsin: Medical Physics Publishing Corporation, 1995.
17. Klein EE, Grigsby PW, Williamson JF, et al. Pre-installation empirical testing of room shielding for high dose rate remote afterloaders. Int J Radiat Oncol Biol Phys 1993;27:927-931.
18. Nath R, Anderson LL, Luxton G, et al. Dosimetry of interstitial brachytherapy sources recommendations of the AAPM Radiation Therapy Committee Task Group 43. Medical Physics 1995;22:209-234.
19. Williamson JF, Li Z. Monte Carlo aided dosimetry of the microSelectron pulsed and high dose-rate Ir-192 sources. Med Physics 1995;22: 809-819.
20. Fessenden KK. Monte Carlo dose calculations about a high intensity Ir-192 source of high dose rate brachytherapy. Med Physics, 1995; 22:903.
21. Mishra V, Waterman FM, Suntharalingam N. Anisotropy of an iridium-192 high dose rate source measured with a miniature ionization chamber. Med Physics 1997;24:751-755.
22. Muller-Runkel R, Cho SH. Anisotropy measurements of a high dose rate Ir-192 source in air and polystyrene. Med Physics 1994;21:1131-1134.
23. Podgorsak MB, DeWerd LA, Paliwal BR, et al. Accuracy of the point source approximation to high dose rate Ir-192 sources. Medical Dosimetry 1995;20:177-181.
24. Bastin KT, Podgorsak MS, Thomadsen B. The transit dose component of high dose-rate brachytherapy: Direct measurements and clinical implications. Int J Radiat Oncol Biol Phys 1993; 26:695-702.
25. Houdek PV, Glasgow GP, Schwade J, et al. Design and implementation of a program for high dose rate brachytherapy. In: Nag S ed. High Dose Rate Brachytherapy: A Textbook. Armonk, New York: Futura Publishing Co, 1994.
26. Houdek PV, Schwade JG, Wu X, et al. Dose determination in high dose rate brachytherapy. Int J Radiat Oncol Biol Phys 1992;24:795-801.
27. Jones B, Bleasdale C, Tan LT, et al. The achievement of isoeffective bronchial mucosal dose during endobronchial brachytherapy. Int J Radiat Oncol Biol Phys 1995;33:195-199.
28. Kolkman-Deruloo IK, Visser AG, Niel CG, et al: Optimization of interstitial volume implants. Radiother Oncol 1994;31:229-234.
29. van der Laarse R. The stepping source dosimetry system as an extension of the Paris system. In: Mould RF, Battermann JJ, Martinez AA, et al, eds. Brachytherapy from Radium to Optimization. Veenendaal, the Netherlands: Nucletron Corporation, 1994.
30. Anderson LL. Treatment optimization with the Gamma-med II Proceedings of the First Symposium on Gamma-med Remote Afterloading. Bronx, NY: Mick Radio-Nuclear Instruments, Inc., 1985:18-27.
31. Anderson LL. Plan optimization and dose evaluation in brachytherapy. Seminars in Radiation Oncology 1993; 3:290-300.
32. van der Laarse R, de Boer RW. Computerized high dose rate brachytherapy treatment planning. In: Martinez AA, Orton CG, Mould RF, eds. Brachytherapy HDR and LDR. Columbia, MD: Nucletron Corporation; 1990:169-183.
33. van der Laarse R, Edmundson GK, Luthmann RW, et al. Optimization of HDR brachytherapy dose distributions. Activity—The Selectron User's Newsletter 1991;5:94-101.
34. van der Laarse R, Prins TPE. Introduction to HDR brachytherapy optimisation. In: Mould RF, Battermann JJ, Martinez AA, et al, eds. Brachytherapy from Radium to Optimization. Veenendaal, the Netherlands: Nucletron Corporation, 1994.
35. Renner WD, O'Conner TP, Bermudez NM. An algorithm for generation of implant plans for high-dose-rate irradiators. Medical Physics 1990;17:35-40.
36. Sloboda RS. Optimization of brachytherapy dose distributions by simulated annealing. Medical Physics 1992;19:955-964.
37. Ezzell GA, Luthmann RW. Clinical implementation of dwell time optimization techniques for single stepping-source remote applicators. In: Williamson J, Thomadsen B, and Nath R, eds. Brachytherapy Physics. Madison, Wisconsin: Medical Physics Publishing Corporation, 1994.
38. Edmundson GK. Geometry based optimization for stepping source implants. In: Martinez AA, Orton CG, and Mould RF, eds. Brachytherapy HDR and LDR. Columbia, MD: Nucletron Corporation, 1990:184-192.
39. Thomadsen BR, Houdek PV, Van der Laarse R, et al. Treatment planning and optimization. In: Nag S ed. High Dose Rate Brachytherapy: A Textbook. Armonk, NY: Futura Publishing Co., 1994.
40. Low DA, Williamson JF. The evaluation of optimized implants for idealized implant geometries. Med Physics 1995;22:1477-1485.
41. Houdek PV, Schwade JG, Abitol AA, et al. Optimization of high dose-rate cervix brachytherapy: Part I: Dose Distribution. Int J Radiat Oncol Biol Phys 1991;21:1621-1625.
42. Niel CG, Koper PC, Visser AG, et al. Optimizing brachytherapy for locally advanced cervical cancer. Int J Radia Oncol Biol Phys 1994; 2:873-877.
43. Stitt JA, Fowler JF, Thomadsen BR, et al: High dose rate intracavitary brachytherapy for carcinoma of the cervix: The Madison system: I. Clinical and radiobiological considerations Int J Radiat Oncol Biol Phys 1992;24:335-348.
44. Thomadsen BR, Shahabi S, Stitt JA, et al: High dose rate intracavitary brachytherapy for carcinoma of the cervix: The Madison system: II. Procedural and physical considerations. Int J Radiat Oncol Biol Phys 1992,24:349-357.
45. Jones B, Tan LT, Freestone G, et al. Non-uniform dwell times in line source high dose rate brachytherapy: physical and radiobiological considerations. Physics in Medicine and Biology 1994;67:1231-1237.
46. Spratling L, Speiser BL. Endoscopic brachytherapy. Chest Surgery Clinics of North America 1996;6:293-304.
47. Edmundson GK, Rizzo NR, Teahan M, et al. Concurrent treatment planning for high dose rate prostate template implants. Int J Radiat Oncol Biol Phys 1993; 27:1215-1223.
48. Edmundson GK, Yan D, Martinez AA. Intraoperative optimization of needle placement and dwell times for conformal prostate brachytherapy. Int J Radiat Oncol Biol Phys 1995; 33: 1257–1263.
49. Aldrich JE, Samant SS. Technical note: an integrated phantom ~ for HDR quality control. Brit J Radiol. 1993; 66:363-365.
50. DeWerd LA, Jursinic P, Kitchen R,. et al. Quality assurance tool for high dose rate brachytherapy. Med Physics 1995; 22:435-440.
51. Ezzell GA. Acceptance testing and quality assurance for high dose-rate remote afterloading systems. In: Martinez AA, Orton CG, Mould RF, eds. Brachytherapy HDR and LDR. Columbia MD: Nucletron Corporation, 1990:138-159.
52. Ezzell GA. Quality assurance in HDR brachytherapy: physical and technical aspects. Selectron Brachytherapy Journal 1991; 5:59-62.
53. Flynn A. Quality assurance checks on a MicroSelectron-HDR. Selectron Brachytherapy Journal 1990;4:112-115.
54. Jones, CH. HDR microSelectron quality-assurance studies using a well-type ionization chamber. Physics in Medicine and Biology 1995; 40:95-101.
55. Kutcher GJ, Cola L, Gillin M, et al. Comprehensive quality assurance for radiation oncology: Report of AAPM Radiation Therapy Committee Task Group 40. Med Phys 1994;21:581-601.
56. Kubo HD, Glasgow GP, Pethel TD, et al. HDR treatment delivery safety: Report of the AAPM Radiation Therapy Committee Task Group 59. Medical Physics. 1998;25:375-403.
57. Nath R, Anderson LL, Meli JA, et al. Code of practice for brachytherapy physics: Report of the AAPM Radiation Therapy Committee Task Group 56. Med Physics. 1997;24:1557-1598.
58. DeWerd LA, Ezzell GA, Williamson JF. Calibration Principle ~ and Techniques. In: Nag S, ed. High Dose Rate Brachytherapy: A Textbook. Armonk. NY. Futura Publishing Co., 1994.
59. DeWerd LA, Thomadsen BR: Source Strength Standards and Calibration of HDR/PDR Sources. In: Williamson J, Thomadsen B, Nath R, eds. Brachytherapy Physics, Madison, WI: Medical Physics Publishing Corporation, 1995.
60. Ezzell GA. Evaluation of calibration techniques for the MicroSelectron HDR. In Mould RF, ed. Brachytherapy 2: Proceedings of the 5th International Selectron User's Meeting. Leersum, The Netherlands: Nucletron International BV, 1989:61-69.
61. Goetsch SJ, Attix FH, Pearson DW, et al. Calibration of Ir-192 high-dose-rate afterloadinq systems. Med Phys 1991;18:462-467.

62. Venselaar JL, Brouwer WF, van Straaten BH, et al. Intercomparison of calibration procedures for Ir-192 HDR sources in The Netherlands and Belgium. Radiother Oncol 1994;30:155-161.
63. Steggerda MJ, Mignheer BJ. Replacement corrections of a Farmer-type ionization chamber for the calibration of Cs-137 and Ir-192 sources in a solid phantom. Radiother Oncol 1994;31:76–84.
64. Goetsch SJ, Attix FH, DeWerd LA, et al. A new re-entrant ionization chamber for the calibration of iridium-192 high dose rate sources. Int J Radiat Oncol Biol Phys 1992;24:167-170.
65. Ho AK, Sibata CH, deSouza CN, et al. Evaluation of a well-type ionization chamber for calibration of HDR and LDR brachytherapy sources. Medical Dosimetry 1995;20:31-34.
66. American Association of Physicists in Medicine, Task Group 32. Specification of brachytherapy source strength. New York: American Institute of Physics, 1987.
67. British Committee on Radiation Units and Measurements. Specification of brachytherapy sources. Brit J Radiol 1984;57:941-942.
68. Comite Francais Mesure des Rayonnements Ionisants. Recommendations pour la determination des doses Absorbees en Curietherapie, CFMRI Report No. 1. Paris: Bureau National de Metrologie, 1983.
69. Williamson JF, Anderson LL, Grigsby PW, et al. American Endocurietherapy Society recommendations for specification of brachytherapy source strength. Endocurietherapy/Hyperthermia Oncol 1993;9: 1-7.
70. Williamson JF, Nath R. Clinical implementation of AAPM Task Group 32 recommendations on brachytherapy source strength specifications. Med Physics 1991;18:439-449.
71. Neblett DL, Wesick JS. Quality Assurance of computer-assisted treatment planning. In: Williamson J, Thomadsen B, and Nath R, eds. Brachytherapy Physics. Madison, WI: Medical Physics Publishing Corporation, 1995.
72. Jones CH. Quality assurance in brachytherapy using the Selectron LDR/MDR and MicroSelectron-HDR. Selectron Brachytherapy Journal 1990;4:48-52.
73. United States Nuclear Regulatory Commission. Quality Management in Remote Afterloading Brachytherapy. United States Nuclear Regulatory Commission, NUREG/CR-6276: Washington, D.C., 1995.
74. Ahmad M, Fontenla DP, Curran J et al. Fast verification of treatment time for single-catheter HDR brachytherapy. Endocurietherapy/Hyperthermia Oncol 1995; 11:179-183.
75. Kubo H, Chin RB. Simple mathematical formulas for quick-checking of single-catheter high dose rate brachytherapy treatment plans. Endocurietherapy/Hyperthermia Oncol. 1992;8:165-169.
76. Miller AV, Davis MG, Horton JL. A method for verifying treatment times for simple high-dose-rate endobronchial brachytherapy procedures. Med Physics 1996;23:1903-1908.
77. Ezzell G. Quality assurance of treatment plans for optimized high dose rate brachytherapy–planar implants. Med Phys 1994; 21:659-661.
78. Venselaar JLM, Bierhuizen HWJ, Klop Rien. A method to check treatment time calculations in Ir-192 high-dose-rate implants. Med Phys, 1995;22:1499-1500.
79. Alecu R, Feldmeier JJ, Court WS et al. A method to avoid misadministrations in high dose rate brachytherapy. Med Phys 1997; 24:259-262.

Chapter 14

Clinical Applications of Low Dose Rate and High Dose Rate Brachytherapy

Judith Anne Stitt and Bruce Robert Thomadsen

DEVELOPMENT OF LOW DOSE RATE AND HIGH DOSE RATE BRACHYTHERAPY

The treatment of cancer with radioactive sources using topical molds and intracavitary radium demonstrated the efficacy of brachytherapy long before external radiation therapy became common practice. Source handling during the infancy of brachytherapy utilized radioisotopes preloaded into the applicator before placement into the patient (1). Liabilities of this type of source handling include exposure not only to the physician who inserted and positioned the applicator and isotope, but also nursing and other personnel in the procedure suite and hospital room. Manual afterloading applicators developed for use with low dose rate (LDR) sources decreased the exposure to personnel since the sources were loaded into the applicator after the positioning was correct and dosimetry films were obtained (2,3). Computer-controlled remote afterloading developed at the Radiumhemmet allowed for complete radiation safety for medical and nursing staff, hospital personnel, and visitors (4). This advance eliminated personnel exposure and expanded the options for customized therapy by remotely controlling the source position.

High Dose Rate Brachytherapy

Remote afterloading with high-intensity sources was introduced by Henschke and Hilaris in the 1960s (2,5). Low dose rate is considered less than 1.2 Gy/hr, while high dose rate (HDR) therapy is considered treatment delivered with durations that are short compared to the half-time of cellular repair of sublethal damage (about 1.5 h), so the duration should be less than 0.5 Gy/hr. With this technology a dose rate of 100-300 cGy/minute approaches that of linear accelerators. Treatment is given in multiple fractions that last minutes instead of continuous treatment which requires several days of inpatient therapy. High dose rate remote afterloading brachytherapy resulted from the development of new computer-controlled treatment units, modification of treatment techniques for outpatient therapy, altered dose schedules of external beam and intracavitary or interstitial irradiation, and revised dose specification definitions (6).

The development of high-intensity sources has promoted the clinical and technologic innovations of HDR brachytherapy (7–9). Clinical advantages of HDR brachytherapy include outpatient treatment, avoidance of general anesthesia for most patients, and elimination of complications resulting from prolonged bed rest. HDR brachytherapy can provide improved physical dose delivery because of the short treatment time and fixed applicator positioning, and optimized dosimetry with a computer-controlled stepping source. Technologic advances include reduced possibility of human error through computer driven afterloading and improved radiation safety and protection with HDR remote afterloading units (10).

Disadvantages of HDR brachytherapy relate to the potential for the large radiation doses that can be delivered if strict attention is not paid to treatment planning and delivery. Early clinical trials of HDR brachytherapy for cervical cancer demonstrated higher bladder and bowel complications if time, dose, and distance effects on normal tissues were not observed (11). An additional risk when moving from LDR to HDR brachytherapy treatment schedules is the potential for decreased tumor control in curative applications, such as for cervical carcinoma. Certain clinical applications of HDR brachytherapy require considerable intensity and time commitment of physics and dosimetry staff to perform simulation and treatment planning in a timely manner. This may increase the demand on physics staffing and availability.

High dose rate brachytherapy is being used more widely for curative treatment of gynecologic and urologic cancer, palliation of endoluminal obstruction from lung and esophageal cancer, and for a variety of interstitial treatments. The technical application ranges from multiple fractions of atlas-generated treatments to customized treatment with computer optimized plans for each fraction. The American Brachytherapy Society published a consensus report of the Clinical Education Committee describing guidelines for HDR brachytherapy for treatment of a variety of clinical sites (12). It is mandatory for each brachytherapy treatment center to develop and follow consistent treatment polices in a controlled fashion with complete documentation of treatment parameters and outcome including efficacy and morbidity.

The development of HDR brachytherapy technology has encouraged integration of external beam therapy and brachytherapy with novel approaches. Because HDR brachytherapy is a daily fractionated treatment the sequence of brachytherapy and external beam can be manipulated to decrease overall treatment time. Several clinical trials in head and neck and cervical cancer demonstrated that prolonged treatment courses lead to decreased tumor control (13–15). Additionally, brachytherapy can be given on the same day as external beam therapy if the isotope treatment volume is shielded. Institutions embarking upon HDR programs are obligated to examine fractionation schemes with regard to the number of HDR fractions, dose per fraction, and the fashion in which isotope and external therapy are integrated.

Low Dose Rate Brachytherapy

Low dose rate brachytherapy has decades of clinical history demonstrating the efficacy of radioactive isotope treatment in the management of cancer as boost therapy for well defined tumor volumes. Moving from LDR to other levels of dose-rate treatment carries the concern that tumor control may not be maintained at the levels achieved with the previous standard. While normal tissue effects may become evident within a short time of treatment, local disease control may take longer to observe.

Low dose rate gynecologic techniques have depended heavily on the "art" of clinical experience in applicator insertion and packing to achieve and maintain the anatomic position needed for appropriate dose distribution. Institutions with large patient numbers and thus greater clinical expertise with insertion techniques have established the standards for toxicity and local control rates in gynecologic cancer treated with LDR therapy (16–18).

Brachytherapy techniques for LDR therapy require a lower concentration of medical, physics, and nursing staff during the insertion and treatment course. Applicator insertion, treatment planning, and treatment are carried out over hours to days rather than minutes to hours as with HDR techniques.

ADVANTAGES AND DISADVANTAGES OF HIGH DOSE RATE BRACHYTHERAPY

HDR brachytherapy offers many advantages over conventional LDR brachytherapy. Advantages are present in clinical aspects of patient management, technical approaches to applicator positioning as well as physics and dosimetry procedures. Some of the major advantages include:

Dose optimization capability: HDR brachytherapy planning allows better optimization of the isodose distributions to the shapes of the treatment volume compared to low dose rate brachytherapy. Because of the relatively large size of many LDR sources and the limited number of source strengths available for a given implant, optimization with conventional LDR brachytherapy is more difficult, and, in most cases less satisfactory, than with HDR brachytherapy. Each HDR dwell position may assume treatment times from zero and 999 seconds in 0.1 second intervals, thus offering the possibility of weighting the dwell times at the various dwell positions to sculpt the dose distribution within the rules of physics. The capability is a double-edged sword as discussed below under disadvantages.

Outpatient treatment: Most HDR procedures last only a few hours. Patients are treated in outpatient facilities, thus eliminating overnight hospital cost, one of the most expensive components of health care.

More stable positioning: The short duration of HDR procedures, particularly gynecologic insertions, allows immobilization of both the patient and the appliance during the important period between localization imaging and the completion of treatment. With LDR brachytherapy, King documented movements of applicators of up to 2 cm over the course of treatment (19). Thomadsen et al studied the movements of the applicator for HDR cervical applications and found an average shift of less than 3 mm at the end of treatment compared with the applicator's location on the localization films (10).

Increased distance to normal tissues: Intracavitary therapy often allows placement of retractors or packing to push normal tissue away from the source dwell positions, thereby lowering the dose to critical structures. While retraction of normal tissues via packing is sometimes possible during LDR treatments, patients tolerate increased distention over the short duration of the HDR treatments compared to the several days' treatment time for LDR.

Smaller applicators: The iridium-192 (Ir-192) source for HDR units approximates the diameter of the nylon ribbon that carries LDR iridium seeds. Some HDR sources are even smaller, passing through a 21-gauge needle. For intracavitary applications, the small size means that intrauterine tandems can be smaller than with LDR Cesium sources. The typical 3-mm diameter HDR tandem passes through the cervical canal without dilatation which is required for the use of a 7-mm LDR tandem.

No treatment delay for source shipment: Not infrequently, interstitial implants change considerably in the operating room compared to the previously calculated plan. Most commonly, the implanted volume increases in size. Using LDR iridium-192 sources requires ordering additional sources following the generation of the new plan. HDR brachytherapy still requires the generation of a new plan, but the patient can be treated immediately following the calculation of new dwell times, thus extending the duration of treatment only minimally.

Better documentation: Because an HDR unit requires programming of the dwell times for activated dwell positions, the printout of the program provides documentation of the treatment intention. During treatment, the HDR unit logs each movement of the source, indicating the dwell position (and the position location, if relevant) and the time the source spends at that location, the time that treatment begins and ends, and any abnormalities occurring during the treatment. Documentation of LDR treatments exist only if someone happens to write in the patient's chart.

Reduction of radiation exposure to health care providers: Because only the patient remains in the shielded treatment room during the delivery of therapy, no staff person receives exposure from this part of the procedure. This reduction not only affects the therapist, physician, and physicist who otherwise would prepare and load the LDR applicator, but also greatly reduces the amount of radiation received by the nursing staff caring for the patient. HDR brachytherapy does not eliminate nursing exposure if the unit is housed close to the procedure table during an insertion. A typical unit with a new source delivers approximately 2.5 uSv/h (0.25 mR/h) at 1 m. A nurse sitting at this distance for 1 h/procedure × 15 procedures/week receives approximately 150 uSv/month (15 mR/month). While just measurable with most personnel dosimeters, this exposure remains below that of nurses attending patients containing LDR radioactive sources. An exposure of this nature can be reduced by judicial placement of the unit with respect to nursing necessities during the insertion. Other personnel still receive some secondary radiation during fluoroscopy performed as part of the HDR procedure, but that remains the same with either HDR or LDR modalities.

LDR remote afterloaders also eliminate radiation exposure to personnel. While available since the early 1970s and common in Europe and Canada, few remote units have been sold in the United States. Thus, the advantage of eliminating personnel exposure apparently did not justify the cost of such units. The capacity for outpatient treatment with HDR units appears to be the advantage that drives the remote afterloader market.

High dose rate brachytherapy also has its down side. Disadvantages relate to the intensity of physics and dosimetry labor and the potential for a serious overdose, and limited follow-up of clinical results compared with LDR therapy. Some of the major disadvantages include:

Potential for increased late radiation injuries: As the dose rate of radiotherapy delivery increases, the biologic effectiveness of the radiation increases, so that 1 Gy delivered over 2 h with conventional LDR brachytherapy produces less biologic damage than that same gray delivered in 2 minutes with an HDR approach. The absolute amount of the increase in biologic effectiveness depends on many variables, but one of the most important is the tissue type. Generally, normal tissues exhibit a larger increase in the effectiveness than tumor cells. This differential in the biologic effectiveness translates into a relative disadvantage in the therapeutic ratio for HDR brachytherapy compared to LDR. The therapeutic ratio reflects the effectiveness of a given treatment to produce a desired endpoint, such as killing tumor cells, compared to the detrimental effect on health tissue.

The effect of dose rate on the therapeutic ratio is shown in Figure 14.1A. The therapeutic ratio becomes difficult to measure in practice because the value for the quantity varies with the exact endpoint used to measure "effectiveness." The figure shows the inverse of the therapeutic ratio (i.e., the worsening of normal tissue response compared to tumor cell kill) with the increase in dose rate. Clearly, therapeutic ratio suffers at the high dose rates (20). The data in Figure 14.1B is the same data as in Figure 14.1A except that the dose rate is plotted logarithmically, making the effects at the lower dose rates more evident. Figure 14.2 shows the percentage of improvement in the therapeutic ratio for each additional fraction added. Changing from one fraction to two produces a 6% improvement (21). However, increasing from six fractions to seven only yields an improvement of 3%. Each additional fraction carries a price with it, both in patient discomfort and inconvenience and in staffing and supplies.

No correct number of fractions exist; each facility must decide on a compromise between the benefits and costs when establishing a treatment regimen. That regimen may differ for various treatment sites. For example, curative cases of cancer of the cervix treated with a tandem and ovoid may need five fractions, while two fractions may suffice for postoperative treatment of the vaginal cuff following hysterectomy for cancer of the corpus. The difference in biologic responsiveness between normal and malignant cells also forces a decision if an institution attempts to match the biologic effects of HDR protocols with established LDR schedules.

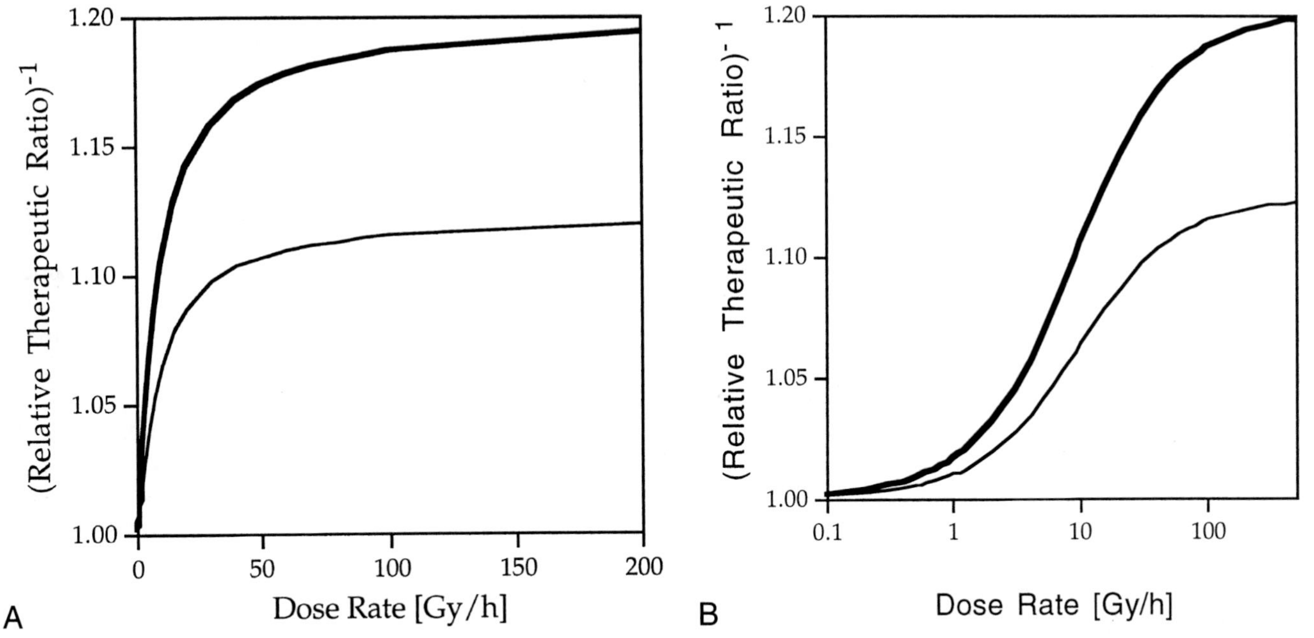

Figure 14.1. **A.** The effect of dose rate (0-200 Gy/h) on the inverse of the therapeutic ratio. The thick line corresponds to the relative effects of irradiation on normal tissue such as spinal cord (α/β = 2, $T_{1/2}$ = 1.5h) versus damage to an aggressive tumor (α/β = 20, $T_{1/2}$ = 0.5h). The thin line compares the effect on normal connective tissue (α/β = 3, $T_{1/2}$ = 1.5h) to that of a fairly typical carcinoma (α/β = 10, $T_{1/2}$ = 1.5h). Normal tissue response worsens with increasing dose rate relative to tumor kill. **B.** The effect of dose rate, plotted logarithmically, on the inverse of the therapeutic ratio. The same data as in **A** is displayed, except with the dose rate plotted logarithmically, making the effects at the lower dose rates more visible. The therapeutic ratio varies little with dose rate in the LDR (less than 1 Gy/h) and HDR (greater than 75 Gy/h) regions, but varies rapidly over the middle dose rate region.

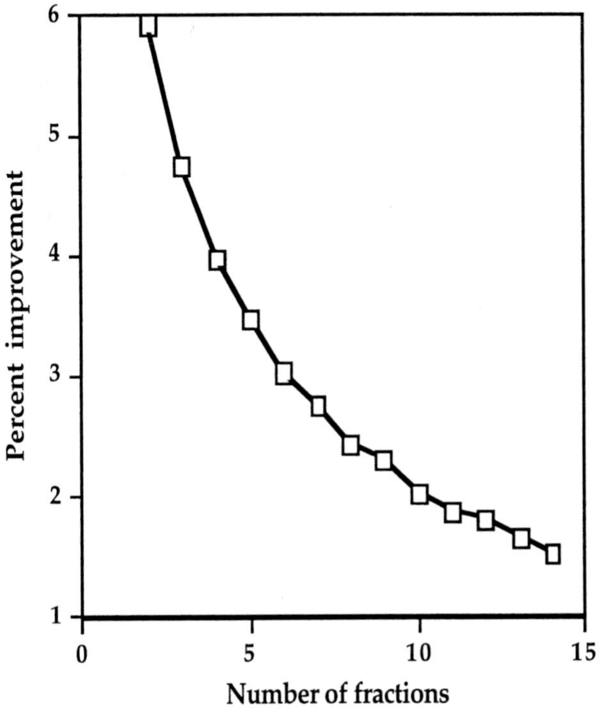

Figure 14.2. Percentage improvement in therapeutic ratio compared to the use of one less fraction. Increasing the number of fractions reduces the relative damage to normal tissue per unit cell kill, but the improvement decreases with each additional fraction added.

Increased need for dosimetric, anatomic, and geometric information: Maintaining doses below levels that would compromise healthy tissues which may be at greater risk with HDR than with LDR brachytherapy requires more accurate anatomic and geometric information. Optimization, as practiced with HDR brachytherapy, requires a better knowledge of the dose distribution desired than most LDR treatments. Use of computer tomography (CT) or magnetic resonance imaging (MRI) can be useful in evaluating the target and tumor volumes.

Relatively complicated treatment systems: Several aspects of HDR treatments add to the complexity of the system. To deliver treatment, a machine is required to move the source to prescribed positions of predetermined times. Thus, there are moving parts and electrical components to consider, computer programs to learn, and a wide variety of connections and interlocks that need to match specific conditions for the treatment to begin. Operating the unit requires considerably more training than the instruction necessary to insert LDR sources into afterloading applicators. Second, the number of positions often exceeds five times the number of low dose rate sources that would be used for the same treatment with low dose rate techniques. Assuring the correct programming of all positions becomes more intensive than checking the identity of the sources for many LDR insertions. Although for large, differentially loaded LDR iridium implants, assuring the correct loading can become more difficult than for the comparable high dose rate application. Additionally, manual verification that the optimization algorithm of the treatment planning system correctly produced the desired dose distribution between the completion of planning and the initiation of treatment becomes difficult to impossible without unduly extending the time the patient waits on the treatment table.

Increased probability of treatment delivery errors: Since each fraction may deliver a large dose, errors can lead to severe consequences. The entire procedure often must proceed quickly to prevent patient movement, to reduce the probability for thrombosis, and in cases using general anesthesia, to minimize the expense to the patient. Often, an HDR unit coexists with an external beam treatment machine in the same room. When either schedule is delayed, it stresses those involved in the HDR and external beam treatments and personnel tend to rush, increasing the probability of errors.

Potential for very high radiation doses to patients and unit operators: High dose rate brachytherapy carries with it an increase in the probability of accidents. Such accidents also have a higher likelihood for serious injury because of the strength of the source involved. An HDR source is about 100 times the strength of the sources comprising a typical LDR application. Thus, a source stuck in an applicator delivers an injurious dose to the patient in a matter of minutes. For personnel in the room responding to a problem with the source, an exposure of 25 rem (250 mSv, a dose at which one might begin to be concerned about health hazards) at half a meter from the source requires approximately an hour, although the maximum permissible dose (MPD) for a year, 5 rem, takes just over 10 minutes. According to as-low-as-reasonably-achievable (ALARA) guides of keeping workers at less than one-tenth of the maximum permissible dose, one year's exposure passes in a minute.

Labor intensive staffing during procedure: In addition to the staff normally in the procedure room during placement of the applicators (radiation oncologists, nurses, anesthesiologists) HDR procedures require imaging immediately after applicator placement (radiographer) and that dosimetry begin as soon as the localization procedures finish (physicist and dosimetrist). Independent verification calls for another physicist. All of these individuals participate in a matter of 1 or 2 hours. With LDR brachytherapy, the localization, dose calculation, and quality assurance phases of the treatment often spread out over hours or days, which does not require the concentration of staffing over a short time period.

Short history of clinical results: LDR brachytherapy has almost 9 decades of patient treatment and clinical outcomes to guide the dose prescriptions of radiation oncologists. While a few HDR cases date to the 1920s, and some cases used the "newer" remote afterloading equipment from the late 1960s, large numbers of patients began receiving HDR brachytherapy only from the mid-1980s.

Distances to normal structures cannot be increased for interstitial implants: While gynecologic and oral applications frequently allow moving some normal structures away from the source, most interstitial implants offer no such protection for healthy tissue. In these cases, the geometric potential for advantage disappears and the radiobiologic disadvantage takes over. For interstitial implants, the use of an HDR afterloader requires some changes in technique including:

1. Extending the margin at the ends of the catheters or needles to allow for the larger source length.
2. Using friction buttons, so as not to block the passage of the source into the catheters.
3. Keeping the total length within the operational limits of the unit.
4. Use of a stiffening filament in the catheter to avoid sharp bends (20).

Total treatment duration may equal LDR brachytherapy for fractionated treatments: An HDR endobronchial insertion treated with four fractions two times a day keeps the patients near the treatment facility for a day and a half; the same overall duration as the treatment delivered using LDR sources. An advantage to the patient, however, is that time need not be spent in radiation isolation as an inpatient.

The dangerous aspects of HDR brachytherapy stem directly from some of its disadvantages. The main characteristics that could lead to an accident include:

1. During lengthy procedures the patient may become uncomfortable and move, thus losing the precision advantage. Immobility during long procedures can contribute to venous thromboses and increased complications of general anesthesia.
2. Large quantities of input data (~350 pieces of information) are required for entry into the computer to perform a treatment plan.
3. Complicated, optimized dwell-time distributions make it difficult to check a plan by hand in a short time period.

Most advantages of HDR brachytherapy fall in the realm of the physical advantages, while the main disadvantage is biologic. The biologic disadvantage of high dose rate brachytherapy is that, as the dose rate goes up, the normal tissues become relatively more sensitive to radiation damage than the tumor tissue. This means that users of HDR brachytherapy must make use of the physical advantages for the treatments to succeed without complications. In cases other than cervical treatments with a tandem and ovoid, such as implants with needles, no distance can be added between the implant and normal tissue, so HDR may have a net disadvantage, depending on the doses used. This becomes particularly important in regions previously irradiated to doses near tissue tolerance, for example, with external beam therapy. Despite all of the relative disadvantages, the advantages of HDR brachytherapy make it a desirable approach in many settings. Successful brachytherapy includes choosing judiciously among the options for specific cases.

DIFFERENCES BETWEEN LDR AND HDR BRACHYTHERAPY PHYSICS

The physical properties of radioactive sources and technologic nature of the procedures separate LDR and HDR brachytherapy. The types of radioactive sources, treatment planning and dose specification techniques, and enhanced quality assurance procedures differentiate LDR and HDR brachytherapy.

Reversal of time and source strength: Low dose rate brachytherapy applications usually leave all the sources in place for a single treatment duration while the strength of the sources may vary at different locations. High dose rate brachytherapy cases use a single source of a given strength that moves through the applicators, usually stopping for calculated durations (dwell times) at specified locations (dwell positions). The dose delivered at any point from a source at a location depends on the number of nuclear transitions, and that varies with the product of the source strength and the time the source resides at the location. Thus, the reversal of the roles between the source strength and the duration creates no physical difference between LDR and HDR brachytherapy.

Optimization of the dose distribution: While "optimization" occurs in LDR brachytherapy by varying the source strengths used in the tandem for cervical cases, or differentially loading a pelvic template, the possibilities for various source strengths are fairly limited. For HDR cases optimization becomes a normal part of the HDR treatment planning procedure. Because dwell times can vary almost continuously, most of the treatment planning programs use inverse planning to deliver conformal therapy. Instead of specifying the time the source dwells at each location, the operator enters the dose desired at various points, and the computer calculates the dwell times to achieve the desired dose distribution.

Need for rapid verification of the treatment plan: The short time between the end of the treatment planning and the completion of the treatment necessitates rapid methods to assure that no errors were entered into the plan or the treatment program. While LDR cases also need such verification, the lack of time constraints with LDR brachytherapy allows the possibility for more direct but longer processes.

Increased need for quality assurance of the delivery system: The delivery system for most low dose rate brachytherapy cases consists of the sources and the hands of the person placing the sources into the applicators. HDR brachytherapy procedures use sophisticated machines to control the movement of the source and the times it resides at each dwell position. The machine requires periodic testing of many parameters each treatment day.

Difference in dose specification: Aside from the need to change the prescribed dose to account for the different biologic effectiveness of HDR applications compared to LDR cases, both physical and biologic factors require further alterations in dose specification to try to obtain the same biologically effective dose distribution one might have used with an LDR treatment. The first change recognizes that the biologic effectiveness of a high dose rate treatment varies with the absolute dose. As a result, recreating the same physical dose distribution with an HDR application as with an LDR application produces a different biologic effectiveness distribution. For example, if a practitioner used an ovoid surface dose equal to 145% of the Point A dose for LDR treatments of cervical cancer, for HDR fractions of 5 Gy to Point A, the ovoid surface should receive 139% to maintain the same relative biologic effectiveness. If the dose to Point A is 7 Gy per fraction, the dose to the ovoid surface should drop to 137%. For simulating a Paris system interstitial implant, where with LDR the Reference Dose equals 85% of the Basal Dose (the equivalent of the mean of the local dose within the implant volume), the HDR equivalent would reduce the differential to about 88% because the varying biologic effectiveness accentuates the difference in dose.

Another needed change in prescription comes from the optimization of most treatments. Using the Paris system interstitial implant, optimization of the implant effectively decreases the highest basal dose points in the interior of the implant, leaving the peripheral-most points alone, and lowering the average basal dose. Using the 85% coefficient with the new, lowered average would extend the treatment volume further from the periphery, expanding the treatment volume. Thus, the factor relating the Basal Dose and the Reference Dose needs to increase. A typical, optimized HDR implant could use the Reference Dose equal to 93% of the Basal Dose.

CLINICAL SITES

High dose rate brachytherapy techniques are used for essentially any anatomic site that is suitable for radioactive isotope treatment. Treatment of endobronchial obstruction by lung cancer, localized prostate cancer, and postoperative vaginal cuff irradiation for endometrial carcinoma are probably the most common uses of HDR technology in the United States.

Endobronchial and Intraluminal Brachytherapy

The endobronchial HDR brachytherapy is most commonly used for palliation of more advanced disease but may play a role in definitive therapy for early stage lung cancer. The greatest efficacy of intrabronchial HDR treatment is for palliation of those who have not received prior irradiation or for patients with recurrence after prior curative-intent external beam therapy. Although LDR endobronchial therapy has been used for decades to treat obstructed bronchi for lung cancer, the enormous interest in HDR therapy stems from the relatively common clinical presentation of an obstructed lung from an endobronchial tumor combined with the ability to perform outpatient treatment with a few fractions. Since sources do not have to be special ordered per case, procedures are more easily scheduled.

Because of the variability in patient selection, reporting of responses, and dose prescription specification, results of endobronchial brachytherapy can be difficult to interpret. Mehta reported that 88% of patients had improved pulmonary symptoms and 85% improved findings on chest x-rays after HDR brachytherapy using 4 Gy/fraction at 20 mm twice a day over 2 days for a total of four fractions (22). Speiser described 85% improved symptoms and 80% improvement at bronchoscopy using 3 HDR fractions of 7.5 Gy/fraction at 10 mm (23).

The most common side effect of endobronchial brachytherapy is radiation bronchitis and stenosis. For those receiving palliative therapy with brachytherapy alone the incidence is 17%. Bronchial complications for patients treated with brachytherapy and concurrent external beam therapy are 10%. The overall incidence of fatal hemoptysis in patients treated with endobronchial brachytherapy is 6% (23).

Intraluminal brachytherapy is used for palliative treatment of malignant obstructions of the esophagus and bile ducts and has been included as part of definitive therapy in certain combined modality protocols. Esophageal brachytherapy to the primary lesion can be administered before or after external beam therapy. To address the question of optimal timing of brachytherapy and external beam treatment a prospective randomized study was performed in Canada. Preliminary results suggest that brachytherapy after external beam therapy may provide a higher rate of pathologically negative specimens (51% versus 38%) compared with brachytherapy given before external beam treatment. Patients were randomized to receive brachytherapy of 15 Gy at 1 cm from the central source either before or following external beam therapy of 40 Gy in 15 fractions over 3 weeks.

HDR Brachytherapy for Prostate Carcinoma

The development of transrectal ultrasound (TRUS) has enhanced the technical aspects of prostate brachytherapy. Ultrasound-guided template techniques of prostate implantation result in more accurate needle and seed placement than prior methods of prostate brachytherapy. Fractionated HDR brachytherapy provides conformal brachytherapy capability and the potential for dose optimization in the prostate. HDR interstitial brachytherapy is used as a prostate boost in combination with external beam therapy or as definitive prostate irradiation. Brachytherapy with transrectal ultrasound is performed with general or spinal anesthesia. Interstitial brachytherapy techniques rely on transrectal ultrasound identification of the prostate volume for afterloading-catheter placement. Computerized treatment planning utilizing computer tomography or ultrasound images obtained during catheter placement can be optimized for conformal brachytherapy dose distribution (24).

Bertermann reported on 171 patients treated with 50 Gy external beam irradiation and two HDR iridium implants given during the external beam therapy without increasing the overall treatment time (25). With mean follow-up of 53 months clinical progression was seen in 21 patients, 14 of which were systemic (66%), 5 local, and 2 patients with local recurrence and systemic disease. The average time between the prostate specific antigen (PSA) nadir and clinical progression was 21 months. Progression occurred in 11% of 112 patients who had carcinoma confined to the prostate gland at the time of diagnosis. Ten of 171 patients died of prostate cancer and 18 died of intercurrent disease. Late gastrointestinal sequelae included five patients with grade 3 proctitis, one requiring colostomy, and three patients with grade 3 urinary late effects. Nine patients with incontinence had all previously been treated with transurethral resection of the prostate.

The Swedish Medical Center Tumor Institute in Seattle uses a single interstitial prostate implant delivering four fractions of 4 Gy at a minimum of 6-hour intervals. Pelvic external beam irradiation to 50 Gy starts 2 to 3 weeks after completion of brachytherapy. Few adverse late genitourinary or rectal effects have been observed with this fractionation scheme. For the 92 implants performed since 1989, no significant intraoperative or perioperative complications have been described. Urethral strictures that developed in 6 patients all responded to dilatation or limited urethrotomy. No case of incontinence has been observed (26).

HDR Brachytherapy for Endometrial Carcinoma

Vaginal cuff irradiation is indicated following total abdominal hysterectomy and bilateral salpingo-oophorectomy (TAH-BSO) for patients who are at risk for local recurrence. At the University of Wisconsin postoperative high dose rate vaginal cuff irradiation alone is prescribed for women with Stage Ia grade 3 and stage Ib grade 1, 2 disease. For women with tumor volume ~ 2 cm and those with Stage Ib grade 3, Stage Ic grade 1, 2, 3 and Stage II disease, whole pelvis irradiation is given before vaginal cuff brachytherapy. No adjuvant therapy is given for Stage Ia grade 1, 2 endometrial cancer. Sixty-three patients were treated with 16.2 Gy/fraction at the vaginal surface for each of two fractions 1 week apart using vaginal ovoids (27). One patient with stage IB, grade 1 disease developed histologically proven local-regional recurrence at the pelvic sidewall 1.2 years after completion of HDR therapy. She is presently without evidence of disease 3 years after completing salvage pelvic irradiation and additional HDR brachytherapy that resulted in the only case of vaginal stenosis. Nineteen patients with minimum follow-up of 2 years and 12 patients with minimum follow-up of 3 years have had no vaginal cuff recurrence. One patient died 2.5 years after HDR therapy from cardiovascular disease without evidence of cancer at her autopsy. Late sequelae include 14 patients (22%) with vaginal cuff fibrosis and one patient with vaginal stenosis following salvage therapy. One patient developed a recto-vaginal fistula with no evidence of recurrent disease.

Nori and associates and Mandell and colleagues describe 330 patients treated with postoperative HDR vaginal cuff brachytherapy (28,29). A total brachytherapy dose of 21 Gy in three fractions of 7 Gy was delivered at 0.5 cm depth at 2-week intervals. Patients with deep myometrial invasion, high histologic grade, or extrauterine extension who are at high risk for pelvic recurrence were treated with external beam pelvic irradiation to 40 Gy. The total pelvic/vaginal recurrence rate was 2.7% with an incidence of 3.7% vaginal complications. The 5-year survival rates were 92% for Stage I and 82% for Stage II disease.

HDR Brachytherapy for Cervical Carcinoma-Dose and Dose Specification

The potential risk of HDR brachytherapy in treating cervical carcinoma lies not so much with normal tissue injury but in not being able to attain the standard of disease control and survival achieved with LDR treatment. HDR brachytherapy has the theoretic advantage of optimizing the dose distribution for each insertion and potentially improving the dose distribution to tumor thereby possibly increasing local control and decreasing the dose to bladder and rectal tissue. However, in the parts of the world where cervical cancer is common, access to treatment facilities is difficult and high stage disease is prevalent. Potential benefits of HDR brachytherapy may be offset by the high cost of HDR treatment and the reduced emphasis on brachytherapy for institutions with patient populations that have high stage and large volume of disease.

Institutions that have developed comprehensive HDR programs have demonstrated it is possible to perform HDR brachytherapy and maintain local control and survival consistent with LDR results. Joslins group in Cardiff, England initiated an HDR brachytherapy program for cervical cancer in the late 1960s using high activity cobalt-60 in a Cathetron unit (30). External beam therapy is initiated before brachytherapy. Prescribed doses are the same for all stages of cervical disease. A central wedge that does not protect the lower vagina is used during external therapy. Treatment philosophy is that early stage disease should be treated with a radical dose limited only by normal tissue tolerance. The rectal dose is recorded at the treatment sessions and can be kept at 60% of the point A dose.

The treatment program at McGill University is derived from Joslin's program. The dose from external beam therapy and intracavitary treatment does not vary by stage. Central blocking of the tissues receiving HDR therapy is not done. The HDR fractionation schedule was developed empirically from time-dose-fractionation calculations of prior low dose rate brachytherapy experience and in keeping with the Joslin dose fractionation system (31).

The Wayne State University gynecologic HDR treatment program uses a highly fractionated HDR treatment course with up to 8 to 12 HDR fractions. Brachytherapy is started 2 to 4 weeks after initiation of external beam therapy. A customized central step wedge is used during the HDR treatment period to shield central pelvic tissue while treating peripheral pelvic lymph nodes (32). The highly fractionated schedule was chosen by using the linear-quadratic model to determine how many HDR fractions would be equivalent to an LDR regimen of 60 Gy at point A (33). This gives a rectal dose 200-250 cGy for each HDR fraction which is considered tolerable for fractionated teletherapy. The intracavitary technique utilizes an intrauterine stent and a tandem and ring applicator so that applicators can be placed quickly without cervical dilatation with little or no sedation and to facilitate reproducibility from one insertion to another. Treatment planning is performed on the initial insertion and is duplicated for all fractions by fluoroscopic verification.

At the University of Wisconsin HDR brachytherapy is integrated into the external beam treatment schedule early in the course of therapy for stage I and II cervical carcinoma patients. External beam dose, intracavitary dose, and use of a central block vary according to the stage and volume of disease. For patients with larger volume of central disease, HDR brachytherapy is started after several weeks of whole pelvis irradiation to allow shrinkage of the cervical disease. Intracavitary therapy may be performed twice weekly after external beam treatment is completed (9).

The dose fractionation schedules developed for HDR therapy were designed to produce equivalent tumor control and, with special attention to treatment geometry, late complication rates as the previous LDR therapy. Schedules were based on the linear quadratic model (10). Brachytherapy is accomplished with conscious sedation as an outpatient. Nursing staff manages the intravenous sedation and vital signs during the procedure. Applicator insertion, radiographs for dosimetry, treatment planning, and HDR treatments are performed in the same room without moving the patient. Optimized treatment planning is performed for each insertion.

HDR Brachytherapy for Cervical Carcinoma—Results and Complications

The large patient population from the Cardiff series and the long duration of follow-up provides important data regarding late effects of HDR brachytherapy combined with external beam treatment for cervical carcinoma. Joslin's group has treated 371 patients over 6 years. The 5-year survival is stage I-94.4%, stage II-62%, and stage III-37.2%. There are very few long term survival rates; for patients treated by the Cardiff group, the 15-year survival rate is stage I-93%, stage II-54.3%, and stage III-33.6%. Central disease recurrence developed in 3 of 95 (3%) stage I patients, in 23 of 170 (14%) stage II disease, and 30 of 106 (28%) patients with stage III disease over 8 years. Recurrent disease developed over a 6- to 10-year period (30).

No case of rectovaginal fistula has been seen at up to 15 years. This is a result of limiting the dose to the rectum to a maximum total dose of less than 45 Gy. Ten patients (2.7%) had one or more episodes of rectal bleeding developing at a median of 17.5 months. Two patients required surgery for sigmoid stricture. Bladder symptoms of hematuria in the absence of recurrent disease was seen in 15 patients (4%) in periods ranging up to 107 months. Cystoscopic findings were usually telangiectasia of the bladder base. No surgical intervention was required. Vaginal stenosis or shortening was noted in 93 cases (25%) and was usually an asymptomatic finding (30).

At McGill University 187 patients have been followed for a minimum of 35 months. Patterns of recurrence show that 26 patients developed pelvic recurrence. Of all patients with distant and local failure, 88% were manifest within 24 months of completing treatment. Five-year actuarial survival is: stage IB-72%, stage IIA-65%, stage IIB-66%, IIIA-66%, and IIIB-45% (31).

Acute complications consisted mainly of grade 1 and 2 gastrointestinal and urinary toxicities. No increase in frequency or the nature of acute toxicities was observed when compared to their low dose rate experience. Late complications were seen in 14.7% of HDR patients, with 7.6% of patients experiencing grade 3 or 4 complications. Late radiation proctitis developed at a median of 15 months. Four patients developed rectal ulceration with 3 requiring colostomy (32).

The results at Wayne State University with 88 patients treated from August, 1988 to December, 1992 show 5-year survival rates for stage IB/IIA-83%, stage IIB/IIIA-69%, and stage IIB/IVA-56%. Local control was achieved in 71 of 88 (80%) of patients. Central and pelvic failure occurred in 12 patients, with distant relapse only in 17, and combination of local and distant disease recurrence in 5 patients. In patients with recurrent and/or distant disease, 82% died within 2 years (33).

Complications attributable to pelvic radiotherapy and HDR brachytherapy in the Wayne State University series occurred in 11 of 88 patients. Those effects included 6 patients with recurring grade 2 diarrhea and 2 patients with grade 2 rectal symptoms. Grade 3 and 4 sequelae occurred in 3 patients (3.4%). These complications included vaginal-vesical fistula following surgery for recurrent tumor, small bowel obstruction, and severe vaginal stenosis (34).

At the University of Wisconsin patients treated with HDR brachytherapy and external beam therapy for cervical cancer were compared with those treated with LDR therapy. One hundred ninety-eight stage IB-IIIB patients treated with LDR from 1977 to 1989 were compared with 40 patients treated with the HDR regime from 1989 to 1991. Both patient groups were comparable with regards to age, weight, stage distribution, bulk of disease, and histology. No significant difference in survival was found between the LDR and HDR groups. Actuarial overall 3-year survival for LDR and HDR groups was 66% and 77% respectively. Disease control in the pelvis was similar for the LDR and HDR patient groups. Three-year actuarial pelvic control was 80% and 77% for LDR and HDR patients respectively. Overall, 74 of 198 (37%) LDR patients and 11 of 40 (28%) HDR patients failed either locally or distantly (35).

Late complications in patients treated with LDR brachytherapy were comparable to patients receiving HDR brachytherapy. No grade 4 small bowel, large bowel, or urinary sequelae developed in the HDR treatment group. One patient developed grade 4 radiation proctitis requiring resection and colostomy (35).

DISCUSSION

High dose rate therapy is moving into a phase of greater sophistication particularly regarding dose specification and integration of brachytherapy with external beam treatment. As institutions proceed with HDR programs they are reporting their past LDR experience of survival and complications compared to their current HDR program results. It is unlikely that multi-institutional randomized controlled trials will be established to evaluate the effectiveness of HDR compared with LDR brachytherapy. Institutions proficient at HDR brachytherapy have developed their own novel approaches for combining external beam irradiation with brachytherapy that may enhance the therapeutic ratio and lead to increased tumor control rates without altering late sequelae. Innovations in treatment unit design and refinement of hardware and software for treatment planning facilitate treatment techniques that advance research in HDR brachytherapy. Evaluation of initial studies of HDR brachytherapy for cervical cancer show that investigators have moved to increase the number of HDR fractions during a treatment course, while decreasing the dose per fraction. This approach should achieve decreased chronic bladder and bowel complications while maintaining or improving local tumor control.

Use of dose equivalency equations to devise new treatment schedules create a myriad of clinical time-dose-fractionation schedules that may be confusing to the practitioner interested in establishing an HDR brachytherapy program. The American Brachytherapy Society published a consensus report of the Clinical Education Committee that provides a focus point (12). It is difficult to compare HDR brachytherapy results from one institution to another because of variation in dose specification, treatment schedules, and toxicity grading. Within the same institution, sequential LDR and HDR studies suggests that the move to HDR brachytherapy can be accomplished in a safe fashion while maintaining excellent disease control and the expected incidence of normal tissue sequelae.

References

1. Tod M, Meredith W. A dosage system for use in the treatment of cancer of the uterine cervix. Br J Radiol 1938;809:824.
2. Suit H. Modification of the Fletcher ovoid system for afterloading using standard sized radium tubes, Radiology 1960;81:126-131.
3. Henschke U. Afterloading application for radiation therapy of carcinoma of the uterus, Radiology 1960;87:834.
4. Sievert RM. Two arrangements for reducing irradiation dangers in teleradium treatment. Acta Radiol 1937;18:157-162.
5. Hilaris BS, Ju H, Lewis JL, et al. Normal and neoplastic tissue effects of high intensity intracavitary irradiation: Cancer of the corpus uteri. Radiology 1974;110:459-492.
6. Stitt JA. High-dose-rate intracavitary brachytherapy for gynecologic malignancies. Oncology 1992;1:59-79.
7. Van't Hooft E. Recent Advances in Brachytherapy Physics, New York: American Institute of Physics, 1981;167-177.
8. Joslin CAF, O'Connell D, Howard N. The treatment of uterine carcinoma using the Cathetron: III. Clinical considerations and preliminary reports on treatment results, Br J Radiol 1967;40:895-904.
9. Stitt JA, Thomadsen BR, Fowler JF. High dose rate brachytherapy in carcinoma of the cervix-Clinical and biological considerations. Int J Radiat Oncol Biol Phys 1992;24:335-348.
10. Thomadsen BR, Shahabi S, Stitt JA. High dose rate brachytherapy in carcinoma of the cervix-Physics and dosimetry considerations. Int J Radiat Oncol Biol Phys 1992;224:349-357.
11. Utley JF, von Essen CF, Horn RA, et al. High dose rate afterloading intracavitary therapy in carcinoma of the cervix. Int J Radiat Oncol Biol Phys 1984;120:2259-2263.
12. Nag S, et al. Consensus guidelines for high dose rate remote brachytherapy in cervical, endometrial, and endobronchial tumors. Int J Radiat Oncol Biol Phys 1993;27:1241-1244.
13. Perez CA, Grigsby PW, Castro-Vita H, et al. Carcinoma of the uterine cervix. I Impact of prolongation of overall treatment time and timing of brachytherapy on outcome of radiation therapy. Int J Radiat Oncol Biol Phys 1995;32:1275-1288.
14. Petereit DG, Sarkaria JN, Chappell R, et al. The adverse effect of treatment prolongation in cervical carcinoma. Int J Radiat Oncol Biol Phys 1995;32:1301-1307.
15. Girinsky T, Rey A, Roche B, et al. Overall treatment time in advanced cervical carcinoma: A critical parameter in treatment outcome. Int J Radiat Oncol Biol Phys 1994;27:1051-1056.
16. Perez CA, Fox S, Lockett MA, et al. Impact of dose in outcome of irradiation alone in carcinoma of the uterine cervix: Analysis of two different methods. Int J Radiat Oncol Biol Phys 1991;21:885-898.
17. Eifel PJ, Thomas WW, Smith TL, et al. The relationship between brachytherapy dose and outcome in patients with bulky endocervical tumors treated with radiation alone. Int J Radiat Oncol Biol Phys 1993;28:113-118.
18. Lanciano RM, Won MA, Coia R, et al. Pretreatment and treatment factors associated with improved outcome in squamous cell carcinoma of the uterine cervix: A Final Report of the 1973 and 1978 Patterns-of-Care Studies. Int J Radiat Oncol Biol Phys 1991;20:667-676.
19. King GC, Stockstill TF, Bloomer WD, et al. Point dose variations with time in brachytherapy for cervical carcinoma. Med Phys 1992;19:777.
20. Thomadsen BR. Clinical Implementation of Remote-Afterloading in Interstitial Brachytherapy. In: Williamson JF, Thomadsen BR, Nath R, eds. Brachytherapy Physics. Madison, WI: Medical Physics Publishing Company, 1995.
21. Thomadsen BR. Clinical Implementation of HDR Intracavitary and transluminal Brachytherapy. In: Williamson JF, Thomadsen BR, Nath R, eds. Brachytherapy Physics. Madison, WI: Medical Physics Publishing Company, 1995.
22. Mehta M, Petereit D, Chosey L, et al. Sequential comparison of low dose-rate and hyperfractionated high dose-rate endobronchial radiation for malignant airway occlusion. Int J Radiat Oncol Biol Phys 1992;23:133-139.
23. Speiser B, Spratling L. High dose-rate brachytherapy for the local control of endobronchial carcinoma. Int J Radiat Oncol Biol Phys 1993;25:579-588.
24. Mate TP, Kovacs G, Martinez A. High dose-rate brachytherapy of the prostate. In: Nag S, ed. High Dose-Rate Brachytherapy: A Textbook, Chapter 16, Armonk, New York, Futura, 1994;355-371.
25. Bertermann H, Brix F. Ultrasonically guided interstitial high dose-rate brachytherapy with Ir-192: Technique and preliminary results in locally confined prostate cancer. In: Martinez AA, Orton CF, Mould RF, eds. Brachytherapy HDR and LDR: Remote afterloading State of the Art, pp 281-303. Leerson, The Netherlands, Nucletron International BV, 1990.
26. Mate TP, Gottesman J. Fractionated high dose-rate Ir-192 conformal prostate brachytherapy. In: Blasko J, ed. Ultrasonically Guided Seed Implantation Syllabus, Pacific Northwest Cancer Foundation, 1996.
27. Noyes WR, Bastin K, Edwards SA, et al. Postoperative vaginal cuff irradiation using high dose-rate remote afterloading: A phase II clinical protocol. Int J Radiat Oncol Biol Phys 1995;32 (5):1439-1443.
28. Nori D, Hilaris BS, Batata MA, et al. Remote afterloading in cancer management II. Clinical applications of remote afterloaders. In: Hilaris BS, Batata MA, eds. Brachytherapy Oncology, New York, NY, Memorial Sloan-Kettering Cancer Center. 1983;101-118.
29. Mandell L, Nori D, Anderson LL, et al. Postoperative vaginal radiation in endometrial cancer using a remote afterloading technique. Int J Radiat Oncol Biol Phys 1985;11:473-478.
30. Joslin CAF. High activity source afterloading in gynecologic cancer and its future prospects, Ulrich Henschke Memorial Lecture. Endo Hyper Oncol 1989;5:69-81.
31. Roman TN, Souhami L, Freeman CR, et al. High dose rate afterloading intracavitary therapy in carcinoma of the cervix. Int J Radiat Oncol Biol Phys 1991;20:921-926.
32. Selke P, Roman TN, Souhami L, et al. Treatment results of high dose rate brachytherapy in patients with carcinoma of the cervix. Int J Radiat Oncol Biol Phys 1993;27:803-809.
33. Ahmad K, Kim YH, Ezzell G, Han G, et al. Reproducibility of multifractionated outpatient high dose rate brachytherapy in carcinoma of the cervix using the Ahmad-Kim positioner. Endo Hyper Oncol 1992;8:171-173.
34. Han I, Malviaya V, Orton C, et al. Multifractionated high dose rate brachytherapy with concurrent daily teletherapy for cervical cancer. Gyn Oncol 1996;63: 71-77.
35. Sarkaria JN, Petereit DG, Stitt JA, et al. A comparison of the efficacy and complication rates of low-dose-rate versus high-dose-rate brachytherapy in the treatment of cervical carcinoma. Int J Radiat Oncol Biol Phys 1994;30:75-82.

PART II

Practical Clinical Applications

Table 15.1. World Health Organization Pathological Classification System for Primary Tumors of the Central Nervous System (2)

Tumors of neuroepithelial tissue	Tumors of the meninges
Astrocytoma (low grade)	Meningioma
Anaplastic (malignant) astrocytoma	Atypical meningioma
Glioblastoma multiforme	Anaplastic (malignant) meningioma
Oligodendroglioma	Hemangiopericytoma
Anaplastic oligodendroglioma	Other tumors
Oligoastrocytoma	Malignant lymphoma
Anaplastic oligoastrocytoma	Germ cell tumors
Ependymoma	Pituitary adenoma
Anaplastic ependymoma	Craniopharyngioma
Medulloblastoma	Chordoma

Table 15.3. Incidence, Treatment, and Survival Figures for Common Primary Central Nervous System Tumors (1)

Tumor Type	Incidence (%)	Treatment	5-Year Survival (%)
Glioblastoma multiforme	30	S, RT, C	5
Anaplastic astrocytoma[a]	10	S, RT, C	20
Low-grade astrocytoma[b]	15–20	S ± RT	50–90
Meningioma	15–20	S ± RT	75
Pituitary adenoma	10	S ± RT	85
Medulloblastoma	4–8	S, RT, C	60
Ependymoma	1–8	S, RT	50
Craniopharyngioma	1	S ± RT	90

[a] Includes anaplastic oligodendroglioma and anaplastic oligoastrocytoma.
[b] Includes low-grade diffuse fibrillary astrocytomas, pilocytic astrocytoma, oligodendroglioma, and oligoastrocytoma.
S, surgery; R, radiation therapy; C, chemotherapy.

Table 15.2. Grading of Astrocytic Tumors (3)

WHO Designation	WHO Grade	Kernohan Grade	St. Anne/Mayo Grade	St. Anne/Mayo Criteria
Pilocytic astrocytoma	I	I	N/A	N/A
Astrocytoma	II	I, II	1	No criteria fulfilled
			2	1 criterion: nuclear atypia
Anaplastic astrocytoma	III	II, III	3	2 criteria: nuclear atypia and mitoses
Glioblastoma	IV	III, IV	4	3 or 4 criteria: above plus endothelial proliferation and/or necrosis

WHO, World Health Organization.

sists of surgery [or radiosurgery] and/or whole brain radiation therapy [WBRT]) is poor, ranging from 3 to 6 months for patients with multiple metastases (5), to 12 months for those with a solitary metastasis (6). Vertebral metastases, resulting in compression of the spinal cord, are most common from primary lung, breast, and prostate cancers. Median survival time following radiation therapy, which may or may not be preceded by laminectomy for surgical decompression, is also in the range of 3 to 6 months (7).

Anatomy

Knowledge of the basic topographical and functional anatomy of the brain is important for accurate communication of tumor location within the CNS as well as defining areas of functional "eloquence" that need to be considered when planning therapy. Generally, the brain can be considered to have three major divisions: the cerebrum, cerebellum, and brain stem. When considering tumor location it is also common to distinguish between supratentorial (cerebral hemispheres and midline structures) versus infratentorial (cerebellum, lower brain stem, and posterior fossa).

The longitudinal cerebral fissure divides the cerebrum into two hemispheres. Each cerebral hemisphere is then divided by the major sulci into six lobes: frontal, parietal, occipital, and temporal, and the midline central and limbic lobes (Figures 15.1a and b). The prominent central sulcus (of Rolando) separates frontal lobe from parietal lobe. The parieto-occipital fissure separates parietal lobe from occipital lobe. The lateral fissure (of Sylvius) defines the temporal lobe boundaries. The cerebral hemispheres are connected by the corpus callosum, beneath which are the midline structures (third ventricle, pineal body, and midbrain) and the deep paramedian structures (lateral ventricles, caudate nucleus, lentiform nucleus, thalamus, and hypothalamus).

A basic understanding of the functional anatomy of the cerebral hemispheres can be approached in three ways. The first is a regional or "lobe by lobe" consideration of function. The occipital lobe is primarily involved with vision and its dependent functions. The temporal lobe processes sound, vestibular sensations, sights, smells, and other perceptions into complex "experiences" important for memory. Wernicke's area is located on the posterior portion of the superior temporal gyrus and plays a critical role in receptive speech. The parietal lobe, specifically the postcentral gyrus is critically involved in somatosensory function. Sensory integration (body image) and gnostic

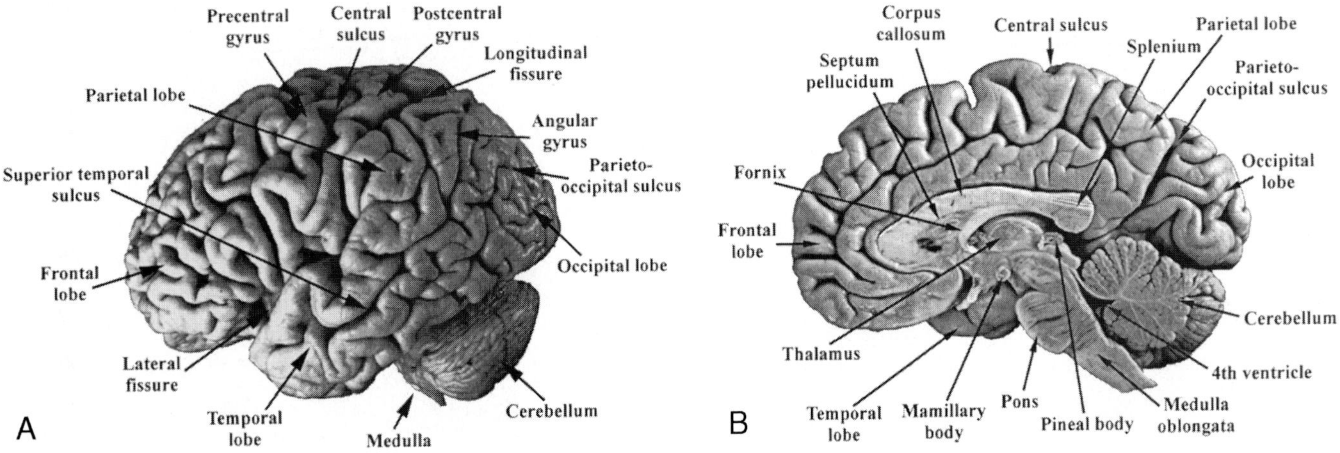

Figure 15.1. **A.** Lateral surface of the left brain including cerebral hemisphere, cerebellum, and brainstem. The major sulci divide the cerebral cortex into four lateral lobes: frontal, parietal, occipital, and temporal. **B.** Medial surface of the left brain demonstrating midline structures of the central and limbic lobes.

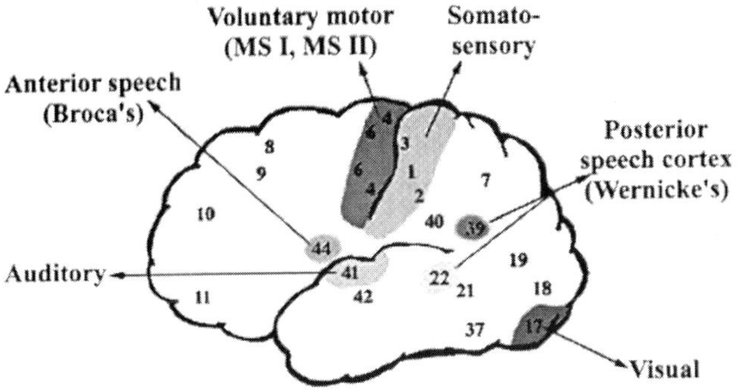

Figure 15.2. Location of the major motor, sensory, and speech areas of the cerebral cortex with reference to Brodmann's area numbers.

(perceptive) functions also reside within the parietal lobe. The frontal lobe is associated with higher level cognitive functions such as reasoning and judgement. The frontal lobes also contain the primary motor cortex (precentral gyrus) and Broca's area (inferior third frontal gyrus), important in expressive speech. The limbic lobe mediates memories, drives, and stimuli. It affects visceral functions central to emotional expression, such as sexual drive. Finally, the central lobe (insula) is important in visceral sensation and motility.

The second approach to functional neuroanatomy is the schema of Brodmann, which numbers areas of structural specialization. These numbered areas, in some cases, correspond to the functional location of important primary sensory and motor areas. The 52 numbered areas provide both an anatomical and functional "road map" of the brain by which tumor location can be described (Figure 15.2).

The final and most eloquent method to describe functional neuroanatomy is through various techniques of functional mapping (Figure 15.3). While classic mapping utilizes microelectrode stimulation of the cortical surface directly, new non-invasive techniques such as functional magnetic resonance imaging (fMRI), positron emission tomography (PET) scanning, and magnetoencephalography (MEG) are rapidly being brought into clinical use (8–13). These procedures allow for precise mapping of function in an individual and can accurately predict deficits related to injury of a given area by tumor or therapy.

The cerebellum is composed of two hemispheres connected by the midline vermis. The vermis, in turn, is composed of the superior, middle, and inferior peduncles, which are important in trafficking information between the cerebrum, brainstem, and spinal cord. The cerebellum is critical for the smooth coordination of motor activity and balance.

Finally, the midbrain, pons, and medulla oblongata comprise the brainstem. This is the most evolutionarily primitive portion of the human brain, and the most crucial. Within the brainstem, nuclei are located which control crit-

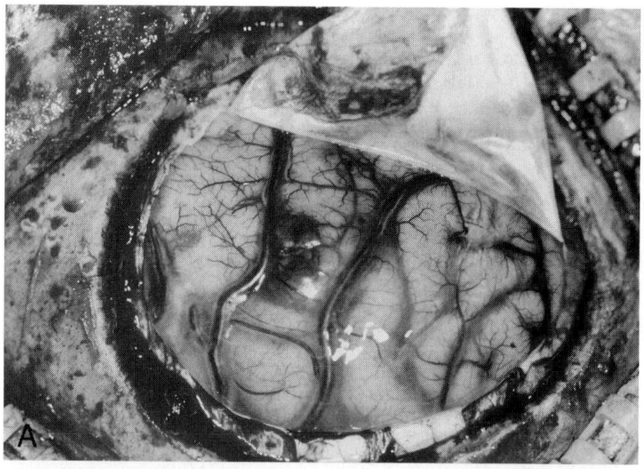

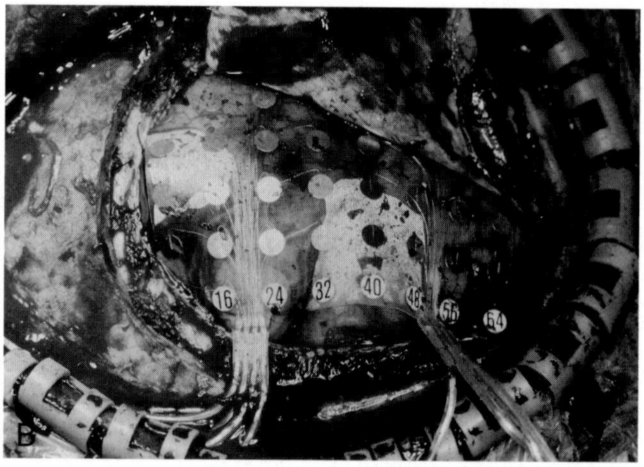

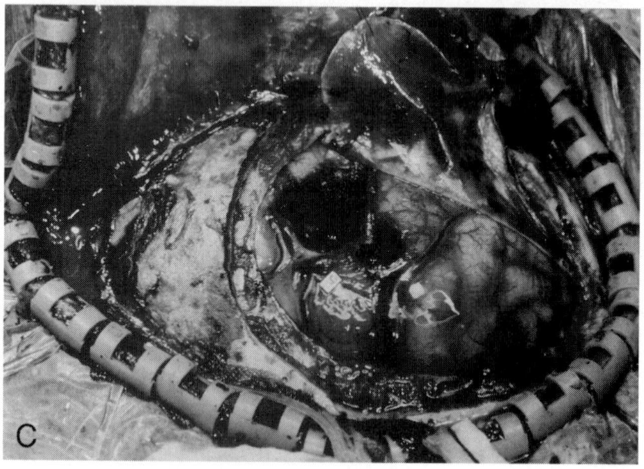

Figure 15.3. Cortical surface electrode mapping of the speech area in a patient undergoing resection of a recurrent glioma. **A.** Exposed cortical surface. **B.** Mapping array in place. **C.** Resection cavity with electrode number 5 demarcating speech area. Patient had normal speech postoperatively.

ical life functions such as heart rate, breathing, and level of alertness. The cranial nerves originate from nuclei within the midbrain, pons, and medulla. Even minute injury to any given part of the brainstem can have devastating consequences. This is one reason why even small or low-grade tumors, when located in the brainstem, may be associated with significant morbidity and mortality.

Imaging Studies

Studies that image CNS tumors serve two purposes. The first is to define the tumor's anatomic extent, which in turn determines and guides therapy, whether surgery, radiation therapy, and/or chemotherapy. The second is to provide information about electron density of the paths traversed by radiation beams to define dose to targets and normal tissues within the treated volumes. As a baseline, almost without exception, patients with a brain and/or spinal cord tumor should undergo an MRI scan and computed tomography (CT) with and without intravenous contrast. Computed tomography, while less expensive than MRI, gives less anatomic detail of the soft tissues but may be more useful in imaging the bony structures, particularly the skull base. Magnetic resonance imaging scans provide the best resolution within soft tissues for distinguishing between tumor, edema, and normal brain.

Central nervous system tumors rarely metastasize outside the CNS, but may spread within it. For example, certain brain tumors, such as medulloblastomas, primitive neuroectodermal tumors, anaplastic ependymomas, choroid plexus carcinomas, pineoblastomas, germ cell tumors, and lymphomas may involve the cerebrospinal fluid (CSF), leptomeninges (i.e., the coverings) of the brain, or spinal cord. Studies that stage or determine the anatomic extent of CNS involvement of these tumors include MRI scans of the brain and spine, and CSF cytology (MRI has largely replaced myelograms/CT myelograms). Other imaging studies, such as MRI spectroscopy, fMRI, PET scans, and single photon emission tomography (SPECT) scans, better reflect biologic characteristics of CNS tumors, such as tumor metabolism, glucose utilization, and blood flow as well as function of surrounding normal brain. Functional and biological imaging data are currently incorporated into decisions as to whether ablative procedures such as surgery, radiosurgery, or brachytherapy can be safely considered. Also, PET scans and MRI spectroscopy (Figure 15.4a –f) may allow for differentiating active tumor

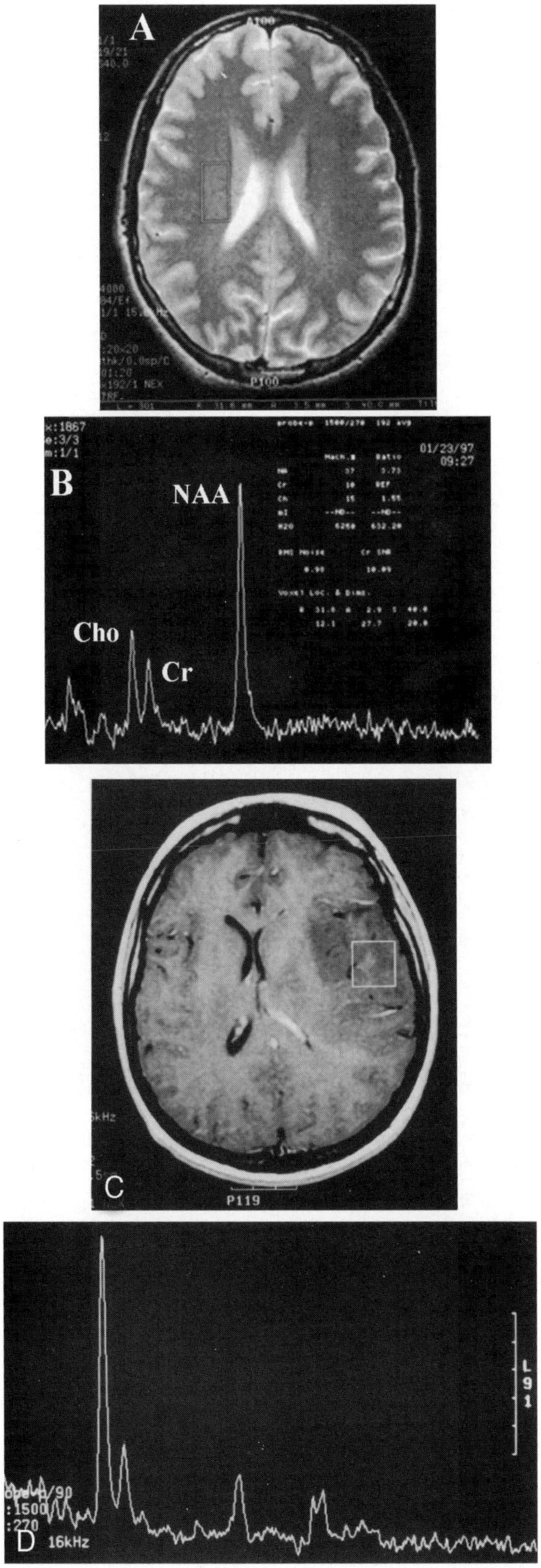

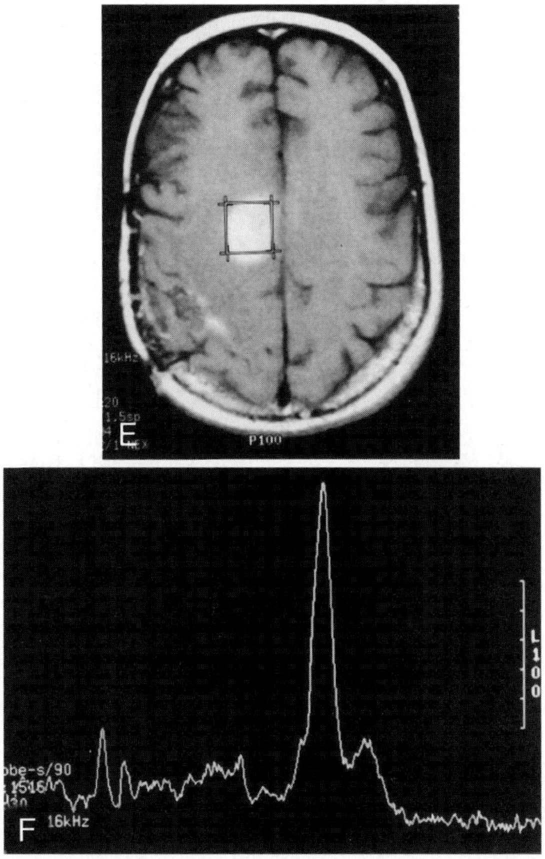

Figure 15.4. Axial MRI images with area of interest outlined and corresponding MRI spectroscopy. Cho, choline; Cr, creatine; NAA, N-acetyl aspartate; L, lactate. **A.** Normal brain **B.** Normal MRI spectroscopy with equal choline:creatine peak. **C.** Recurrent glioblastoma multiforme postirradiation. **D.** MRI spectroscopy with increased choline:creatine ratio consistent with recurrent tumor. **E.** Radiation necrosis. **F.** MRI spectroscopy with increased lactate signal consistent with edema and necrosis.

Table 15.4. Definitions of Gross, Clinical, and Planning Tumor Volume as Related to Central Nervous System (CNS) Tumors

Abbreviation	Represents	Definition
GTV	Gross tumor volume	Gross (often enhancing) tumor seen on MRI, CT, or other imaging study
CTV	Clinical target volume	Other CNS tissue with suspected microscopic tumor; contains and usually extends 1–3 cm beyond the GTV
PTV	Planning target volume	Margin beyond the GTV and CTV accounting for factors such as internal organ motion, setup variation, and patient movement; contains and usually extends 0.5 to 1 cm beyond the GTV and CTV
TV	Targeted volume	Volume enclosed by the desired prescription isodose line (usually ≥90%); contains the GTV, CTV, and PTV
IV	Irradiated volume	Tissue volume that receives a significant dose of radiation; contains the GTV, CTV, PTV, and TV

MRI, magnetic resonance imaging; CT, computed tomography.

versus radionecrosis after radiation therapy (14–17). These types of studies have a less clear role in treatment planning for external beam radiotherapy, but are an active topic of research.

RADIATION THERAPY TREATMENT GUIDELINES FOR CNS TUMORS

Target Volume and Dose Determinations

For the purposes of this chapter, the nomenclature described in the physics publication Report 50 of the International Commission on Radiation Units and Measurements (ICRU-50) (18) will be used, including gross tumor volume (GTV), clinical target volume (CTV), planning target volume (PTV), treated volume (TV), and irradiated volume (IV). These volumes are defined for CNS tumors in Table 15.4. The initial step in the treatment planning process is the identification of the GTV. Typically, the GTV is the enhancing gross tumor seen on an MRI or CT scan with contrast. However, not all tumor is enhancing. For example, edematous brain or non-enhancing "normal" CNS tissue surrounding the enhancing gross lesion often contains microscopic tumor. Therefore, the CTV extends 1-3 cm beyond the GTV and represents the volume of tissue at risk for harboring microscopic tumor. The PTV, which usually extends 0.5 to 1 cm beyond the margin of the GTV and CTV, accounts for factors such as internal organ motion, set-up variation, and patient movement.

Most primary gliomas of the brain can be classified as circumscribed and non-infiltrative tumors, or non-circumscribed and infiltrative (into surrounding normal brain tissue) tumors, or a combination of both (19). Figure 15.5a shows the MRI scan of a cerebral pilocytic astrocytoma, which is a circumscribed, non-infiltrative tumor. The scan shows a well-defined contrast-enhancing tumor without surrounding edema. Biopsy of the enhancement would reveal pure tumor tissue, whereas biopsy beyond the enhancement would reveal normal brain tissue. Tumors like

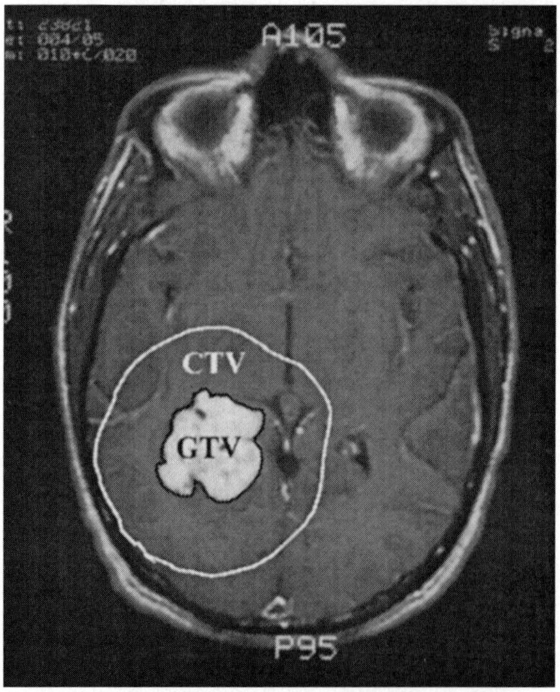

Figure 15.5. Axial MRI image (T1 with contrast) of a right parietal pilocytic astrocytoma showing the GTV and a 2 cm-expansion for CTV.

these are amenable to cure with complete surgical removal. Alternatively, radiosurgery and brachytherapy, modalities which deliver highly focal doses of radiation to lesions with minimal dose to the surrounding normal tissues (see Chapter 10), may also represent curative treatment. Other examples of circumscribed, non-infiltrative tumors include meningiomas, pituitary adenomas, and craniopharyngiomas. In cases like the pilocytic astrocytoma and the other circumscribed non-infiltrative tumors, the GTV is the enhancing tumor. The CTV and the GTV are the same in these cases, and the PTV should add only a 1-2 cm margin beyond the GTV (Figure 15.5b).

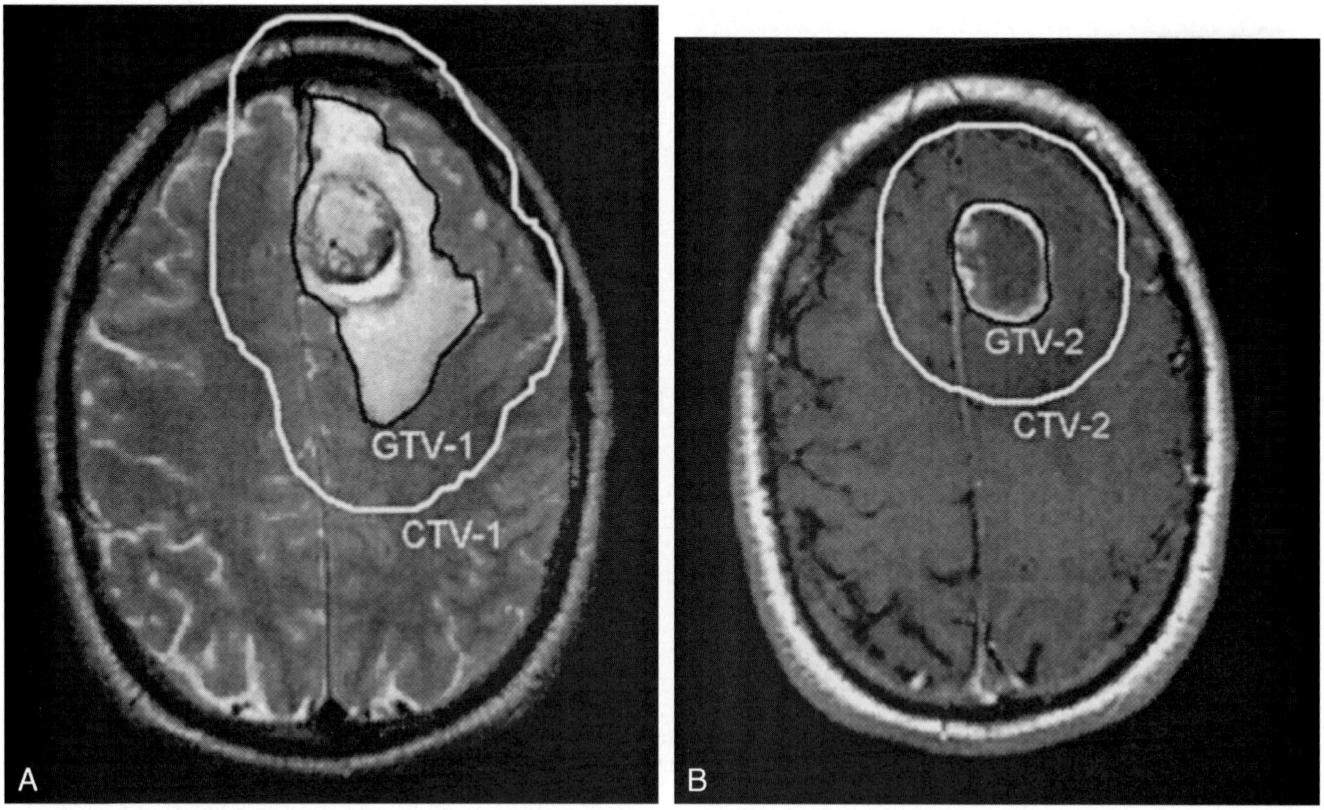

Figure 15.6. **A.** Axial MRI image (T2-weighted) of a left frontoparietal glioblastoma multiforme with GTV-1 and CTV-1 outlined. **B.** Corresponding T1-weighted with gadolinium image of A. Boost GTV-2 and CTV-2 outlined.

Figure 15.6 shows the MRI scan of a cerebral glioblastoma multiforme, which is a non-circumscribed, infiltrative tumor. The T-1 weighted images with contrast (Figure 15.6b) show a well defined, enhancing tumor, with a necrotic center, surrounded by edema (better seen on the T-2 weighted images, Figure 15.6a). Biopsy of the enhancement would again show pure tumor tissue, whereas biopsy of the edema would reveal normal brain tissue interspersed with rare tumor cells. Such tumors are not likely to be cured by complete surgical removal (or radiosurgery) alone, since tumor may even be present several centimeters beyond the MRI defined extent of the edema (20). Furthermore, surgical removal (or radiosurgery) of the edematous brain tissue, which contains both normal brain and tumor tissue, may result in neurologic deficit if the tumor is located in a functionally critical area of the brain. In this example of a glioblastoma multiforme, the initial GTV is the enhancing tumor plus surrounding edema as seen on T-2 weighted images. The initial CTV adds a 2- to 3-cm margin beyond the GTV (Figure 15.6a). This large volume is usually treated to a dose sufficient to address microscopic disease. A smaller, boost volume consisting of the enhancing tumor (GTV-2) is then treated with a 1-2 cm margin (CTV-2) to a higher or "definitive" dose (Figure 15.6b).

Non-circumscribed, infiltrative tumors do not always have an enhancing component on CT or MRI scans with contrast, as in the case of cerebral low-grade gliomas (diffuse fibrillary astrocytomas, oligodendrogliomas, or oligoastrocytomas). In this setting, the GTV is the T-2 weighted high signal lesion corresponding to tumor plus edema. The initial CTV extends 2-3 cm beyond the GTV, and if there is a boost, the margin is reduced to 1-2 cm. Computed tomography scans (Figure 15.7a) often underestimate the GTV and, therefore, the CTV, compared to T-2 weighted MRI scans (Figure 15.7b). Furthermore, MRI scans show greater detail in terms of the normal brain anatomy, specifically the critical normal structures that need to be dose-limited or avoided in the processes of treatment planning and delivery. Thus, except for circumscribed, non-infiltrative tumors that enhance comparably on CT and MRI scans, MRI is the treatment planning study of choice for determination of anatomic extent of most brain and spinal cord tumors. Computed tomography scans, however, remain important for providing electron density data, allowing calculation of accurate dose distribution within the target and nearby critical structures.

Table 15.5 shows the GTVs and CTVs, as well as general dose/fractionation guidelines, for the more common primary CNS tumors as well as for metastatic disease to

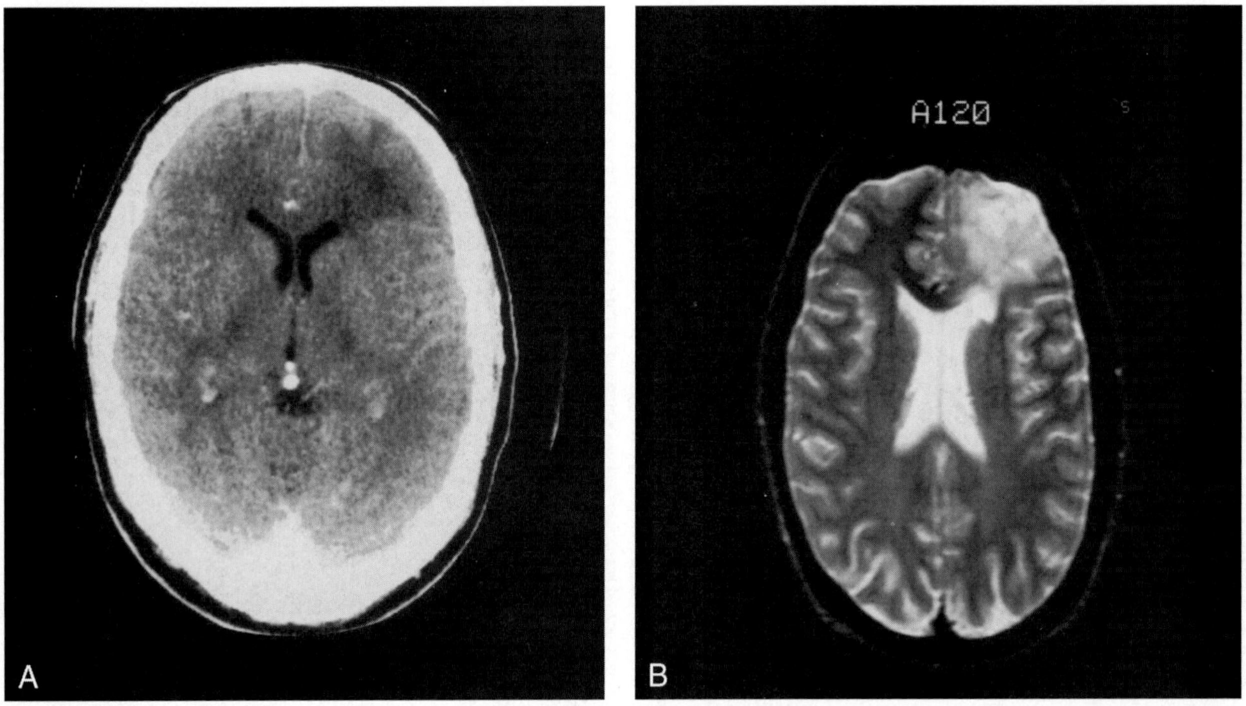

Figure 15.7. A. Axial CT scan with contrast of a left frontal low-grade glioma. **B.** Corresponding axial MRI image (T2-weighted) demonstrating tumor.

Table 15.5. Treatment Guidelines for Common Central Nervous System Tumors (1,24–26)

Tumor Type	GTV	CTV	Total Dose (Gy/# Fractions)
Glioblastoma multiforme, anaplastic, astrocytoma[a]			60/30 or 64.8/36
Initial field	Edema and enhancing tumor	GTV + 2–3 cm margin	46/23 or 50.4/28
Boost field	Enhancing tumor	GTV + 2–2.5 cm margin	14/7 or 14.4/8
Low-grade diffuse fibrillary astrocytoma[b,c]	Edema (and enhancing tumor if present)	GTV + 1–2 cm margin[c]	50.4/28 to 59.4/33
Low-grade pilocytic astrocytoma	Enhancing tumor	GTV + 1–2 cm margin[c]	50.4/28 to 55.8/31
Meningioma	Enhancing tumor	GTV + 1–2 cm margin[c]	50.4/28 to 59.4/33
Pituitary adenoma	Enhancing tumor	GTV + 1–2 cm margin[c]	45/25 to 55.8/31
Medulloblastoma and anaplastic ependymoma			
Initial volume	Entire brain and spine	GTV + 1–2 cm margin[e]	30.6/17 to 36/24
Boost volume	Enhancing tumor	GTV + 1–2 cm margin	19.8/11 to 25.2/14
Ependymoma	Enhancing tumor	GTV + 1–2 cm margin[c]	50.4/28 to 59.4/33
Craniopharyngioma	Enhancing tumor	GTV + 1–2 cm margin[c]	50.4/28 to 59.4/33
Brain metastases	Whole brain	GTV + 1–2 cm margin[f]	30/10[g]
Spinal cord compression	Spinal cord and bony elements at same vertebral levels	1–2 vertebral levels above and below the compression	30/10

[a] For anaplastic astrocytoma that are nonenhancing, plan similarly to a low-grade diffuse astrocytoma.
[b] Most low-grade diffuse fibrillary astrocytomas are nonenhancing. The tumor (i.e., edema) is best seen on the T2-weighted MRI.
[c] Reduce to a 1-cm margin after 50.4 Gy if total dose exceeds 50.4 Gy.
[d] Malignant meningiomas should be planned similarly to glioblastoma multiforme. For meningeal hemangiopericytoma, the CTV should include the GTV + 2–3 cm margin.
[e] Margin at skull base should be about 1 cm, including cribform plate. Margin on spinal canal should be 2 cm except inferior border of lower spine field, which should be a bottom of S3. See section in chapter on craniospinal axis irradiation.
[f] Margin at skull base should be 1 cm. Otherwise there should be flash anteriorly, superiorly, and posteriorly.
[g] Exception would be a solitary metastasis status post complete resection, in which case the dose would be 45–50 Gy in 25–28 fractions.
[h] Include bony elements only when the spinal cord compression is associated with bone metastasis (i.e., vertebral bodies or bony elements involved).

the brain and spinal cord (1,24–26). It is clear that the radiation doses being recommended do not cure the majority of patients with primary or metastatic CNS tumors. Patients with metastatic disease may temporarily obtain local control, but will eventually succumb to systemic disease, new brain metastases, or local progression of their treated lesions. Patients with primary CNS tumors, with few exceptions, fail locally and die of local disease. Examination of patterns of local failures in both low- and high-grade gliomas has demonstrated that the majority of recurrences are within the central, enhancing region of the GTV (21,22). These data have led some to adopt the philosophy of limiting the GTV to the enhancing tumor as seen on T-1 with gadolinium images (23). This allows for escalation of dose to the tumor while limiting toxicity to normal brain tissue. It remains to be seen if this strategy will result in better local control, change patterns of failure, or impact survival in patients with primary CNS neoplasms.

Normal Tissue Tolerance and Radiation Injury of the Brain and Spinal Cord

Radiation tolerance of any normal tissues, including those of the CNS, are dependent on a number of factors, including total dose, fractionation, volume, host factors, organ specific characteristics, the radiation quality (linear energy transfer or LET), and adjunctive therapies. It is beyond the scope of this chapter to discuss the relative contributions of each to radiation induced toxicity, but these principles are addressed in Chapter 1. Table 15.6 shows partial and whole organ tolerance doses for the brain and spinal cord, and includes doses which are predicted to result in a 5% and 50% probability of injury 5 years following treatment with radiation (TD 5/5 and TD 50/5, respectively). These values are based on clinical data describing instances of radiation injury and the total doses and fraction sizes at which they occurred (29,30). Although the TD 50/5 for spinal cord is reportedly lower than that of brain, there are not good data to support this difference. Rather, the sequelae of spinal cord radiation injury are perceived as greater than those of brain injury, therefore tolerance doses have been arbitrarily lowered. In clinical practice, TD 5/5's of 70 Gy for partial brain and 50 Gy for a limited segment of spinal cord are commonly used. The TD 5/5's given for brain and spinal cord tolerance assume a fraction size of 180-200 cGy per day. For CNS tumor patients being treated with curative intent, fraction size should rarely exceed 200 cGy daily, and in most situations, should be 180 cGy. Fraction sizes greater than 200 cGy daily (usually 250-400 cGy) are commonly used for palliation of brain metastases and spinal cord compression, but only because such patients are not expected to live long enough to manifest normal tissue injury.

Table 15.6. Tolerance Doses for Normal Central Nervous System Tissues (29,30)

CNS Tissue	TD 5/5 (GY)	TD 50/5 (GY)	End Point
Rubin et al (15)			Infarction, necrosis
Brain			
Whole	60	70	
Partial (25%)	70	80	
Spinal cord			Infarction, necrosis
Partial (10-cm length)	45	55	
Emani et al (16)			
Brain			Infarction, necrosis
One-third	60	75	
Two-thirds	50	65	
Whole	40	60	
Brainstem			Infarction, necrosis
One-third	60	—	
Two-thirds	53	—	
Whole	50	65	
Spinal cord			Myelitis, necrosis
5 cm	50	70	
10 cm	50	70	
20 cm	47	—	
Cauda equina	60	75	Clinically apparent nerve damage
Brachial plexus			Clinically apparent nerve damage
One-third	62	77	
Two-thirds	61	76	
Whole	60	75	

Radiation injury is usually described in terms of its time course and severity. Acute injury is defined as occurring during the course of brain and spinal cord. These acute toxicities are relatively uncommon and usually only consist of increasing needs for steroids or antiseizure medications related to peri-tumoral edema. More common are the early delayed reactions, which occur several weeks to months after radiation has been completed, and the late delayed reactions, which occur beyond several months (and usually between 1 and 2 years) following treatment.

Early delayed reactions occur because of radiation effects to the oligodendroglial or myelin producing cells, resulting in demyelination. In the brain, this is clinically manifested as somnolence, irritability, loss of appetite, and sometimes an exacerbation of tumor-associated symptoms or signs. When these symptoms occur in children, usually following whole brain radiation, it is called the "somnolence syndrome." In the spinal cord, clinical findings include electric shock-like paresthesias that occur with flexion of the neck, or Lhermitte's sign. These early delayed reactions are nearly always transient (lasting several weeks to months) and do not predict for subsequent injury.

Late delayed reactions, on the other hand, are usually irreversible. The underlying mechanisms of late delayed reactions are two-fold, and include injury to the capillary endothelium leading to narrowing or obliteration of the small vessels supplying blood to the brain or spinal cord, and/or direct damage to CNS tissues. In both cases, the result is radiation necrosis, which is tissue damage to the substance or white matter of the brain or spinal cord. The clinical symptoms are directly related to this tissue damage, or indirectly from swelling of the adjacent normal tissues in response to necrosis. Brain necrosis may be asymptomatic if occurring in a non-critical area, but usually is associated with symptoms that are location specific (e.g., necrosis in the right motor strip would result in a left hemiparesis). Radiation induced necrosis involving the brain stem may have devastating results, including coma or death from loss of critical life functions. Spinal cord necrosis (radiation myelitis) is usually symptomatic and, depending on the level of the injury, may include sensory and motor loss in the legs or arms and legs, sphincter impairment of the bowel and bladder, and impotence in men. While certain treatments of cerebral radiation necrosis have been anecdotally described as being helpful to arrest or reverse the process, such as hyperbaric oxygen or drugs like warfarin or pentoxifylline, there is no proven value to such interventions (27,28).

Identification of critical normal tissues within treatment fields is also an important part of the treatment planning process. For brain tumors, this would include the optic chiasm, optic nerves, eyes, pituitary gland, and brainstem. For spinal cord tumors, critical normal tissues would be location dependent, and include the surrounding normal spinal cord as well as tissues and organs located anterior and lateral to the volume being treated. Table 15.7 shows the tolerance doses for critical normal tissues of the CNS, including the brainstem, eye, ear, optic chiasm, optic nerve, and pituitary gland, and the clinical manifestations of severe injury to these structures (30).

Table 15.7. Tolerance Doses for Miscellaneous Normal Tissues of the Cranium (30,43–45)

Normal Tissue	TD 5/5 (Gy)	TD 50/5 (Gy)	Manifestations of Severe Injury
Brainstem	50	65	Cardiorespiratory failure leading to death
Ear (middle/external)	30–55	40–65	Acute or chronic serous otitis
Eye			
Retina	45	65	Blindness
Lens	10	18	Cataract formation
Optic nerve or chiasm	50	65	Blindness

GENERAL CONSIDERATIONS OF CNS TUMOR TREATMENT PLANNING

Positioning and Immobilization

The first step in the treatment process is the decision of how to position the patient for simulation and treatment. There are two positioning issues for brain tumor patients, the first is whether to have the patient lie supine or prone, and second, whether to have the head and neck in a neutral, flexed, or extended position. In general, the supine position is the most stable and used when treating the majority of brain tumors. Exceptions include tumors located posteriorly, such as those in the occipital lobes or posterior fossa, and patients requiring craniospinal axis irradiation. In these situations, prone position is preferred, as it is for most spinal cord tumor patients. Head and neck positioning is an issue when limited by 2-dimensional radiation treatment planning (2DRTP). Neutral head and neck position may not be optimal for brain tumors in certain locations. For example, anteroposterior (AP) or posteroanterior (PA) beams would enter or exit through the eyes when treating a centrally located target like a pituitary tumor (Figure 15.8a). Flexion rotates the eyes inferiorly relative to the target (Figure 15.8b), thus allowing utilization of AP and PA beams. When treating brain tumors located in the posterior fossa, such as a pontine glioma, the supine position with neck extension allows a PA beam to be utilized, since the eyes are rotated superiorly and out of the exit of the beam (Figure 15.9a and b). Three-dimensional radiation treatment planning (3DRTP) allows for neutral head and neck position in most situations as non-coplanar beams can be used to avoid entry and exit dose to critical structures. Lastly, positioning of the head, neck, and body should be such that the anterior and lateral setup marks are in locatable and reproducible positions. Marks on steeply sloping surfaces, the ears, nose, lips, and chin should be avoided when possible.

Once positioned, the patient must be immobilized. There are a variety of commercially available custom-made head immobilization devices, most of which utilize thermoplastic (Figure 15.10a), plaster casting (Figure 15.10b), or other materials such as expandable foam or plastic beads in a vacuum bag. They are adaptable for flexion or extension when the patient is in the supine position. Similar devices can be used for brain tumor patients requiring the prone position (Figure 15.11). When more rigid head immobilization is desired, such as for fractionated stereotactic radiation therapy or radiosurgery, a modified stereotactic head frame with non-invasive multiple-point head fixation is utilized, examples of which can be found in Chapter 10. Generally, special immobilization devices are not used for patients with spinal cord tumors, although custom devices made of thermoplastic (Figure 15.12), expandable foam, or plastic beads in vacuum bags are avail-

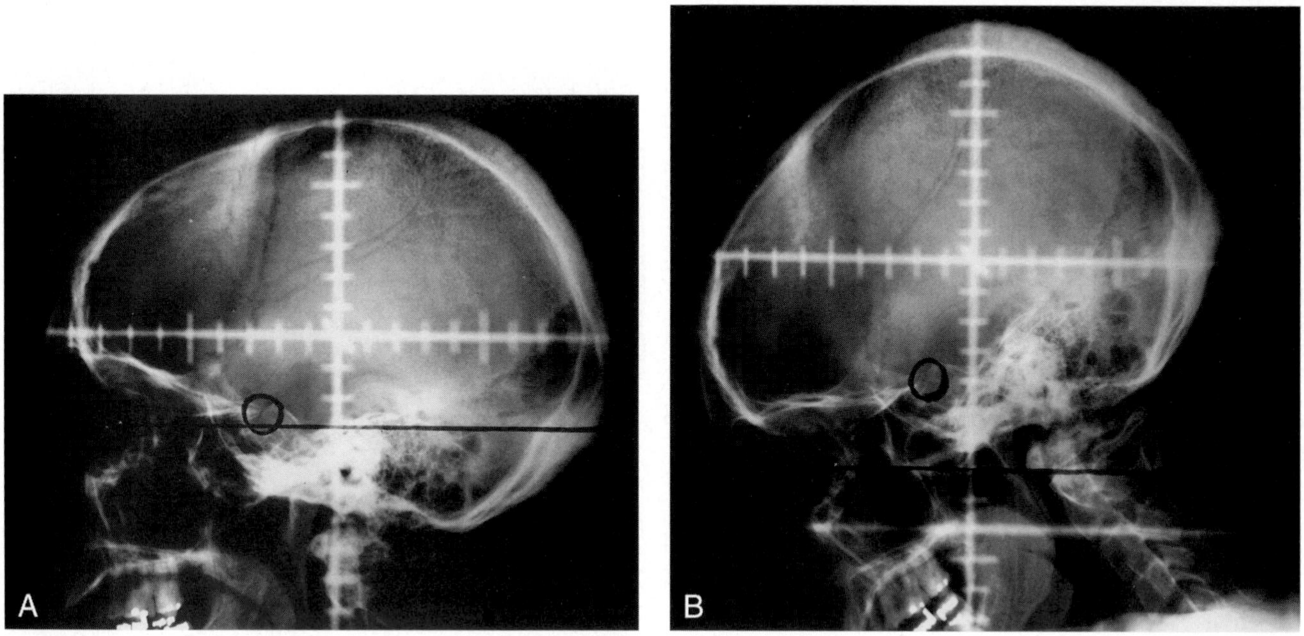

Figure 15.8. Lateral views of the skull with varying head tilt. A horizontal line is drawn through the orbits. The outlined target is representative of a typical pituitary adenoma. **A.** Head in neutral position. **B.** Head and neck flexed (chin tuck).

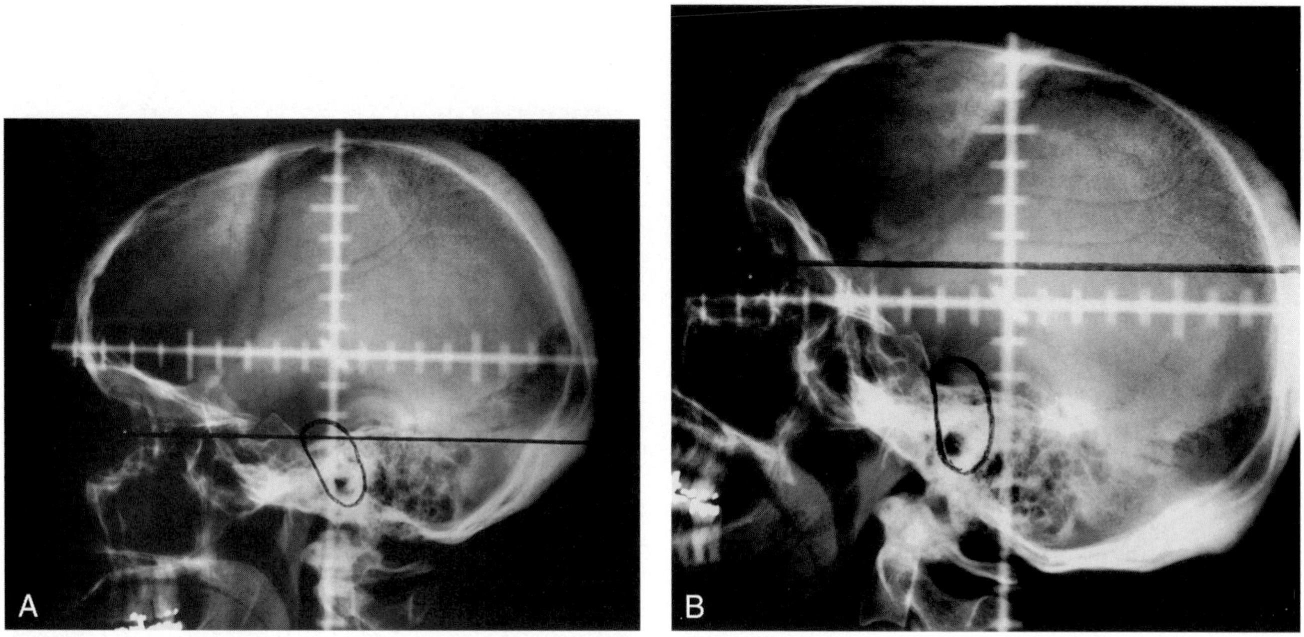

Figure 15.9. Lateral views of the skull as in Figure 15.8. The outlined target is representative of a typical pontine tumor. **A.** Head in neutral position. **B.** Head and neck extended (chin up).

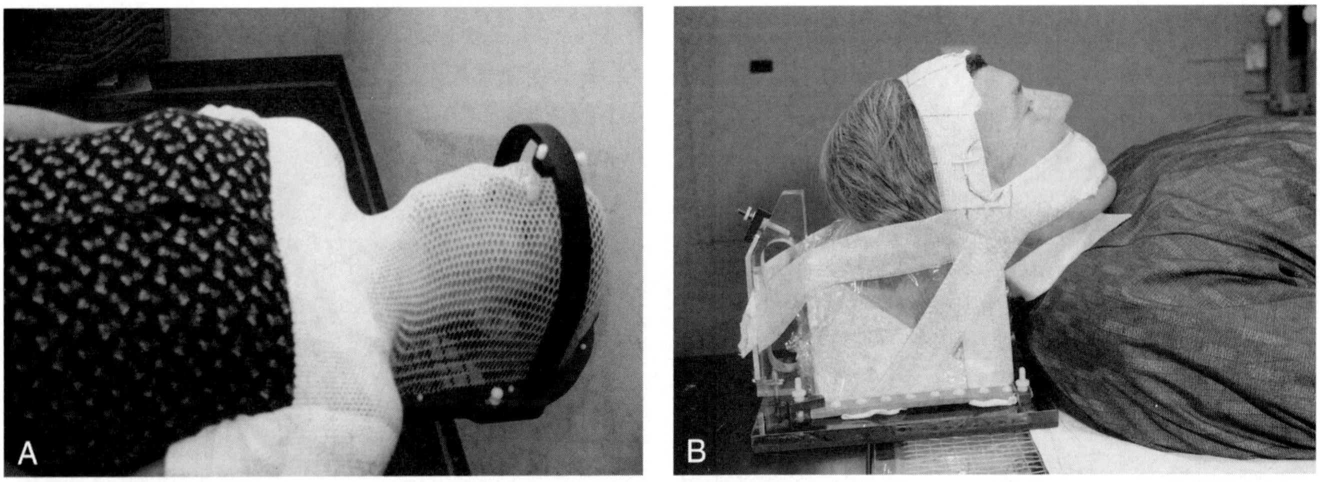

Figure 15.10. A. Supine head immobilization device made of thermoplastic (Courtesy of Med-Tec, Orange City, IA). **B.** Supine head immobilization device made of plaster cast material.

Figure 15.11. Thermoplastic prone head immobilization device used for craniospinal axis irradiation (Courtesy of Med-Tec, Orange City, IA).

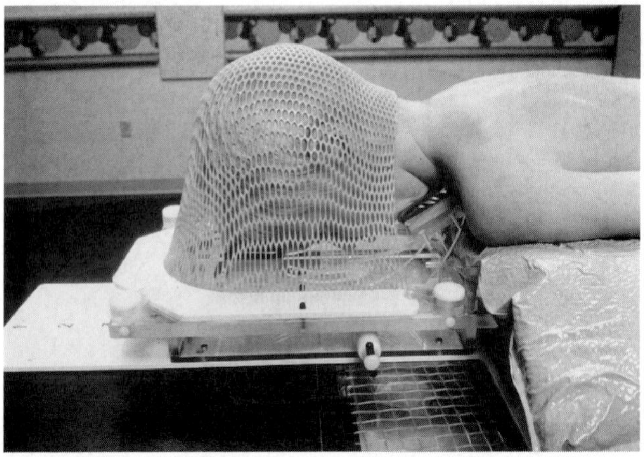

Figure 15.12. Prone trunk immobilization device made of thermoplastic (Courtesy of Med-Tec, Orange City, IA).

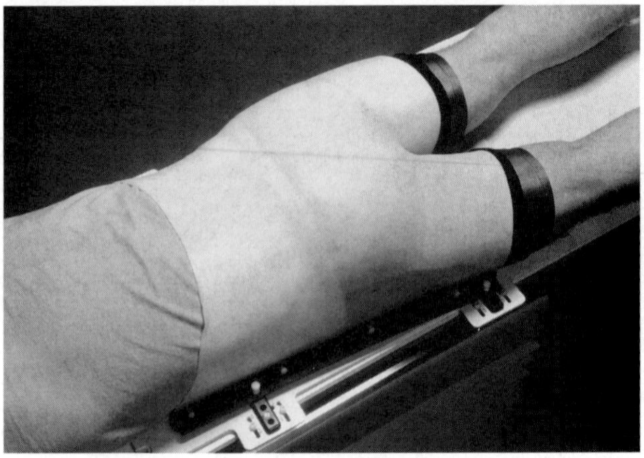

able. Regardless of the immobilization device chosen, it must be designed to fit the physical dimensions of the CT or MRI scanner, and constructed of materials that are compatible with the imaging modality to prevent image artifact or distortion.

Imaging Modalities in 2D and 3D Radiation Treatment Planning

Once immobilized, the patient is ready to have a treatment planning imaging study. Isocenter(s) can be established either before or after the study is obtained. If done before, diagnostic imaging studies can be used to aid placement of the isocenter on the orthogonal simulation films as close to the geometric center of the tumor as possible. Plastic afterloading catheters or gel capsules (e.g. Vitamin E) can be taped on the patient's skin or immobilization device along the axial, coronal, and sagittal planes through the three points used to define the isocenter (Figure 15.13a). This allows relatively precise visualization of the simulated isocenter on the treatment planning imaging study (Figure 15.13b). When 3D treatment planning or CT simulation is not available, this process facilitates the transfer of the GTV onto the simulation films, which in turn aids treatment field placement and custom block definition.

Three-dimensional RTP takes advantage of computer technology which allows reconstruction of 3-D images from the stacked 2-D slices of CT or MRI studies. CT scans were the original imaging studies used in the development of 3DRTP and, in most cases, provide adequate anatomic detail as well as the electron density differences between bone, air cavities, and soft tissue, which are needed for accurate dosimetry. Because of their widespread availability and relatively low cost, CT scans remain an important imaging modality in 3DRTP.

Magnetic resonance imaging, however, has clear advantages as an imaging modality for the 3DRTP of CNS tumors. As stated above, it provides superior anatomic detail and resolution within soft tissues, improved visualization of non-enhancing lesions, and freedom from bone artifact (critical in planning of tumors in and about the base of skull). The disadvantages of MRI are poor visualization of bony anatomy and/or calcifications with standard spin-echo techniques, inability to distinguish tumor from edema on T2-weighted images, and its relatively high cost (31). Magnetic resonance images are potentially subject to geometric distortions that may be machine and time dependent and, therefore, difficult to control. Thus, information relating to patient positioning and localization of structures can be difficult to interpret. Finally, while MRI based dosimetry is an active topic of research, dose calculations taking into account tissue inhomogeneities can routinely be done only with CT data.

To take full advantage of both imaging modalities, the MRI data set can be registered (fused) onto a CT data set, thereby providing superior anatomic resolution in a format amenable to accurate dosimetry and localization. Image registration may be done manually by matching easily defined anatomic constructs (anastructs) common to both MRI and CT, such as the ventricles and globes. The anastructs can be translated along their orthogonal axes and rotated until they are visually matched. The remainder of the data sets are then registered. Automated methods for

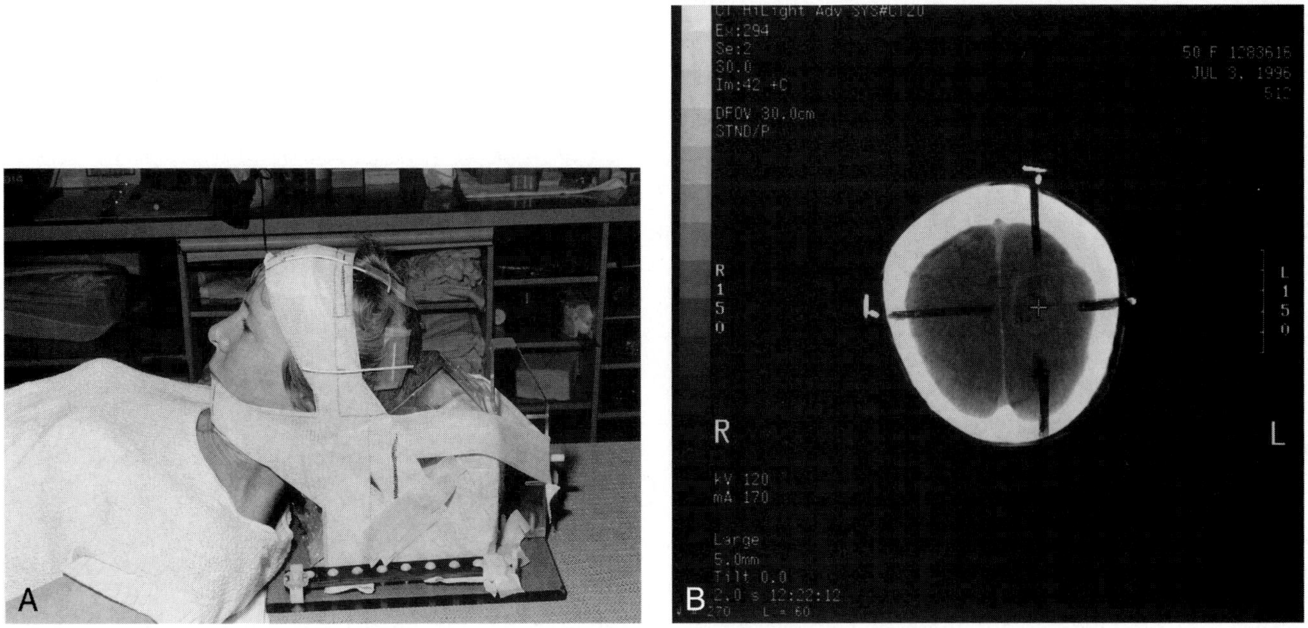

Figure 15.13. **A.** Plastic afterloading catheters taped along the horizontal and vertical axes of three points on the immobilization device that indicate isocenter. **B.** Axial CT slice at isocenter showing the afterloading catheters.

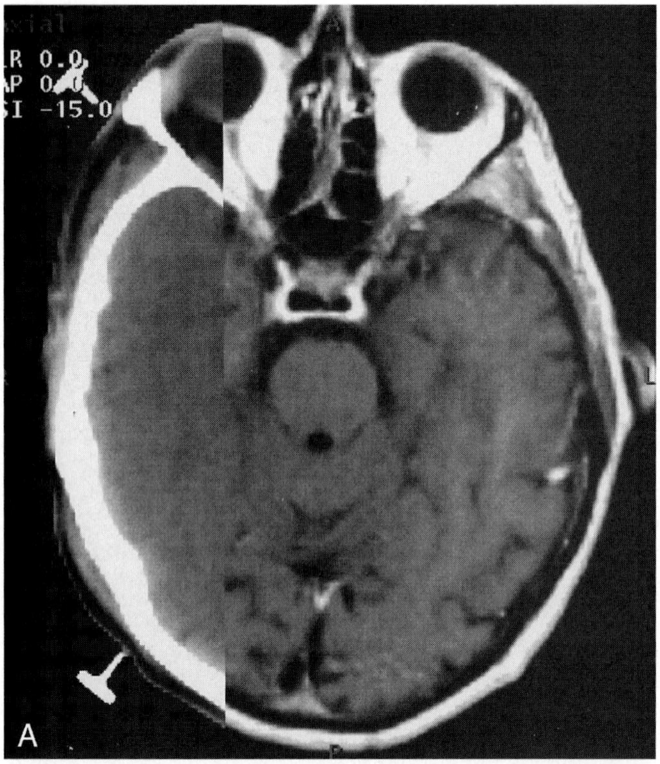

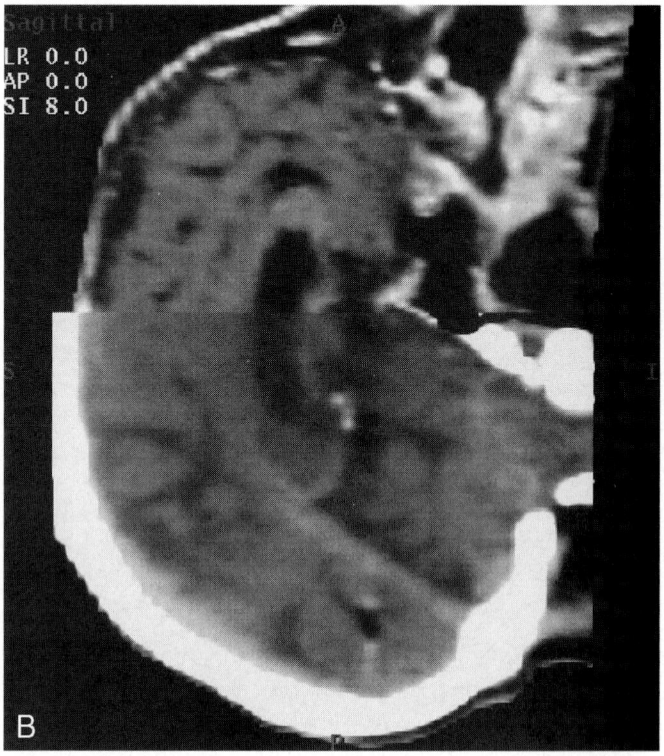

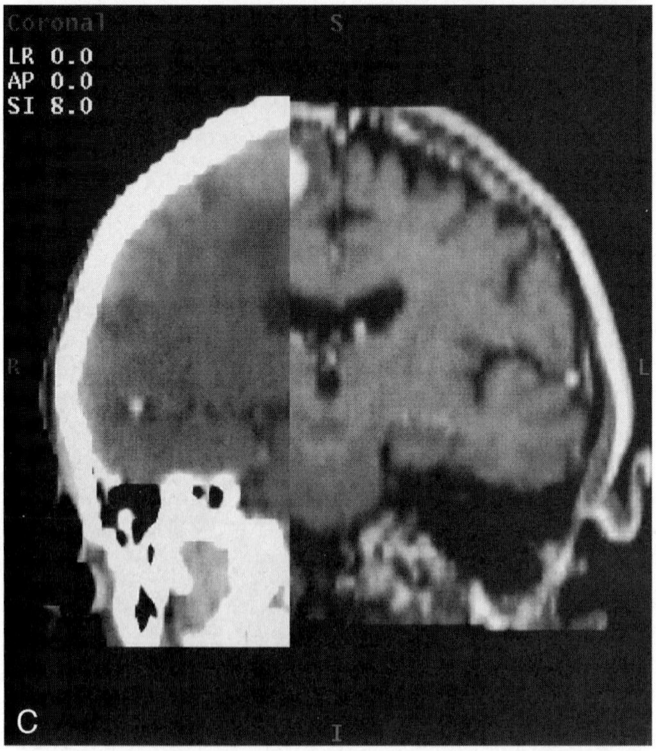

Figure 15.14. CT and MRI image fusions through easily definable anastructs. **A.** Axial plane showing match through the globe. **B.** Sagittal plane showing match through corpus callosum and ventricle. **C.** Coronal plane showing match through ventricles and tumor.

accomplishing the same anatomic registration have been developed by Chen and Pelizzari (32) and by Fraas and McShan (33). Both these methods rely on identification of points, surfaces, objects, or object moments common to the imaging studies. These defining volumes are then translated and rotated until the error in their registration is minimized. The remainder of the data sets are then fused (Figure 15.14a–c). The final step is to identify and contour the GTV and CTV as well as any critical or dose-limiting structures that may be within a treatment field.

General Principles of Treatment Planning for Brain Tumors

Whole Brain Irradiation

There are several techniques that can be utilized for whole brain irradiation. A "clinical" setup involves the use of external anatomic landmarks, usually the canthus and mastoid process, to place a rectangular treatment field over the cranial vault (Figure 15.15). No simulation is needed for the clinical setup as the superior, anterior, and posterior borders are simply set with a light border "flashing" over the skull. The inferior (caudal) border is set with the collimator rotated to produce a field edge 1-2 cm below a line from the canthus to the mastoid tips. A small block is then carefully placed to shield the globes while still allowing adequate coverage of the anterior-inferior extent of the cranial contents.

Alternatively, a "custom" setup can be designed with a shaped block that follows the contour of the base of the brain with a 1-2 cm margin (Figure 15.16). When drawing the custom block, the following structures should be identified: floor of the anterior cranial fossa, including the cribiform plate, middle cranial fossa, posterior fossa, and the skull base, including the foramina through which the cranial nerves exit. The patient should be simulated in the supine position and the head immobilized, usually with a thermoplastic cast. Radiopaque markers should be placed on each lateral canthus to document eye position with respect to the radiation field. If the isocenter is chosen to be centrally located in the cranium, the canthus markers will not be aligned due to beam divergence. The opposite eye will receive dose from each lateral beam unless this divergence is corrected. Three methods are routinely used for this purpose (Figure 15.17). The gantry can be angled an appropriate number of degrees to compensate for beam divergence using the formula:

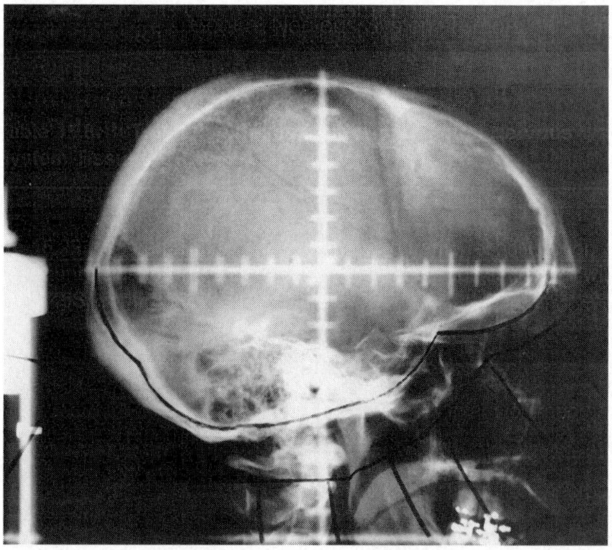

Figure 15.16. Simulation film of a custom setup for whole brain irradiation. Base of skull is outlined and a 2-cm margin is used to define borders of the custom block. Anteriorly, the margin is reduced to 1 cm to allow shielding of the eyes.

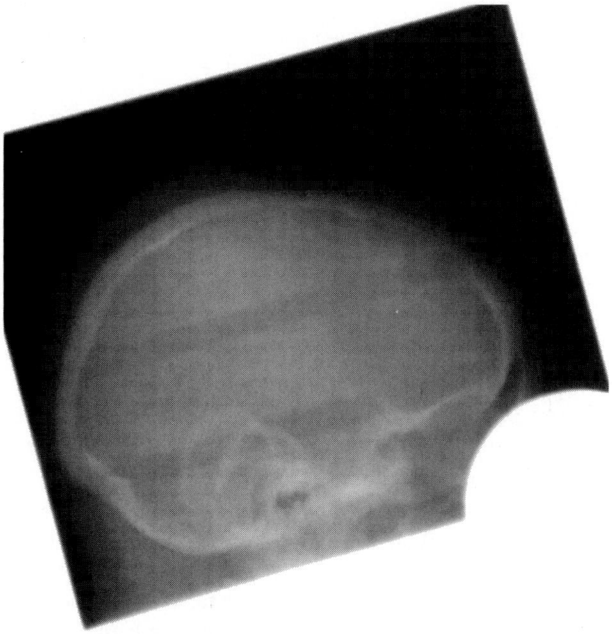

Figure 15.15. Port film of a clinical setup for whole brain irradiation with hand-place eye block.

$$\theta = \tan^{-1}(CL_1/SAD) \qquad (15.1)$$

CL_1 equals the distance from the isocenter to the canthus and SAD is the source-axis distance. Alternatively, the gantry can be rotated under fluoroscopic guidance until the canthus markers are superimposed for each lateral beam. The degree of gantry rotation should be identical whether using the geometric calculation or the manual procedure. The final method for addressing beam divergence through the eyes is to place the central axis on the canthus using asymmetric collimator jaws, or a large anterior block. As long as the patient's head has been set up relatively straight, the canthi should be superimposed and there will be no beam divergence at central axis.

The selection of beam energy is also an issue for whole brain irradiation. Figures 15.18a–c show the isodose curves for whole brain irradiation utilizing 4, 6, and 18 MV photons. With the higher energies (> 10MV), the peripheral tissues of the brain and the meninges may be underdosed, depending on the thickness of the scalp and skull. Conversely, due to the curvature of the skull, there will be relative high dose regions towards the top of the skull. This inhomogeneity is increased with lower energies.

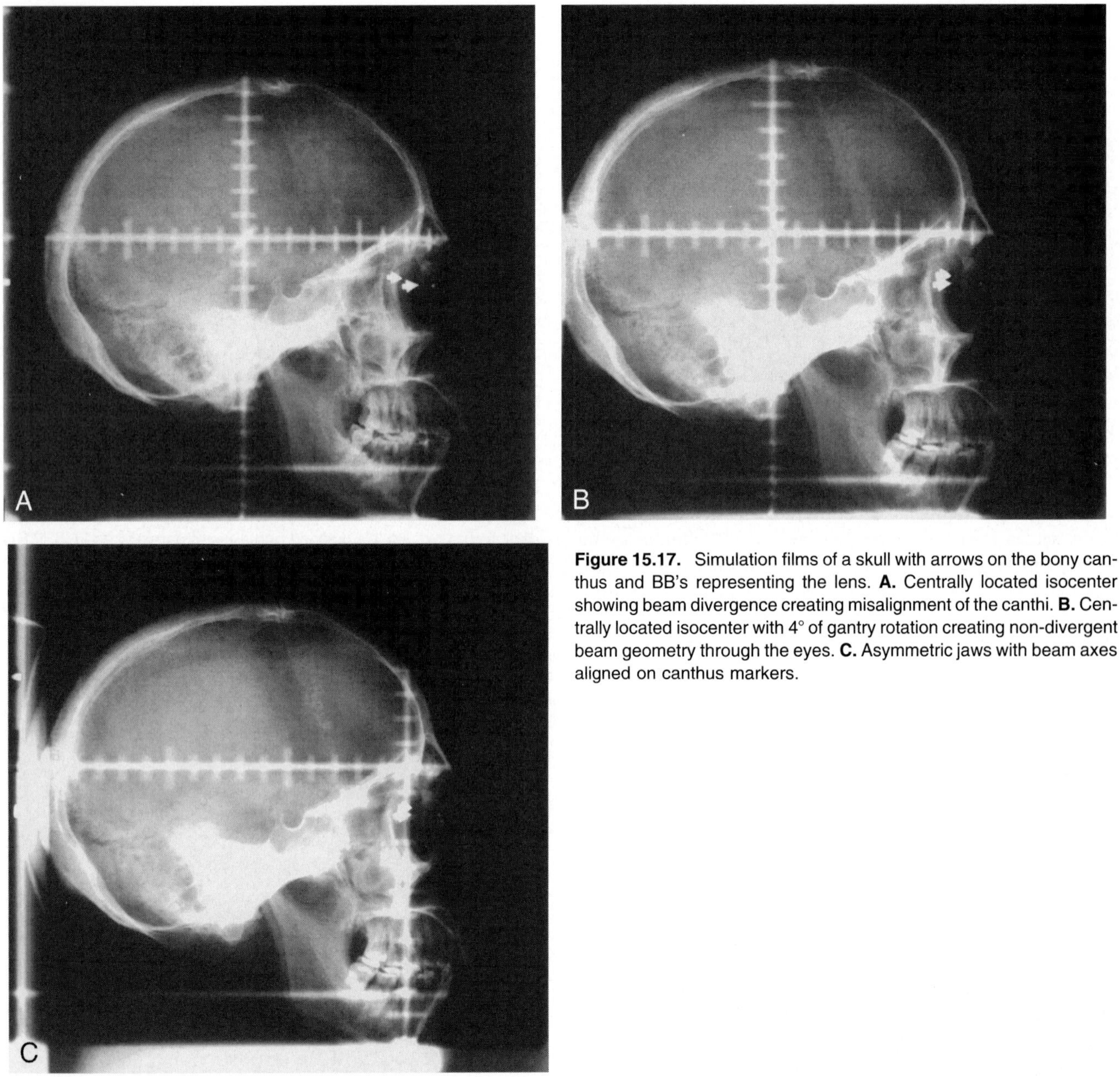

Figure 15.17. Simulation films of a skull with arrows on the bony canthus and BB's representing the lens. **A.** Centrally located isocenter showing beam divergence creating misalignment of the canthi. **B.** Centrally located isocenter with 4° of gantry rotation creating non-divergent beam geometry through the eyes. **C.** Asymmetric jaws with beam axes aligned on canthus markers.

When treating whole brain fields, the clinically relevant issue is to provide a set minimum dose to the entirety of the cranial contents. The relatively overdosed regions are usually not clinically relevant. Therefore, photon energies of ≤ 6MV are recommended.

Custom Fields

There is one general principle that applies for the treatment of all brain tumors not requiring whole brain irradiation: multiple field treatment plans should routinely be used to provide acceptable dose homogeneity within the target while limiting dose to normal brain. These multi-field plans may be generated using standard 2D planning, or, optimally, 3D planning algorithms. Two-dimensional planning involves the use of beams which are coplanar, i.e., oriented in the same plane, whereas 3D planning allows utilization of beams which are non-coplanar, i.e., oriented in different planes. Three-dimensional RTP has the advantage of using an essentially infinite number of beam trajectories, permitting greater sparing of critical normal tissues and allowing higher tumor doses to the GTV and CTV to be given. Figures 15.19a–d show contours from an axial (transverse) slice of a treatment planning imaging

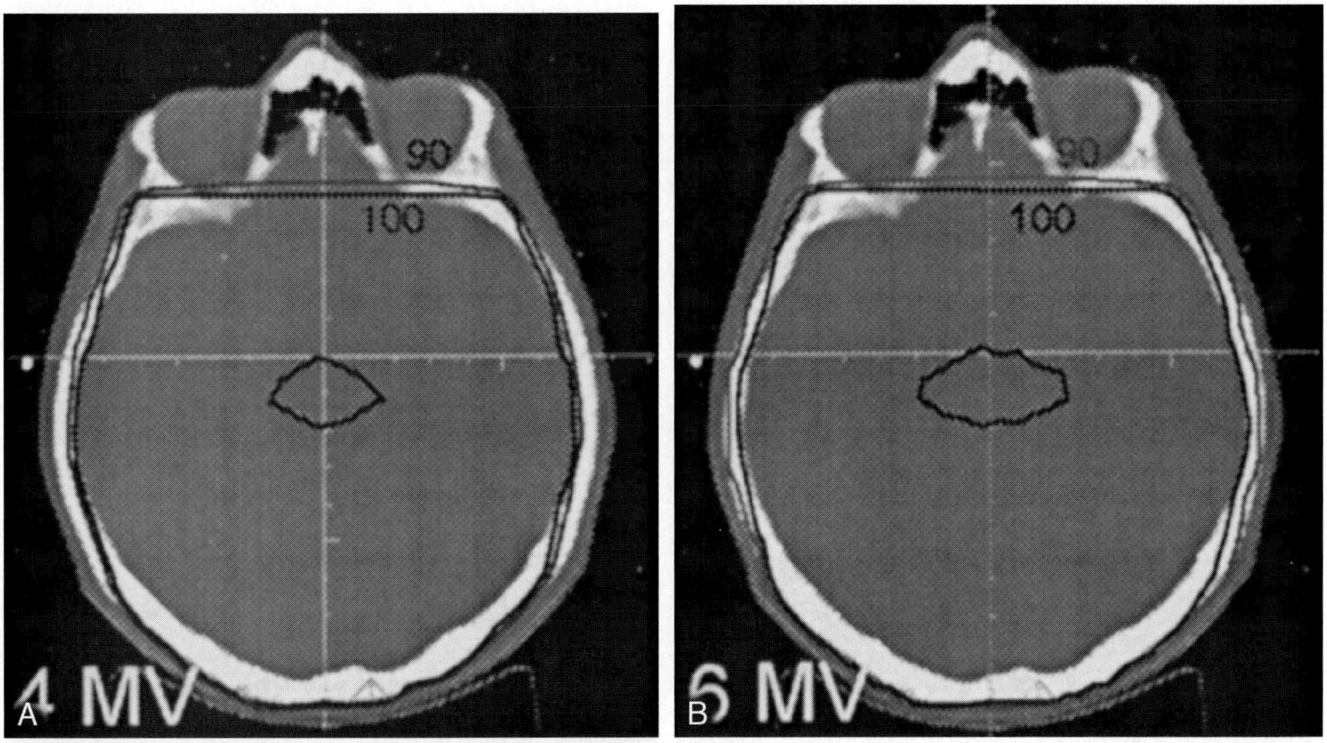

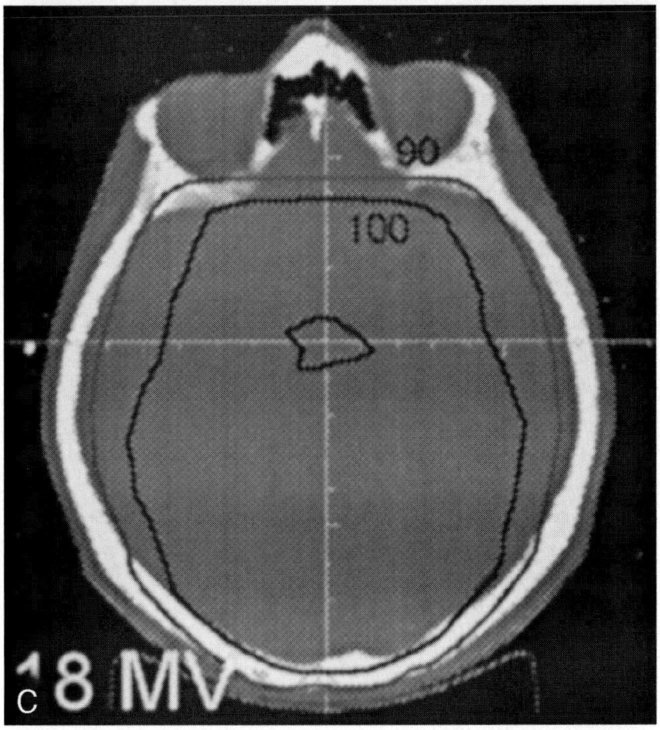

Figure 15.18. Isodose curves on axial CT images for whole brain irradiation. The 100% and 90% lines are highlighted. **A.** 4 MV. **B.** 6 MV. **C.** 18 MV.

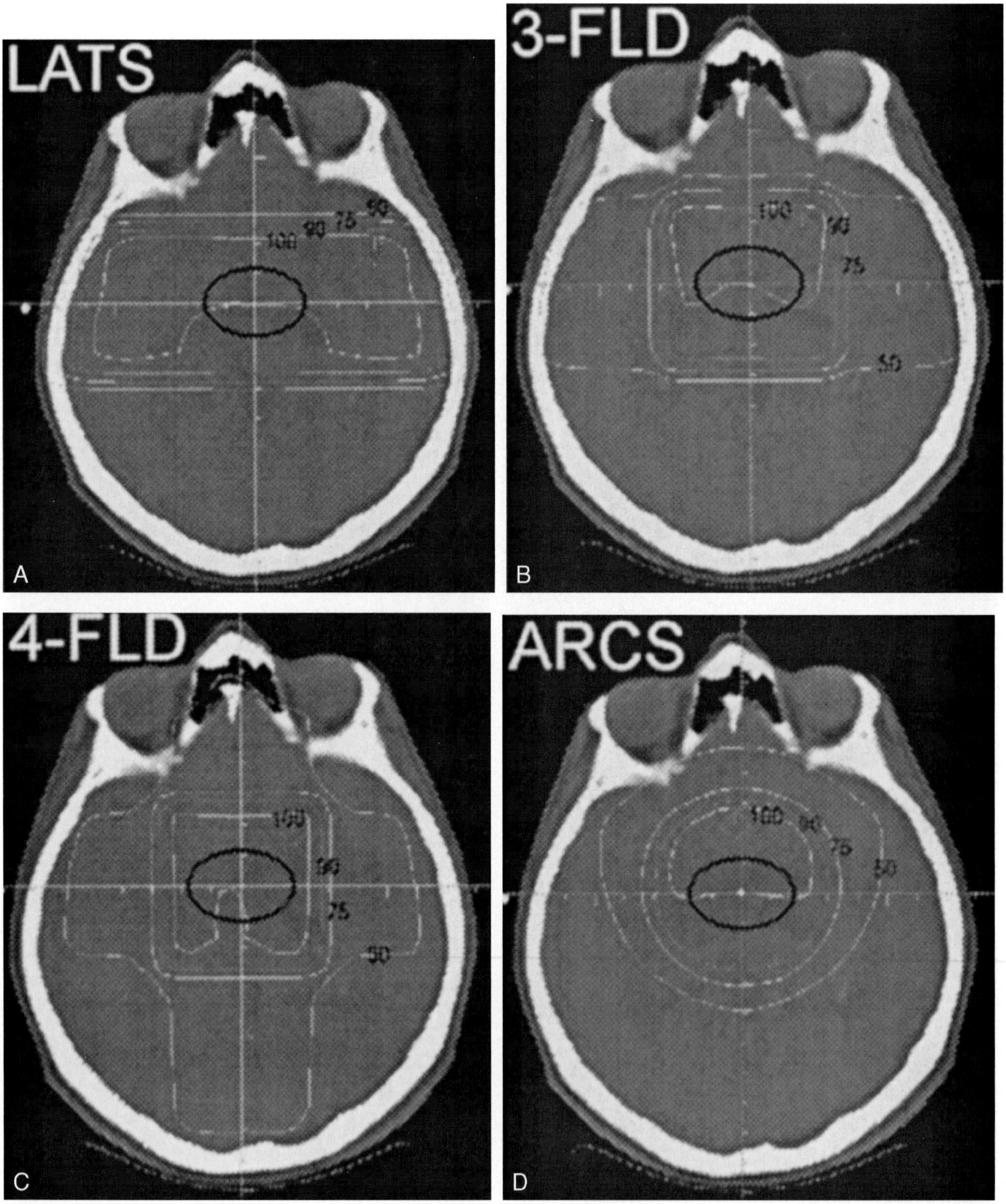

Figure 15.19. Axial CT images with a sphero-elliptical target centrally located. Isodose lines are drawn normalized to 100% at isocenter. **A.** Opposed lateral fields. **B.** AP and opposed laterals. **C.** AP-PA and opposed laterals. **D.** 360° arc rotation.

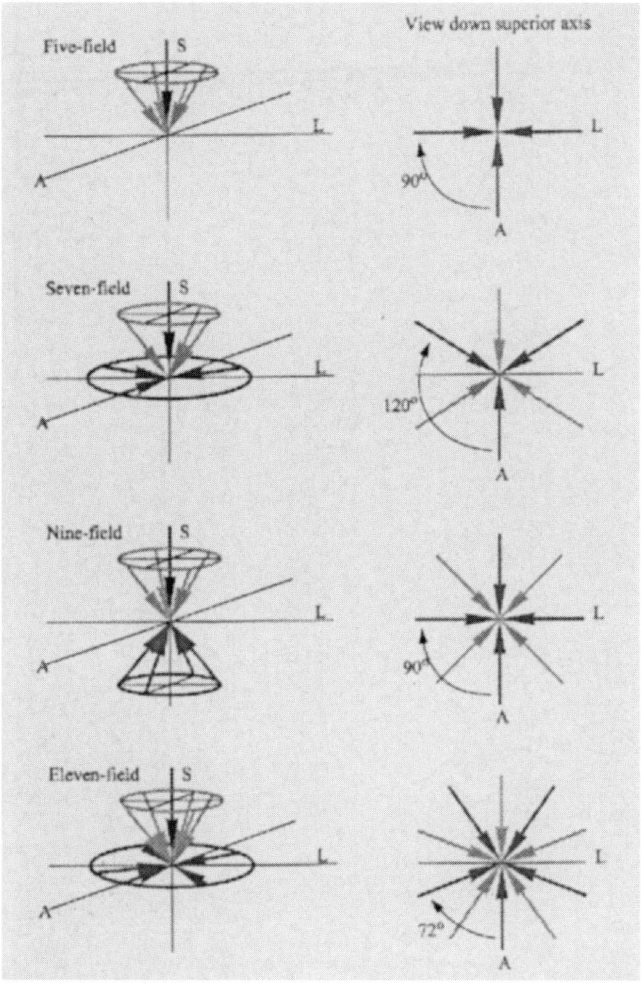

Figure 15.20. Template for static, noncoplanar approaches using 5, 7, 9, and 11 fields. Orientation of fields are shown in the axial plane and from above.

study. The isocenter is located in the middle of a central sphero-elliptical target. Four hypothetical 2D plans are shown, each delivering 100% to isocenter utilizing high energy photon beams, including two fields (opposed laterals), three fields (AP plus opposed laterals), four fields (AP, PA, plus opposed laterals), and a 360° arc rotation. The disadvantage of opposed fields is obvious—the normal tissues lateral to the target receive the same dose as the target itself. As the number of treatment fields is increased, the dose distribution improves, and the dose to the surrounding normal brain tissue decreases, being optimal for the 360° arc rotation. An alternative approach using 3DRTP involves the use of multiple (5, 7, 9, or 11) static non-opposed fields, as described by Bourland et al. (Figure 15.20) (34). This technique results in a sharp beam edge or penumbra, mimicking the approaches of linear accelerator based stereotactic radiotherapy (35) and radiosurgery, as described in Chapter 10.

General Principles of Treatment Planning for Spinal Cord Tumors

The most common approach to the spinal cord tumor patient, primary or metastatic, is with a single PA treatment field. Figure 15.21 shows axial CT images at the level of the middle lumbar spine. Two hypothetical treatment plans are shown, each delivering 100% to isocenter utilizing high energy photon beams, including a single PA field, and a wedged pair (angled posterior obliques). While the single PA field has an inhomogeneous dose distribution (Figure 15.21a), it does have the advantage of sparing normal tissues laterally, which are the kidneys in this case. On the other hand, the two field approach provides a more homogeneous dose distribution, but it spreads out the radiation dose to more anterior normal tissues, such as the small intestine and transverse colon (Figure 15.21b). Kidney tolerance, if a significant portion is encompassed

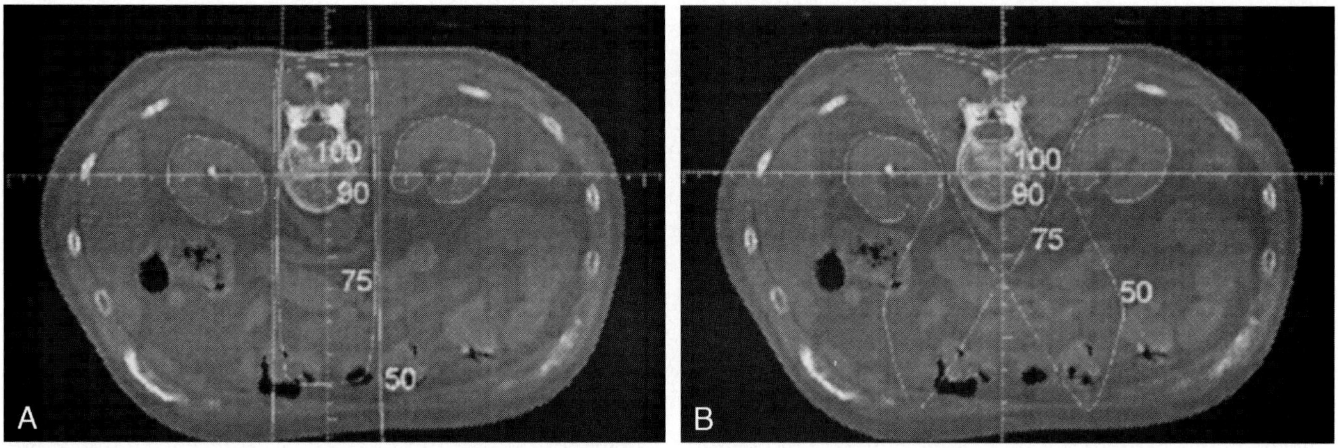

Figure 15.21. Axial CT image through the middle lumbar spine with isodose curves for an isocenter located in the posterior aspect of the spinal cord. **A.** Single PA field. **B.** Two-field, wedged obliques.

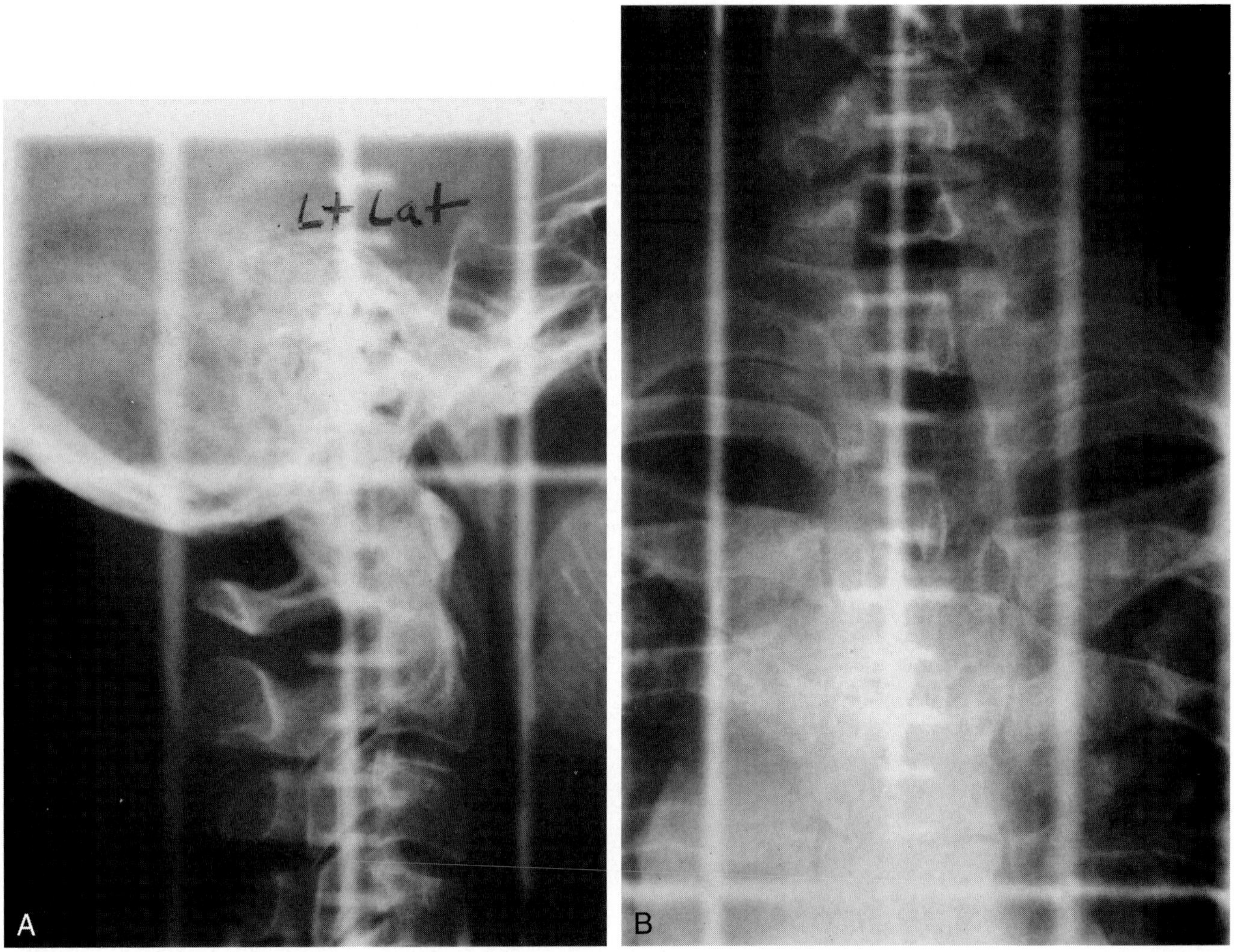

Figure 15.22. Simulation films of the beam split technique for cervicothoracic irradiation. The central axis is placed just above the shoulders (C4). **A.** Opposed lateral fields for the mid and upper spine. **B.** Single PA field for the low cervical and upper thoracic spine. Potential overlap of the abutting fields must be addressed.

(whole organ TD 5/5 = 23 Gy) (30), must be kept in mind when utilizing this approach in the region of the upper lumbar spine. There are situations where single and multiple field approaches can be combined to either minimize normal tissue toxicity or improve the dose distribution. In the case of cervicothoracic irradiation, a single PA field would exit through the oral cavity, oropharynx and larynx superiorly. An alternative approach uses a "split beam." The central axis is placed just above the shoulders. Opposed lateral treatment fields are used for the cervical spine, and a PA field for the thoracic spine (Figure 15.22a and b). The lower lumbar spine and sacrum are often located close to midplane in the AP-PA dimension such that a single PA beam would deliver excessive dose to overlying soft tissues. An AP-PA beam arrangement is most commonly used for this region. Alternatives include a 3- or 4-field approach (PA plus opposed laterals or AP-PA plus opposed laterals), or a "split beam" approach using a PA field to treat the upper lumbar spine and three or four fields to treat the sacrum or pelvis.

Objective Criteria for Evaluating Treatment Plans in CNS Tumor Patients

Once a treatment plan has been generated, it must be critically evaluated by the team of dosimetrists, physicists, and physicians involved in the care of the patient. There are simple ways in which differences in the dose distributions on various treatment plans can be compared. One method is to define areas or volumes of increased dose ("hot spots") and decreased dose ("cold spots"). ICRU-50 defines a "hot spot" as a volume >15 mm in minimum diameter outside the PTV which receives >100% of the specified PTV dose (18). For most of their non-3D brain tumor protocols, the RTOG defines hot and cold spots as those which are <95% and >105%, respectively, of the prescribed total dose, implying that total dose variations of +/- 5% are acceptable. These criteria should also apply to the daily dose distributions as well. The location of hot and cold spots also needs to be taken into account. This is particularly important in CNS tumor radiation therapy in which "acceptable" areas or volumes of increased dose may be in skin, subcutaneous tissue, muscle, bone, or CSF, all normal tissues that are unlikely to manifest clinically significant radiation injury. Conversely, unacceptable hot spots could occur in critical structures such as optic nerve/chiasm, brain stem, or auditory apparatus.

Dose-volume histogram (DVH) analysis can be used to graphically represent dose distribution to targets and surrounding tissues (36). Calculation of DVHs involves volumetric analysis of dose to structures and, therefore, requires 3-D planning capabilities. These analyses allow comparison of competing treatment plans with respect to tumor coverage and dose to critical structures. If the competing treatment plans adequately cover the target volume, the plan that treats a lesser volume of normal tissue to high dose should be superior based on lower toxicity. One can attempt to visually compare DVHs to select an optimal plan. This subjective method of plan "optimization" is to be discouraged, especially if the DVHs overlap.

Mathematical models have been developed by Lyman (37) and Withers (38) that attempt to calculate the probability of normal tissue complications (NTCP) using organ or tissue DVHs. The Lyman model incorporates the variables of dose, volume of the organ treated, and relative radiosensitivity of the tissue. The statistical model proposed by Withers also includes basic information regarding the functional architecture of the tissue. A limited number of investigators have attempted to retrospectively validate these models in patients with CNS malignancies (39–41). However, due to the functional complexity of the brain's neural network, it should be realized that these models, at best, are rough estimates of complication probabilities.

EXAMPLES OF SPECIFIC TREATMENT APPROACHES AND PLANS

Pituitary Adenoma

Figure 15.23 shows a coronal MRI image (T1-weighted plus gadolinium) of a patient following subtotal resection of a pituitary adenoma. The GTV is the residual enhancing tumor, the CTV is the entire sella plus a 1-cm margin. The prescription dose is 50.4 Gy in 28 fractions. The patient is placed in the supine position, with maximum neck flexion, to allow for the use of anteriorly and posteriorly directed beams that will not enter or exit through the eyes. Figures 15.24a and b show the isodose distributions from two acceptable 2-D treatment plans; a 3-field approach (AP plus

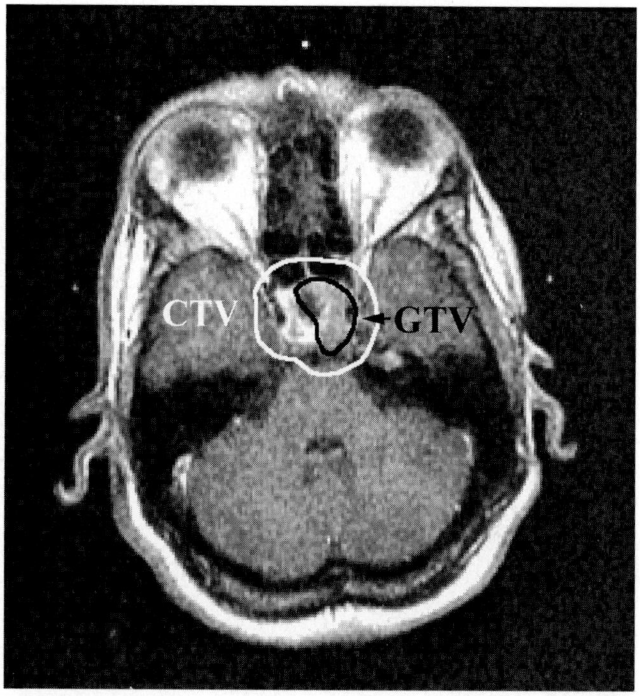

Figure 15.23. Coronal MRI image (T1 with contrast) of a subtotally resected pituitary macroadenoma in a patient with elevated growth hormone (GH) and acromegaly.

wedged opposed laterals), and a 360° arc rotation. The rotational arc plan minimizes dose to the adjacent temporal lobes. Orthogonal simulation films of the rotational arc plan are necessary for weekly isocenter verification since port films cannot otherwise be taken.

Three-dimensional planning allows for the use of multiple non-coplanar beam arrangements to limit dose to the temporal lobes and adjacent structures such as optic chiasm and optic nerves. These structures are easily identified on MRI scans and can sometimes be excluded from high dose regions. Representative 5- and 7-beam arrangements are shown in Figures 15.24c and d with surface rendered reconstructions demonstrating entry and exit dose. The 5-field plan utilizes an AG30S (AP with gantry angled 30° superiorly), SG15A/T32L (vertex with 15° gantry angled anteriorly and couch rotated 32° left), RG15A/T32S (right lateral with gantry angled 15° anteriorly and couch rotated 32° superiorly), LT20I (left lateral with couch rotated 20° inferiorly) and RT20I (right lateral with couch rotated 20° inferiorly). The 7-field plans include all fields just described plus an SG30A (vertex with gantry angled 30° anteriorly) and an SG40P (vertex with gantry angled 40 ° posteriorly). Dose volume histograms for target, optic nerves, and temporal lobes are shown in Figure 15.25. All plans provide adequate dose to the target. The advantage of the 5- and 7-field plans is in limiting dose to surrounding normal structures, in this case optic chiasm, nerves, and temporal

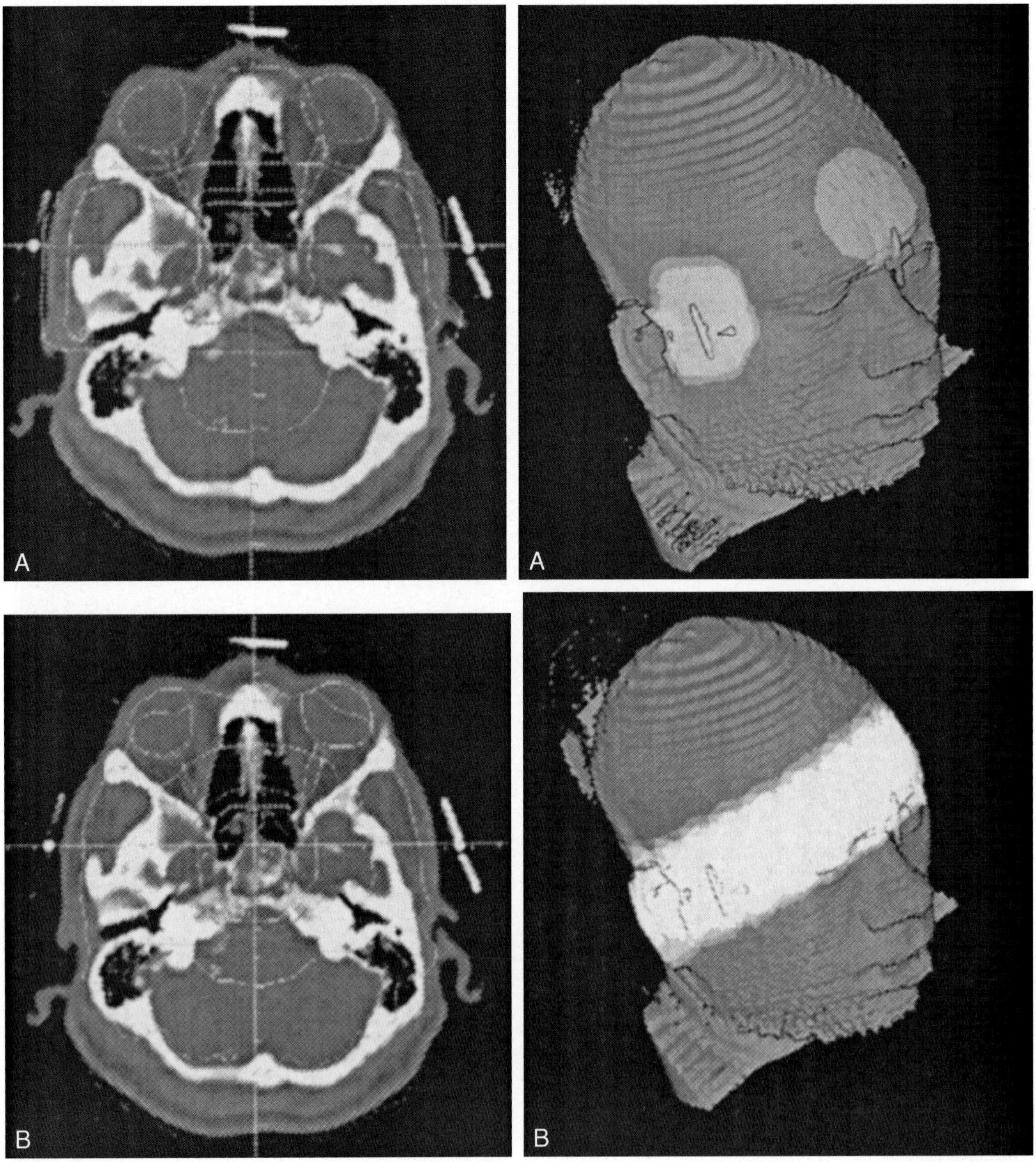

Figure 15.24. Isodose distributions and surface rendered reconstructions of multiple field plans for treatment of the patient shown in Figure 15.23. **A.** Three-field plan (AP and wedged opposed laterals). **B.** 360° arc rotation.

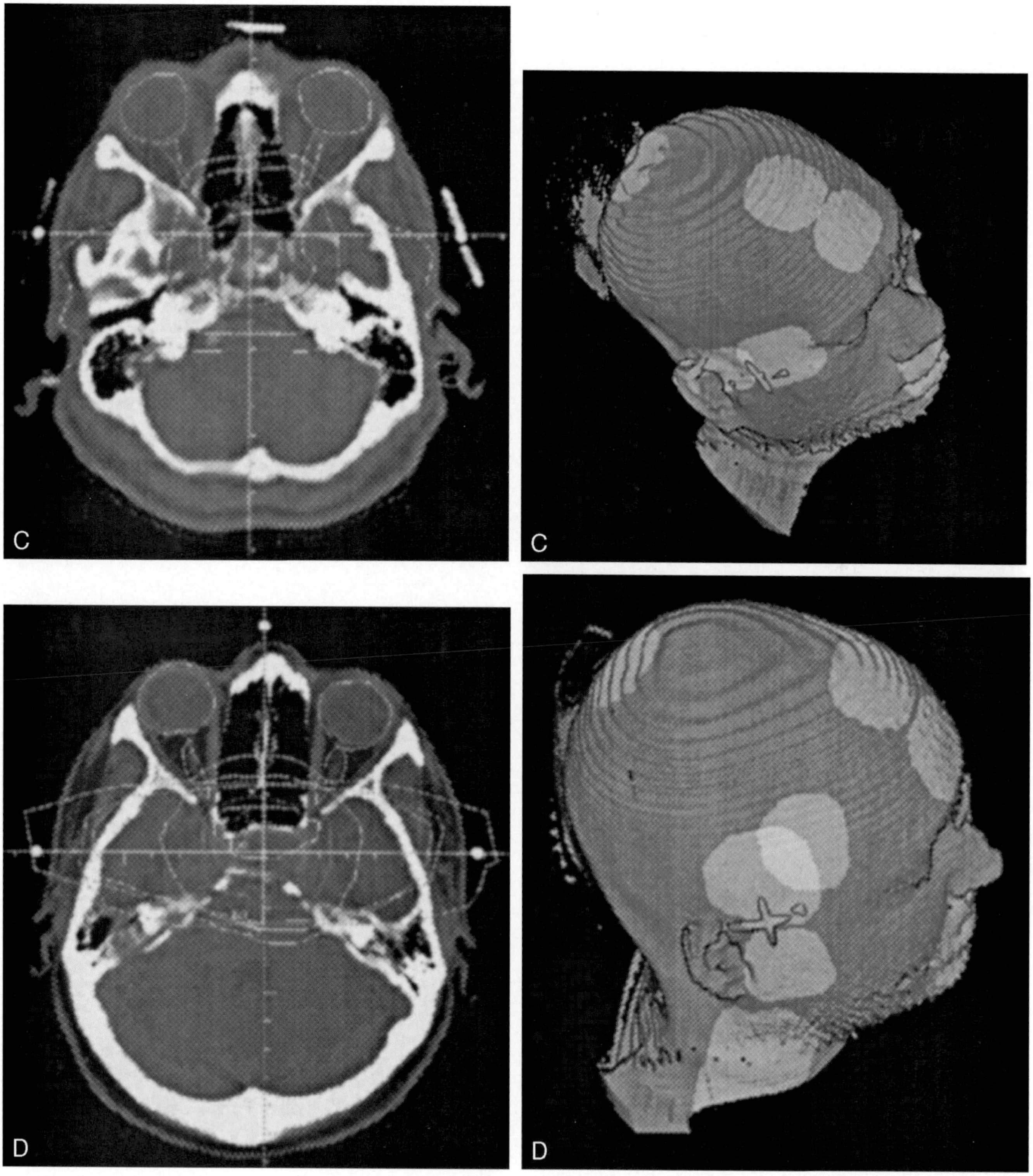

Figure 15.24. *(continued)* **C.** Five-field noncoplanar plan (fields) **D.** Seven-field noncoplanar plan (fields).

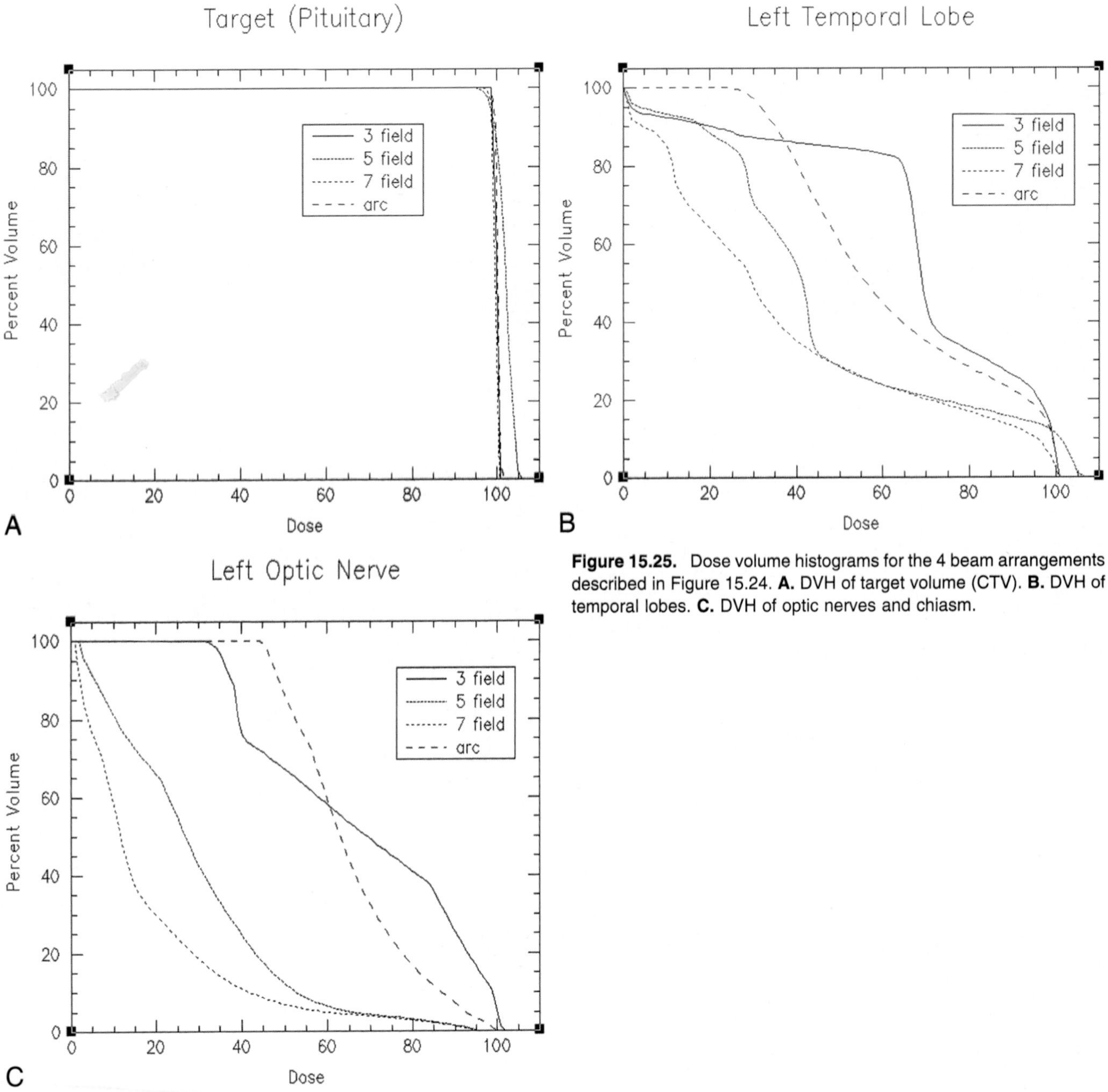

Figure 15.25. Dose volume histograms for the 4 beam arrangements described in Figure 15.24. **A.** DVH of target volume (CTV). **B.** DVH of temporal lobes. **C.** DVH of optic nerves and chiasm.

lobes. Alternatives to the 2-D and 3-D plans described above include stereotactic radiosurgery or fractionated stereotactic radiotherapy as described in Chapter 10.

Temporal Lobe Lesions

Figures 15.26a and b shows the MRI scan of a patient following subtotal resection of a right temporal glioblastoma multiforme. The initial GTV is the resection cavity, residual enhancing tumor, and the surrounding edema. The initial CTV adds a 2-cm margin. The boost GTV is the residual enhancing tumor, and the boost CTV adds 2 cm. The prescription dose is 50.4 Gy in 28 fractions to the initial volume and 14.4 Gy in 8 fractions to the boost volume, for a total dose of 64.8 Gy in 36 fractions. The patient is placed in supine position with the neck in a neutral position. Figure 15.27 shows the daily dose distribution for the initial tumor volume from an acceptable treatment plan that includes wedged opposed laterals and a vertex field. The vertex field permits blocking of the adjacent midline normal tissues (brainstem, pituitary gland, and optic chiasm) and the contralateral temporal lobe. This 3-field plan is superior to a plan utilizing opposed laterals, even if differential beam weighting and beam energies are used (42).

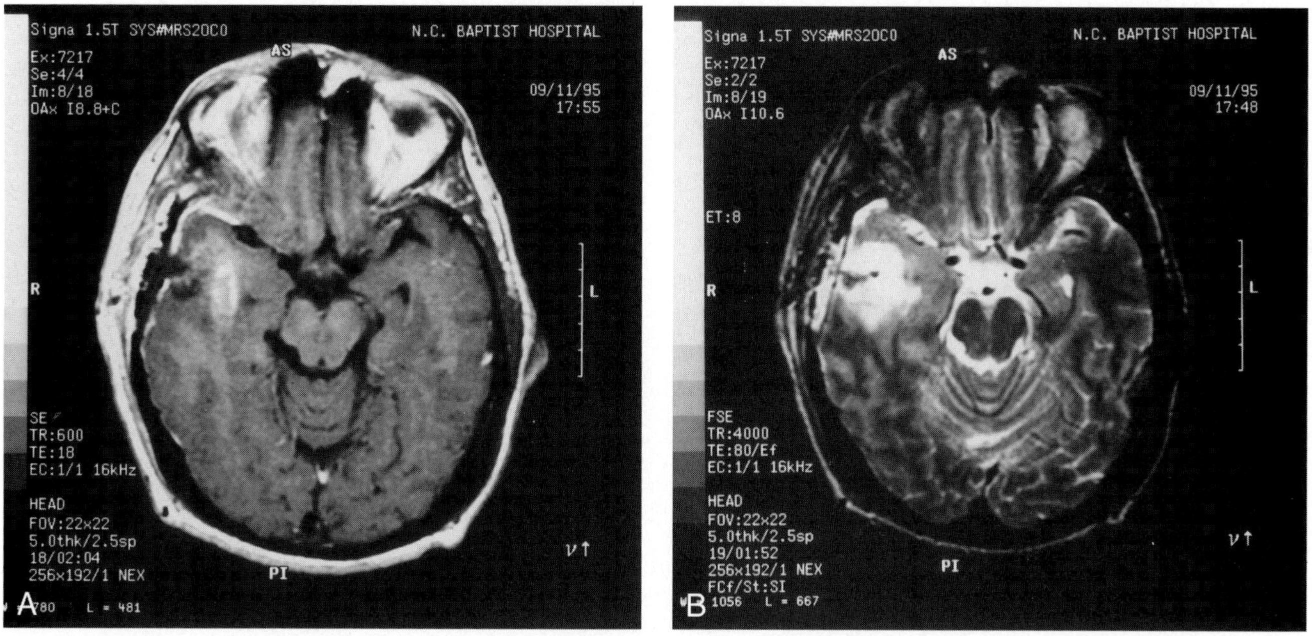

Figure 15.26. Axial MRI of patient after subtotal resection of a right temporal glioblastoma multiforme. **A.** T1-weighted plus contrast. **B.** T2-weighted image.

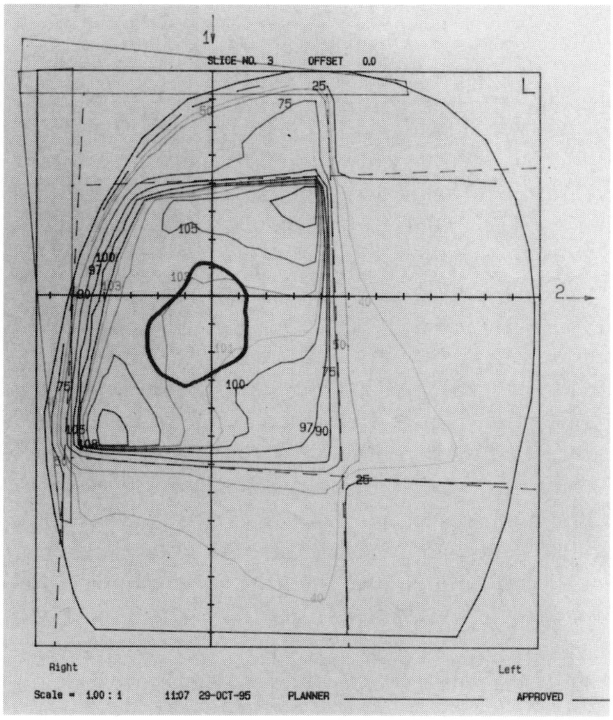

Figure 15.27. Isodose distributions on a coronal contour of a 3-field plan (wedged opposed lateral fields plus a vertex).

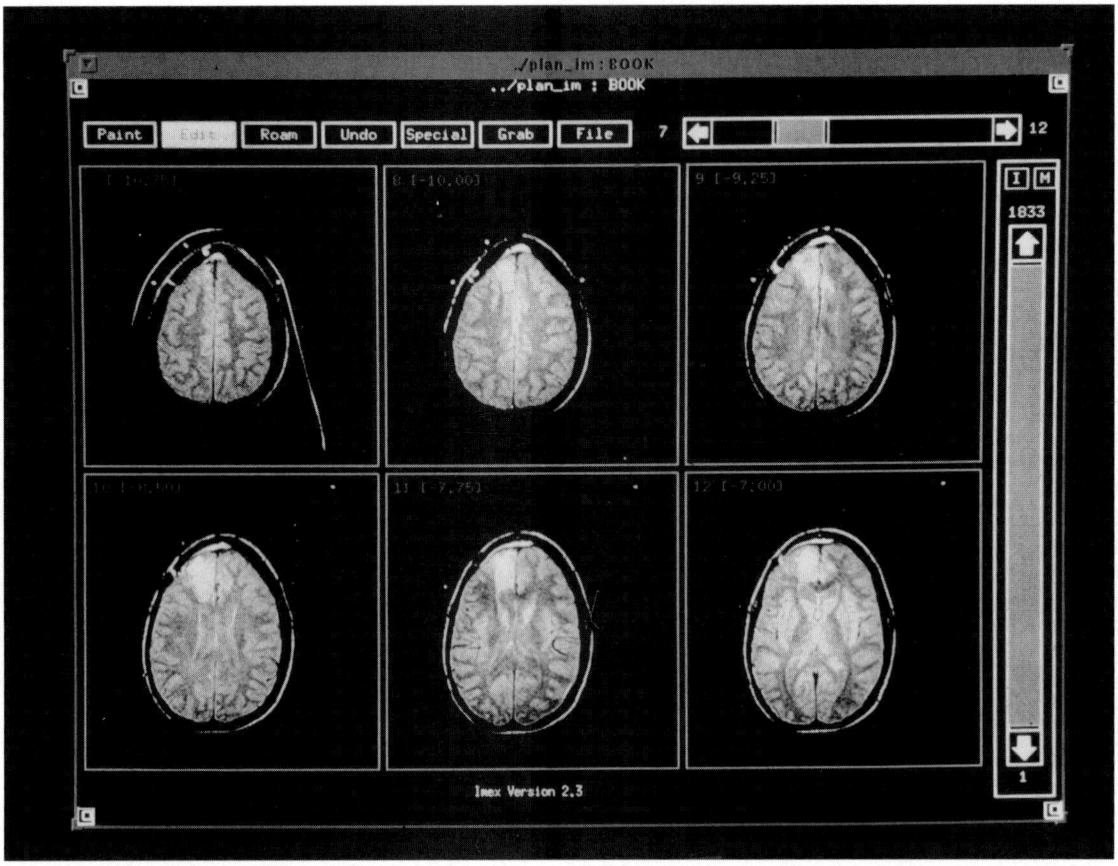

Figure 15.28. Treatment planning axial MRI scans (T2-weighted) of a patient following biopsy of a right frontal low-grade astrocytoma.

Frontal and Parietal Lobe Lesions

Figure 15.28 shows the MRI scan of a patient following subtotal resection of a low-grade astrocytoma of the anterior right frontal lobe. The initial GTV is the area of increased signal on the T-2 weighted MRI images. The initial CTV adds a 2-cm margin, except medially, where only 1 cm is used since the tumor does not cross midline or involve the corpus callosum. The boost GTV is the same as the initial GTV, and the boost CTV reduces the margin to 1 cm in all dimensions. The patient is placed in supine position with the neck in a neutral position. The prescription dose is 50.4 Gy in 28 fractions to the initial volume and 5.4 Gy in 3 fractions to the boost, for a total dose of 55.8 Gy in 31 fractions. One acceptable 2D (coplanar) treatment plan is a 2-field approach utilizing wedged AP and right lateral fields. The contralateral frontal lobe receives exit dose from the right lateral field. An alternative 3D (non-coplanar) approach would be a 3-field plan with non-opposed beams oriented along the sagittal plane, completely sparing the contralateral frontal lobe. Figure 15.29 shows the three fields on the screen of the GRATIS 3D Treatment Planning System (University of North Carolina, 1991, Sherouse Systems, Inc.), including an AP, A45S (i.e., an anterior field with a 45° gantry angle superiorly), and P30S (posterior field with a 30° gantry angle superiorly) treatment fields. Figure 15.30 illustrates how dose extends just to midline on the axial isodose distributions.

A similar approach was used in a patient with a partially resected left frontoparietal glioblastoma multiforme (Figure 15.31). The 4-field non-coplanar plan utilizes an AG15I (anterior with a 15° gantry angle inferiorly), SG15A (vertex with a 15° gantry angle anteriorly), L15S (left lateral with gantry angled 15° superiorly), and R15S (right lateral with gantry angled 15° superiorly) as seen in Figure 15.32. Digitally reconstructed radiographs of beam's eye views for each field are shown in Figure 15.33, along with corresponding gantry and couch rotations necessary for treatment delivery. Differential energy and weighting of the beams (AG15I = 1.0[6 MV]; L15S = 1.56[10 MV]; R15S = 0.48[10 MV]; SG15A = 1.04[10 MV]) as well as appropriate wedge placement allows for more homogenous dose distribution while minimizing dose to optic chiasm and opposite hemisphere. A dose of 46 Gy in 23 fractions is prescribed to the initial CTV followed by 14 Gy in 7 fractions to CTV-2 for 60 Gy total dose.

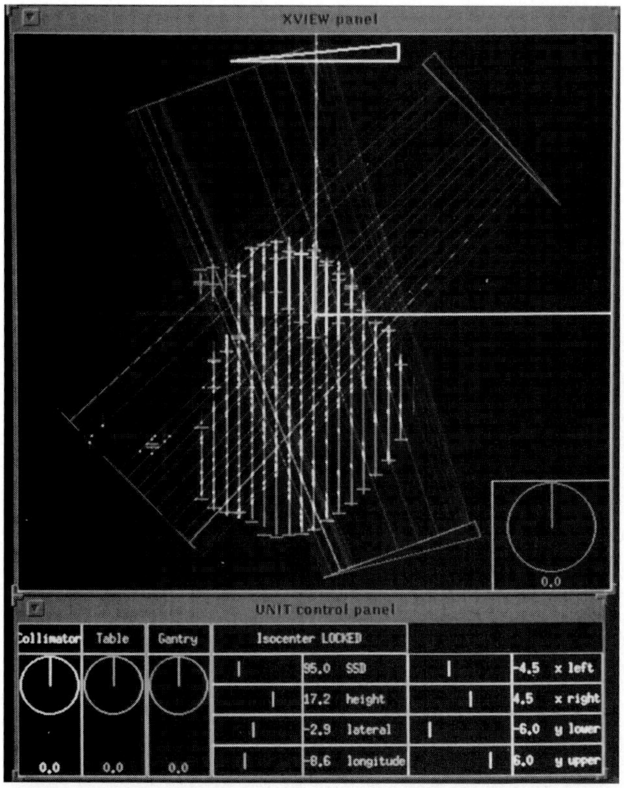

Figure 15.29. Screen display showing the wire frame reconstruction of the treatment fields for the patient in Figure 15.28. Sagittal contour with the AP, A45S, and P30S wedged fields.

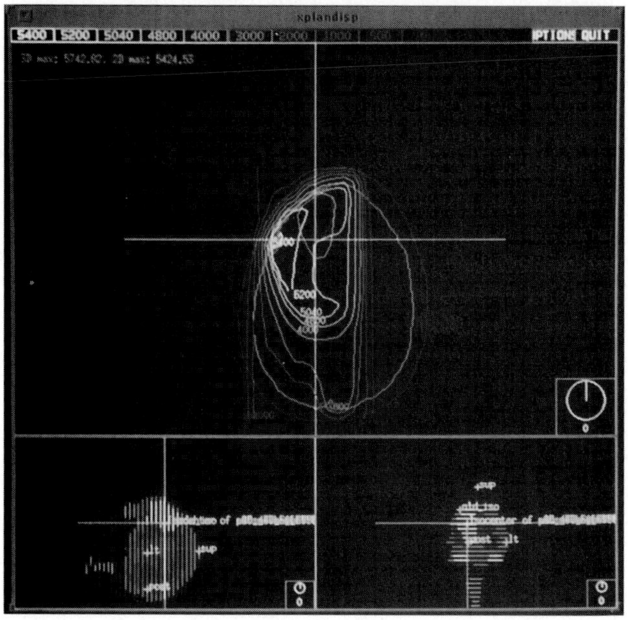

Figure 15.30. Axial isodose distribution of the 3-field plan as seen in Figure 15.29.

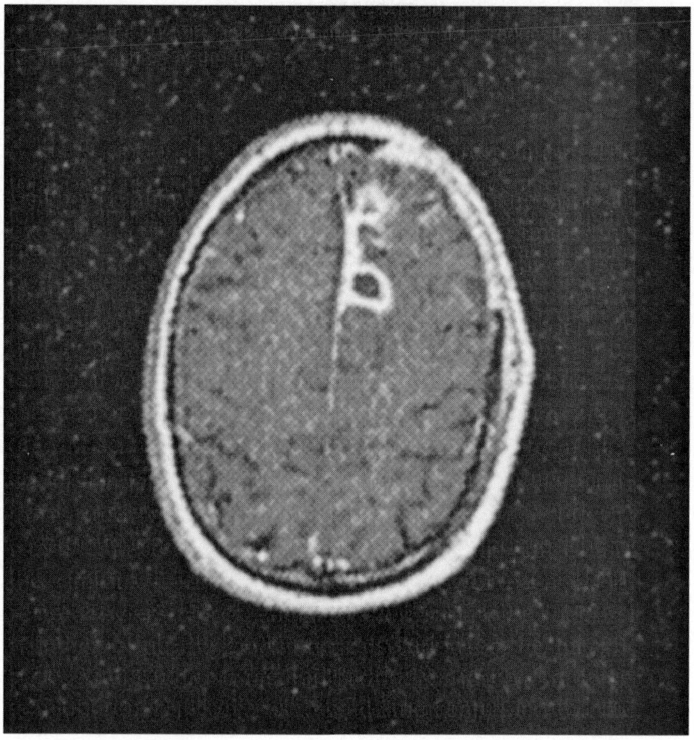

Figure 15.31. Axial MRI (T1-weighted with gadolinium) of a patient with a subtotally resected left frontoparietal glioblastoma multiforme.

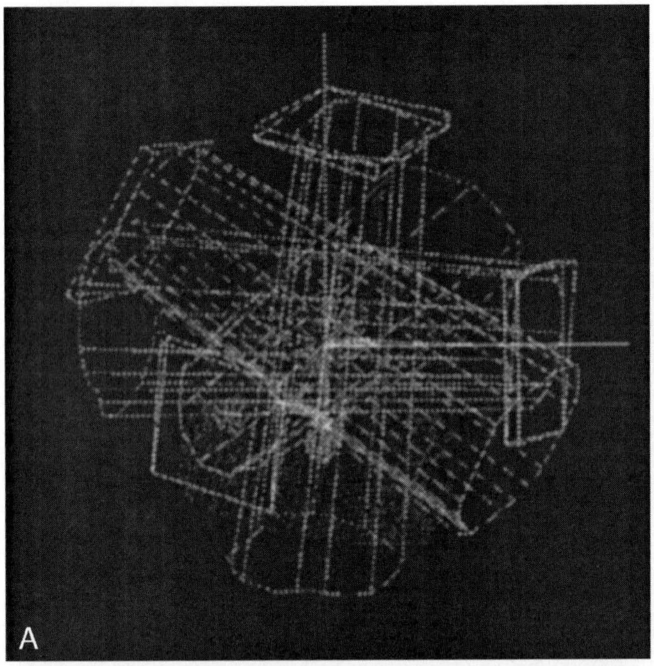

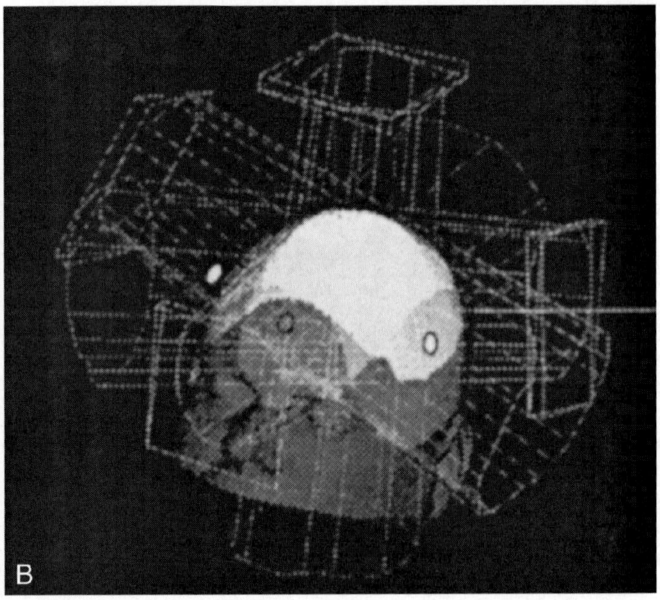

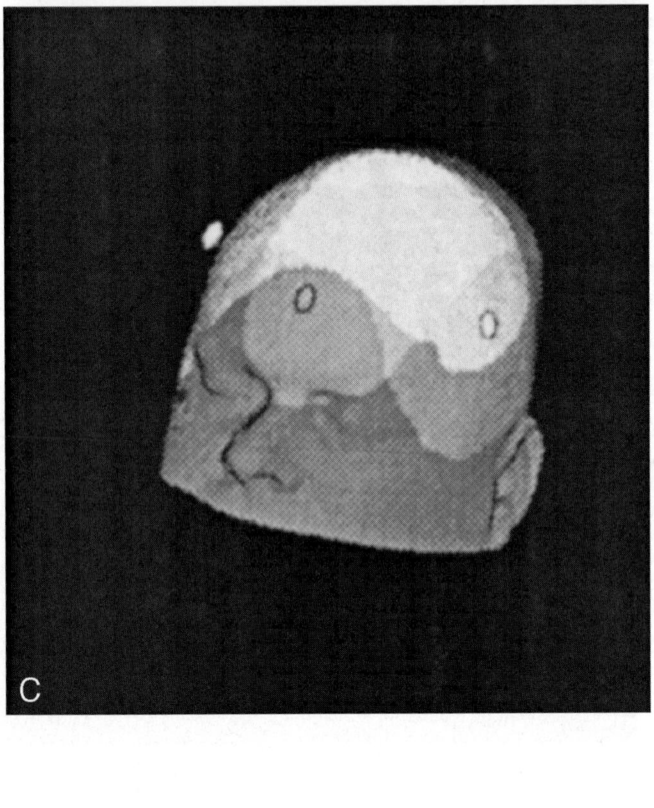

Figure 15.32. Wire-frame and surface rendered views of the 4-field noncoplanar plan designed for the patient in Figure 15.31. Beam arrangement is an AG15I, SG15A, L15S, and R15S. **A.** Wire-frame view with beam arrangement. **B.** Fusion of wire-frame and surface rendered views. **C.** Surface rendered image showing beam entry and exit (light areas).

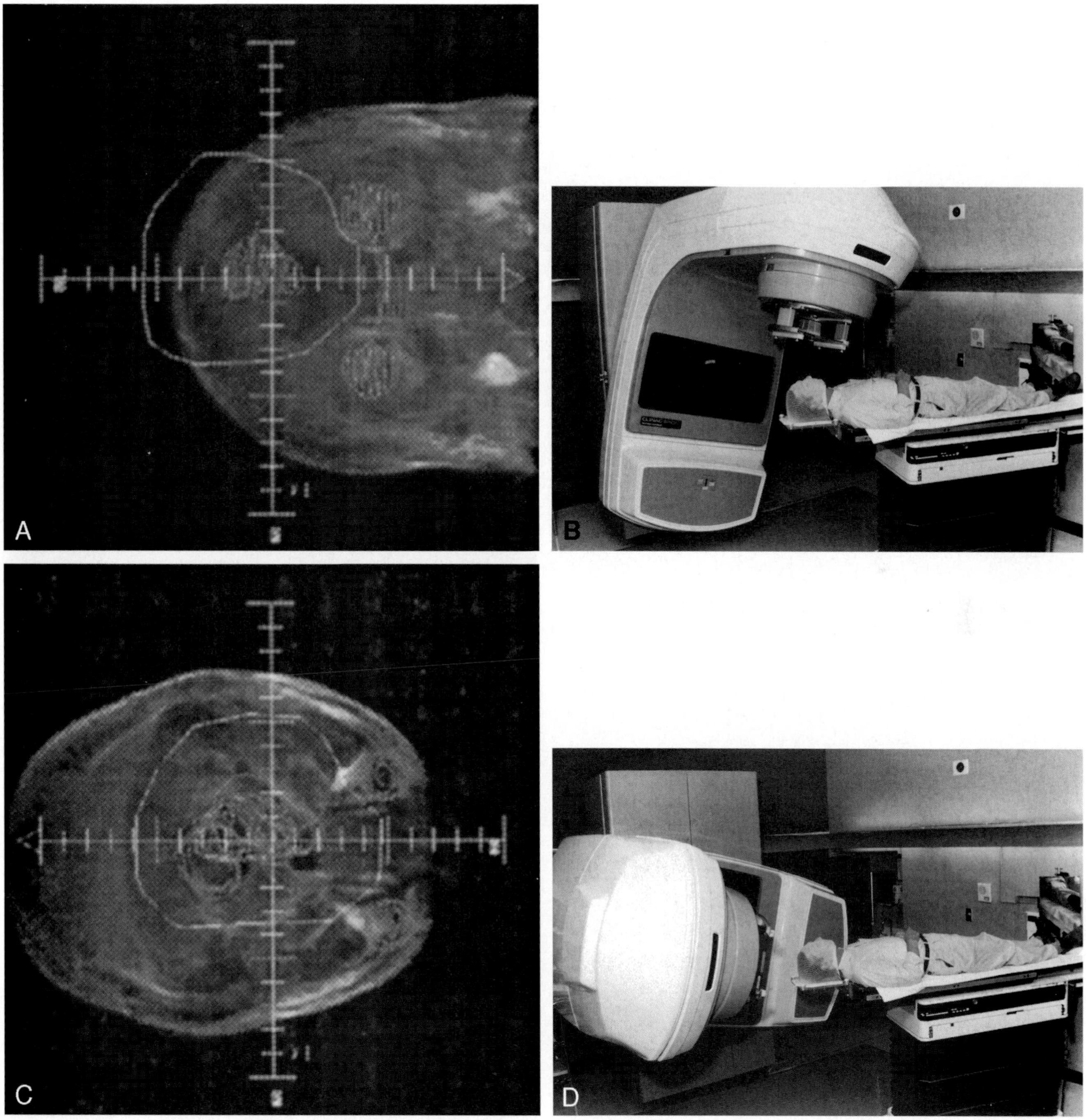

Figure 15.33. A. Digitally reconstructed radiograph (DRR) of the AG15I used in Figure 15.32. **B.** Corresponding view of couch and gantry rotation for delivery of the AG15I. **C.** DRR of the SG15A. **D.** Corresponding couch and gantry. **E.** DRR of the L15S. **F.** Corresponding couch and gantry. **G.** DRR of the R15S. **H.** Corresponding couch and gantry.

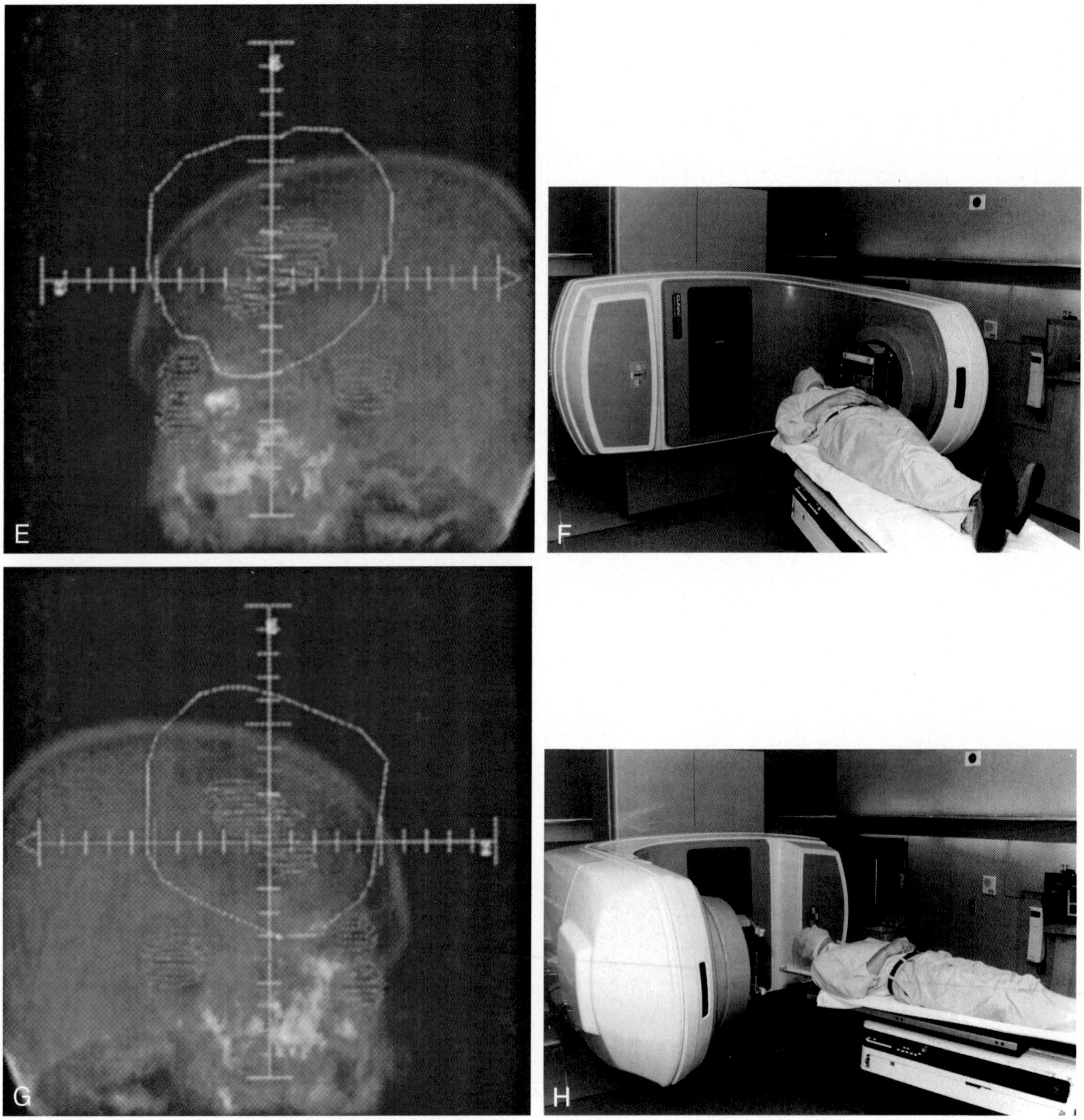

Figure 15.33. *(continued)*

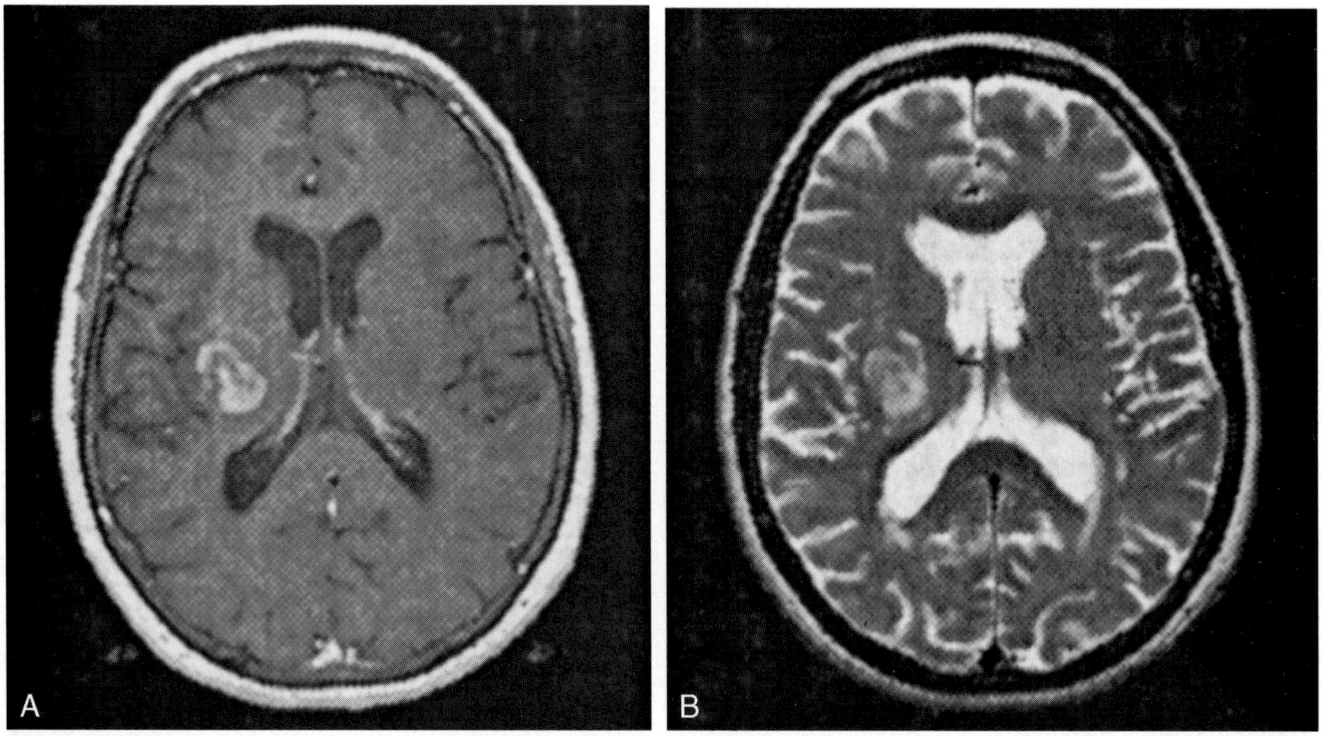

Figure 15.34. Axial MRI images (**A.** T1-weighted with contrast and **B.** T2-weighted) from a patient with a right internal capsule anaplastic astrocytoma.

Central and Thalamic Lesions

Figure 15.34 shows the MRI scan from a patient following stereotactic biopsy of a right internal capsule anaplastic astrocytoma. The initial CTV was treated to 46 Gy in 23 fractions, followed by the boost to CTV-2 to a total of 60 Gy in 30 fractions. A 4-field non-coplanar beam arrangement was used to minimize dose to the contralateral hemisphere (Figure 15.35). The beams included an AG40R (anterior with gantry rotated 40° right), PG40R (posterior with gantry rotated 40° right), SG45A/T25R (superior with gantry rotated 45° anterior and table 25° right), and PG30R/T20I (posterior with gantry rotated 30° right and table 20° in). Beam weighting was 1.4 (AG40R) : 1 (all others) with optimal wedges in place. DVH analysis of the plan revealed $\leq$ 3% dose heterogeneity to the CTVs and $\leq$ 15% of dose to significant portions of contralateral hemisphere or brainstem.

Posterior Fossa Tumors

Figure 15.36 shows the MRI scan of a patient with recurrent meningeal hemangiopericytoma of the left occipital meninges. The GTV is the enhancing tumor. The CTV adds a 2-cm margin to encompass the adjacent meninges. The patient is placed in prone position with neck extension to allow for the use of a PA beam that will not exit through the eyes. The prescription dose is 52.2 Gy in 29 fractions (a radiosurgical boost of 15 Gy in 1 fraction to the GTV preceded the external beam radiation). Figure 15.37 shows the daily dose distribution from an acceptable treatment plan, utilizing a coplanar 3-field approach with wedged opposed laterals and a PA field. The PA has been modified to spare the lenses from its exit dose (simulation films shown in Figures 15.38a and b). Alternative plans include 2-field plans such as opposed laterals or wedged right posterior and left posterior oblique fields, and other 3-field arrangements such as wedged opposed laterals and a vertex field.

Figure 15.39 shows the MRI scan of a patient with a low-grade astrocytoma of the midline cerebellum. The initial GTV includes the enhancing tumor and surrounding edema; the initial PTV adds a 2-cm margin. The boost GTV includes only the enhancing tumor. There is a 2-cm margin for the boost PTV. The prescription dose is 50.4 Gy in 28 fractions to the initial volume and 9 Gy in 5 fractions to the boost volume, for a total dose of 59.4 Gy in 33 fractions. The patient is placed in supine position with the neck in a neutral position. Figure 15.40 shows the isodose curves from an acceptable treatment plan, which includes opposed lateral, P30S (posterior field with the gantry angled 30° superiorly), and vertex fields (simulation and port films shown in Figures 15.41a–c).

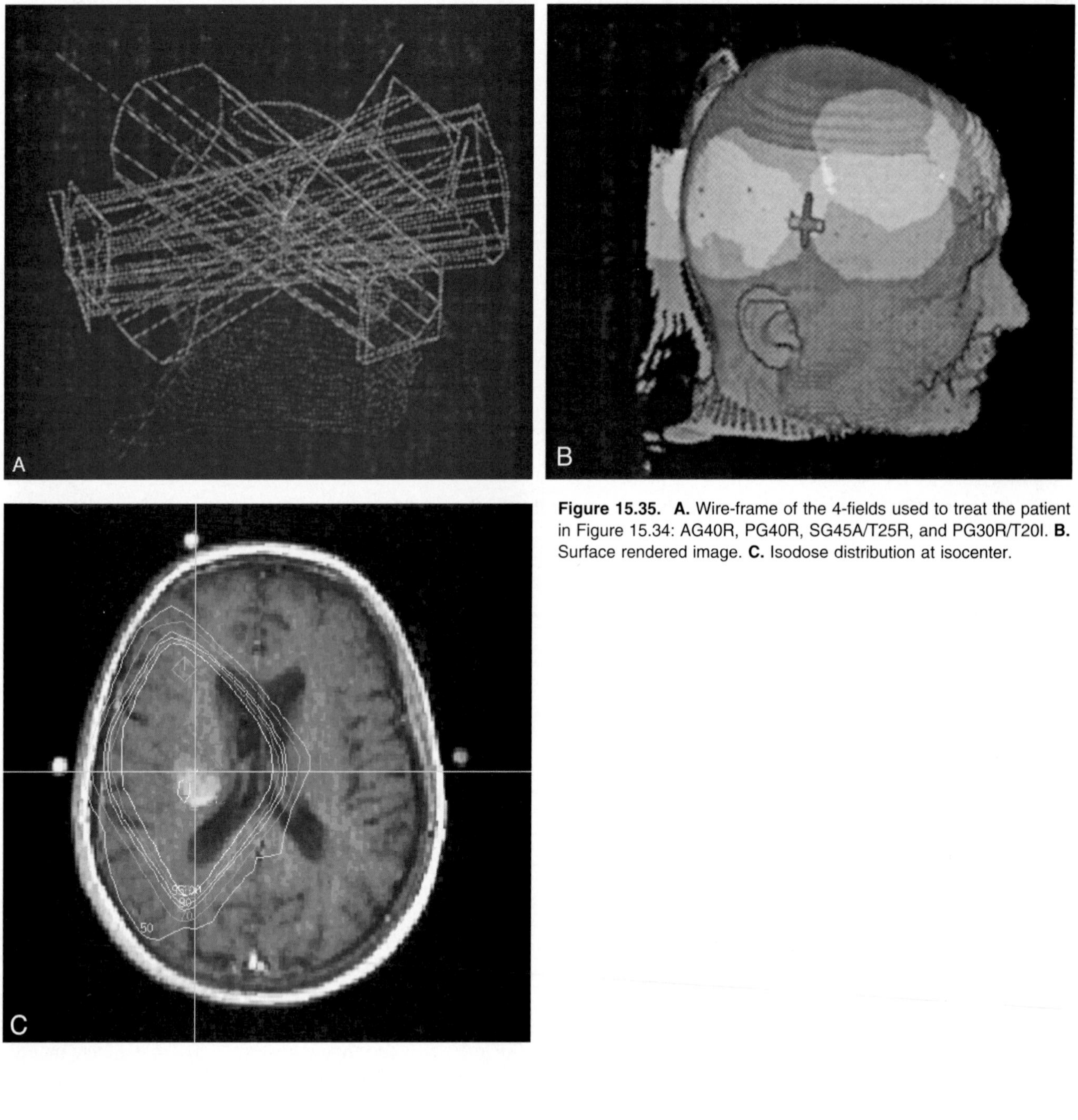

Figure 15.35. A. Wire-frame of the 4-fields used to treat the patient in Figure 15.34: AG40R, PG40R, SG45A/T25R, and PG30R/T20I. **B.** Surface rendered image. **C.** Isodose distribution at isocenter.

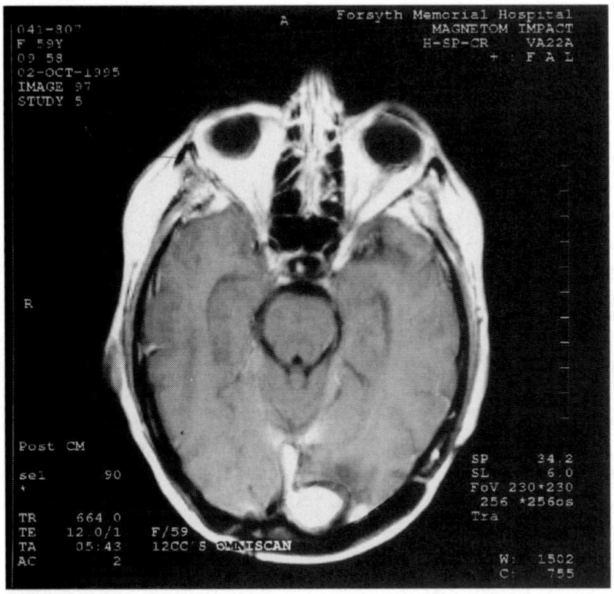

Figure 15.36. Axial MRI image (T1-weighted with gadolinium) of a patient with a recurrent meningeal hemangiopericytoma of the left occipital meninges.

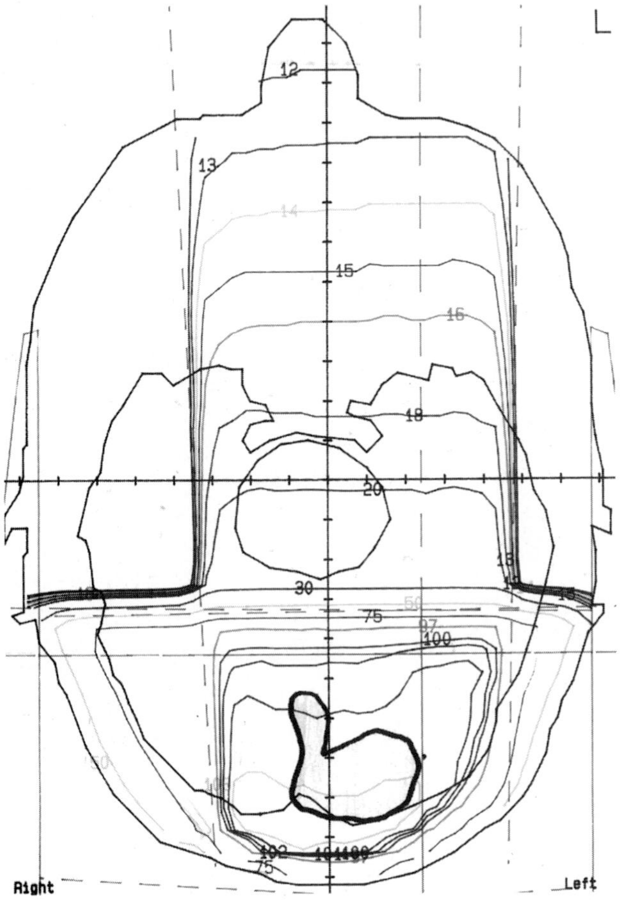

Figure 15.37. Axial isodose distribution of the 3-field treatment plan used for the patient shown in Figure 15.36.

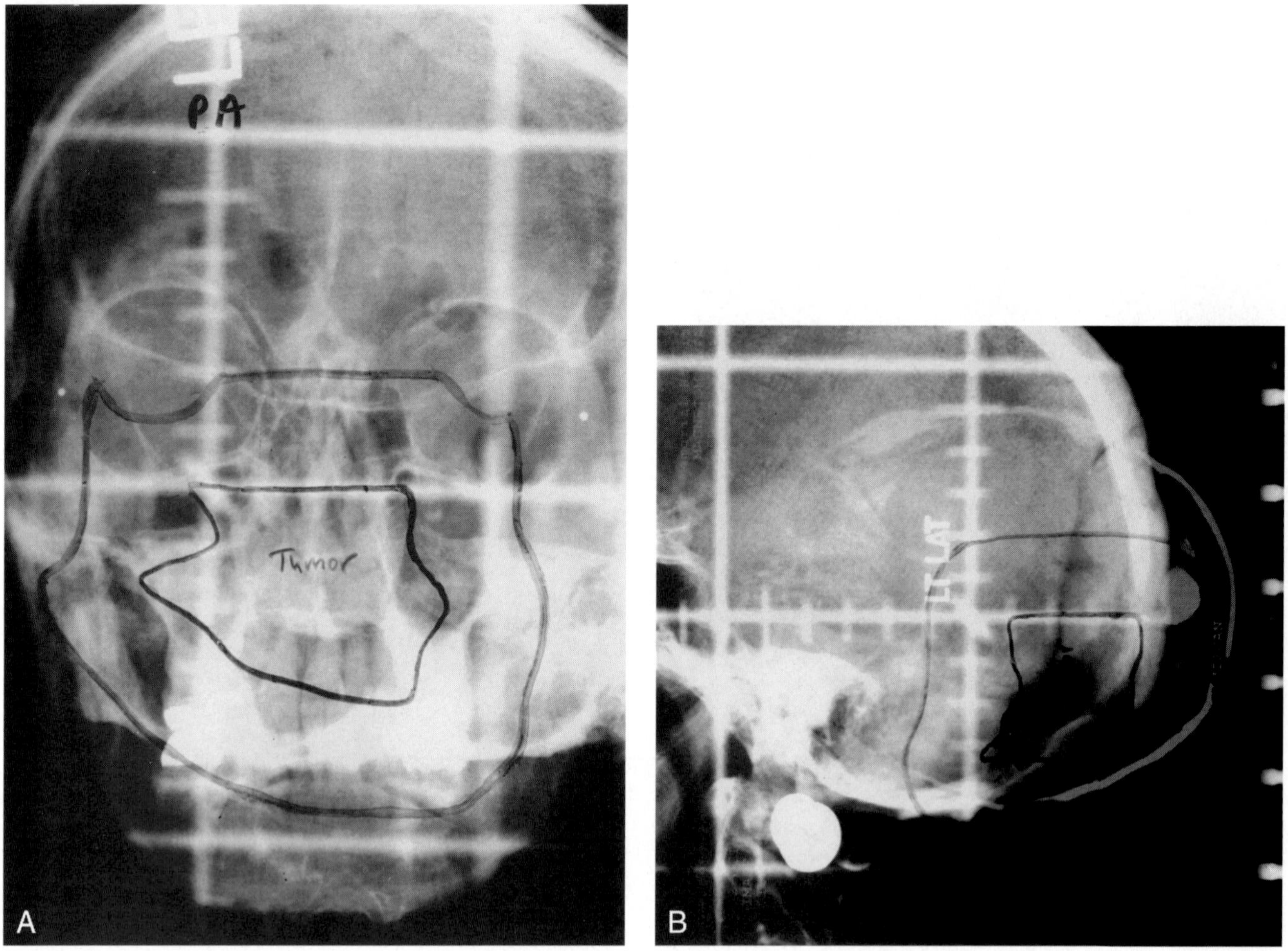

Figure 15.38. A. PA simulation film of the treatment fields used for the treatment plan shown in Figure 15.37. Note the modification of the block to shield the eyes. **B.** Lateral simulation film of the treatment fields.

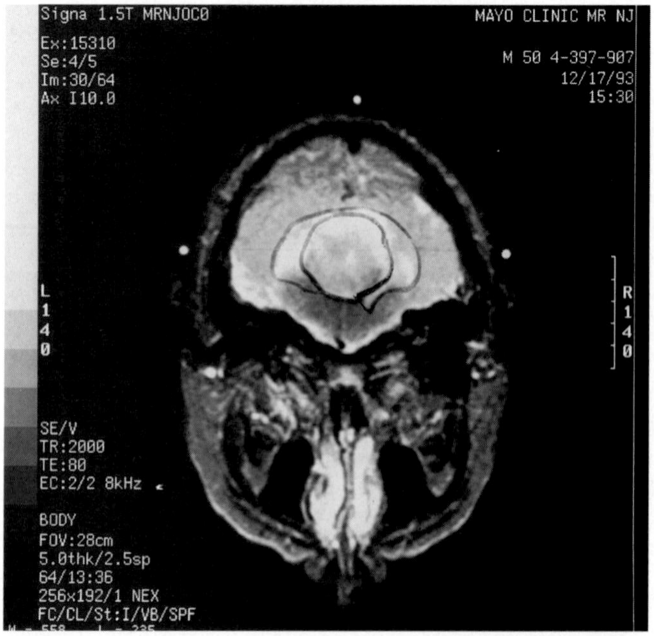

Figure 15.39. Treatment planning axial MRI image (T2-weighted) of a patient with a low-grade midline cerebellar astrocytoma.

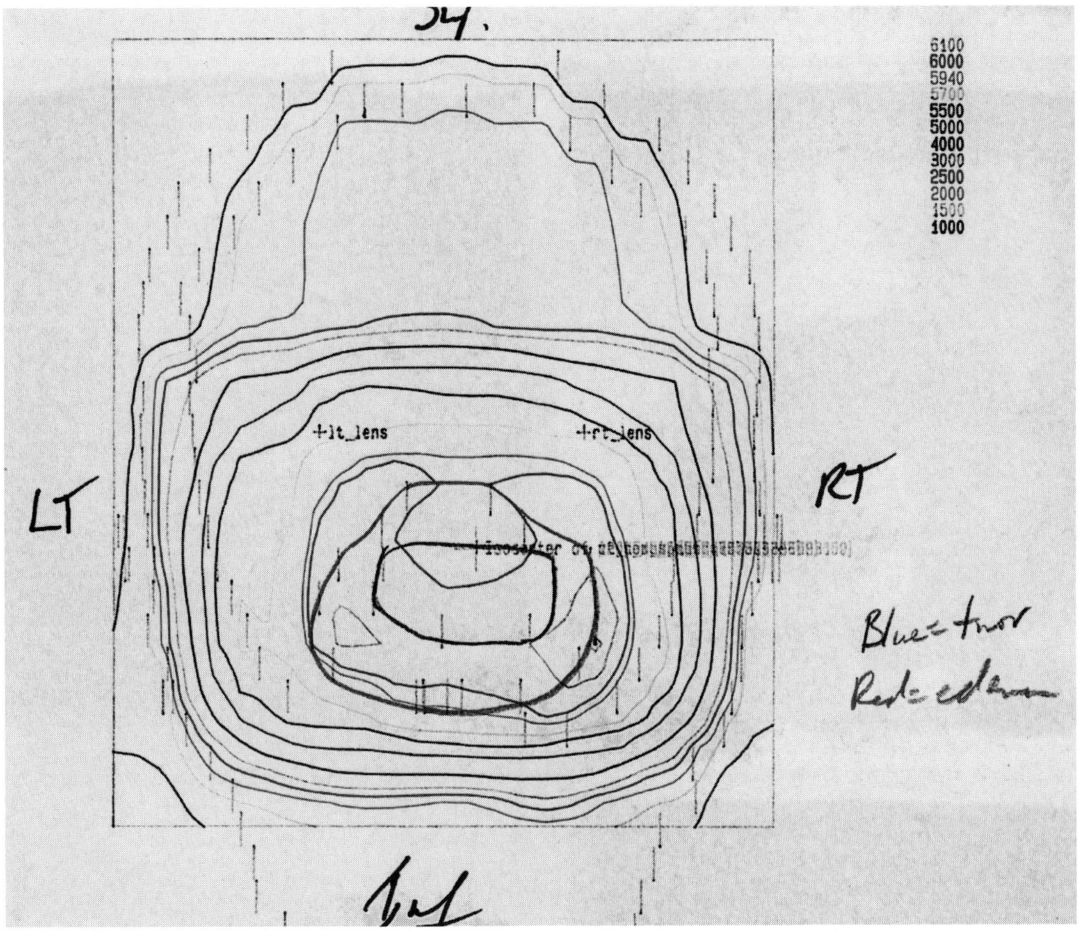

Figure 15.40. Coronal isodose distribution of the noncoplanar 4-field treatment plan used for the patient shown in Figure 15.39.

Figures 15.42a and b show the MRI scan of a patient with a presumed low-grade astrocytoma of the brainstem. The initial GTV is the area of increased signal on the T2 weighted MRI images. The initial CTV includes the adjacent portions of the brainstem (thalamus, basal ganglia, midbrain, and medulla) that are likely to contain microscopic tumor, plus a 2-cm margin. The boost GTV is the same as the initial GTV; the boost CTV adds a 1-cm margin to the boost GTV in all dimensions. The prescription dose is 45 Gy in 25 fractions to the initial volume and 10.8 Gy in 6 fractions to the boost volume, for a total dose of 55.8 Gy in 31 fractions. The patient is placed in supine position with the neck in a neutral position. Figure 15.43 shows the isodose curves from an acceptable 3D (non-coplanar) treatment plan, which includes RT15S and LT15S treatment fields (right and left lateral beams angled 15° superiorly so they are unopposed), along with a SG20P field (vertex field with the gantry angles 20° posteriorly) and an AG40S field (AP field with gantry rotated 40° superiorly) (Figure 15.44a–d). In the two prior examples, the 3D non-coplanar 4-field treatment plans are superior to the alternative using only opposed lateral fields because they spare dose to the ears and auditory apparatus.

Craniospinal Axis Irradiation

Figure 15.45 shows the preoperative MRI scan of a child with a medulloblastoma. As with other brain tumors in which all of the craniospinal meninges are at risk, appropriate radiation therapy includes craniospinal irradiation with a localized boost. The initial GTV is the posterior fossa, and the initial CTV includes the whole brain and entire spinal cord with a 1- to 2-cm margin to insure adequate coverage of the meninges over the brain (including skull base and cribiform plate) and spinal cord. The boost GTV is the posterior fossa. The corresponding boost CTV adds a 2-cm margin. Typical prescription doses are 36 Gy in 20-24 fractions to the initial craniospinal volume and 18 to 19.8 Gy in 10-11 fractions to the posterior fossa for a total dose of 54 to 55.8 Gy in 31 fractions. Lower doses to the craniospinal axis may be used if the patient receives

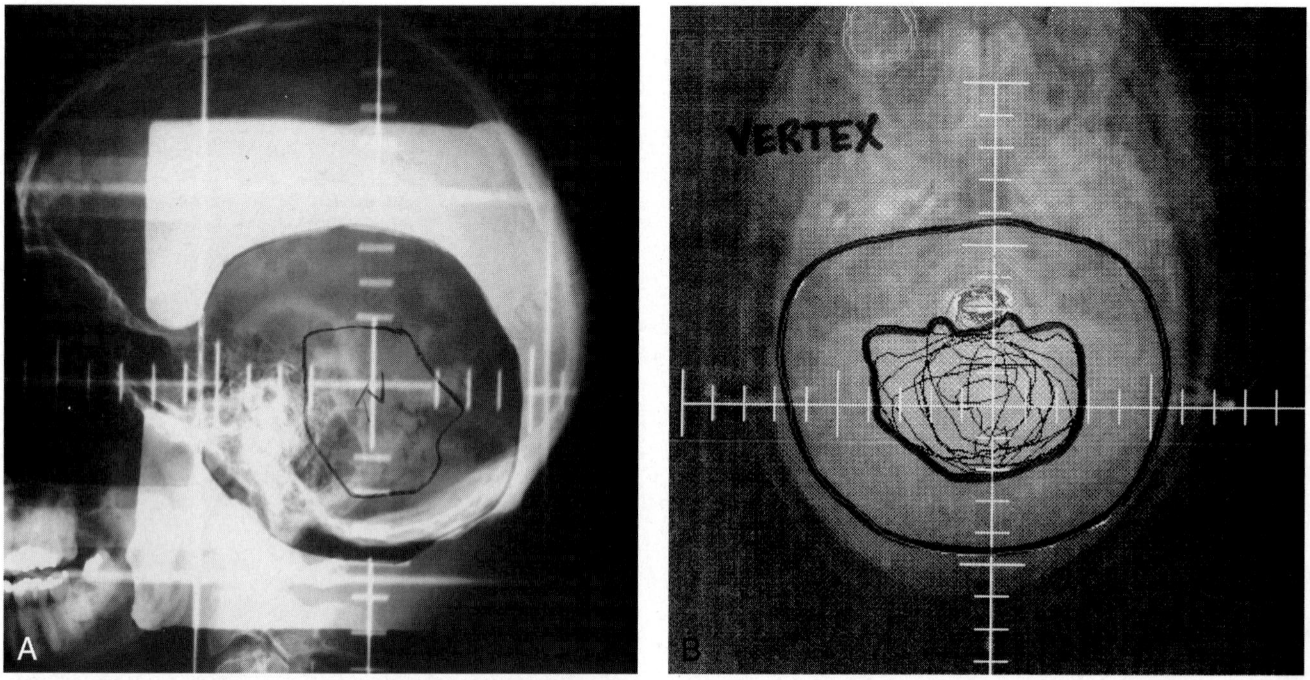

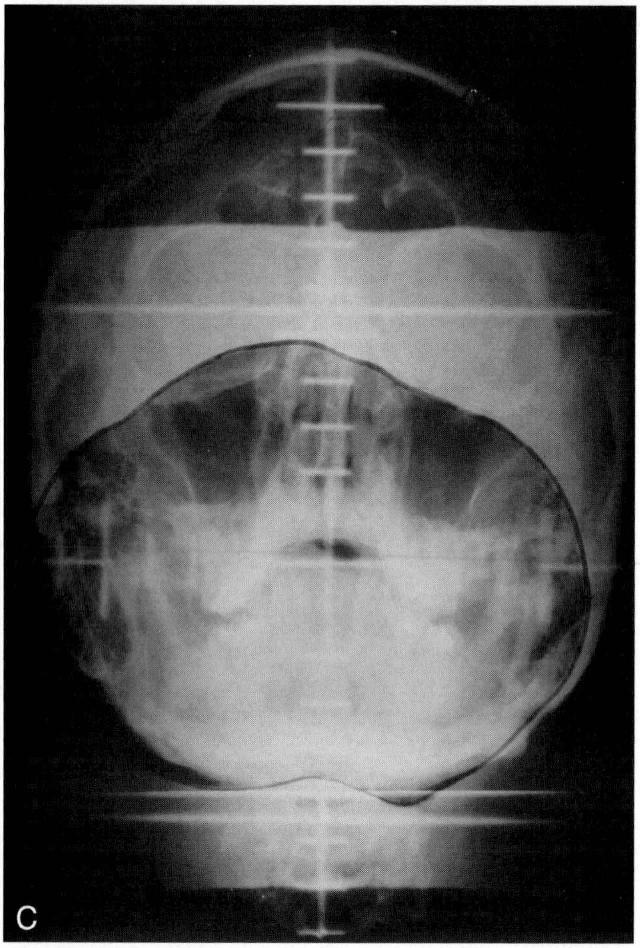

Figure 15.41. **A.** Simulation (block check) film of the lateral treatment field used to treat the patient shown in Figure 15.39. **B.** Digitally reconstructed radiograph (DRR) of the vertex field. **C.** Simulation (block check) film of the P30S treatment field.

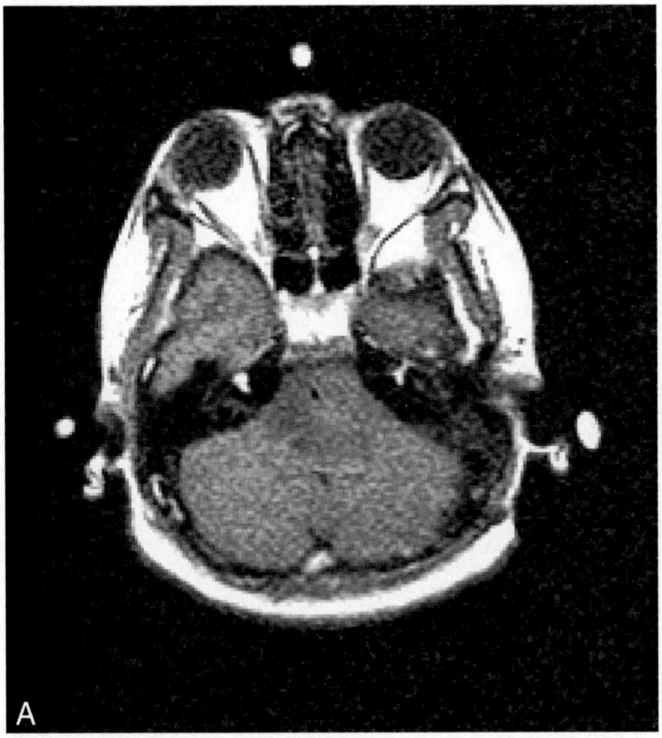

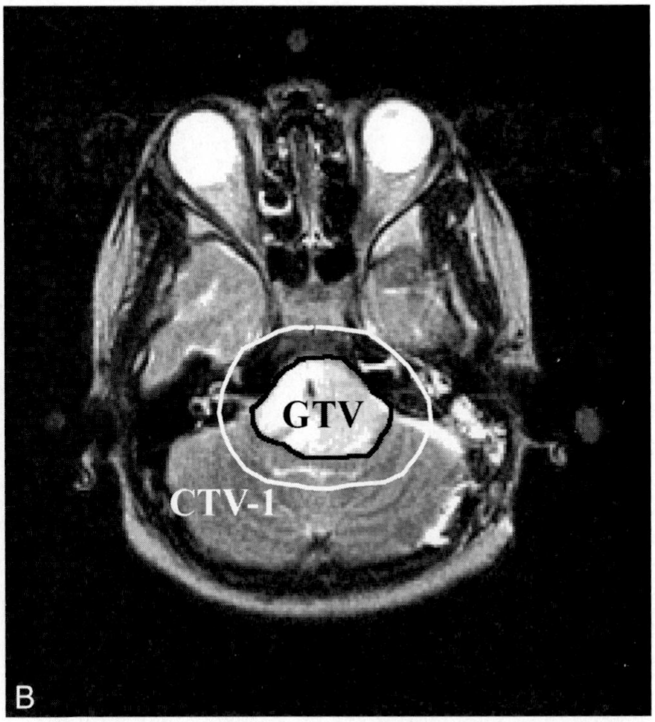

Figure 15.42. Treatment planning MRI images of a patient with a presumed low-grade glioma of the brainstem. **A.** Axial T1–weighted with gadolinium **B.** Axial T2-weighted image with tumor (GTV) and CTV-1 outlined.

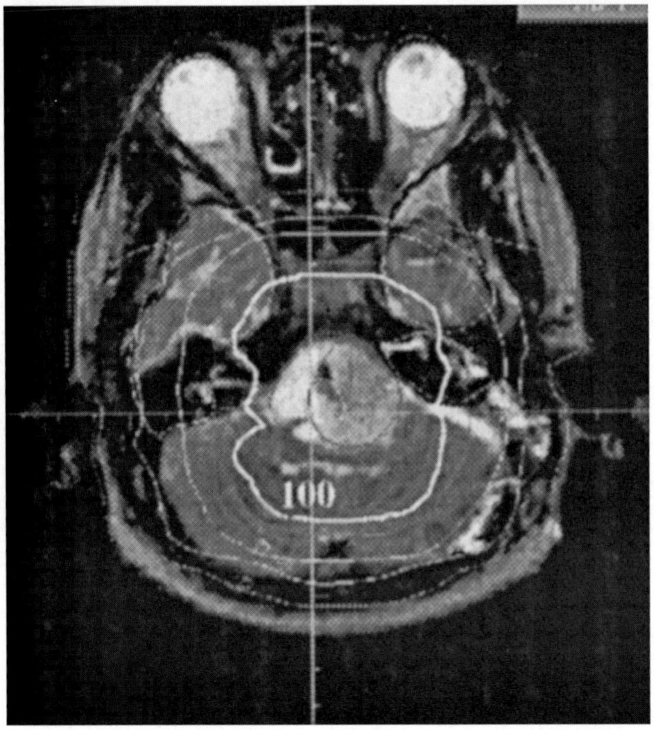

Figure 15.43. Axial isodose distribution of the noncoplanar 4-field treatment plan used for the patient shown in Figure 15.42.

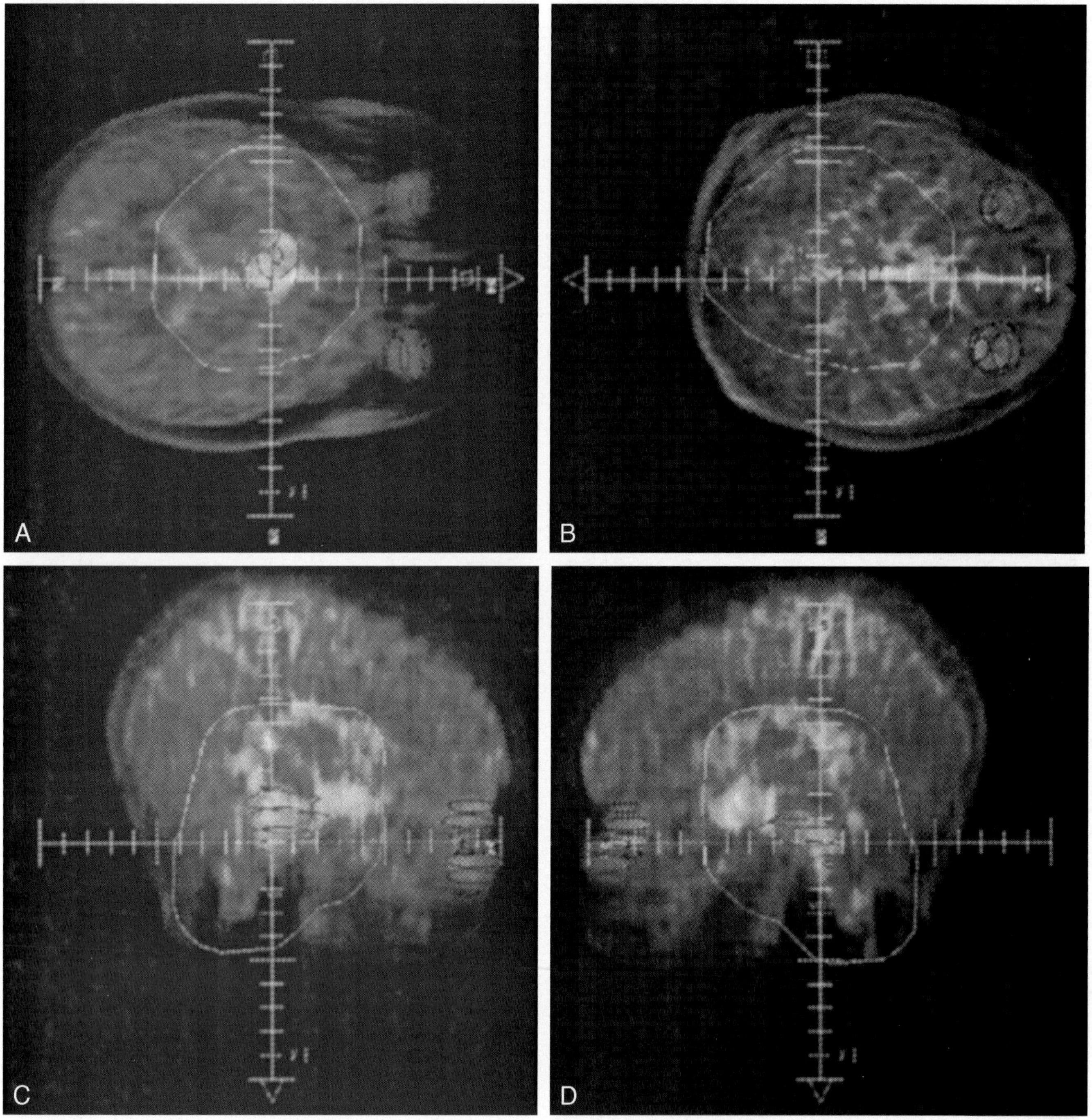

Figure 15.44. A. DRR of the AG40S treatment field used for the plan shown in Figure 15.43. **B.** DRR of the SG20P treatment field. **C.** DRR of the RT15S treatment field. **D.** DRR of the LT15S treatment field.

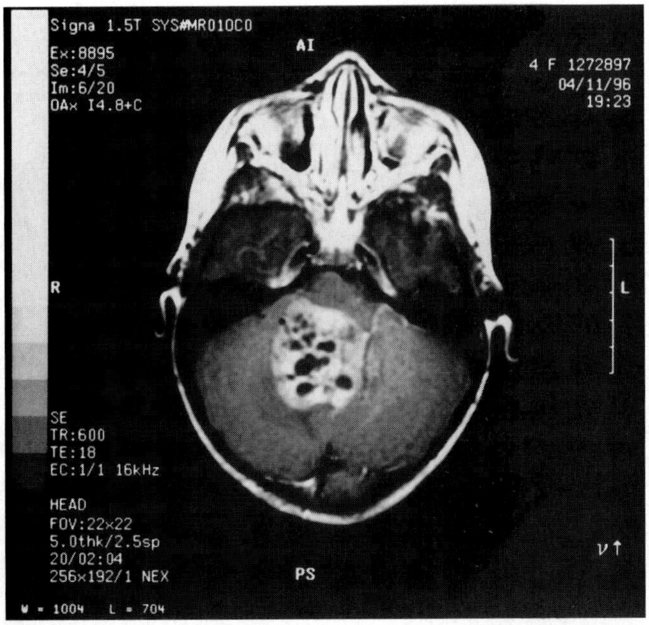

Figure 15.45. Axial MRI image (T1-weighted with gadolinium) of a child with medulloblastoma.

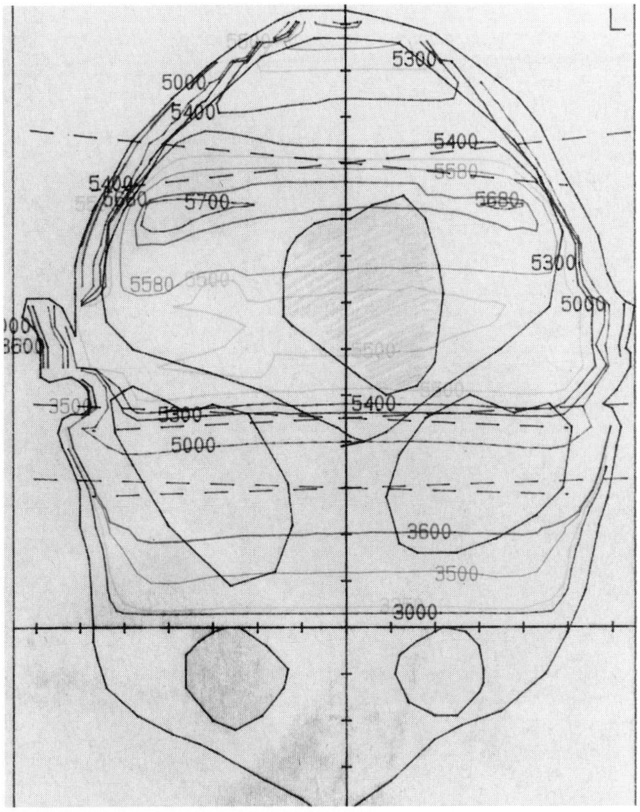

Figure 15.46. Axial isodose distribution of the plan used to treat the patient in Figure 15.45, using opposed laterals for the initial whole brain followed by a posterior fossa boost.

chemotherapy as part of the treatment. Figure 15.46 shows isodose curves through the midposterior fossa for the treatment plan used in this patient, which included opposed laterals for the initial whole brain treatment fields as well as the boost fields (Figure 15.47a). Usually, the whole brain and upper cervical spinal cord are treated with one set of treatment fields, while the spine is treated separately in one or two fields (simulation films of spinal fields shown in Figures 15.47b and c).

The technical approach described herein is that used at the Wake Forest University School of Medicine Department of Radiation Oncology. For craniospinal irradiation, the patient is placed in the prone position, with the neck in a somewhat flexed position (the mandible, maxilla, and oral cavity should not be in the exit of the upper spine field). The lateral brain fields are simulated first. The opposed fields are positioned such that isocenter is at midline with the beam axes passing through the lateral canthi. The fleshy canthi are visualized fluoroscopically by placing radiopaque lead markers on the patient's skin. The fields are positioned in this manner to minimize beam divergence, and, thereby, dose to the patient's lenses. The anterior, superior, and posterior borders of the cranial field "flash" outside of the skull surface. The "short" inferior border is placed around C2-3, leaving adequate room for subsequent shifts in the match with the upper spine field (see below).

Next, the issue of how to abut the lateral brain fields with the PA upper spine must be addressed. This is the most critical aspect of the craniospinal axis irradiation setup. The brain and upper spine fields, being divergent and orthogonal, have field edges that project through the patient at different angles. If these fields overlap, they will create a region of high dose which may threaten the upper cervical spinal cord. The first step to avoid this is to introduce a collimator rotation to the lateral brain fields. This rotation must be of an angle equal to the divergent angle of the superior border of the upper PA spine field, which is a function of the length of the upper PA spine field (Figure 15.48 and formula 15.1). The lateral brain and PA upper spine fields are now matched at midline, from skin to depth, and do not overlap at the spinal cord. However, the collimator rotation does not prevent the inferior border of the lateral brain fields from diverging across midline into the superior border of the upper PA spine field. This results in overlap of dose in the soft tissues of the neck lateral to the spinal cord, as shown in Figures 15.49.

Figure 15.50 demonstrates with radiographic film exposures the match technique described above. Figure 15.50a shows the expected result of the field abutment

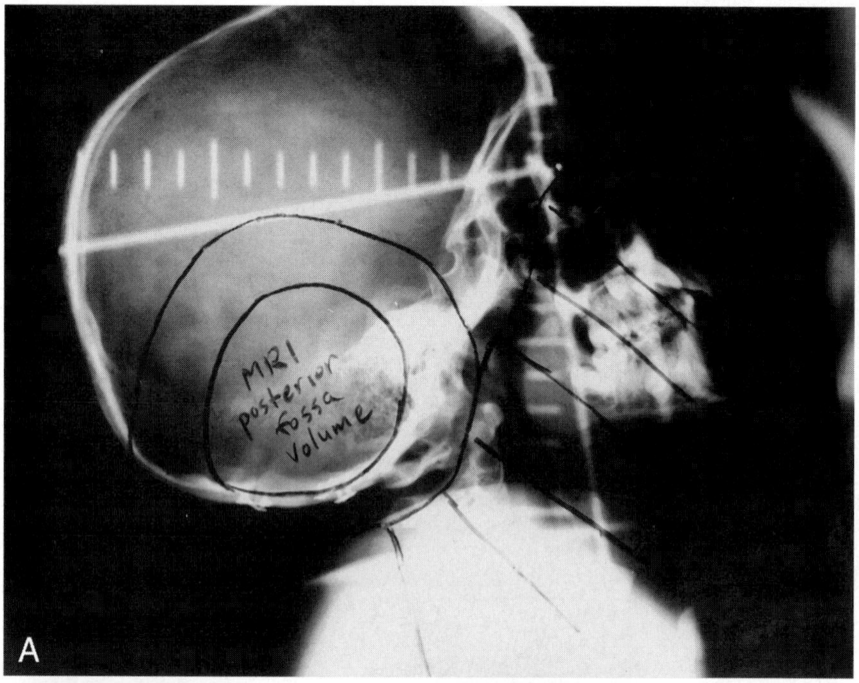

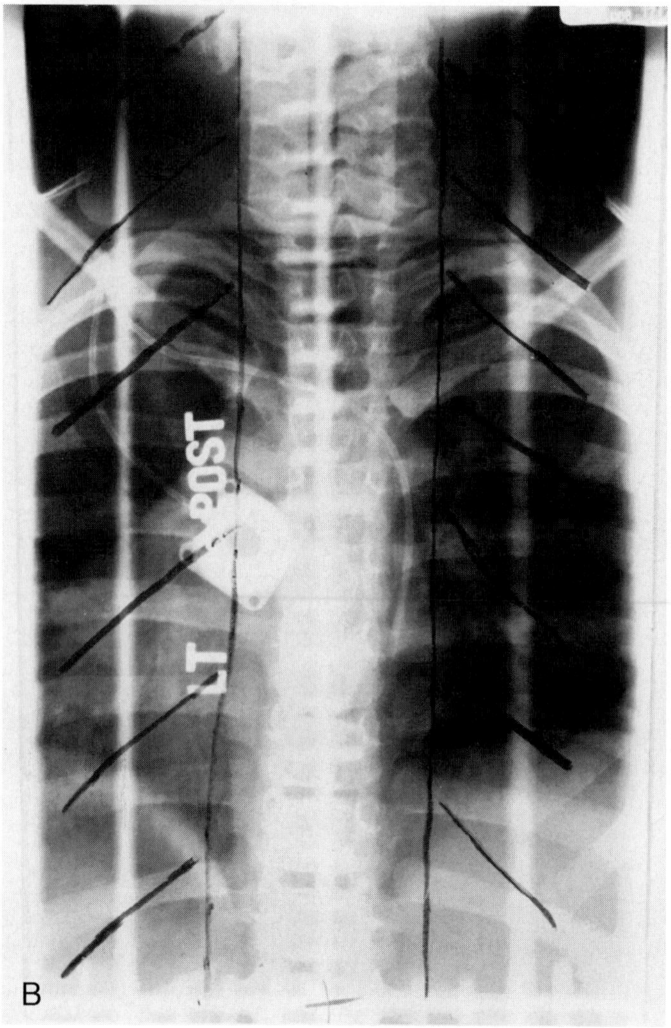

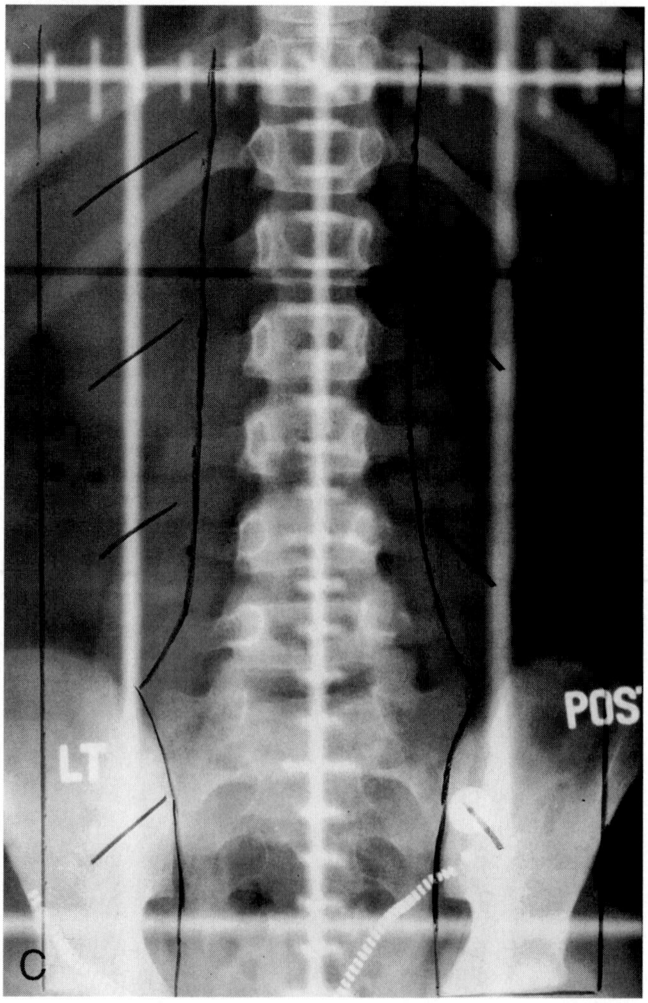

Figure 15.47. A. Simulation film of the lateral whole brain and boost fields used in the treatment of the patient in Figure 15.45. **B.** Simulation film of the upper half of the PA spine field. **C.** Simulation film of the lower half of the PA spine field.

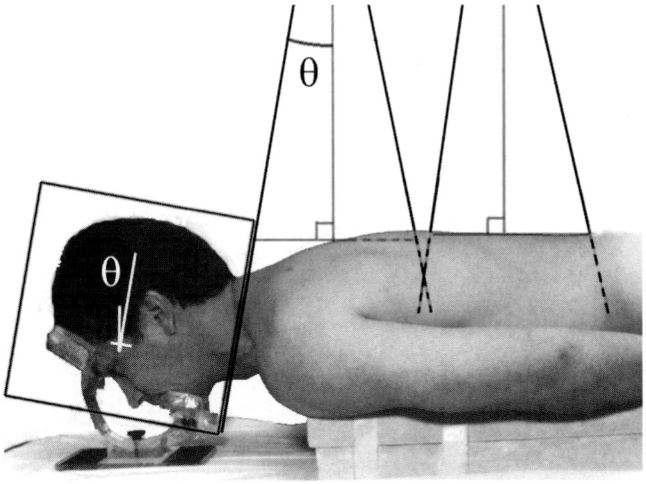

Figure 15.48. Lateral view of the treatment fields used for craniospinal axis irradiation. The collimator of the lateral brain fields must be rotated by the angle shown to match the divergence of the upper spine field.

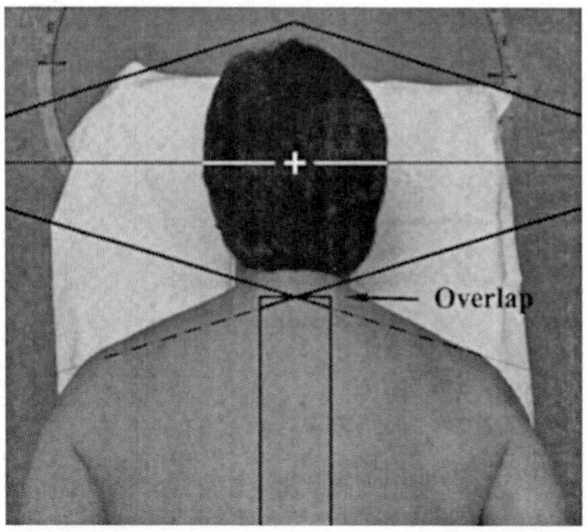

Figure 15.49. PA view of the match between the lateral brain fields and the upper spine field. Note the areas of overlap and gap between the inferior border of the brain fields and the superior border of the upper spine field.

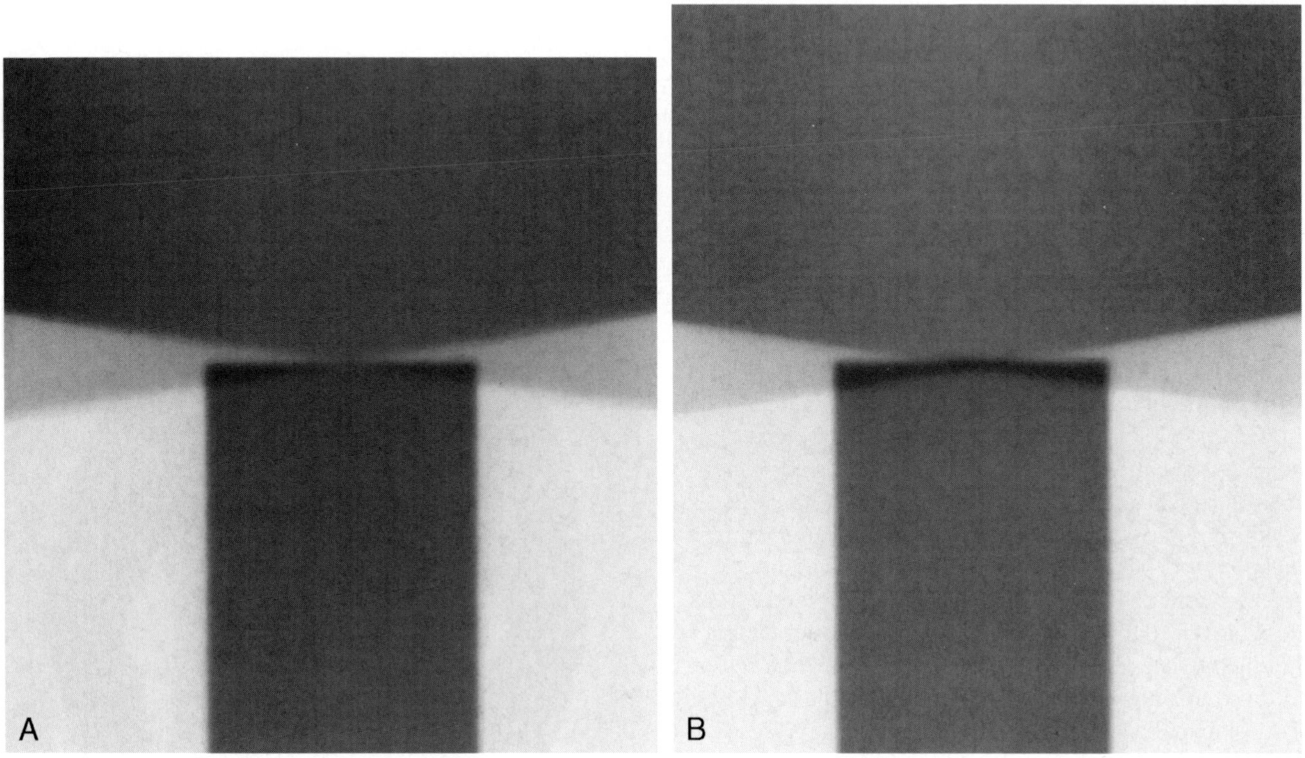

Figure 15.50. **A.** A film study of a "perfect" match between the lateral brain fields and the upper spine field. Note the areas of overlap and gap between the inferior border of the brain fields and the superior border of the upper spine field. **B.** Film study of an "imperfect" match (1- to 2-mm overlap) between the lateral brain fields and the upper spine field. Note the increased areas of overlap and decreased areas of gap between the inferior border of the brain fields and the superior border of the upper spine field when compared with **A.**

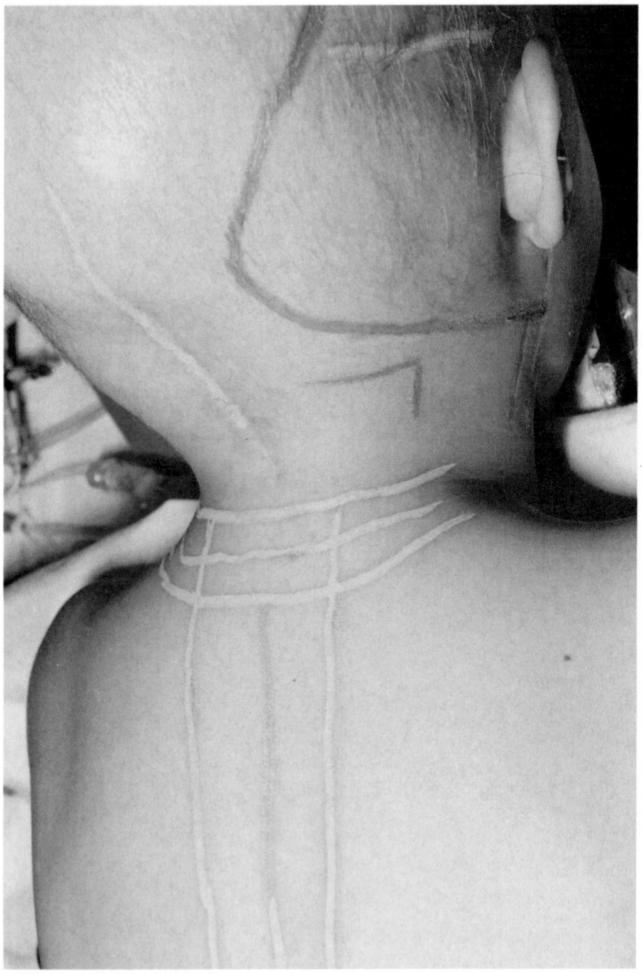

Figure 15.51. Drawn on the patient's skin are the match lines from the inferior border of the lateral brain fields and the superior border of the PA upper spine field.

between the brain and upper spine fields. Figure 15.50b shows a possible result where misalignment between the radiation field and light field creates a small overlap in the spinal cord. The misalignment, while small (on the order of 1-2 mm), is well within a linear accelerator manufacturer's tolerance for the light and radiation field congruence of large treatment fields. The effect of this potential (and probable) overlap is minimized by the technique of twice shifting the field abutment. For added safety, when setting up these treatment fields clinically, we use the thickness of the skin marks which serve as "miniature gaps" separating the light field edges of the two fields. Alternatively, a 0.5-cm gap can be placed between the two fields with the knowledge that the small area of underdosing will be spread over the two field shifts.

The inferior border of the brain field and superior border of the upper PA spine field are drawn on the patient's skin and abut at the midline of the patient's posterior neck (Figure 15.51). Three transverse marks are used to indicate the "short, medium, and long" brain field borders and the complementary "long, medium, and short" PA upper spine field borders (Figure 15.52).

It is customary to maximize the field length of the upper spine field (40 cm at 100 cm SSD) and minimize the length of the lower spinal field. If 40 cm or less of length covers the entire spine inclusive of S3 (the end of the thecal sac), a lower PA spine field is not necessary. Should a lower PA spine field be needed, it must be designed taking into account the two shifts used to "feather" all abutting fields. The amount of each shift is arbitrary but is typically accomplished by a 1-2 cm reduction in the upper spine field with compensatory increase in the size of the cranial and lower spine fields. All fields' central axes remain fixed. Only the field lengths are changed. Therefore, the caudal border of the lower PA spine field should be set inferior to S3 by a length equal to the two field shifts, then blocked back to S3 using asymmetric collimators or a cerrobend block.

The upper and lower PA spine fields are separated by a calculated gap at the skin to produce a dosimetric match at the depth of the spinal cord. The size of the skin gap is dependent upon the collimated length of the PA spine

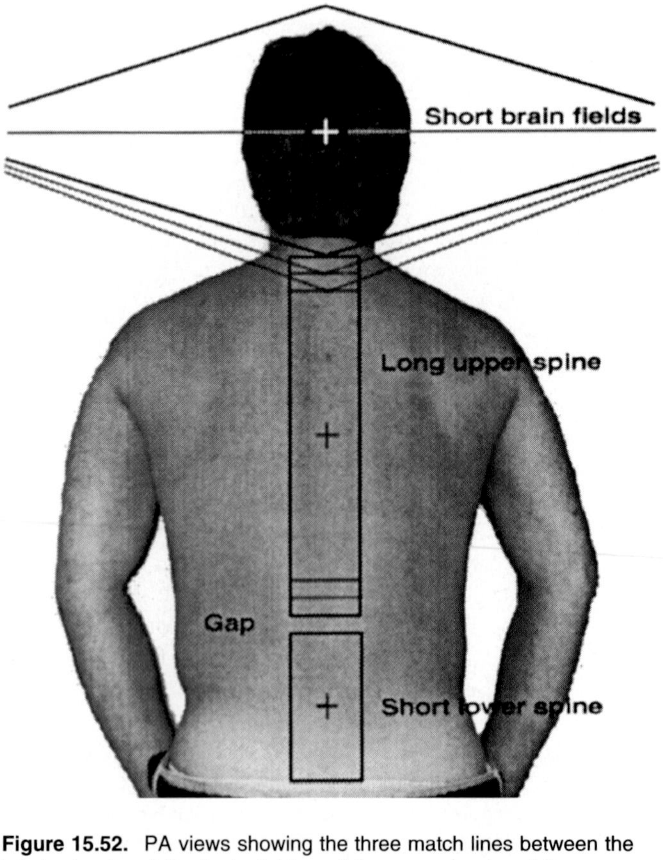

Figure 15.52. PA views showing the three match lines between the inferior border of the brain fields and the upper border of the upper spine field as well as the three match lines between the inferior border of the upper spine field and the superior border of the lower spine field.

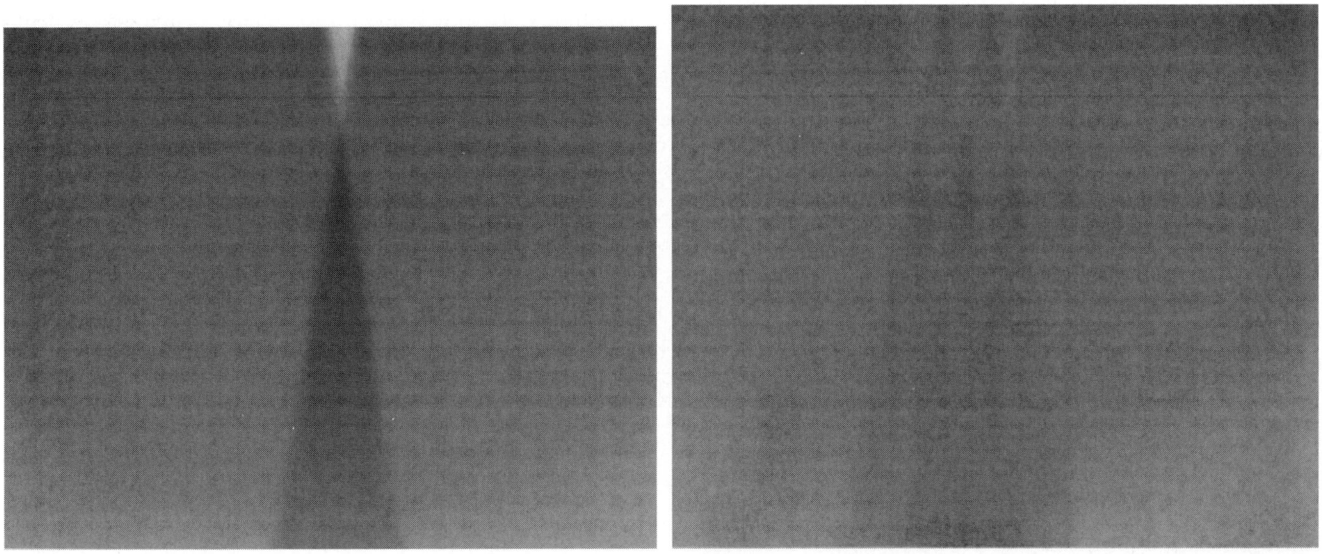

Figure 15.53. A. Film study of the surface gap created by the match at depth of the upper and lower spine fields. Note the area of overlap deep to the match point. **B.** Film study of the skin gap shifting (i.e., match point shifting at depth) between the PA upper and lower spine fields. Note the reduction of the degree of overlap deep to the match points compared with **A.**

fields (CL_1, CL_2), the source-axis distance (SAD) of the linear accelerator, and the cord depth (d). The cord depth is measured directly off a lateral verification film or from a diagnostic CT or MRI scan, when available. The total gap (G) is calculated using the formula:

$$G = \frac{1/2(CL_1 + CL_2) \times d}{SAD} \qquad (15.2)$$

The location of the gap is arbitrary (depending on the lengths of the spine fields), and is usually located in the lower thoracic or upper lumbar spine. As described above, it is moved twice during the course of craniospinal treatment. Figure 15.53a shows how the two PA spine fields, separated by a skin gap, diverge toward each other, match at the depth of the spinal cord, and overlap beyond (i.e., anterior to) the cord and the structures of the thoracic and abdominal cavities. Figure 15.53b shows the effect of shifting the gap twice during the course of craniospinal treatment, and how it reduces the dose in the anterior overlap regions by spreading it out over a larger area. Our practice is to make each shift equal to the size of the skin gap, thus minimizing the number of field markings on the patient's back. As described above, the upper spine field is reduced at each shift and the lower PA spine field is increased in size to maintain a match at depth. The caudal border of the lower spine field remains fixed using asymmetric collimators or blocks (Figure 15.52).

A variation of the technique above improves the dosimetry in the region where the brain and upper spine fields abut. The inferior or caudal borders of opposed brain fields have been shown to diverge across the patient's neck at an angle, creating hot and cold spots lateral to midline. These dose perturbations can be eliminated by angling the foot of the treatment couch toward the collimator for each lateral field, by an amount equal to the divergent angle of the lateral brain fields (see equation 15.1). The brain fields would be unopposed, and their inferior borders would project along the transverse marks, perpendicular to the patient's long axis. In combination with a collimator rotation, all divergent mismatches are eliminated and a perfect abutment results.

There are two problems with this approach. Angling the table for the lateral fields will cause the proximal canthus (and the lens of the proximal eye) to project superiorly, closer to the open field block edge. This makes it more difficult to shield the lens with the custom block while providing adequate margin about the cribiform plate (a midline structure unaffected by the table angulation). The radiograph in Figure 15.54a was obtained with no table rotation. The radiograph in Figure 15.54b was obtained with a table angulation of 8° (appropriate for a lateral brain field length). Radiopaque markers indicate the position of the cribiform plate, lateral canthi, and the approximate positions of the lens of the eyes. In the table angulation technique, the proximal lens does indeed project marginally closer to the cribiform plate. A second problem concerns the uniformity of dose in the brain fields, specifically at midline along the patient's long axis. The prescribed dose is delivered off-axis, at mid-brain, where the patient is thickest. The patient's neck, being thinner, will receive a higher dose regardless of technique. This dose is increased further by the table rotation technique which pivots the neck closer to the beam source,

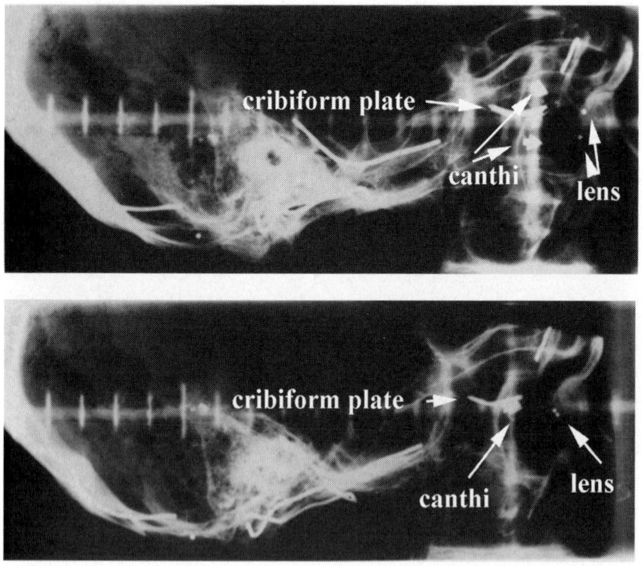

Figure 15.54. Lateral radiographs of a skull with arrows placed on the bony canthi. BB's are placed on the lens. A piece of solder wire was placed in the cribiform plate and is visible at the intersection of the beam axes. **A.** Neutral table angle showing beam divergence and misalignment of the canthi and lens. **B.** As above with 8° of couch rotation. Note alignment of canthi and lens. Also, note closer proximity of lens to cribiform plate, making adequate coverage of the cribiform plate, or shielding of the lens difficult.

decreasing the treatment distance in this area. For these two reasons we elect to treat with opposed brain fields with no table angulation.

SUMMARY

Radiation therapy treatment planning for CNS tumors has developed as a complex interplay between the relatively aggressive nature of many CNS neoplasms and the eloquent functional nature of the brain and spinal cord. The ability to deliver tumoricidal doses of ionizing radiation using external beam therapy is limited by sensitivity of normal CNS tissues to potentially devastating toxicities. Thus, targeting of CNS tumors has become a critical issue in the delivery of external beam radiotherapy. Computer technology has allowed for the use of CT and MRI to accurately describe, in three dimensions, the location of CNS tumors and critical normal tissues. This has led to a proliferation of 3DRTP systems that can accurately target lesions and use complex beam geometries to provide homogeneous dose distribution within the tumor and minimize dose to normal tissues.

Unfortunately, the development and implementation of 3DRTP have not yet resulted in a demonstrable improvement in survival for patients with CNS tumors. This is the impetus for the external beam dose escalation studies being performed at a number of institutions. Combinations of external beam radiotherapy plus brachytherapy or radiosurgery are also being investigated as methods of dose escalation. Fractionated stereotactic radiation therapy, a hybrid of the EBRT and stereotactic radiosurgery (SRS), combines the biological advantage of fractionation with the precise target localization of SRS, the ultimate goal of 3DRTP. Proton beam therapy and boron neutron capture therapy, two methods which take advantage of "controlled" energy deposition, are also being actively studied at institutions where these modalities are available.

Ultimately, the successful treatment of patients with CNS tumors will likely involve multi-modality therapy including surgery and/or radiation for local control, and some form of "systemic" CNS therapy for microscopic disease. New developments in the understanding of the biology and genetics of CNS tumors will be necessary for the development of these novel strategies. Customized therapies targeted for an individual's specific tumor type and location will, hopefully, allow for better control and cure in the future.

References

1. Levin VA, Gutin PH, Leibel S. Neoplasms of the central nervous system. In: DeVita VT, Hellman S, Rosenberg SA, eds. Cancer: principles and practice of oncology. 4th ed. Philadelphia: JB Lippincott, 1993.
2. Kleihues P, Burger PC, Scheithauer BW, eds. Histological typing of tumours of the central nervous system. 2nd ed. Berlin: New York, Springer-Verlag, 1993.
3. Kleihues P, Burger PC, Scheithauer BW. The new WHO classification of brain tumors. Brain Pathology 1993;3:255–268.
4. Posner JB, Chernik NL. Intracranial metastases from systemic cancer. In: Schoenberg BS, ed. Advances in neurology, Vol. 19. New York: Raven Press, 1978.
5. Borgelt B, Gelber R, Kramer S, et al. The palliation of brain metastases: final results of the first two studies by the Radiation Therapy Oncology Group. Int J Radiat Oncol Biol Phys 1980;6:1–9.
6. Loeffler JS, Shrieve DC, Wen PY, et al. The palliation of brain metastases: final results of the first two studies by the Radiation Therapy Oncology Group. Int J Radiat Oncol 1995;5:225–234.
7. Carabell SC, Goodman RL. Oncologic emergencies. Spinal cord compression. In: DeVita VT, Hellman S, Rosenberg SA, eds. Cancer: principles and practice of oncology. 4th ed. Philadelphia: JB Lippincott, 1993.
8. Schad L, Lott S, Schmitt F. Correction of spatial distortion in MR imaging: a prerequisite for accurate stereotaxy. J Comput Assist Tomogr 1987;11:499–503.
9. Kahn T, Schwabe B, Bettag M, et al. Mapping of the cortical motor hand area with functional MR imaging and MR imaging-guided laser-induced interstitial thermotherapy of brain tumors. Works in progress. Radiology 1996;200:149–157.
10. McCarthy G, Puce A, Luby M, Belgar A, Allison T. MR imaging studies of functional brain activation: analysis and interpretation. Electroenceph & Clin Neurophys 1996;547:15–31.
11. Yetkin FZ, Mueller WM, Morris GL, et al. Functional MR activation correlated with intraoperative cortical mapping. AJNR 1997;18:1311–1315.
12. Rezai AR, Mogilner AY, Cappell J, et al. Integration of functional brain mapping in image-guided neurosurgery. Acta Neurochir 1997;568:85–89.
13. Hund M, Rezai AR, Kronberg E, et al. Magnetoencephalographic mapping: basics of a new functional risk profile in the selection of patients with cortical brain lesions. Neurosurg 1997;40:936–942.
14. Vins FC, Zomorano L, Mueller RA, et al. [150]-water PET and intraoperative brain mapping: a comparison in the localization of eloquent cortex. Neuro Res 1997;19:601–608.

15. Nelson SJ, Huhn S, Vigneron DB, et al. Volume MRI and MRSI techniques for the quantitation of treatment response in brain tumors: presentation of a detailed case study. J Magn Res Imaging 1997;7: 1146–1152.
16. Slosman DO, Lazeyras F. Metabolic imaging in the diagnosis of brain tumors. Curr Opin Neurol 1996;9:429–435.
17. Kizu O, Naruse S, Furuya S, et al. Application of proton chemical shift imaging in monitoring of gamma knife radiosurgery on brain tumors. Magn Res Imaging 1998;16:197–204.
18. Prescribing, recording, and reporting photon beam therapy. International Commission on Radiation Units and Measurements, Report 50. Washington, 1993.
19. Daumas-Duport C, Monsaingeon V, Szenthe L, et al. Serial stereotactic biopsies—a double histological code of gliomas according to malignancy and 3-D configuration as an aid to therapeutic decision and assessment of results. Appl Neurophysiol 1982;45:431–437.
20. Kelly PJ, Daumas-Duport C, Scheithauer BW, et al. Stereotactic histologic correlations of CT and MRI defined abnormalities in patients with glial neoplasms. Mayo Clinic Proceedings 1987;62:450–459.
21. Lian BC, Thornton A Jr, Sandler HM, Greenberg HS. Malignant astrocytomas: focal tumor recurrence after focal external beam radiation therapy. J Neurosurg 1990;18:559–563.
22. Wallner K, Galicich J, Krol G. Patterns of failure following treatment for glioblastoma multiforme and anaplastic astrocytoma. Int J Radiat Oncol Biol Phys 1989;16:1405–1409.
23. Sandler HM. 3-D conformal radiotherapy for brain tumors. In: Meyers JL, Purdy JA, eds. 3-D conformal radiotherapy. Front Radiat Ther Oncol. 1996:250–254.
24. Karlsson UL, Leibel SA, Wallner K, Davis LW, Brady LW. Brain. In: Perez CA, Brady LW, eds. Principles and practice of radiation oncology. 2nd ed. Philadelphia: JB Lippincott, 1992.
25. Kun LE. The brain and spinal cord. In: Cox JD, ed. Moss' radiation oncology. Rationale, technique, results. 7th ed. St. Louis: Mosby, 1994.
26. Halperin EC, Constine LS, Tarbell NJ, Kun LE, eds. Pediatric radiation oncology. 2nd ed. New York: Raven Press, 1994.
27. Gutin P, Leibel SA, Sheline GE. Radiation injury to the nervous system. 1st ed. New York: Raven Press, 1991.
28. Schueltheiss TE, Kun LE, Ang KK, Stephens LC. Radiation response of the central nervous system. Int J Radiat Oncol Biol Phys 1995;31: 1093–1112.
29. Rubin P, ed. Radiation biology and radiation pathology syllabus. American College of Radiology: Chicago, 1975.
30. Emami B, Lyman J, Brown A, et al. Tolerance of normal tissues to therapeutic irradiation. Int J Radiat Oncol Biol Phys 1991;21:109–122.
31. Munroff LR, Runge VM. The use of MR contrast in neoplastic disease of the brain. Topics in Mag Res Imag 1995;7:137–157.
32. Pelizzari CA, Chen GTY, Spelbring DR, Weichselbaum RR, Chen CT. Accurate three-dimensional registration of CT, PET and/or MR images of the brain. J Comput Assist Tomogr 1989;13:20–26.
33. Ten Haken RK, Thornton AF Jr, Sandler HM, et al. A quantitative assessment of the addition of MRI to CT-based, 3-D treatment planning of brain tumors. Radiother Oncol 1992;25:21–33.
34. Bourland JD, McCollough KP. Static field conformal sterotactic radiosurgery: physical techniques. Int J Radiat Oncol Biol Phys 1994;28: 471–479.
35. Shrieve DC, Tarbell NJ, Alexander E, et al. Stereotactic radiotherapy: a technique for dose optimization and escalation for intracranial tumors. Acta Neurochirurgica 1994;62(suppl):118–123.
36. Niemieriko A. Treatment plan optimization. In: Purdy JA, Emami B, eds. 3D radiation treatment planning and conformal therapy. Madison: Medical Physics Publishing, 1995.
37. Lyman JT, Wolbarst AB. Optimization of radiation therapy: 3. A method for assessing complication probabilities from dose-volume histograms. Int J Radiat Oncol Biol Phys 1987;13:103–109.
38. Withers HR, Taylor JMG, Maciejewski B. Treatment volumes and tissue tolerance. Int J Radiat Oncol Biol Phys 1988;14:751–759.
39. Hamilton RJ, Kuchnir FT, Sweeney P, et al. Comparison of static conformal field with multiple noncoplanar arc techniques for stereotactic radiosurgery or stereotactic radiotherapy. Int J Radiat Oncol Biol Phys 1995;33:1221–1228.
40. Hamilton RJ, Sweeney PJ, Pelizzari CA, et al. Functional imaging in treatment planning of brain lesions. Int J Radiat Oncol Biol Phys 1997; 37:181–188.
41. Smith V, Verhey L, Serago CF. Comparison of radiosurgery treatment modalities based on complication and control probabilities. Int J Radiat Oncol Biol Phys 1998;40:507–513.
42. Cooley G, Gillin MT, Murray KJ, Wilson JF, Janjan JA. Improved dose localization with dual energy photon irradiation in treatment of lateralized intracranial malignancies. Int J Radiat Oncol Biol Phys 1991; 20:815–821.
43. Sklar CA, Constine LS. Chronic neuroendocrinological sequelae of radiation therapy. Int J Radiat Oncol Biol Phys 1995;31:1113–1122.
44. Gordon KB, Char DH, Sagerman RH. Late effects of radiation on the eye and ocular adnexa. Int J Radiat Oncol Biol Phys 1995;31: 1123–1140.
45. Cooper JS, Fu K, Marks J, Silverman S. Late effects of radiation in the head and neck region. Int J Radiat Oncol Biol Phys 1995;31: 1141–1164.

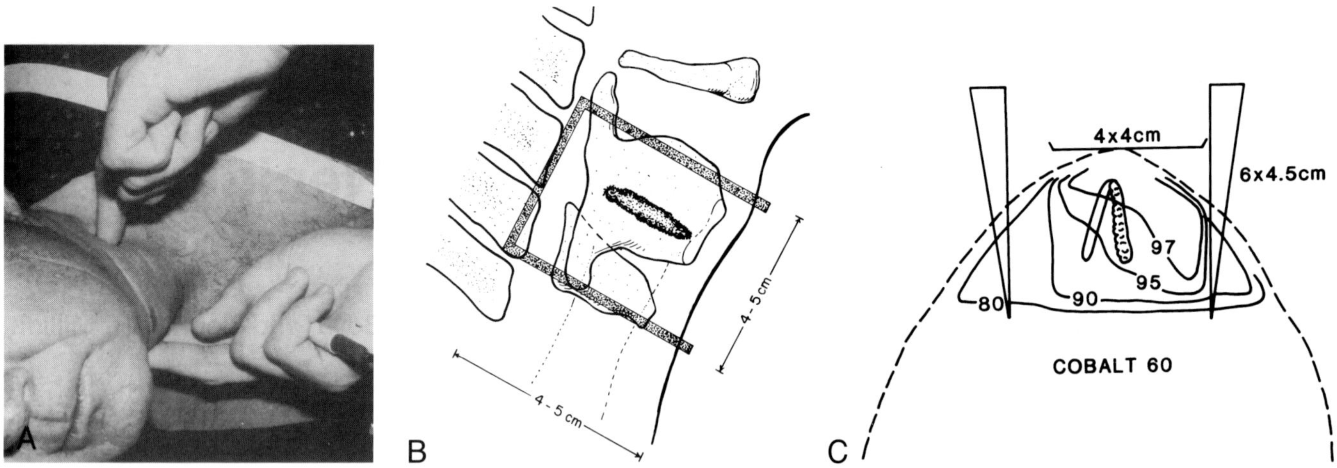

Figure 16.1. Radiation treatment technique for carcinoma of glottic larynx, stage T1-T2. **A.** Patient is in lateral decubitus position. To locate posterior border of thyroid cartilage, fingers of one hand are positioned under patient's neck and larynx is lifted gently a few millimeters while index finger of other hand simultaneously locates posterior edge of thyroid lamina. **B.** For T1 cancer, superior border of field usually is at mid-thyroid notch (height of notch typically is about 1.0 cm or slightly more in male adults; for minimal lesions (e.g., carcinoma in situ), bottom of thyroid notch is chosen. If ventricle or false vocal cords are minimally involved, top of notch (which corresponds to cephalad portion of thyroid lamina as palpated just off midline) is often selected; more advanced lesions call for greater superior coverage. If only anterior one-half of vocal cord is involved, posterior border is placed at back of midportion of thyroid lamina. If posterior portion of cord is involved, border is 1.0 cm behind lamina. If anterior face of arytenoid is also involved, posterior border is placed 1.5 cm behind cartilage. If no subglottic extension is detected, inferior border of irradiation portal is at bottom of cricoid arch as palpated at midline. If computed tomography demonstrates subglottic extension, portal is adjusted accordingly. Anteriorly, beam falls off (by 1.5 cm) over patient's skin. **C,** Three-field technique (two lateral wedge fields and an anterior open field) is used commonly to treat vocal cord cancer at University of Florida. Lateral fields are differentially weighted to involved side. Anterior field, which usually measures 4 $\times$ 4 cm, is centered approximately 0.5 cm lateral to midline in patients with one cord involved and typically delivers about 5% of total tumor dose (usually on last 2 treatment days) after treatment from lateral portals is completed. Anterior portal is essentially reduced portal that centers high dose to the tumor. Isodose line at which dose is specified is that which covers gross disease. By appropriate field weightings, encompassing the tumor within 95 to 97% of maximum isodose line is virtually always possible. (**B** reprinted with permission from Million RR, Cassisi NJ, Mancuso AA. Larynx. In Million RR, Cassisi NJ, eds. Management of head and neck cancer: a multidisciplinary approach. 2nd ed. Philadelphia: J.B. Lippincott; 1994:431–497.)

sues and muscles down to and including the perichondrium of the laryngeal cartilages, while leaving the vocal cords in place (9). The distance between the lowest portion of the thyroid notch and the superior surface of the cords at the anterior commissure averaged 7 mm (range, 5 to 11 mm), and the attachment of the anterior commissure by its tendon was approximately 1 cm above the lower free edge of the thyroid cartilage in the midline. The posterior border of the thyroid cartilage may be difficult to locate, especially in obese or muscular patients (Figure 16.1A). In women or in massively obese men, all of the landmarks may be difficult to identify, and the setup should be verified and/or designed on the simulator; if the landmarks cannot be palpated, the patient is treated supine. Cobalt-60 (Co-60), 4 MV, or 6 MV photon beams are acceptable. When Co-60 is used, the light field is opened approximately 1 cm wider than the lines that are drawn on the patient's skin, and the beam is secondarily collimated by lead blocks stacked on a wire mesh tray that is positioned approximately 15 cm above the patient.

Computed tomography (CT) helps determine tumor extent and therefore portal design in patients with large T2 cancers. It is useful in detecting subglottic spread, which may be submucosal and difficult to detect by direct laryngoscopy. Computed tomography is not obtained for T1 or early T2 cancers.

Stage T3

The initial portals for T3N0 true vocal cord cancer at the University of Florida are shown in Figure 16.2 (10). Because of a 20 to 25% risk of subclinical involvement of the jugulodigastric or midjugular lymph nodes, these areas are electively treated with 45.6 to 50 Gy tumor dose. A small low-neck portal treats the low jugular lymph nodes with 50 Gy given dose (at Dmax [the dose at maximum buildup]) over 5 weeks (see subsequent section, Design of the Low Neck Portal). Primary fields are then reduced, and the treatment is continued to the final tumor dose with fields that are usually slightly larger than those described for early vocal cord cancer. Most patients currently receive 74.4 Gy at 1.2 Gy twice a day.

Preliminary data suggest that local control rates are dependent on tumor volume in cubic centimeters (cm^3) (11).

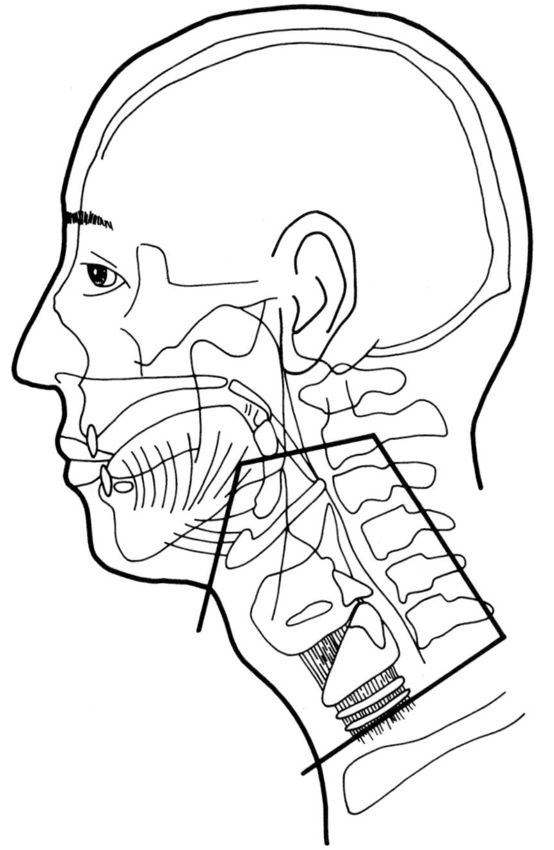

Figure 16.2. Radiation treatment technique for carcinoma of glottic larynx, stage T3-T4N0. Patient is treated supine, and field is shaped with Lipowitz's metal. Anteriorly, field is allowed to fall off. Entire pre-epiglottic space is included by encompassing hyoid bone and epiglottis. Superior border (just above angle of mandible) includes jugulodigastric lymph nodes. Posteriorly, portion of spinal cord must be included within field to ensure adequate coverage of midjugular lymph nodes; spinal accessory lymph nodes themselves are at little risk of involvement. Lower border is slanted (1) to facilitate matching with low neck field and (2) to reduce length of spinal cord in high-dose field. Inferior border is placed at bottom of cricoid cartilage if patient has no subglottic spread; in presence of subglottic extension, inferior border must be lowered according to disease extent. (Reprinted with permission from Parsons JT, et al. Twice-a-day radiotherapy for squamous cell carcinoma of the glottic larynx. Head Neck 1989;11:123.)

Supraglottic Larynx, T1-T3

Radiation therapy alone produces high control rates for T1, T2, and selected T3 supraglottic cancers. Control rates depend on tumor volume in cubic centimeters (cm^3) (12). The treatment volume is similar to that shown in Figure 16.2, with the exception that the beam generally is not allowed to "fall off" over the anterior skin surface, except in patients who are very thin, have extensive spread of tumor into the preepiglottic space, have very bulky lymphadenopathy that extends anteriorly, or have lesions involving the infrahyoid epiglottis near the anterior commissure. Shielding even a few millimeters of the anterior skin, subcutaneous tissues, and lymphatic vessels may lessen the risk of serious laryngeal edema. The situation may be analogous to that of extremity sarcomas, in which sparing of a strip of skin, subcutaneous tissues, and dermal lymphatics preserves a route of egress for lymph.

The inferior border of the portal is adjusted according to disease extent. For a false cord or infrahyoid epiglottic cancer, the middle or bottom of the cricoid cartilage commonly is chosen. For an epiglottic tip cancer, the lower border may be placed at or above the level of the true cords, depending on the extent and growth pattern (infiltrative versus exophytic) of disease.

If the neck is clinically negative and tumor does not extend beyond the larynx, only the jugulodigastric and midjugular areas are treated. If the base of tongue or pyriform sinus is involved or if neck disease is extensive, the primary portal includes the entire jugular chain and spinal accessory chain. In all situations, the low neck is treated with an anterior en face portal, the size and shape of which vary according to the N stage and laterality of disease (see subsequent section, "Design of the Low Neck Portal").

HYPOPHARNYX

Pyriform Sinus

The portals used for the initial treatment volume of early and moderately advanced pyriform sinus cancer are shown in Figure 16.3. In addition to the entire jugular lymphatic chain, the lateral retropharyngeal lymph nodes (medial to the carotid arteries, usually located just in front of the C1-C2 vertebral bodies) and spinal accessory nodes are also at risk and are treated even if the neck is clinically negative. The pyriform sinus lies posteriorly in the pharynx, extending from its upper limit on the pharyngoepiglottic fold to its apex at or just below the level of the cricoid cartilage. It is rarely necessary to allow anterior "falloff" over the anterior skin of the midline. If the lesion is so extensive as to require falloff anteriorly to achieve adequate coverage, total laryngopharyngectomy is usually the treatment of choice.

Pharyngeal Wall

Most pharyngeal wall lesions involve only the posterior wall. With CT, some lesions are seen to extend posterolaterally, in effect wrapping around the anterior vertebral body (Figure 16.4) (13). If the posterior edge of the reduced portal splits the middle of the vertebral body, geographic miss may result. The initial treatment volume is much like that shown in Figure 16.3 for pyriform sinus cancer. The upper margin of the port should be at the base of the skull, to include all retropharyngeal tissues. The initial lower portal margin should include the entire pharyngeal wall because of these tumors' propensity to

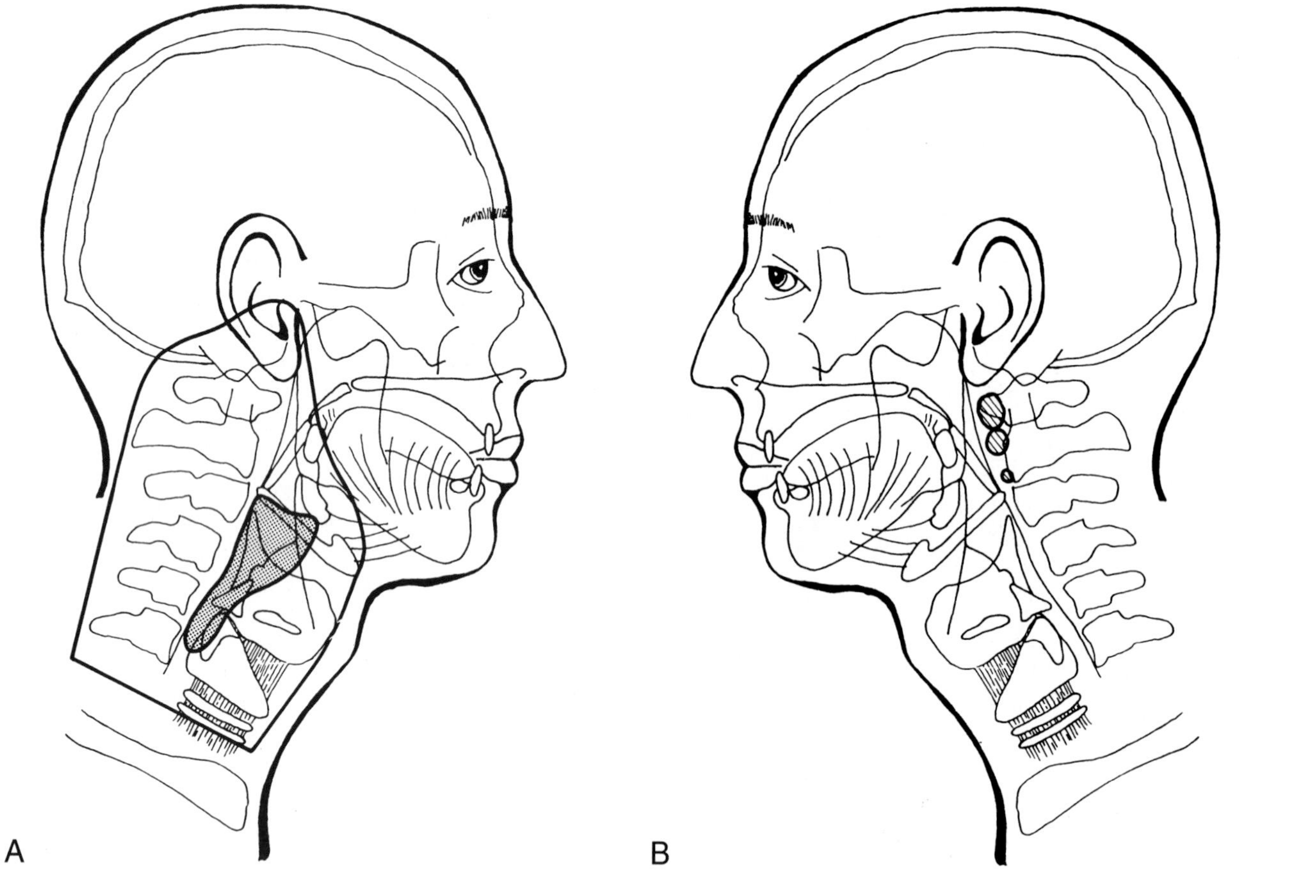

Figure 16.3. **A.** Portals used for initial treatment volume in patient with carcinoma *(stippled area)* of pyriform sinus. Superiorly, portal covers lymph nodes at base of skull, then sweeps anteroinferiorly to cover posterior tongue base and jugulodigastric lymph nodes. Anteriorly, at least 1 cm of skin and subcutaneous tissues (as viewed from lateral projection) is usually spared. Inferior border is 2 to 3 cm below bottom of cricoid cartilage and is slanted to facilitate matching with low neck portal and to avoid irradiating shoulders. Posterior field edge usually encompasses spinous process of C2 vertebral body. As treatment progresses, several field reductions are made (to shield spinal cord and to limit volume of mucosa that receives high dose irradiation). **B.** Location of lateral retropharyngeal lymph nodes in relation to C1-C2 vertebral bodies.

have "skip lesions." The reduced portals are shown in Figure 16.4. The posterior field edge is placed at the posterior vertebral body; daily portal films are obtained to ensure reproducibility.

POSTOPERATIVE IRRADIATION OF LARYNGEAL AND HYPOPHARNYGEAL TUMORS

In this situation, the larynx has been removed. The primary fields are treated through lateral parallel-opposed Co-60 portals (Figure 16.5A) (14) to include the anterior and posterior neck from the base of skull to the top of the tracheal stoma. Techniques with either anterior or anterior and posterior portals have the disadvantages of underdosage of lymph nodes at the base of the skull in the region of the mastoid and unnecessary irradiation of a large volume of brain tissue in the posterior cranial fossa. After the administration of 45 to 50 Gy, the field is reduced so that the spinal cord is no longer in the treatment field; the dose to high-risk areas behind the plane of the spinal cord may be boosted with 8 to 10 MeV electrons.

The low-neck portal, which usually includes the stoma, is treated as shown in Figure 16.5B (14). The dose at Dmax in most patients is 50 Gy in 25 fractions. In patients at high risk for recurrence in the low neck (i.e., who have positive low jugular nodes), a boost dose occasionally is given through a reduced field. In patients with subglottic extension, the dose to the stomal and peristomal tissues is boosted with electrons, usually 12 to 14 MeV. The energy selected should be high enough to deliver an adequate dose to the paratracheal and tracheoesophageal lymph nodes.

Cobalt-60 is the beam of choice because of its buildup characteristics; higher energy beams are less desirable because of underdosage of superficial tissues. Petrolatum gauze bolus is placed on all scars and over drain sites. All scars, suture holes, and drain sites are treated with generous (2 to 3 cm) margins.

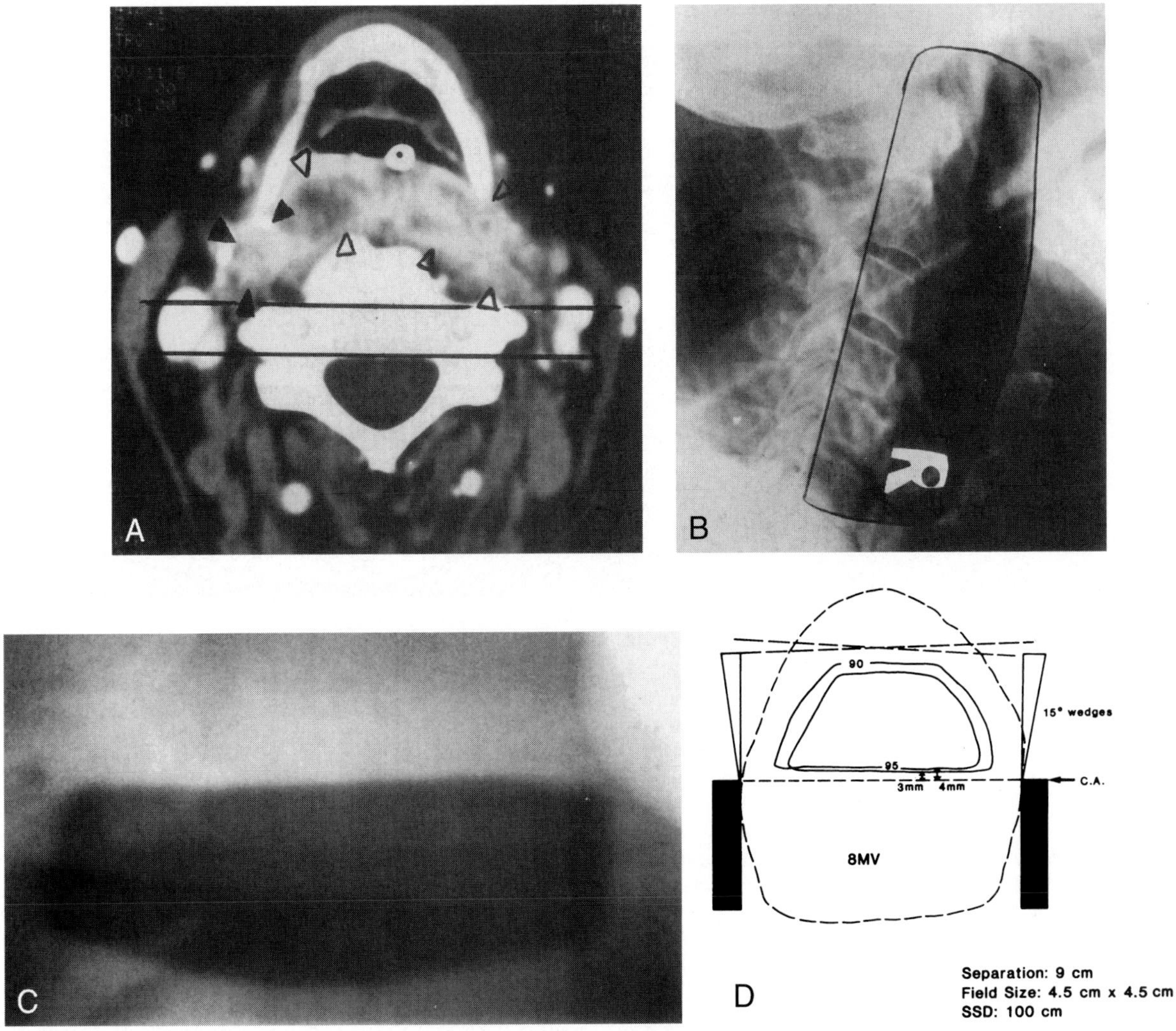

Figure 16.4. Radiation treatment techniques for carcinoma of posterior pharyngeal wall. **A.** Computed tomogram of T3 posterior pharyngeal wall cancer *(arrowheads)*. Horizontal lines represent two possible placements of posterior field edge. If field edge bisects vertebral body when spinal cord is shielded, part of cancer will be in penumbra or altogether outside irradiated volume. Entire width of vertebral body is always treated in patients with posterior pharyngeal wall tumors. **B.** Simulation film shows first field reduction (to shield spinal cord) for a patient with T3N0 cancer. **C.** Portal films are taken each day because margin for error (and thereby spinal cord injury) is tiny. Note that with reduced portals, little of larynx remains within treatment volume. Only epiglottis and part of arytenoids and aryepiglottic folds cannot be excluded. **D.** Isodose plots for reduced portals. In our practice, 6 MV or 8 MV photons are ideal energy. Because of characteristics of high-energy (e.g., 17 MV) photons near field edge, isodose distributions are constricted compared with 8 MV. (2) Result is reduced dosage to cancer near posterior field edge, which is undesirable in treatment of posterior pharyngeal wall cancer. Central axis (CA) is placed at posterior field edge to provide nondivergent posterior field edge. Wedges are used to reduce dose anteriorly and to pull isodose distribution slightly posteriorly. SSD, source-to-surface distance. (Parts **A** and **B** reprinted with permission from Mendenhall WM, et al. Squamous cell carcinoma of the pharyngeal wall treated with irradiation. Radiother Oncol 1988; 11:205.)

OROPHARYNX

Important points in the design of portals for the oropharynx are as follows: 1) The risk of lymph node metastases in both the upper and lower neck is significant, and both areas should be treated even when the neck is clinically disease-free (stage N0); 2) The use of long lateral primary fields that include the larynx and a longer length of spinal cord than necessary is inappropriate. Dividing the treatment volume into upper (primary) and anterior low-neck fields is essential so that the larynx can be shielded from irradiation and the spinal cord dose is reduced; this is true even in the presence of a large lymph node that is bisected by the lower border of the primary field. Although many radiation oncologists explain that treating the larynx with 50 Gy is acceptable because "it can tolerate it," there is little excuse for exposing a vital structure to a moderately high dose of irradiation when it is avoidable. Inclusion of the larynx within the primary portals causes more severe mucositis, which often leads

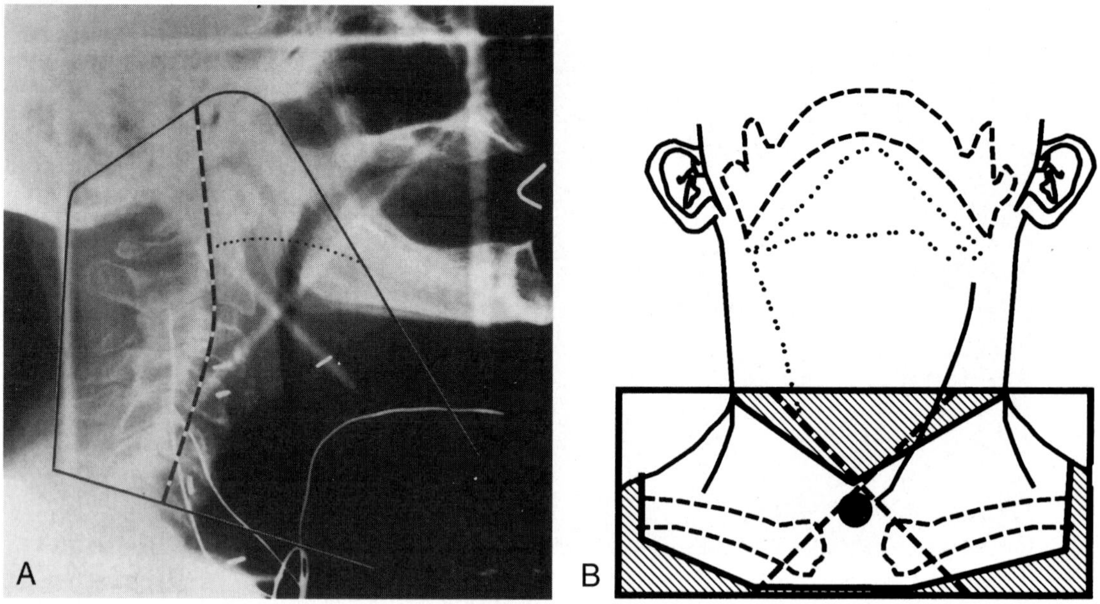

Figure 16.5. **A.** Typical postoperative simulation film of patient with advanced-stage cancer of laryngopharynx. *Dashed line,* initial field reduction (after 50 Gy, to shield spinal cord); *dotted line,* final reduction (after 60 Gy). Wires mark surgical scars and stoma. Slanting line used on lower border reduces length of spinal cord treated by primary field, allows better caudal coverage of mucosal surfaces while simultaneously bypassing shoulders, and facilitates matching with low neck field. **B.** Low neck field. Beam is vertical (0°). Rectangle *(solid line)* represents light field. *Dashed line,* central axis; *shaded areas,* blocked portions of field (stacked lead blocks). Superior border of neck field is inferior border of primary field. Actual line is treated only with primary field. Upper border of low neck field assumes V shape. In midline of patient, apex of V generally is at or close to central axis, so portion of beam that irradiates the spinal cord is nondivergent. At junction of the three fields, short (2 to 3 cm) segment of spinal cord remains untreated through any of fields. (Reprinted with permission from Amdur RJ, et al. Postoperative irradiation for squamous cell carcinoma of the head and neck: An analysis of treatment results and complications. Int J Radiat Oncol Biol Phys 1989;16:25–36.)

to unplanned treatment interruptions or requires treatment with low total daily doses, either of which results in poor tumor control. Treatment of the larynx also produces some edema and dries the mucous membranes. The larynx is endowed with a rich supply of mucous glands, which are particularly abundant on the arytenoids, laryngeal sacculus, and epiglottis. Irradiation of this minor salivary tissue, whose function is to maintain a lubricated mucosal surface, results in unnecessary chronic morbidity (15). Such treatment also complicates the management of the patient who later develops a second primary cancer in the larynx. We are aware of at least one patient (with cancer of the nasopharynx) treated at another institution who died as a result of severe laryngeal edema after a course of treatment in which the larynx unfortunately was included within the primary portals.

Base of Tongue

Typical initial and reduced portals for treating a cancer of the base of the tongue are shown in Figure 16.6 (16). A variety of ways are used to administer the final "boost" dose. All lesions currently are managed by external beam irradiation alone, except for small, discrete lesions on the anterolateral base of the tongue, where an interstitial transoral implant can be readily accomplished; this type of lesion is unusual.

Iridium-192 (Ir-192) implantation is a popular boost technique in some treatment centers. Local control rates after continuous-course, external-beam therapy alone at the University of Florida and at M. D. Anderson Hospital were compared with the results from five centers in which Ir-192 implants were used. No convincing evidence is available at this time that the implant produces superior local control rates or reduced complications when compared with the results of external beam irradiation alone (17,18).

Two ways to deliver the final dose by external beam are by using reduced lateral fields (Figure 16.6 [16]) or the submental technique (Figure 16.7 [19,20]). The submental portal is particularly useful for lesions in the posterior base of the tongue because it allows delivery of additional irradiation to the primary lesion without irradiating the mandible. If extensive invasion into the tonsillar fossa has occurred, the submental boost technique is not used. Anterior lesions and lesions with major extension into the oral tongue are not well suited to the submental technique,

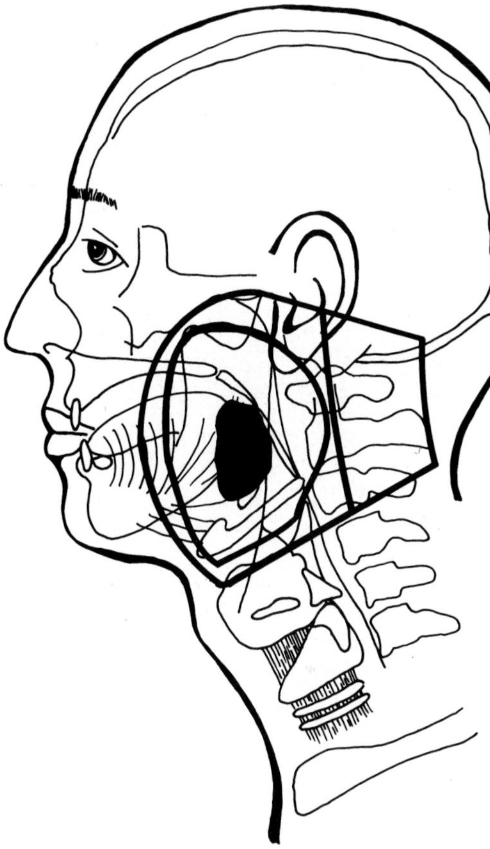

Figure 16.6. Radiation treatment technique for carcinoma of base of tongue. Superiorly, portal treats jugular and spinal accessory lymph nodes to base of skull. Posterior border is behind spinous process of C2. Inferior border is at or just below thyroid notch, depending on disease extent. Anteroinferiorly, skin and subcutaneous tissues of submentum are shielded, except in case of advanced disease, especially if submental boost technique is used. Anterior tongue margin is set by palpation. Placing a small stainless steel pin in anteriormost extent of palpable disease is useful for identification on simulation film. If tumor is too posterior to pin, point at which anterior tonsillar pillar inserts into tongue is pinned for orientation purposes. Two portal reductions are shown. (Reprinted with permission from Parsons JT, Mendenhall WM, Moore GJ, Million, RR. Radiotherapy of tumors of the oropharynx. In: Thawley SE, Panje WR, eds. Comprehensive management of head and neck tumors. 2nd ed. Philadelphia: W.B. Saunders [in press].)

because the treatment distance makes dose delivery inefficient.

Tonsillar Area

The minimum initial treatment volume for early cancers of the tonsillar region includes the retromolar trigone, tonsillar pillars, soft palate, base of the tongue, and entire tonsillar fossa. The anterior margin of the portal varies according to the anterior extent of disease; in patients with cancer at an early stage, it is at the level of the third molar tooth. If the buccal mucosa is invaded, anterior coverage should be generous for the first 50 Gy to avoid geographic miss. Anterior extension into the oral tongue is sought by digital palpation. For early, well-lateralized lesions of the tonsillar region with no tongue invasion, ipsilateral treatment with a combination of high energy photons and electrons is sometimes used to preserve salivary flow on the contralateral side (Figure 16.8 [21,22]). A wedge pair is also acceptable, and with the availability of three-dimensional simulation and treatment planning, it has become easier to plan the appropriate treatment volume, avoid geographic miss, and shape the fields.

The technique of irradiation for more advanced tonsillar cancers is by parallel-opposed portals, similar to those shown in Figure 16.6, that are used for lesions of the base of the tongue. Portals are usually weighted 3:2 or 1:1, depending on the anatomic distribution of disease. The pterygoid plates up to the base of the skull should be irradiated in patients with advanced disease; if trismus is present, the pterygoids should remain within the treatment volume for the entire course of irradiation. Nasopharyngeal or hypopharyngeal extension must be recognized to avoid geographic miss with the reduced fields.

The dose to tongue nodules usually is boosted by implant after external-beam irradiation, even if the nodule has disappeared during the treatment course. If the primary lesion is large, and especially if palpable nodularity in the tonsillar fossa persists after external-beam irradiation, the pterygoid region also is implanted (Figure 16.9) (16). The boost dose usually is 10 to 15 Gy after full-dose, external-beam irradiation. The entire extent of the original lesion usually is not covered by the implant; only the area of heaviest tumor infestation and/or areas of residual nodularity receive a boost dose.

The failure rate after irradiation alone for T1-T2 lesions of the anterior tonsillar pillar is higher than for tonsillar fossa lesions. External beam (45 Gy) plus iridium implantation (30 Gy) has produced a high rate of success (15 of 15) in a report by Mazeron et al (23). In selected early-stage pillar lesions, the dose may be boosted with an intraoral cone rather than by implant (e.g., 20 Gy in 8 fractions via intraoral cone, followed by 50 Gy via external beam).

Soft Palate

The irradiation technique by parallel opposed fields for soft palate cancer is demonstrated in Figure 16.10 [16]). Figure 16.11 (16) depicts the treatment of early, discrete lesions that can be encompassed by an intraoral cone. Intraoral cone treatment has the advantage of delivering a high dose to a limited tissue volume in a short overall treatment time. Intraoral cone treatment is administered before the start of external beam treatment, while the lesion is still clearly visible and before the onset of mucositis; it is not recommended as the sole treatment because of the risk of lymph node metastases.

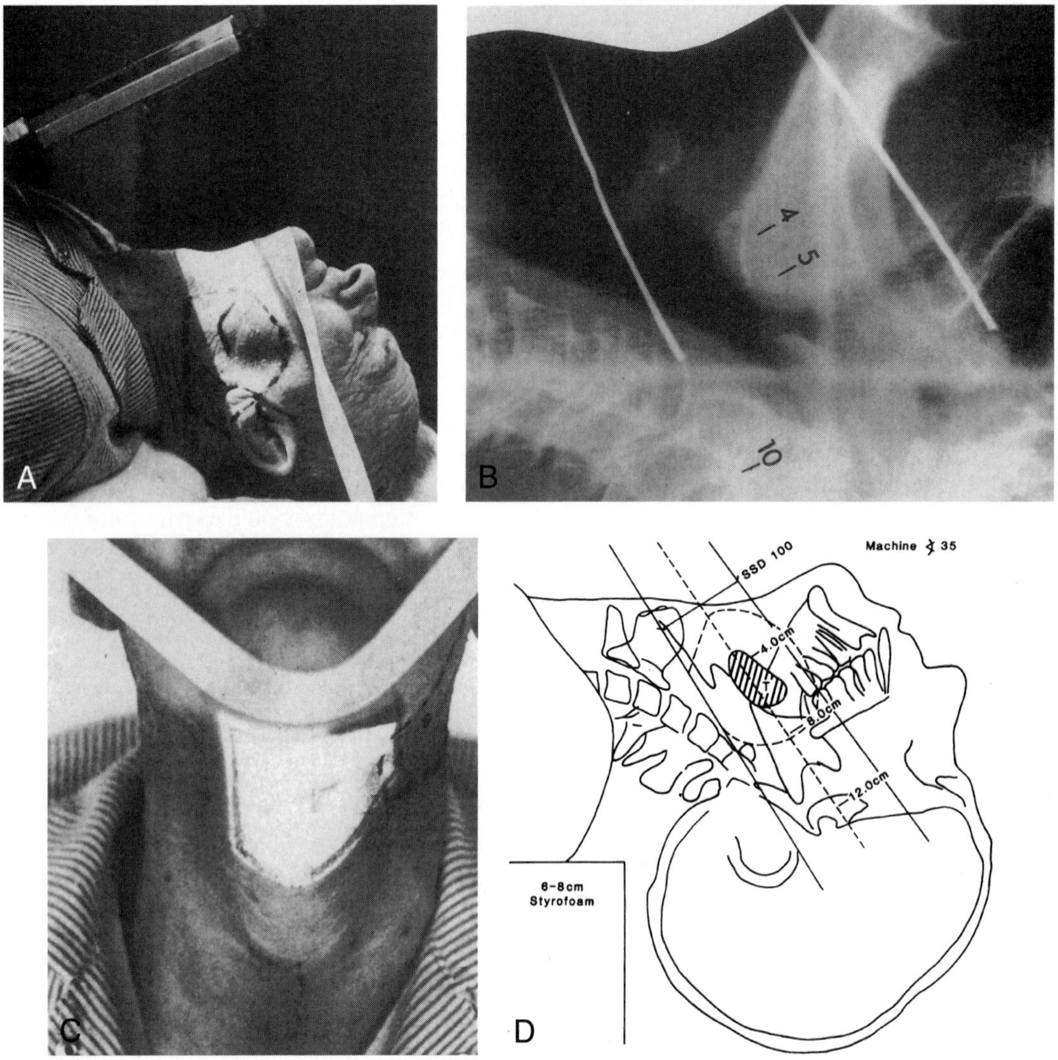

Figure 16.7. Submental boost technique for carcinoma of base of tongue. **A.** Final 10 to 15 Gy may be delivered to base of tongue by submental route, thereby reducing dose to mandible and lateral soft tissues of neck. Boost may be delivered with high energy electrons or photons. Cobalt 60 or 6 MV photons have been used at University of Florida more commonly than electrons and have definite advantages for tumors that extend anteriorly, toward oral tongue, because distance from submental skin may be greater than can be efficiently covered by 20 MeV electrons. If submental boost portal is used, anterior submental skin must be shielded on lateral portals to avoid excessive fibrosis and telangiectasis. Head of table is stepped down or torso is raised approximately 6 cm to hyperextend patient's neck. Machine head is tilted cephalad 30° to 35°. Collimators are opened wide to adjust superior tilt so that little or no overlap occurs at portion of spinal cord that was irradiated by lateral portals. (*Dashed lines,* initial lateral treatment portal and reduced lateral treatment portal.) Once beam is properly aligned, patient's head is secured with one or two strips of masking tape. Note angle of mandible marked in this patient ("hockey stick" line). Spinal cord is generally shielded from lateral portals at 45 Gy tumor dose, because for each 10 Gy tumor dose (at 4-cm depth, ^{60}Co), upper cervical cord would receive an additional 5 to 5.5 Gy (at 10 to 11 cm depth) if some overlap occurred. No instances of transverse myelitis have occurred in patients treated with this technique at University of Florida. **B.** To verify adequate tumor coverage and spinal cord exclusion, patient is positioned on simulator table (as in Figure 16.6A). Wires are taped on patient along superior and inferior edges of beam, and cross-table lateral radiograph is obtained. Dorsum of base of tongue lies 4 to 5 cm from skin along central axis. Spinal cord lies approximately 10 cm from skin along lower edge of portal. **C.** Lower border of submental boost portal usually is slightly below thyroid notch. Field width is adjusted to allow generous coverage because understaging of base of tongue cancers occurs frequently. Portal may be shaped by secondary collimation to include unilateral or bilateral upper neck nodes (inverted L or inverted U). **D.** Submental technique. *Dashed lines,* final lateral portal reduction, useful in verifying adequacy of submental treatment volume. SSD, source-to-surface distance. (**A** and **C** reprinted with permission from Parsons JT, Million RR, Cassisi NJ. Carcinoma of the base of the tongue: Results of radical irradiation with surgery reserved for irradiation failure. Laryngoscope 1982;92: 689–696.) (**B** reprinted with permission from Million RR, Cassisi NJ, Mancuso AA. Oropharynx. In: Million RR, Cassisi NJ, eds. Management of head and neck cancer: a multidisciplinary approach. 2nd ed. Philadelphia: J.B. Lippincott; 1994:401–429.)

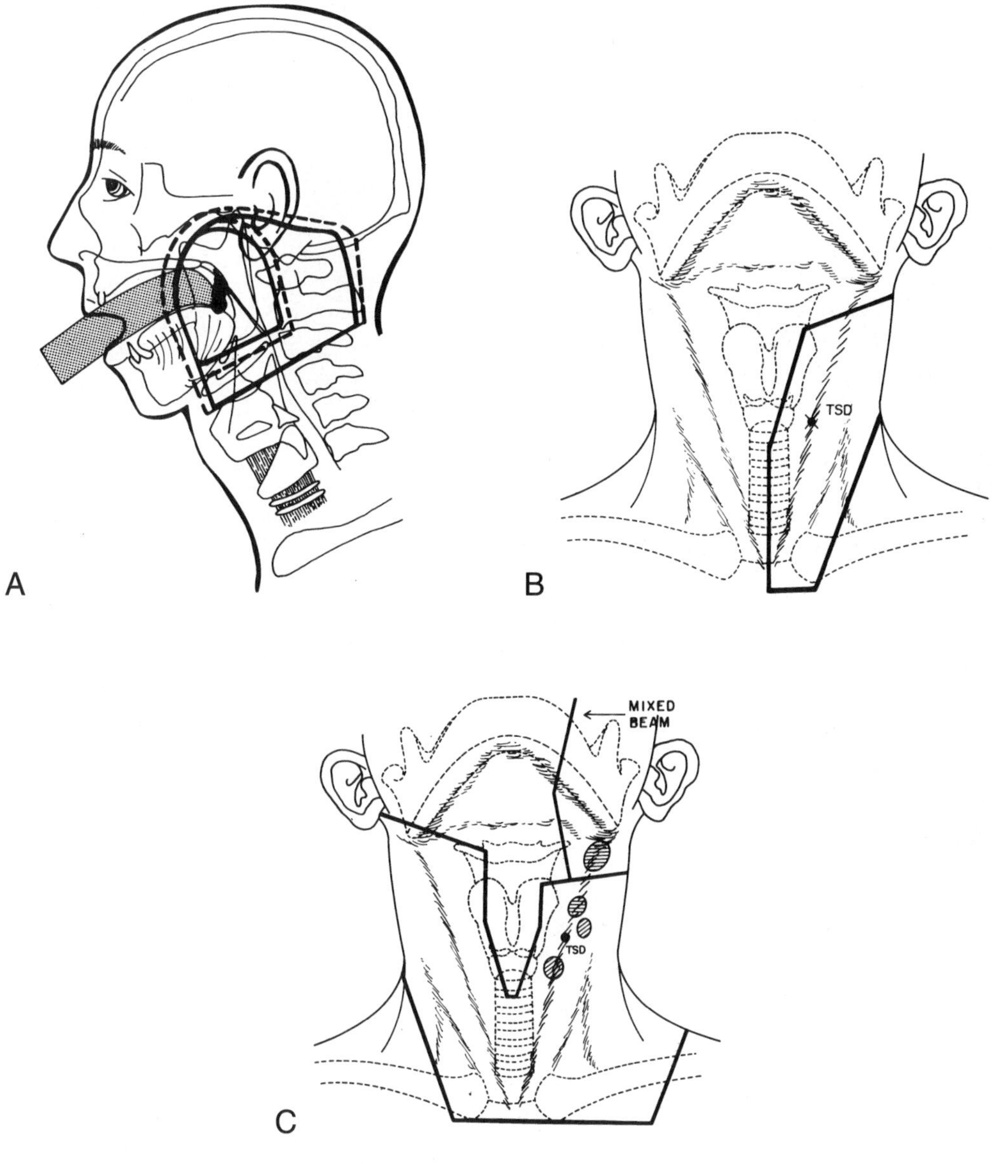

Figure 16.8. "Mixed beam" irradiation portals for tonsillar cancer. **A.** Early lesions of tonsillar region that do not extend near the midline may be treated by ipsilateral technique using both high energy electron and high energy photon treatments. Advantage of technique is delivering low dose to contralateral parotid gland and contralateral mucosal surfaces. Intraoral lead block further reduces irradiation dose to contralateral mucosa and shields some minor salivary glands from beam. Because of constriction of effective treatment area with electrons compared with photons, perimeter of electron beam portals *(dashed lines)* is larger by 1 cm, except at inferior border, which adjoins lower neck field. Because these lesions lie behind dense mandible, 1.0 to 1.5 cm is added for depth dose calculations for electron portion of treatment to compensate for shadowing of tumor by mandible. **B.** Portal used to irradiate neck in conjunction with mixed beam therapy to primary. If neck is not involved clinically, only ipsilateral nodes require irradiation (50 Gy given dose at Dmax in 25 fractions). TSD, tumor-to-source distance. **C.** Portal arrangement for irradiating both sides of neck in conjunction with mixed beam therapy in patient with ipsilateral clinically positive nodes. Even if primary lesion does not extend near the midline, risk of contralateral subclinical disease particularly in subdigastric region is about 30% in presence of ipsilateral clinically positive nodes or base of tongue invasion. Dose contribution to contralateral subdigastric region from treatment of primary portals must be calculated so superior border of contralateral neck field can be reduced at appropriate time. For example, if treatment of primary mixed beam portals delivers 30 Gy to contralateral subdigastric lymph nodes, upper border of low neck portal on contralateral side is reduced to top of thyroid notch after 20-Gy dose to low neck portal so total dose to subdigastric area does not exceed 50 Gy. TSD, tumor-to-source distance. (**A** and **B** reprinted with permission from Parsons JT, Million RR. Radiotherapy of tumors of the oropharynx: In: Thawley SE, Panje WR, eds. Comprehensive management of head and neck tumors. 2nd ed. Philadelphia: W.B. Saunders [in press]). (**C,** reprinted with permission from Million RR, Cassisi NJ, Mancuso AA, et al. Management of the neck for squamous cell carcinoma. In: Million RR, Cassisi NJ, eds. Management of head and neck cancer: a multidisciplinary approach. 2nd ed. Philadelphia: J.B. Lippincott; 1994:75–142.)

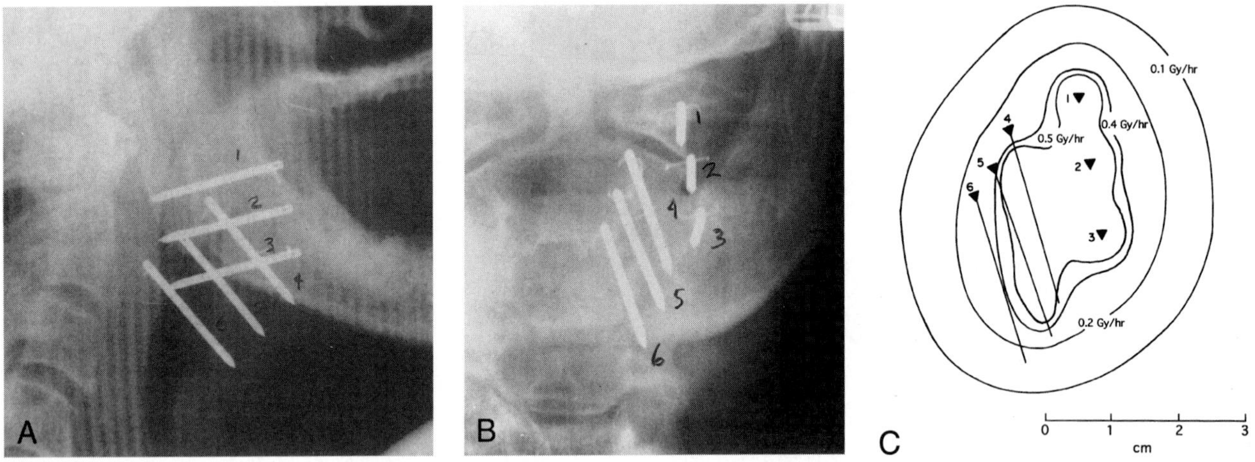

Figure 16.9. Lateral (**A**) and anteroposterior (**B**) radiographs of tongue-pterygoid implant used to boost dose to tumor in tonsillar fossa and base of tongue after external beam irradiation. Three radium (or cesium) needles (2.0 cm active length, 3.2 cm actual length) are attached to each of two rigid (nylon) implant devices (not visible). Use of rigid implant devices shortens overall operating time, ensures adequate spacing between needles, and helps make planes parallel. Approach to pterygoid implantation (needles 1 to 3) is through lateral floor of mouth; needles are inserted perpendicularly through mucosa between retromolar trigone and free edge anterior tonsillar pillar, entering region of internal pterygoid muscle and parapharyngeal and pterygomandibular spaces. Plane of needles in base of tongue (needles 4 to 6) is approximately 1.0 cm medial to that in pterygoid region. Usually no crossing needles are required. Bars are sutured into place with 2-0 silk. Anteroposterior and lateral radiographs are obtained to verify proper positioning of needles before patient leaves operating room. **C.** Orthogonal radiographs are obtained on way from recovery room to patient's room. Computer dosimetry is performed. Orientation of dosimetry is as shown in anteroposterior view in Figure 15.9B. Plane of calculation is perpendicular to and through middle of needle 2. Dose of 15 Gy is delivered to 0.4 Gy per hour line (implant time: 37.5 hours). Implanted needles are removed in patient's room. (Reprinted with permission from Parsons JT, Mendenhall WM, Moore GJ, Million RR. Radiotherapy of tumors of the oropharynx. In: Thawley SE, Panje WR, eds. Comprehensive management of head and neck tumors. 2nd ed. Philadelphia: W.B. Saunders [in press].)

Figure 16.10. Initial and reduced lateral fields for treatment of carcinoma of soft palate. Usual technique involves parallel opposed portals. Minimum treatment volume for early-stage disease includes entire soft palate and adjacent pillars. Timing and extent of field reductions after 50 Gy depend on status of neck as well as extent of primary lesion. If primary lesion extends to midline or if clinically positive lymph nodes are present, both sides of lower neck are irradiated. (Reprinted with permission from Parsons JT, Mendenhall WM, Moore GJ, Million RR. Radiotherapy of tumors of the oropharynx. In: Thawley SE, Panje WR, eds. Comprehensive management of head and neck tumors. 2nd ed. Philadelphia: W.B. Saunders [in press].)

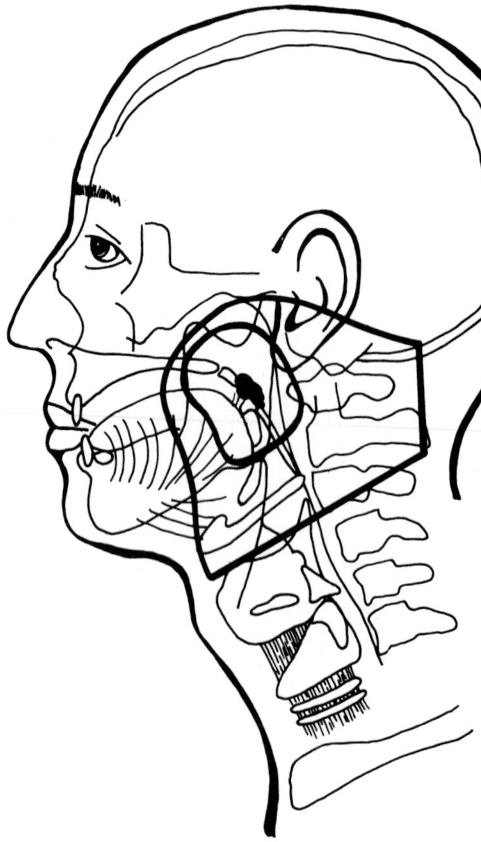

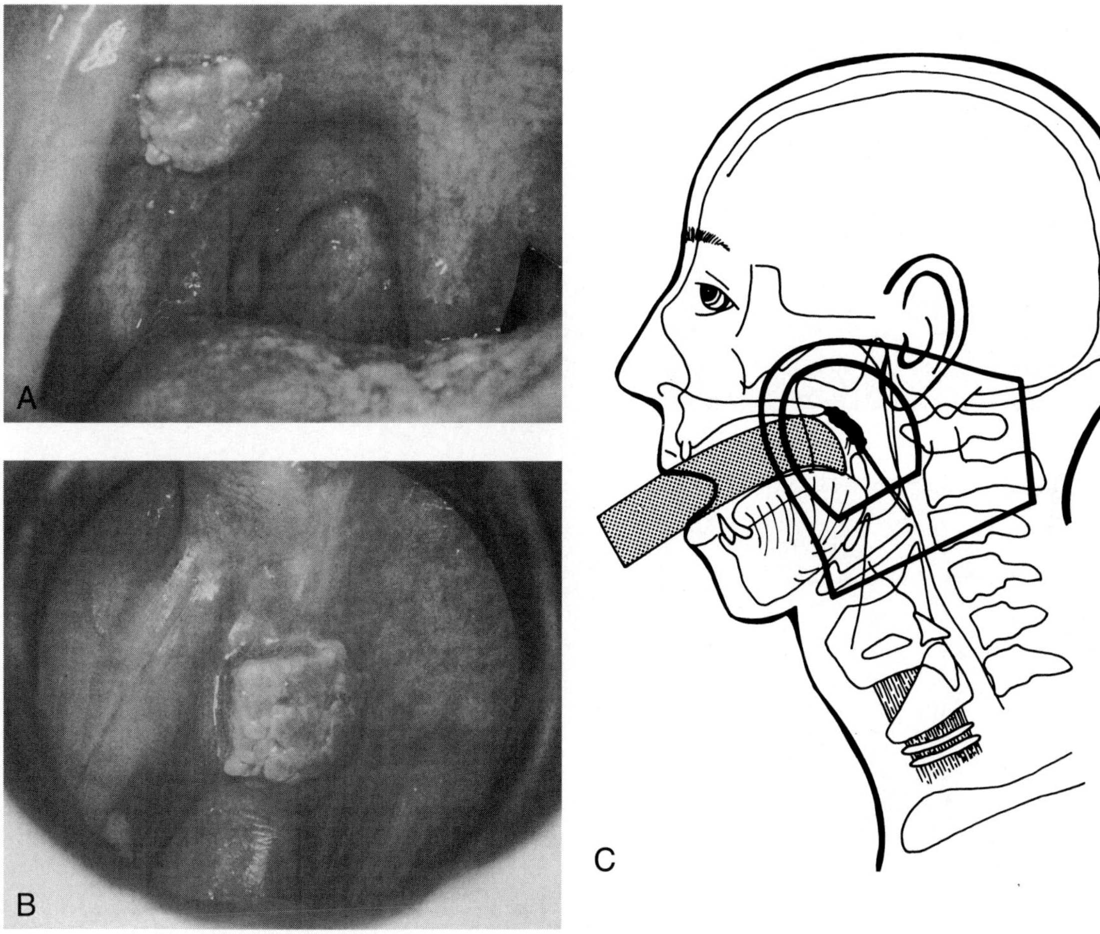

Figure 16.11. Intraoral cone treatment technique. **A.** Exophytic invasive squamous cell carcinoma, 1.5 cm, of right side of soft palate. Discrete lesions in cooperative patients receive 15 to 20 Gy (2.5 to 3 Gy per fraction) with intraoral cone before external beam irradiation. **B.** View through intraoral cone shows adequate coverage of lesion. **C.** If lesion is well lateralized and neck shows no evidence of involvement, treatment is completed by ipsilateral ^{60}Co portal that encompasses primary lesion and upper neck nodes, plus low neck portal as shown in Figure 16.8**B.** After jugulodigastric lymph nodes receive approximately 50 Gy tumor dose at depth of 2 cm, primary portal is reduced to encompass only primary lesion for last few treatment days. Use of intraoral lead block reduces irradiation to contralateral mucosa and contralateral parotid gland. Treatment with both high energy photons and electrons is suitable alternative to ^{60}Co. (Reprinted with permission from Parsons JT, Mendenhall WM, Moore GJ, Million RR. Radiotherapy of tumors of the oropharynx. In: Thawley SE, Panje WR, eds. Comprehensive management of head and neck tumors. 2nd ed. Philadelphia: W.B. Saunders [in press].)

NASOPHARYNX

A typical portal for a patient with an advanced-stage cancer of the nasopharynx is outlined in Figure 16.12. The basic plan must be individualized according to disease extent. The retropharyngeal lymph nodes usually are involved and are best seen by magnetic resonance imaging (MRI). They incidentally fall within the treatment volume. Because of the high density of capillary lymphatics in the nasopharynx, the spinal accessory and jugular lymph node chains are irradiated in their entirety, even in the N0 setting.

After shielding the spinal cord, the final dose may be administered via parallel-opposed lateral portals, oblique portals, antral fields (Figure 16.13 [24,25]), a cephalically tilted anterior field, or rotational fields. Planning the appropriate boost technique for the nasopharyngeal cancer is perhaps the single most challenging task that the radiation oncologist faces in the treatment of head and neck cancer. The boost must be designed to encompass all areas of primary disease and retropharyngeal lymphadenopathy, while sparing as much normal tissue as possible. Treatment is highly individualized; high-quality CT and/or MRI are essential. Use of CT for simulation and treatment planning facilitates the planning of oblique-entry portals. Techniques other than lateral fields have some advantages in terms of dose-sparing to the pterygoid musculature, mandible, temporomandibular joints, and temporal lobes. Treatment planning for the boost portals is highly individualized.

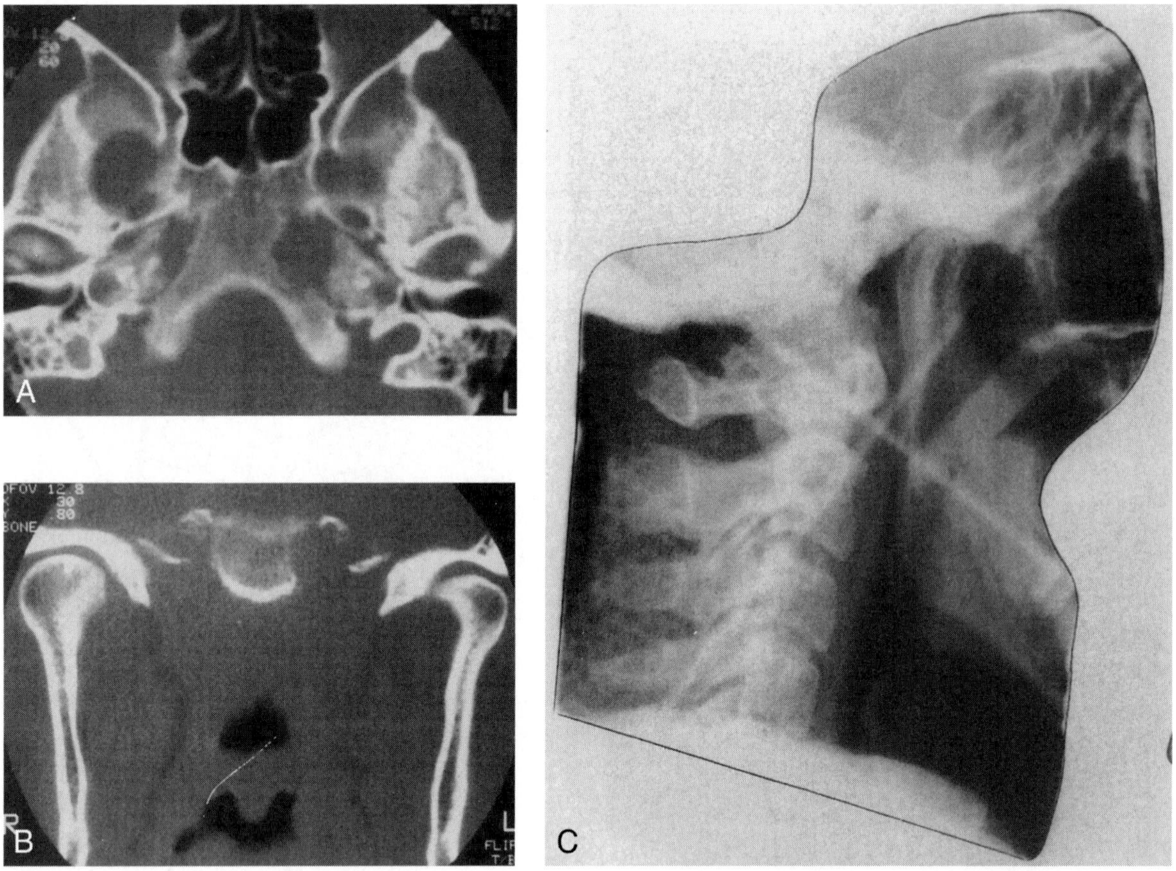

Figure 16.12. Radiation treatment technique for carcinoma of nasopharynx. Axial (**A**) and coronal (**B**) computed tomograms of patient with T4N3B squamous cell carcinoma of nasopharynx. Note bone destruction at petroclival junction. **C.** Beam angled 5° posteriorly to avoid exit irradiation through posterior pole of contralateral eye. Because of destruction of base of skull, superior border of treatment volume is above pituitary fossa; in less advanced presentations, superior border often passes through anterior and posterior clinoid processes, thereby placing optic nerve in penumbra or out of radiation beam. Portal reductions are made so that the optic nerves are either shielded or receive a reduced dose of radiation whenever it is possible to do so based on tumor extent. Lymph nodes are included up to jugular foramen or about 2 cm above tip of mastoid. Posteriorly, spinal accessory chain is irradiated; in presence of large or multiple lymph nodes, posterior coverage can be more generous. Inferior border excludes larynx, except in rare circumstance of tumor extension down lateral pharyngeal wall into hypopharynx. Submandibular lymph nodes are at risk in patients with extensive lymph node metastases. Anterior border is designed to shield segment of posterior mandible while still encompassing tonsillar area. Posterior 2 cm of nasal cavity is included by portals. If necessary, portal may be bowed anteriorly to cover more of nasal cavity.

A supplemental dose of 5 Gy is usually administered through small fields (e.g., 5 × 4 cm) to the base of the skull to compensate for underdosage caused by bone absorption and field edge effect (Figure 16.14).

ORAL CAVITY

Lip

Lip cancer may be treated by external beam, interstitial implant, or both. External-beam techniques use orthovoltage x-rays or electrons. A lead shield placed behind the lip limits irradiation to the mandible and oral cavity. The shield consists of two sheets of lead (each ⅛ inch thick), overlaid with one sheet of aluminum ($\frac{1}{64}$ inch) and is coated with wax or vinyl to prevent excessive exposure from low-energy scattered electrons to tissue adjacent to the shield. Dose schemes are similar to those for skin cancer. Protracted treatment schedules (4 to 6 weeks) are preferred over short regimens because short courses are more likely to cause progressive radiation changes with passing years.

Bulky cancers are often treated first by external beam (30 to 50 Gy), followed by interstitial cesium or Ir-192 implant once the lesion has flattened (Figure 16.15 [26]). We prefer preloaded implant devices that allow rapid, accurate positioning (27). Iridium has a slight advantage because it can be afterloaded.

The regional lymphatics are not electively treated in patients with cancer in its early stages because the risk of metastasis is low. Patients with advanced, poorly differen-

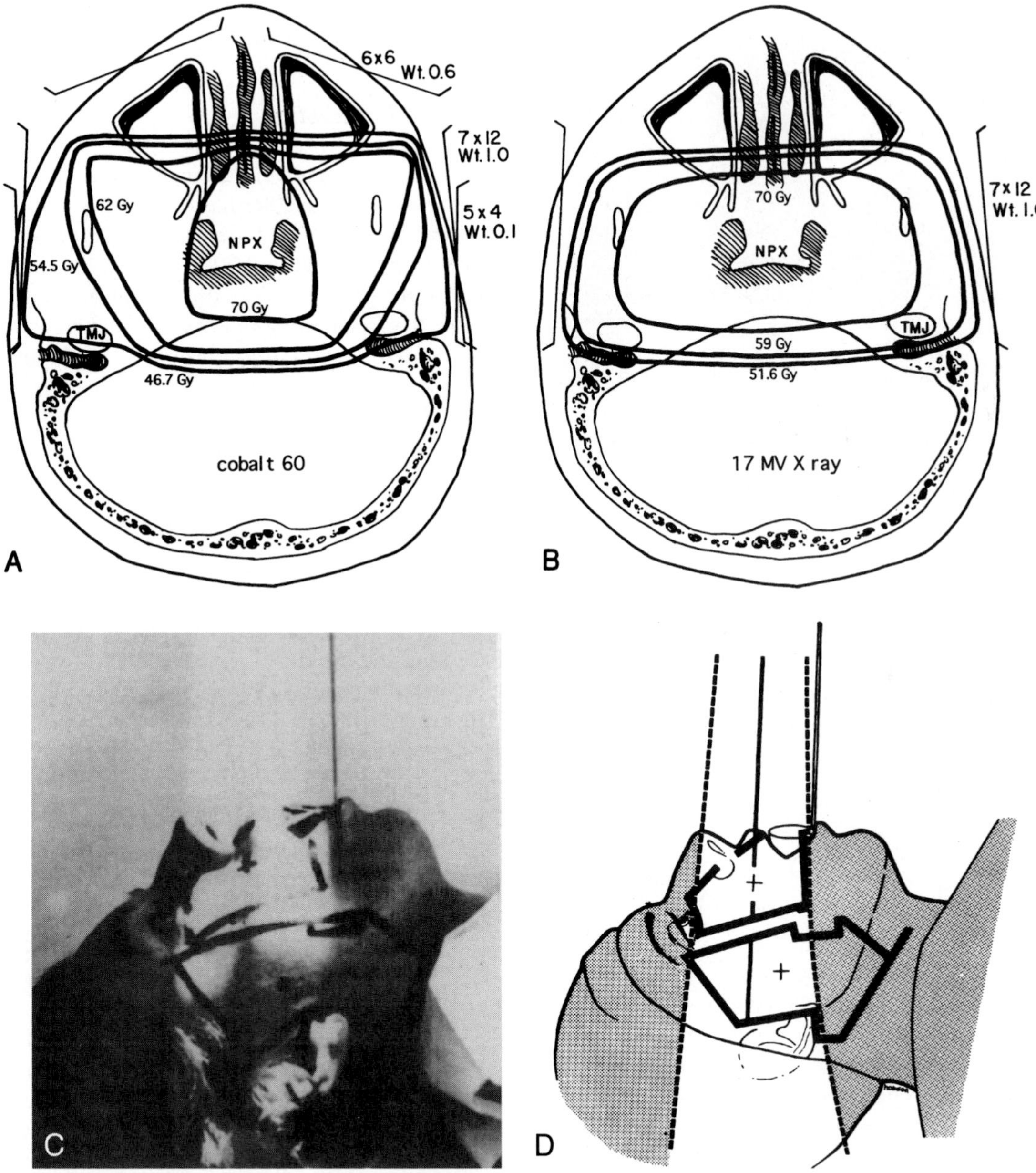

Figure 16.13. Comparison of dose distribution from four-field technique with ^{60}Co (**A**) and from two-field technique with 17 MV photons (**B**) for irradiation of nasopharyngeal (NPX) cancer. For tumor dose of 70 Gy, four-field technique delivers dose to temporomandibular joint (TMJ), tympanic cavity, and pterygoid musculature that is 5 to 6 Gy less than that delivered by high energy, two-field technique. Weight (Wt.) refers to relative given dose (at Dmax) to each field. **C** and **D.** Antral portal. Cork and tongue blade depress tongue as far as possible out of treatment volume. Beam is tilted medially an average of 20 to 30° and aimed superiorly with aid of collimator light (**D**). Superior margins glance eyeballs. Medial margins are usually 1 cm from midline. Inferior borders are normally at commissure of lip, and fields are about 6 cm wide. Portal films are useless. (**A** and **B** reprinted with permission from Parsons JT. The effect of radiation on normal tissues of the head and neck. In: Million RR, Cassisi NJ, eds. Management of head and neck cancer: a multidisciplinary approach. Philadelphia: J.B. Lippincott; 1984.) (**C** and **D** from Fletcher GH, Million RR. Nasopharynx. In: Fletcher GH, ed. Textbook of radiotherapy. 3rd ed. Philadelphia: Lea & Febiger; 1980:364–383.)

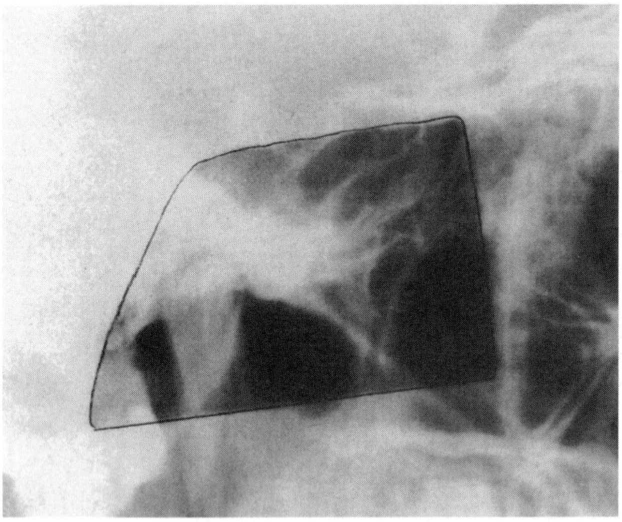

Figure 16.14. Simulation film of small portal used in patients with nasopharyngeal carcinoma to compensate for underdosage to base of skull. Field is shaped to exclude optic nerves and brain stem and is centered on floor of middle cranial fossa and sphenoid sinus. Portal is not intended to cover entire initial extent of disease.

tiated, or recurrent cancers should receive elective neck treatment because the risk of lymphatic involvement is substantial. The risk of involvement also increases in patients with tumors that extend onto the wet mucosa of the lip or the buccal mucosa. Lymphatic spread is to the submental, submandibular, or subdigastric lymph nodes and rarely to a facial node.

Floor of the Mouth

At the University of Florida, most floor of the mouth cancers are treated with resection. If irradiation is used, availability of intraoral cone or interstitial therapy is essential to obtain maximum local control rates. Intraoral cone therapy is preferred when the lesion is suitable. Megavoltage external beam alone gives inferior control results, even for T1 lesions.

External Beam Irradiation

External beam portals for cancer of the anterior floor of the mouth usually are opposed lateral portals. If the lesion is small and confined to the floor of the mouth, the tip of the tongue is elevated out of the portal with a cork (Figure 16.16 [28]). If the lesion has grown into the tongue, the tongue is flattened to reduce the superior border of the portal (Figure 16.17 [28]). A small stainless steel pin is inserted into the posterior border of the tumor and serves as a marker on the treatment planning (simulation) film for external beam therapy and for confirmation of coverage at the time of interstitial implantation. About 1 cm of skin and subcutaneous tissue can usually be shielded in the submental area; the submental lymph nodes are at little risk of involvement. In advanced cases, direct invasion of the skin and subcutaneous tissues of the mental and submental areas requires inclusion of these areas.

Interstitial Irradiation

A preloaded, custom-designed, metal or nylon implant device for cesium needles has been in use at the University of Florida since 1976 (Figures 16.18 [29] and 16.19 [26]) (27). It is used for T1 and T2 lesions and holds the cesium needles in a fixed position, thus ensuring near-perfect geometry. The location of the needles relative to the gingiva is tailored according to the distribution of tumor. The arrangement of needles for early stage lesions is usually a modified, curved, teardrop-shaped, two-plane implant with a single crossing needle that lies close to the mucosal surface. Homogeneity of dose is better than can generally be achieved by freehand implantation with either active sources or afterloading techniques, because the computer implant dosimetry is available before implantation so the arrangement of sources can be modified as necessary. Use of the implant device avoids piercing and unnecessarily irradiating the tongue, as was necessary when free-hand techniques were used. Implantation is completed in less than 1 minute with minimal exposure to personnel and minimal implant trauma. The operating time is substantially reduced compared with that required for freehand techniques.

Intraoral Cone Irradiation

An orthovoltage intraoral cone can be used instead of an interstitial implant for small, anterior, superficial lesions in the edentulous patient with a low alveolar ridge. Tiny lesions can be treated solely by cone (e.g., 50 Gy over 3 weeks or 60 Gy over 4 weeks). Larger lesions receive 20 to 25 Gy (2.5 to 3 Gy per treatment) via intraoral cone, followed by external-beam irradiation (45 to 50 Gy) to the primary tumor and first-echelon lymph nodes. The technique has the advantages of delivering a smaller dose to the mandible than an implant and avoiding hospitalization. Lesions more than 1 cm thick may be underdosed because of the rapid falloff in depth dose from short treatment-distance orthovoltage cones. The cones used at the University of Florida are poured from lead and can be trimmed individually to adapt the cone to the anatomy. A variety of cone sizes, with straight or beveled edges, must be available. Intraoral cone therapy requires daily, meticulous positioning by the physician, because the margin for error is less than with other techniques of irradiation. The patient must be cooperative. After the treatment cone is centered on the tumor, its position is verified with the use of a peri-

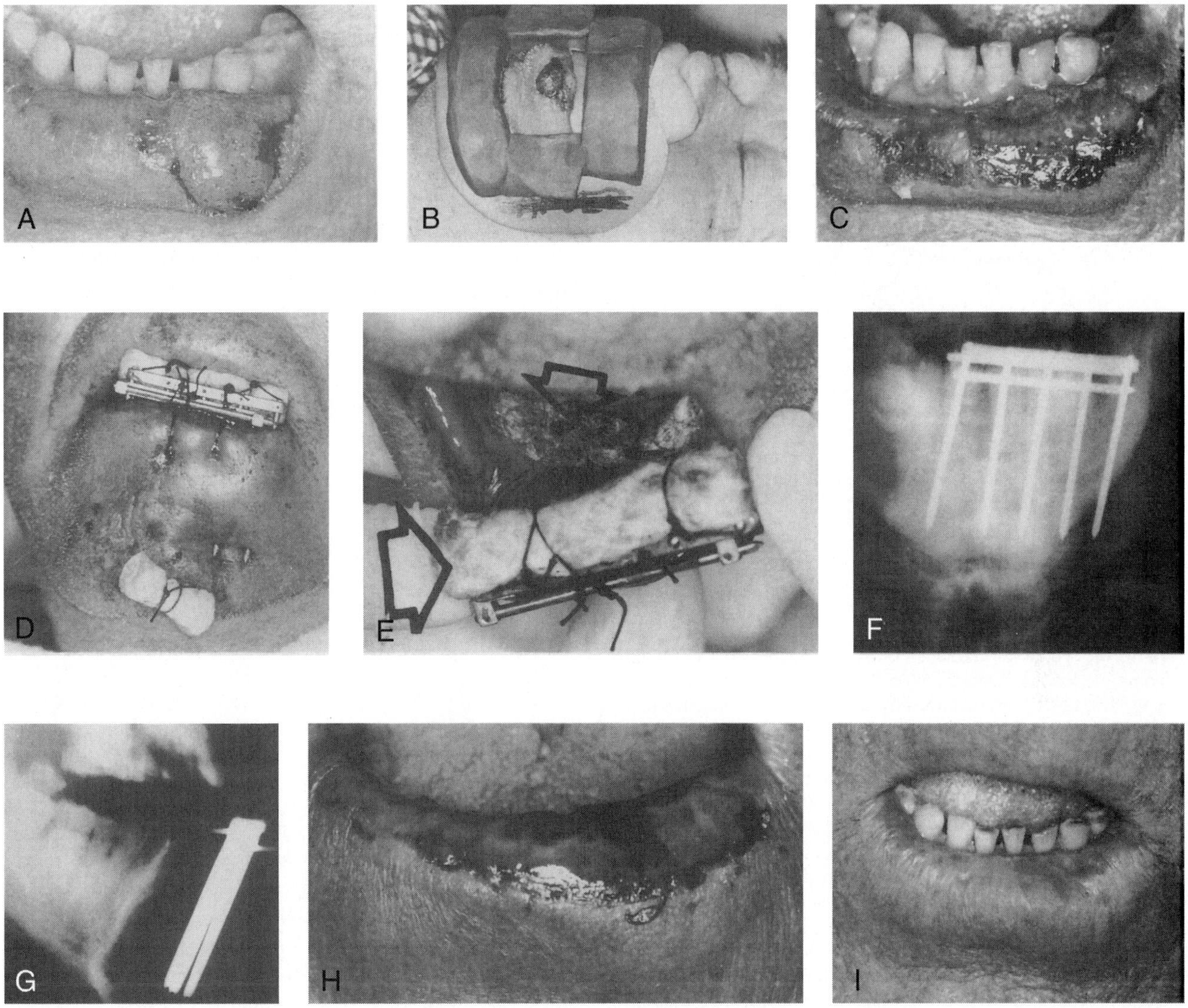

Figure 16.15. A 67-year-old man had T2N0 squamous cell carcinoma of lower lip. **A.** Lesion measured 3.0 × 2.0 × 1.5 cm. Radiation therapy was elected because of functional deficit likely to result from excision of large lesion. **B.** Lead mask, 2 mm thick, designed to outline portal. Lead putty was added to shield to reduce transit irradiation to less than 1%. Separate lead shield covered with beeswax was inserted behind lower lip. Patient received 30 Gy in 2 weeks, 3 Gy per fraction, 250 kV (0.5 mm Cu). **C.** By completion of 30 Gy, he had brisk mucositis of lip and approximately 60 to 70% regression of obvious tumor. **D.** Single-plane radium needle implant with double crossing. Pack was tied to top of bar to displace upper lip away from radiation, and chin pack anchored gingivolabial pack in place (see **E**). **E.** Gauze pack *(arrows)* sewn into gingivolabial gutter to displace radium from mandible, teeth, and gums. **F** and **G.** Anteroposterior and lateral views of implant. Implant added 35 Gy at 0.5 cm. **H.** 2.5 weeks after implantation. Note superficial ulceration. **I.** 22 months after treatment. No evidence of disease, and lip was completely healed. Nine-year follow-up revealed no evidence of disease. (Reprinted with permission from Million RR, Cassisi NJ, Mancuso AA. Oral cavity. In: Million RR, Cassisi NJ, eds. Management of head and neck cancer: a multidisciplinary approach. 2nd ed. Philadelphia: J.B. Lippincott; 1994:321–400.)

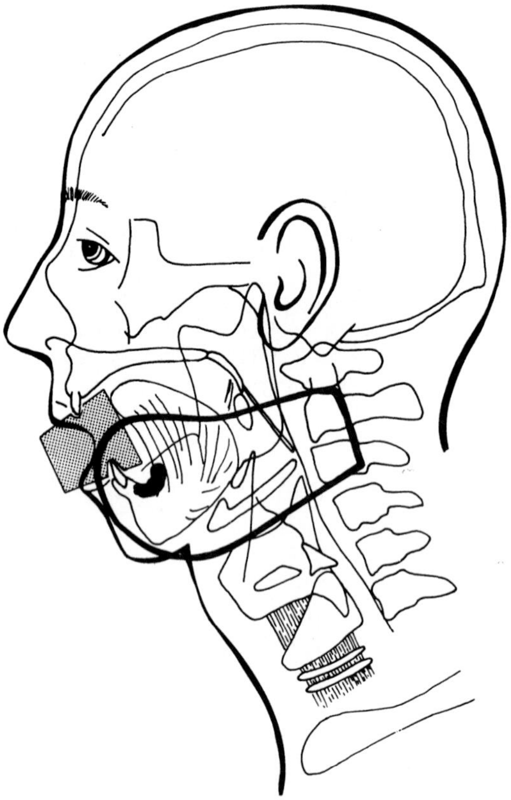

Figure 16.16. Portal for irradiation of limited anterior floor of mouth carcinoma (no tongue invasion; N0 or N1 neck disease) by parallel-opposed ^{60}Co fields. Two notches on a cork ensure it is held in same position between upper and lower incisors during every treatment session; tip of tongue is displaced from treatment field. Anterior border of field covers full thickness of mandibular arch. Lower field edge is at thyroid cartilage, ensuring adequate coverage of submandibular lymph nodes. Subdigastric lymph nodes are covered adequately by including entire width of vertebral bodies posteriorly. Superior border is shaped so oropharynx, much of oral cavity, and parotid glands are out of portal. Minimum tumor dose is specified at primary site (i.e., not along central axis of portal) with aid of computer dosimetry. (Reprinted with permission from Parsons JT, Million RR. Radiotherapy of tumors of the oral cavity. In: Thawley SE, Panje WR, eds. Comprehensive management of head and neck tumors. 2nd ed. Philadelphia: W.B. Saunders [in press].)

scopic localizer to ensure adequacy of coverage (Figure 16.20 [30]). The end of the cone is in contact with the oral mucosa during treatment. A dental appliance is often used to ensure reproducibility of the treatment setup.

Oral Tongue

The ability to control the primary tumor is enhanced by giving all or part of the treatment by either interstitial implant or intraoral cone. Megavoltage external beam irradiation alone produces poor results, even for T1 lesions. Patients referred after excisional biopsy of small lesions (TX) or with T1 lesions measuring less than 1.0 cm often are treated by interstitial or intraoral cone therapy alone. More advanced lesions receive a component of the treatment from external beam.

External Beam Irradiation

Before external beam irradiation, the cancer is photographed and diagramed to document its extent at the of time of the implant. Sometimes, the anterior and posterior borders of the lesion are tattooed with two tiny (1 to 2 mm) marks. Under no circumstances should the ink that is used to tattoo the patient be injected under pressure (e.g., with a syringe), because the ink may diffuse over a large area.

Portals usually are shaped to exclude part of the parotid gland. If teeth with metal fillings lie against the tongue or buccal mucosa, a thin layer of gauze (a few millimeters thick) is inserted between the teeth and tongue or buccal mucosa to prevent a high-dose effect secondary to scat-

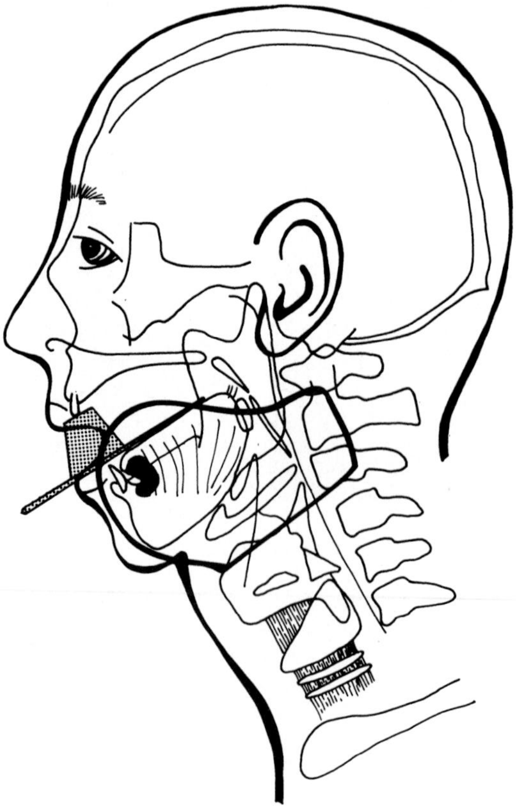

Figure 16.17. Treatment portal for carcinoma of floor of mouth with tongue invasion. Tongue is depressed into floor of mouth with tongue blade and cork. (Reprinted with permission from Parsons JT, Mendenhall WM, Million RR. Radiotherapy of tumors of the oral cavity. In: Thawley SE, Panje WR, eds. Comprehensive management of head and neck tumors. 2nd ed. Philadelphia: W.B. Saunders [in press].)

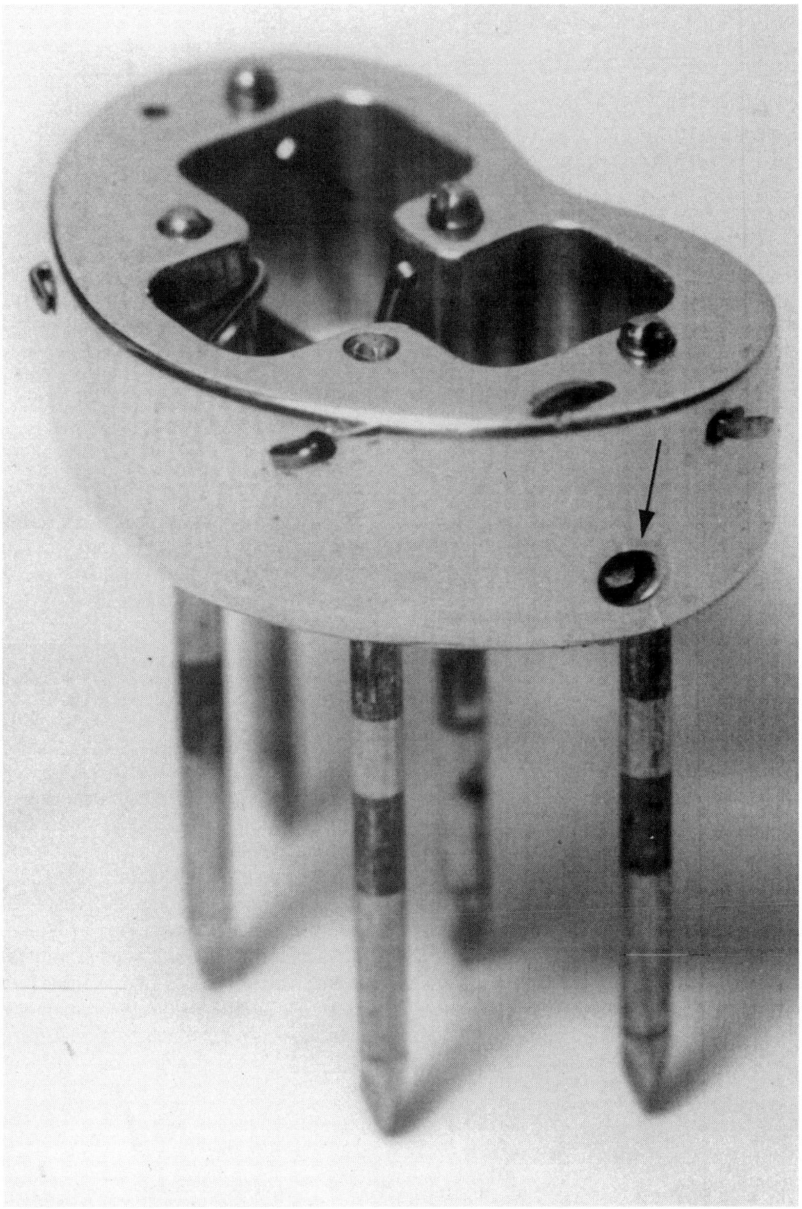

Figure 16.18. Custom-made implant device for stage T1-T2 cancers of floor of mouth. Note single crossing needle (*arrow*) through center. Devices machined from nylon also are available. Cesium needles usually are used (2.0 cm active length, 3.2 cm actual length). Intensity of needles is adjusted so dose rate is approximately 0.4 Gy per hour to area of gross disease. To ensure adequate surface dose, height of implant device (9 mm) is such that 3 mm of active ends of cesium needles extend above mucosal surface. Crossing needle is also 3 mm above mucosal surface (i.e., at active ends of needles). (Reprinted with permission from Marcus RB Jr, Million RR, Mitchell TP. A preloaded, custom-designed implantation device for stage T1-T2 carcinoma of the floor of mouth. Int J Radiat Oncol Biol Phys 1980;6:111–112.)

tered low-energy electrons. Common dose schedules for T1 or T2 lesions consist of 32 Gy in 20 fractions (1.6 Gy twice a day) followed (after 3 to 5 days) by an interstitial implant (35 to 40 Gy). If the intraoral cone is used, generally the dose is 25 Gy in 10 fractions with the cone, followed by 32 to 38.4 Gy at 1.6 Gy twice a day, depending on the lesion size and presence or absence of infiltrating characteristics.

N0 Situation If the lesion is well lateralized, it is treated with a single ipsilateral portal with an intraoral lead block to reduce the dose to contralateral minor salivary glands and mucosa. The subdigastric and submandibular lymph nodes are included in the primary portal, and the ipsilateral low neck nodes receive 35 Gy (at Dmax) in 10 fractions via a separate *en face* field (Figure 16.21) (28).

If tumor extends near the midline of the tongue, the upper neck is irradiated on both sides through parallel opposed fields, and the low neck, on both sides, is encompassed by an *en face* field.

N+ Situation In general, the submandibular and subdigastric lymph nodes are irradiated bilaterally and both sides of the low neck are treated; a neck dissection is added 4 to 6 weeks after irradiation.

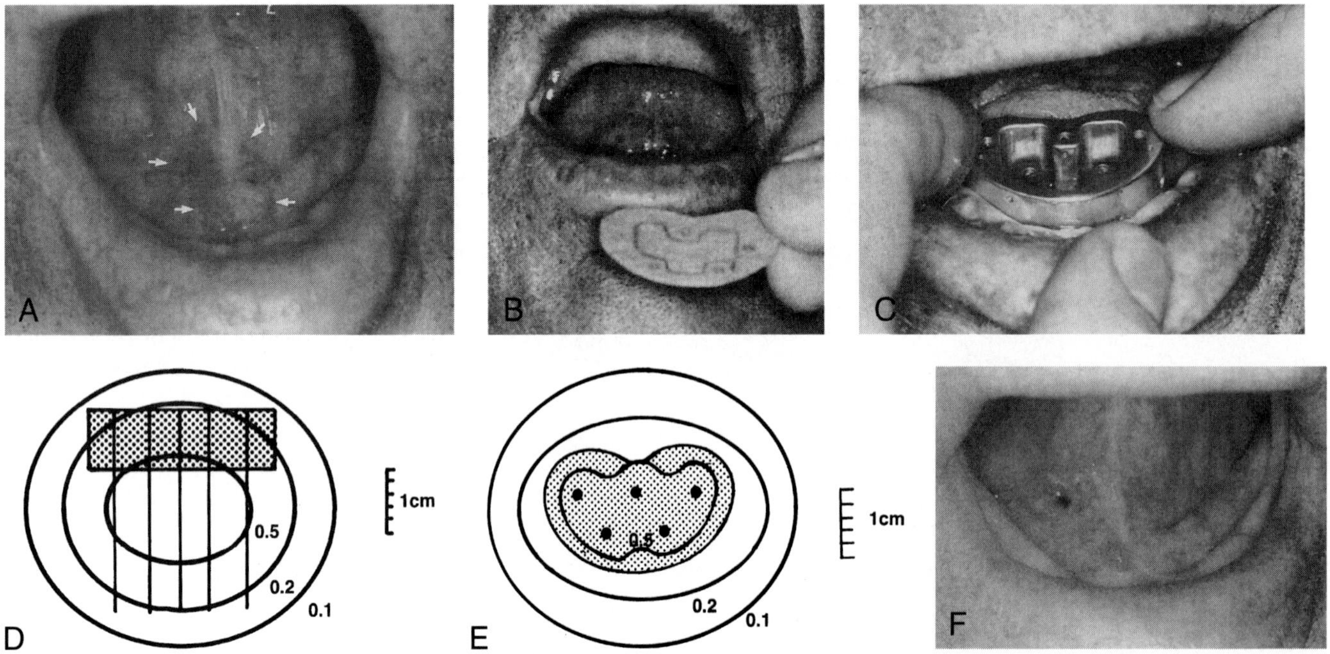

Figure 16.19. Radiation treatment technique for squamous cell carcinoma of floor of mouth (T2N0). **A.** Lesion measuring 2.5 × 2.5 cm *(arrows),* including induration, and tethered to periosteum at midline. Treatment plan is 50 Gy over 5 weeks with parallel-opposed portals that include submandibular and subdigastric lymph nodes. Midjugular lymph nodes are treated with anterior portal. Implant is planned to add 15 Gy. **B.** Cardboard template for design of cesium needle holder. **C.** One day preoperatively, before securing cesium needles to implant device, implant holder is placed into floor of mouth to ensure adequate fit and check adequacy of tumor coverage. At surgery, device is sutured with two 1-0 silk sutures passed on long curved needle through submentum into floor of mouth. Five, 2.0-cm active length, full-intensity (0.66 mg/cm) radium needles without crossing are used. **D.** Coronal isodose distribution. The 0.5 Gy per hour line is selected for specification of dose; implant remains in place for 30 hours. *Stippled area,* implant device. **E.** Transverse isodose distribution through middle of needles. The 0.5 Gy per hour isodose line is approximately 2 mm outside needles. Highest dose rate to anterior lingual gingiva would be about 0.3 to 0.35 Gy per hour, or at least 4.5 Gy lower than minimum tumor dose. **F.** Patient is free of disease at 4 years, 8 months with no complications. (Reprinted with permission from Million RR, Cassisi NJ, Mancuso AA. Oral cavity. In: Million RR, Cassisi NJ, eds. Management of head and neck cancer: a multidisciplinary approach. 2nd ed. Philadelphia; J.B. Lippincott; 1994:321–400.)

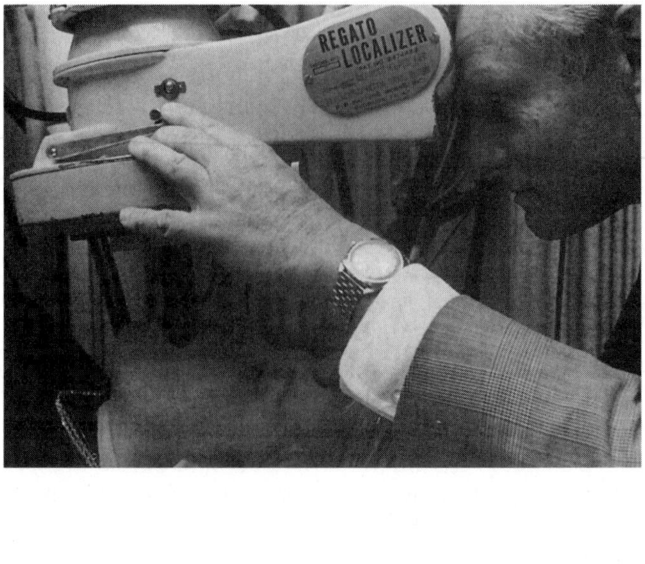

Figure 16.20. Positioning of lead cone used for orthovoltage intraoral therapy is checked each day by physician. A good localizer is essential for final positioning. (Reprinted with permission from Million RR, Cassisi NJ. General principles for treatment of cancers in the head and neck: radiation therapy. In: Million RR, Cassisi NJ, eds. Management of head and neck cancer: a multidisciplinary approach. Philadelphia: J.B. Lippincott; 1984.)

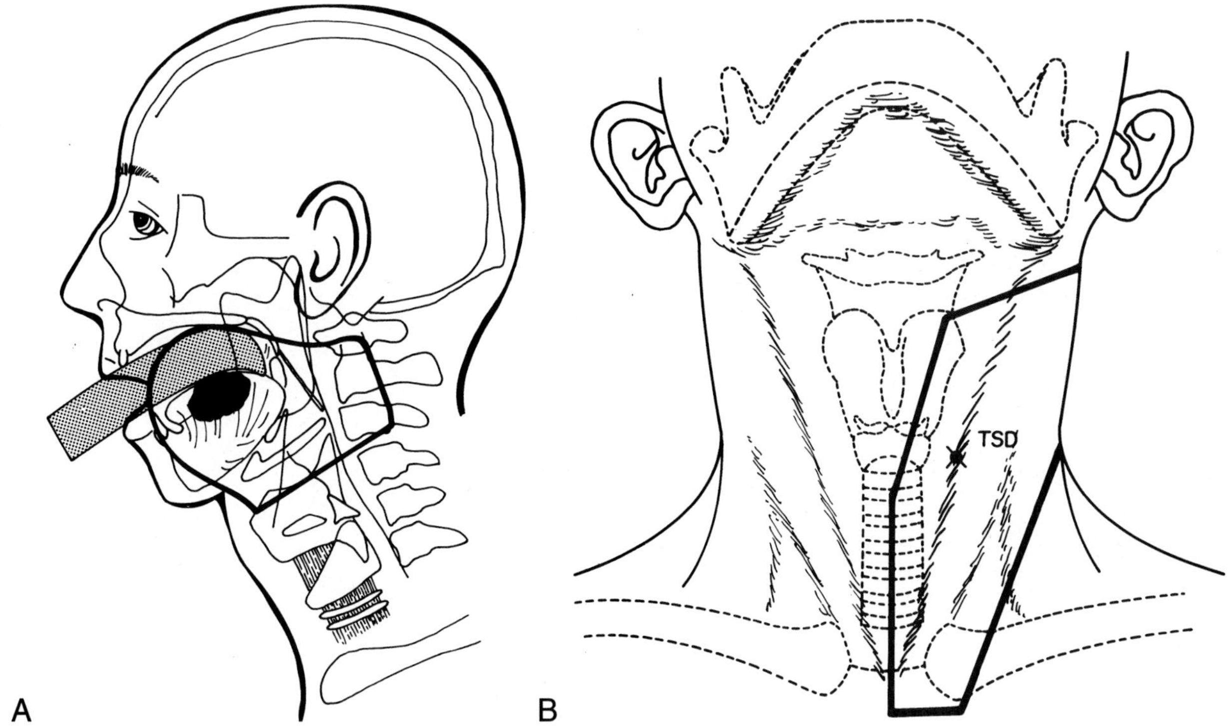

Figure 16.21. Superficial squamous cell carcinoma of oral tongue; NO neck. **A.** Single ipsilateral field encompasses submandibular and subdigastric lymph nodes; entire width of vertebral body is included to ensure adequate posterior coverage of subdigastric lymph nodes. Stainless steel pins inserted into most anterior and posterior aspects of lesion aid in localizing cancer on treatment planning (simulation) radiograph and confirm coverage by interstitial implant. Larynx is excluded from radiation field. Anterior submental skin and subcutaneous tissues are shielded when possible. Upper border is shaped to exclude most of parotid gland. Intraoral lead block *(stippled area)* shields contralateral mucosa and is coated with beeswax to prevent high dose effect on adjacent mucosa from scattered low energy electrons from metal surface. Usual preinterstitial tumor dose is 30 Gy over 10 fractions (or 32 Gy given with 1.6 Gy twice a day) with ^{60}Co. For larger lesions that extend near midline, treatment is by parallel opposed portals without intraoral lead block. **B.** For patients with clinically negative necks, only ipsilateral low neck field is irradiated when the primary is treated only with an ipsilateral field. If the primary is irradiated with bilateral portals, then the low neck is also irradiated bilaterally. TSD, tumor-to-source distance. (Reprinted with permission from Parson JT, Mendenhall WM, Million RR. Radiotherapy of tumors of the oral cavity. In: Thalli SE, Pane WR, eds. Comprehensive management of head and neck tumors. 2nd ed. Philadelphia: W.B. Saunders, [in press].)

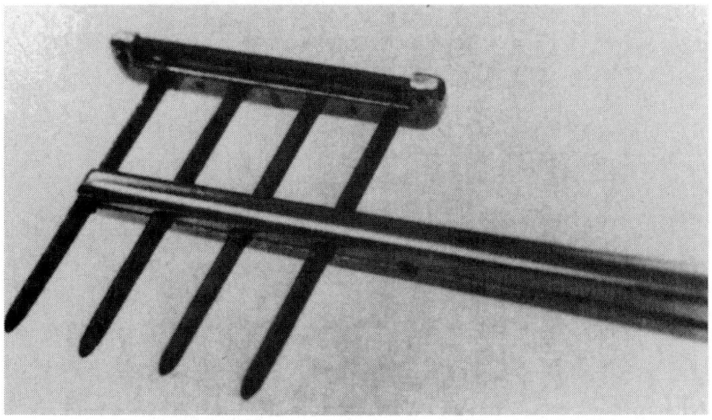

Figure 16.22. Cesium needles mounted in rigid device for single-plane implantation of oral tongue cancer. Note single crossing needle. Holders originally were of stainless steel or aluminum; nylon has proved more satisfactory. Needles are secured to bar with half-hard stainless steel wire passed through eyelets. Allen forceps has been drilled at 1-cm intervals to grasp needles during surgery. (Reprinted with permission from Ellingwood KE, Million RR, Mitchell TP. A preloaded radium needle implant device for maintenance of needle spacing. Cancer 1976;37:2858–2860.)

Interstitial Irradiation

Small-volume implants are readily performed with cesium needles on rigid implant devices (Figure 16.22 [27]). The implants are virtually always double plane; because of frequent subclinical infiltrative extensions of tumor that occur even in apparently superficial lesions, single-plane implants are not recommended. The implant is performed after the administration of general anesthesia with a short operating time and minimal exposure to operating personnel. The dose to the mandible and gingiva can be reduced significantly by inserting a pack into the floor of the mouth to displace the tongue medially (Figure 16.23) (26).

For larger volume implants, rigid cesium implant devices are difficult to manipulate (particularly the medial plane, if it contains more than three needles). We prefer to use iridium hairpins under fluoroscopic control (Figure 16.24). Iridium implants may be performed under general anesthesia or a combination of regional and local anesthesia, with the patient sedated and in a sitting position. If

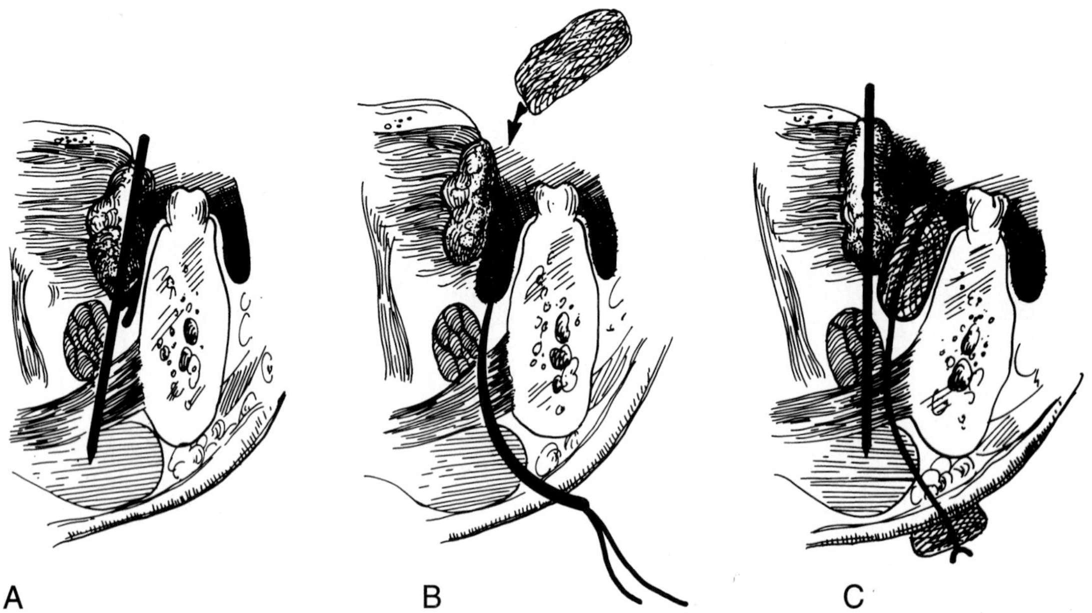

Figure 16.23. Cesium needle implant for cancer of lateral border of oral tongue. Gauze packing displaces tongue from mandible and thus reduces dose to bone. **A.** Implant without packing; **B.** Large curved needle inserted through skin into lateral floor of mouth; **C.** Gauze pack tied to suture and secured between mandible and tongue after implant is completed. (Reprinted with permission from Million RR, Cassisi NJ, Mancuso AA. Oral cavity. In: Million RR, Cassisi NJ, eds. Management of head and neck cancer: a multidisciplinary approach. 2nd ed. Philadelphia: J.B. Lippincott; 1994:321–400.)

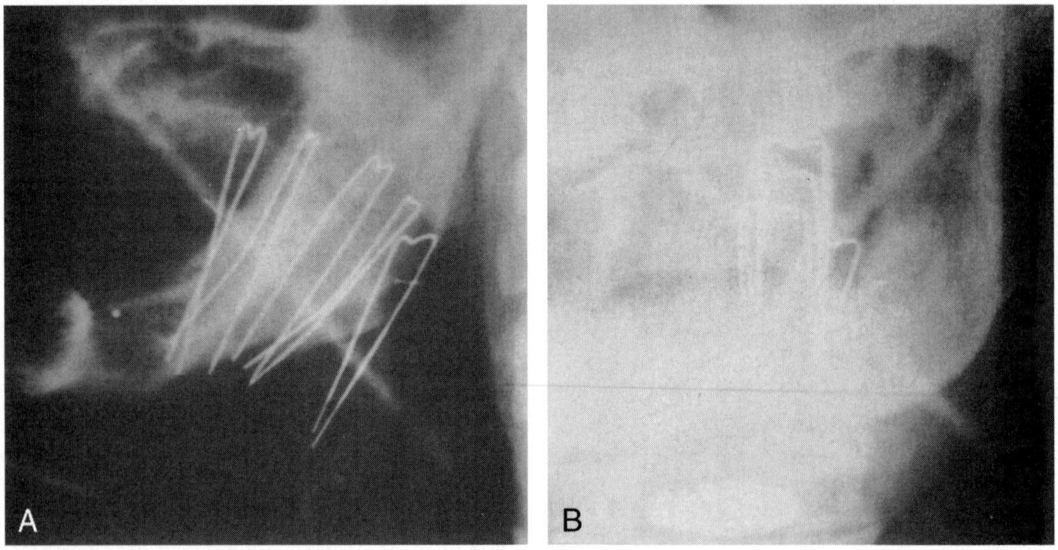

Figure 16.24. Lateral (**A**) and anteroposterior (**B**) views of ^{192}Ir implant for carcinoma of left side of oral tongue, stage T2N0, measuring 3.5 × 2.0 × 2.0 cm, with submucosal extension to within 0.5 cm of midline of tongue. Treatment consisted of 30 Gy in 10 fractions, followed by ^{192}Ir implant the next week. Gutter-guide technique was used with patient sitting; local anesthesia and regional nerve block were administered. Fluoroscopy in the operating room verified accurate source spacing and alignment. Implant sources are 4 cm in length. Gauze pack secured into lateral floor of mouth displaces tongue medially away from mandible. Implant remained in place for 73 hours and delivered 40 Gy tumor dose to area of gross disease (0.55 Gy/hour).

hairpins are unavailable, then either small-caliber iridium needles or the plastic tube technique are used.

Intraoral Cone Irradiation

Intraoral cone treatment is useful in well-selected lesions and may be used instead of an implant. When intraoral cone therapy is used, our preference is to administer this treatment before the external beam treatment, while the lesion is clearly visible and before the mouth becomes sore.

POSTOPERATIVE IRRADIATION FOR TUMORS OF THE ORAL CAVITY AND OROPHARYNX

In this situation, the larynx is intact, and the portal arrangements are similar to those used when radiation therapy is the primary treatment. The primary fields are parallel opposed portals (Figure 16.25A) (14), and the low neck is treated by a single anterior *en face* portal [Figure 16.25B) (14). The junction of the primary and low neck portals facilitates shielding the larynx by a midline block.

The choice of beam, the bolus technique, and details of treatment volume are similar to those described for the larynx and hypopharynx (see Postoperative Irradiation for Tumors of the Larynx and Hypopharynx).

NASAL CAVITY, PARANASAL SINUSES, AND NASAL VESTIBULE

The external-beam techniques for nasal cavity, ethmoid sinus, and maxillary sinus cancers are similar. Treatment emphasizes an anterior portal with one or two lateral portals that are angled 5° posteriorly (frequently with the use of wedges). Even when the lesion is considered to be of limited extent, treating a large initial volume is preferable to relying too greatly on the findings of radiography and physical examination. Fields may be reduced to the area of initial gross disease, with a margin, after 50 Gy.

For limited cancers of the nasal cavity, the initial treatment volume includes the medial maxillary sinus, ethmoid sinus, medial portion of the orbit, nasopharynx, sphenoid sinus, and base of skull (31).

Ethmoid sinus and advanced nasal cavity cancers are similarly managed (Figure 16.26) (32-34). Treatment is heavily weighted toward the anterior field. The weighting of tumor doses administered to the anterior versus the lateral fields is usually 8:1 or 10:1 in favor of the anterior portal. Wedges are used to achieve a satisfactory dose distribution. A reduced anterior open field often is incorporated into the treatment plan to concentrate the dose to the major bulk of disease. Orbital invasion is common when tumor involves the ethmoid sinus. When such invasion is minimal, the major lacrimal gland and lateral upper eyelid are shielded on the anterior portal; more advanced orbital invasion requires irradiation of all of the orbital contents. An example of a two-field technique for advanced nasal cavity or ethmoid sinus cancers with invasion of the orbit is shown in Figure 16.27 (3,35-37). In recent years, the patient's head has usually been immobilized with slight neck extension, so that the orbital floor parallels the angle of entry of the anterior portal, thus allowing greater sparing of the intraorbital contents (34). The patient is treated with

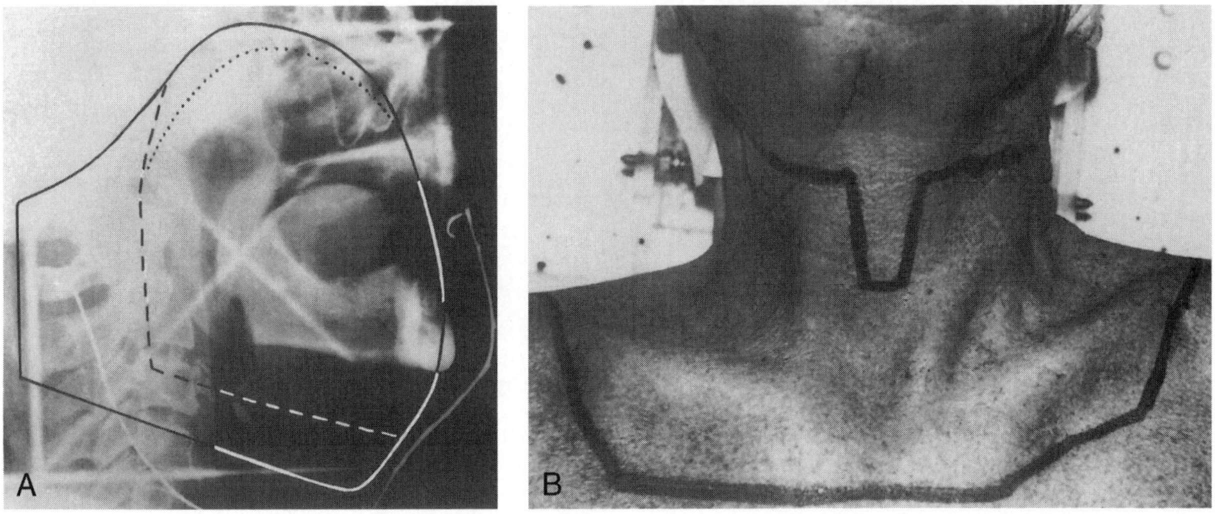

Figure 16.25. Typical portal for irradiation after hemimandibulectomy, partial maxillectomy, and radical neck dissection for pathologic stage T4N0 retromolar trigone lesion. **A.** Field reductions made at 45 Gy *(dashed line)* and 60 Gy *(dotted line)*. **B.** Low neck receives 50 Gy given dose (at Dmax) in 25 fractions. Larynx and a segment of spinal cord are shielded by tapered midline block. (Reprinted with permission from Amdur RJ, et al. Postoperative irradiation for squamous cell carcinoma of the head and neck: an analysis of treatment results and complications. Int J Radiat Oncol Biol Phys 1989;16:25–36).

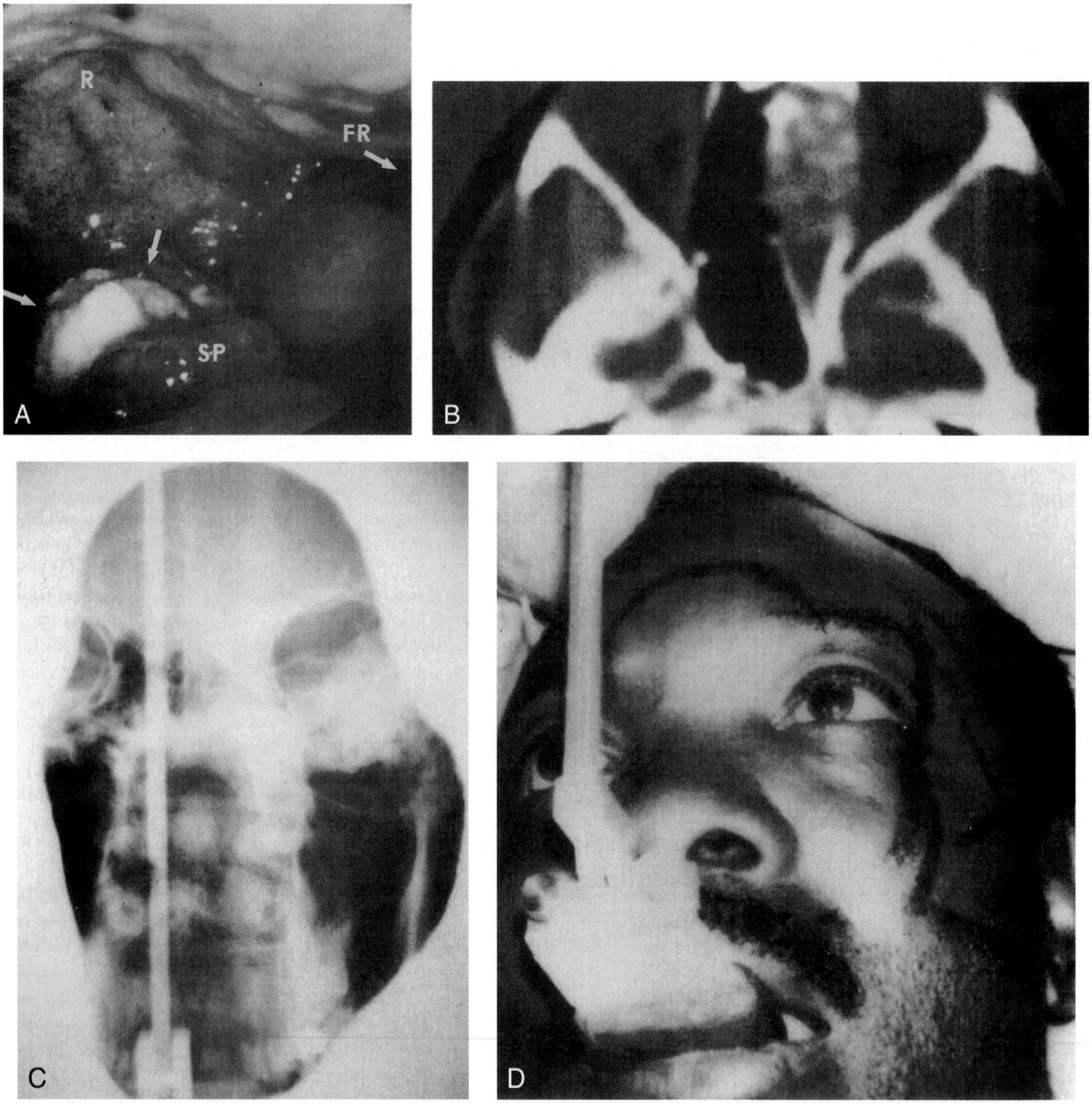

Figure 16.26. Radiation treatment technique for squamous cell carcinoma filling entire nasal cavity and extending into nasopharynx. **A.** Tumor mass extends into nasopharynx *(arrows)*. R, roof; SP, soft palate; FR, right fossa of Rosenmüller. **B.** Computed tomogram at level of orbit and ethmoids. Mass bulges into medial aspect of left orbit. Additional views showed opacification of left sphenoid sinus and left maxillary sinus, erosion of left pterygoid plates, and possible erosion of cribriform plate. Site of origin could have been nasal cavity or maxillary antrum. Tumor is considered unresectable because of involvement of nasopharynx and possible sphenoid sinus invasion. **C.** Anteroposterior view (simulation) of anterior portal. Straight white line is aluminum support for bite block. Patients can be immobilized with customized Aquaplast7 masks from which windows for portals are cut to accomplish skin sparing (WFR/Aquaplast Corp, Wyckoff, NJ). **D.** Radiation is delivered through anterior and left and right lateral portals. Left upper lateral eyelid and lacrimal gland are shielded because only medial orbit is involved by tumor.

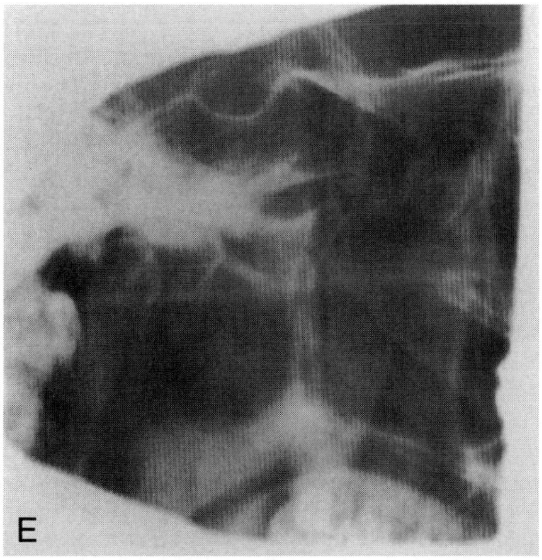

E

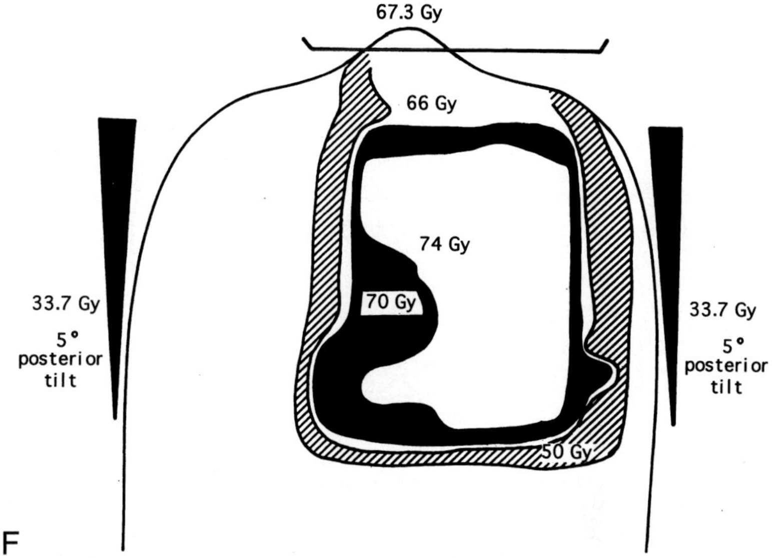

F

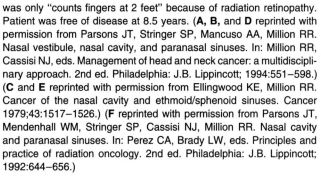

Figure 16.26. *(continued)* **E.** Simulation film of lateral portal (5° posterior tilt). Treatment volume encompasses base of skull, posterior ethmoid and maxillary sinuses, posterior nasal cavity, sphenoid sinus, nasopharynx, posterior one-third of both orbits, pterygoid plates, infratemporal fossa, and parapharyngeal lymph nodes. Posterior border of portal is just anterior to external auditory canal, thereby excluding cervical spinal cord and brain stem. **F.** Treatment plan was 70 Gy minimum (77 Gy maximum) tumor dose over 7 weeks. Weighting of given doses was 2 to 1 in favor of anterior portal. Right and left upper neck received 40.5 Gy over 3 weeks through anterior portal with midline shielding. Visible tumor disappeared during therapy in this patient. Patient returned to full-time work as a truck driver at 4 months. A cataract developed in left eye at 36 months. After cataract extraction, visual acuity was only "counts fingers at 2 feet" because of radiation retinopathy. Patient was free of disease at 8.5 years. (**A, B,** and **D** reprinted with permission from Parsons JT, Stringer SP, Mancuso AA, Million RR. Nasal vestibule, nasal cavity, and paranasal sinuses. In: Million RR, Cassisi NJ, eds. Management of head and neck cancer: a multidisciplinary approach. 2nd ed. Philadelphia: J.B. Lippincott; 1994:551–598.) (**C** and **E** reprinted with permission from Ellingwood KE, Million RR. Cancer of the nasal cavity and ethmoid/sphenoid sinuses. Cancer 1979;43:1517–1526.) (**F** reprinted with permission from Parsons JT, Mendenhall WM, Stringer SP, Cassisi NJ, Million RR. Nasal cavity and paranasal sinuses. In: Perez CA, Brady LW, eds. Principles and practice of radiation oncology. 2nd ed. Philadelphia: J.B. Lippincott; 1992:644–656.)

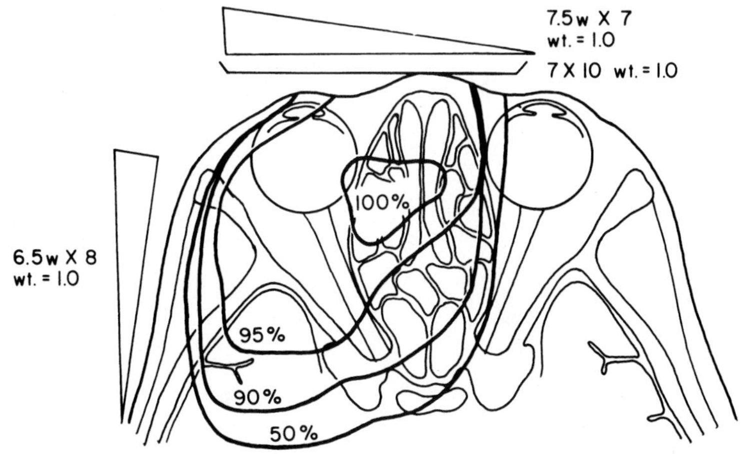

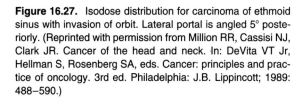

Figure 16.27. Isodose distribution for carcinoma of ethmoid sinus with invasion of orbit. Lateral portal is angled 5° posteriorly. (Reprinted with permission from Million RR, Cassisi NJ, Clark JR. Cancer of the head and neck. In: DeVita VT Jr, Hellman S, Rosenberg SA, eds. Cancer: principles and practice of oncology. 3rd ed. Philadelphia: J.B. Lippincott; 1989: 488–590.)

the eyes open. In patients receiving extensive orbital irradiation, an eyelid retractor is sometimes useful to displace some of the upper lateral lid from the treatment field. Too narrow margins around the eye may result in geographic miss. The anterior portal extends 1.5 to 2.0 cm across the midline to encompass the entire nasal cavity and ethmoid-sphenoid complex and the medial aspect of the contralateral orbit. The superior margin encompasses the roof of the ethmoid sinuses, the cribriform plate, and all or part of the frontal sinus. The inferior margin is low enough to cover the floor of the nose, the maxillary antrum, and the upper gum; the inferior border generally extends to the lip commissure. The tongue is displaced out of the treatment field by a tongue blade and cork (Figure 16.28 (34).

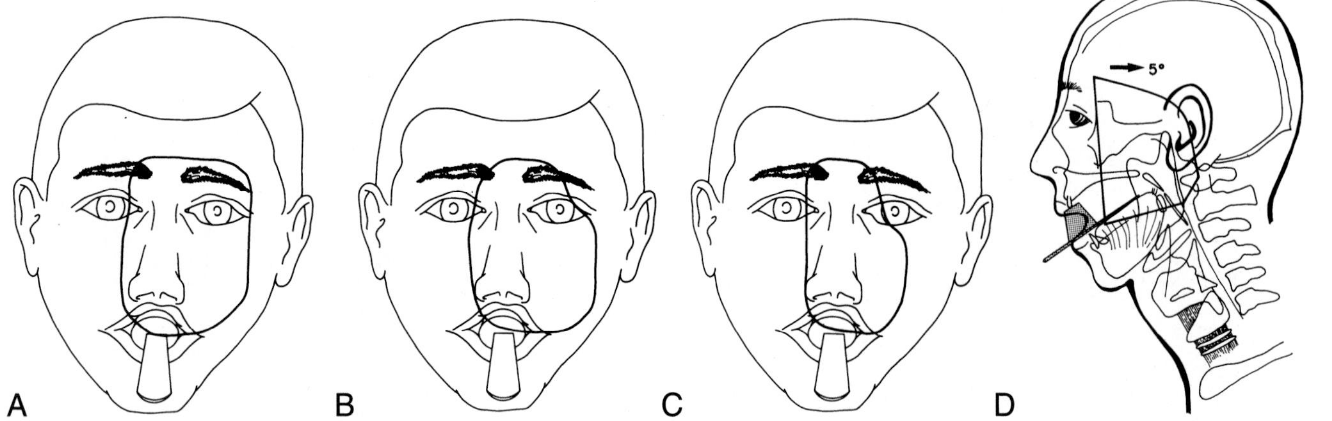

Figure 16.28. Portals used to treat patients with tumors of nasal cavity and paranasal sinuses. **A.** In patients with extensive orbital invasion (palpable orbital mass, proptosis, or blindness), all orbital contents are irradiated. **B.** In patients with limited orbital invasion, at least the major lacrimal gland is shielded. In recent years, the head is often tilted back so that the orbital floor parallels the beam, often allowing greater sparing of intraorbital contents. **C.** Portal primarily used for limited lesions of nasal cavity or as reduced field for ethmoid sinus primary lesion. In patients with lesions of nasal cavity without orbital invasion, field edge is placed at medial limbus. With evidence of gross disease in ethmoid sinuses, field is reduced with great caution because of both high incidence of subclinical tumor extension through lamina papyracea and anatomic configuration of sinus relative to orbit. Although upper lateral walls of ethmoid sinuses are parallel, inferiorly and posteriorly they diverge to conform to cone-shaped orbit. If eyeball is totally shielded from anterior portal, some posteroinferior ethmoid air cells also are shielded. The same principle applies to roof of maxillary sinus, which slopes upward as it proceeds from anterior to posterior. **D.** Typical lateral portal for treatment of paranasal sinus and nasal cavity tumors. Beam is angled 5° posteriorly to avoid exit irradiation to contralateral eye. Anterior border is at lateral bony canthus; thus some of posterior pole of ipsilateral eyeball is included within treatment volume. Superior border is adjusted according to extent of disease, generally 1.0 cm above roof of ethmoid sinuses, but may be raised to cover known or suspected intracranial extension. Inferior border is usually at level of lip commissure, covering floor of antrum, which is below floor of nasal cavity. Cork and tongue blade are used to depress tongue out of field. Posterior and posterosuperior borders are shaped to exclude spinal cord and brain stem, respectively. Usually, posterior border is at or near tragus and bisects vertebral bodies. Posterosuperior border is usually 2 to 3 mm posterior to clivus. If spinal cord and brain stem are encompassed by lateral portal(s) for initial 50 Gy, total dose to these structures exceeds 50 Gy at completion of "typical" course of irradiation (e.g., 65 to 70 Gy); shielding brain stem from reduced anterior field after 50 Gy is not possible. These structures should be encompassed within lateral portals only if tumor extension involves area posterior to plane of cord. Patient must then be apprised of increased risk of neurologic sequelae. (**D** reprinted with permission from Parsons JT, Mendenhall WM, Stringer SP, Cassisi NJ, Million RR. Nasal cavity and paranasal sinuses. In: Perez CA, Brady LW, eds. Principles and practice of radiation oncology. 2nd ed. Philadelphia: J.B. Lippincott; 1992: 644–656.)

The anterior portal for maxillary sinus cancers resembles that used for nasal cavity and ethmoid sinus lesions. The inferior border must be shaped to cover the lowest extent of disease (e.g., tumor tracking down the buccal mucosa from the gingivobuccal sulcus or tumor in the low parapharyngeal or tonsillar regions must be recognized). If the temporal fossa is grossly invaded, the lateral border (of the anterior portal) usually is allowed to fall off.

The lateral fields for nasal cavity, ethmoid sinus, and maxillary sinus lesions are similar (see Figure 16.26). The superior border is at least 1.0 cm above the base of the skull. If intracranial extension is demonstrated or suspected, the superior border is raised 2 to 3 cm.

Radiation therapy to the nasal vestibule may be delivered by external-beam therapy (Figures 16.29 [3] and 16.30 [38]), interstitial therapy (cesium or iridium) (Figure 16.31 [39]), or a combination of the techniques. Currently, the most common external beam technique at the University of Florida uses both high energy electrons and photons. Virtually all patients at the University of Florida receive

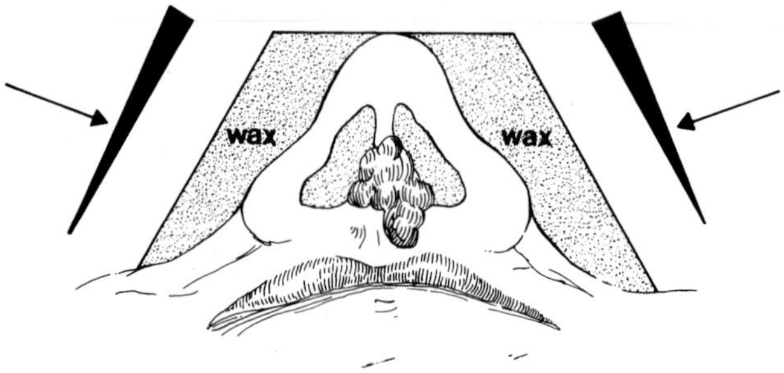

Figure 16.29. Treatment plan for external-beam irradiation of nasal vestibule carcinoma. (Reprinted with permission from Million RR, Cassisi NJ, Wittes RE. Cancer of the head and neck. In: DeVita VT Jr, Hellman S, Rosenberg SA, eds. Cancer: principles and practice of oncology. 2nd ed. Philadelphia: J.B. Lippincott; 1985:407–506.)

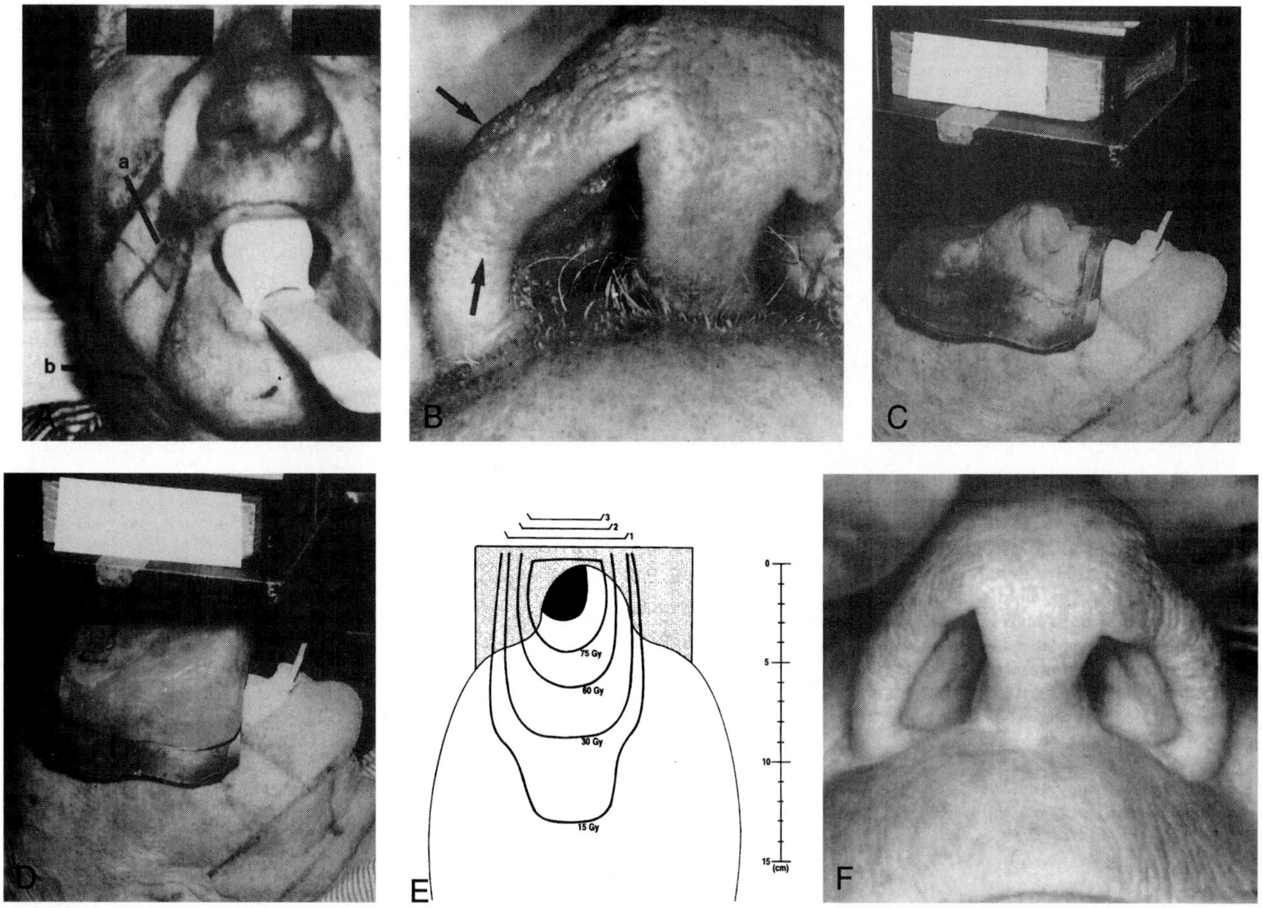

Figure 16.30. An 84-year-old man with 3-month history of nosebleeds had 1.5-cm tumor on right lateral nasal vestibule with erythema and induration extending to overlying skin of tip and ala of nose and just into lip. Invasion of lateral alar cartilage was likely. He also had squamous cell carcinoma of vocal cord (T1N0). **A.** Squamous cell carcinoma of right lateral wall of nasal vestibule (arrows indicate skin invasion). **B.** Outline of treatment portals. Transit lymphatics and facial lymph nodes were treated with electrons a), and submandibular lymph nodes are treated electively b) because of significant dermal extension and undesirability of neck dissection in 84-year-old patient.). **C.** Treatment setup with lead shield, wax plugs in nose, and tongue depressor. **D,** Wax bolus in place. Electron beam is used, collimated by Lipowitz's metal block on tray. Treatment plan is 75 Gy over 8 weeks using both photons and electrons. Usually, no bolus is applied over tip of nose unless skin at this site is infiltrated by tumor. **E.** Isodose distribution. *Lightly stippled area,* beeswax bolus/compensator; *darker stippled area,* extent of gross tumor. **F.** At 2 years, no evidence of disease. Patient remained free of disease at 8 years, 4 months. (Reprinted with permission from Million RR, Cassisi NJ, Hamlin DJ. Nasal vestibule, nasal cavity, and paranasal sinuses. In: Million RR, Cassisi NJ, eds. Management of head and neck cancer: a multidisciplinary approach. Philadelphia: J.B. Lippincott; 1984:407–444.)

external-beam irradiation (e.g., 50 Gy) followed by an implant (20 to 25 Gy).

MAJOR SALIVARY GLAND

Parotid Gland

Radiation therapy plays its major role as an adjunct to surgery and is usually administered postoperatively, although preoperative treatment may be considered in special situations. The minimum treatment volume includes the parotid bed and upper neck nodes. The entire ipsilateral neck is electively irradiated for high-grade lesions or when tumor is found in lymph nodes in the radical neck dissection specimen.

External Beam Irradiation Treatment is administered by one of three external beam techniques. One technique involves a wedge pair, with the portals aimed either superiorly and inferiorly (to direct the exit dose away from the orbits and oral cavity) or anteriorly and posteriorly (with the portals angled so that the beams pass below the level of the eyes). The latter technique facilitates matching the low-neck portal to the primary fields. The wedge pair technique can treat a generous portion of the base of skull in a homogeneous manner and is particularly useful when perineural spread is present or suspected, as in adenoid cystic carcinoma. Fields are best designed with the aid of three-dimensional simulation and treatment planning.

A second basic technique uses ipsilateral portals

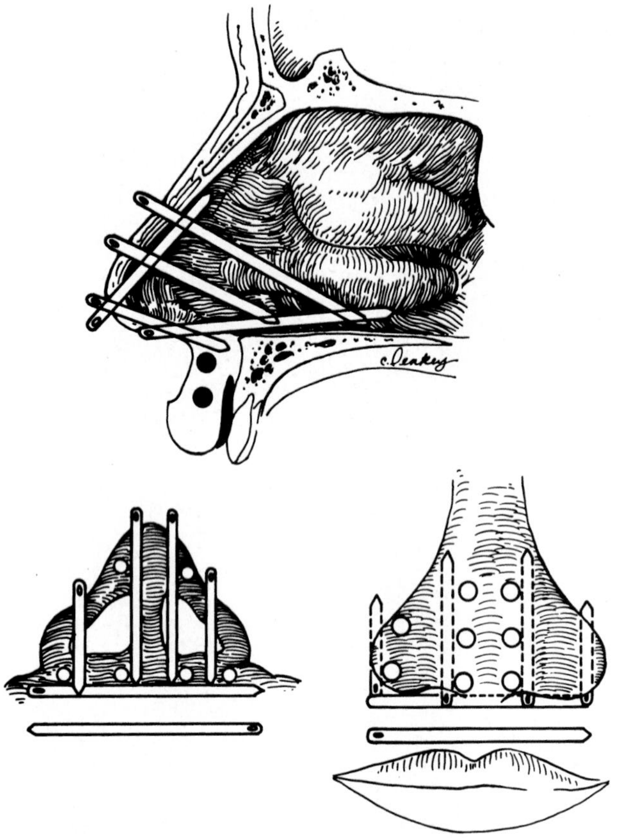

Figure 16.31. Interstitial implant for carcinoma of nasal vestibule. (Reprinted with permission from Million RR, Cassisi NJ, Clark JR. Cancer of the head and neck. In: DeVita VT, Jr, Hellman S, Rosenberg SA, eds. Cancer: principles and practice of oncology. 3rd ed. Philadelphia: J.B. Lippincott; 1989:488–590.)

shaped to fit the anatomy (Figure 16.32). A treatment scheme using a combination of photons and high-energy electrons produces a homogeneous dose distribution and delivers 30 Gy or less to the opposite salivary glands. The advantages of the technique are the ability to shape and reduce the fields easily and the ease with which an ipsilateral low neck field may be adjoined to the primary portal. A disadvantage, especially in patients with adenoid cystic carcinoma, is underdosage of possible perineural tumor extensions deep in the temporal bone because of inadequate penetration of electrons in dense bone. Because electrons are subject to perturbations from tissue inhomogeneity, the risk of deep geographic miss must always be kept in mind.

When tumor involves the deep lobe or otherwise extends near the midline, a third technique, parallel opposed photon portals weighted to the side of the lesion, is necessary.

Calculation of the brain stem–spinal cord dose must be precise in all three techniques. Field reductions are highly individualized.

Interstitial Irradiation

Interstitial implants may be added if the primary tumor is located in the preauricular portion of the superficial lobe, or when there are positive margins or unresectable or locally recurrent disease. A modified two-plane cesium needle implant (the deep plane extends into the retromandibular area) will cover the tumor bed, but may give inadequate coverage of the retromandibular portion of the parotid bed. To ensure an adequate treatment margin along the external ear canal, the needles usually penetrate the tragal cartilage. The implantation of the retromandibular deep lobe area is a "blind" procedure, but can be done safely and with relative ease (Figure 16.33 [40]); a preoperative CT scan can be used to help plan the implant and avoid major blood vessel injury.

Submandibular Gland

Ipsilateral external beam portals are tailored to the extent of disease found in the surgical specimen. The possi-

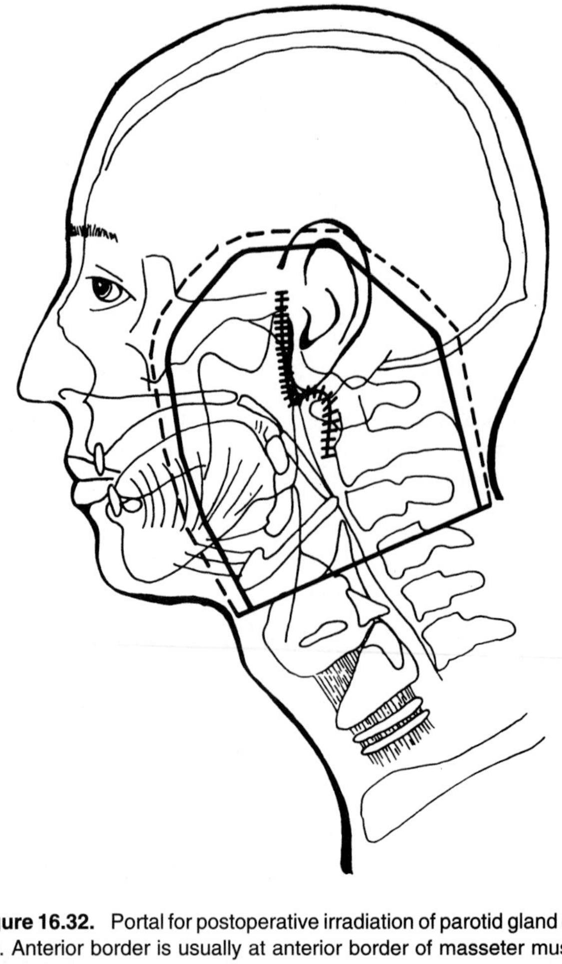

Figure 16.32. Portal for postoperative irradiation of parotid gland cancer. Anterior border is usually at anterior border of masseter muscle; inferior border is at top of thyroid cartilage. Superiorly and posteriorly, entire parotid and surgical bed are included. Electron portal *(dashed lines)* is 1.0 cm larger than photon portal, because of constriction of electron isodose lines at depth.

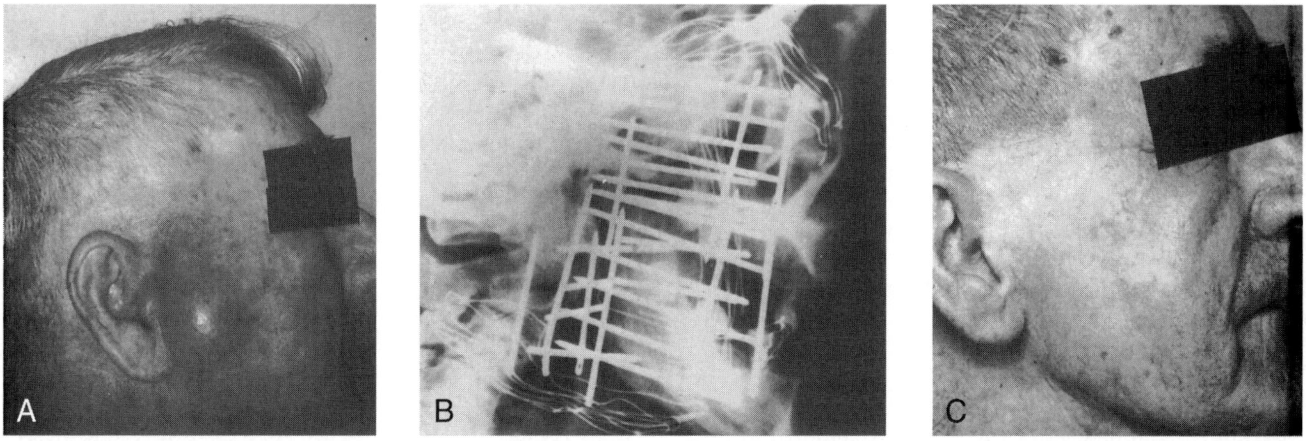

Figure 16.33. A. Squamous cell carcinoma metastatic to parotid lymph node. (Squamous cell carcinoma of skin of temple had been treated 2 years previously.) Note tragal involvement. **B.** Modified three-plane radium needle implant. One plane (four needles) is in retromandibular deep lobe. **C.** Complete healing at 1 year (no evidence of disease at 9 years). (Courtesy of Lindberg RL, MD, Department of Radiation Therapy, M. D. Anderson Hospital and Tumor Institute, Houston, Texas.) (Reprinted with permission from Mendenhall WM, Million RR, Mancuso AA, Cassisi NJ, Flowers FP. Carcinoma of the skin. In: Million RR, Cassisi NJ, eds. Management of head and neck cancer: a multidisciplinary approach. 2nd ed. Philadelphia: J.B. Lippincott; 1994: 643–691.)

ble sites of local recurrence include the submandibular triangle, adjacent oral cavity, pterygomaxillary fossa, base of the skull, parotid gland, and neck. The entire ipsilateral neck is always included; the opposite side of the neck usually is not treated. The energy used depends on the depth at risk. An electron beam, photon beam, or a combination of both is selected, depending on the situation.

UNKNOWN PRIMARY

Treatment planning for the patient with metastases to the nodes in the neck from a primary site that cannot be located after multiple physical examinations, CT, and direct laryngoscopy with biopsies depends on the location of the lymph nodes; occasionally histology also plays a role in determining the treatment volume. Involvement of the upper and midjugular lymph nodes indicates elective irradiation of the nasopharynx, oropharynx, supraglottic larynx, and hypopharynx via parallel opposed portals (Figure 16.34), and low neck irradiation to the level of the clavicles via an anterior field. The neck is usually thinner than the head, and this difference must be accounted for by the use of compensators or portal reductions at appropriate times. If the clinician suspects a primary focus but has no proof, an extra boost dose may be added to this specific site. Sparing a midline strip of skin on the neck is important to avoid lymphedema. A node in the upper neck with histologic findings suggestive of lymphoepithelioma indicates treatment to the nasopharynx, oropharynx, and low neck. When a solitary submandibular lymph node is involved, treatment with neck dissection and observation is preferred because irradiation of the entire oral cavity plus the neck causes major morbidity. A preauricular

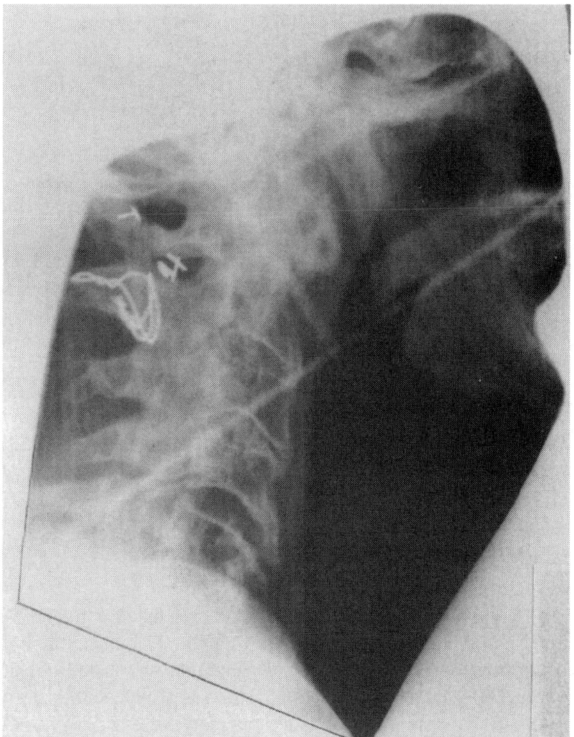

Figure 16.34. Simulation film with treatment volume for patient with unknown primary tumor, metastatic to jugulodigastric lymph nodes. Initial volume includes nasopharyngeal, oropharyngeal, hypopharyngeal, and laryngeal mucosa as well as jugular and spinal accessory lymph node chains. Indentation on anterior margin of field spares part of mandible. Anteroinferiorly, approximately 1.0 cm of skin and subcutaneous tissue is shielded. Inferior border is about 2.0 cm below bottom of cricoid cartilage so entire length of pyriform sinus is covered with a margin. Superiorly, field design is similar to that for early nasopharyngeal carcinoma.

lymph node(s) containing squamous cell carcinoma typically represents metastasis from a skin cancer and is treated by a combination of parotidectomy and radiation therapy or radiation therapy alone. Supraclavicular nodes are irradiated through a generous regional portal, which should include the adjacent apex of the axilla.

DESIGN OF THE LOW NECK PORTAL

Oropharynx, Nasopharynx, and Oral Cavity Cancers

The low neck portal is designed according to external anatomic landmarks and findings from the clinical and radiographic examination of the neck. No simulation films or portal verification films are taken. The lines are drawn on the patient's skin, and lead blocks are stacked freehand on a wire mesh tray positioned approximately 15 cm above the patient to shape the beam to the desired volume.

For all base of tongue, midline soft palate, advanced tonsil, nasopharyngeal, and oral cavity cancers that require parallel opposed portals, both sides of the neck are irradiated, even in the N0 situation. Failure to irradiate the low neck in patients with the lesions just listed will result in at least a 10% rate of failure in the mid and low jugular areas, even when the upper neck is clinically negative. The low neck is irradiated through an anterior field only. The basic portal design in all of these situations is similar (Figure 16.35 [16,22]).

For patients with early-stage cancer of the tonsillar region or lateralized tumors of the oral tongue, retromolar trigone, or soft palate, only the ipsilateral upper and lower neck require irradiation in the N0 situation (the low-neck portal is shown in Figure 16.8B). When the ipsilateral neck is clinically positive, our policy is to irradiate the neck bilaterally. Although the exact risk of subclinical involvement of the contralateral side of the neck is difficult to determine

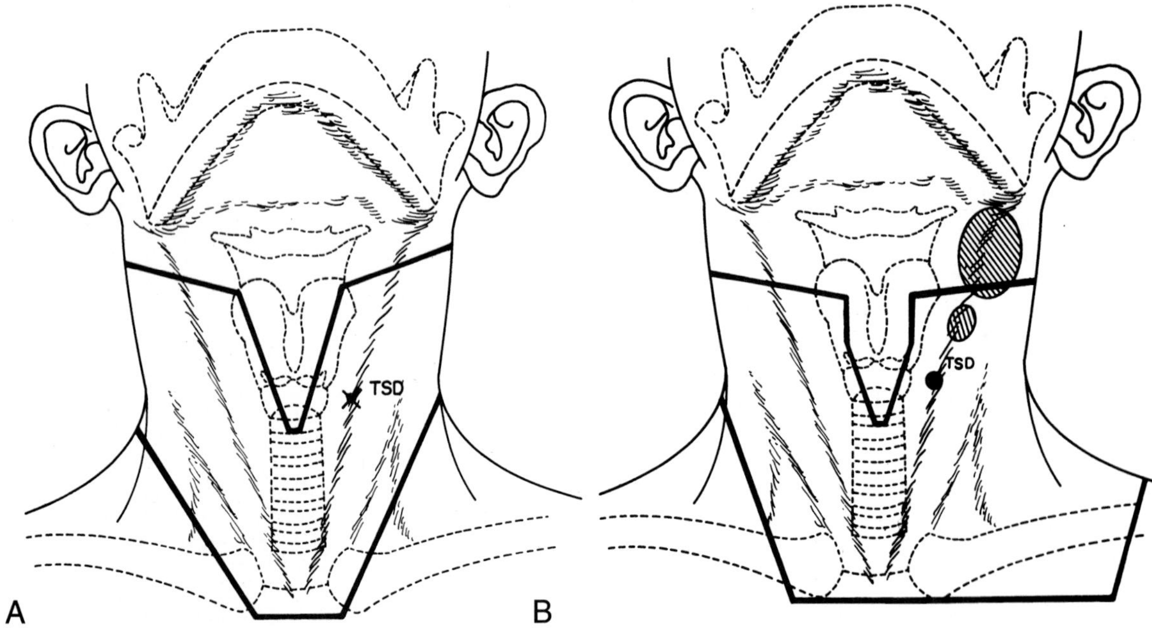

Figure 16.35. Fields for bilateral lower neck irradiation in patients with base of tongue, midline soft palate, advanced tonsil, nasopharynx, or advanced oral cavity cancers. **A.** N0 neck. Larynx shield design is important. Because midjugular lymph nodes lie adjacent to posterolateral margin of thyroid cartilage, attempts to shield entire thyroid cartilage with 4- to 5-cm wide block produce low dose area in these nodes. Inferior extent of larynx shield is usually at cricoid cartilage or first or second tracheal ring; shield is tapered; nodes in low neck may lie close to midline. If larynx block is extended for entire length of low neck portal, it should probably cast a shadow no wider than 1.0 to 1.5 cm in suprasternal notch region. TSD, tumor-to-source distance. In N0 setting, lateral supraclavicular lymph nodes are at little risk of involvement, except possibly for patients with cancer of nasopharynx. Usually, only root of neck is included. The most common error observed in design of low neck portal is actually a combination of mistakes that results in underdosage of high risk areas and unnecessary treatment of low risk zones by 1) shielding larynx with large, square or rectangular block, 2) blocking midline with wide (3 to 4 cm) block down to level of suprasternal notch, and 3) irradiating entire supraclavicular fossa bilaterally. **B.** Neck with clinical evidence of disease. Treatment to each side of neck is individualized. If extensive neck disease is limited to one side, entire neck, including all supraclavicular lymph nodes (out to junction of trapezius muscle and clavicle), is irradiated on that side. If both sides are involved, treatment on each side is modified according to disease extent. (**A,** reprinted with permission from Parsons JT, Mendenhall WM, Moore GJ, Million RR. Radiotherapy of tumors of the oropharynx In: Thawley SE, Panje WR, eds. Comprehensive management of head and neck tumors. 2nd ed. Philadelphia: W.B. Saunders [in press].) (**B,** reprinted with permission from Million RR, Cassisi NJ, Stringer SP, Mendenhall WM, Parsons JT. Management of the neck for squamous cell carcinoma. In: Million RR, Cassisi NJ, eds. Management of head and neck cancer: a multidisciplinary approach. 2nd ed. Philadelphia: J.B. Lippincott; 1994:75–142.)

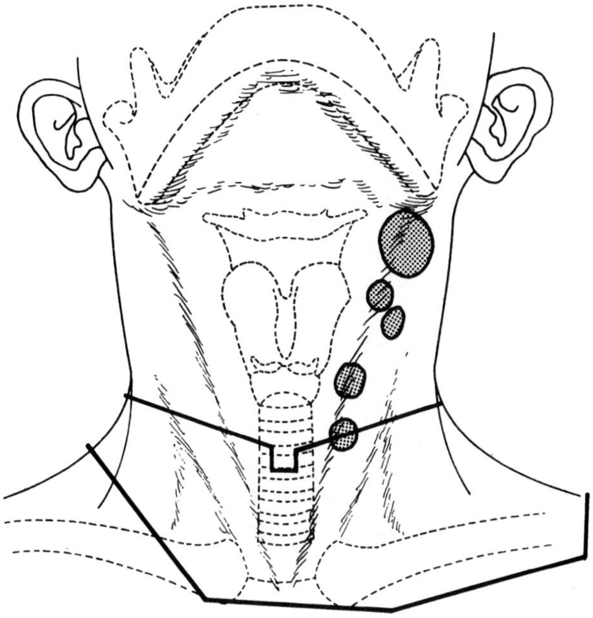

Figure 16.36. Anterior portal for treatment of low neck in patients with hypopharyngeal or laryngeal cancer. Low neck is irradiated bilaterally. Level of superior border of portal varies according to primary lesion treated and may be as high as cricothyroid membrane (e.g., lesion of suprahyoid epiglottis) or as low as 2 to 3 cm below inferior border of cricoid cartilage (e.g., for advanced pyriform sinus cancer). Matchline is treated in primary portals but excluded from low neck field. Usually, a 1 × 1 cm midline block is introduced at upper edge of field, except in postoperative patients in whom tracheal stoma is at risk (14). Each side of low neck portal is individualized according to risk and/or presence of lymph node metastases on that side.

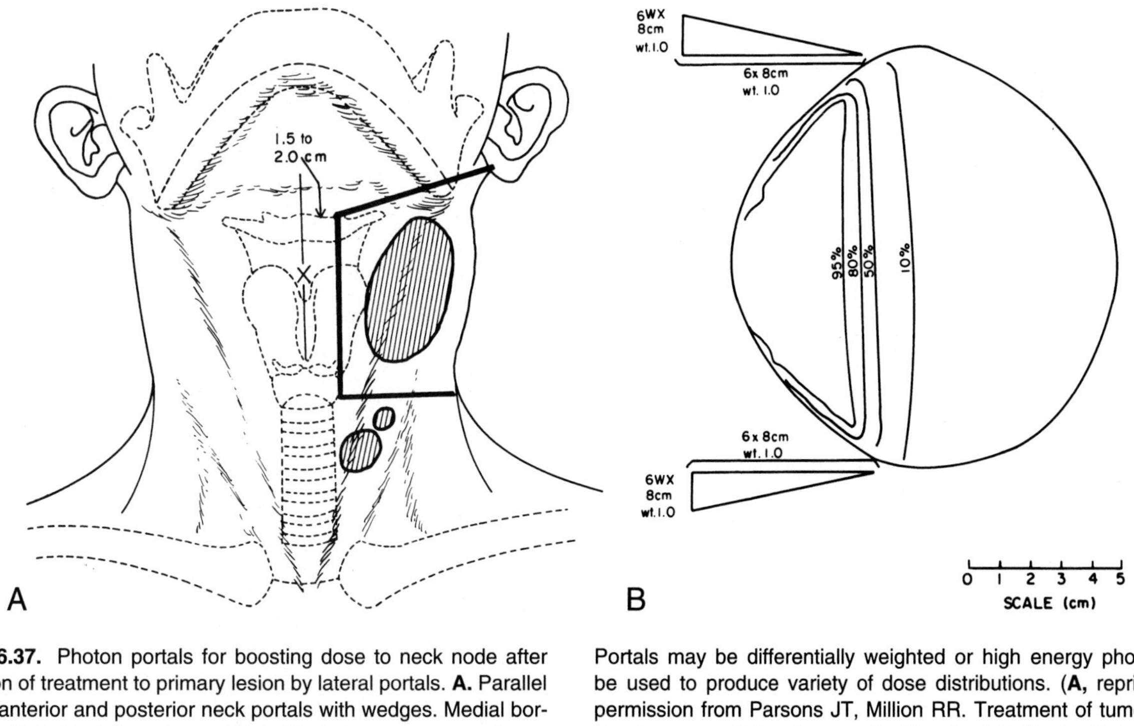

Figure 16.37. Photon portals for boosting dose to neck node after completion of treatment to primary lesion by lateral portals. **A.** Parallel opposed anterior and posterior neck portals with wedges. Medial border is usually 1.5 to 2.0 cm from midline. Technique spares much normal mucosa and cervical spinal cord from high dose irradiation and is particularly useful in patient with small primary cancer (e.g., T1) that requires dose of 60 Gy and a large neck node (e.g., N3A) that requires a high dose (e.g., 70 to 75 Gy). **B.** Dose distribution produced by anterior and posterior portals with equally weighted ^{60}Co wedge pair. Portals may be differentially weighted or high energy photons may be used to produce variety of dose distributions. (**A,** reprinted with permission from Parsons JT, Million RR. Treatment of tumors of the oropharynx: radiation therapy. In: Thawley SE, Panje WR, eds. Comprehensive management of head and neck tumors, Vol. 1. Philadelphia: W.B. Saunders, 1987.) (**B,** reprinted with permission from Million RR, Cassisi NJ, Mancuso AA. The unknown primary. In: Million RR, Cassisi NJ, eds. Management of head and neck cancer: a Multidisciplinary approach. 2nd ed. Philadelphia: J.B. Lippincott; 1994:311–320.)

from previous reports, and probably varies according to primary site, a ballpark figure of 25 to 30% is our best estimate under most circumstances. The mechanism of metastasis to the contralateral neck from a well-lateralized primary lesion with ipsilateral nodal involvement is not well defined. One possibility is that shunting of lymph occurs via submental pathways because of relative obstruction of lymph flow by grossly involved lymph nodes; such shunting is observed when lymphatic pathways are surgically interrupted (41).

Larynx and Hypopharynx Cancers

The principles of portal design are the same as those described in the previous section (Figure 16.36).

Boost Technique for Large or Fixed Lymph Nodes

Some patients have small or unknown primary lesions that require only 55 to 60 Gy, but have a large, fixed nodal mass (e.g., 7 to 8 cm or more in size) that requires a higher dose, e.g., 70 to 80 Gy even when neck dissection is planned. In many treatment centers, the common practice is to treat the neck node with electrons after the primary lesion has been irradiated. We prefer to use anterior and posterior parallel opposed wedged portals to spare the mucosal surfaces and to avoid the excessive skin reaction and fibrosis produced by high energy electrons (Figure 16.37 [21,42]). Only the large mass, and not the entire neck, receives the high-dose boost, even if there are other involved lymph nodes in the neck. Radical neck dissection usually is performed 6 weeks after irradiation, unless the nodal mass is a lymphoepithelioma. We believe that wound healing after neck dissection is less likely to be a problem when the patient has been irradiated with photons rather than electrons.

References

1. Fletcher GH. Textbook of radiotherapy. 3rd ed. Philadelphia: Lea and Febiger; 1980.
2. Million RR, Cassisi NJ, eds. Management of head and neck cancer: a multidisciplinary approach. 2nd ed. Philadelphia: J.B. Lippincott; 1994.
3. Million RR, Cassisi NJ, Clark JR. Cancer of the head and neck. In: DeVita VT Jr, Hellman S, Rosenberg SA, eds. Cancer: principles and practice of oncology. 3rd ed. Philadelphia: J.B. Lippincott, 1989.
4. American Joint Committee on Cancer. Manual for staging of cancer. 2nd ed. Philadelphia: J.B. Lippincott Company; 1983:37–42.
5. Million RR, Cassisi NJ, Mancuso AA. Larynx. In: Million RR, Cassisi NJ, eds. Management of head and neck cancer: a multidisciplinary approach. 2nd ed. Philadelphia: J.B. Lippincott; 1994:431–497.
6. Mendenhall WM, Parsons JT, Brant TA, Stringer SP, Cassisi NJ, Million RR. Is elective neck treatment indicated for T2N0 squamous cell carcinoma of the glottic larynx? Radiother Oncol 1989;14(3):199-202.
7. Mendenhall WM, Parsons JT, Million RR, Fletcher GH. T1-T2 squamous cell carcinoma of the glottic larynx treated with radiation therapy: relationship of dose-fractionation factors to local control and complications. Int J Radiat Oncol Biol Phys 1988;15:1267–1273.
8. Parsons JT. Time-dose-volume relationship in radiation therapy. In: Million RR, Cassisi NJ, eds. Management of head and neck cancer: a multidisciplinary approach. Philadelphia: J.B. Lippincott; 1984: 137–172.
9. Pantoja E. Relation of the vocal cord to the thyroid cartilage. An aid for checking localization of radiation fields in the treatment of glottic lesions. Radiology 1967;89:513–514.
10. Parsons JT, Mendenhall WM, Mancuso AA, Cassisi NJ, Million RR. Twice-a-day radiotherapy for T3 squamous cell carcinoma of the glottic larynx. Head Neck 1989;11:123–128.
11. Lee WR, Mancuso AA, Saleh EM, Mendenhall WM, Parsons JT, Million RR. Can pretreatment computed tomography findings predict local control in T3 squamous cell carcinoma of the glottic larynx treated with radiotherapy alone. Int J Radiat Oncol Biol Phys 1993;25: 683–687.
12. Freeman DE, Mancuso AA, Parsons JT, Mendenhall WM, Million RR. Irradiation alone for supraglottic larynx carcinoma: can CT findings predict treatment results? Int J Radiat Oncol Biol Phys 1990;19: 485–490.
13. Mendenhall WM, Parsons JT, Mancuso AA, Cassisi NJ, Million RR. Squamous cell carcinoma of the pharyngeal wall treated with irradiation. Radiother Oncol 1988;11:205–212.
14. Amdur RJ, Parsons JT, Mendenhall WM, Million RR, Stringer SP, Cassisi NJ. Postoperative irradiation for squamous cell carcinoma of the head and neck: an analysis of treatment results and complications. Int J Radiat Oncol Biol Phys 1989;16(1):25–36.
15. Nassar VH, Bridger GP. Topography of the laryngeal mucous glands. Arch Otolaryngol 1971;94:490–498.
16. Parsons JT, Mendenhall WM, Moore GJ, Million RR. Radiotherapy of tumors of the oropharynx. In: Thawley SE, Panje WR, eds. Comprehensive management of head and neck tumors. 2nd ed. Philadelphia: W.B. Saunders; 1997.
17. Foote RL, Parsons JT, Mendenhall WM, Million RR, Cassisi NJ, Stringer SP. Is interstitial implantation essential for successful radiotherapeutic treatment of base of tongue carcinoma. Int J Radiat Oncol Biol Phys 1990;18:1293–1298.
18. Parsons JT, Million RR. Interstitial implantation is essential [letter]. Int J Radiat Oncol Biol Phys 1988;14:597–598.
19. Parsons JT, Million RR, Cassisi NJ. Carcinoma of the base of the tongue: results of radical irradiation with surgery reserved for irradiation failure. Laryngoscope 1982;92:689–696.
20. Million RR, Cassisi NJ, Mancuso AA. Oropharynx. In: Million RR, Cassisi NJ, eds. Management of head and neck cancer: a multidisciplinary approach. 2nd ed. Philadelphia: J.B. Lippincott; 1994:401–429.
21. Parsons JT, Million RR. Treatment of tumors of the oropharynx: radiation therapy. In: Thawley SE, Panje WR, eds. Comprehensive management of head and neck tumors. Philadelphia: W.B. Saunders; 1987:684–699.
22. Million RR, Cassisi NJ, Mancuso AA, Stringer SP, Mendenhall WM, Parsons JT. Management of the neck for squamous cell carcinoma. In: Million RR, Cassisi NJ, eds. Management of head and neck cancer: a multidisciplinary approach. 2nd ed. Philadelphia: J.B. Lippincott; 1994:75–142.
23. Mazeron JJ. Interstitial radiation therapy for squamous cell carcinoma of the tonsillar region: The Creteil experience (1971–1981). Int J Radiat Oncol Biol Phys 1986;12:895–900.
24. Parsons JT. The effect of radiation on normal tissues of the head and neck. In: Million RR, Cassisi NJ, eds. Management of head and neck cancer: a multidisciplinary approach. Philadelphia: J.B. Lippincott; 1984:173–207.
25. Fletcher GH, Million RR. Nasopharynx. In: Fletcher GH, ed. Textbook of radiotherapy. 3rd ed. Philadelphia: Lea & Febiger; 1980:364–383.
26. Million RR, Cassisi NJ, Mancuso AA. Oral cavity. In: Million RR, Cassisi NJ, eds. Management of head and neck cancer: a multidisciplinary approach. 2nd ed. Philadelphia: J.B. Lippincott; 1994:321–400.
27. Ellingwood KE, Million RR, Mitchell TP. A preloaded radium needle implant device for maintenance of needle spacing. Cancer 1976;37: 2858–2860.
28. Parsons JT, Mendenhall WM, Million RR. Radiotherapy of tumors of the oral cavity. In: Thawley SE, Panje WR, eds. Comprehensive management of head and neck tumors. 2nd ed. Philadelphia: W.B. Saunders; 1997.
29. Marcus RB Jr, Million RR, Mitchell TP. A preloaded, custom-designed implantation device for stage T1-T2 carcinoma of the floor of the mouth. Int J Radiat Oncol Biol Phys 1980;6:111–113.
30. Million RR, Cassisi NJ. General principles for treatment of cancers in the head and neck: Radiation therapy. In: Million RR, Cassisi NJ, eds.

Management of head and neck cancer: a multidisciplinary approach. Philadelphia: J.B. Lippincott; 1984.

31. Parsons JT, Mendenhall WM, Mancuso AA, Cassisi NJ, Million RR. Malignant tumors of the nasal cavity and ethmoid and sphenoid sinuses. Int J Radiat Oncol Biol Phys 1988;14(1):11–22.
32. Parsons JT, Stringer SP, Mancuso AA, Million RR. Nasal vestibule, nasal cavity, and paranasal sinuses. In: Million RR, Cassisi NJ, eds. Management of head and neck: a multidisciplinary approach. 2nd ed. Philadelphia: J.B. Lippincott; 1994:551–598.
33. Ellingwood KE, Million RR. Cancer of the nasal cavity and ethmoid/ sphenoid sinuses. Cancer 1979;43:1517–1526.
34. Parsons JT, Mendenhall WM, Stringer SP, Cassisi NJ, Million RR. Nasal cavity and paranasal sinuses. In: Perez CA, Brady LW, eds. Principles and practice of radiation oncology. 2nd ed. Philadelphia: J.B. Lippincott; 1992:644–656.
35. Parsons JT, Bova FJ, Fitzgerald CR, Mendenhall WM, Million RR. Radiation optic neuropathy after megavoltage external-beam irradiation: analysis of time-dose factors. Int J Radiat Oncol Biol Phys 1994; 30:755–763.
36. Parsons JT, Bova FJ, Fitzgerald CR, Mendenhall WM, Million RR. Radiation retinopathy after external-beam irradiation: analysis of time-dose factors. Int J Radiat Oncol Biol Phys 1994;30:765–773.
37. Parsons JT, Bova FJ, Fitzgerald CR, Mendenhall WM, Million RR. Severe dry-eye syndrome following external beam irradiation. Int J Radiat Oncol Biol Phys 1994;30:775–780.
38. Million RR, Cassisi NJ, Hamlin DJ. Nasal vestibule, nasal cavity, and paranasal sinuses. In: Million RR, Cassisi NJ, eds. Management of head and neck cancer: a multidisciplinary approach. Philadelphia: J.B. Lippincott; 1984.
39. Million RR, Cassisi NJ, Wittes RE. Cancer of the head and neck. In: DeVita VT Jr, Hellman S, Rosenberg SA, eds. Cancer: principles and practice of oncology. 2nd ed. Philadelphia: J.B. Lippincott; 1985: 407–506.
40. Mendenhall WM, Million RR, Mancuso AA, Cassisi NJ, Flowers FP. Carcinoma of the skin. In: Million RR, Cassisi NJ, eds. Management of head and neck cancer: a multidisciplinary approach. 2nd ed. Philadelphia: J.B. Lippincott; 1994:643–691.
41. Fisch U. Lymphography of the cervical lymphatic system. Translated by M. Tobias. Philadelphia: W.B. Saunders; 1968.
42. Million RR, Cassisi NJ, Mancuso AA. The unknown primary. In: Million RR, Cassisi NJ, eds. Management of head and cancer: a multidisciplinary approach. 2nd ed. Philadelphia: J.B. Lippincott; 1994: 311–320.

Chapter 17

Breast Cancer

Marsha D. McNeese, Eric A. Strom, Thomas A. Buchholz, Seymour H. Levitt, and Faiz M. Khan

Regardless of the surgical procedure that precedes irradiation, the radiation oncologist may be called on to treat part or all of the following areas in patients with breast cancer: chest wall or breast, axilla, internal mammary nodes, and supraclavicular nodes. In this chapter, we present pertinent anatomic information, describe treatment areas, and suggest a variety of treatment techniques—the choice of technique depending on the prior surgical procedure, the stage of the disease, and the equipment available.

ANATOMY

Breast

The protuberant breast extends from the second or third to the sixth or seventh costal cartilage and from the edge of the sternum to the anterior axillary line. Mammary tissue, however, is found as a thin layer below the clavicle from the midline laterally to the edge of the latissimus dorsi muscle. The thickest part of the breast is in the upper outer quadrant, which usually contains a greater bulk of mammary tissue than other parts of the breast. The axillary tail of the breast can become so large that it forms a visible axillary mass and frequently is the site of the primary tumor. The lymphatic drainage is shown in Figure 17.1 (1).

All the draining lymphatics of the breast, including those of the pectoral musculature and chest wall, empty into the confluence of the internal jugular and subclavian veins in the base of the neck under the insertion of the sternocleidomastoid muscle to the head of the clavicle. The lymphatic trunks are therefore located in the medial portion of the supraclavicular area (Figure 17.1). Three trunks are of primary importance: the subclavian trunk from the axilla, the jugular trunk from the neck and supraclavicular area, and the bronchomediastinal trunks (2). All connecting trunks combine in a variety of ways to empty, on the right side, into a short common trunk, the right lymphatic duct, and on the left side, into the internal jugular vein, the subclavian vein, or the thoracic duct.

This investigation was supported in part by grant CA06294 and CA16672 awarded by the National Cancer Institute, DHEW.

Axilla

The axillary lymph nodes are divided into three levels according to certain anatomic guidelines (Figure 17.2) (3).

Level I (proximal) — nodes located under the lower part of the pectoralis minor muscle

Level II (middle) — nodes directly under the pectoralis minor muscle

Level III (distal) — nodes superior to the pectoralis minor muscle

These nodes provide the major drainage of the breast tissue, and analysis of histologic involvement of these nodes by metastases provides the most important single prognostic factor for breast carcinoma (2,4–6). Often the level I nodes alone are removed for staging purposes in a lateral axillary dissection. In a series of 539 patients, Veronesi et al showed that the incidence of skip metastasis was quite low, with only 20 patients having a skip distribution. Conversely, when the nodes at level I were positive, approximately 40% of higher level nodes were also involved (7). The distribution of node metastases by level is shown in Table 17.1.

Internal Mammary Nodes

The internal mammary lymph nodes are small, 2 to 5 mm in diameter, and can be either structural nodes or collections of lymphocytes in areolar tissue. They are lo-

Figure 17.1. Distribution of lymphatic trunks draining breast and chest wall musculature. Intercostal lymphatics are probably also direct route of spread. (Reprinted with permission from Haagensen CD. Diseases of the breast. 3rd ed. Philadelphia: W.B. Saunders, 1986.)

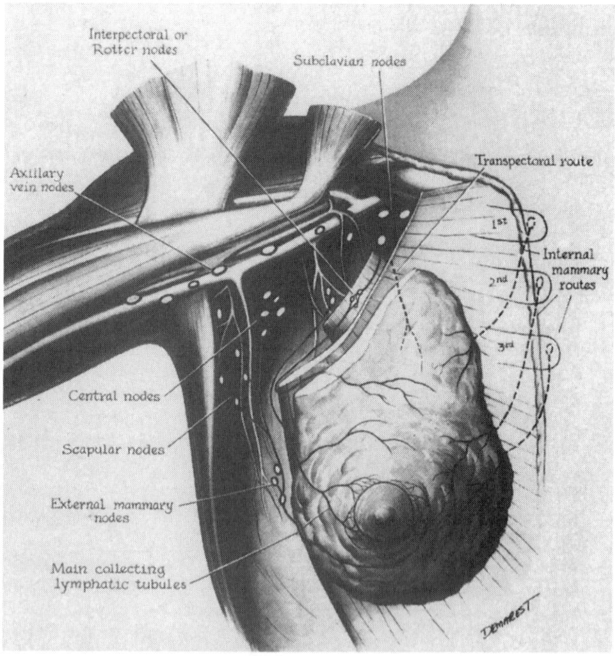

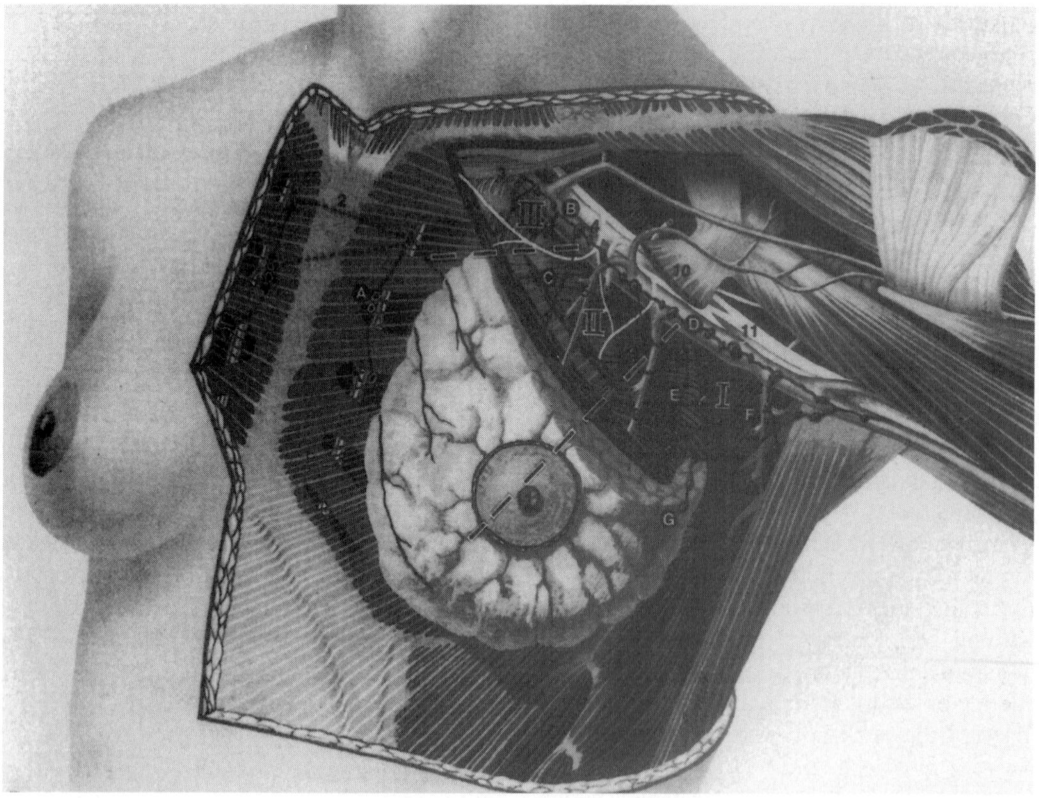

Figure 17.2. Anatomy of axilla (pectoralis major and minor muscles partially removed to demonstrate anatomic levels of lymph nodes). 1) Internal mammary artery and vein, 2) Substernal cross drainage to contralateral internal mammary lymphatic chain; 3) Subclavius muscle and Halsted's ligament; 4) Lateral pectoral nerve (from lateral cord); 5) Pectoral branch from thoracoacromial vein; 6) Pectoralis minor muscle; 7) Pectoralis major muscle; 8) Lateral thoracic vein; 9) Medial pectoral nerve (from medial cord); 10) Pectoralis minor muscle; 11) Median nerve; 12) Subscapular vein; 13) Thoracodorsal vein; A) Internal mammary lymph nodes; B) Apical lymph nodes; C) Interpectoral (Rotter's) lymph nodes; D) Axillary vein lymph nodes; E) Central lymph nodes; F) Scapular lymph nodes; G) External mammary lymph nodes; Level I lymph nodes, lateral to lateral border of pectoralis minor muscle; Level II lymph nodes, behind pectoralis minor muscle; Level III lymph nodes, medial to medial border of pectoralis minor muscle. (Reprinted with permission from Osborne MP. Breast development and anatomy. In: Harris JR, Hellman S, Henderson IC, Kinne DW, eds. Breast disease. Philadelphia: J.B. Lippincott, 1987.)

cated along the course of the internal mammary lymphatic trunks, generally within 3 cm of the lateral margin of the sternum. Rarely is a node located under the edge of the costal cartilage; they usually lie on the endothoracic fascia in the interspaces between the costal cartilages. The greatest concentration of nodes is in the upper three interspaces. Between the left and right lymphatic trunks at the level of the first interspace, retromanubrial connecting lymphatics have been described in autopsied patients. Ultrasonography has provided a means of determining the depth of the pleural reflection on which the lymph nodes are found. In addition, lymphoscintigraphy demonstrates lymph nodes in the internal mammary node spaces so that their location lateral to the midline can be determined accurately; crossover is demonstrated in about 20% of patients. Figures 17.3A and B show venograms that demonstrate variations in individual anatomy in two patients (1).

Table 17.1. Distribution of Node Metastases by Level

Level	Number (%)
I	314 (58.2)
I + II	117 (21.7)
I + II + III	88 (16.3)
Total number of cases with regular distribution	519 (96.2)
II	6 (1.2)
III	2 (0.4)
I + III	12 (2.2)
II + III	0
Total number of cases with "skip" distribution	20 (100)

Reprinted with permission from Veronesi U. et al. Distribution of axillary node metastases by level of invastion: an analysis of 539 cases. Cancer 1987; 59:682.

POSTMASTECTOMY

Indications

Regional lymphatic and chest wall irradiation is indicated after mastectomy when more than four of the axillary nodes are histologically positive and/or gross (>2 mm) extranodal extension into axillary connective tissues is seen, when the primary tumor is greater than 5 cm and is associated with grave signs, or when the tumor is located in the central or inner quadrant of the breast and is associated with positive axillary nodes (5,8–22). Mastectomy scar extensions onto the opposite breast, upper abdomen, or arm can be treated with electrons. Drain sites are included if possible; however, recurrences are rarely noted at these sites. Figure 17.4A and B show the electron beam peripheral lymphatic and chest wall portals. The fields are as described subsequently.

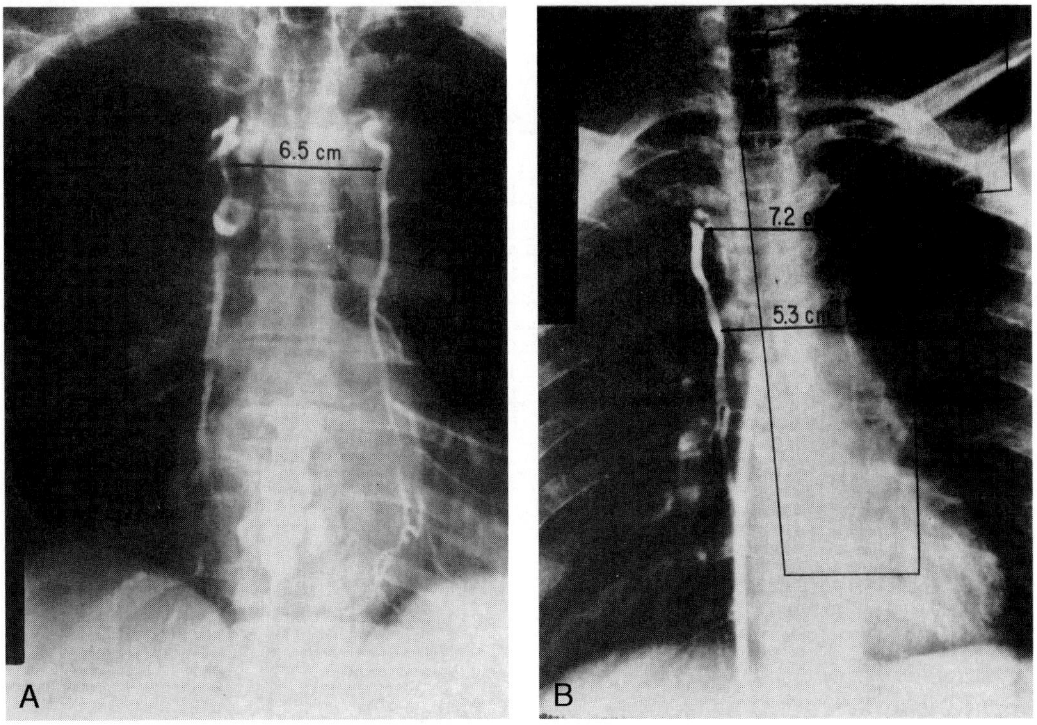

Figure 17.3. A, and B, Internal mammary venograms. Normal anatomic variation in two different patients. (Reprinted with permission from Fletcher GH, Montague ED. Does adequate irradiation of the internal mammary chain and supraclavicular nodes improve survival rates? Int J Radiat Oncol Biol Phys 1978;4:481.)

Figure 17.4. Chest wall and lymphatic fields in a patient with fairly curved chest wall. Two separate low energy fields are used with the anterior field treated straight on and the lateral field at a 35° lateral tilt, with junctions moved weekly. A, Shows the appearance of the two fields at the beginning of treatment. B, Shows a patient after 5 weeks of treatment, with junctions moved weekly.

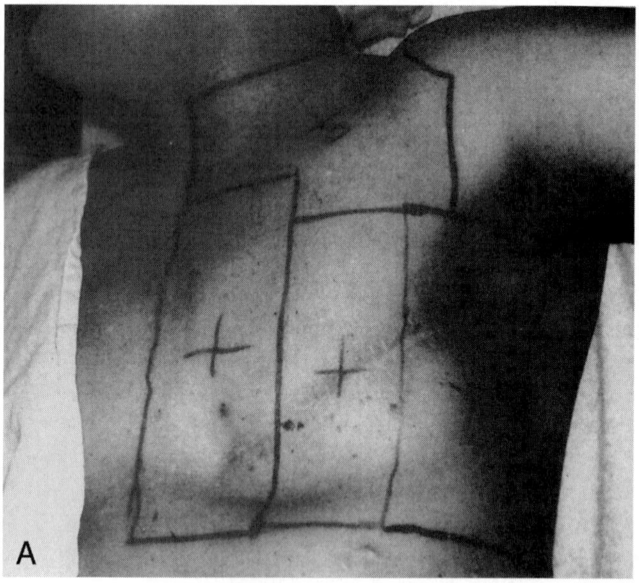

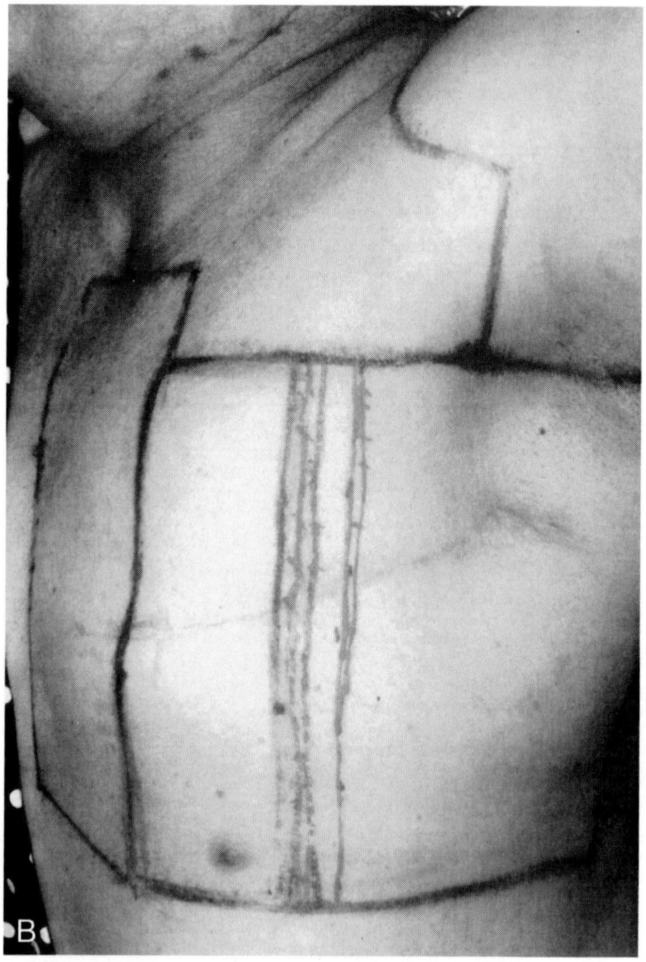

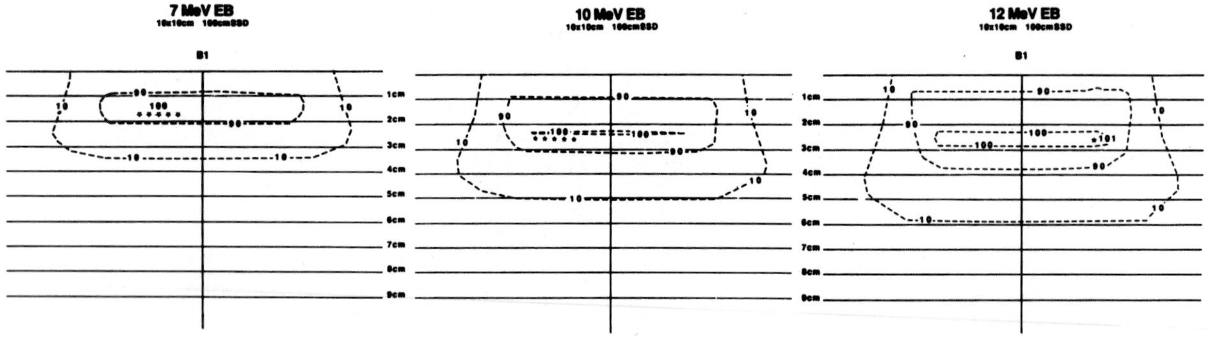

Figure 17.5. Isodose distributions for 10 × 10 cm field at 100 SSD (source-surface distance) for various electron beam (EB) energies using Siemens Mevatron-80. Low energy beams (5 to 8 MeV) are used to treat postoperative chest wall, with slightly higher energies (9 to 11 MeV) to treat supraclavicular field and axillary apex. Energies of 11 to 13 MeV are usually required to reach depth of internal mammary nodes.

Internal Mammary Fields

Treatment to the internal mammary chain (IMC) nodes is given with electron beam irradiation to avoid underlying cardiac and mediastinal tissues (10,23,24) (see isodose curves, Figure 17.5). Our policy does not include bilateral internal mammary node irradiation for the following reasons:

1. Experience with internal mammary node metastases has been gained with ipsilateral surgical dissection, and contralateral parasternal nodules are extremely rare.
2. Adequate irradiation to nodes of both internal mammary chains would entail a portal 12 cm wide, which substantially increases the volume of

mediastinal irradiation, even with electron beam.

3. Contralateral internal mammary node irradiation would interfere with future irradiation in those patients who develop a contralateral breast cancer.

The patient is supine, the upper arm is abducted, usually with an immobilization device such as a Vaculock cast (Bionix Corp, Toledo, Ohio), and the head is turned to the contralateral side (2).

The portal consists of a single rectangular electron beam field, usually 7 cm in width, covering the ipsilateral internal mammary nodes and the confluence of venous drainage under the insertion of the sternocleidomastoid muscle into the head of the clavicle. The medial border is 1 cm across the midline because of constriction of electron isodose curves at depth. Thus, the upper border includes the head of the clavicle and the lower border is usually at the same level as the lower border of the chest wall.

Dose

When using electrons, the dose is 50 Gy to d_{max} (depth of maximum dose) over 5 weeks, 5 fractions/week. It may not be possible to give the entire treatment with electrons alone, depending on the skin doses, which vary according to the type of accelerator used. In such cases, a combination of electrons and photons may be necessary to achieve a lower dose to the skin. At least 50% of total dose delivered should be given with electrons. Energy is sufficient for approximately 90% depth dose at 3 to 4 cm (usually 10- to 13-MeV electrons). Computed tomography (CT) planning or ultrasound to measure the depth to the pleural interface is highly desirable.

Supraclavicular Nodal Irradiation

Close attention must be given to the medial border of the supraclavicular field because involved nodes may be located under the junction of the sternocleidomastoid muscle and the head of the clavicle. The upper medial border of the field should be 1 cm on the opposite side of the midline. The field covers the supraclavicular, subclavicular apical, and low jugular nodes. For electron beam radiation, separate fields are used for the supraclavicular and internal mammary nodes because the depth of the target volume determines the energy to be used. The patient is placed on a slant board on the treatment table so that the plane of the sternum is relatively parallel to the treatment table (the angle of the tilt is documented for daily duplication of treatment).

Supraclavicular and Axillary Apex Field (Electron Beam Technique)

The medial border extends superiorly from the superomedial corner of the internal mammary field 1 cm across the midline to the level of the thyrocricoid groove. The superior border extends laterally across the neck and the trapezius to the acromial process. The lateral border crosses the acromioclavicular joint and extends to meet the inferior border. The inferior border is a horizontal line extending laterally at the level of the second intercostal space.

Electron beam energy is sufficient for 90% depth dose at 2 to 2.5 cm depth (usually 9 to 10 MeV). The dose is 50 Gy to d_{max} over 5 weeks, 5 fractions per week. A combination of electrons and photons (usually 4:1) may be substituted to achieve less skin reaction. Patients with thicker body habitus who would require higher electron energies are probably better treated with photons alone to avoid a geographic miss of apical nodes and to allow for more skin sparing.

Electron Beam Chest Wall Fields

The entire chest wall sometimes is treated with electron beam fields. The medial border is contiguous with the lateral border of the internal mammary field. The superior border is contiguous with the inferior border of the supraclavicular field, at the level of the second costal cartilage. The inferior border is a horizontal line at the level of the xiphoid. The lateral border follows the midaxillary line. Because of the slope of the chest wall, it is usually divided into two fields, medial and lateral, with the lateral field angled about 35°. The medial field is not angled in order to avoid too large a "hot spot" from overlap into the higher-energy IMC field. To avoid dose buildup at the junction of the medial and lateral chest wall fields, the junction is moved 0.5 cm laterally each week (see Figure 17.4B).

Dose

The dose is 50 Gy to dmax over 5 weeks followed by a 10-Gy boost to a reduced field, which generously encompasses the scar and original tumor bed.

Energy

Usually, 5 to 8 MeV is sufficient for most chest wall tissue after modified radical mastectomy. Ultrasonography or CT is mandatory for determining chest wall thickness to avoid a high lung dose. With the increased skin-sparing ability of the newer accelerators, the chest wall fields require bolus, usually 0.5 cm in thickness, for the first 5 days of treatment, increasing the energy to 8- or 9-MeV electrons for those few days and re-evaluating the skin reaction at the fourth week of treatment. Bolus is also used during the boost treatment, unless the patient has already developed brisk erythema in the reduced field.

Anterior Supraclavicular-Axillary Photon Field

The anterior supraclavicular-axillary field covers the low and central axilla, subclavicular/axillary apex nodes, and the supraclavicular fossa, including the deep inferior cervical nodes and low jugular nodes. The medial border is a vertical line 1 cm across the midline extending from the second costal cartilage to the thyrocricoid groove, following the inner border of the sternocleidomastoid muscle. The superior border extends laterally across the neck and the trapezius, just avoiding falloff, to the acromial process. The lateral border is at the acromioclavicular joint and is drawn across the shoulder to exclude the shoulder joint. The line then follows the pectoral fold, just avoiding fall off. The inferior border is a horizontal line at the level of the second costal cartilage, abutting the medial edge of the internal mammary field, which extends upward to over the first intercostal space. The junction of the inferior supraclavicular-anterior axillary field and the chest wall is set up using a rod and chain and a half-beam block to avoid divergence (25).

The beam is tilted 15° laterally to avoid irradiating part of the trachea, esophagus, and spinal cord and to irradiate the deep inferior cervical nodes medial to the sternocleidomastoid muscle. The angulation additionally ensures that nodes close to the margin of the pectoral muscle are included without requiring falloff of the beam, which may produce moist desquamation in the axilla.

Dose

The dose is 50 Gy to dmax over 5 weeks in 25 fractions, usually with 6 MV photons.

AXILLARY IRRADIATION

Indications

This technique is used 1) any time the axilla requires irradiation after simple or segmental mastectomy or excisional biopsy without axillary dissection, 2) for preoperative irradiation (reserved for inoperable (N2) patients), or 3) in patients who require axillary irradiation because of inadequate axillary dissection (only a few nodes are recovered and are positive), gross (>2 mm) extranodal axillary disease, or matted or fixed axillary nodes (N2 disease) at presentation.

Posterior Axillary Field

The machine is rotated 180° without moving the patient, and the thickness of the Vaculock device is taken into account. The superior border splits the clavicle, extending medially to inside the spine of the scapula. The verification film should show a small amount of lung in the upper inner portion of the field. The lateral superior border goes to the humoral head, as in the anterior field. The lateral and inferior borders match the anterior field (Figure 17.6).

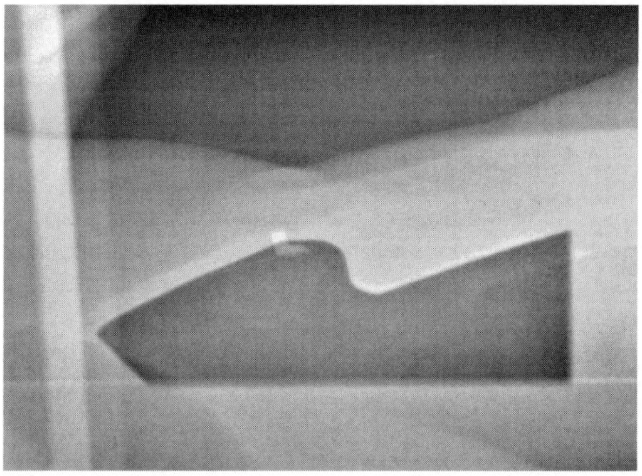

Figure 17.6. Localization radiograph of posterior axillary portal indicates inclusion of upper chest wall and part of lung medially and soft tissues of axilla bounded by clavicle and humerus.

Beam

The beam is vertical.

Dose

The posterior axillary portal supplements the dose from the anterior portal to deliver the tumor dose to the thickest part of the axilla. Dose contribution from both the AP and PA fields should not exceed 2.0 Gy per fraction at midplane to minimize risk of arm edema or other late effects.

For preoperative treatment (designed to reduce matted or fixed nodes to facilitate axillary dissection), a midplane dose of 50 Gy is necessary. For postoperative patients in whom extranodal extension in the axilla is found but no gross residual disease remains, the midaxillary dose is reduced to 40 to 45 Gy in an attempt to decrease the risk of arm edema. Those patients with small involved nodes without extracapsular extension do not need the posterior supplement if they have had adequate dissection (10 or more nodes obtained), as axillary failure in this group is rare.

Postoperative Chest Wall Tangential Photon Fields

Tangential fields are used if the chest wall flaps are too thick or too irregular for electron beam therapy. These fields usually abut an internal mammary field, the use of which not only treats nodes but also decreases the amount of lung and/or heart in the tangents. Figure 17.7 shows a patient with thick, irregular flaps who would be best treated with tangent photon fields.

The medial border coincides with the lateral border of the internal mammary field. Because of chest wall curvature and tangential angle of the beam, the medial border

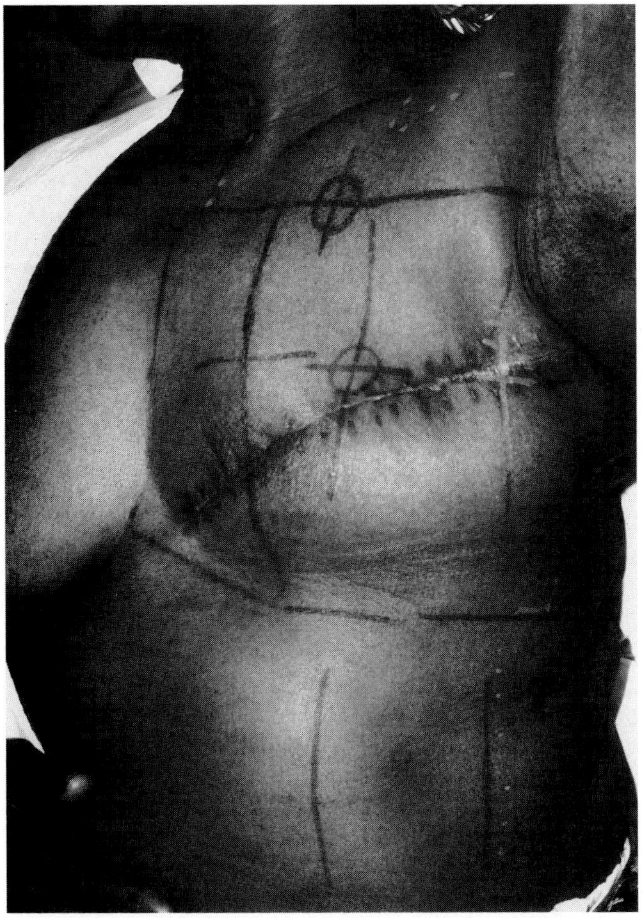

Figure 17.7. Postmastectomy patient with thick, irregular flaps which are best treated by photons. Lines on abdomen are for laser setup. Note curve of matchline of the internal mammary chain and chest wall fields and the dotted lines indicating the supraclavicular field.

rarely is a straight line. On most patients, the lateral border of the internal mammary field is shaped to match this curvature. An overlap of up to 0.5 cm is acceptable to avoid a cold spot, and the internal mammary electron field can be angled if necessary.

The lateral border is at the midaxillary line. If the surgical scar extends to or beyond the midaxillary line, the lateral border is moved posteriorly to obtain adequate margins, or if moving the lateral border would require excessive radiation to lung or heart, an additional appositional electron-beam field may be used for the portion of the scar beyond the midaxillary line.

The superior border coincides with the lower border of the supraclavicular field. Since postmastectomy patients have been selected for irradiation because of high risk of locoregional recurrence, the contiguous line is treated by both chest wall and supraclavicular fields, which may result in a slight overdose. However, with current techniques and equipment and careful field-matching, this has not resulted in significant problems.

The inferior border is a horizontal line at the level of the tip of the xiphoid, including scar extension with a 1- to 2-cm margin. For scars that extend further inferiorly than the level of the xiphoid, a separate electron beam field is used to treat that portion of the scar.

At simulation, a half-beam block is used so that the isocenter is set up on the medial and lateral field edges. Otherwise, the technique is essentially that described for simulation of the intact breast.

Dose

50 Gy is delivered over 5 weeks at 2.0 Gy per fraction, usually with 6 MV photons. The energy is increased if medial lateral field separation for tangent fields exceeds 24 cm. Both medial and lateral fields are treated each day. The tumor depth dose percentage is determined from either contour distributions of the chest wall or by CT-based dosimetry to a point specified as two-thirds the distance from the skin to the lung/chest wall interface. Treatments with bolus are required to increase the skin dose, usually every other day for the first 2 weeks and then re-evaluated beginning after the next week. The chest wall adjacent to the scar is boosted with an additional 10 Gy with electrons to include at least 3 cm on either side of the scar, again using bolus as necessary to achieve a brisk erythema.

IRRADIATION OF THE INTACT BREAST

Indications

The purpose of irradiation in this patient group is to eradicate microscopic residual disease at the original site as well as to eliminate multicentric disease. Because 80% of treatment failures in this patient group are in the same quadrant as the original primary, achieving adequate coverage in that area is imperative. The risk of multicentric disease is a function of the volume of breast tissue; it is low if a small volume of breast tissue is left unirradiated, if that volume is well away from the primary site. However, it is unwise to have adjacent fields at or near the tumor bed, as cold spots in that area can result in treatment failure.

Computerized tomography (CT) scanning is used for more accurate dosimetry and to gather more information about depth of nodes, coverage of breast, and pulmonary tissue. The treatment techniques continue to evolve to achieve better cosmetic results and local control.

Treatment to Breast Only

Irradiation is administered to the breast alone in patients who have excision ("lumpectomy" or segmental resection) of a noninvasive intraductal carcinoma, or an invasive tumor with nodes that are histologically negative as determined by axillary node dissection. If no axillary histology is available, whether or not irradiation should be given to the breast, axilla, internal mammary nodes, and supraclavicular nodes is controversial. Also, the increasing use of sentinel node biopsy to replace axillary dissection will inevitably lead to disagreement as to whether the breast alone should be irradiated using "high" tangents to include the low axilla or whether to treat regional nodes with separate fields. This may be addressed in the future by randomized trials.

If the tumor is in the upper breast and close to the superior border of the tangential fields, or if the patient has large breasts with significant breast tissue above the tangential fields, the breast tissue extending beyond the superior border of the tangential field to the clavicle can be treated with electrons. For other patients with smaller breasts, the risk of failure outside the tangential fields is low and the additional infraclavicular field is not necessary (26–28).

Throughout the various adaptations of technique for treating an intact breast, close teamwork between the surgeon and radiation oncologist is necessary. Clips placed at the time of surgery to delineate the tumor extent and depth are extremely helpful in treatment planning, even though postoperative changes or bleeding may decrease their reliability.

Simulation—University of Minnesota and University of Texas MDACC Method

Although slight differences exist in the techniques at these two institutions, they are not significant and therefore will not be described separately. The basic technique is described in the literature (29). The patient is positioned on the treatment couch in a stable and reproducible manner. A supine position meets these requirements and is preferable to other possible angled positions, unless special problems arise related to patient comfort, anatomy, or location of the target volume.

Gantry angles are set relative to a reference plane (e.g., a horizontal plane represented by the table top), and therefore the patient's body must be leveled relative to that plane. A sagittal laser beam passing over certain anatomic landmarks such as the nasion, middle of the chin, sternal notch, and the xiphoid tip will provide most of the leveling, although a bubble level is necessary for confirmation in the transverse plane (Figure 17.8). Thus, in a "leveled" patient, the transverse plane is perpendicular to the table top.

The arm is positioned in such a way that it is not in the path of the tangential beams. Another important consideration is that the arm position should not distort the anatomy such that it becomes difficult to treat the nodal sites. We prefer the arm abducted to 90 to 120° with the help of an immobilization device, as recommended previously in this chapter. A change in this angle may be necessary because of a special problem posed by an individual patient, but the important criteria are that the arm remains outside the beams and that its position does not significantly distort the rib cage or the supraclavicular axillary region or change appreciably from day to day.

The sternum in most patients slopes superiorly, which creates difficulty in adequately covering the entire breast and chest wall in the tangential beams. When this problem is encountered, an inclined board may be used to level the patient in the cephalad-caudad direction. It is important to

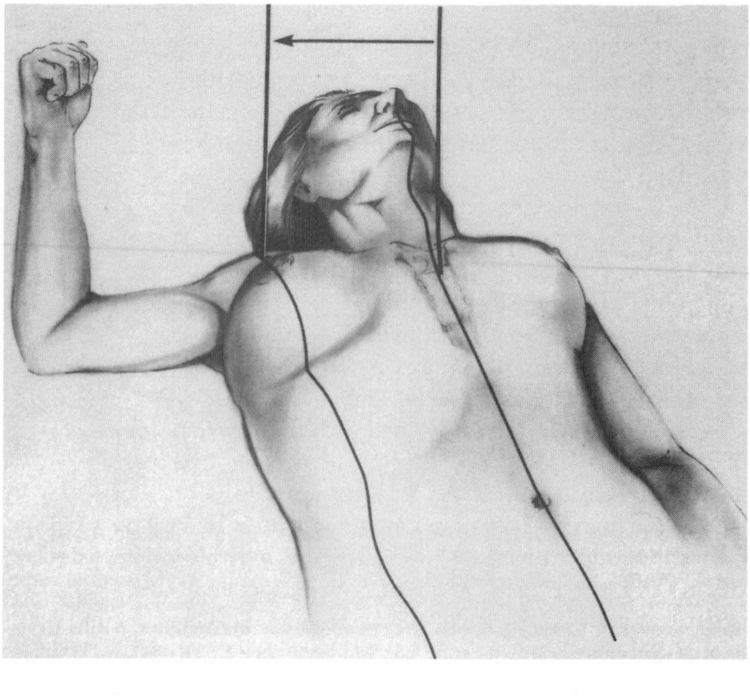

Figure 17.8. Sagittal laser beam used for setting up patient relative to anatomic landmarks. Isocenter point first positioned in sagittal plane and then shifted laterally through precalculated distance to position within breast to define treatment isocenter.

record the angle of the inclined board and the distance from the top of the head to the superior edge of the board for routine reproducibility.

The breast is a mobile structure and its position may change from day to day, especially if it is pendulous. Some radiation oncologists try to immobilize the breast by using a netted brassiere or masking tapes. None of these solutions are perfect, however, and they may pose problems with regard to increased skin dose, lack of reproducibility, or interference with the clinical observation of the field borders. We prefer the breast to lie in its natural position dictated by the position of the patient. Any day-to-day changes in the breast position would not significantly change the dosimetry if isocentric beams are used. In other words, because the total thickness of the breast in the path of the isocentric parallel opposed beams remains the same, no change in dose calculation is required if the individual treatment source-to-skin distances (SSD) change slightly from one day to another.

When the breast is so pendulous that it creates a fold, the increased skin dose under the inframammary fold may present a problem. Again, no perfect solution exists. In some cases, we have used Styrofoam wedges (density of 0.03 g/cm^3) under the breast to prop it up, but we have not as yet assessed the benefit of this procedure in terms of decrease in skin dose or the skin reaction. Other institutions are evaluating treating such patients in a prone position, with the breast hanging down. One drawback of this approach is that it is more difficult to abut fields to treat regional nodes.

Setup Parameters

Tangential Fields With the patient positioned appropriately as discussed previously, the medial and lateral tangential field borders, as well as the superior and inferior borders, are marked on the patient. For an intact breast, the field borders can be marked to include all the breast tissue with appropriate margins (e.g., about 1 to 2 cm beyond the clinically discernable breast tissue). The superior border is drawn perpendicular to the sagittal plane, at a level just inferior to the arm. If this border does not adequately cover the superior extent of the breast and if a supraclavicular field is not planned, a contiguous infraclavicular field (suprabreast field) may be added for treatment with a single vertical electron portal.

To determine the tangential beam border radiographically, a solder wire is laid on the patient along the entire length of the medial border. A short piece of solder wire is taped on the skin to delineate the lateral field border. Using the fluoroscopic view and adjusting the table position (vertical and lateral) as well as the gantry angle, the central axis of the beam is made to align exactly with the medial and lateral field markers (Figure 17.9A and B). The extent of lung in the field is noted; if needed, an adjustment may be made in the lateral border position. This alignment procedure is repeated until the field placement is radiographically acceptable. Approximately 2 cm of lung between the medial border (solder wire image) and the chest wall is considered appropriate to provide an adequate field margin for chest wall irradiation. The extent of lung in the beam, however, depends on many conditions, such as the breast span, positions of the medial and the lateral field borders, and the chest wall curvature. When the fluoroscopic view shows an acceptable beam arrangement, a radiograph is taken for a more quantitative assessment. If the radiographic findings also are acceptable, the gantry angle is recorded on the setup sheet.

With the patient in the same position as described previously, three external transverse contours of the breast are taken using a mechanical pantograph-type device; one contour is at midfield level and the other two are near the superior and inferior borders of the fields. Various landmarks, such as the midsternal line, medial border, lateral border, and table top are marked on these contours. On the central contour, the beam geometry is reconstructed to determine the rest of the setup parameters: lateral couch shift and the setup SSD.

In Figure 17.10, AB is the line joining the points on the medial and lateral borders. Angle θ is defined by the vertical line AB as shown. This angle must be equal to the gantry angle determined in the simulation procedure. Next, a midpoint, C, is taken on the line AB, and a line, CG, is drawn perpendicular to AB. The line CG designates the field width and is set sufficiently long to include the apex of the breast with a clearance of 1 to 2 cm. The midpoint O of the line CG is the isocenter position for the tangential beams. This isocenter point is then shifted horizontally to the midsternal line to define the isocenter position for setup only. The lateral shift L is recorded as well as the setup SSD at the sternum (SSD_{setup}).

The gantry angle θ is increased slightly by an amount equal to $\tan^{-1}$ (OC/SAD) so that the rays that would normally diverge into the lung are now aligned along the baseline AB. The gantry angle for the lateral field is also changed by the same amount to align its rays along AB. Thus, by making the two tangential fields slightly nonparallel opposed, the divergence of the beams into the lungs is eliminated. This procedure achieves the same effect as a beam splitter traditionally used to block off the lower one-half of the field to shield the lung.

These parameters can also be determined mathematically. Referring to Figure 17.10,

$$SSD_{setup} = SAD - d \qquad (1)$$

$$d = S\cos\theta - W\sin\theta - g \qquad (2)$$

$$L = W\cos\theta + S\sin\theta + a \qquad (3)$$

where SAD is source-to-axis distance (usually 100 cm), d is the depth of isocenter at midline sternum, S is half the

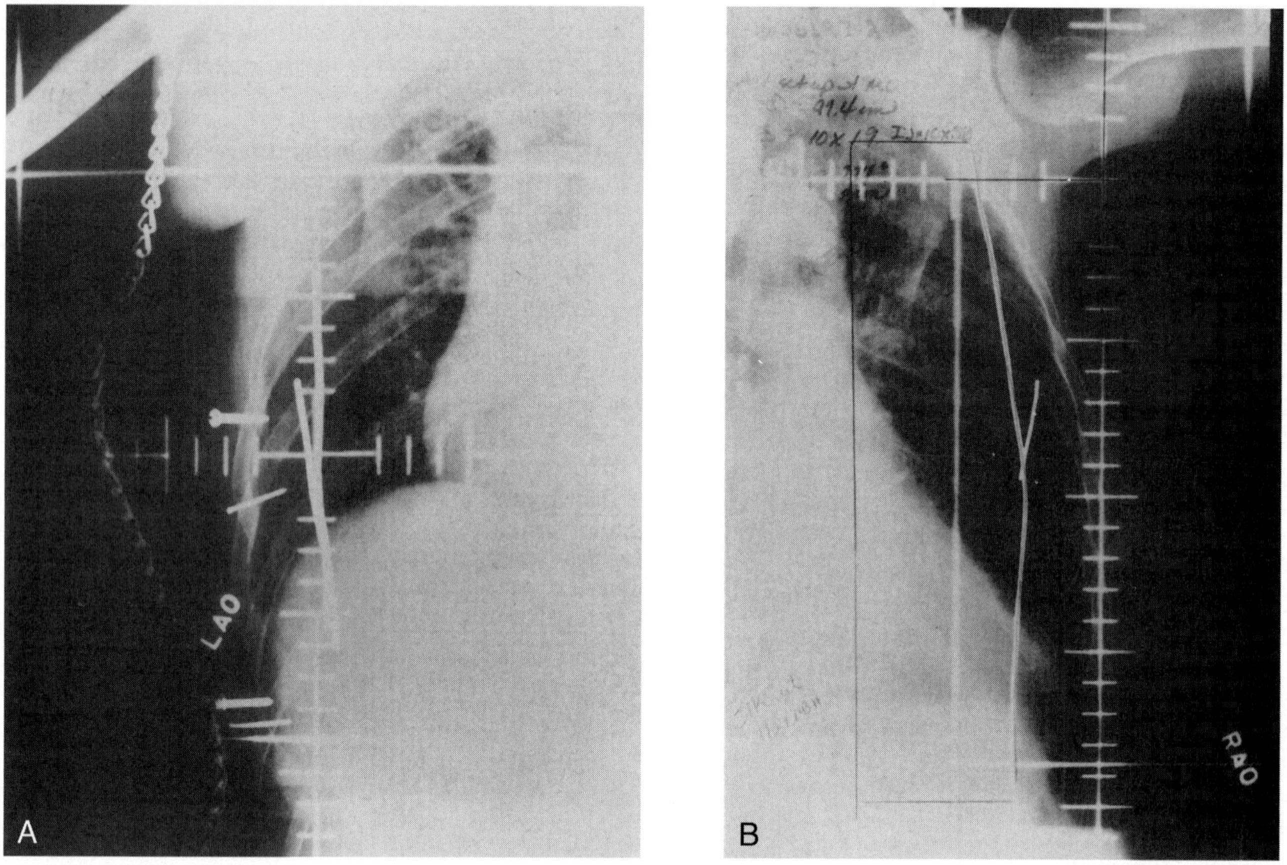

Figure 17.9. A, Initial simulation to set medial and lateral borders of tangential fields and to assess amount of lung permitted in beam. B, Final simulation indicates medial border, lateral border, and position of central axis at superior border of tangential fields (simulating independent jaw position). Custom blocks are then cut to define medial and lateral borders of tangential fields.

chest wall span, (1/2AB), θ is the angle that the line AB makes with the vertical (using International Electrotechnical Commission [IEC] convention of angles in which vertically downward directed beam is incident at angle 0° and increases to 360° as the gantry moves clockwise through one rotation), W is half the field width (1/2 CG), g is height of the entrance point A of the medial tangential field above midline, L is the lateral shift of isocenter from midline, and a is the lateral separation of the medial point A of beam entry from the midline.

Custom Blocking

Because of the curvature of the sternum in the cephalad-caudad direction, the medial field border as projected on the surface becomes crooked and often falls short of covering the breast tissue superiorly along the marked border. To overcome this problem, a custom block is made from the simulator film to define the medial field border along the solder wire image (Figure 17.9B). The same film is used upside-down to make the block for the lateral border, with the solder wire line as was used for the medial border. On the first day of treatment, the field width is increased, without changing the isocenter position, to cover all the breast tissue, and the excess field up to the marked medial border is blocked off using the medial custom block. The lateral field border is defined by using the lateral custom block.

This custom block procedure eliminates the need for tilting the collimator to straighten the field border on the surface, a procedure that often fails because the sternum slope does not follow a perfect triangle. However, the block is shaped appropriately to provide visual breast coverage in accordance with the field border marked on the surface as well as radiographically as shown by the simulator film.

Infraclavicular Breast Field

The superior border follows the clavicle. The medial border is at midline. The inferior border is contiguous with the superior border of the tangential fields. The lateral border follows the curve of the pectoralis major muscle, avoiding falloff.

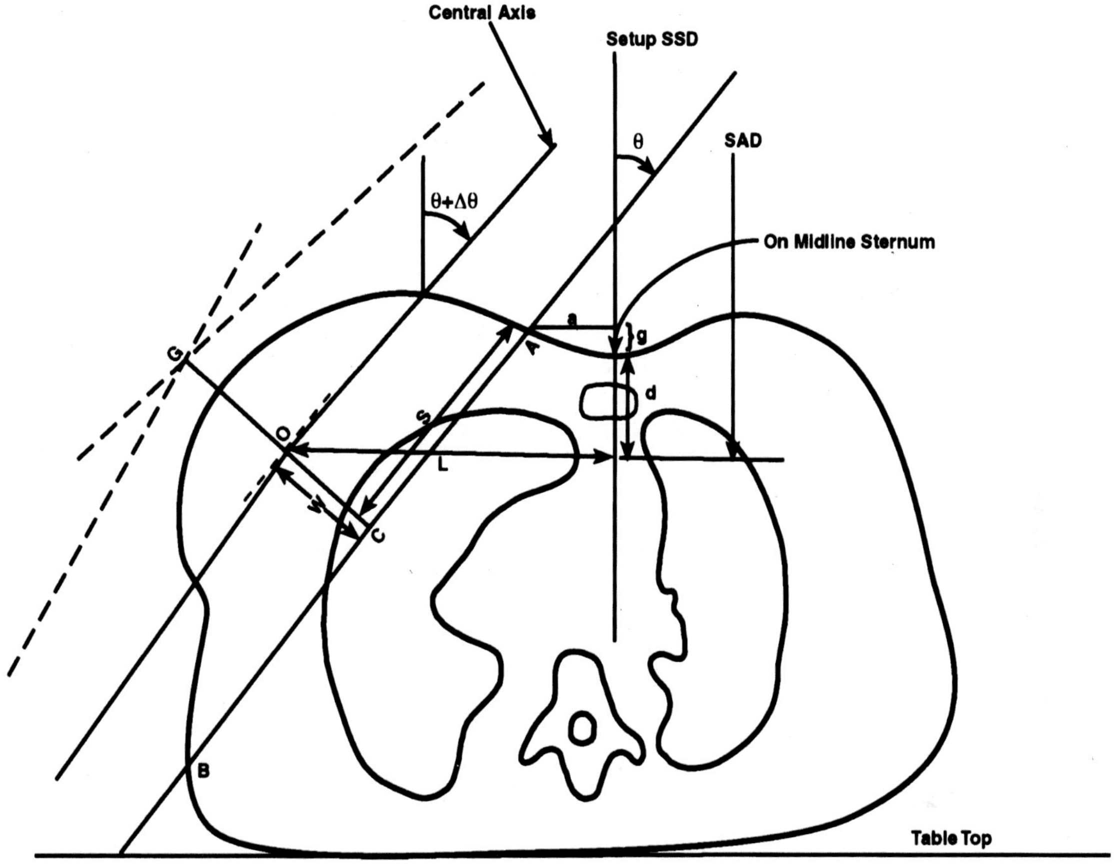

Figure 17.10. Determination of isocenter point, O, setup SSD, lateral isocenter shift, L, and angle O med. source axis distance: SSD, source-surface distance: IM, internal mammary.

Dose

Dosage is 50 Gy in 25 fractions over 5 weeks.

Boost to Primary Site

If margins are close or unknown, re-excision should be done, provided the amount of breast tissue is sufficient, to insure the lowest failure rate and avoid the consequences of higher doses of irradiation (30–35).

With noninvasive unifocal breast cancer with clear margins >5 mm, no boost is delivered. With larger invasive carcinoma, with any extensive or multifocal intraductal component, lymphatic invasion, or anaplastic nuclear grade, or any patient who has irradiation deferred until after chemotherapy, the field is reduced after 50 Gy, and an additional 10 Gy in five fractions with electrons is delivered to include the site and scar of the excision biopsy. The choice of voltage depends on the thickness of the breast in treatment position. Figure 17.11 demonstrates an electron beam field used to boost a tumor bed in a patient with a T2 inner quadrant primary. If the tumor bed is more than 4 to 5 cm deep within the breast, an interstitial implant may be preferable because of decreased dose to the skin with the implant compared to the dose that would be delivered by electrons. Use of a staggered double-plane technique usually is best because of the possibility of a geographic miss with a single-plane implant.

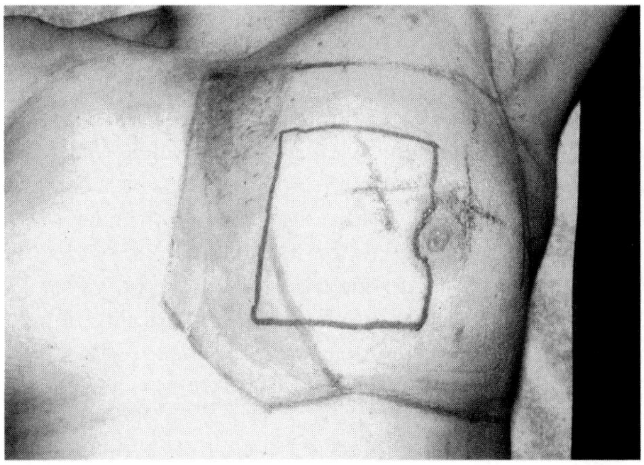

Figure 17.11. Electron boost field (12 MEV) in a patient with a T2 inner quadrant primary. Note that the nipple is blocked when possible.

For patients with tumors close to the chest wall, additional external irradiation may be delivered by means of compression technique, turning the patient into the prone oblique position for the lateral field and the anterior oblique position for the medial field; an additional 10 Gy tumor dose is delivered in 5 fractions with photons.

TREATMENT TO BREAST, INTERNAL MAMMARY NODES, AND SUPRACLAVICULAR AREAS

Indications

At the University of Minnesota and University of Texas MDACC, after conservation surgery for invasive carcinoma medially in the breast when axillary nodes are histologically positive, the internal mammary and supraclavicular nodes are treated in addition to the breast.

At the University of Minnesota, treatment is delivered to these three sites when the dissected axillary nodes are involved, regardless of the location of the primary tumor, whereas at University of Texas MDACC the internal mammary nodes may not be treated if the primary was in the outer portion of the breast. If the axillary nodes are small and levels I and II have been dissected, the mid-axilla is not treated. The treatment technique is the same as that described previously (chest-wall tangential fields).

If too much lung is included in the breast tangential fields when trying to include internal mammary nodes, an appositional electron or a combination of photons and electrons can be used to irradiate these nodes through a separate portal. To avoid cardiac toxicity, photons alone should not be used.

The position and depth of the internal mammary nodes should be evaluated, particularly when the nodes are to be included within the tangential portals. Lymphoscintigraphy allows measurement of the distance of the nodes from the midline at each interspace, and ultrasonography or CT gives the accurate depth of the nodes. When the internal mammary nodes are to be treated with a separate field, field junctions should not overlie the primary site. A lateral tilt may be added to the internal mammary electron beam field to avoid a dosimetric "cold" area; however, the scatter dose to the lung along with the possibility of missing the targeted lymph nodes because of beam constriction at depth must be taken into account when planning this technique.

Dose

The dosage is 50 Gy in 25 to 28 fractions, depending on breast size, delivered to all areas, followed in some cases by a boost to the tumor site as described previously.

Fields

The internal mammary and supraclavicular fields are the same as those described previously; the breast is also treated with tangential fields, usually using equally loaded open and 45° wedged fields.

If a patient has large breasts with breast tissue extending above what can be adequately covered in the tangential fields, the breast tissue above the tangential fields can be treated with low energy (9- to 10-MeV) electrons as described previously.

References

1. Haagensen CD. Disease of the Breast. 3rd ed. Philadelphia: W. B. Saunders, 1986.
2. Osborne MP. Breast development and anatomy. In: Harris JR, Hellman S, Henderson IC, Kinne DW, eds. Breast diseases. Philadelphia: J.B. Lippincott, 1987.
3. Valagussa P, Bonadonna G, Veronesi U. Patterns of relapse and survival in operable breast carcinoma with positive and negative axillary nodes. Tumori 1978;64:241-258.
4. Strom EA, McNeese MD, Fletcher GH. Treatment of the peripheral lymphatics: rationale, indications, and techniques. In: Fletcher GH, Levitt SH, eds. Non-disseminated breast cancer: controversial issues in management. Berlin: Springer-Verlag, 1993.
5. Fowble B, Gray R, Gilchrist K, Goodman RL, Taylor S, Tormey DC. Identification of a subgroup of patients with breast cancer and histologically positive axillary nodes receiving adjuvant chemotherapy who may benefit from postoperative radiotherapy. J Clin Oncol 1988; 6:1107-1117.
6. Ragaz J, Jackson SM, Le N, et al. Adjuvant radiotherapy and chemotherapy in node-positive premenopausal women with breast cancer. N Engl J Med 1997;337:956-962.
7. Veronesi U, Rilke F, Luini A, et al. Distribution of axillary node metastases by level of invasion: an analysis of 539 cases. Cancer 1987;59: 682–687.
8. Ahern V, Barraclough B, Bosch C, Langlands A, Boyages J. Locally advanced breast cancer: defining an optimum treatment regimen. Int J Radiat Oncol Biol Phys 1994;28:867-875.
9. Auquier A, Rutqvist L, Höst H, Rotstein S, Arriagada R. Post-mastectomy megavoltage radiotherapy: the Oslo and Stockholm trials. Eur J Can 1992;28:433-437.
10. Cuzick J, Stewart H, Rutqvist L, et al. Cause-specific mortality in long-term survivors of breast cancer who participated in trials of radiotherapy. J Clin Oncol 1994;12:447-453.
11. Griem KL, Henderson IC, Gelman R, et al. The 5-year results of a randomized trial of adjuvant radiation therapy after chemotherapy in breast cancer patients treated with mastectomy. J Clin Oncol 1987; 5:1546-1555.
12. Gröhn P, Heinonen E, Klefström P, Tarkkanen J. Adjuvant postoperative radiotherapy, chemotherapy, and immunotherapy in Stage III breast cancer. Cancer 1984;54:670-674.
13. Klefstrom P, Grohn P, Heinonen E, Holsti L, Holsti P. Adjuvant postoperative radiotherapy, chemotherapy, and immunotherapy in stage III breast cancer: II, 5-year results and influence of levamisole. Cancer 1987;60:936-942.
14. Lê MG, Arriagada R, de Vathaire F, et al. Can internal mammary chain treatment decrease the risk of death for patients with medical breast cancer and positive axillary lymph nodes? Cancer 1990;66:2313-2318.
15. Levitt SH, Potish RA, Lindgren B. Assessing the role of adjuvant radiation therapy in the treatment of breast cancer. Int J Radiat Oncol Biol Phys 1988;15:787-790.
16. Levitt S. The importance of locoregional control in the treatment of breast cancer and its impact on survival. Cancer 1994;74:1840-1846.
17. Overgaard M, Hansen PS, Overgaard J, et al. Postoperative radiotherapy in high-risk premenopausal women with breast cancer who receive adjuvant chemotherapy. Danish Breast Cancer Cooperative Group 82b Trial. N Engl J Med 1997;237:949-966.
18. Pierce LJ, Lippman M, Ben-Baruch N, et al. Local-regional recurrence in breast cancer after mastectomy and adriamycin-based adjuvant chemotherapy: evaluation of the role of postoperative radiotherapy. Int J Radiat Oncol Biol Phys 1992;23:949-960.

19. Pierce LJ, Lichter AS. Postmastectomy radiotherapy: more than locoregional control. J Clin Oncol 1994;12:444-446.
20. Sykes HF, Sim DA, Wong CJ, Cassady JR, Salmon SE. Local-regional recurrence in breast cancer after mastectomy and adriamycin-based adjuvant chemotherapy: evaluation of the role of postoperative radiotherapy. Int J Radiat Oncol Biol Phys 1989;16:641-647.
21. Fletcher GH, Montague ED. Does adequate irradiation of the internal mammary chain and supraclavicular nodes improve survival rates? Int J Radiat Oncol Biol Phys 1978;4:481.
22. Fletcher GH, Montague ED, Tapley, N duV, Barker, JL. Radiotherapy in the management of nondisseminated breast cancer. In: Fletcher GH, ed. Textbook of radiotherapy. Philadelphia: Lea & Febiger, 1980: 527–579.
23. Janjan N, Gillin M, Prows J, et al. Dose to the cardiac vascular and conduction systems in primary breast irradiation [published erratum appears in Med Dosim 1989;14(4):305]. Med Dosim 1989;14:81-87.
24. Rutqvist LE, Lax I, Fornander T, Johansson H. Cardiovascular mortality in a randomized trial of adjuvant radiation therapy versus surgery alone in primary breast cancer. Int J Radiat Oncol Biol Phys 1992; 22:887-896.
25. Chu JC, Solin LJ, Hwang CC, Fowble B, Hanks GE, Goodman RL. A nondivergent three field matching technique for breast irradiation. Int J Radiat Oncol Biol Phys 1990;19:1037-1040.
26. McNeese MD, Fletcher GH, Levitt SH, Khan FM. Breast cancer. In: Levitt SH, Khan FM, Potish RA, eds. Levitt and Tapley's technological basis of radiation therapy: practical clinical applications. Philadelphia: Lea and Febiger, 1992:232–247.
27. Montague ED, Spanos WJ Jr, Ames FC, et al. Conservative treatment of states I and II breast cancer. In: Feig SA, McLelland R, eds. Breast carcinoma: current diagnosis and treatment. Philadelphia: J.B. Lippincott, 1983:439–443.
28. Montague ED, Spanos WJ Jr, Ames FC, et al. Conservative treatment of noninvasive and small-volume invasive breast cancer. In: Geig SA, McLelland R, eds. Breast carcinoma: current diagnosis and treatment. New York: Masson, 1983:429–432.
29. Hiramatsu H, Bornstein BA, Recht A, et al. Local recurrence after conservative surgery and radiation therapy for ductal carcinoma in situ. Cancer J Sci Am 1995;1:55.
30. Renton SC, Gazet JC, Ford HT, Corbishley C, Sutcliffe R. The importance of the resection margin in conservative surgery for breast cancer. Eur J Surg Oncol 1996;22:17-22.
31. Holland R, Connolly JL, Gelman R, et al. The presence of an extensive intraductal component following a limited excision correlates with prominent residual disease in the remainder of the breast. J Clin Oncol 1990;8:113-118.
32. Hurd TC, Sneige N, Allen PK, et al. Impact of extensive intraductal component on recurrence and survival in patients with stage I or II breast cancer treated with breast conservation therapy. Ann Surg Oncol 1997;4:119-124.
33. Schnitt SJ, Abner A, Gelman R, et al. The relationship between microscopic margins of resection and the risk of local recurrence in patients with breast cancer treated with breast-conserving surgery and radiation therapy. Cancer 1994;74:1746-1751.
34. van Dongen JA, Bartelink H, Fentiman IS, et al. Factors influencing local relapse and survival and results of salvage treatment after breast-conserving therapy in operable breast cancer: EORTC trial 10801, breast conservation compared with mastectomy in TNM stage I and II breast cancer. Eur J Cancer 1992;801-805.
35. Veronesi U, Luini A, Del Vecchio M, et al. Radiotherapy after breast-preserving surgery in women with localized cancer of the breast [see comments]. N Engl J Med 1993;328:1587-1591.

Chapter 18

Carcinoma of the Lung and Esophagus

Mary V. Graham

BRONCHOGENIC CARCINOMA OF THE LUNG

Lung cancer will be diagnosed in approximately 171,000 persons in the United States in 1998 (1). Despite technologic advances that have resulted in improved diagnostics and therapy, the overall cure rate of patients with lung cancer is still disappointingly low (less than 15% at 5 years) (1–3). Recent reports, however, cite progress in certain subsets of patients with therapeutic approaches involving a combination of methods (4–9).

Anatomy

The right lung is composed of the upper, middle, and lower lobes, which are separated by the oblique or major and the horizontal or minor fissures. The left lung is composed of two lobes separateded by a single fissure. The lingular portion of the left upper lobe corresponds to the middle lobe on the right. The trachea enters the superior mediastinum and bifurcates approximately at the level of the fifth thoracic vertebra. The hila contain the bronchi, pulmonary arteries, and veins, various branches from the pulmonary plexus, bronchial arteries and veins, and lymphatics.

The lung has a rich network of lymphatic vessels throughout its loose interstitial connective tissue, ultimately draining into various lymph node stations: the intrapulmonary lymph nodes, along the secondary bronchi, or in the bifurcation of branches of the pulmonary artery; the bronchopulmonary lymph nodes, situated either alongside the lower portions of the main bronchi (hilar lymph nodes) or at the bifurcations of the main bronchi into lobar bronchi (interlobar nodes); the mediastinal lymph nodes, which are divided in the superior, above the bifurcation of the trachea (carina), including the upper paratracheal, pretracheal, retrotracheal, and lower paratracheal nodes (azygos nodes), and a group of nodes located in the aortic window and the inferior, situated in the subcarinal region and inferior mediastinum, including the subcarinal, paraesophageal, and pulmonary ligament nodes (Figure 18.1).

Lymph from the right upper lobe flows to the hilar and tracheobronchial lymph nodes. Lymph from the left upper lobe flows to the venous angle of the same side and to the right superior mediastinum. The right and left lower lobe lymphatics drain into the inferior mediastinal and subcarinal nodes and from there to the right superior mediastinum (left lower lobe also may drain into left superior mediastinum).

Natural History and Pathologic Features

Bronchogenic carcinoma usually originates in secondary to tertiary bronchial divisions or, in the case of adenocarcinoma, in the periphery of the lung. Even before the tumor has reached a clinically detectable size, invasion of the regional lymphatics and the blood vessels may occur, resulting in widespread lymphatic and hematogenous dissemination (10). The pattern of spread in lung cancer may be divided into three different pathways: 1) local (intrathoracic), 2) regional (lymphatic), and 3) distant (hematogenous). The pattern of lymphatic spread of lung cancer is shown in Figure 18.2. This information is important in designing radiation therapy portals. Ipsilateral hilar node metastasis occurs in between 50 and 60% of patients (11,12,13). Mediastinal adenopathy is noted in 40 to 50% of operative specimens (6). Metastasis to the scalene (supraclavicular) nodes is predominantly from primary sites in ipsilateral upper lobes or from superior mediastinal lesions (Table 18.1). Many patients with lung cancer, and most of those with advanced disease, have distant metastasis (10). Matthews et al., however, studied a group of 131 patients with epidermoid carcinoma of the lung; autopsies were

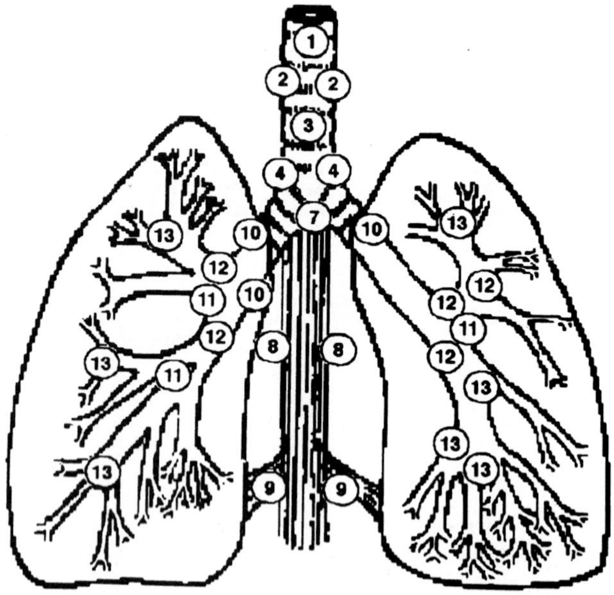

Figure 18.1. Sites of lymph nodes in lungs and mediastinum. N2 nodes include the superior and inferior mediastinal nodes and the aortic nodes. Superior mediastinal nodes: 1, highest mediastinal; 2, upper paratracheal, 3, pretracheal and retrotracheal; 4, lower paratracheal (including azygous nodes). Aortic nodes: 5, subaortic (aortic window); 6, paraaortic (ascending aorta or phrenic). Inferior mediastinal node. 7, subcarinal; 8, paraesophageal (below carina); 9, pulmonary ligament. N1 nodes: 10, hilar; 11, interlobar; 12, lobar; 13, segmental (proximal). NO node 14 and 15, segmental (distal). (Reprinted with permission from Emami B, Graham MV. Lung. In: Perez CA, Brady LW, eds. Principles and practice of radiation oncology, 3rd ed. Philadelphia: Lippincott-Raven, 1998:1181-1220.)

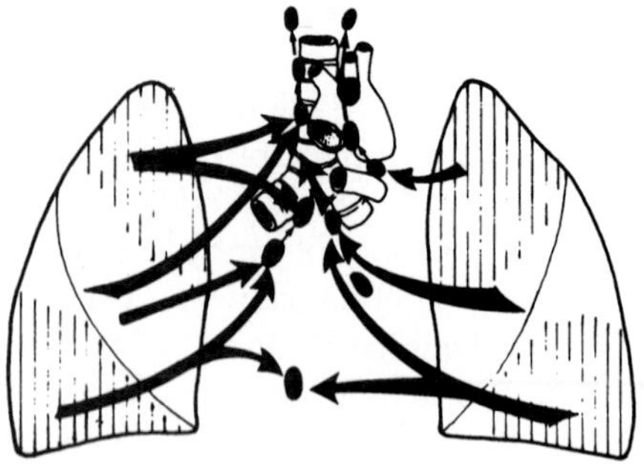

Figure 18.2. Lymphatic drainage of various lobes of lung. Almost all lobes drain to subcarinal nodes and then the right superior mediastinum.

performed within 30 days after curative surgical procedures. Forty-four patients had persistent disease, but only 22 (50%) had distant metastasis (14). Further, two large clinical trials of chemotherapy and radiotherapy for inoperable lung cancer documented local failure or persistence of tumor in 85–90% of patients, while documenting distant metastasis in only 40–45% (5,15). This limited spread be-

Table 18.1. Supraclavicular Nodal Metastasis in Lung Cancer

	Incidence of Supraclavicular Nodal Involvement	
Primary Site	Right	Left
Right upper lobe	31.0% (11–37.5%)[a]	8.5% (0.1–10%)
Right middle lobe	2.0% (2–9%)	1.0% (0–7%)
Right lower lobe	7.0% (0.4–7%)	0.5% (0–3.5%)
Left upper lobe	1.7% (0–9%)	17.0% (12–32%)
Lingula	1.0% (0–7%)	0.5% (0–3.5%)
Left lower lobe	2.0% (0–5%)	4.5% (0–7%)

[a] Numbers in parentheses are the lowest and highest reported in the literature. (Data from Baird JA. The pathways of lymphatic spread of carcinoma of the lung. Br J Surg 1965;52:868; Brantigan OC, Moszkowski E. Bilateral biopsy of non-palpable cervical lymph nodes. Diagnosis and prognosis of carcinoma of the lung. Dis Chest 1966;50:464; Emami B, Perez CA. Carcinoma of the lung. In: Brady L, Perez CA, eds. Principles and practice of radiation oncology. Philadelphia JB Lippincott, 1987.)

comes a compelling argument for more aggressive surgical or radiotherapeutic management of patients with clinically localized bronchogenic carcinoma. Also, to increase the cure rates in these patients, effective systemic adjuvant therapy to control metastasis is needed.

The pathologic classification of carcinoma of the lung is broadly divided into non-small cell (80%) and small cell (20%) categories, based on the natural histories and differing common presentations. Untreated small cell lung cancer is rapidly metastatic and fatal; indeed two-thirds of patients present with metastatic disease. The remaining minority (approximately one-third) usually present with bulky centrally-located tumors confined to the chest. Currently, the staging of small cell lung cancer is either extensive or limited, respectively.

The majority of lung cancer patients have non-small cell lung cancer. This is divided into pathologic subcategories of squamous cell carcinoma, adenocarcinoma, large cell carcinoma, undifferentiated and unspecified. These pathologic subcategories do not currently significantly impact on treatment choice decision making. Treatment for non-small cell lung cancer should be made based on the TNM staging, performance status, absence or presence of weight loss, and operability. These factors have significant prognostic importance (16,17).

Staging

It is critical that one identify those patients in whom local control by irradiation is possible from those with advanced disease for whom palliation is the only goal. All patients must be staged according to the extent of disease. The American Joint Committee on cancer staging has recently revised the TNM classifications, originally proposed by Mountain (18,19), which was primarily based on surgical findings (20).

Table 18.2. TNM Classification of Carcinoma of the Lung

Primary Tumor (T)

- TX Primary tumor cannot be assessed, or tumor proven by presence of malignant cells in sputum or bronchial washings but not visualized by imaging or bronchoscopy
- TO No evidence of primary tumor
- Tis Carcinoma in situ
- T1 Tumor 3 cm or less in greatest dimension, surrounded by lung or visceral pleura, without bronchoscopic evidence of invasion more proximal than the lobar bronchus
- T2 Tumor with any of the following features of size or extent:
  - More than 3 cm in greatest dimension
  - Involves main bronchus, 2 cm or more distal to the carina
  - Invades the visceral pleura
  - Associated with atelectasis or obstructive pneumonitis that extends to the hilar region but does not involve the entire lung
- T3 Tumor of any size that directly invades any of the following: chest wall (including superior sulcus tumors), diaphragm, mediastinal pleura, parietal pericardium; or tumor in the main bronchus less than 2 cm distal to the carina but without involvement of the carina; or associated atelectasis or obstructive pneumonitis of the entire lung
- T4 Tumor of any size that invades any of the following: mediastinum, heart, great vessels, trachea, esophagus, vertebral body, carina, or separate tumor nodules in the same lobe; or tumor with a malignant pleura

Lymph Node (N)

- NX Regional lymph nodes cannot be assessed
- NO No regional lymph node metastasis
- N1 Metastasis to ipsilateral peribronchial and/or ipsilateral hilar lymph nodes, and intrapulmonary nodes involved by direct extension of the primary tumor
- N2 Metastasis in ipsilateral mediastinal and/or subcarinal lymph node(s)
- N3 Metastasis in contralateral mediastinal, contralateral hilar, ipsilateral or contralateral scalene or supraclavicular lymph node(s)

Distant Metastases (M)

- MX Presence of distant metastasis cannot be assessed
- MO No distant metastasis
- M1 Distant metastasis

Major changes in the 1998 staging include the subdivisions of stage IA and IB based on primary tumor size, and IIA and IIB with the inclusion of T3NO patients among stage IIB. Staging grouping by T, N, and M with five-year survivals are shown in Tables 18.2 and 18.3. It should be noted that the survival results of the new staging system are based primarily upon surgical staging and treatment. Patient outcome and survival may be significantly affected by surgical procedure and additional combined modality therapy (21–23).

General Management of Non-Small Cell Lung Cancer (NSCLC)

The generally accepted treatments of choice by stage are shown in Table 18.4. All newly diagnosed patients

Table 18.3. 1998 AJCC Staging and 5-Year Survival

Overall Stage	T	N	M	5-Year Survival (%) (as read from survival curve)
0	Tis	NO	MO	—
IA	T1	NO	MO	60–70%
IB	T2	NO	MO	~40%
IIA	T1	N1	MO	~35%
IIB	T2	N1	MO	25–35%
	T3	NO	MO	
IIIA	T1	N2	MO	~10%
	T2	N2	MO	
	T3	N1–2	MO	
IIIB	T1–4	N3	MO	~5%
	T4	NO–3	MO	
IV	Any T	Any N	M1	~2%

(Adapted from: Mountain CF, Libshitz HF, Hermes KE. In: Clifton F, ed. Lung cancer handbook for staging and imaging, 2nd ed. Houston: Mountain Foundation, 1997.)

should be evaluated for surgical resection. However, it is estimated that only about 20% of all newly diagnosed patients will be appropriate for surgical resection based on stage and/or medical inoperability secondary to comorbid disease(s).

Definitive radiation therapy is an appropriate alternative to surgery for early stage patients who have medical contraindications to surgery. Several series have reported three-year survivals of 17% to 55% (24–31). Recent studies support the treatment of the primary tumor only (no elective nodal therapy) to doses of ≥65 Gy, conventionally fractionated (32–34).

For stage IIIA patients who have a good performance status and absence of weight loss, the standard of care is chemotherapy and radiation therapy ± surgical resection (4,6,7,9). Controversy still revolves around which chemotherapeutic agents to use (such as cisplatin-based, Taxol-based, Taxotere, Gemcitibine), how to combine them with radiation (sequential versus concurrent), and the role of surgical resection. We await the results of well-designed prospective randomized studies to sort out these issues.

The role of postoperative radiation therapy has been diminishing because randomized trials have failed to show a survival advantage. However, none of the trials reported to date have had the statistical power to prove or disprove a survival effect in N2 patients (35,36). Many have shown a significant local tumor control and disease-free survival improvement (35,36). The RTOG recently completed a comparison of postradiation therapy versus postoperative radiation therapy + cisplatin and VP-16 for N1 and N2 patients. The results of this study have not yet been reported. We recommend postoperative radiation therapy to all completely resected patients with N2 disease, and/or positive margins and T3 or T4 tumors.

Table 18.4. Accepted Treatment Options

Stage	Treatment of Choice	Alternative Treatment	Experimental Treatment
IA	Surgical resection (lobectomy)	Definitive radiation	Adjuvant chemotherapy before or after surgery
IB	Surgical resection (lobectomy)	Definitive radiation therapy	Chemotherapy before or after surgery
IIA	Surgical resection (lobectomy)	Definitive radiation therapy	Chemotherapy before or after surgery
IIB	Surgical resection (lobectomy) ± postop RT	Definitive radiation therapy	Chemotherapy before or after surgery
IIIA	Chemotherapy + RT	Surgical resection with postop RT or CT-RT (selected patients)	• Altered fractionation RT ± CT • Chemotherapy + RT + surgical resection
IIIB	Chemotherapy + RT	CT-RT-Surgery (selected patients)	
IV	Chemotherapy	Supportive care palliative RT, surgical resection (selected patients)	Experimental chemotherapy

Definitive Radiation Therapy

Central issues regarding definitive radiation therapy are 1) selection of appropriate patients, and 2) treatment planning considerations, which include optimal tumor dose, fractionation, and volume to be irradiated. Major additional issues are the integration and timing of irradiation with chemotherapy and surgery, and how the radiation therapy may need to be altered in combination with other modalities.

Patient Selection

Virtually any stage patient may be appropriately referred for radiation therapy. The first determination should be whether they are candidates for palliation or definitive treatment. Palliative patients are those thought to have a survival of less than 6 to 12 months. These people should be treated with the minimal effective dose to relieve a symptom(s) (37,38). Patients with early stage (I-II) NSCLC but who are medically inoperable, should be treated with definitive radiation therapy (8,24,26,27,29,31,39). Patients with stage IIIA/B with a KPS of ≥70 and <5% weight loss may also be treated definitively. Their median survival may be 14 to 20 months (6,40) and up to 20% may survive longer than 5 years.

Treatment Planning

The treatment of cancer of the lung with radiation is complex. Errors in dose delivery or portal design resulting in inadequate coverage of the primary tumor and the potential area of spread will decrease significantly the probability of tumor control and survival. It is important to pay critical attention to the details of the radiotherapeutic techniques and dose delivery to ensure maximum dosage to the tumor, adequate coverage of the tumor and potentially high risk areas, and finally, a minimum dose of radiation to normal structures, especially critical structures. Sophisticated treatment plans utilizing shaped fields, compensating filters, angled beams, and patient repositioning aids are required to deliver high doses of radiation to the tumor while keeping the normal structures below tolerance levels. Optimizing such treatment plans is difficult for several reasons: 1) difficulty in delineating the target volume; 2) proximity of sensitive structures (spinal cord, heart, and lung) to the tumor; 3) sloping surface of the chest with decreased diameter at the thoracic inlet; 4) presence of tissues with nonuniform densities, such as lung and bone, in the treatment volume; 5) frequent requirement for irregular field dose calculations; and 6) motion of the target and normal structures (i.e., heart and lung) associated with respiration. The standard of care requires that delineation of target volume be performed with computed tomography (CT) imaging for all but the most palliative of patients, in whom a simulation chest x-ray may suffice. There has been an explosion of available technology to the radiation oncologist that facilitate the process by which CT data is analyzed and converted into radiation targets and portals. Radiation oncologists are called upon to have an increased ability to interpret CT data and define tumor targets versus normal anatomy on CT images (41). Newer imaging modalities may have increasing importance in the delineation of tumor including positron-emission tomography (PET) and ventilation perfusion scans (42,43).

Emami et al. published a consensus opinion on radiation tolerance doses and volumes based upon clinical experience (32). Since that time, several authors have reported their experience with lung tolerance to radiation therapy and the development of pneumonitis (44–49).

Martel et al. (49) described the stratification of patients for their development of pneumonitis on the effective volume (V_{eff}) and normal tissue complication probability (NTCP) from lung dose volume histograms (49). Their data was subsequently confirmed by Oetzel et al (50). Graham et al. reported the percent volume of the total lung exceeding 20 Gy to be the best predictor of the development of pneumonitis (45,46). Marks similarly reported the V_{30} (% volume > 30 Gy) to be most predictive of the development of pneumonitis (48). Kwa et al. related the incidence of pneumonitis with the total lung mean dose (47). Each of these parameters gives clinicians newer guidelines to use and develop improved radiation treatment plans. In the future it is anticipated that there will be similar guidelines developed to guide clinicians with partial volume irradiation of esophagus, heart and possibly spinal cord. Until that time, conservative estimates of Emami et al. may guide clinicians in keeping doses to normal organs within tolerable limits (51). With traditional treatment planning, planners are cautioned to keep portals to ≤ 1.0–2.0 cm around the primary and nodal disease to keep toxicity within acceptable limits (52).

The choice of appropriate beam energies and loadings, are crucial to the delivery of adequate doses of irradiation to the tumor without producing injury to the adjacent normal tissues. Controversy weighs in the choice of beam energies in intrathoracic tumors (31,53–57). Because of the large diameter of most patients chest, many people prefer higher energy photons (≥10 MeV) for this population of patients. These energy photons allow reduced hot spots in the chest wall and surrounding critical other organs such as spinal cord and heart. However, the negative effects of the high energy photons may be several. High energy photons may have problems with equilibrium re-establishment (55,58). This may result in underdosing to periphery of tumor primaries within the low density parenchyma of the lung. High energy photons also result in a widened penumbra within low density lungs (53,59). This phenomenon may increase the risk of pneumonitis and not be reflected in current treatment planning isodose displays (60). Lastly, Yoke et al. (31) have demonstrated the effects of small fields for 10 MV where tumors have a 10% lower dose at the periphery versus the center. This problem is a result of the loss of electronic equilibrium of tumors embedded within the periphery of the lung, but is most significant when small field sizes are used. Klein et al. (59) recommended caution when applying corrections for lung cancer radiotherapy planned with 3D RTP. The authors reported overestimation of correction factors, especially at tumor borders. At Washington University, we initially prescribe dose and assess PTV coverage, on unit density planning, without heterogeneity corrections. Beam arrangement and irradiated organ doses are then interactively optimized using heterogeneity corrected isodoses.

An additional problem encountered in treatment planning for bronchogenic cancer is the sloping surface of the chest with decreased diameter at the thoracic inlet. The sloping surface of the chest results in varying source-tumor distances over the treatment field and produces a nonuniform dose distribution. One method of compensating for this problem is to use the decreasing-field technique or "poor man's wedge," which achieves an effective isodose distribution by decreasing the field size when a desired tumor dose is achieved at a given point. A disadvantage of its use is that it requires setups for varying field sizes, complicated prescriptions, and multiple calculations at various points.

The sloping-surface effect may be corrected by the use of compensating filters. Several of these devices have been described, and some are commercially available. At our institution, a Lucite step-wedge compensating filter is used routinely in the treatment of chest portals. This filter is relatively inexpensive and can be assembled easily. This device is, however, a special-purpose filter that compensates for only the midsagittal plane and for surfaces sloping in the cephalocaudad direction only.

A method of compensating for sloping surfaces and tissue heterogeneities over a volume was outlined by Ellis in 1960 (61). He indicated that information on the inhomogeneity of thoracic tissue (obtained by transverse axial tomography at several levels), when used in conjunction with the information derived from standard isodose curves for tumor dose beyond the inhomogeneity, could provide the basis for avoiding errors as large as 30% in dosage to the esophagus. This method, although sound in principle, is difficult in practice without adequate radiographic facilities and a mould-room staff. In a more recent report, Ellis and Lescrenier describe a technique in which film is used to measure transmitted-beam parameters on which the construction of individual compensators can be based (62). The method requires the use of diametrically opposed beams. A densitometer is used to monitor the photographic image of the high-energy treatment beam after passage through the patient; this device allows one to estimate the amount of matter traversed at each point, whether modified by surface irregularities or tissue inhomogeneities. By compensating for these variations, the entire tissue volume can be covered.

A 45 Gy tumor dose is relatively easy to deliver to the midplane of the mediastinum with AP-PA ports, particularly when high-energy beams are used, but special attention should be paid to the dose delivered to the spinal cord. In the past, it was common practice to decrease the spinal cord dose by inserting a 1.5- to 2-cm wide shielding block of the posterior port with varying degrees of thickness (1 to 5 HVL). Use of this technique should be abandoned because it reduces the dose delivered to the midplane of the mediastinum and thus underdoses the target for most lung and or esophageal tumors.

To adequately deliver tumoricidal doses to the mediastinum, oblique ports that spare the spinal cord are preferred. When the treatment plan indicates, wedges may be used (Figures 18.3 and 18.4). The radiation oncologist should be familiar with the anatomy of the chest in oblique-beam arrangements. A useful technique is to identify the volume of interest and outline the appropriate port under fluoroscopic conditions using the simulator on the AP projection. Once accomplished, the beam can be rotated with frequent fluoroscopic observation. The physi-

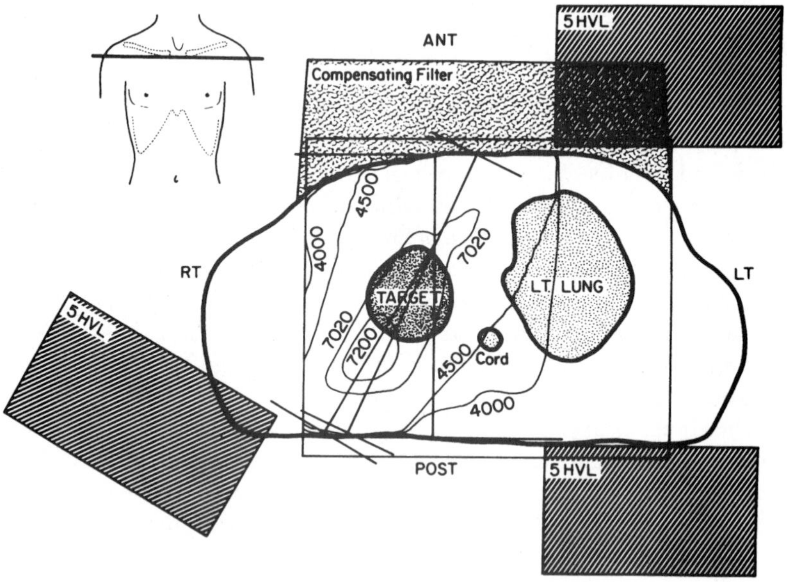

Figure 18.3. Optimized treatment plan for right lower lobe tumor.

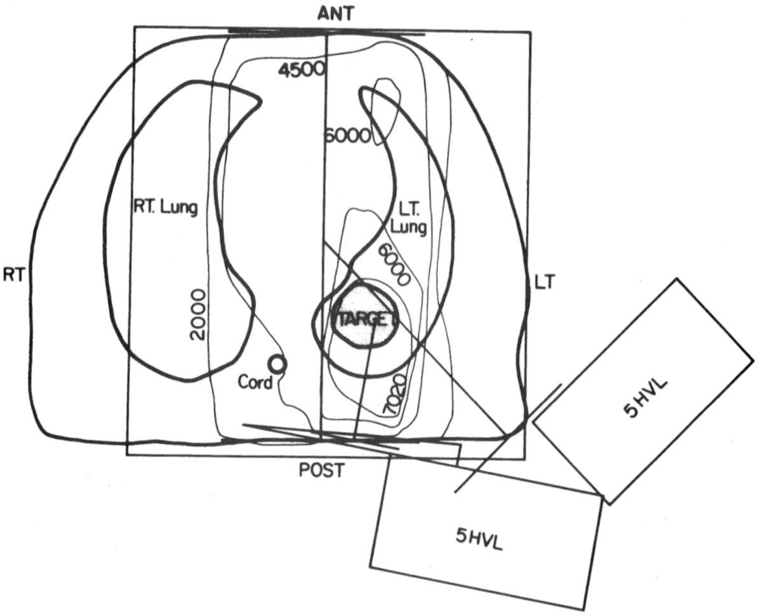

Figure 18.4. Optimized treatment plan for left lower lobe tumor.

cian can then observe the progressive distortion of the anatomy with the rotation of the beam. When using simulator films to block the spinal cord from oblique beams, placement of the field edge at the anterior border of the vertebral body pedicles allows sufficient margin to account for unexpected differences in positional variations (63). Sparing the spinal cord with oblique beams may also be easily accomplished using beam's eye view (BEV) with 3-D treatment systems.

The large, irregularly shaped treatment fields commonly used for carcinoma of the lung necessitate the calculation of dose by an approximation method or by using the scatter-calculations method described by Clarkson (64). Two commonly used approximation methods involve either a geometric approximation, in which the irregular treatment field is approximated by a rectangular field, or empirically determined correction factors, which give the variation of the treatment setup from a standard phantom setup. The accuracy of these approximations depends on the particular type of radiation unit, field size and shape used for measurement, and the points chosen for calculation.

Clarkson's more general approach using either scatter functions or scatter-air ratios has been explained in detail for manual calculations by Cundiff et al. (65) and Johns and Cunningham (66). With this approach, the dose to any point within the patient is calculated as a summation of the primary and scattered radiation contributions to that point. If the variation in source-skin distances and the variation of dose rate across the field are taken into consideration, the Clarkson method is reasonably accurate.

Tumor Dose Standard of treatment for patients with advanced disease localized to the chest and with good performance status should be treated with 65 to 70 cGy to the primary tumor, at least 60 cGy in 6 to 7 weeks to the regional nodes harboring gross disease seen on computed tomographic (CT) scans, and 50 cGy to other thoracic nodal regions in an effort to sterilize both the primary tumor and metastatic regional nodes. A critical relationship exists between the dose of radiation administered to the tumor and the probability of controlling the lesion.

Definitive doses of radiation therapy currently are approximately ≥66–70 Gy with conventional fractionation. However, the optimal dose of radiation for treatment of non-oat cell bronchogenic carcinoma has not been well defined. Considering the advanced status of lung cancer seen in patients treated in radiation therapy departments, modest doses of radiation are inadequate for tumor control. On the basis of basic principles advocated by Fletcher (67), an obvious conclusion is that doses in the range of 80 to 100 cGy would be required to sterilize tumors of the size frequently treated in bronchogenic carcinoma. Some authors, such as Salazar et al. (68), Choi and Doucette (2), Mantravadi et al. (69), and Perez and colleagues (70), have shown improved survival rates in patients receiving higher doses of radiation up to 3 years after radiation. Two retrospective studies have shown improved 5-year survival with ≥70 Gy/7 weeks versus lower doses (71,72).

In the 1970s, the Radiation Therapy Oncology Group (RTOG) conducted randomized studies in which different doses of radiation were investigated. Their results showed better 3-year survival rates (15%) with 60 Gy than with lower doses of radiation (40 or 50 Gy) (70). Intrathoracic failure rate was evaluated clinically 33% at 3 years for 60 Gy as compared with 42% for 50 Gy and 52% for patients receiving 40 Gy. Although 3-year survival rates and median survival were better with a higher dose of radiation, the 5-year survival rate for various radiation doses was not statistically significant.

Intrathoracic tumor control was associated with increased survival in patients surviving 6 or 12 months. In this group, radiation dose of 50 to 60 Gy resulted in a 3-year survival rate of 22% when intrathoracic tumor growth was controlled versus 10% if such attempts failed. Similar results for 40 Gy were 25% versus 5%. An interesting observation was the relation of tumor size with tumor control. In RTOG protocol 7301, tumors less than 3 cm in diameter had a tumor control of 60% as opposed to only 40% for larger lesions (73). These observations support the need for higher doses of radiation in order to control larger tumors, although this increase must be tempered by the effect of large doses of radiation on surrounding normal tissues and the possibilities of serious complications. In another RTOG study, with the use of CT scans, computerized treatment planning, and dose optimizations, it was possible to deliver 75 Gy in 28 fractions to the gross tumor while the normal tissue doses were limited to the tolerance level (74,75). Of 44 patients analyzed in this study, the tumor control was 38%.

The RTOG completed a large dose escalation trial with hyperfractionated radiotherapy (1.2 Gy BID). Total tumor doses ranged from 60 Gy to 79.2 Gy (76). In patients with good prognostic factors, 69.6 Gy emerged as a dose level with improved survival. Although the level of pneumonitis increased modestly with higher doses, the reason for lack of improvement with higher doses was never clearly delineated. In a follow-up randomized trial, 69.6 Gy (hyperfractionated) did *not* prove better (in terms of survival) compared to chemotherapy + 60 Gy/30 fx(9).

With the availability of 3-D treatment planning, the base of maximum tolerable *and* maximum benefit dose has again been raised. Several treatment planning studies have reported the feasibility of increasing doses to NSCLC without increasing toxicity (77–79). Graham et al. found that pneumonitis could be best predicted by dose volume histogram (DVH) analysis of the total lung volume (46,80). The percent volume of the total lung exceeding 20 Gy (V_{20}) has been highly predictive in assessing risk of pneumonitis and is the basis on which patients are stratified for an ongoing RTOG dose escalation trial. A similar trial based on the effective volume (V_{eff}) of Kutcher and Burman (81) is ongoing at the University of Michigan (82). At least two other dose escalation trials have also been initiated, one stratifies patients based on the lung NTCP (77) and the other upon the mean lung dose (47). The results of these trials should provide answers to the question of what is the optimal dose for NSCLC.

Fractionation Multiple daily fractions have been advocated for the delivery of higher doses of radiation to the tumor without enhancing morbidity in the normal tissue (83). Theoretically, repair of sublethal damage occurs between the fractions, when separated by 4 to 6 hours. Because the total dose of radiation is given in a shorter period of time, and higher doses can be delivered, a greater biologic effect is anticipated. The RTOG conducted a multi-institutional prospective dose-escalation study evaluating the effect of hyperfractionation (HFX) in tumor control and the survival of patients with non-small cell lung cancer(84). Fractions of 1.2 Gy were administered twice daily (at 4- to 6-hour intervals). Patients were randomized to escalating doses between 60 Gy to 79.2 Gy. Among 519 patients, 248 had favorable prognosis (performance status 70 to 100 and weight loss of less than 5%) and 271 had an unfavorable prognosis (performance status 50 to 69 or weight loss more than 5%). No significant difference in disease-free survival was found among the five arms in the group of patients with an unfavorable prognosis. Patients with a favorable prognosis showed significant benefit (P = .04) in survival and disease-free survival with 69.6 Gy compared to the lower total doses (median 14.8 months and 2-year survival of 33%). No further benefit was found with hyperfractionation at 7440 and 7920 Gy. There was an increased incidence of pneumonitis with higher doses though the differences did not achieve statistical significance. It is unclear why higher doses did not result in increased survival.

Subsequent to this large phase II trial the hyperfractionated regimen (69.6 Gy) was compared in a randomized fashion to 60 Gy/30 fx of chemotherapy followed by 60 Gy/30 fx (40). Although 69.6 Gy was slightly better than 60 Gy/30 fx it was inferior to chemotherapy/60 Gy RT. Currently, the RTOG is testing hyperfractionation with chemotherapy versus correctional fractionation plus chemotherapy.

Jeremic et al. (39) randomized 169 patients with stage IIIA NSCLC to investigate the maximum tolerable dose of chemotherapy with HFX radiation therapy. The authors found that the addition of carboplatin/etoposide chemotherapy and HFX RT (64.8 Gy) carried a high risk of acute and late complications. The local control and median survival, however, was statistically significantly improved in the concurrent chemotherapy plus HFX RT arm (P = .02).

Saunders et al. reported results of a large prospective trial of continuous hyperfractionated accelerated radiotherapy (CHART) versus conventional 60 Gy/30 fx for inoperable NSCLC. The CHART regimen delivery schema was 1.5 Gy three times daily for 36 fractions (total dose 54 Gy). This CHART regimen resulted in an improved overall 2 year survival (85). Subgroup analysis suggested the greatest benefit for squamous cell carcinoma primaries. However, the development of severe dysphagia was significantly increased (19% versus 3%).

The results of these recent altered fractionation regimens are substantial enough to warrant further evaluations including further dose escalation and combinations with modern chemotherapy.

Volume The volume of the chest to be treated with definitive radiotherapy has come under close scrutiny. Traditional portals are depicted in Figure 18.5. With three dimensional radiotherapy treatment planning systems and Beam's eye view (BEV) techniques the delineated of gross disease has improved (78) (Figure 18.6). Many have challenged the traditional ideas that electively irradiating the mediastinum and hilar lymph node is necessary (33,34). Ongoing dose escalation trials are proceeding with the exclusion of and any electively irradiated areas (15,82). Prospective studies are indicated to define whether and which electively irradiated regions are important to treat with radiation therapy.

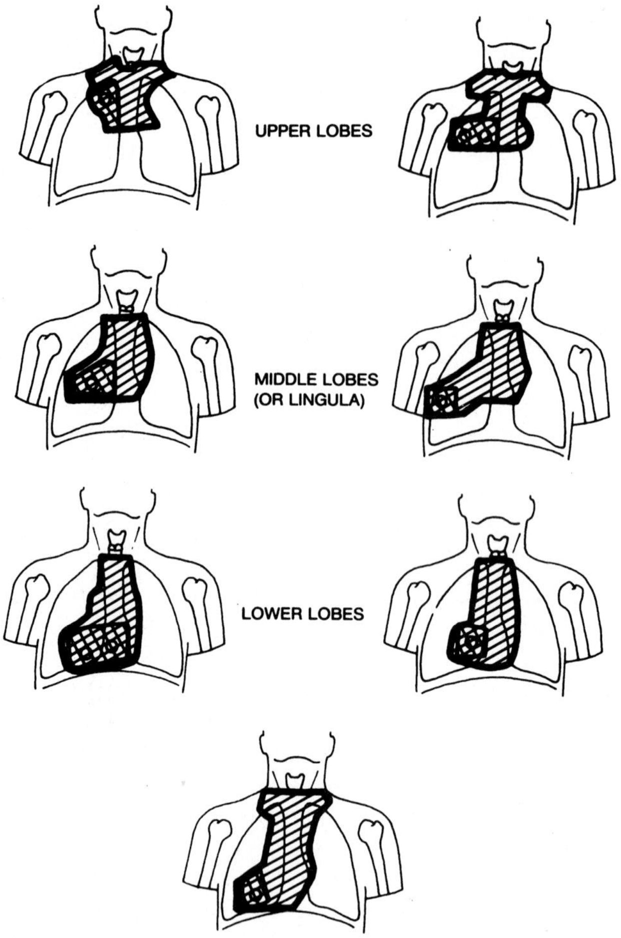

Figure 18.5. Portals used for irradiation of non-oat cell carcinoma of lung, depending on anatomic location of primary tumor. Tumor and grossly enlarged lymph nodes are treated to higher doses (cross-hatched area).

Integrating Radiation Therapy in Multimodality Treatment

Current management of most lung cancer patients is a multimodality effort. The combination of radiation therapy with chemotherapy and/or surgery requires the understanding of the potential gains and the expected potential for increased toxicity. When radiation therapy is combined with chemotherapy, improved survival has been demonstrated for stage IIIA and B patients (6,7,9). In the early trials that demonstrated benefit, the two modalities were employed sequentially (6,7,9). Toxicities increased when the two modalities were used, but not excessively. When chemotherapy and radiation therapy are given concurrently, there may be additional therapeutic benefit (39) but the toxicity increases also (42). The main toxicity that has often become dose limiting is esophagitis (86).

Hyperfractionation and accelerated fractionation with chemotherapy clearly increases acute toxicity—including esophageal, pulmonary, and spinal cord toxicities (87,88).

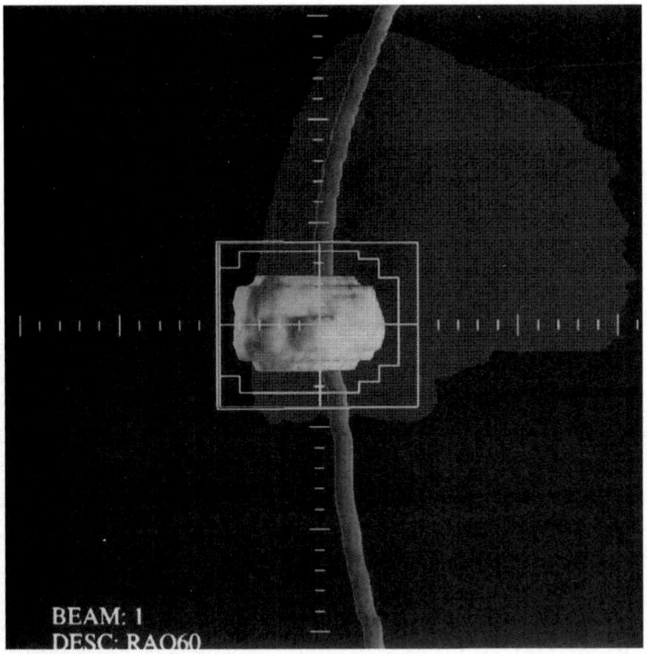

Figure 18.6. Nontraditional beam's eye view (BEV) portal for NSCLC for 3D CRT.

Further investigations into radiation therapy modifications are in order—including altered fractionation, 3-D treatment techniques, and various sequencing alternatives.

When radiation therapy has been used preoperatively with chemotherapy, the dose has usually been limited (≤50 Gy) in an effort to keep surgical complications at an acceptable rate (4). Altered fractionation may be used and may also improve efficacy but increases toxicity in this group of patients also (89,90).

As new chemotherapeutic agents are incorporated into multimodality regimens, the traditional parameters of radiation therapy dose, fractionation and volume will need to be addressed. Caution needs to be used as increased and unexpected toxicities may arise (91–95).

Postoperative radiation therapy has declined in popularity over the last few years because randomized trials to show a survival advantage (96,97). Postoperative radiation therapy to the mediastinum of 50–60 Gy is indicated to reduce loco-regional failures. This may be particularly important for resected patients, those with T3 or T4 primaries and patients with positive margins. Our recommendation is for 60–66 Gy to this later group of patients. None of the randomized trials to date have had the power to prove or disprove a survival advantage in this group of patients.

Patterns of Failure Perez et al. reported results of an early RTOG trial that the tumor failure rate within the irradiated volume was 48% with 40 Gy delivered continuously, 38% with 40 split course or 50 Gy continuously, and 27% with 60 Gy continuously (98). The failure rate in the nonirradiated lung ranged from 25 to 30% in various groups (99). The site of first failure, according to initial tumor stage, is shown in Table 18.5.

Table 18.5. Non-Oat Cell Carcinoma of the Lung: Anatomic Site of First Failure Correlated with Tumor Stage

Characteristic	Total Evaluable	Intrathoracic (%)	Intrathoracic and Distant Metastasis (%)	Distant Metastases (%)
T1–T2/N0	10	1 (0)	5 (50)	3 (30)
T3/N0	61	25 (41)	12 (20)	17 (28)
T4/N0	34	13 (38)	5 (15)	14 (41)
T–1,2,3/N1	59	26 (44)	13 (22)	19 (32)
T4/N1	27	8 (30)	8 (30)	11 (41)
T–1,2,3/N2	200	81 (40)	41 (21)	71 (36)
T4/N2	69	29 (42)	15 (22)	24 (35)
T4–1,2,3,/N3	65	40 (62)	10 (15)	13 (20)
T4/N3	26	14 (54)	5 (19)	6 (23)

(Reprinted with permission from: Perez CA, et al. Long-term observations of the patterns of failure in patients with unresectable non-oat cell carcinoma of the lung treated with definitive radiotherapy: Report by the Radiation Therapy Oncology Group. Cancer 1987;9:1874).

More sobering, however, were the results of trials where biopsy by bronchoscopy was required after combined chemotherapy and radiation therapy (65 Gy) (7). Local control was only 15 to 17%. In patients achieving complete or partial response, the incidence of brain metastasis was 16% for squamous cell carcinoma and 30 to 40% for adenocarcinoma and large-cell undifferentiated carcinoma. The frequency of brain metastasis suggests that, in non-oat cell carcinoma as in small cell carcinoma of the lung, elective radiation of the brain (PCI) may be necessary, if not to improve survival, to enhance the quality of life of those patients. However, the RTOG a large randomized trial of prophylactic cranial irradiation for inoperable adenocarcinoma and large cell lung carcinoma (100). No survival difference was observed between patients who did or did not receive prophylactic cranial irradiation. However, if local control improves (with better technology) and systemic control of metastasis improves (with chemotherapy), the tissue of PCI may need to be revisited.

Management of Small Cell Carcinoma

Role of Radiation Therapy

Radiation therapy has an important role in the curative treatment of limited stage small cell lung cancer (SCLC) (101–103). In extensive stage disease the role is limited to palliative treatment of symptomatic disease failing to respond to systemic therapy. In limited disease the central issues include: 1) thoracic radiation therapy, 2) dose, 3) fractionation, 4) treatment volume and timing with systemic therapy, and 5) prophylactic cranial irradiation (PCI).

Thoracic Radiotherapy (TRT)

In the 1970s and 1980s, several small phase III trials compared chemotherapy (CT) alone versus TRT plus CT (101,104–108). The small size of the trials resulted in unclear benefit and small differences in outcome. In 1992, two meta-analyses were published and both concluded that the addition of TRT to systemic therapy resulted in improved local control and overall survival compared to systemic chemotherapy alone (109,110). Pignon et al. reported an improved 3-year survival for 14.3% with CT plus TRT versus 8.9% with CT alone. Local control is also improved with TRT plus CT. Perry et al. (105), reported 50% 3-year actuarial local control with 50 Gy concurrent TRT versus 10% without TRT.

Dose

Choi and Carey (111) in a retrospective review reported only 50% local control with 30 to 35 Gy and 70% local control with doses of 40 to 50 Gy. These data suffer from their retrospective nature and inherent biases of patient selection, era of treatment, etc. Perry et al. reported 3-year actuarial local control notes of only 50% with 50 Gy TRT. The NCI trial reported by Coy et al. reported delayed time to intrathoracic future with higher doses, but *not* ultimate local control (112). Twenty-five Gy/10 fx resulted in only 20% 2-year local control. The Aarhus Lung Cancer Group (110) compared 40 Gy versus 45 Gy (prospectively, but not randomized to this parameter) with chemotherapy interdigitated with early versus late TRT. They reported local infield recurrence rates at 2 years of 60% and 70%, respectively. Perry et al. (105) reported similar local failure rates with 50 Gy TRT. Common practice of the era used posterior spinal cord blocks to protect the spinal cord, though it is clear this resulted in underdosing to the mediastinum and probably tumor. This practice is no longer considered acceptable. The results of these reports plus those of accelerated fractionation, suggest still rather high local failure patterns and that there may be further benefit to dose escalation trials in the future.

Fractionation

Laboratory studies have suggested typical SCLC cell lines have radiation survival curves with little to no shoulders and have suggested that accelerated fractionation schemas would, therefore, be advantageous. Several phase II trials combining BID TRT with cisplatin and etoposide were performed. The favored regimen administered 45 Gy/30 fractions. Median survivals of 18 to 27 months were reported with 2-year survivals of 19 to 60% (113–118). A multi-institutional trial compared cisplatin/etoposide (4 cycles) with once daily TRT (45 Gy/35 fx/5 weeks) versus TRT 45 Gy (30 fx/3 weeks)(88). Local control appeared significantly improved in the BID TRT regimen. Both study arms resulted in a 40% 2-year overall survival. The accelerated fractionation regimen showed a trend toward improved survival, but at the cost of increased esophageal complications.

Treatment Volume and Timing With Systemic Therapy

The issue of early (and concurrent) TRT with CT versus delayed (until after CT completed) versus interdigitated is hotly debated and no clear directive is available (40,105,110,119–123). Table 18.6 summarizes the compar-

Table 18.6. Trials Addressing Early Versus Delayed TRT

Institution (ref)	TRT	MST (months)	2-Year Survival	Is early TRT better?
Danish Cancer Society (110)	Early wk 1 (40–45 Gy split),	10.5	20	NO
	Late wk 18 (40–45 Gy split)	12.0	19	
CALGB (105)	50 Gy/6 wks (day 1)	13.1	15	NO
	50 Gy/6 wk (day 64)	14.6	25	
NCIC (121)	40 Gy/15 fx/3 wk (1st PE cycle)	16	25 (4 yr)	YES
	40 Gy 15 fx/3 wks (3rd PE cycle)	12.2	15 (4 yr)	
Shultz (123)	TRT (40 Gy/22 fx/4.5 Gy) day 1 vs day 120	10.7	NR	NO
	(45 Gy/22 fx/split course)	12.9	NR	
Japanese Clinical Oncology Group (122)	TRT (1st cycle PE)	31.3	NR	YES
	TRT (4th cycle PE)	20.8	NR	
Jeremic (119)	54 Gy/36 fx/3.6 wk			YES
	TRT wk 1–4	34	30% (5 yr)	
	TRT wk 6–9	26	15% (5 yr)	

TRT, thoracic radiation therapy, MST, median survival time; PE, cisplatin-etoposide chemotherapy; NR, not reported.

ison trials of early versus late TRT in limited stage SCLC. Three trials reported a survival benefit, but not necessarily local control advantage (one did not report local control, the other showed no difference), which raises the issue of the mechanism by which early TRT conveys a survival benefit. Three trials reported no survival advantage. Murray et al. (121) has proposed that accelerated repopulation and the emergence of drug resistant clones occur with late TRT and that early TRT mitigates this occurrence. Similar good survival results (40–50% 2 year survival) with BID early AHFRT TRT regimens (119) is the one randomized study of early versus late accelerated, hyperfractionated TRT and it strongly supports early TRT.

If TRT is delayed until after chemotherapy, the issue arises of whether to treat the prechemotherapy volume of disease versus the smaller postchemotherapy volume. Some authors advocate generous portals that would include the primary with generous margins as well as both hilar regions, the entire mediastinum, and both supraclavicular areas. Other authors, however, argue that only limited portals encompassing the prechemotherapy primary tumor with a 1-cm margin and high risk nodal areas are adequate, because effective chemotherapy takes care of subclinical or microscopic and thus eliminates the need for generous portals. Moreover, the use of limited portals may reduce complications resulting from a combined therapeutic approach with radiation and chemotherapy. The Southwest Oncology Group (SWOG) addressed this question in the only randomized trial of its nature. Patients achieving a partial response without CT were randomized to initial versus postchemotherapy volume (104). No benefit was seen for the larger target volume. In a retrospective review, Liengswangwong et al. found no benefit to larger volume TRT and no negative impact on survival to postchemotherapy TRT volumes (124). A typical AP port for early treatment of SCLC is shown in (Figure 18.7).

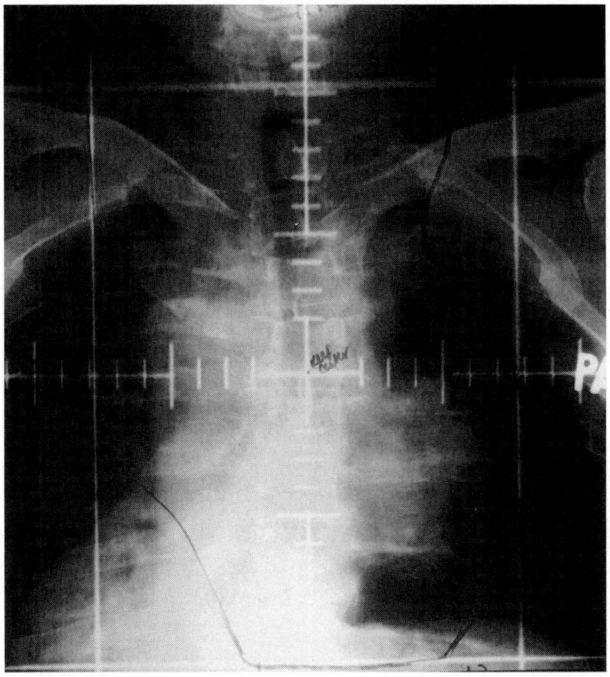

Figure 18.7. Traditional small cell portal.

Prophylactic Cranial Irradiation (PCI)

The issue of whether or not to prophylactically treat the brain of SCLC patients has been hotly debated for many years. The primary concern is that the brain remains a very common site of failure, particularly for complete responders. The risk of brain metastasis for 2 year survivors may be as high as 80% (125). PCI reduces the brain failure rate but has never shown any survival advantage (126,127). Much of the controversy centers about in neuropsychological sequelae after PCI in long term survivors (128). The frequency of mental deterioration including memory deficits, cognitive decline and language difficulties was reported in as many as 86% of survivors living 6 to 13 years after treatment (129). Retrospective studies have reported late neurologic abnormalities ranging from 19% (130) to 63% (131). However, Komaki et al (132) reported fully 97% of patients with small cell lung cancer demonstrated evidence of cognitive dysfunction *prior* to PCI including impairment of memory, frontal lobe dysfunction and fine motor coordination raising the question of whether the PCI causes neurologic dysfunction *or* the underlying small cell lung cancer disease. The authors further commented that with follow-up of 6 to 20 months, no significant neurologic deterioration in 30 patients receiving PCI were seen. Two recent large randomized prospective trials were both concluded that modern therapy with PCI is indicated. The first by Ohonshi et al (133) randomized 46 patients with SCLC who achieved a complete response to receive PCI or not. With a median follow-up of 8.5 years the incidence of brain metastases was 22% for the PCI group versus 52% for those receiving no PCI. In addition, 5-year survival was better for the PCI group (22% versus 13%, $P = .097$). They reported infrequent late neurological toxicity.

In a larger trial of 314 SCLC patients (134) with complete response to induction therapy, PCI again significantly reduced the incidence of brain metastasis but not overall survival. While there was evidence of cognitive impairment after treatment, there was no difference between patients receiving PCI or not.

Doses of PCI range from 8 Gy in a single fraction to 36 Gy in 18 fractions. There currently seems to be no consensus on what is the best dose nor if there is any clear relationship between hypofractionated regimens or total dose and neurologic sequelae.

Sequelae

Acute and late side effects of combined chemotherapy and concurrent and hyperfractionated thoracic radiation therapy can be considerable. High grade, severe acute esophagitis occurs in approximately 27%. Dose limiting neutropenia occurs in approximately 17 to 24% (119,135). Symptomatic pneumonitis occurs in approximately 4%. Late sequelae of symptomatic pulmonary fibrosis, esophageal stricture, pleural effusion, myelopathy appear to be less than 0.5 to 1%.

CARCINOMA OF THE ESOPHAGUS

New cases of carcinoma of the esophagus are expected to total 12,300 in the United States in 1998. An estimated 11,900 patients will die (1). This is approximately 1% of new cases and 2% of cancer deaths. There are no significant differences between the races and death rates or stage at diagnosis for esophageal cancer (1).

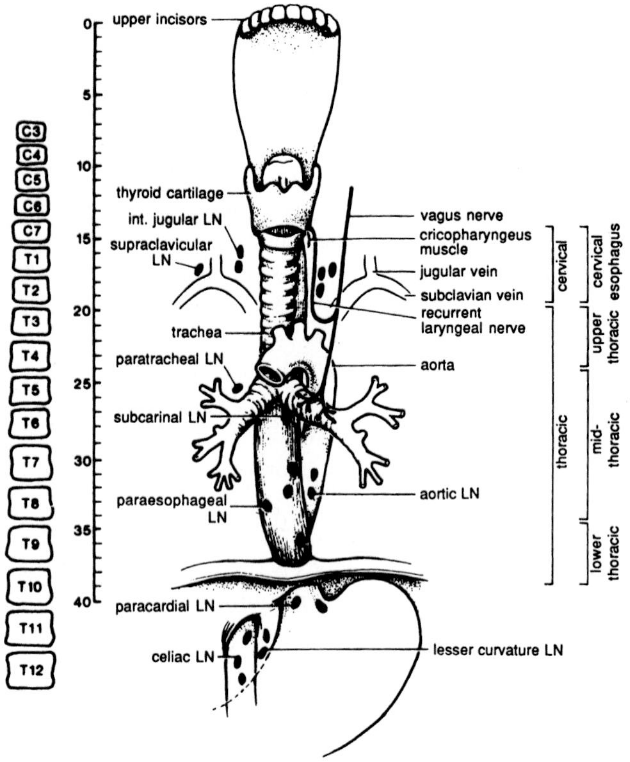

Figure 18.8. Basic anatomy of the esophagus. Note the lengths of the various segments of the esophagus from the upper central lesions and the two classification schemes for subdividing the esophagus. LN, lymph node. (Reprinted with permission from Emami B, Graham MV. Lung. In: Perez CA, Brady LW, eds. Principles and practice of radiation oncology, 3rd ed. Philadelphia: Lippincott-Raven, 1998:1181-1220.)

Anatomy

The esophagus is a thin-walled, hollow tube with an average length of 25 cm. The normal esophagus is lined with stratified squamous epithelium similar to the buccal mucosa. There are many methods of subdividing the esophagus, all of which are arbitrary. The cervical esophagus begins at the cricopharyngeal muscle (C7) and extends to the thoracic inlet (T3). The thoracic esophagus represents the remainder of the organ, going from T3 to T10 or T11.

The American Joint Committee (AJC) divides the esophagus into four regions: cervical, upper thoracic, midthoracic, and lower thoracic (Figure 18.8) correlates the basic anatomy of the esophagus with the subdivision schemes described above. The esophagus has a dual longitudinal interconnecting system of lymphatics. As a result of this system, lymph fluid can travel the entire length of the esophagus before draining into the lymph nodes, so that the entire esophagus is at risk for lymphatic metastasis. In "skip areas," up to 8 cm of normal tissue can exist between gross tumor and micrometastasis within lymph fluid traveling in the esophagus. Lymphatics of the esophagus drain into nodes that usually follow arteries, including the inferior thyroid artery, the bronchial and esophageal arteries from the aorta, and the left gastric artery (celiac axis). Lymph node metastases are found in about 70% of patients at autopsy.

Natural History and Pathologic Features

While previously up to 20% of esophageal cancers occurred in the cervical esophagus versus 80% in the thoracic esophagus, this is true only for squamous cell histology. The relative incidence of squamous cell carcinomas has fallen dramatically as the incidence in adenocarcinomas and lower esophageal and gastroesophageal (GE) junction tumors have risen (136,58). The cause of this occurrence is unknown and unrelated to alcohol or smoking behavior. Barrett's esophagus is a high risk factor for the development of adenocarcinoma of the esophagus (137). Carcinoma of the esophagus commonly exhibits submucosal spread along the muscular layers and frequently extends to lengths of 10 cm or more, forming a scirrhous lesion. Spread by direct contiguity to structures in the neck and mediastinum is common, facilitated by the absence of serosa. Lesions of the cervical esophagus may extend to the carotid arteries, pleura, recurrent laryngeal nerves, and trachea. Lesions of the middle one third may invade the mainstem bronchi, thoracic duct, aortic arch, subclavian artery, intercostal vessels, azygos vein, and the right pleura. Tumors of the lower one third may extend into pericardium, left pleura, and descending aorta. These tumors can spread and perforate the mediastinum, causing mediastinitis, or they can spread into the tracheobronchial tree, causing tracheobronchial fistulas and bronchopneumonia.

The esophagus has a rich lymphatic supply, and spread of the lesion in the upper one-third of the esophagus leads to involvement of the lymph nodes of the anterior jugular chain and supraclavicular region; tumors of the lower one third of the esophagus often metastasize to the celiac and perigastric lymph nodes. Hematogeneous metastases, noted in 40% of patients with primary carcinoma of the esophagus at presentation are mainly to the liver, lung, bones, and kidneys.

Staging

Dynamic examinations while the patient is drinking barium are useful in showing a fixed nondistensible esophagus (19). Esophagoscopy and biopsy definitively establish the diagnosis (endoscopy is accurate in about 96% of the cases) (138). Bronchoscopy is indicated in patients with tumors in the upper and middle thoracic esophagus. Distant metastasis may be detected with chest radiographs, bone scans, CT scans, and so forth.

Although esophageal carcinomas may extend over wide areas of mucosal surface, the 1998 AJCC Staging Manual (20) only recognizes depth of penetration and metastasis in staging. Thus, the current staging system is primarily applicable to surgical staging only. This makes accurate, reproducible staging for inoperable patients difficult. The 1998 staging is shown in Table 18.7. The T-stage is based on depth of primary tumor invasion. Regional lymph nodes are defined relative to the primary tumor location. For cervical esophagus primary, regional lymph node areas include scalene, internal jugular, upper cervical, periesophageal and, supraclavicular. Any other lymph node involvement should be considered distant metastasis (MI). For upper, middle or lower esophageal primaries, regional lymph node groups include tracheobronchial, superior mediastinal, peritracheal, carinal, hilar, periesophageal perigastric and paracardial. All others for these locations should be considered distant metastasis (MI) including supraclavicular and celiac axis.

Table 18.7. AJC 1998 TNM Staging and Stage Groupings for Esophageal Cancer

Primary Tumor			
TX	Primary tumor cannot be assessed		
T0	No evidence of primary tumor		
Tis	Carcinoma in situ		
T1	Tumor invades lamina propria or submucosa		
T2	Tumor invades muscularis propria		
T3	Tumor invades adventitia		
T4	Tumor invades adjacent structures		
Regional Lymph Nodes (N)			
NX	Regional lymph nodes cannot be assessed		
N0	No regional lymph node metastasis		
N1	Regional lymph node metastasis		
Distant Metastasis (M)			
MX	Distant metastasis cannot be assessed		
M0	No distant metastasis		
M1	Distant metastasis		
Stage Grouping			
Stage 0	Tis	N0	M0
Stage I	T1	N0	M0
Stage IIA	T2	N0	M0
	T3	N0	M0
Stage IIB	T1	N1	M0
	T2	N1	M0
	T3	N1	M0
Stage III	T3	N1	M0
	T4	Any N	M0
Stage IV	Any T	Any N	M1
Stage IVA	Any T	Any N	M1a
Stage IVB	Any T	Any N	M1b

(From: American Joint Commission: Manual for Staging of Cancer, 6th ed., 1998.)

General Management

Although the prognosis for most patients esophageal carcinoma is very poor, patients presenting with localized or loco-regional disease (N1) may be offered potentially curative treatment. Patients with M1 presentations should be treated with palliative intent only. This may include chemotherapy, external beam radiation therapy, intraluminal endoesophageal brachytherapy, esophageal dilation, esophageal laser treatment and photodynamic therapy.

Definitive Treatment

Surgical Approaches Many consider surgical resection of esophageal carcinoma to be the standard of care for local or locoregional disease. However, surgical resection alone generally results in cure in less than 15%. The results of surgery are highly dependent upon present staging. Most patients in the United States present with stage III or IV disease. In retrospective series, the 5-year survival for stage III disease, completely resected was 13.3 and 15.2% (35,139,140).

There have been several phase II trials of preoperative chemotherapy and radiation therapy. These studies are summarized in Table 18.8. Two randomized trials of surgery alone versus chemotherapy + radiation therapy followed by surgery reported no survival advantage to the combined modality treatment (145,146). However, one randomized study by Walsh et al. (147) reported significant survival improvement with 5FU, cisplatin and 40 Gy RT followed by surgical resection compared to surgery alone. The reported 3-year survival were 32% versus 6%, $P = .01$). This trial was limited to patients with adenocarcinoma. Confirmatory results may be forthcoming from large cooperative group trials in progress (148).

Nonsurgical Approaches The selection of patients for nonsurgical therapy varies from one institution to another

Table 18.8. Phase II Trials of Preoperative Chemotherapy and Thoracic Radiation Therapy for Operative Esophageal Cancer

Institution (ref)	Preoperative Tx Regimen	Median Survival (mo)	Survival (%) 2 Yr	Survival (%) 3 Yr
RTOG (141)	Cisplatin 5FU 30 Gy RT	13	15	8
SWOG (142)	Cisplatin 5FU 30 Gy	14	28	16
St. Louis University (143)	Cisplatin 5FU 30–36 Gy	23	—	40
University of MI (45)	5FU (CI) Cisplatin Vinblastine 37.5–45 Gy	29	—	34[a]
Fox Chase (144) (adenoca only)	5FU Mitomycin C 60 Gy	—	33	25

[a] 5-yr survival
Tx, treatment, CI, continuous infusion; 5FU, 5-fluorouracil; RT, radiation therapy; Gy, Gray.

(149). A randomized comparison of nonsurgical treatment versus surgery has not yet been performed but was initiated via an intergroup trial in 1998. The standard treatment for nonsurgical is the combination of chemotherapy and radiation therapy. The randomized trials have been performed of radiation therapy alone versus concurrent chemotherapy plus radiation therapy. These are summarized in Table 18.9.

Controversy remains regarding the nonsurgical treatment of cervical esophageal carcinomas and GE junction carcinomas. These specific locations were excluded from the intergroup trial. In our experience the response rates and long term survival appear similar with concurrent chemoradiotherapy in these populations of esophageal cancer patients. It is often technically feasible to deliver higher RT doses in the cervical and upper thoracic lesions. Whether this will result in improved outcomes is the study question of an ongoing Radiation Therapy Oncology Group (RTOG) trial comparing chemotherapy plus 64 Gy versus 50 Gy.

RADIATION TECHNIQUES: VOLUME, PORTALS, AND BEAM ARRANGEMENT

Special consideration must be given to the location of the primary tumor, the extent of the involvement of the adjacent esophagus, and the location of the mediastinal lymph nodes. Treatment of the supraclavicular lymph nodes (in cervical or proximal thoracic lesions) and the gastroesophageal junction and celiac axis (in distal thoracic-esophagus tumors) also warrants careful consideration.

Table 18.9. Randomized Trials of Radiation Therapy Plus or Minus Chemotherapy for Localized Inoperable Esophageal Carcinoma

Institution (ref)	Treatment Regimen	No. of Median Patients	5-Year Survival (mo)	Survival (%)
Brazilian Trial (150)	RT (50 Gy)	31	—	6
	RT + 5FU, Mitomycin (50 Gy) Bleomycin	28	—	16
ECOG (151)	RT (40 Gy)	59	9.1	NR
	RT (40 Gy) + 5 FU + Mitomycin	60	14.8 (P = .03)	NR
Intergroup (152, 153)	RT (64 Gy)	60	8.9	0
	RT (50 Gy) + 5 FU + Cisplatin	61	12.5	30

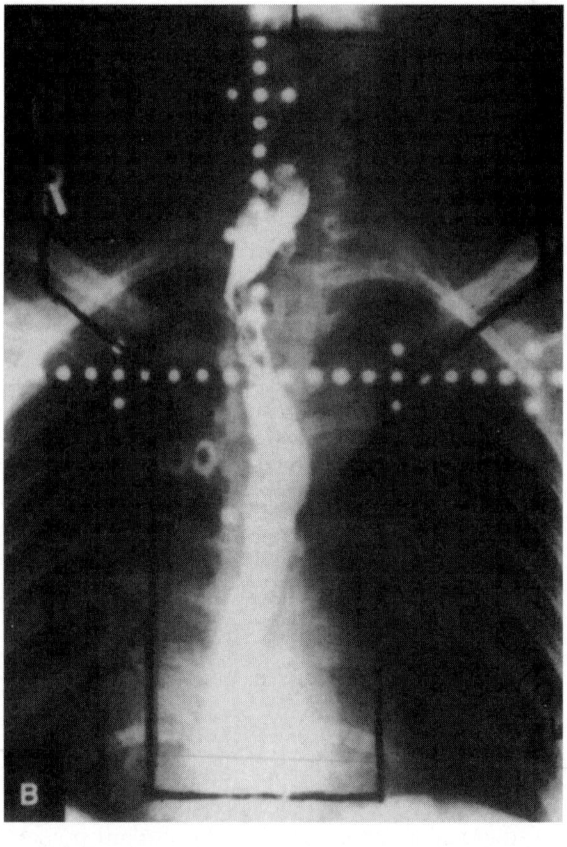

Figure 18.9. Simulation film of volume irradiated in patient with carcinoma of thoracic esophagus. (Reprinted with permission from Radiation Therapy Oncology Group, S. Kramer, Chairman: Standard treatment planning summary: Dosimetry guidelines for cancer of the esophagus, stomach and pancreas, No. 6, p. 34).

For tumors in the cervical esophagus, the ports extend from the laryngopharynx to the junction of the upper and middle two thirds of the thoracic esophagus. The anterior

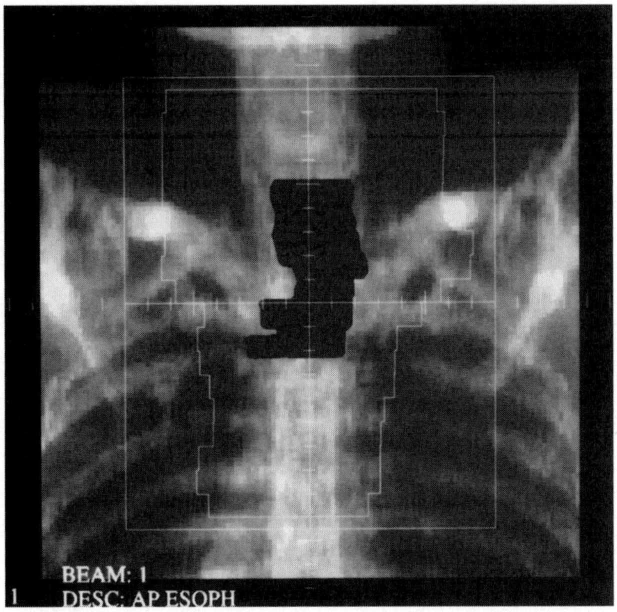

Figure 18.10. Digital Reconstructed Radiograph (DRR) for esophageal cancer portal with tumor delineated.

cervical and superior mediastinal lymph nodes should be included in the irradiated volume. For cervical or upper thoracic-esophagus tumors, the portals should include the supraclavicular lymph nodes. In patients with tumors in the middle or distal thoracic esophagus the supraclavicular regions need not be treated unless palpable. For lesions of the thoracic esophagus, the entire length of the thoracic esophagus is included in the irradiated volume typically, a larger port (up to 10 cm above and below the primary). A 5-cm margin beyond the gross tumor is then boosted to 50 to 64 Gy. The portals thus include some of the cervical esophagus in the treatment field for tumors in the upper thoracic esophagus (Figure 18.9). In patients with tumors in the distal one third of the thoracic esophagus, the gastroesophageal junction and celiac-axis lymph nodes may be included.

We have recently found CT simulation to be highly useful in the design of esophageal portals. Patients are given oral contrast to delineate the esophagus. On a slice by slice basis, the extent of the tumor primary and enlarged lymph nodes are contoured and portals defined accordingly (Figure 18.10). This method has the advantage of ensuring coverage for bulky tumors (and lymph nodes)

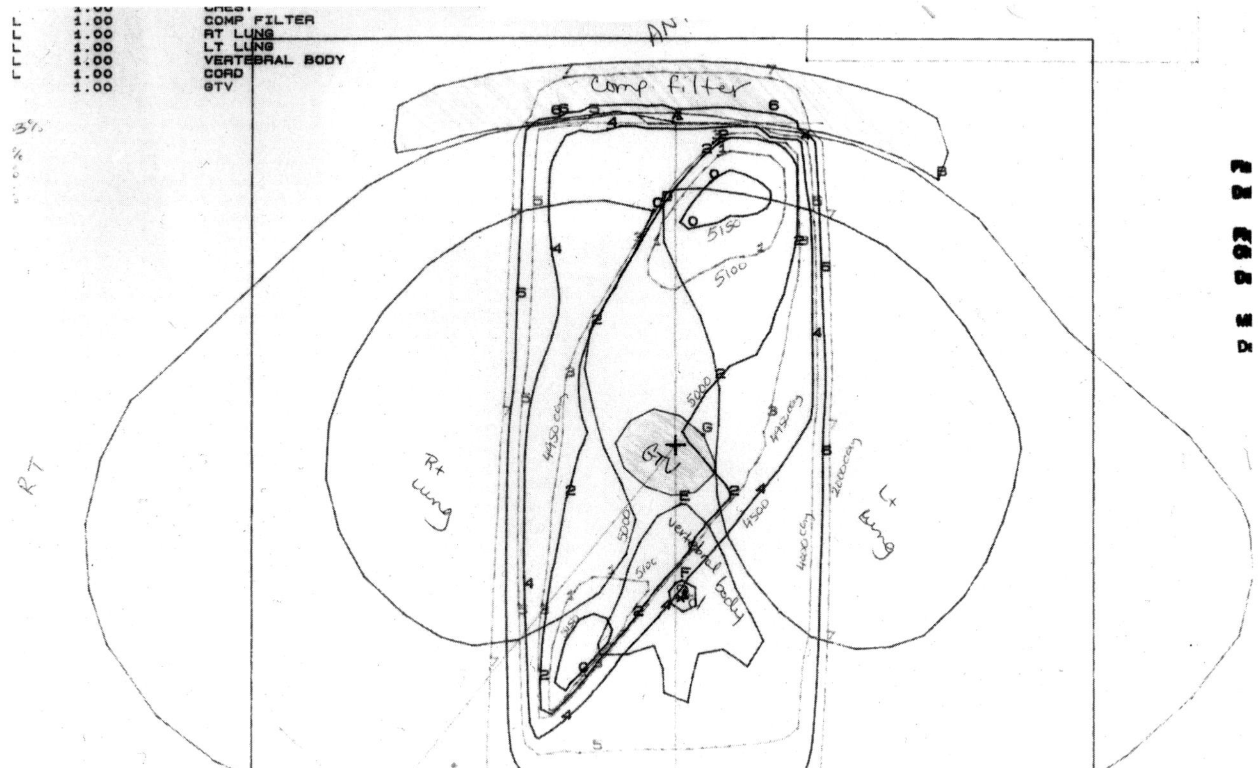

Figure 18.11. Isodose curve for esophageal cancer.

that are not easily seen on conventional simulation with radiopaque substance in the esophagus. We have also increasingly used positron emission tomography (PET) to determine portal volumes. We have seen anecdotal cases where CT scans have missed regional lymph node involvement and PET scan identified it.

Portal arrangement is similar to lung cancers in that AP/PA portals are used to core tolerance ($\leq$ 45 Gy) and then oblique angled fields (typically $<$ 60°) used to boost the tumor to the desired dose (Figure 18.11). The cervical esophageal lesions where the boost portals may be improved by using an anterior wedge pair or even lateral beams. The ideal tumor coverage is probably best determined using 3D simulation for these patients.

Sequelae

Sequelae of surgical resection and/or chemotherapy-radiation therapy can be significant. In centers where surgical resection is performed frequently, the mortality of esophagectomy should be less than 2-5%. However, postoperative complications including anastomotic leaks, pneumouria, arrhythmias, and wound infections may occur in up to 20%. Sequelae after definitive chemotherapy and radiation therapy include neutropenia (30–40%) and neutropenic fever, severe esophagitis (10–30%), weight loss, and pneumonitis ($<$1%).

References

1. Landis SH, Murray T, Bolden S, Wingo PA. Cancer statistics, 1998. CA Cancer J Clin 1998;48:6.
2. Choi NC, Doucette JA. Improved survival of patients with unresectable non-small-cell bronchogenic carcinoma by an innovated high-dose en-bloc radiotherapeutic approach. Cancer 1981;48:101.
3. Parker S, Tong T, Bolden S, et al. Cancer statistics. CA J Clin 1996; 65:5–27.
4. Albain KS, Rusch WV, Crowley JJ, et al. Concurrent cisplatin/etoposide plus clust radiotherapy followed by surgery for stages IIIA (N2) and IIIB non-small-cell lung cancer: mature results of the Southwest Oncology Group Phase II study 88-05. J Clin Oncol 1995;13:1880.
5. Dillman R, Seagren S, Propert K, et al. A randomized trial of induction chemotherapy plus high-dose radiation versus radiation alone in stage III non-small-cell lung cancer. N Engl J Med 1990;323: 940–945.
6. Dillman RO, Herndon J, Seagren SL, Eaton WL Jr, Green MR. Improved survival in stage III nonsmall cell lung cancer: seven-year follow-up of cancer and leukemia group B (CALGB) 8433. J Natl Cancer Inst 1996;88:1210.
7. LeChevalier T, Arriagada R, Quoix E, et al. Radiotherapy alone versus combined chemotherapy and radiotherapy in unresectable non-small cell lung carcinoma. Lung Cancer 1994;10:S239.
8. Rusch VW. Resection of stage III non-small cell lung cancer following induction therapy. World J Surg 1995;19:817.
9. Sause WT, Scott C, Taylor S, et al. Radiation Therapy Oncology Group (RTOG) 88-08 and Eastern Cooperative Oncology Group (ECOG) 4588: preliminary results of a phase III trial in regionally advanced, unresectable non-small-cell lung cancer. J Natl Cancer Inst 1995;87:198.
10. Line DH, Deeley TJ. The necropsy findings in carcinoma of the bronchus. Br J Dis Chest 1971;64:238.
11. Carter D, Eggleston JC. Tumors of the lower respiratory tract. Washington, DC, Armed Forces Institute of Pathology, 1980.
12. Goldberg EM, Shapiro CM, Glicksman AS. Mediastinoscopy for assessing mediastinal spread in clinical staging of lung carcinoma. Semin Oncol 1974;1:205.
13. Baird JA. The pathways of lymphatic spread of carcinoma of the lung. Br J Surg 1965;52:868.
14. Matthews MJ, Kanhouwa S, Pickren J. Frequency of residual and metastatic tumor in patients undergoing curative resection for lung cancer. Cancer Chemother Rep 1973;4(suppl 4):63.
15. LeChevalier T, Arriagada R, Quoix E, et al. Radiotherapy alone versus combined chemotherapy and radiotherapy in nonresectable non-small-cell lung cancer: first analysis of a randomized trial in 353 patients. J Natl Cancer Inst 1991;83:417–423.
16. Capewell S, Sudlow MF. Performance and prognosis in patietns with lung cancer. The Edinburgh Lung Cancer Group. Thorax 1990;45: 951.
17. Scott C, Sause WT, Byhardt R, et al. Recursive partitioning analysis of 1592 patients on four Radiation Therapy Oncology Group studies in inoperable non-small-cell lung cancer. Lung Cancer 1997;17:S59.
18. Mountain CF. The new international staging system for lung cancer. Surg Clin North Am 1987;67:925.
19. Mountain CF. A new international staging system for lung cancer. Chest 1989;4S:225S.
20. American Joint Committee on Cancer. Manual for Staging of Cancer, 6th ed. Philadelphia: JB Lippincott, 1998.
21. Ginsberg RJ, Rubinstein LV. Randomized trial of lobectomy versus limited resection for T1N0 non-small cell lung cancer. Lung Cancer Study Group. Ann Thorac Surg 1995;60:615.
22. Kris MG, Pister KM, Ginsberg RJ, et al. Effectiveness and toxicity of preoperative therapy in stage IIIA non-small cell lung cancer including the Memorial Sloan-Kettering experience with induction MVP in patients with bulky mediastinal lymph node metastasis (clinical N2). Lung Cancer 1995;12:S47.
23. Martini N, Kris MG, Ginsberg RJ. The role of multimodality therapy in locoregional non-small cell lung cancer. Surg Oncol Clin North Am 1997;6:769.
24. Dosoretz D, Katin M, Blitzer P, et al. Radiation therapy in the management of medically inoperable carcinoma of the lung: results and implications for future treatment strategies. Int J Radiat Oncol Biol Phys 1992;24:3–9.
25. Haffty B, Goldberg N, Gerstley J. Results of radical radiation therapy in clinical stage I, technically operable non-small cell lung cancer. Int J Radiat Oncol Biol Phys 1988;15:69.
26. Hayakawa K, Mitsuhashi N, Furuta M, et al. High-dose radiation therapy for inoperable non-small cell lung cancer without mediastinal involvement (Clinical Stage N_0N_1). Strahlentherapie and Onkologie 1996;172:489.
27. Kaskowitz L, Graham M, Emami B, et al. Radiation therapy alone for stage I non-small cell lung cancer. Int J Radiat Oncol Biol Phys 1993;27:517.
28. Noordijk E, Poest-Clement E, Weaver A, et al. Radiotherapy as an alternative to surgery in elderly patients with resectable lung cancer. Radiothera Oncol 1988;13:83.
29. Rosenthal S, Curran WJ, Herbert S, et al. Clinical stage II non-small cell lung cancer treated with radiation therapy alone: the significance of clinically staged ipsilateral hilar adenopathy (N1 disease). Cancer 1992;70:2410.
30. Sandler H, Curran W, Turrisi A. The influence of tumor size and pretreatment staging on outcome following radiation therapy alone for stage I non-small cell lung cancer. Int J Radiat Oncol Biol Phys 1990;19:9.
31. Yorke E, Harisiadis L, Wessels B, Aghdam H, Altemus R. Dosimetric considerations in radiation therapy of coin lesions of the lung. Int J Radiat Oncol Biol Phys 1996;34:481.
32. Emami B. Management of hilar and mediastinal lymph nodes with radiation therapy in the treatment of lung cancer. In: Meyer JL, ed. The lymphatic system and cancer. Basel, Switzerland: S. Karger, 1994.
33. Krol ADG, Aussems P, Noorduk V, Hermans J, Leer JWH. Local irradiation alone for peripheral stage I lung cancer: cound we omit the elective regional nodal irradiation. Int J Radiat Oncol Biol Phys 1996;34:297.
34. Slotman BJ, Antonisse IE, Jno KH. Limited field irradiation in early stage ($T_{1-2}N_0$) non-small cell lung cancer. Radiother Oncol 1996;41: 41.

35. Dautzenberg B, Chastang C, Arriagada R, et al. Adjuvant radiotherapy versus combined sequential chemotherapy followed by radiotherapy in the treatment of resected non-small cell lung carcinoma. A randomized trial of 267 patients. G.E.T.C.B. Cancer 1995;76:779.
36. The Lung Cancer Study Group. Effects of postoperative mediastinal radiation on competely resected stage II and stage III epidermoid cancer of the lung. N Engl J Med 1986;315:1377.
37. Simpson JR, et al. Palliative radiotherapy for inoperable carcinoma of the lung: final report of a RTOG multi-institutional trial. Int J Radiat Oncol Biol Phys 1985;11:751.
38. Slotman BJ, et al. Hypofractionated radiation therapy in unresectable stage III non-small cell lung cancer. Cancer 1993;72:1885.
39. Jeremic B, Shibamoto Y, Acimoyic L, Milisavljevic S. Hyperfractionated radiation therapy with or without concurrent low dose daily carboplatin etoposide for stage III non-small cell lung cancer: a randomized trial. J Clin Oncol 1996;14:1065.
40. Sause W, Scott C, Taylor S, et al. RTOG 8808 ECOG 4588, prelimianry analysis of a phase II trial in regionally advanced unresectable non-small cell lung cancer. Am J Clin Oncol 1994;13:325.
41. Vijayakumar S, Myrianthopoulos LC, Rosenberg I, Halpern HJ, Low N, Chen GTY. Optimization of radical radiotherapy with beam's eye view techniquest for non-small cell cancer. Int J Radiat Oncol Biol Phys 1991;21:779.
42. Blanke C, DeVore R, Shyr Y, et al. A pilot study of protracted low dose cisplatin and etoposide with concurrent thoracic radiotherapy in unresectable stage III nonsmall cell lung cancer. Int J Radiat Oncol Biol Phys 1997;37:111.
43. Marks B, Spencer DP, Bentel GC, et al. The utility of SPECT lung perfusion scans in minimizing and assessing the physiological consequences of thoracic irradiation. Int J Radiat Oncol Biol Phys 1993; 26:659.
44. Boersma LJ, Damen EMF, de Boer RW, et al. Three-dimensional superimposition of SPECT and CT data to quantify radiation-induced ventilation and perfusion changes of the lung; as a function of the locally delivered dose. In: Schmidt HA, Hofer R, eds. Proceedings of European Nuclear Medicine Congress, Vienna. New York: Schattauer, 1992.
45. Forastiere AA, Orringer MB, Perez-Tamayo C, et al. Preoperative chemoradiation followed by transhiatal esophagectomy for carcinoma of the esophagus: final report. J Clin Oncol 1993;11:1118.
46. Graham MV. Predicting radiation response [editorial]. Int J Radiat Oncol Biol Phys 1997;39:561.
47. Kwa SLS, Lebesque JV, Theuws JCM, et al. Radiation pneumonitis as a function of mean lung dose: an analysis of pooled data of 540 patients. (Accepted for publication to Int J Radiat Oncol Biol Phys, 1997).
48. Marks LB, Munley MT, Bentel GC, et al. Physical and biological predictors of changes in whole-lung function following thoracic irradiation. Int J Radiat Oncol Biol Phys 1997;39:563.
49. Martel MK, Ten Haken RK, Hazuka MB, Turrisi AT, Fraass BA, Lichter AS. Dose-volume histogram and 3D treatment planning evaluation of patients with pneumonitis. Int J Radiat Oncol Biol Phys 1994;28: 575.
50. Oetzel D, Schraube P, Hensley F, Sroka-Perez G, Menke M, Flentje M. Estimation of pneumonitis risk in three-dimensional treatment planning using dose-volume histogram analysis. Int J Radiat Oncol Biol Phys 1995;33:455.
51. Emami B, Lyman J, Brown A, et al. Tolerance of normal tissue to therapeutic irradiation. Int J Radiat Oncol Biol Phys 1991;21:109.
52. Byhardt RW, Martin L, Pajak TF, Shin K H, Emami B, Cox JD. The influence of field size and other treatment factors in pulmonary toxicity following hyperfractionated irraduatuib for inoperable non-small cell lung cancer (NSCLC)—analysis of a Radiation Therapy Oncology Group (RTOG) Protocol. Int J Radiat Oncol Biol Phys 1993;27:537.
53. Ekstrand KE, Barnes WH. Pitfalls in the use of high energy x-rays to treat tumors in the lung. Int J Radiat Oncol Biol Phys 1990;18: 249–252.
54. MacDonald SC, Keller BE, Rubin P. Method for calculating dose when lung tissue lies in the treatment field. Med Phys 1976;3:210.
55. Mackie TR, El-Khatib E, Battista J, Scrimger J, Van Dyk J, Cunningham JR. Lung dose corrections for 6- and 15-MV x-rays. Med Phys 1985;12:327.
56. Rice RK, Mijnheer BJ, Chin LM. Benchmark measurements for lung dose corrections for x-ray beams. Int J Radiat Oncol Biol Phys 1988; 15:399.
57. White PJ, Zwicker RD, Haung DT. Comparison of dose homogeneity effects due to electron equilibrium loss in lung for 6 MV and 18 MV photons. Int J Radiat Oncol Biol Phys 1996;34:1141.
58. Powell J, McConkey CC. Increasing incidence of adenocarcinoma of the gastric cardiac and adjacent sites. Br J Cancer 1990;62:440.
59. Klein ER, Morrison A, Purdy JA, Graham MV, Matthews J. A volumetric study of measurements and calculations of lung density corrections for 6 and 18 MV photons. Int J Radiat Oncol Biol Phys 1997; 37:1163.
60. Kan MW, Wong TP, Young EC, Chan CL, Yu PK. A comparison of two photon planning algorithms for 8 MV and 25 MV x-ray beams in lung. Aust Phys and Eng Sci in Med 1995;18:95.
61. Ellis F. Accuracy in compensation for tissue heterogeneity in treatment by x-rays, supervoltage x-rays and electron beams. Br J Radiol 1960;33:404.
62. Ellis F, Lescrenier C. Combined compensator for contours and heterogeneity. Radiology 1973;106:191.
63. Miller RC, Bonner JA, Wenger DE, Foote RL, Kisrow KL, Shaw EG. Spinal cord localization in the treatment of lng cancer: use of radiographic land markers. Int J Radiat Oncol Biol Phys 1998;40:347.
64. Clarkson JR. A note on depth doses in fields of irregular shape. Br J Radiol 1941;14:265.
65. Cundiff JH, et al. A method for the calculation of dose in the radiation treatment of Hodgkin's disease. AJR 1973;117:30.
66. Johns HE, Cunningham JR. The physics of radiology. 3rd ed. Springfield, IL: Charles C. Thomas, 1971.
67. Fletcher GH. Clinical dose-response curves of human malignant epithelial tumours. Br J Radiol 1973;46:1.
68. Salazar OM, et al. The assessment of tumor response to irradiation of lung cancer: Continuous versus split-course regimes. Int J Radiat Oncol Biol Phys 1976;1:1107.
69. Mantravadi RVP, et al. Unresectable non-oat cell carcinoma of the lung: definitive radiation therapy. Radiology 1989;172:851.
70. Perez CA, et al. Impact of irradiation technique and tumor extent in tumor control and survival of patients with unresectable non-oat cell carcinoma of the lung. Cancer 1982;50:1091.
71. Ball D, et al. Longer survival with higher doses of thoracic radiotherapy in patients with limited non-small cell lung cancer. Int J Radiat Oncol Biol Phys 1993;25:599.
72. Wurschmidt F, et al. Inoperable non-small-cell lung cancer: a retrospective analysis of 427 patients treated with high-dose radiotherapy. Int J Radiat Oncol Biol Phys 1994;28:583.
73. Perez CA, et al. Long-term observations of the patterns of failure in patients with unresectable non-oat cell carcinoma of the lung treated with definitive radiotherapy: Report by the Radiation Therapy Oncology Group. Cancer 1987;59:1874.
74. Emami B, Perez CA, Herskovic A, Hederman MA. Phase I/II study of treatment of locally advanced (T3 T4) non-oat cell lung cancer with high dose radiotherapy (rapid fractionation): Radiation Therapy Oncology Group Study. Int J Radiat Oncol Biol Phys 1988;15: 1021.
75. Graham MV, Purdy JA, Emami B, Matthews JW, Harms WB. Preliminary results of a prospective trial using three-dimensional radiotherapy for lung cancer. Int J Radiat Oncol Biol Phys 1995;33:993.
76. Cox JD, Azarnia N, Byhardt RW, Shin KH, Emami B, Pajak TF. A randomized phase I/II trial of hyperfractionated radiation therapy with total doses of 660.0 Gy to 79.2 Gy: Possible survival benefit with greater than or equal to 69.9 Gy in favorable patients with radiation oncology group stage III non-small cell lung carcinoma: Report of Radiation Therapy Oncology Group 83-11. J Clin Oncol 1990;8:1543.
77. Armstrong JG, Burman C, Leibel S, et al. Three-dimensional conformal radiation therapy may improve the therapeutic ratio of high dose radiation therapy for lung cancer. Int J Radiat Oncol Biol Phys 1993;26:685.
78. Graham MV, Matthews JW, Harms WB, Emami B, Glazer HS, Purdy JA. Three-dimensional radiation treatment planning study for patients with carcinoma of the lung. Int J Radiat Oncol Biol Phys 1994; 29:1105.

79. Ha CS, Kijewski PK, Langer MP. Gain in target dose from using computer controlled radiation therapy (CCRT) in the treatment of non-small cell lung cancer. Int J Radiat Oncol Biol Phys 1993;26: 335.
80. Graham MV. Three-dimensional conformal radiotherapy for lung cancer: the Washington University Experience. In: Meyer JL, Purdy, JA, eds. Frontiers of radiation therapy and oncology. Basel, Switzerland: S. Karger, 1996.
81. Kutcher GJ, Burman C. Calculation of complication probability factors for non-uniform normal tissue irradiation: the effective volume method. Int J Radiat Oncol Biol Phys 1989;16:1623.
82. Robertson JM, Ten Haken RK, et al. Dose escalation for non-small-cell lung cancer using conformal radiation therapy. Int J Radiat Oncol Biol Phys. 1997;37:1079.
83. Cox JD, Bauer M. Therapeutic ratio and fractionation in cancer of the lung. Front Radiat Ther Oncol 1988;22:121.
84. Cox JD, Azarnia N, Byhardt RW, Shin KH, Emani B, Pajak TF. A randomized phase I/II trial of hypofractionated radiation therapy with total doses of 60.0 Gy to 79.2 Gy possible survival benefit with greater than or equal to 69.6 Gy in favorable patients with Radiation Therapy Oncology Group Stage III non-small-cell lung carcinoma: report of Radiation Therapy Oncology Group 83-11. J Clin Oncol 1990;8:1543–1555.
85. Saunders M, Dische S, Barrett A, Harvey A, Gibson D, Pasmar M. Continuous hyperfractionated accelerated radiotherapy (CHART) versus conventional radiotherapy in non-small-cell lung cancer: a randomized multicentre trial, CHART Steering Committee. Lancet 1997;350:161.
86. Kelly K, Hazuka M, Pan Z, et al. Phase I study of daily carboplastin and simultaneous accelerated hyperfractionated chest irradiation in patients with regionally inoperable non-small cell lung ancer. Int J Radiat Oncol Biol Phys 1998;40:559.
87. Komaki R, Scott C, Lee JS, et al. Impact of adding concurrent chemotherapy to hyperfractionated radiotherapy for locally advanced non-small cell lung cancer (NSCLC): comparison of RTOG 83-11 and RTOG 91-06. Am J Clin Oncol 1997;20:435.
88. Kunitoh H, Watanabe K, Nagatomo A, Okamoto H, Kimbara K. Concurrent daily carboplatin and accelerated hyperfractionated thoracic radiotherapy in locally advanced nonsmall cell lung cancer. Int J Radiat Oncol Biol Phys 1997;37(1):103–109.
89. Choi NC, Carey RW, Daly W, et al. Potential impact on survival of improved tumor downstaging and resection rate by preoperative twice-daily radiation and concurrent chemotherapy in stage III non-small cell lung cancer. J Clin Oncol 1997;15:712.
90. Eberhardt W, Wilke H, Stamatis G, et al. Preoperative chemotherapy followed by concurrent chemoradiation therapy based on hyperfractionated accelerated radiotherapy and definitive surgery in locally advanced nonsmall cell lung cancer: mature results of a phase III trial. J Clin Oncol 1998;16;622.
91. Choy H, DeVore RF III, Hande KR, et al. Preliminary analysis of a phase II study of paclitaxel, carboplatin and hyperfractionated radiation therapy for locally advanced inoperable nonsmall cell lung cancer. Semin Oncol 1997;24:S12.
92. Graham MV, Jahanzeb M, Dresler CM, Cooper JD, Emami B, Mortimer JE. Results of a trial with Topotecan dose escalation and concurrent thoracic radiation therapy for locally advanced, inoperable non-small cell lung cancer. Int J Radiat Oncol Biol Phys 1996;36:1215.
93. Gregor A. Gentabine plus radiotherapy for nonsmall cell lung cancer. Semin Oncol 1997;24:88.
94. Langer CJ, Mouvas B, Hudes R, et al. Induction paclitaxel and carboplatin followed by concurrent chemoradiotherapy in patients with unresectable, locally advanced nonsmall cell lung carcinoma: report of Fox Chase Cancer Center study 94-001. Semin Oncol 1997; 24:S12–S89.
95. Rosenthal DI, Okani O, et al. Seven-week continuous-infusion paclitaxel plus concurrent radiation therapy for locally advanced non-small cell lung cancer: a phase I study. Semin Oncol 1997;24:S12.
96. Smolle-Juettner FM, Mayer R, Pinter H, et al. Adjuvant external beam radiation of the mediastinum in radically resected non-small cell lung cancer. Eur J Cardiothorac Surg 1996;10:947.
97. The Lung Cancer Study Group. The benefits of adjuvant treatment for resected locally advanced non-small cell lung cancer. J Clin Oncol 1988;6:9.
98. Perez CA, et al. Randomized trial of radiotherapy to the thorax in limited small cell carcinoma of the lung treated with multiagent chemotherapy and elective brain irradiation: a preliminary report. J Clin Oncol 1984;2:1200.
99. Tucker MA, Murray N, Shaw EG, et al. Secondary primary cancers related to smoking and treatment of small cell lung cancer. Lung cancer working cadre. J Nat Cancer Inst 1997;89:1782.
100. Russell AH, Pajak TE, Selim HM, et al. Prophylactic cranial irradiation for lung cancer patients at high risk for development of cerebral metastasis: results of a prospective randomized trial conducted by the radiation therapy oncology group. Int J Radiat Oncol Biol Phys 1991;21:637.
101. Chute JP, Venzon DJ, et al. Outcome of patients with small cell lung cancer during 20 years of clinical research at the U.S. National Cancer Institute. Mayo Clinic Proceedings 1997;72:901.
102. Looper JD, Hornback NB. The role of chest irradiation in limited small cell carcinoma of the lung treated with combination chemotherapy. Int J Radiat Oncol Biol Phys 1984;10:1855–1860.
103. Turrisi AT, et al. Concurrent chemoradiotherapy for limited samll-cell lung cancer. Oncology 1997;11:31.
104. Kies MS, et al. Multimodal therapy for limited small-cell lung cancer: a randomized study of induction combination chemotherapy with or without thoracic radiation in complete responders; and with wide-field versus reduced-field radiation in partial responders: A Southwest Oncology Group Study. J Clin Oncol 1987;5:592–600.
105. Perry MC, et al. Chemotherapy with or without radiation therapy in limited small-cell carcinoma of the lung. N Engl J Med 1987;316: 912.
106. Deleted.
107. Warde P, Payne D. Does thoracic irradiation improve survival and local conrol in limited-stage small-cell carcinoma of the lung. J Clin Oncol 1992;10:890.
108. Mira JG, et al. Influence of chest radiotherapy in frequency and patterns of chest relapse in disseminated small cell lung. (A Southwest Oncology Group Study). Cancer 1982;50:1266.
109. Pignon JP, Arriagada R, et al. A meta-analysis of thoracic radiotherapy for small-cell lung cancer. N Engl J Med 1992;327:1618.
110. Work E, Nielsen OS, Bertzen SM, Fode K, Palshof T. Randomized study of initial versus late chest irradiation combined with chemotherapy in limited-stage small-cell lung cancer. Aarhus Lung Cancer Group. J Clin Oncol 1997;15:3030.
111. Choi NC, Carey RW. Importance of radiation dose in achieving improved loco-regional tumor control in limited stage small-cell lung carcinoma: an update. Int J Radiat Oncol Biol Phys 1989;17:307.
112. Coy P, et al. The effect of dose of thoracic irradiation on recurrence in patients with limited stage small cell lung cancer initial results of a Canadian multicenter randomized trial. Int J Radiat Oncol Biol Phys 1988;14:219.
113. Johnson B, Salem C, et al. Limited (LTD) stage small cell lung cancer (SCLC) treated with concurrent bid chest radiotherapy (RT) and etoposide/cisplatin (VP-PT) followed by chemotherapy (CT) selected by in vitro drug sensitivity testing (DST) (Abstract). Lung Cancer 1991;7:151.
114. Johnson D, Turrisi A, et al. Alternating chemotherapy and twice-daily thoracic radiotherapy inlimited-stage small-cell lung cancer: a pilot study of the Eastern Cooperative Oncology Group. J Clin Oncol 1993;11:879.
115. Johnson BE, Bridges JD, Sobczeck M, et al. Patients with limited stage small-cell lung cancer treated with concurrant twice daily chest radiotherapy and etoposide/cisplatin followed by cyclophosphamide, doxorubicin, and vincristine. J Clin Oncol 1996;14:806.
116. Johnson DH, Kim K, Turrisi AT, et al. Cisplatin (P) etoposide (E) + thoracic radiotherapy (TRT) administered once vs twice daily (BID) in limited stage (LS) small cell lung cancer (SCLC): final report of inrgroup trial 0096 (Abstract). Proc Am Soc Clin Oncol 1996;15: 374.
117. McCracken J, Janaki L, et al. Concurrent chemotherapy/radiotherapy for limited small cell lung carcinoma: a Southwest Oncology Group study. J Clin Oncol 1990;8:892.
118. Turrisi AT, Glover DJ, Mason BA. A preliminary report: concurrent twice-daily radiotherapy plus platinum-etoposide chemotherapy for limited small cell lung cancer. Int J Radiat Oncol Biol Phys 1988; 15:183.

119. Jeremic B, Shibamoto Y, Acimoyic L, Milisavljevic S. Initial versus delayed accelerated hypfractionated radiation therapy and concurrent chemotherapy in limited stage small-cell lung cancer: a randomized study. J Clin Oncol 1997;15:893.
120. Lebeau B, Chastang C, et al. A randomized trial of delayed thoracic radiotherapy in complete responder patients with small cell lung cancer. Chest 1993;104:726.
121. Murray N, Coy P, et al. Importance of timing for thoracic irradiation in the combined modality treatment of limited-stage small-cell lung cancer. J Clin Oncol 1993;11:336.
122. Takada M, et al. Phase III study of concurrent versus sequential thoracic radiotherapy (TRT) ihn combination with cisplatin (C) and etoposide (E) for limited-stage (LS) small cell lung cancer: preliminary results of the Japanese Clinical Oncology Group (Abstract). Proc ASCO 1996;15:1103.
123. Schultz H, Nielson O, et al. Timing of ch est irradiation with respect to combination chemotherapy in small cell lung cancer, limited disease. Lung Cancer 1988;4:153.
124. Liengswangwong V, Bonner JA, Shaw EG, et al. Limited-stage small-cell lung cancer: patterns of intrathoracic recurrence and the implications for thoracic radiotherapy. J Clin Oncol 1994;12:496.
125. Komaki R, Cox JD, Whitson W. Risk of brain metastasis in small cell carcinoma of the lung related to length of survival and prophylactic irradiation. Cancer Treat Rep 1981;65:811.
126. Komaki R. Prophylactic cranial irradiation for small cell carcinoma of the lung. Cancer Treat Symp 1985;2:35.
127. Rosenstein M, Armstrong J, Kris M, et al. A reappraisal of the role of prophylactic cranial irradiation in limited small cell carcinoma of the lung. Int J Radiat Oncol Biol Phys 1991;24:43.
128. VanOosterhout AG, Boon PJ, Hoox PJ, tenVelde GP, Twinjstra A. Follow-up of cognitive functioning in patients with small cell lung cancer. Int J Radiat Oncol Biol Phys 1995;31:911.
129. Johnson BE, Patronas N, Hayes W, et al. Neurologic computed cranial tomographic, and magnetic resonance imaging abnormalities in patients with small-cell lung cancer: further follow-up of 6- to 13-year survivors. J Clin Oncol 1990;8:48.
130. Lishner M, Feld R, Payne DG, et al. Late neurologic complications after prophylactic cranial irradiation in patients with small-cell lung cancer: the Toronto experience. J Clin Oncol 1990;8:215.
131. Fleck JF, Einhorn LH, Lauer RC, Schulz SM, Miller ME. Is prophylactic cranial irradiatio indicated in small-cell lung cancer? J Clin Oncol 1990;8:209–214.
132. Komaki R, Meyers CA, Shin DM, et al. Evaluation of cognitive function in patients with limited small cell lung cancer prior to and shortly following prophylactic cranial irradiation. Int J Radiat Oncol Biol Phys 1995;33:179.
133. Ohonoshi T, Ueoka H, Kawahara S, et al. Comparative study of prophylactic cranial irradiation in patients with small cell lung cancer achieving a complete response: a long-term follow-up result. Lung Cancer 1993;10:47.
134. Gregor A, Coll A, Stephens RJ, et al. Prophylactic cranial irradiation is indicated following complete response to induction therapy in small cell lung cancer: results of a multicentre randomized trial. United Kingdom Coordinating Committee for Cancer Research (UK CCRC) and the European Organization for Research and Treatment of Cancer (EORTC). Eur J Cancer 1997;33:1752.
135. Martini N, Flehinger BJ, Nagasaki F, Hart B. Prognostic sign of N1 disease in carcinoma of the lung. J Thorac Cardiovasc Surg 1983; 86:646.
136. Blot J, Devesa SS, Kneller RW, et al. Increasing incidence of adenocarcinoma of the esophagus and gastric cardia. JAMA 1991;265: 1287.
137. Pera M, Cameron AJ, et al. Increasing incidence of adenocarcinoma of the esophagus and esophagogastric junction. Gastroenterol 1993; 104:510.
138. Rice TW, Adelstein DJ. Precise clinical staging allows treatment modification of patients with esophageal carcinoma. Oncology 1997;11:58.
139. King MR, Pairolero PC, et al. Ivor Lewis esophagectomy for carcinoma of the esophagus: early and late functional results. Ann Thorac Surg 1987;44:119.
140. Ellis FH, Gibb SP, et al. Limited esophagogastrectomy for carcinoma of the cardiac. Ann Surg 1988;208:354.
141. Seydel HG, Leichman L, Byhard R, et al. Preoperative radiation and chemotherapy for localized squamous cell carcinoma of the esophagus: An RTOG study. Int J Radiat Oncol Biol Phys 1988;14:33.
142. Poplin E, Fleming T, Leichman L, et al. Combined therapies for squamous-cell carcinoma of the esophagus. A Southwest Oncology Group study (SWOG-8037). J Clin Oncol 1987;5:622.
143. Naunheim KS, Petruska PJ, Roy TS, et al. Preoperative chemotherapy and radiotherapy for esophageal carcinoma. J Thorac Cardiovasc Surg 1992;103:887.
144. Sauter ER, Coia LR, Keller SM. Preoperative high-dose radiation and chemothrapy in adenocarcinoma of the esophagus and esophapgogastric junction. Ann Surg Oncol 1994;1:5.
145. LePrise E, Etienne P, Meunier B, et al. A randomized study of chemotherapy, radiation therapy, and surgery versus surgery for localized squamous cell carcinoma of the esophagus. Cancer 1994;73:1779.
146. Urba S, Orringer M, Turrisi A, et al. A randomized trial comparing transhiatal esophagectomy to preoperative concurrent chemoradiation followed by esophagecto in locoregional esophageal carcinoma (Abstract). Proc Am Soc Clin Oncol 1995;14:1995.
147. Walsh T, Noonan N, Hollywood D, et al. A comparison of multimodal therapy and surgery for esophageal adenocarcinoma. N Engl J Med 1996;335:462.
148. Bossett JF, Gignoux M, Triboulet JP, et al. Randomized phase III clinical trial comparing surgery alone vs preoperative combined radiochemotherapy in stage I-II epidermoid cancer of the thoracic esophagus: preliminary snalysis, a study of the FFCD (French Group) no. 8805 and EORTC no. 40881 (Abstract). Proc Am Soc Clin Oncol 1994;13:576.
149. Coia LR. Esophageal cancer: is esophagectomy necessary? Oncology 1989;3:101.
150. Araujo C, Souhami L, Gil R, et al. A randomized trial comparing radiation therapy vs. concomitant radiation therapy and chemotherapy in carcinoma of the thoracic esophagus. Cancer 1991;67: 2258.
151. Sischy B, Ryan L, Haller D, et al. Interim report of EST 1282 phase III protocol for the evaluation of combined modalities in the treatment of patients with carcinoma of the esophagus, stage I and II (Abstract). Proc Am Soc Clin Oncol 1990;9:105.
152. al-Sarraf M, Martz K, Herskovic A, et al. Superiority of chemoradiotherapy vs. radiotherapy in patients with esophageal cancer. Final report of an Intergroup randomized and confirmed study (Abstract). Proc Am Soc Clin Oncol 1996;15:464.
153. Herskovic A, Martz K, al-Sarraf M, et al. Combined chemotherapy and radiotherapy compared with radiotherapy alone in patients with cancer of the esophagus. N Engl J Med 1992;326:1593.

Chapter 19

Cancers of the Colon, Rectum, and Anus

James A. Martenson, Jr., Michael G. Haddock, and Leonard L. Gunderson

Combined radiation therapy and chemotherapy is often used as an adjuvant to surgical resection in selected patients with rectal cancer. Radiation therapy and chemotherapy are also used as the definitive procedures in patients with locally advanced rectal and colon cancer. Combined radiation therapy and chemotherapy has replaced abdominal perineal resection as the principal form of treatment for anal cancer. Appropriate radiotherapeutic management of the patient with lower gastrointestinal cancer includes proper patient selection and diagnostic evaluation, close cooperation by all physicians participating in the patient's care, and utilization of proper radiotherapeutic techniques.

DIAGNOSTIC EVALUATION

Colon and Rectal Cancer

The diagnostic evaluation of the patient with colorectal cancer begins with a history and physical examination. In taking a history from a patient with large bowel cancer, particular attention should be given to rectal bleeding, change in bowel habits, and abdominal pain (1). Other presenting features of large bowel cancer include nausea, vomiting, weakness, and abdominal mass. Loss in performance status, fatigue, weight loss, anorexia, and sweats may indicate distant metastatic disease. Patients found incidentally to have microcytic anemia should be considered to have large bowel cancer until some other cause can be proven.

Laboratory studies should consist of liver function tests and a complete blood cell count. The preoperative carcinoembryonic antigen (CEA) value is an independent prognostic factor. Some physicians obtain a baseline value preoperatively so that serial measurement can be used postoperatively to identify disease progression in asymptomatic patients (2,3). The value of CEA in this situation is limited because most patients with recurrence have symptoms before the CEA value increases (4) and most patients with recurrence do not have an increased CEA value (5). Moreover, patients found to have recurrent disease on the basis of serial CEA measurements are unlikely to be cured (2,6–11).

The radiation oncologist often is consulted after a patient's malignant tumor has been resected. In this situation, it is necessary to use information from preoperative studies as well as operative and pathologic findings in the design of radiation therapy fields. Preoperative studies that are helpful in the evaluation of local disease include digital examination, proctoscopy or colonoscopy (or both), and a barium enema study, including cross-table lateral views. Although endoscopic procedures are of value in diagnosis, a barium enema study is more helpful to the radiation oncologist in determining the preoperative tumor volume. When endoscopy is performed, a description of the lesion should be provided, including its position on the bowel wall, its distance from the anal verge, its size, the degree of circumference involved, and whether the lesion is exophytic or ulcerative.

If the lesion is palpable, the physician should note the inferior extent relative to the anal verge, the location of the tumor on the bowel wall, the degree of circumference involved, and whether the lesion is clinically mobile or fixed to extrarectal structures. If lesions are immobile or fixed, computed tomography (CT) or magnetic resonance imaging (MRI) of the pelvis may be helpful in assessing resectability. If CT or MRI findings demonstrate that the tumor is unresectable for cure, consultation with a radiation oncologist is appropriate for consideration of moderate-dose preoperative irradiation (that is, approximately 5040 cGy in 28 fractions) combined with simultaneous 5-

fluorouracil (5-FU)-based chemotherapy, with the goal of shrinking the tumor so that it becomes resectable.

Anal Cancer

Evaluation of a patient with anal cancer begins with a thorough history. The patient should be questioned about the common presenting symptoms, including a mass sensation in the anal region, pain, or bleeding. The majority of patients with anal cancer are elderly women. Most patients do not have a history of multiple recent sex partners, intravenous drug abuse, or other factors that place them at risk for human immunodeficiency virus (HIV) infection or sexually transmitted disease. A sexual and drug abuse history should be obtained in all patients, however, because anal cancer may develop in a minority of patients because of these risk factors.

The physical examination should give particular attention to evaluation of the abdomen, inguinal lymph nodes, anus, and rectum. In addition, a pelvic examination should be performed in female patients. During examination of the anus and rectum, the size and location of the tumor and whether any perirectal lymph nodes are palpable should be noted.

Laboratory studies should include liver function tests and a complete blood cell count. Routine testing for HIV is unnecessary in most cases but should be done in all patients with a history that places them at risk for this infection. Identification of patients with overt acquired immunodeficiency syndrome (AIDS) is important, since these patients may not tolerate conventional combined modality therapy for anal cancer.

Imaging studies should include a chest radiograph and a CT scan of the abdomen and pelvis. Except in patients with very large lesions, the CT scan is inferior to physical examination for assessment of the primary lesion. Nevertheless, CT scans are useful for assessment of regional and para-aortic lymph nodes and for evaluation of the liver.

ANATOMY

Rectum

The rectum begins in the upper to middle presacrum as a continuation of the sigmoid colon. Whereas the sigmoid colon has a complete peritoneal covering and mesentery, the upper rectum is covered by peritoneum only anteriorly and laterally. The lower one-half to two-thirds of the rectum is not covered by peritoneum and is surrounded by fibrofatty tissue and by organs and structures that can be involved by direct tumor extension, including the bladder, prostate, ureters, vagina, sacrum, nerves, and vessels.

Lymphatic and venous drainage of lesions limited to the rectum depends on the level of the lesion. The lymphatic system of the upper rectum follows the inferior mesenteric system via the superior hemorrhoidal veins. The middle and lower rectum can, in addition, drain directly to internal iliac and presacral nodes. Lesions that extend to the anal canal can spread to inguinal nodes, and lesions that extend beyond the rectal wall may theoretically spread through the lymphatic system of the invaded tissue or organ.

Colon

The ascending and descending colon, as well as splenic and hepatic flexures, share some anatomical features with the rectum. They are relatively immobile structures that lack a mesentery and usually do not have a peritoneal covering on the posterior and lateral surfaces. Lesions that extend through the entire bowel wall in these locations may have narrow radial operative margins, especially in patients with tumors that invade through the posterior or lateral colonic wall. Lesions on the anterior wall or medial wall of the retroperitoneal colon have closer access to a free peritoneal surface.

The sigmoid and transverse colons are intraperitoneal organs with a complete mesentery and serosa. Each is freely mobile except for its proximal and distal segments, where extracolonic extension may result in narrow surgical margins. If the lesion is in the midtransverse or midsigmoid colon, excellent surgical margins can usually be obtained unless tumor is adherent to or invades adjacent organs or structures.

The cecum has a variable mesentery and some mobility. When cecal lesions extend posteriorly, it may be difficult in some patients to obtain tumor-free surgical margins in the region of the iliac wing with its associated musculature and blood vessels.

The lymphatic and venous drainage of the colon is by the inferior mesenteric system for the left colon and superior mesenteric system for the right colon. If organs or structures adjacent to the primary lesion are involved, the lymphatic drainage of these areas may also be at risk for development of regional metastatic lesions. For example, if lesions in the sigmoid colon invade the bladder, the iliac nodes may be at risk. When extrapelvic lesions involve the posterior abdominal wall, direct spread to periaortic lymph nodes can occur. If the anterior abdominal wall is involved at or below the level of the umbilicus, inguinal nodes may be at risk for metastatic involvement.

PATHWAYS OF SPREAD

Colorectal Cancer

Colorectal cancers can metastasize hematogenously, by surgical implantation, to the peritoneum, or to regional lymph nodes. Peritoneal spread is relatively rare with rectal lesions because most of the rectum is below the peritoneal reflection. With colonic lesions, direct extension to a free peritoneal surface can occur more easily.

Tumor extension within the bowel wall is unusual. In one analysis, for example, only 4 of 103 patients had microscopic intramural spread greater than 0.5 cm from the gross lesion, and the maximum extent of longitudinal spread was 1.2 cm (12). Because primary venous and lymphatic channels originate in submucosal layers of the bowel, lesions limited to the mucosa are at little risk for either venous or lymphatic dissemination.

Lymph node involvement is found in about 50% of patients and is usually orderly and predictable. Skip metastasis or retrograde spread is associated with an ominous prognosis. It occurs in only 1 to 3% of these patients and usually is related to lymphatic blockage (13). The major spread through lymphatic channels is cephalad, except for lesions 8 cm or less above the anal verge, where both lateral and distal flow can occur. In female patients, this latter pattern of flow places the posterior vaginal wall at risk for involvement by tumor (14).

Anal Cancer

The anal canal extends from the dentate line to the anal verge. It has an average length of 2.1 cm (15). The dentate line is located at the lower border of the anal valves (16,17). Lymphatic drainage from the anal region is to the inguinal nodes, to the lateral pelvic sidewall nodes along the path of the middle hemorrhoidal vessels, and into the inferior mesenteric nodes (16). The most distal portion of the rectum and the proximal anal canal share a plexus that drains to lymphatics that accompany the inferior rectal and internal pudendal blood vessels and ultimately drain to internal iliac nodes. Carcinomas of the lower rectum or those that extend into the anal canal may metastasize to superficial inguinal nodes via connections to efferent lymphatics draining the lower anus. Tumors below the anal verge drain primarily to the inguinal system.

PATTERNS OF FAILURE AFTER POTENTIALLY CURATIVE RESECTION

Rectal Cancer

The risk of local recurrence after complete surgical resection is related to the degree of disease extension beyond the rectal wall and to the extent of nodal involvement. The incidence of local recurrence for lesions with involved nodes but with tumor confined to the wall varies in most studies from 20 to 40%. This is similar to the local recurrence risk in patients without nodal involvement who have extension beyond the wall. Lesions that have *both* tumor extension beyond the rectal wall and lymph node involvement have nearly an additive risk of local recurrence, 40 to 65% in clinical studies (18-21) and 70% in a reoperative series (22).

Colon Cancer

The study of patterns of failure in patients with colon cancer is of interest because of the possibility that future randomized trials may define a role for adjuvant radiation treatment in high-risk patients who have undergone surgical resection.

Data from clinical studies of patterns of failure suggest that one-third of patients in whom tumor relapse develops after curative resection have failures solely in the liver (23). Patterns-of-failure studies that do not routinely use reoperation or autopsy, however, may underestimate the incidence of local-regional failure in patients with colon cancer. Autopsy and reoperative series suggest that liver-only relapse occurs in fewer than 10% of cases (24,25). Data from autopsy and reoperative patterns-of-failure studies must also be interpreted with caution, because only a subset of patients who undergo a potentially curative operation subsequently undergo reoperation or autopsy.

Patterns of failure in colon cancer may have been analyzed in autopsy, clinical, and reoperation series (23,24,26–31). Data from these series suggest that local failure is a significant problem after resection of colon cancer in selected patients. Local failure is highest among patients with tumors adhering to surrounding structures and among patients who have both tumor extension beyond the bowel wall and metastatic involvement of lymph nodes. In one retrospective study, the local recurrence rate among patients with these pathologic characteristics was 42% (32).

In a colorectal reoperative series from the University of Minnesota, failures in the tumor bed or lymph nodes were most common with rectal lesions but did occur with primary lesions at other bowel sites (24). Peritoneal seeding was least common with primary lesions of the rectum, probably because these tumors are less accessible to the peritoneal cavity than most colon cancers. The incidence of hematogenous spread was similar for all sites, although the distribution differed. With primary rectal lesions, hematogenous failures were fairly evenly divided between liver and lung. This distribution is explained by the pattern of venous drainage through both the inferior mesenteric system, which drains to the liver via the portal vein, and the internal iliac system, which ultimately drains to the lungs via the inferior vena cava. With primary tumors of the colon, initial hematogenous failures usually were in the liver. This is consistent with the colon's pattern of venous drainage, which is initially to the liver via the portal system.

Anal Cancer

Although primary surgical management of anal cancer has largely been replaced by sphincter-sparing therapy, analysis of patterns of failure from surgically treated patients is informative for treatment planning. Approximately 35% of patients treated by abdominal-perineal resection have metastatic involvement of pelvic lymph nodes, and approximately 13% of patients treated by abdominal-perineal resection have recurrence in the inguinal lymph nodes (33). A patterns-of-failure analysis in 118 patients treated by abdominal-perineal resection with curative intent determined that 46 patients (39%) had recurrence subsequent to surgery. Local-regional failure occurred in 23% of the 118 patients treated with a potentially curative operation. Five percent experienced both local and distant recurrence, and 6% had distant metastasis without local failure. In 7% of patients, the site of tumor recurrence could not be determined (33).

ADJUVANT IRRADIATION FOR COLON AND RECTAL CANCER

Rectal Cancer

The foundation of treatment for patients with resectable rectal cancer is surgery. When radiation therapy, with or without chemotherapy, is offered as an adjuvant to patients who are candidates for surgical resection or who have undergone a potentially curative surgical resection, it is, by definition, being used in a person who may already be cured by surgery alone. A high standard of scientific evidence for the efficacy of adjuvant treatment, which is potentially toxic, expensive, and inconvenient, should therefore be provided before its use in routine clinical practice can be justified. Although randomized clinical trials comparing preoperative radiation therapy with surgery alone have demonstrated improved local control, most scientific studies have not demonstrated a survival advantage for a preoperative approach to adjuvant treatment. In contrast, several randomized trials of postoperative adjuvant radiation therapy and chemotherapy have demonstrated improved local control and survival compared with surgery alone or surgery followed by adjuvant radiation therapy without chemotherapy (34-36). Combined modality postoperative chemotherapy and radiation therapy, therefore, should be the standard of care in the adjuvant treatment of rectal cancer. Continuous-infusion 5-FU during radiation therapy has been found to be more effective than bolus 5-FU during radiation therapy (37).

Radiation therapy fields used in the adjuvant treatment of rectal cancer should include the primary tumor or tumor bed, with 3- to 5-cm margins, and the regional lymph nodes. In most institutions, internal iliac and presacral nodes are not routinely dissected during surgery for rectal cancer. These lymph nodes should be included in the initial irradiation volume. External iliac nodes are not a primary nodal drainage site and should not be included unless pelvic organs with major external iliac drainage, such as the prostate, bladder, vagina, cervix, and uterus, are involved by direct extension.

Most tumor bed recurrences are in the posterior one-half to two-thirds of the true pelvis (38). The internal iliac and presacral nodes are located posteriorly in the pelvis (39). Therefore, it is possible to use lateral fields for a portion of the treatment to reduce the dose of radiation to anterior normal tissues, such as the small bowel (Figure 19.1). Bladder distention and prone position are useful techniques for providing additional displacement of the small bowel out of the high-dose radiation field. A shrinking-field technique is used, with initial radiation therapy fields designed to treat the primary tumor volume and regional lymph nodes to a dose of 4500 cGy in 25 fractions.

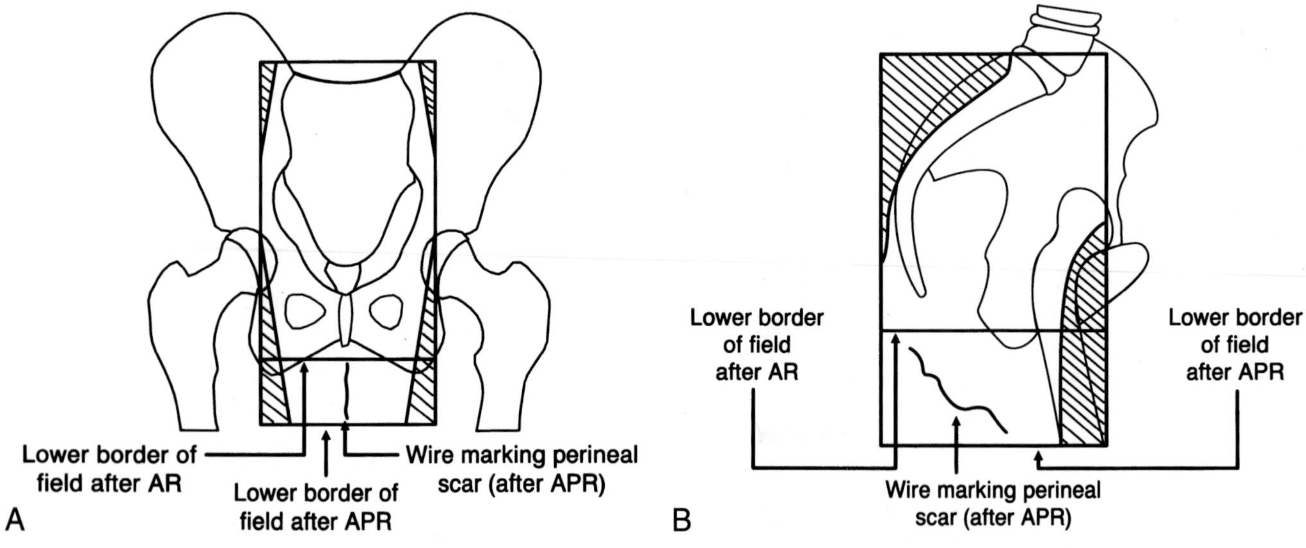

Figure 19.1. Posteroanterior **(A)** and lateral **(B)** pelvic radiation therapy fields used in adjuvant radiation therapy for rectal cancer. In patients with tumor adherence to organs drained by external iliac lymph nodes, the anterior border of the lateral field is modified to place it anterior to the symphysis pubis. AR, anterior resection; APR, abdominal perineal resection. (Reprinted with permission from Martenson JA, Schild SE, Haddock MG. Cancers of the Gastrointestinal Tract. In: Khan FM, Potish RA, eds. Treatment Planning in Radiation Oncology. Baltimore: Williams & Wilkins, 1998:319-342. By permission of Williams & Wilkins.)

Smaller fields can then be used to treat the primary tumor bed to an additional 540 to 900 cGy in three to five fractions, as clinically indicated. Isodose curves for anterior, posterior, and opposed lateral fields are shown in Figure 19.2. Simulation films obtained after the use of oral contrast medium can be used to demonstrate the amount of small bowel in the radiation field and are particularly helpful in the design of radiation boost fields. Films with contrast in the small bowel are often helpful in assessing the utility

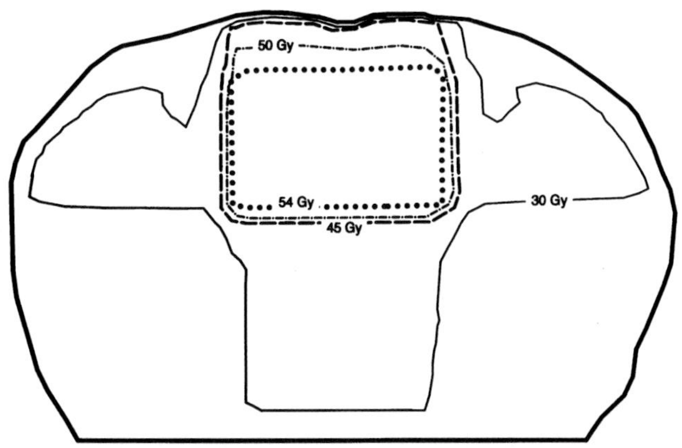

Figure 19.2. Isodose curves for adjuvant pelvic radiation therapy for rectal cancer with use of anterior, posterior, and opposed lateral fields. The total dose at isocenter is 5400 cGy in 30 fractions. (Reprinted with permission from Martenson JA, Schild SE, Haddock MG. Cancers of the Gastrointestinal Tract. In: Khan FM, Potish RA, eds. Treatment Planning in Radiation Oncology. Baltimore: Williams & Wilkins, 1998: 319-342. By permission of Williams & Wilkins.)

of bladder distention (39) or other measures (40) to decrease the volume of intestine in radiation fields.

Anterior and posterior radiation therapy fields (see Figure 19.1) should cover the pelvic inlet with a 2-cm margin. The superior margin is usually 1.5 cm above the level of the sacral promontory. In patients who have had an anterior resection, the usual inferior margin is below the obturator foramina, or approximately 3 cm below the most inferior portion of the tumor bed.

The posterior field margin for lateral fields is critical, because the rectum and perirectal tissues lie just anterior to the sacrum and coccyx. Accordingly, the posterior field margin should be at least 1.5 to 2 cm behind the anterior bony sacral margin (Figure 19.1, 19.3, and 19.4). The entire sacral canal with a 1.5-cm margin should be included in patients with locally advanced disease to avoid sacral recurrence from tumor spread along nerve roots. The anterior margin sometimes can be shaped to decrease the amount of radiation to the femoral head and bladder inferiorly and small bowel superiorly. Anteriorly, the lower one-third of the rectum abuts the posterior vaginal wall and prostate, and the posterior portion of these structures should be included in the radiation therapy field. In female patients, inclusion of the vagina can be verified at simulation by use of a contrast-soaked gauze pad or tampon during simulation (see Figure 19.3).

After abdominoperineal resection, the perineum should be included with the tumor bed and nodal x-irradiation volumes to prevent marginal recurrences from surgical implantation of tumor (22,41–43). In a study from Massa-

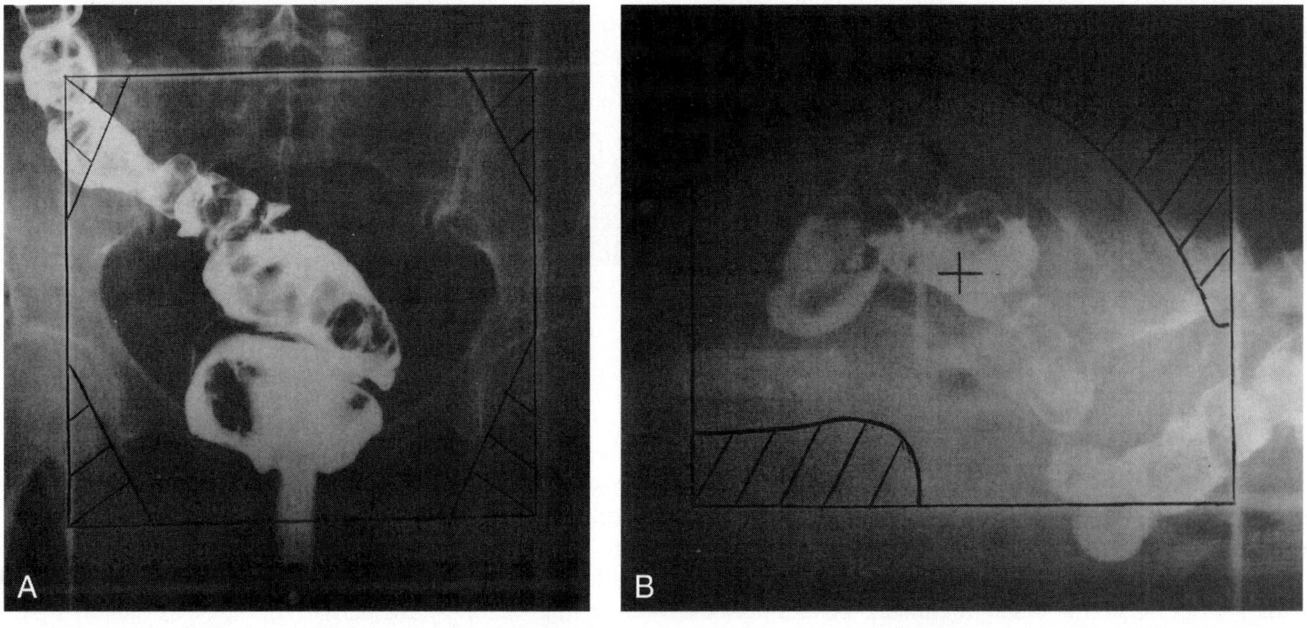

Figure 19.3. Postoperative radiation therapy posteroanterior **(A)** and lateral **(B)** fields with a four-field technique after anterior resection of the rectum and reanastomosis. Patient is simulated in the prone position with contrast material in the rectum, a tampon with contrast material in the vagina, and a lead radiopaque marker on the anal verge.

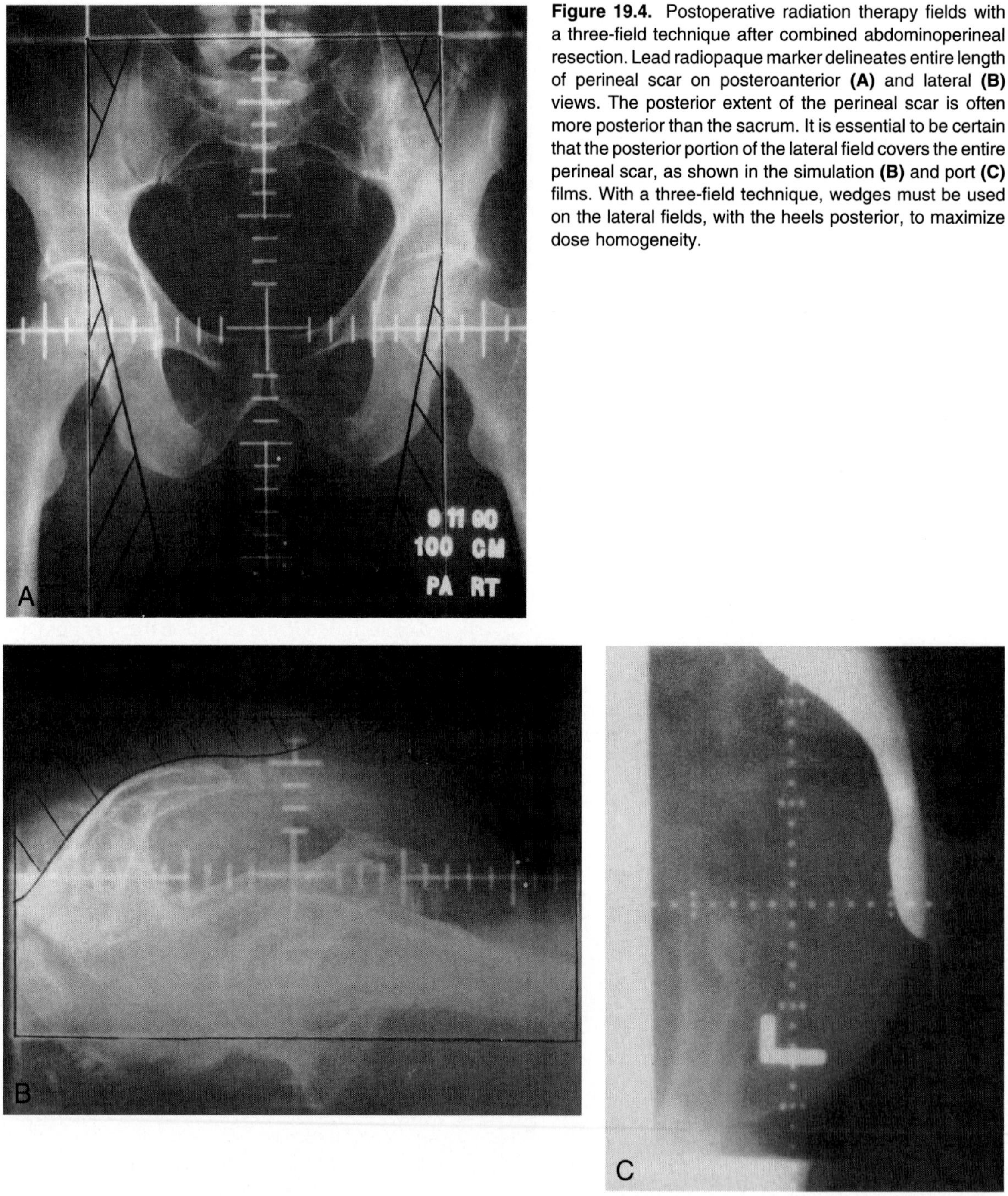

Figure 19.4. Postoperative radiation therapy fields with a three-field technique after combined abdominoperineal resection. Lead radiopaque marker delineates entire length of perineal scar on posteroanterior **(A)** and lateral **(B)** views. The posterior extent of the perineal scar is often more posterior than the sacrum. It is essential to be certain that the posterior portion of the lateral field covers the entire perineal scar, as shown in the simulation **(B)** and port **(C)** films. With a three-field technique, wedges must be used on the lateral fields, with the heels posterior, to maximize dose homogeneity.

chusetts General Hospital, the incidence of perineal recurrence with surgery alone was 8.5% (42). The incidence of perineal recurrence was only 1.7% in patients who were treated with postoperative irradiation (41). In a Mayo Clinic analysis of patients with rectal cancer who were treated with postoperative irradiation, the incidence of a perineal component of failure was 2% after abdominoperineal resection followed by ≥4000 cGy to the perineum but was 23% when the perineum was not adequately irradiated after abdominoperineal resection ($P < .05$) (43). Lead shot or wire should be used to mark the entire extent of the perineal scar when simulation films are obtained (see Figure 19.4). The inferior and posterior field edges should include a margin extending 1.5 cm beyond the perineal scar. Inferolaterally, the margin should be the lateral aspect of the ischial tuberosities. For treatment of the posterior field, the buttocks should be taped apart, and bolus material should be placed over the perineal incision (thickness

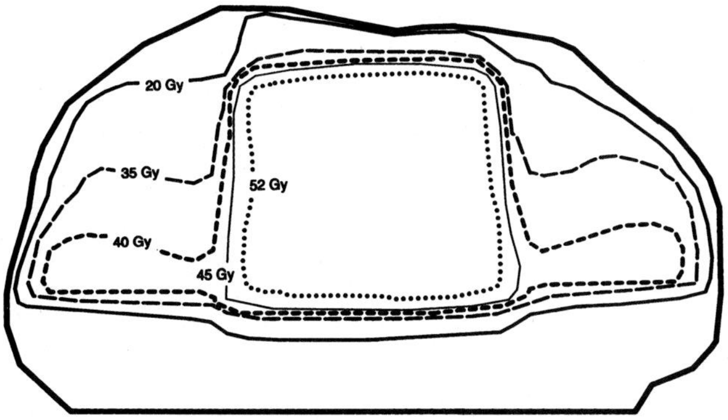

Figure 19.5. Isodose curves for adjuvant pelvic radiation therapy for rectal cancer with use of posterior and opposed lateral fields. The total dose at isocenter 5220 cGy in 29 fractions. Wedges, with heels posterior, are used on the lateral fields to increase dose homogeneity. (Reprinted with permission from Martenson JA, Schild SE, Haddock MG. Cancers of the Gastrointestinal Tract. In: Khan FM, Potish RA, eds. Treatment Planning in Radiation Oncology. Baltimore: Williams & Wilkins, 1998:319-342. By permission of Williams & Wilkins.)

depends on beam energy) to allow delivery of an adequate dose to the scar surface. If pelvic drains exited through the buttocks instead of the perineal wound, the drain sites should also be bolused. All patients in whom the perineum is included within radiation fields experience perineal discomfort during treatment. This can be mitigated by a three-field technique with posterior and lateral fields. Wedges are used on the lateral fields with heels posteriorly in a three-field technique to increase dose homogeneity (Figure 19.5).

The perineum usually can be treated to a dose level of 4500 cGy in 25 fractions over 5 weeks with acceptable short- and long-term tolerance. Because of skin reactions, patients occasionally require a 7- to 10-day rest during treatment, sitz baths, and protective ointments, such as Aquaphor. Most patients finish on schedule, and limited skin reactions generally improve markedly within 1 to 2 weeks of completion.

Colon Cancer

No mature, randomized clinical trials have examined the value of postoperative adjuvant radiation therapy for large bowel cancer above the rectum. However, several retrospective studies suggest that this may be a fruitful avenue for research (13,27,32,44–46). Because of positive results with adjuvant systemic therapy in high-risk patients with colon cancer (47,48), a randomized trial was begun to compare radiation therapy, 5-FU, and levamisole with 5-FU and levamisole alone after resection in high-risk patients with colon cancer. Until the results of this or other prospective clinical trials are available, adjuvant radiation therapy for colon cancer should not be used except in a prospective clinical trial. Potential radiation therapy fields for the adjuvant treatment of colon cancer in clinical trials are similar to those used for locally advanced colon cancer (Figure 19.6).

Dose

The dose to the extended tumor bed and nodal fields should be 4500 cGy in 25 fractions. A boost of 540 to 900 cGy in three to five fractions is then given, depending on the location of the small bowel in relation to the boost fields. The volume of the boost fields is defined in part by information available on the tumor bed, including the original preoperative description of the tumor by physical examination and endoscopy, results of preoperative imaging studies, such as the barium enema or CT scan, the description of the tumor from the operative notes and pathology report, and placement of surgical clips. A small bowel series should be performed on the simulator with the patient in treatment position. Information from this study can be used to verify that all small bowel is excluded from boost fields that receive doses of more than 5040 cGy.

LOCALLY ADVANCED AND LOCALLY RECURRENT COLORECTAL CANCER

Patients are generally treated with 4500 to 5040 cGy in 25 to 28 fractions to a field designed to cover the tumor and the regional lymph nodes. This treatment can be followed by a boost of 540 to 900 cGy in 3 to 5 fractions in selected patients. Doses greater than 5040 cGy are rarely administered in external radiation therapy unless the small bowel can be completely excluded from the radiation therapy field after 5040 cGy. Boost pelvic fields usually are treated with opposed lateral fields or three fields (posteroanterior and lateral with wedges on the laterals, heels posterior). Field shaping of the lateral boost fields can often be used to reduce or eliminate the volume of small intestine in the radiation therapy field anteriorly and superiorly. Bladder distention may be extremely useful in displacing small bowel loops superiorly and anteriorly out of both large and boost fields (39,49–52). Small bowel films can help to identify patients in whom immobile loops remain in an area at high risk (39,49–54). In such instances, the radiation oncologist must limit the dose to conform to small bowel tolerance.

For patients with residual, recurrent, or fixed pelvic lesions in posterior or lateral locations, it is important to include the sacral canal as target volume for the initial 4500 to 5000 cGy (39). Including this area is indicated because of the increased risk of tumor spread along nerve roots. Failure to do so may result in a marginal recurrence in the sacral canal (52).

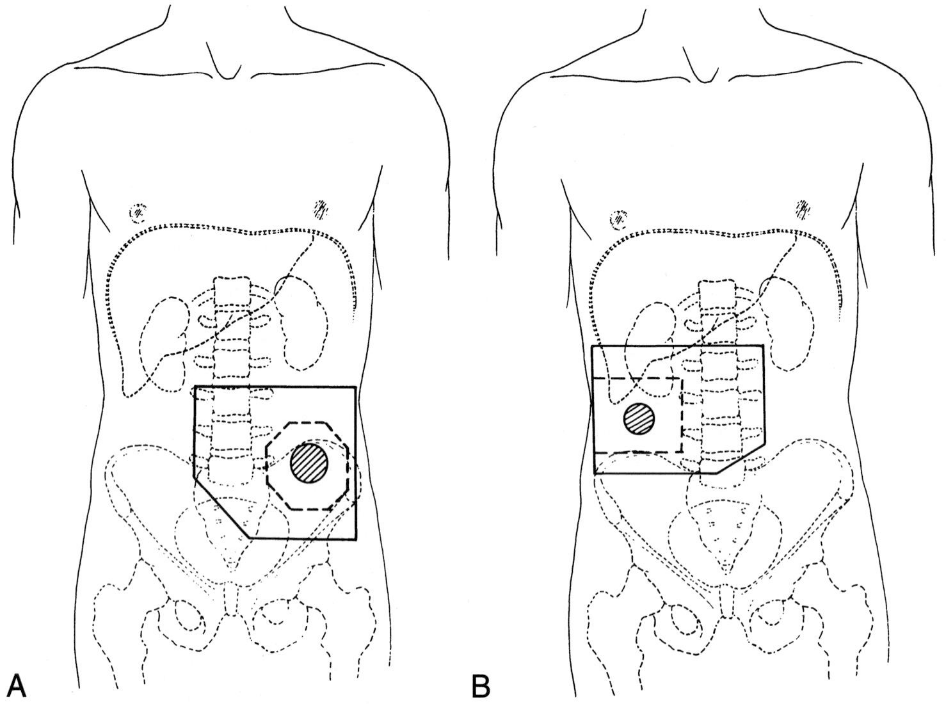

Figure 19.6. Idealized anteroposterior external radiation therapy fields used in the treatment of locally advanced or locally recurrent colon cancer. After 4500 cGy in 25 fractions to the large field, a boost field (*broken lines*) is used for the delivery of an additional 540 to 900 cGy in 3 to 5 fractions. **A.** A field designed to treat a lesion in the distal descending colon includes the ipsilateral iliac and para-aortic nodes. **B.** A field designed to treat a lesion in the midascending color includes the immediately adjacent regional nodes and the para-aortic nodes.

For patients with locally advanced or recurrent colon cancer, initial external beam radiation therapy fields should include the primary tumor, immediately adjacent lymph nodes, and adjacent para-aortic nodes (see Figure 19.6). These fields should receive 4500 cGy in 25 fractions. Smaller boost fields can then be considered for an additional 540 to 900 cGy in three to five fractions. In general, total cumulative doses above 5040 cGy are not recommended unless all small bowel can be excluded from fields considered for such doses. A small bowel study obtained on the simulator with the patient in treatment position is helpful for determining the position of the small bowel for this purpose. These films sometimes demonstrate that a lateral decubitus position for a portion of the treatment may be useful to decrease exposure or exclude small bowel from boost fields.

After administration of 4500 to 5040 cGy of external beam radiation, a boost of 1000 to 2000 cGy to areas of residual tumor can be given with the use of an intraoperative electron beam. In patients who completed a course of external beam radiation therapy, surgical debulking, and an intraoperative electron boost, 5-year survival rates of approximately 20% for locally recurrent disease and 45% for primary locally advanced disease were reported by Massachusetts General Hospital and the Mayo Clinic (55–57).

PRIMARY TREATMENT OF ANAL CANCER

The results of several recently published clinical trials have substantially added to our understanding of appropriate treatment planning for anal cancer. The Radiation Therapy Oncology Group (RTOG) and Eastern Cooperative Oncology Group (ECOG) conducted a randomized, intergroup clinical trial comparing radiation therapy and 5-FU with radiation therapy, 5-FU, and mitomycin-C (58). A continuous 5-FU intravenous infusion, 1000 mg/m^2/day, was given on days 1 through 4 of radiation therapy and was repeated on days 29 through 32 of radiation therapy. Mitomycin-C, 10 mg/m2 intravenously, was given on days 1 and 29 of radiation therapy in patients who were randomized to receive this drug. All patients received 3600 cGy in 20 fractions to the primary tumor, pelvic lymph nodes, and inguinal lymph nodes, followed by a field reduction to include the primary tumor with a 10- × 10-cm field, which was then treated to an additional 900 cGy in 5 fractions for a total dose of 4500 cGy in 25 fractions. In patients thought to have residual tumor after 4500 cGy, the final boost field was continued to a total cumulative dose of 5040 cGy in 28 fractions.

The combination of radiation therapy, 5-FU, and mitomycin-C resulted in a lower colostomy rate than radiation therapy and 5-FU without mitomycin-C. At 4 years, the colostomy rate was 9% in patients who received mitomycin-C and 23% in patients who did not receive mitomycin-C ($P = .002$). Persistent or recurrent tumor was by far the most common cause of colostomy: residual tumor was found in the surgical specimen in 97% of the colostomy patients who did not receive mitomycin-C and in 85% of the colostomy patients who received mitomycin-C. A statistically significant difference in survival between patients who received mitomycin-C and those who did not was not observed. The RTOG-ECOG study demonstrates that mitomycin-C is an important component of combined modality therapy for anal cancer.

Although the RTOG-ECOG trial provided critical information about combined modality therapy for anal cancer, it did not definitively address whether this form of treatment is superior to high-dose radiation therapy alone. Two randomized trials comparing radiation alone with radiation therapy, 5-FU, and mitomycin-C for cancer of the anal canal recently provided important data in this regard. A phase III trial, reported by the United Kingdom Coordinating Committee on Cancer Research (UKCCCR), compared radiation therapy alone with radiation therapy combined with a regimen of 5-FU and mitomycin-C (59). All patients in this study received 4500 cGy in 4 to 5 weeks, and most received a boost of 1500 to 2500 cGy after a 6-week break. Patients randomized to combined modality therapy generally received 5-FU, 1000 mg/m^2 per day, on the first 4 days of radiation therapy and for 4 days during the fourth or fifth week of radiation therapy. A single dose of mitomycin-C, 12 mg/m^2, was generally given on the first day of radiation therapy in the combined modality therapy group. Some variation on these standard doses was allowed in selected patients (59). The local failure rate at 3 years was 61% in patients randomized to radiation therapy alone and 39% in patients randomized to combined modality therapy. There was no difference in overall survival between patients treated with radiation therapy and those treated with combined modality therapy.

The European Organization for the Research and Treatment of Cancer (EORTC) randomized trial compared radiation therapy alone with radiation therapy, 5-FU, and mitomycin-C in patients with T3, T4, or lymph-node-positive anal cancer. The treatment program was very similar to that used in the UKCCCR study. An early report of this study indicated that the 3-year local control and colostomy-free survival rates were superior in the patients randomized to combined modality therapy (60).

These randomized studies provide strong evidence that combined modality therapy should be used in patients with anal cancer, with the goal of sphincter preservation and cure. Radiation therapy without chemotherapy (61) should be reserved for patients who are unable to tolerate combined modality therapy, such as those with serious comorbid illnesses. Because most patients with anal cancer are treated with mitomycin-C and an initial 4-day infusion of 5-FU, concurrent with initiation of radiation therapy, close coordination with the patient's medical oncologist is needed before treatment begins. The patient should receive a treatment with radiation on each of the days that 5-FU is infused to maximize the interaction of radiation therapy and chemotherapy. Accordingly, it is preferable to begin treatment on a Monday or Tuesday. Alternatively, special arrangements can be made for the patient to receive radiation treatments on the first weekend after initiation of radiation therapy if treatment is started later in the week.

Radiation therapy fields should be designed to include the primary lesion and regional pelvic and inguinal lymph nodes. A portion of the inguinal lymph node chain is superficial to the femoral head and neck. Radiation therapy fields should be designed to avoid giving full dose to these structures. Anteroposterior and posteroanterior fields or four-field box techniques that include the inguinal lymph nodes with the femoral head and neck may place patients at risk for subsequent treatment-induced fracture (61). Factors increasing the chance of this complication are of particular concern in a population of patients that includes a large number of elderly women, many of whom are already at risk for this problem because of osteoporosis. Radiation techniques should be used that minimize the dose to the femoral head and neck by treating lateral superficial inguinal nodes through anterior fields only. This can be accomplished by treating the primary tumor, pelvic nodes, and inguinal nodes with an anterior photon field that encompasses all these structures (Figure 19.7A). The posterior photon field includes only the primary tumor and pelvic lymph nodes (Figure 19.7B). Electron fields are used to supplement the dose to the portion of the lateral superficial inguinal nodes not included in the posterior photon field (Figure 19.7C). The medial borders of the lateral electron fields are the same as the lateral border of the posterior photon field at its exit point on the patient's anterior abdominal wall. This border is determined with the aid of radiopaque markers placed on the anterior abdominal wall under fluoroscopic guidance while the posteroanterior photon field is being simulated (Figure 19.7B and 19.7C). Isodose curves for this technique are shown in Figure 19.8.

The radiation treatment regimen used in the most effective arm of the RTOG-ECOG study was different from that used in the EORTC and UKCCCR studies because the RTOG-ECOG study used a lower total radiation dose without a treatment break, together with a somewhat more intensive chemotherapy regimen, whereas the EORTC and UKCCCR studies used a higher total dose with a 6-week treatment break after 4500 cGy. Definitive recommendations are not possible for the preferred treatment regimen, because a direct scientific comparison of these regimens has not been performed. Data from a preliminary RTOG study of high-dose radiation therapy, however, suggest that the use of a treatment regimen that includes a planned treatment break may result in an inferior outcome (62).

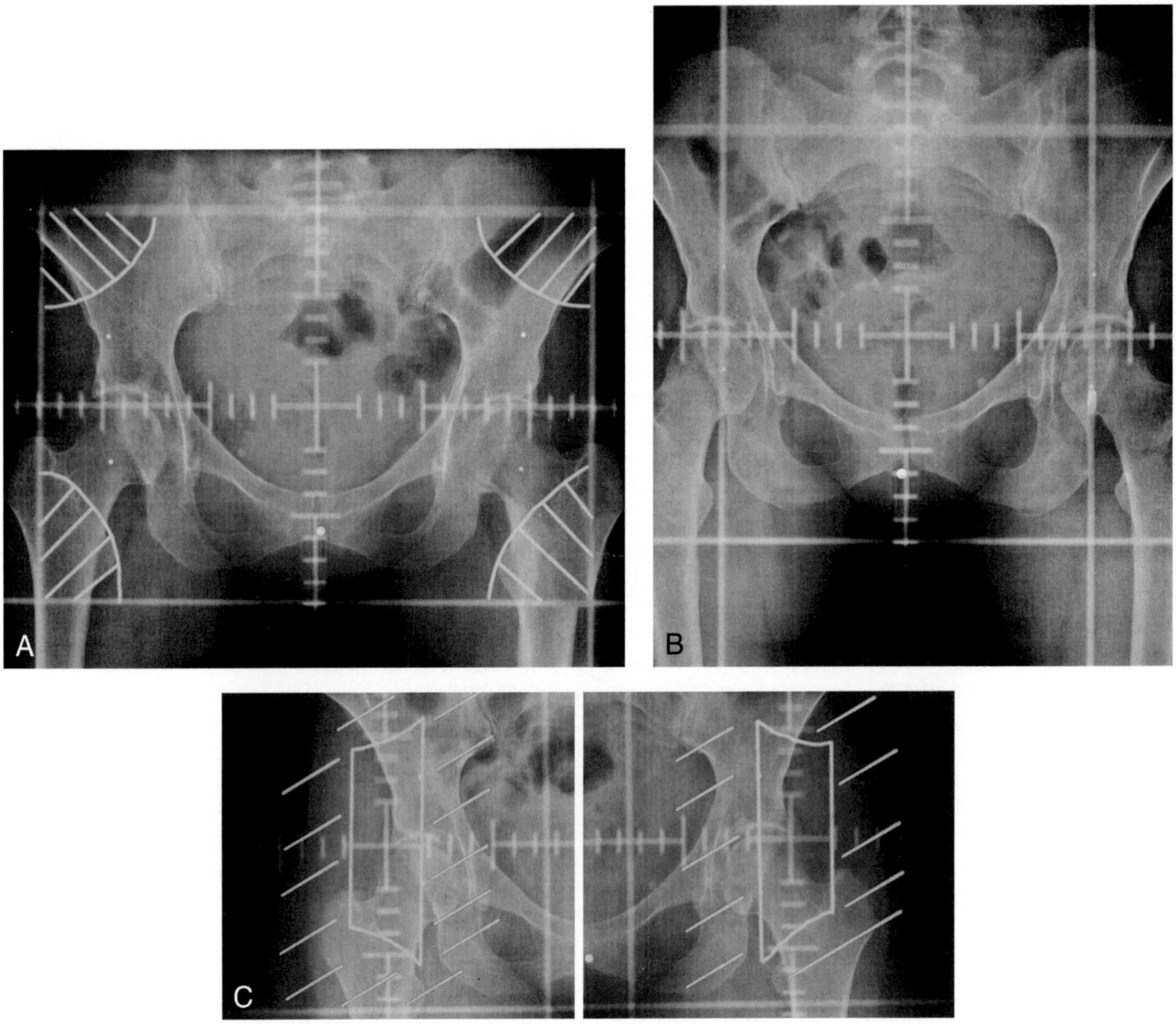

Figure 19.7. **(A)** anterior and **(B)** posterior radiation therapy photon fields used for anal cancer. **(C)** electron fields are used to supplement lateral inguinal nodes not included in the posterior photon field. The medial borders of the electron fields are determined by placing radiopaque markers on the anterior abdominal wall at the exit point of the lateral border of the posterior photon field. (Reprinted with permission from Martenson JA, Schild SE, Haddock MG. Cancers of the Gastrointestinal Tract. In: Khan FM, Potish RA, eds. Treatment Planning in Radiation Oncology. Baltimore: Williams & Wilkins, 1998:319-342. By permission of Williams & Wilkins.)

Accordingly, a treatment regimen based on the one used in the RTOG-ECOG randomized trial, with total radiation doses of approximately 4500 to 5040 cGy in 25 to 28 fractions, together with two courses of 5-FU and mitomycin-C, is generally accepted as the standard of care in the United States. Treatment programs that use substantially higher radiation doses or different chemotherapy combinations (63) should be confined to peer-reviewed clinical trials.

THERAPEUTIC RATIO

The potential for optimizing the therapeutic ratio is enhanced by close cooperation among surgeon, medical oncologist, and radiation oncologist (50,64). The use of radiopaque clips to mark the tumor or tumor bed areas is particularly helpful in the design of high-dose boost volumes. Reconstruction techniques that exclude or minimize the volume of small bowel in the irradiated field are also helpful.

A number of techniques can be used by the radiation oncologist to potentially improve the therapeutic ratio. For both rectal and colon cancers, shrinking-field techniques should be used after a dose of 4500 cGy. With rectal cancers and proximal sigmoid cancers, lateral fields should be used for a portion of the treatment to avoid as much small bowel as possible. Treatment with bladder distention is

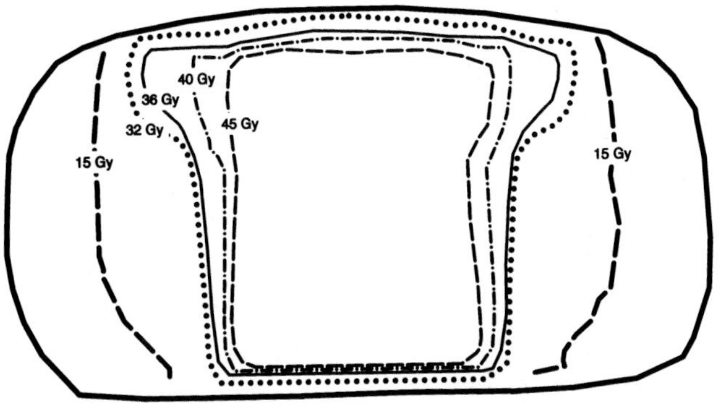

Figure 19.8. Isodose curves for pelvic radiation therapy fields used in the primary treatment of anal cancer. The total dose at the isocenter for the photon fields is 4500 cGy. Lateral inguinal nodes receive 3600 cGy through a combination of the anterior photon field and supplementary electron fields (see Figure 19.7). (Reprinted with permission from Martenson JA, Schild SE, Haddock MG. Cancers of the Gastrointestinal Tract. In: Khan FM, Potish RA, eds. Treatment Planning in Radiation Oncology. Baltimore: Williams & Wilkins, 1998:319-342. By permission of Williams & Wilkins.)

appropriate unless the result is displacement of tumor outside the radiation field. In patients with colon cancer, it may be possible to reduce the volume of small bowel within the field, often by placing the patient in the lateral decubitus position for a portion of treatment.

In studies of patients with rectal cancer given postoperative radiation as adjuvant therapy, the risk of small bowel obstruction requiring reoperation seems to be affected by treatment technique. When pelvic and para-aortic fields were treated with an anterior and posterior opposed technique at M.D. Anderson Hospital, the incidence of small bowel obstruction requiring reoperation was 17.5%, compared with 5% with surgery alone (65,66). When the superior extent of the field was shifted down to L-5, the incidence of complications requiring operative intervention decreased to about 12%. At Massachusetts General Hospital, multifield techniques and bladder distention were used. The incidence of small bowel obstruction requiring surgical intervention in patients receiving postoperative radiation therapy was 6%, which was essentially equal to that in the patients treated with operation alone.

When multiple-field irradiation techniques are used in combination with chemotherapy in the adjuvant treatment of rectal cancer, no apparent increase occurs in the risk of severe small bowel complications (67). In an analysis of the North Central Cancer Treatment Group randomized trial, with minimum 3-year follow-up, the incidence of severe small bowel complications was less than 5% with either irradiation alone or irradiation plus chemotherapy.

A large retrospective analysis of patients who received radiation therapy for high-risk, completely resected colon cancer or for incompletely resected colon cancer found that acute enteritis resulting in hospitalization or a break from treatment occurred in 16 of 203 patients (8%). Long-term toxicity requiring surgery was observed in nine patients (4.5%). Nonsurgical complications, such as chronic abdominal pain, were not assessed (46). The lack of data on serious nonsurgical complications and the potential for significant toxicity requiring surgical intervention underscore the importance of avoiding adjuvant radiation therapy for large bowel cancer outside a clinical trial until there is evidence from a scientific prospective study demonstrating that adjuvant radiation therapy is effective.

Some reassurance about the risk of surgical complications resulting from radiation therapy is provided by the above data from the Mayo Clinic, MD Anderson Hospital, and Massachusetts General Hospital. Until recently, however, little information was available about the risk of serious nonsurgical complications. A recent study suggests that the risk of functionally significant long-term toxicity, not requiring surgical correction, after pelvic radiation therapy and chemotherapy is high. Functional assessment of bowel function was undertaken in patients who either had or had not received postoperative adjuvant treatment with radiation and chemotherapy after anterior resection for rectal cancer. Consistently worse bowel function was found in the patients who had received radiation therapy and chemotherapy. For example, 56% of the patients who had received adjuvant treatment reported at least occasional fecal incontinence, in contrast to only 7% of patients who did not receive adjuvant treatment ($P < .001$) (68).

No treatment has been clearly demonstrated to be effective in the management of radiation therapy complications. Decreasing the risk and severity of complications by minimizing the volume of normal tissue within the radiation therapy field is therefore very important. Clinical trials to assess the value of olsalazine and cholestyramine in mitigating radiation-related side effects have demonstrated that these agents are associated with unacceptable toxicity (69,70). Sucralfate is a more promising agent. A European study has suggested that sucralfate may reduce both acute and long-term adverse effects of pelvic radiation therapy (71). A confirmatory randomized trial has been undertaken by the North Central Cancer Treatment Group. Further clinical trials of measures to reduce toxicity are needed. Continued studies of methods to improve tumor control and survival are also needed. The oncology community will have the best chance of improving the therapeutic ratio for patients with lower gastrointestinal cancer if radiation oncologists and other oncologists are committed to entering patients into well-designed prospective studies to assess promising new ways of improving treatment.

References

1. Postlethwait RW. Malignant tumors of colon and rectum. Ann Surg 1949;129:34-46.
2. Martin EW Jr, James KK, Hurtubise PE, Catalano P, Minton JP. The

use of CEA as an early indicator for gastrointestinal tumor recurrence and second-look procedures. Cancer 1977;39:440-446.
3. Wanebo HJ, Rao B, Pinsky CM, Hoffman RG, Stearns M, Schwartz MK, Oettgen HF. Preoperative carcinoembryonic antigen level as a prognostic indicator in colorectal cancer. N Engl J Med 1978;299:448-451.
4. Beart RW Jr, O'Connell MJ. Postoperative follow-up of patients with carcinoma of the colon. Mayo Clin Proc 1983;58:361-363.
5. Moertel CG, Schutt AJ, Go VL. Carcinoembryonic antigen test for recurrent colorectal carcinoma. Inadequacy for early detection. JAMA 1978;239:1065-1066.
6. Patterson DJ, Alpert E. Tumour Markers of the Gastrointestinal Tract. In: Hodgson HJF, Bloom SR, eds. Gastrointestinal and Hepatobiliary Cancer. Boston: Butterworths, 1983:189.
7. Moertel CG, Fleming TR, Macdonald JS, Haller DG, Laurie JA, Tangen C. An evaluation of the carcinoembryonic antigen (CEA) test for monitoring patients with resected colon cancer. JAMA 1993;270:943-947.
8. Fletcher RH. CEA monitoring after surgery for colorectal cancer. When is the evidence sufficient? [Editorial]. JAMA 1993;270:987-988.
9. Minton JP, Hoehn JL, Gerber DM, Horsley JS, Connolly DP, Salwan F, Fletcher WS, Cruz AB Jr, Gatchell FG, Oviedo M, Meyer KK, Leffall LD Jr, Berk RS, Stewart PA, Kurucz SE. Results of a 400-patient carcinoembryonic antigen second-look colorectal cancer study. Cancer 1985;55:1284-1290.
10. Fletcher RH. Carcinoembryonic antigen. Ann Intern Med 1986;104: 66-73.
11. Northover J, Houghton J, Lennon T. CEA to detect recurrence of colon cancer [Letter to the editor]. JAMA 1994;272:31.
12. Black WA, Waugh JM. Intramural extension of carcinoma of descending color, sigmoid, and rectosigmoid: pathologic study. Surg Gynecol Obstet 1948;84:457-464.
13. Grinnell RS. Lymphatic block with atypical and retrograde lymphatic metastasis and spread in carcinoma of the colon and rectum. Ann Surg 1966;163:272-280.
14. Enquist IF, Block IR. Rectal cancer in the female: selection of proper operation based upon anatomic studies of rectal lymphatics. Prog Clin Cancer 1966;2:73-85.
15. Nivatvongs S, Stern HS, Fryd DS. The length of the anal canal. Dis Colon Rectum 1981;24:600-601.
16. Stearns MW Jr, Urmacher C, Sternberg SS, Woodruff J, Attiyeh F. Cancer of the anal canal. Curr Probl Cancer 1980;4:1-44.
17. Morson BC. The pathology and results of treatment of squamous cell carcinoma of the anal canal and anal margin. Proc R Soc Med 1960; 53:416-420.
18. Gilbert SG. Symptomatic local tumor failure following abdominoperineal resection. Int J Radiat Oncol Biol Phys 1978;4:801-807.
19. Gunderson LL, Tepper JE, Dosoretz DE, Kopelson G, Hoskins RB, Rich TA, Russell AH. Patterns of failure after treatment of gastrointestinal cancer. Cancer Treat Symp 1983;2:181-197.
20. Mendenhall WM, Million RR, Pfaff WW. Patterns of recurrence in adenocarcinoma of the rectum and rectosigmoid treated with surgery alone: implications in treatment planning with adjuvant radiation therapy. Int J Radiat Oncol Biol Phys 1983;9:977-985.
21. Walz BJ, Green MR, Lindstrom ER, Butcher HR Jr. Anatomical prognostic factors after abdominal perineal resection. Int J Radiat Oncol Biol Phys 1981:7:477-484.
22. Gunderson LL, Sosin H. Areas of failure found at reoperation (second or symptomatic look) following "curative surgery" for adenocarcinoma of the rectum. Clinicopathologic correlation and implications for adjuvant therapy. Cancer 1974;34:1278-1292.
23. Welch JP, Donaldson GA. Detection and treatment of recurrent cancer of the colon and rectum. Am J Surg 1978;135:505-511.
24. Gunderson LL, Sosin H, Levitt S. Extrapelvic colon—areas of failure in a reoperation series: implications for adjuvant therapy. Int J Radiat Oncol Biol Phys 1985;11:731-741.
25. Welch JP, Donaldson GA. The clinical correlation of an autopsy study of recurrent colorectal cancer. Ann Surg 1979;189:496-502.
26. Cass AW, Million RR, Pfaff WW. Patterns of recurrence following surgery alone for adenocarcinoma of the colon and rectum. Cancer 1976;37:2861-2865.
27. Russell AH, Pelton J, Reheis CE, Wisbeck WM, Tong DY, Dawson LE. Adenocarcinoma of the colon: an autopsy study with implications for new therapeutic strategies. Cancer 1985;56:1446-1451.
28. Willett CG, Tepper JE, Cohen AM, Orlow E, Welch CE. Failure patterns following curative resection of colonic carcinoma. Ann Surg 1984;200:685-690.
29. Willett C, Tepper JE, Cohen A, Orlow E, Welch C, Donaldson G. Local failure following curative resection of colonic adenocarcinoma. Int J Radiat Oncol Biol Phys 1984;10:645-651.
30. Minsky BD, Mies C, Rich TA, Recht A, Chaffey JT. Potentially curative surgery of colon cancer: patterns of failure and survival. J Clin Oncol 1988;6:106-118.
31. Russell AH, Tong D, Dawson LE, Wisbeck W. Adenocarcinoma of the proximal colon. Sites of initial dissemination and patterns of recurrence following surgery alone. Cancer 1984;53:360-367.
32. Willett CG, Tepper JE, Skates SJ, Wood WC, Orlow EC, Duttenhaver JR. Adjuvant postoperative radiation therapy for colonic carcinoma. Ann Surg 1987;206:694-698.
33. Boman BM, Moertel CG, O'Connell MJ, Scott M, Weiland LH, Beart RW, Gunderson LL, Spencer RJ. Carcinoma of the anal canal. A clinical and pathologic study of 188 cases. Cancer 1984;54:114-125.
34. Krook JE, Moertel CG, Gunderson LL, Wieand HS, Collins RT, Beart RW, Kubista TP, Poon MA, Meyers WC, Mailliard JA, Twito DI, Morton RF, Veeder MH, Witzig TE, Cha S, Vidyarthi SC. Effective surgical adjuvant therapy for high-risk rectal carcinoma. N Engl J Med 1991; 324:709-715.
35. Gastrointestinal Tumor Study Group. Prolongation of the disease-free interval in surgically treated rectal carcinoma. N Engl J Med 1985; 312:1465-1472.
36. Douglass HO Jr, Moertel CG, Mayer RJ, Thomas PR, Lindblad AS, Mittleman A, Stablein DM, Bruckner HW. Survival after postoperative combination treatment of rectal cancer [Letter]. N Engl J Med 1986; 315:1294-1295.
37. O'Connell MJ, Martenson JA, Wieand HS, Krook JE, Macdonald JS, Haller DG, Mayer RJ, Gunderson LL, Rich TA. Improving adjuvant therapy for rectal cancer by combining protracted-infusion fluorouracil with radiation therapy after curative surgery. N Engl J Med 1994; 331:502-507.
38. Gilbertsen VA. Adenocarcinoma of the rectum: incidence and locations of recurrent tumor following present-day operations performed for cure. Ann Surg 1960;151:340-348.
39. Gunderson LL, Russell AH, Llewellyn HJ, Doppke KP, Tepper JE. Treatment planning for colorectal cancer: radiation and surgical techniques and value of small-bowel films. Int J Radiat Oncol Biol Phys 1985;11:1379-1393.
40. Shanahan TG, Mehta MP, Gehring MA, Buchler DA, Kubsad SS, Kinsella TJ. Minimization of small bowel volume utilizing customized "belly board" mold [Abstract]. Int J Radiat Oncol Biol Phys 1989;17 Suppl 1:187-188.
41. Hoskins RB, Gunderson LL, Dosoretz DE, Rich TA, Galdabini J, Donaldson G. Cohen AM. Adjuvant postoperative radiotherapy in carcinoma of the rectum and rectosigmoid. Cancer 1985;55:61-71.
42. Rich T, Gunderson LL, Lew R, Galdibini JJ, Cohen AM, Donaldson G. Patterns of recurrence of rectal cancer after potentially curative surgery. Cancer 1983;52:1317-1329.
43. Schild SE, Martenson JA Jr, Gunderson LL, Ilstrup DM, Berg KK, O'Connell MJ, Weiland LH. Postoperative adjuvant therapy of rectal cancer: an analysis of disease control, survival, and prognostic factors. Int J Radiat Oncol Biol Phys 1989;17:55-62.
44. Duttenhaver JR, Hoskins RB, Gunderson LL, Tepper JE. Adjuvant postoperative radiation therapy in the management of adenocarcinoma of the colon. Cancer 1986;57:955-963.
45. Fabian CJ, Reddy E. Jewell W, Trowbridge AA, McCracken D, Vogel S, Goodwin JW, Fletcher WS. Phase I-II pilot of whole abdominal radiation and concomitant 5-FU as an adjuvant in colon cancer: a Southwest Oncology Group Study. Int J Radiat Oncol Biol Phys 1988; 15:885-892.
46. Willett CG, Fung CY, Kaufman DS, Efird J, Shellito PC. Postoperative radiation therapy for high-risk colon carcinoma. J Clin Oncol 1993; 11:1112-1117.
47. Moertel CG, Fleming TR, Macdonald JS, Haller DG, Laurie JA, Goodman PJ, Ungerleider JS, Emerson WA, Tormey DC, Glick JH, Veeder MH, Mailliard JA. Levamisole and fluorouracil for adjuvant therapy of resected colon carcinoma. N Engl J Med 1990;322:352-358.
48. Moertel CG. Fleming TR, Macdonald JS, Haller DG, Laurie JA, Tangen CM, Ungerleider JS, Emerson WA, Tormey DC, Glick JH, Veeder MH,

Mailliard JA. Fluorouracil plus levamisole as effective adjuvant therapy after resection of stage III colon carcinoma: a final report. Ann Intern Med 1995;122:321-326.
49. Gallagher MJ, Brereton HD, Rostock RA, Zero JM, Zekoski DA, Poyss LF, Richter MP, Kligerman MM. A prospective study of treatment techniques to minimize the volume of pelvic small bowel with reduction of acute and late effects associated with pelvic irradiation. Int J Radiat Oncol Biol Phys 1986;12:1565-1573.
50. Gunderson LL, Cohen AM, Welch CE. Residual, inoperable or recurrent colorectal cancer. Interaction of surgery and radiotherapy. Am J Surg 1980;139:518-525.
51. Gunderson LL, Meyer JE, Sheedy PF, Munzenrider JE. Radiation Oncology. In: Margulis AR, Burhenne JH, eds. Alimentary Tract Radiology. 3rd ed. St. Louis: CV Mosby, 1983:2409-2446.
52. Gunderson LL, Cohen AC, Dosoretz DD, Shipley WU, Hedberg SE, Wood WC, Rodkey GV, Suit HD. Residual unresectable, or recurrent colorectal cancer: external beam irradiation and intraoperative electron beam boost ± resection. Int J Radiat Oncol Biol Phys 1983;9: 1597-1606.
53. Green N. The avoidance of small intestine injury in gynecologic cancer. Int J Radiat Oncol Biol Phys 1983;9:1385-1390.
54. Green N, Iba G, Smith WR. Measures to minimize small intestine injury in the irradiated pelvis. Cancer 1975;35:1633-1640.
55. Suzuki K, Gunderson LL, Devine RM, Weaver AL, Dozois RR, Ilstrup DM, Martenson JA, O'Connell MJ. Intraoperative irrradiation after palliative surgery for locally recurrent rectal cancer. Cancer 1995;75:939-952.
56. Gunderson LL, Nelson H, Martenson JA, Cha S, Haddock M, Devine R, Fieck JM, Wolff B, Dozois R, O'Connell MJ. Intraoperative electron and external beam irradiation with or without 5-fluorouracil and maximum surgical resection for previously unirradiated, locally recurrent colorectal cancer. Dis Colon Rectum 1996;39:1379-1395.
57. Gunderson LL, Martenson JA, Haddock MG. Indications for and results of irradiation ± chemotherapy for rectal cancer. Ann Acad Med Singapore 1996;25:448-459.
58. Flam M, John M, Pajak TF, Petrelli N, Myerson R, Doggett S, Quivey J, Rotman M, Kerman H, Coia L, Murray K. Role of mitomycin in combination with fluorouracil and radiotherapy, and of salvage chemoradiation in the definitive nonsurgical treatment of epidermoid carcinoma of the anal canal: results of a phase III randomized intergroup study. J Clin Oncol 1996;14:2527-2539.
59. UKCCCR Anal Cancer Trial Working Party. Epidermoid anal cancer: results from the UKCCCR randomised trial of radiotherapy alone versus radiotherapy, 5-fluorouracil, and mitomycin. Lancet 1996;348: 1049-1054.
60. Roelofsen F, Bosset JF, Eschwege F, Pfeiffer, van Glabbeke M, Bartelink H. Concomitant radiotherapy and chemotherapy superior to radiotherapy alone in the treatment of locally advanced anal cancer. Results of a phase III randomized trial of the EORTC Radiotherapy and Gastrointestinal Cooperative Groups [Abstract]. Proc Am Soc Clin Oncol 1995;14:194.
61. Martenson JA Jr, Gunderson LL. External radiation therapy without chemotherapy in the management of anal cancer. Cancer 1993;71: 1736-1740.
62. John MJ, Pajak TH, Flam MS, Hoffman JP, Markoe AM, Wolkov HB, Paris KJ. Dose acceleration in chemoradiation (CRX) for anal cancer: preliminary results of RTOG 92-08 [Abstract]. Int J Radiat Oncol Biol Phys 1995;32 Suppl 1:157.
63. Martenson JA, Lipsitz SR, Wagner H Jr, Kaplan EH, Otteman LA, Schuchter LM, Mansour EG, Talamonti MS, Benson AB III. Initial results of a phase II trial of high dose radiation therapy, 5-fluorouracil, and cisplatin for patients with anal cancer (E4292): an Eastern Cooperative Oncology Group Study. Int J Radiat Oncol Biol Phys 1996; 35:745-749.
64. Cohen AM, Gunderson LL, Welch CE. Selective use of adjuvant radiation therapy in resectable colorectal adenocarcinoma. Dis Colon Rectum 1981;24:247-251.
65. Romsdahl MM, Withers HR. Radiotherapy combined with curative surgery. Its use as therapy for carcinoma of the sigmoid colon and rectum. Arch Surg 1978;113:446-453.
66. Withers HR, Cuasay L, Mason KA, Romsdahl MM, Saxton J. Elective radiation therapy in the curative treatment of cancer of the rectum and rectosigmoid colon. In: Stroehlein JR, Romsdahl MM, eds. Gastrointestinal Cancer. New York: Raven Press, 1981:351-362.
67. Gunderson LL, Collins R, Earle JD, Wieand HS, Moertel C, Krook J, Martenson J, Beart RW, Kubista T. Adjuvant treatment of rectal cancer: randomized prospective study of irradiation ± chemotherapy: a NCCTG, Mayo Clinic Study [Abstract]. Int J Radiat Oncol Biol Phys 1986;12 Suppl 1:169.
68. Kollmorgen CF, Meagher AP, Wolff BG, Pemberton JH, Martenson JA, Ilstrup DM. The long-term effect of adjuvant postoperative chemoradiotherapy for rectal carcinoma on bowel function. Ann Surg 1994;220:676-682.
69. Martenson JA Jr, Hyand G, Moertel CG, Mailliard JA, O'Fallon JR, Collins RT, Morton RF, Tewfik HH, Moore RL, Frank AR, Urias RE, Deming RL. Olsalazine is contraindicated during pelvic radiation therapy: results of a double-blind, randomized clinical trial. Int J Radiat Oncol Biol Phys 1996;35:299-303.
70. Chary S, Thomson DH. A clinical trial evaluating cholestyramine to prevent diarrhea in patients maintained on low-fat diets during pelvic radiation therapy. Int J Radiat Oncol Biol Phys 1984;10:1885-1890.
71. Henriksson R, Franzen L, Littbrand B. Effects of sucralfate on acute and late bowel discomfort following radiotherapy of pelvic cancer. J Clin Oncol 1992;10:969-975.

Chapter 20

Bladder Cancer

Alan R. Schulsinger, Ron Allison, Chul K. Sohn, Vinceno Valentini, and Marvin Rotman

INTRODUCTION

Bladder cancer is the sixth most common cancer in the United States (1). It comprises approximately 6% of all cancers, which translates into 50,000 new cases a year. The 12,000 deaths per year attributable to bladder malignancies are comparable to the yearly mortality rate of ovarian, stomach, and gastric cancers. Over the last 2 decades, we have witnessed a nearly two-fold increase in the incidence of bladder cancer, but overall survival rates have remained essentially unchanged.

Risk factors for transitional cell cancer of the bladder include exposure to chemical carcinogens (i.e., aniline dyes), tobacco (estimated to account for half of all cases that occur in men in the United States and one-third of all cases that occur in women), coffee, artificial sweeteners, and phenacetin containing analgesics (2). Chronic irritation by foreign bodies (i.e., indwelling Foley catheters, calculi, Schistosoma hematobium in endemic areas) are risk factors for squamous cell cancers. Extrophy of the bladder is the main risk factor for adenocarcinoma (3).

For nonmuscle-invading disease [stage 0 (Tis), and stage A (T1)], acceptable local control rates and 5-year survival rates have been obtained with a variety of interventions including transurethral resection (TUR) and fulguration of the bladder, partial cystectomy, interstitial implants, intraoperative irradiation, intravesicular chemotherapy, and Bacillus Calmette Guerin (BCG) following TUR. For muscle-invasive bladder cancers, survival results and morbidity remain poor with cystectomy. This surgery usually includes permanent ileal conduit with loss of sexual potency and is considered "standard treatment" in the United States. Although preoperative external beam irradiation may improve outcome (4), and the combination of chemotherapy with irradiation may allow for organ preservation, only a fraction of patients are offered these options.

ANATOMY

The bladder is a hollow muscular organ that lies in the anterior half of the pelvis. When full, it contains about half a liter of urine. It occupies a triangular space bounded anteriorly and laterally by the symphysis pubis and the diverging walls of the pelvis, respectively. The posterior border is the rectum/rectovaginal septum. The lateral and inferior portion of the bladder are supported by the obturator internus muscles and levator ani muscles, respectively. In males, the prostate lies between the levator ani and the bladder. The superior surface of the bladder is covered by peritoneum.

The interior inferior surface of the bladder is lined by a loosely attached mucus membrane except in the trigone region where the mucus membrane is firmly attached. The trigone region that leads into the bladder neck is defined by the urethral orifices posterolaterally and by the urethral aperture at the inferior/anterior angle. Transitional cell epithelium lines the bladder and is contiguous into the ureters (urothelium).

The bladder contains a submucosal plexus of lymphatics that are most abundant in the region of the trigone. These lymphatics usually drain into channels that pierce the muscular layers and then organize from the superior and inferolateral surfaces of the bladder to ultimately drain into the external iliac lymph nodes. From the posterior surface of the bladder, lymphatic channels drain to both the external iliac and internal iliac lymph node chains. Lymphatic vessels from the bladder neck may combine with some prostatic lymphatic vessels in males, which can ultimately drain to the presacral and common iliac lymph nodes.

Clinical Presentation and Prognostic Factors

Some of the more common clinical presentations of bladder cancer include 1) painless hematuria, which occurs in up to 80% of patients; 2) bladder irritability, such as urinary frequency, urgency, and dysuria (all of which are suggestive of muscle-invasive disease); and 3) recurrent urinary tract infections, particularly in men. Some of the less common clinical presentations include 1) flank pain or anemia associated with a pelvic mass and 2) pelvic mass associated with lower extremity weakness, weight loss, abdominal pain, or bone pain.

Approximately 70% of patients have Tis, Ta, or T1 disease at presentation. Approximately 20% have stage T2 to T4 disease and another 10% present with metastatic disease. Even though the majority of tumors are superficial, they can behave aggressively and locally recur repeatedly, often with further and deeper invasion. Eventually, penetration of the bladder muscular layers occurs. Once muscle is involved, lymphatic and blood vessel invasion is common. It is generally reported that pathologic T2 disease has a 30% risk of nodal involvement, as does early T3 disease. Patients with advanced T3 or T4 tumors have a 50 to 80% risk of nodal metastasis (5). As nodal metastasis is in part an indicator of potential for systemic spread, a similar frequency of distant metastasis is eventually noted for these patients as well. The most common sites of spread are lung, bone, and liver. Poor prognostic factors at presentation include deeply invasive tumors, associated carcinoma in-situ (CIS), vascular invasion, positive lymph nodes, tumors of size greater than 6 cm, urethral obstruction/obstructive uropathy, solid tumor morphology, and multiple tumors (5).

Workup and Staging

The basis of the workup in bladder cancer is to determine if the disease is a superficial noninvasive cancer, a locally invasive lesion, or metastatic disease. In addition to evaluating the bladder, the ureters and kidneys are also examined for lesions as well since multiple tumors are not uncommon. Perhaps this is related to common carcinogen exposure.

Cystoscopy and urethroscopy allow for excellent visualization and biopsy of lesions. A bladder diagram should be completed at the time of cystoscopy to record pertinent findings (Figure 20.1). In addition, computed tomography (CT) and/or magnetic resonance imaging (MRI) can be used to evaluate for bladder wall thickening and invasion as well as for lymphadenopathy. All patients should also have a chest x-ray, complete blood count, and serum chemistries including liver functions, as these may offer clues to systemic spread (Table 20.1).

Bimanual examination under anesthesia should be performed both before and after transurethral bladder resection of the visualized lesion to get a better appreciation of the size, consistency, and location of the tumor. This allows for estimation of the extent of local infiltration into the surrounding tissue by assessing whether the mass is freely mobile, tethered or fixed, before and after maximal transurethral bladder resection.

Determination of muscular wall invasion is the most important aspect of staging. It is often not possible for the pathologist examining TUR specimens to determine if the tumor is confined to the superficial muscle layers or has involved the deep muscle. For this reason, clinical understaging is a frequent problem. These limitations to accurate staging have undoubtedly compounded the difficulty of showing the benefit of effective bladder-sparing treatments.

A further difficulty to accurate staging is the use of both clinical and pathological staging systems in clinical trials. Caution is therefore required in the interpretation and comparisons of trial results. The two most widely used staging systems are presented in Table 20.2. In the Ameri-

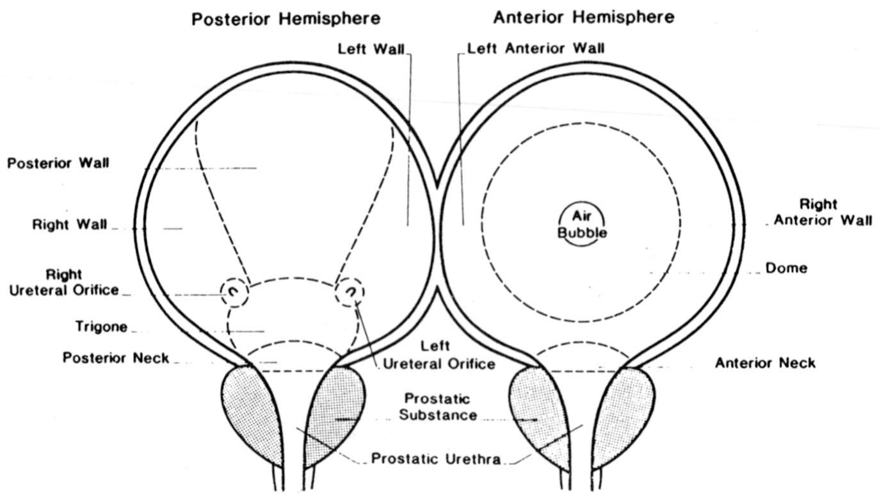

Figure 20.1. A bladder diagram is completed at the time of cystoscopy and used to record the cystoscopy findings, biopsy information, and tumor characteristics.

can Joint Committee on Cancer (AJCC) system, if staging is based on evaluation of the cystectomy specimen, the stages are preceded by the lower case letter p.

Pathology

The most common histology in the United States is transitional cell carcinoma, which comprises approximately 90% of cases, followed by squamous cell (7%), and adenocarcinoma (less than 1%) (6). Sarcomas, lymphomas, carcinoid, and small cell tumors are rarely seen. About 30% of bladder cancers present as multiple lesions. Adjacent CIS is also common.

Tumors of the bladder may be papillary in appearance, which generally are not deeply invasive, or solid in appearance, which generally are deeply invasive. Most transitional cell tumors are found at the trigone, followed in frequency by the lateral and posterior walls and then the neck (7). Adenocarcinoma also most frequently arises at the trigone (8).

Tumors progress by further muscle invasion and by lymphatic involvement to the external iliac lymph nodes. About 40% of patients with muscle-invasive cancers have involved lymph nodes at presentation (9). Almost all of these patients will ultimately die of distant metastasis (9). Of note is that the squamous cell histology rarely metastasizes.

Table 20.1. Diagnostic Workup for Bladder Cancer

Routine
- History and physical examination
- Pelvic/rectal examination

Laboratory studies
- Complete blood cell count
- Live function tests and chemistries
- Urinalysis and Urine Cytology

Imaging
- Computed tomography or magnetic resonance scan of pelvis and abdomen
- Intravenous pyelography
- Chest radiograph
- Radioisotope bone scan

Cystourethroscopy

Bimanual pelvic/rectal examination under anesthesia

Biopsies of bladder and urethra

Transurethral resection, if indicated

Treatment Options

Optimal therapeutic options for bladder cancer depend on histology and stage of disease. Patients with squamous cell cancer tend to fail locally. Management for these individuals should be by a course of preoperative radiation

Table 20.2. Comparison of Marshall and AJC Staging System for Bladder Cancer

	Marshall Modification of Jewett-Strong Classification	AJCC
Tumor Extent		
Confined to Mucosa	0	
• nonpapillary, noninvasive		TIS
• papillary, noninvasive		Ta
Not Beyone Lamina Propria (no mass palpable after complete TUR)	A	T1
Invasion of superficial muscle (inner half) (no duration after complete TUR)	B1	T2a
Invasion of deep muscle (outer half) (induration after complete TUR)	B2	T2b
Invasion into perivesical fat (mobile mass after TUR)—microscopic	C	T3a
—macroscopic		T3b
Invasion of neighboring structures: Muscle invasion present		
Substance of prostate, vagina, uterus	D1[a]	T4a
Pelvic sidewall fixation or invading abdominal wall	D1[a]	T4b
Nodal involvement (N)		
Minimum requirements to assess the regional nodes cannot be met		Nx
No involvement of regional lymph nodes		No
Involvement of a single lymph node, 2 cm or less in size		N1
Involvement of a single lymph node >2 cm or less but ≤5 cm or multiple lymph nodes measuring ≤5 cm		N2
Lymph node mestastasis >5 cm in diameter		N3
Distant metastasis (M)		
Minimum requirements to assess the presence of distant metastasis cannot be met		Mx
No distant metastasis		Mo
Distant metastasis		M1

[a] In the Marshall modification of the Jewett-Strong staging system, D1 disease may involve lymph nodes below the sacral promontory (bifurcation of the common iliac artery). D2 implies distant metastases or more extensive lymph node metastases.
TUR, transurethral resection.

therapy to the pelvis followed by radical cystectomy. This approach yields an approximately 50% 5-year survival rate and is generally considered to offer the best chance for cure (10,11). The management of transitional cell cancers should be based on whether the patient has nonmuscle- or muscle-invasive disease. Early stage patients (Tis, Ta, T1) with nonmuscle-invasive disease are generally managed by maximal TUR followed by intravesicular BCG instillation. Patients are then closely followed cystoscopically to monitor for recurrence. Perhaps due to the inherent inadequacies of clinical staging, the optimal management for muscle invasive disease remains unclear. Treatment options include cystectomy (partial in selected cases) and combined modality therapy with a view to bladder preservation (i.e., maximal TUR followed by irradiation with chemotherapy).

Surgery

For most patients, surgical options mean either radical cystectomy or TUR. Radical cystectomy includes resection of the bladder, distal ureters, perivesicular fat, and the regional peritoneum. In men, the prostate, seminal vesicles, vas deferens, and proximal urethra are removed as well. In women, the uterus, fallopian tubes, ovaries, anterior vaginal wall, and urethra are resected. Urinary diversion may be by ileal conduit with external appliance or an internal stomal reservoir that may even maintain continence.

A small minority of patients may be eligible for partial cystectomy. These are individuals with solitary well defined tumors that allow at least 2 cm of margin all around the resection plane. Preoperative pelvic irradiation should be considered when there is a significant likelihood of microscopically involved pelvic lymph nodes.

Transurethral resection is often an outpatient procedure in which transurethral visualization of the lesion(s) in question is obtained and a biopsy, if not a resection, is accomplished. Tumor removal may be by scalpel, heat, or laser source. The goal is to remove tumor down to uninvolved tissue.

Chemotherapy/Immunotherapy

Chemotherapy has been successful in improving outcome for both early and advanced patients. As compared to TUR alone, single agents instilled into the bladder, or more recently BCG employment for early stage patients following maximal transurethral bladder resection, clearly increases local control. For patients with muscle-invasive disease, chemotherapy plays an important role in enhancing the effects of radiation therapy. Numerous trials demonstrate that the addition of radiosensitizing doses of chemotherapy (i.e., 5-fluorouracil [5FU], cisplatinum, etc.) improve complete response rates by more than 50% compared to the efficacy of radiation therapy alone (12–16).

Incorporation of chemotherapy into the management paradigm of muscle-invasive bladder cancer offers the theoretical advantage of "spatial cooperation" where the primary role of chemotherapy is to control micrometastasis at distant sites while either surgery, irradiation, or irradiation with radiosensitizing doses of chemotherapy are used to address the localized primary tumor.

Irradiation

Irradiation has been employed in all stages of muscle-invasive bladder cancer both by external beam and less commonly by brachytherapy techniques. In addition to its use as a principal modality, irradiation has also been used in neoadjuvant and adjuvant roles generally with various chemotherapeutic agents.

Situations in which surgically managed patients should be considered for radiation therapy are based on the assumption that a certain percentage of patients will have microscopically involved pelvic lymph nodes and/or residual disease without distant metastasis. Sterilization of this microscopic disease with radiation may improve survival. With this in mind, pelvic irradiation should be considered in the following clinical situations: 1) prior to radical cystectomy for resectable T3 and T4a tumors; 2) large /T2 tumors (>4 cm); 3) high grade lesions; or 4) tumors with lymphovascular invasion. In each of these clinical situations, the risk of micrometastasis to the regional lymph nodes is significant.

Radiation Therapy Treatment Techniques

A wide variety of planning, dosing, and actual therapy techniques are available in the treatment of bladder cancer. The ultimate goal for each of these is to optimally define the tumor volume, while at the same time minimizing dose to normal tissues. This requires accurate definition of the critical normal structures in relation to the tumor volume so that uninvolved organs can be maximally shielded during treatment to minimize morbidity. Diagnostic studies such as treatment position CT scans are invaluable in this process. The following section outlines the techniques that are more commonly employed to accomplish this.

Simulation

Preparation One must always remember that patient comfort is a priority when setting up a treatment (i.e., simulation). One half-hour prior to simulation, the patient may be given an oral contrast to drink so that the small bowel can be adequately visualized during the simulation process. Patients may be treated supine or prone. When the regional lymph nodes are to be covered for the initial 4500 cGy of treatment, we recommend that the patient be treated prone on a belly board with the bladder fully distended. If this pushes the small bowel out of the lateral treatment portals, one may minimize small bowel toxicity, otherwise supine treatment may be more comfortable to the patient. During simulation, an alpha cradle is fashioned, or landmarks are identified, for each patient so that the individual can be optimally and accurately repositioned for precise daily treatment setup. Once positioned, a Foley catheter is inserted into the bladder with a sterile technique and 7 cc of hypaque is used to inflate the Foley catheter balloon. The Foley catheter is pulled down to ensure that the balloon is at the base of the bladder. This critical step is required to ensure identification of the location of the bladder base. A solution of hypaque mixed with saline in a one to two ratio is then instilled into the bladder. Generally, 25 cc of this mixture is instilled. Subsequent to this, approximately 25 cc of air is also injected into the bladder and the Foley catheter is clamped. Patients should be informed that a small quantity of air will be injected into their bladders so that they will not become alarmed when, after the procedure is over, they note that air is being passed from their bladder. The information obtained from this air contrast cystogram is combined with information previously obtained from examination under anesthesia, CT scan, and possibly cystogram, if previously performed, to optimally define the bladder location and the tumor and target volume for treatment. At some institutions, a rectal tube is inserted into the patient's rectum and an anal marker is placed at the distal end of the anal canal to identify this anatomy. The rectal tube is then connected to a Tomey syringe that has been previously filled with 25 cc of barium paste mixed with 25 cc of water. Please note that the rectal tube should be inserted into the rectum empty; No barium should be injected into the rectum until later during the procedure when the lateral fields are simulated. The barium may obscure the outline of the bladder on anterior posterior simulation films. An anal canal marker should be placed at the distal end of the anal canal.

At this point, patient positioning should be reverified by fluoroscopy as these manipulations may have induced misalignment.

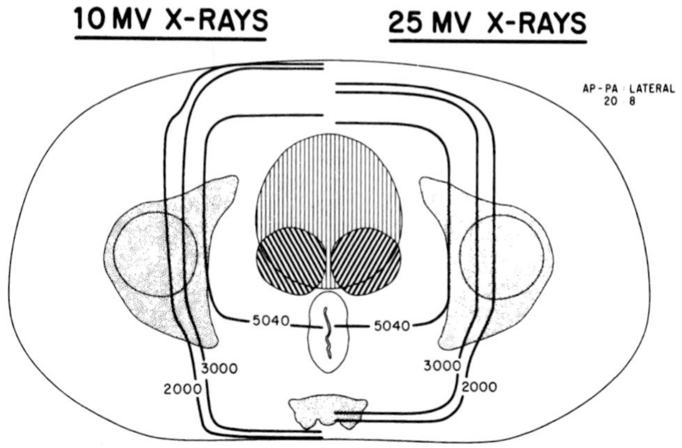

Figure 20.2. Composite isodose curves for whole pelvic irradiation (isocentric four field) to 50.4 Gy. Compares 10 MV with 25 MV photons.

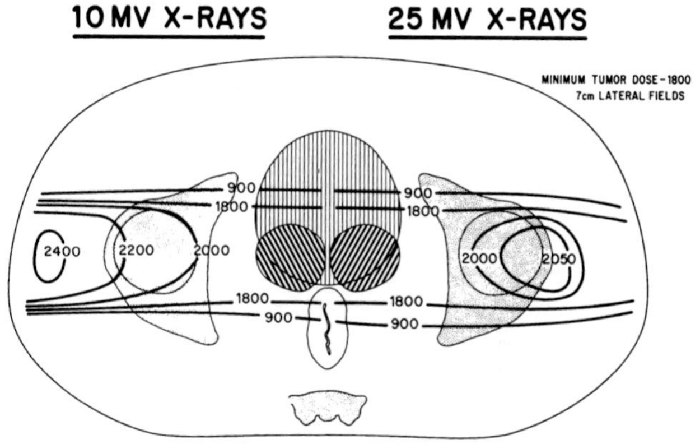

Figure 20.3. Isodose distributions for boost portion of treatment delivered through opposed lateral fields. These do not reflect effects of beam width improving device. Compares 10 MV with 25 MV photons.

Design of Anterior and Posterior Fields External beam therapy is most commonly delivered by a four-field box technique (Figures 20.2 through 20.4); however, multiple conformal fields outlining the bladder can also be employed. In a four-field treatment plan, matched anterior/posterior and lateral portals are employed. The anteroposterior-posteroanterior (AP/PA) field encompasses the bladder as outlined by the information obtained from both diagnostic studies and during simulation, and may be expanded to cover the regional lymph nodes if needed. When the regional lymph nodes are covered for the initial 4500 cGy of treatment, the patient should be treated prone on the belly board with the bladder full to push the small bowel out of the field, minimizing small bowel toxicity. In general, these fields are defined superiorly by the S1/S2 interspace (midsacroiliac joint) to cover pelvic nodes up to the level of the common iliac lymph nodes.

If this volume will encompass a significant amount of small bowel despite the patient being prone and on a belly board, then the upper border should be lowered accordingly to minimize the volume of small bowel in the treatment field. This generally requires the upper border to be placed at the lower sacroiliac joints. However, it must be kept in mind that to adequately cover the bladder, the upper border should extend approximately 2 cm above the dome of the bladder as visualized by the air contrast cystogram. The inferior border of the AP/PA field is placed at the lower border of the obturator foramen, which allows for good nodal and bladder coverage. The lower border of the field should be placed at the lower border of the obturator foramen only when there is no clinical suspicion or cystoscopic evidence of involvement at the base of the bladder or proximal urethra.

In cases where the tumor is at the bladder neck or

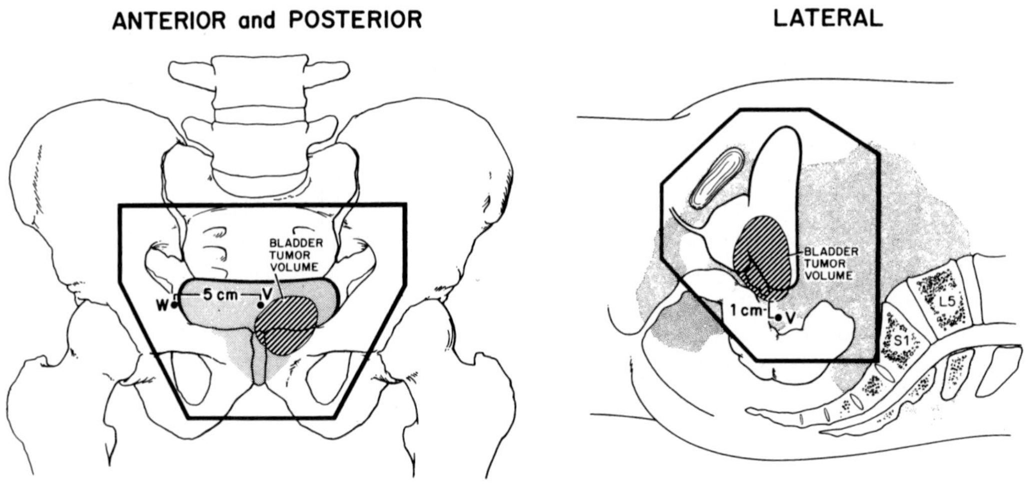

Figure 20.4. Radiation fields for initial whole pelvic treatment. A, anterior/posterior; B, laterals.

disease is noted near or involving the proximal urethra, the border should be extended inferiorly, generally to the level of the ischial tuberosity, to adequately cover disease in this region. If there is any suspicion of urethral involvement, the entire length of the proximal urethra should be covered. Frequently in this situation, the lower border will be at the bottom of the ischial tuberosities.

Laterally, the anterior field borders are placed 1.5 to 2 cm lateral to the bony pelvis to allow coverage of the iliac lymph nodes. Custom blocking is employed to shield the femoral heads and prepubertal soft tissues. If the lymphatics are not to be included, these fields should be diminished to outline the bladder with a 2-cm margin. In this clinical situation, the patient should be treated with an empty bladder to minimize the treatment volume.

Design of the Paired Right and Left Lateral Fields The lateral fields superior and inferior borders are set at the same anatomical levels of the AP/PA fields, hence the term four-field box technique. The anterior border on the lateral field should be placed 2 cm above the bladder as outlined on the air contrast cystogram and also include the external iliac lymph nodes on the lateral fields. The only way to accurately locate these external iliac lymph nodes is to perform a bipedal lymphangiogram prior to simulation. This technique is not frequently employed, but we have found that the external iliac lymph nodes are adequately covered if the anterior border on the lateral field is defined by a line extending from the tip of the pubic symphysis to a point 2.5 cm anterior to the bony sacral promontory. After 4500 cGy of therapy has been delivered, an attempt to shield a portion of the pubic symphysis on the lateral films should be made to prevent later osteoradionecrosis or fracture from developing. The posterior border of the lateral field is also determined by the air contrast cystogram and placed 2 cm beyond where the bladder is outlined. During lateral simulation, the barium paste mixed with saline should be injected into the rectum so that it can be accurately defined on the lateral simulation field and optimally blocked by custom blocking. Also note that the small bowel, which is opacified by the oral contrast given to the patient prior to simulation, should be shielded as outlined on the lateral field. The entire anal canal as well as the soft tissue anterior/inferior to the pubic symphysis should also be shielded. During design of these custom blockings to shield both the rectum and the small bowel, care should be taken so that the tumor is not inadvertently blocked. After AP/PA and lateral radiographs have been obtained and reviewed to the satisfaction of the attending radiation oncologist, the field borders and field centers of the AP and lateral fields are marked on the patient.

Treatment Plan If available, we recommend obtaining a computer treatment plan to optimize dose homogeneity. To accomplish this, generally a treatment position CT scan cut is obtained at the isocenters of the field. A physicist will use the CT scan to optimally select appropriate wedges and field weighting to minimize dose inhomogeneity to less than 5 to 10% around the target volume while also minimizing the dose to the normal surrounding critical organs. A typical four-field box technique isodose is shown in Figure 20.2. In general, these large fields are treated to 4500 to 5040 cGy at 180 cGy per day. If the patient is being treated by chemoradiation and any small bowel is present in the treatment fields, we routinely reduce the fields by employing custom blocking to shield the small bowel after 4000 cGy. This minimizes the chance of small bowel toxicity even if it means potentially blocking the external iliac lymph nodes. Further, if chemotherapy is used during treatment, we generally limit our treatment to the bladder and lymphatics to 4500 cGy in 5 weeks. After this dose has been delivered, a boost field is constructed to encompass regions at risk such as residual disease or premaximal TUR tumor volume.

Planning the Boost Field Information obtained from pre-TUR CT scan, examination under anesthesia, and cystoscopy findings are used to optimally define the boost volume for treatment planning (Figure 20.5). This volume is taken to be the tumor bed with margin. In some institutions, boost is delivered with bilateral 120° arc rotations as seen in Figure 20.6. Several composite examples of radiation treatment techniques are provided in Figures 20.7 and 20.8. The boost fields are generally treated to a total dose of 6500 cGy.

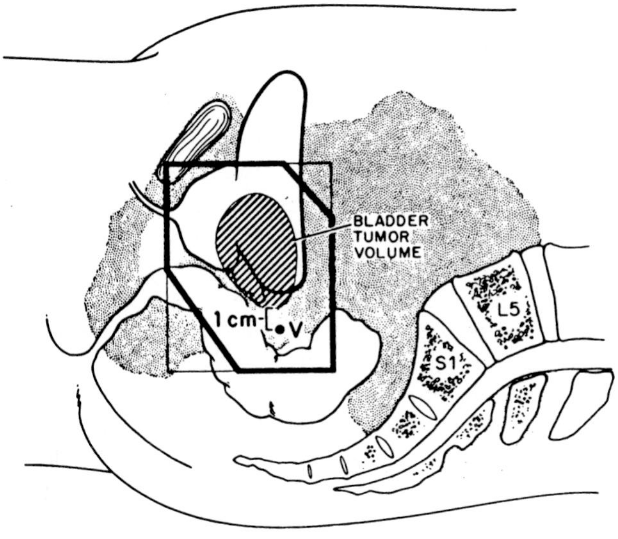

Figure 20.5. Lateral boost field.

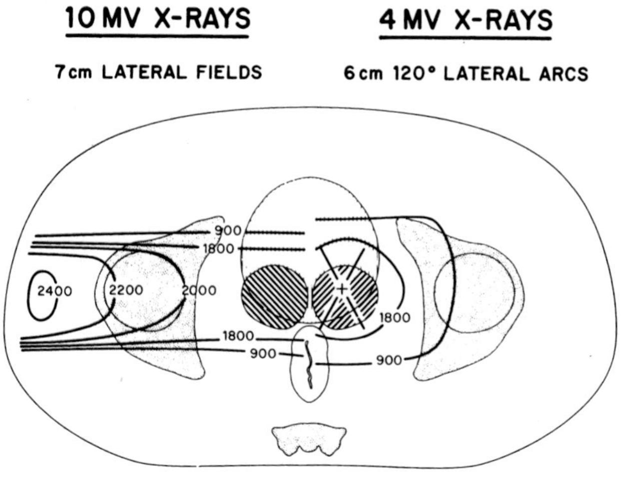

Figure 20.6. Isodose distribution for boost portion of treatment compares 120° arc rotation using 4 MV photons with opposed lateral fields using 10 MV photons.

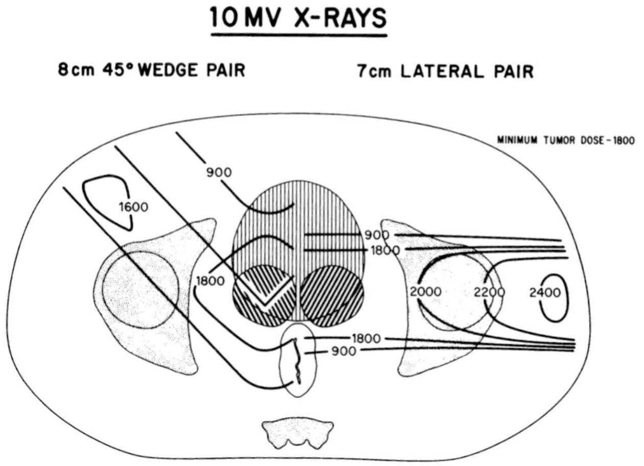

Figure 20.7. Isodose distribution for boost portion of treatment using 10 MV photons delivered through opposed laterals or an anterior wedged pair.

It is of utmost importance that the normal tissue tolerances of critical organs such as the rectum, small bowel, and femoral heads, be respected. We regard the tolerance of the entire rectum to be 6000 cGy (6 ½ weeks) and try to limit our dose to the rectum to no more than 5500 cGy, especially when chemotherapy is employed. We also keep the dose to the femoral head and small bowel below 45 Gy. As previously mentioned, we limit the dose to the small bowel to 4000 cGy when chemotherapy is employed.

As part of the entire radiation treatment or as part of the boost field, conformal three-dimensional (3D) radiation therapy is an option if it is available. Figure 20.9 is an example of a 3D Beam's eye view treatment plan for fields conformally outlining the bladder. Normal tissues such as bowel, rectum, prostate, and femoral bones are outlined as is the bladder. With the resultant anatomical information and localization, a treatment plan can be created that offers high precision and dosing to the bladder while constructing appropriate and precise blocks to shield as much normal anatomy as possible. Since this anatomical information is readily available in all dimensions, not just AP/PA and lateral as is the usual for a box field simulation, the flexibility to create an improved course of therapy using multiple noncoplanar portals is at hand.

In summary, multiple CT scan slices are obtained from the pelvis in the treatment position. The bladder is outlined on each slice and digitized into an appropriate 3D conformal treatment planning computer. At that point custom blocks are created based on the reconstructed digitized bladder anatomy so that four, six, and possibly eight or more fields can be employed to treat the bladder and spare a maximal amount of normal surrounding tissues. Many

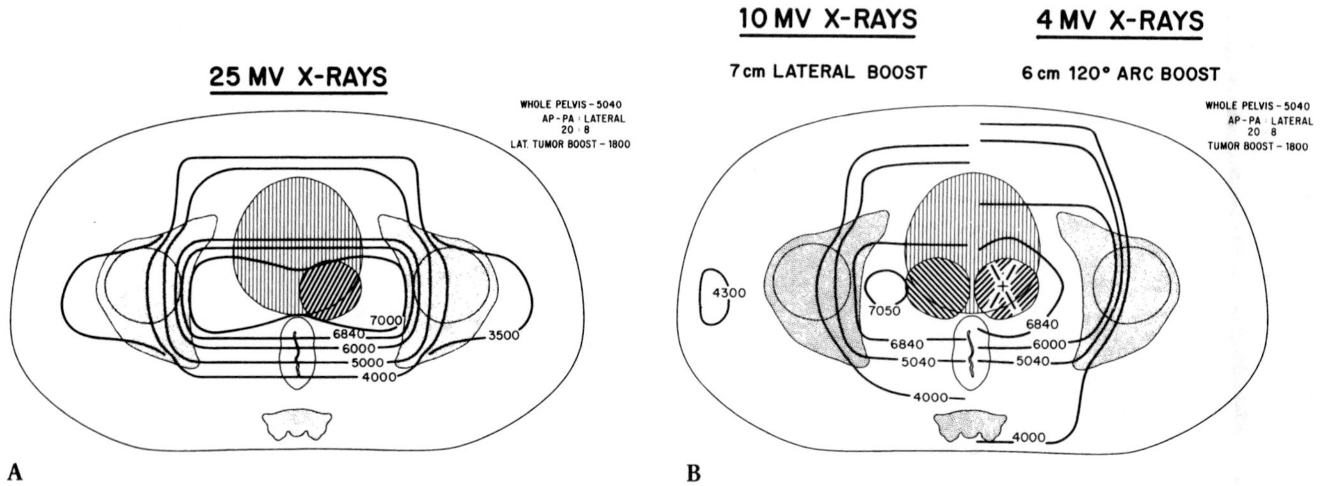

A B

Figure 20.8. Composite isodose distributions for whole pelvic irradiation through four-field technique (50.4 Gy) plus various boost methods (18 Gy) in definitive plan for T2-T3 bladder carcinoma.

linear accelerators are directly linked to the 3D treatment planning device and create the blocking necessary using multi-leaf collimators.

Radiation Fractionation

Fractionation is important to outcome as well as to morbidity in the treatment of bladder cancer. Large daily fractions in the range of 225 to 250 cGy often result in severe morbidity. In a series reported by Duncan et al. where the fraction sizes used were 250 cGy, close to 50% of patients suffered severe bladder morbidity and approximately 10% of patients developed small bowel toxicity (17). In addition, severe late and chronic reactions were noted in an additional 40%, with some of these complications actually leading to death. Based on these data, doses of 180 to 200 cGy given daily have become standard, with most studies employing 180 cGy per fraction. With these fraction sizes and the above outlined treatment techniques, acute morbidity is expected to be tolerable in most patients, while chronic morbidity can be minimized to less than 10% of patients. A more current application at some institutions is multiple daily fractions (hyperfractionation), this appears to decrease morbidity and possibly improve outcomes as described in the following section.

Results

Following are fairly standard treatment results based on disease stage. Although a wide variety of treatment combinations as discussed above is used to treat bladder cancer, there is still no optimal or accepted "gold standard" for therapy.

Stage Tis/TA/T1

Most of these patients undergo one or more TUR generally followed by intravesicular BCG. Local control rates of 60 to 80% are obtained (18). A significant minority of patients will go on to develop invasive bladder cancer or a second urethral malignancy. For this reason, close follow-up with cystoscopy performed at 3- to 4-month intervals is recommended. Interstitial and intraoperative radiation treatment of bladder cancer has excellent outcome for selected patients, but is rarely employed in the United States. Matsumoto, using intraoperative radiation therapy delivered by an electron beam, achieved an impressive 95% local control rate for early stage solitary lesions (19). Van der Werf-Messing et al. (20) implanted the bladder by brachytherapy, and reported 80 to 85% local control rates.

Stage T2

For these patients, TUR alone is unacceptable due to high local failure rates. Most commonly, cystectomy alone is employed and offers a 60% survival in pathologically staged patients (21,22). The role of radiation in this stage of disease is not yet well defined; however, Van der Werf-Messing reported on selected T2 patients implanted with radium needles who achieved an 80% disease-free survival at 5 years (23). These results were replicated by Batterman and Denue (24). External beam radiation series for stage T2 disease is composed mainly of clinically staged patients. Clinical staging is inherently inaccurate and often includes individuals with pathologically more advanced tumors. Further, these outcomes are generally based on medically inoperable or elderly and frail patients. Despite these shortcomings, good local control and survival rates are possible as summarized in Table 20.3.

Stage T3

A significant number of patients undergoing cystectomy for clinical stage T3 lesions are found to have T4

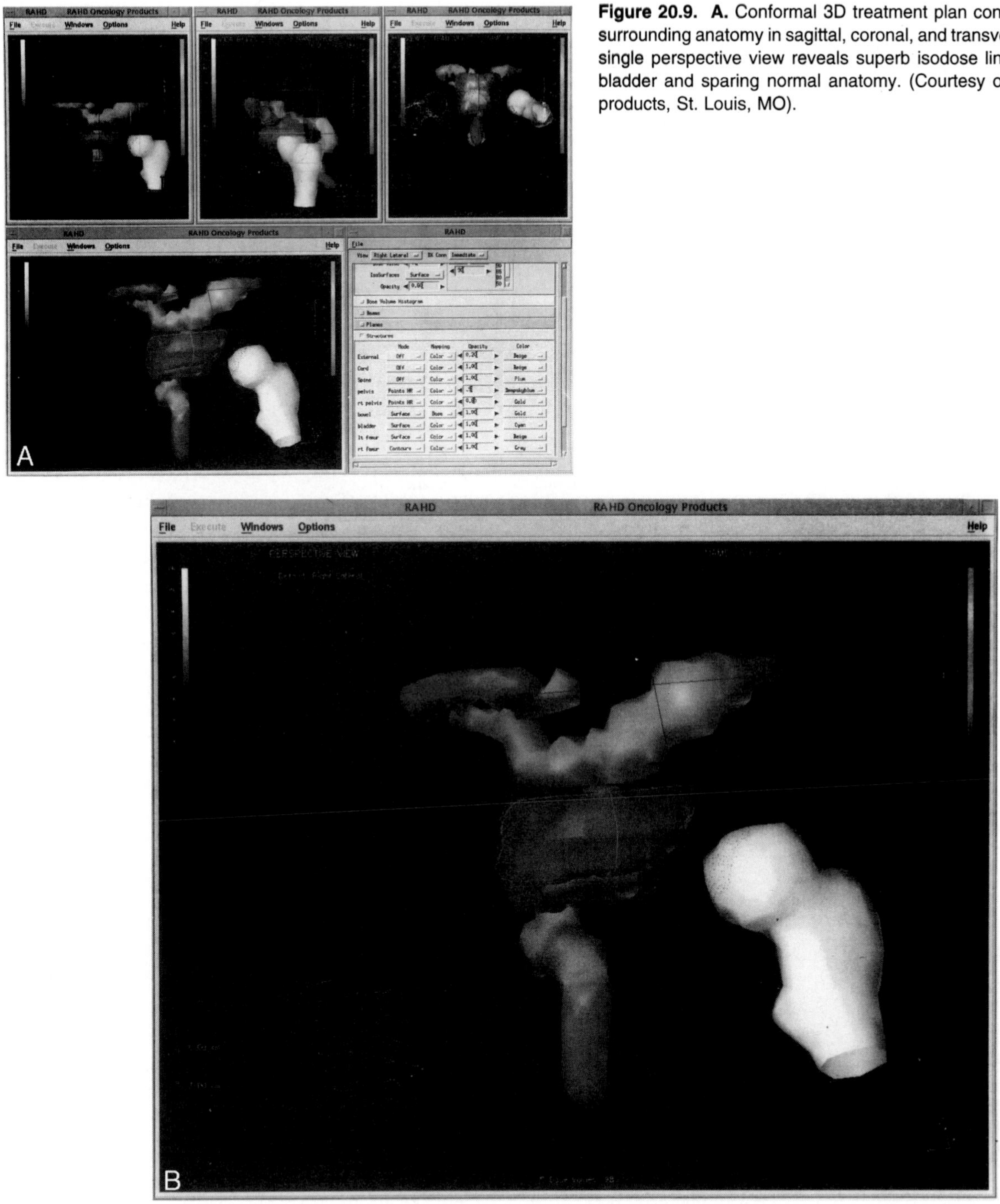

Figure 20.9. A. Conformal 3D treatment plan contours bladder and surrounding anatomy in sagittal, coronal, and transverse views. **B.** The single perspective view reveals superb isodose lines contouring the bladder and sparing normal anatomy. (Courtesy of RAHD oncology products, St. Louis, MO).

lesions on pathological analysis (25–27). A significant minority are also down staged (25–27). For this reason, comparing results from clinically staged patients to patients who are pathologically staged is difficult. Cystectomy alone offers a 20 to 40% 5-year survival and similar local control rates (28–32). In an attempt to improve results, several randomized studies involving preoperative external beam radiation therapy have been employed. In general, 4500 cGy are delivered (33–36). Despite the fact that these studies have shown improved local control and survival rates, most patients undergoing radical cystectomy do not receive preoperative radiation therapy in the United States.

Radiation therapy alone is usually unsuccessful, with 5-year survivals reported in the 20% range (33,37–41). This may be due, in part, to the fact that many of the patients who are chosen for "definitive radiation therapy" are often patients who initially failed multiple TURs with BCG and either refused salvage cystectomies or were deemed medically inoperable. These patients typically have scarred, contracted bladders to begin with, and perhaps have biologically more aggressive tumors as evidenced by their history of recurrences. Some radiation series do reveal fair pelvic local control rates (Table 20.3) but often it is based on salvage cystectomy in patients able to undergo this procedure.

Numerous clinical trials suggest that bladder cancer is a chemoresponsive tumor. Recent reports of chemotherapy integrated with radiation therapy suggest that results can be improved over radiation therapy alone, and may obviate the need for radical cystectomy with its resultant compromised quality of life.

As distant metastases remain the most common course of treatment failures for patients with muscle-invasive bladder carcinoma, it seems reasonable to try to incorporate a systemic component into the treatment regimen in an attempt to control micrometastases at distant sites. In studies reported by Rotman et al., patients with clinically staged bladder cancer underwent high doses of external beam radiation therapy in combination with sensitizing doses of chemotherapy (42). The majority of patients retained functioning bladders and minimal toxicities were noted. More importantly, survival rates were excellent. When transurethral resection of bladder tumor (TURBT), radiation, and multiagent chemotherapy are combined, complete response rates of 70% or greater have been obtained (43–46).

Table 20.3. Outcomes of Trials of Radiation Alone to Treat Bladder Cancer

		Complete Response	
Series (ref)	No. of Patients	T2 (%)	T3 (%)
Blandy et al (47)	704	48	42
Duncan et al (48)	889	49	41
Smaaland (49)	146	69	36
Greven et al (50)	116	36	18
Vale et al (51)	60	79	46

Table 20.3 summarizes the complete response rates for various studies employing the use of radiation therapy alone (47–51). Table 20.4 summarizes the results of studies combining chemotherapy and radiation therapy and aggressive TURBT (52–57). Comparison of these results strongly suggest that the addition of chemotherapy improves results over standard radiation therapy alone.

Hyperfractionation trials draw from the encouraging results from the Royal Marsden Hospital where local control for muscle-invading bladder cancer was enhanced by accelerated multiple daily treatments (58,59). Incorporating this benefit into combined modality therapy with maximal TURBT and chemotherapy has resulted in impressive results in both French and Italian trials (60,61).

Arcangeli et al. recently reported on a phase I/II trial in which a series of invasive bladder carcinomas were treated with or without an initial two cycles of MCV followed by concomitant continuous infusion Cisplatin and continuous infusion 5FU and irradiation (61). Treatment consisted of three 100 cGy fractions per day of radiation, 5 days per week, for a total dose of 5000 cGy in 4½ weeks. If required, due to residual disease, a consolidative dose of 2000 cGy was given in 1 week. A complete response rate of 90% was obtained in a series of 34 patients. High grade toxicity was uncommon. With a median follow-up of 26 months, 26 of 28 with complete response were still alive, and 24 of these patients remain with a tumor free bladder.

Stage T4

Patients with T4 disease have poor survival no matter what treatment is employed. Radical surgery has few 5-year survivals and preoperative irradiation, delivered prior to radical cystectomy, has not improved on this. Some investigators have examined multiagent chemotherapy for these patients. However, long-term results are not yet available. Possibly organ preservation chemoradiation protocols may be an option (Table 20.4).

Table 20.4. Outcomes of Trials of Chemotherapy and Radiation to Treat Bladder Cancer.

Series (ref)	Stage	Patients	Treatment	Sequence	% CR
Erlangen (52)	T2–4	67	50 Gy + C	Conc	75% + −
SUNY (53)	T1–4	18	60–65 Gy + 5FU	Conc	61%
Innsbruck (54)	T3–4	22	60 Gy + C ± MV	Conc	77% +
RTOG-8802 (55)	T2–4	92	CMV, 40 Gy + C	Neo + Conc	79%
Yorkshire (56)	T-3	55	60Gy, A + 5FU	Adjuvant	51%
Ljubljana (57)	T2–4	45	CMV + 40 − 60 Gy	Neo	62% +

C, cisplatin; M, mitomycin; CMV, cisplatin, mitomycin, vinblastin; A, adriamycin; Conc, concurrent; Neo, neoadjuvant; CR, complete response.

MORBIDITY

Transurethral Bladder Resection (TUR)

Transurethral bladder resection is a well tolerated procedure; however, after multiple TURs have been performed, the bladder is typically fibrotic and contracted. Perforations are rare, although at times they do occur and they may require surgical repair.

Cystectomy

Operative mortality is about 1% and the major consequences are the change in lifestyle brought about by this procedure including vaginal dryness, incontinence (depending on the method of reconstruction), and the loss of sexual function.

External Beam Radiation Therapy

The radiation therapist, when considering morbidity related to treatment, should think in terms of both acute and chronic morbidity. As previously mentioned, with optimal treatment planning, acute morbidity can be minimized to less than 10%, and long-term morbidity to the normal surrounding structures can be brought down to less than 5%.

Morbidity should also be analyzed by envisioning the tissues that will be traversed by the treatment beams. Consider the consequences of the beam as it passes through skin, bowel and rectum, bone, and especially bladder. Acute skin reactions including dry and moist desquamation are seen in most patients and heal with applications of Biafine cream. Bowel morbidity is generally acute diarrhea which usually responds to treatment with Imodium. In our experience, we have found that if patients are started on one dose of Metamucil taken each day, and two to three doses of Pepto Bismol taken each day, that small bowel acute morbidity (i.e., diarrhea) is often prevented and eliminates the need for patients being placed on Imodium.

The bladder itself is subject to the effects of radiation and often patients develop a radiation cystitis with symptoms of urgency, frequency, and dysuria. These symptoms are relieved quickly with Pyridium given to the patients (100 to 200 mg of Pyridium by mouth three times a day) along with instructions that they should not become alarmed at the orange color of their urine. Patients must also be informed that the Pyridium may stain their clothes orange. Urised may also be employed. In our clinical experience, we have found that in patients who do develop moderate symptoms of cystitis, despite negative urine cultures for bacterial growth, antibiotics empirically given during part of their treatment will increase their response to Pyridium. These acute side effects to the skin, bladder, and small bowel generally subside within 2 to 4 weeks after radiation therapy has been completed.

Both acute and long-term radiation proctitis are also potential complications. Again, we have found that prophylactically starting patients on a combination of Metamucil and Pepto Bismol, prior to treatment, significantly reduces the chance of the patient developing radiation proctitis. Chronic radiation proctitis is generally conservatively managed. Patients are instructed to avoid straining and this often means placing patients on a high fiber diet or daily Metamucil for extended periods. We also encourage them to drink at least 6 8-ounce glasses of water to avoid constipation. In those few patients who do develop chronic radiation proctitis, we have found that the majority respond either to Rowasa suppositories or ProctoFoam cream. If patients do not respond to these conservative measures, they are referred to experienced colorectal surgeons.

Chemotherapy

The major side effect of chemotherapy is generally hematological toxicity. Also, many patients who were referred for radiation therapy with chemotherapy are often sent because they are medically inoperable. Frequently, these patients have coronary artery disease, and certain chemotherapeutic agents may cause coronary artery spasm (i.e., 5FU) (43). Although it is unclear whether or not the addition of chemotherapy will ultimately increase the rate of long-term complications, to the best of our knowledge, this has not yet been reported in any prospective randomized studies. There may be increased frequency of diarrhea in patients who are treated with concomitant 5FU, but these side effects are frequently prevented by prophylactically placing patients on a combination of Metamucil and Pepto Bismol prior to initiation of treatment.

CONCLUSION

Optimal therapy for bladder cancer has yet to be defined. Accurate staging without extensive surgery is generally unavailable, making outcome analysis difficult for clinically evaluated patients. As such, comparing surgical series with nonsurgical series to determine strategies that improve results is fraught with uncertainty. Bladder conserving protocols offer obvious benefit to patients, and should be more vigorously pursued. This will require a true team approach.

References

1. Cancer Statistics. 1995 Jan/Feb Vol. 45 No. 1.
2. Whitmore WF Jr, Batata MA, Ghoneim MA, et al. Radical cystectomy with or without prior radiation in the treatment of bladder cancer. General Urology 1977;188:184–187.
3. Morison AS, Cole P. Epidemiology of bladder cancer. Urol Clin North Am 1976;3:13–29.
4. Silverman OT, Hartage P, Morrison S, et al. Epidemiology of bladder cancer. Hematol Oncol Clin North Am 1992;10:1–30.

5. Shipey WU, Rose MA, Perrone TL, et al. Full dose irradiation for patients with invasive bladder carcinoma. Clinical and histologic factors prognostic of improved survival. J Urol 1985;134:679.
6. Pearse HD. The urinary bladder. In: Cox JD, ed. Moss' radiation oncology: rationale, technique results. St. Louis: Mosby, 1994:522.
7. Mostofi FK, Davis CJ Jr, Sesterhenn IA. Pathology of tumors of the urinary tract. In: Skinner DG, Lieskovskky G, eds. Diagnosis and management of genitourinary cancer. Philadelphia: WB Saunders, 1988:83–117.
8. Johnson DE, Hogan JM, Ayala AG. Primary adenocarcinoma of the urinary bladder. South Med J 1972;65:527–530.
9. Skinner DG, Tift JP, Kaufman JJJ. High dose, short course preoperative radiation therapy and immediate single stage radical cystectomy with pelvic node dissection in the management of bladder cancer. J Urol 1982;127:671.
10. Awwad H, Abd El, Baki HA El, et al. Preoperative irradiation of T3 carcinoma in bilharzial bladder. A comparison between hyperfractionation and conventional fractionation. Int J Radiat Oncol Biol Phys 1979;5:787.
11. Ghoneim MA, Ashaella AC, Awaad HK, et al. Randomized trial of cystectomy with or without pre-operative radiotherapy for carcinoma of the bilharzial bladder. J Urol 1985;134:266.
12. Rotman M, Macchia R, Silverstein R. Treatment of advanced bladder cancer with irradiation and 5 Fluorouracil infusion. Cancer 1987;59: 710–714.
13. Reibischung JL, Vannetjel ZM, Fournier F. Cyclic concomitant chemoradiotherapy for invasive bladder cancer. Phase II study with organ preservation. Proc Am Soc Clin Oncol 1992;11:208.
14. Tester W, Porter A, Asbell S. Combined modality program with possible organ preservation for invasive bladder cancer: Results of RTOG protocol 85-12. Int J Radiat Oncol Biol Phys 1993;25:783–790.
15. Cervak J, Cufer T, Kragelj B. Sequential transurethral surgery, multiple drug, and radiation therapy for invasive bladder carcinoma. Int J Radiat Oncol Biol Phys 1993;25:777–782.
16. Dunst J, Sauer R, Shrott KM, et al. Organ sparing treatment of advanced bladder cancer; a ten year experience. Int J Radiat Oncol Biol Phys 1994;30:264.
17. Duncan W, Arnott SJ, Jack WJL, et al. A report of a randomized trial of d(13) + Be neutrons compared with megavoltage x-ray therapy of bladder cancer. Int J Radiat Oncol Biol Phys 1985;11:2043–2049.
18. Herr HW, Schwalb DM, Zhaang ZF, et al. Intravesical bacillus Calmette-Guerin therapy prevents tumor progression and death from superficial bladder cancer. Ten year follow-up of a prospective randomized trial. J Clin Oncol 1995;13:1404–1408.
19. Matsumoto K, Kakizoe T, Mikuriya S, et al. Clinical evaluation of intraoperative radiotherapy for carcinoma of the urinary bladder. Cancer 1981;47:509–513.
20. Van der Werf-Messing B, Hop WCJ. Carcinoma of the urinary bladder (category $T1N_XMO$) treated either by radium implant or by transurethral resection only. Int J Radiat Oncol Biol Phys 1981;7:199–303.
21. Resnick MI, O'Conor VJ Jr. Segmental resection for carcinoma of the bladder: review of 102 patients. J Urol 1973;109:1007–1010.
22. Brannan W, Ochsner MG, Fuselier HA Jr, et al. Partial cystectomy in the treatment of transitional cell carcinoma of the bladder. J Urol 1978;119:213–215.
23. Van der Werf-Messing B, Menon RS, Hop WCJ. Cancer of the urinary bladder category $T^{2,}$ T^3 ($N^XM^{0)}$ treated by interstitial radium implant: Second report. Int J Radiat Oncol Biol Phys 1983;9:481–485.
24. Battermann JJ, Tierie AH. Results of implantation for T_1 and T_2 bladder tumors. Radiother Oncol 1986;5:85–90.
25. Marshall VF. The relation of the preoperative estimate to the pathologic demonstration of the extent of vesical neoplasms. J Urol 1952; 68:714.
26. Richie JP, Skinner DG, Kaufman JJ. Radical cystectomy for carcinoma of the bladder: 16 years of experience. J Urol 1975;113:186.
27. Whitmore WF, Batat MA, Ghoneim MA, et al. Radical cystectomy with or without prior irradiation in the treatment of bladder cancer. J Urol 1977;118:184.
28. Greven KM, Spera JA, Solin LJ, et al. Local recurrence after cystectomy alone for bladder carcinoma. Cancer 1992;69:2767–2770.
29. Montie JE, Straffon RA, Stewart BH. Radical cystectomy without radiation therapy for carcinoma of the bladder. J Urol 1984;131:477–482.
30. Morabito RA, Kandzari SJ, Milam DF. Invasive bladder carcinoma treated by radical cystectomy: survival of patients. Urology 1979;14: 478–481.
31. Drago JR, Rohner TJ Jr. Bladder cancer: results of radical cystectomy for invasive and recurrent superficial tumors. J Urol 1983;130: 460–462.
32. Marshall VF, McCarron JP Jr. The curability of vesical cancer: greater now or then? Cancer Res 1977;37:2753–2755.
33. Bloom JJG, Hendry WF, Wallace DM, et al. Treatment of T3 bladder cancer: controlled trial of pre-operative radiotherapy and radical cystectomy versus radical radiotherapy. Second report and review (for the Clinical Trials Group, Institute of Urology) Br J Urol 1982;54: 136–151.
34. Batata MA, Chu FCH, Hilaris BS, et al. Pre-operative whole pelvis versus true pelvis irradiation and/or cystectomy for bladder cancer. Int J Radiat Oncol Biol Phys 1981;7:1349–1355.
35. Timmer PR, Hartlief HA, Hooijkass JAP. Bladder cancer: pattern of recurrence in 142 patients. Int J Radiat Oncol Biol Phys 1985;11: 899–905.
36. Woehre H, Ous S, Klevmark B, et al. A bladder cancer multi-institutional experience with total cystectomy for muscle-invasive bladder cancer. Cancer 1993;72:3044–3051.
37. Goffinet DR, Schneider MJ, Glatstein EJ, et al. Bladder cancer: results of radiation therapy in 384 patients. Radiology 1975;117:149–153.
38. Quilty PM, Duncan W. Primary radical radiotherapy for T3 transitional cell cancer of the bladder: an analysis of survival and control. Int J Radiat Oncol Biol Phys 1986;12:853–860.
39. Pollack A, Zagars GK, Swanson DA. Muscle-invasive bladder cancer treated with external beam radiotherapy: prognostic factors. Int J Radiat Oncol Biol Phys 1994;30:267–277.
40. Edsmyr F, Anderson L, Esposti PL, et al. Irradiation therapy with multiple small fractions per day in urinary bladder cancer. Radiother Oncol 1985;4:197–203.
41. DeWeerd JH, Colby MY Jr. Bladder carcinoma treated by irradiation and surgery: Interval report. J Urol 1973;109:409–413.
42. Rotman M, Aziz H, Porrazo M, et al. Treatment of advanced transitional cell carcinoma of the bladder with irradiation and concomitant 5-FU infusion. Int J Radiat Oncol Biol Physics 1990;18:1131–1137.
43. Devita V, Hellman S, Rosenberg S. Cancer principles and practice of oncology, 3rd ed. Philadelphia: JB Lippincott, 1989:P361–362.
44. Dunst J, Saur R, Schrott KM, et al. An organ-sparing treatment of advanced bladder cancer: a 10 year experience. Int J Radiat Oncol Biol Phys 1994;30:261–266.
45. Eapen L, Stewart D, Danjoux C, et al. Intraarterial cisplatin and concurrent radiation for locally advanced bladder cancer. J Clin Oncol 1989;7:230–235.
46. Housset M, Maulard C, Chretien YC, et al. Combined radiation and chemotherapy for invasive transitional-cell carcinoma of the bladder. A prospective study. J Clin Oncol 1993;11:2150–2157.
47. Blandy JP, England HR, Evans SJW, et al. T3 bladder cancer, the case for salvage cystectomy. Br J Urol 1980;52:502–506.
48. Duncan W, Quilty PM. The results of a series of 963 patients with transitional cell carcinoma of the bladder primarily treated by radical megavoltage x-ray therapy. Radiother Oncol 1986;7:299–310.
49. Smaaland R, Aksle A, Tonder B, Mehus A, Lote K, Albrektsen G. Radical radiation treatment of invasive and locally advanced bladder carcinoma in elderly patients. Br J Urol 1991;67:61–69.
50. Greven KM, Solin Hanks GE. Prognostic factors in patients with bladder carcinoma treated with definitive irradiation. Cancer 1990;65: 908–912.
51. Vale JA, A'hern Liu K, et al. Predicting the outcome of radical radiotherapy for invasive bladder cancer. Eur Urol 1993;24:48–51.
52. Saver R, Dunst J, Alternddor F, et al. Radiotherapy with and without Cisplatin in bladder cancer. Int J Radiat Oncol Biol Phys 1990;19: 687–691.
53. Rotman M, Macchia R, Silverstein R. Treatment of advanced bladder cancer with irradiation and 5 Fluorouracil infusion. Cancer 1987;59: 710–714.
54. Jakse G, Fromhold H, Zurmedden D. Combined radiation and chemotherapy or locally advanced transitional cell carcinoma of the urinary bladder. Cancer 1985;55:1659–1664.
55. Tester W, Porter A, Asbell S. Combined modality program with possible organ preservation for invasive bladder cancer: results of RTOG protocol 85-12. Int J Radiat Oncol Biol Phys 1993;25:783–790.

56. Richards B, Bastabla JR, Freedman L, et al. Adjuvant chemotherapy in T3NxM0 bladder cancer treated with radiotherapy. Br J Urol 1983; 55:386–391.
57. Cervak J, Cufer T, Kragelj B. Sequential transurethral surgery, multiple drug, and radiation therapy for invasive bladder carcinoma. Int J Radiat Oncol Biol Phys 1993;25:777–782.
58. Cole D, Durrant K, Robert J, et al. A pilot study of accelerated fractionation in the radiotherapy of invasive carcinoma of the bladder. Br J Radiol 1992;65:792–798.
59. Horwich A, Pendlebury S, Dearnaley DP. Organ conservation in bladder cancer. Eur J Cancer 1995;31(suppl 5):208.
60. Housset M, Maulard C, Chretien Y, et al. Combined radiation and chemotherapy for invasive transitional-cell carcinoma of the bladder: a prospective study. J Clin Oncol 1993;11:2150–2157.
61. Arcangeli G, Tirindelli Danesi D, Mecozzi A, Saracino B, Crucianni E. Combined hyperfractionated irradiation and protracted infusion chemotherapy in invasive bladder cancer with conservative intent. Phase I study. Int J Radiat Oncol Biol Phys 1996;36:314.

Chapter 21

Low-Dose Rate-Brachytherapy for Carcinoma of the Cervix

Kathryn E. Dusenbery and Bruce J. Gerbi

INTRODUCTION

Megavoltage external beam radiation therapy (EBRT) combined with intracavitary brachytherapy (BT) is the standard radiotherapeutic management for patients with carcinoma of the cervix. Low-dose-rate (LDR) brachytherapy has been used since the early 1900s, but starting in the late 1950s with the cathetron cobalt ^{60}, high-dose-rate (HDR) brachytherapy has become an acceptable treatment modality (1–3). Although there are few randomized trials comparing the advantages and disadvantages of each approach, one major advantage to LDR is the extensive clinical experience and accumulated data that exists which demonstrates its efficacy and safety. Additionally, radiobiological data suggests that LDR may enhance the therapeutic ratio, possibly sparing the late effects in the bowel or bladder. This is particularly important for patients with gynecologic malignancies since most of these patients will be cured of their cancer and will survive long enough to be at risk for developing late complications. This chapter focuses on the medical and technical considerations of LDR brachytherapy in cervical cancer. The relative advantages of LDR and HDR therapy are not discussed, but are outlined in Table 21.1.

Anatomy

The uterus is located in the midplane of the true pelvis, in an anteverted position, behind the bladder and in front of the rectum. It is partially covered by peritoneum in its fundal portion and posteriorly; its lateral surfaces are related to the parametria and the broad ligaments. The two main regions are the corpus and cervix; the cervix is separated from the corpus by the isthmus and is divided into a supravaginal portion above the ring containing the endocervical canal and the vaginal portion, which projects into the vault.

The uterus is attached to the surrounding structures in the pelvis by the broad and the round ligaments. The broad ligament is a double layer of peritoneum extending from the lateral margin of the uterus to the lateral wall of the pelvis and the pelvic floor. It contains the fallopian tubes. The round ligament extends from its attachment in the anterolateral portion of the uterus to the lateral pelvic wall; it crosses the pelvic brim and reaches the abdominoinguinal ring through which it traverses the inguinal canal and terminates in the superficial fascia. The cardinal ligaments, also called the transverse cervical ligaments (Mackenrodt's), arise at the upper lateral margins of the cervix and insert into the pelvic diaphragm.

The uterus has a rich lymphatic network that drains principally into the paracervical lymph nodes; from there it goes to the external iliac (of which the obturator nodes are the innermost component) and the hypogastric lymph nodes (Figure 21.1). The pelvic lymphatics drain into the common iliac and the periaortic lymph nodes. Lymphatics from the fundus pass laterally across the broad ligament continuous with those of the ovary, ascending along the ovarian vessels into the periaortic lymph nodes. Some of the fundal lymphatics also drain into the external and internal common iliac lymph nodes.

Overview of the Treatment Plan

Design of the radiation treatment program depends on the extent and volume of the tumor. Staging (clinical or surgical) consists of a complete history and physical examination, a number of laboratory studies (complete blood

Table 21.1. Advantages of Low- and High-Dose-Rate Brachytherapy

Low-Dose-Rate Advantages	
Patient	Long history of use
	Ability to predict rate of late complications
Clinical	Improves chances of catching tumors in sensitive phase of cell cycle
Physical	Longer treatment times allow for leisurely review of and potential modifications to the treatment
	Plan prior to the delivery of a significant portion of treatment
	Favorable dose-rate effect on repair of normal tissues
	Infrequent replacement and calibration of sources because of long isotope half-life
High-Dose-Rate Advantages	
Patient	No short- or long-term confinement to bed
	No indwelling bladder catheters
	Not labeled "radiation risk zone" to relatives, visitors, and staff
	Avoid several anesthesias (possibly)
Clinical	Maintain position of the sources during the brief treatment
	Patient preparation
	No specialized nursing
	Ability to treat greater patient loads (high output of patients on each machine)
Physical	Short treatment times and minimal radiation protection problems
	Possibility of optimizing dose distribution by altering the dwell times of the source at different locations

Modified from Joslin, C.A. (60)

count, blood chemistry, and urinalysis), a chest x-ray, and either an intravenous pyelogram or computed tomography (CT) scan of the abdomen and pelvis along with an examination under anesthesia (EUA). The EUA allows the radiation oncologist to physically determine the size and consistency of the cervix, as well as any extension beyond the cervix to the parametrium, pelvic side wall, or vagina. Disease extent should be carefully documented with detailed notes or diagrams. These diagrams can be referred to at the time of the first brachytherapy application, when significant tumor shrinkage may have occurred and the full extent of disease is not so obvious. During the EUA, a cystoscopy and proctoscopy may be done to determine if there is extension to the bladder or rectum. Additionally, some institutions add an extraperitoneal pelvic and periaortic lymph node sampling (4,5), which provides prognostic information and may help in designing the limits of the EBRT fields.

Most patients receive a combination of external beam and brachytherapy, although very early lesions may be treated with brachytherapy alone. The ratio of external beam dose relative to brachytherapy dose can be determined by general guidelines, although experience provides optimal treatment determinations. In general, advanced tumors require more external beam therapy because the rapid decrease in dose occurring at a distance from the brachytherapy implant may result in inadequate treatment of the peripheries of large tumors. For advanced tumors, most or all of the external beam therapy is given prior to brachytherapy to shrink the tumor. This leads to a technically superior brachytherapy application and may result in radiobiologic advantages (6), such as better oxygenated and, therefore, more radiosensitive tumor cells. Therefore, the first brachytherapy application is performed 3 to 4 weeks after the start of EBRT and the second application is performed 2 weeks later. Two implants are generally considered to be superior to a single implant (7). During the intervening 2 weeks between brachytherapy applications, the remainder of the whole pelvis (with or without periaortic nodal chain) and split pelvis irradiation may be given. The entire course of treatment, including both brachytherapy applications, usually takes 6 to 7 weeks. Protracted treatment times are associated with decreased local control and survival rates.

Design of External Beam Field

Design of the external beam fields takes into account the predictable manner in which cancer of the uterine cervix usually spreads, first laterally into the paracervical nodes, then to the internal iliac, common iliac, and finally

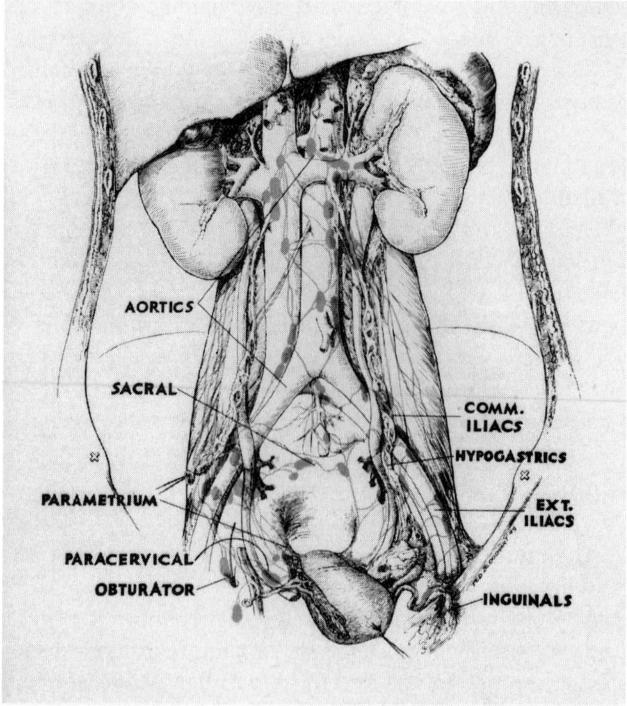

Figure 21.1. Lymph vessels and lymph nodes of the cervix and the body of the uterus (Henrikson E. Am J Obstet Gynecol 1949;58:924-942.)

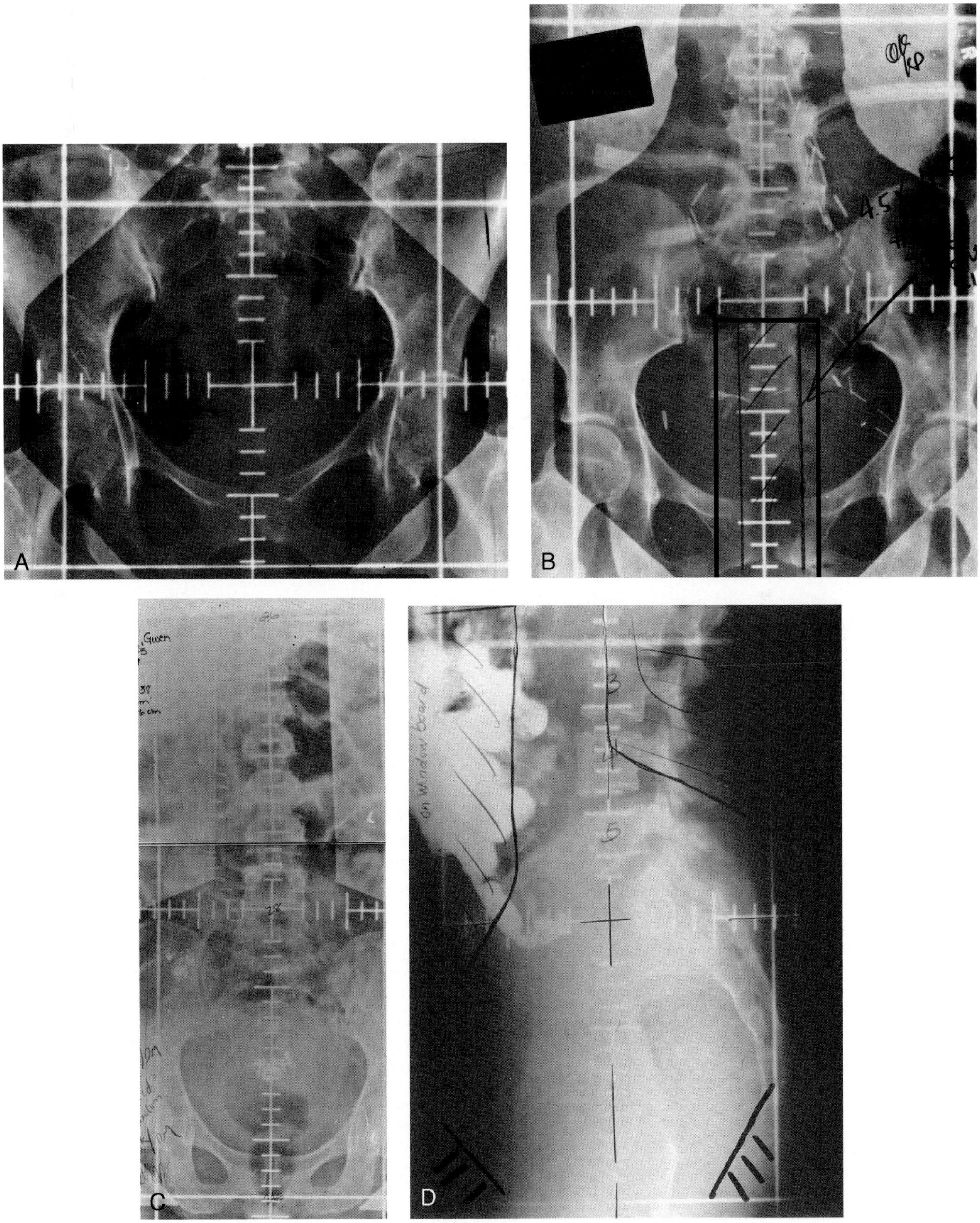

Figure 21.2. A. External beam field for surgically staged patient with *no* nodal spread documented. B. External beam field for surgically staged patient with low pelvic nodal spread, but not common iliac or periaortic node. C. External beam field for surgically staged patient with periaortic nodal spread. D. Lateral field for surgically staged patient with periaortic nodal spread.

into the periaortic nodes. In patients with early disease, the nodes are often not involved. For larger tumors, the risk of nodal spread beyond the pelvis increases. Knowledge of nodal involvement is important when designing EBRT fields. At the University of Minnesota, most patients undergo extraperitoneal lymph node sampling. This allows us to know the number and distribution of involved nodes with some certainty. For patients with no nodal involvement, our external beam includes the pelvic nodes (to approximately the bottom of L5), (Figure 21.2a). For patients with pathologically confirmed spread to the pelvic (but not periaortic) nodes we usually extend the field to include the low periaortic nodes (to the level of the second lumbar vertebrae) (Figure 21.2b). For patients with periaortic nodal spread, we include the entire periaortic chain (to the level of the tenth thoracic vertebra) (Figure 21.2c) (8–11). A four field arrangement is generally preferred for patients treated to the pelvis or pelvis and low periaortic areas (Figure 21.2d).

In patients who are not surgically staged and have no clinical evidence of pelvic or periaortic nodal spread, the limits of the EBRT are individualized. For patients with large cervical tumors or extension into the parametrium, we generally extended the EBRT field to at least the low periaortic nodal area. The prophylactic use of extended fields remains controversial, although a recent update of the Radiation Therapy Oncology Group (RTOG) trial continues to show a superior survival for patients with either bulky FIGO stage Ib, or II, or III disease randomized to receive pelvic and periaortic irradiation, compared to pelvic only irradiation (12–14).

In addition to the initial whole pelvic EBRT or whole pelvic and periaortic EBRT, it is often desirable to continue to treat the nodal areas while blocking the central area where the high dose from the brachytherapy application is concentrated. Fields that have the central area blocked are called "split pelvis" fields. Some institutions design partial transmission blocks that correspond to the isodose lines of the brachytherapy application. At the University of Minnesota, our split pelvis block is generally 4.5 cm wide. The height of the block is determined by the height of the tandem and roughly corresponds to the height of the 30 cGy/ hour isodose line (Figure 21.2b).

Low-Dose-Rate Brachytherapy

Patients undergo a preoperative history and physical examination just prior to the application of brachytherapy, since medical conditions may have changed since initiating the external beam therapy and may influence the brachytherapy application. A complete blood count, electrolyte profile, and creatinine are obtained. For patients older than 40 years, a recent EKG is recommended. Patients should have had a chest x-ray at the time of diagnosis, so this is not repeated unless an abnormality was seen. If the patient is on coumadin, the anticoagulation is usually not reversed, but the level of anticoagulation is ascertained and adjusted as necessary. The majority of patients will be candidates for an intrauterine tandem with vaginal ovoids.

Table 21.2 outlines the major types of gynecological brachytherapy implants, (and the indications for using them) that are used at the University of Minnesota.

Equipment

Manual afterloading Fletcher Suit Delclos Applicators are used for the majority of cervical cancer patients at the University of Minnesota (Figure 21.3). Over 100 other applicators are available worldwide. Low-dose-rate remote afterloading systems, which minimize the exposure to medical personnel, are available from manufacturers in several countries. For both manual and remote afterloading, the clinical, radiobiological, and physics principles of LDR are the same. Only the size of the applicators, radiation protection features and possibly the ability to limit applicator movement during treatment differs. Integral to

Table 21.2. Types of Brachytherapy Applications Used for Cervix Cancer

Implant Type	Indication
Intrauterine tandem + ovoids	Preferred application for the majority of patients
Intrauterine tandem + Protruding vaginal source	Insufficient space to accommodate ovoids (other option is miniovoids)
Intrauterine tandem + Vaginal cylinder	Proximal vaginal extension more than 2 cm from the cervix *and* the bulk of tumor extending into the vagina is ≤0.5 cm thick
Intrauterine tandem + Parametrial interstitial iridium	Poor parametrial tumor regression at the time of brachytherapy application if confined to one side or in patients with large IIB or IIIB disease.
Intrauterine tandem + Paracopal (vaginal) interstitial iridium	Proximal vaginal extension more than 2 cm in length from cervix and the bulk of the vaginal extent of tumor is >0.5 cm thick
Vaginal ovoids (only)	Consider in post Type I or II hysterectomy with + or − margin. Post type III with RH positive vaginal cuff margin (also consider vaginal cylinder to treat a longer length of vagina).
Interstitial iridium (uterine, parametrial, +/or paracolpos)	Extensive disease or unable to locate intrauterine canal. Recurrent cervix cancer after hysterectomy. Cervical stump cancer with short (<4 cm) intrauterine canal.

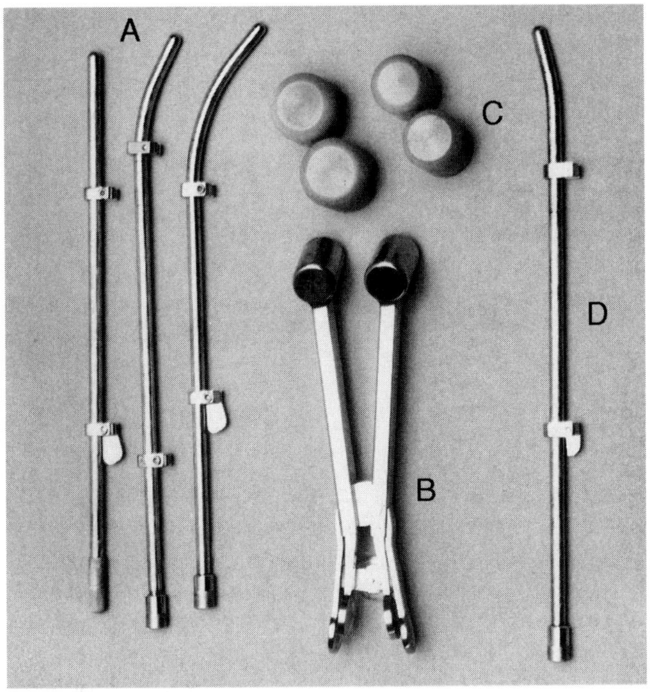

Figure 21.3. Fletcher-Suit-Delclos tandems, ovoids, and caps for ovoids. A. Tandems are available curved or without curvature. B. Rectangular handled ovoids. Each ovoid has a 2.0 cm diameter. C. Caps available in two sizes resulting in ovoid diameters of 2.5 and 3 cm, respectively. D. Most frequently used tandem (#1 curvature), embossed at 2 cm intervals corresponding to eventual location of the cesium. Isodose distribution at 1.5 cm above and of effect of shielding around the colpostats.

the applicator itself is an implantation system that has evolved around the use of those applicators. Table 21.2 outlines types of brachytherapy applicators used for different situations.

Fletcher-Suit-Delclos Colpostats. The original Fletcher colpostats were introduced in the early 1950s to replace the then standard Manchester radium tubes and ovoid applicators. Rectal and bladder shielding were provided but the colpostats needed to be preloaded. A subsequent modification by Suit in the later 1950s (Fletcher-Suit rectangular handled after loading colpostat) allowed for afterloading, but modifications to the shielding were needed because of mechanical difficulties. These mechanical difficulties were corrected and the original shielding design is available for afterloading use (Fletcher-Suit round handled after loading colpostat). Figure 21.4 illustrates the position of the tungsten shields and the resultant isodose distribution at 1.2 cm above and 1.0 cm below the ovoids (15). The clinical significance of these shielding differences has not been determined.

Fletcher Intrauterine Tandems. The stainless steel intrauterine tandems are available without curvature (#0) or with 3 curvatures (#1, #2, and #3) that fit the majority of uterine cavities. The #1 curvature is most often used, but the more curved #2 or #3 tandems are appropriate for a significantly anteverted uterus or for a long intrauterine canal. Embossed lines are present at 2 cm intervals along the tandem, corresponding to the eventual location of the cesium sources that will be loaded into the tandem. The stainless steel collar (flange) is placed at the line corresponding to the length of the intrauterine canal. When sutured to the external os, it prevents the tandem from sliding further into the uterus (therefore preventing fundal perforation). It also serves as a radiographic marker of the position of the cervix.

Vaginal Cylinders. Vaginal cylinders are used in conjunction with an intrauterine tandem to irradiate the vagina when the disease extends from the uterine cervix along the vaginal walls (Figure 21.5). A cylinder alone may be used after a radical hysterectomy if there is a close or positive vaginal margin. A vaginal cylinder is also useful for a patient with a very narrow vagina in whom it is technically difficult to secure the collar on the intrauterine tandem to the cervix. A small vaginal cylinder may be used for these patients, since the ring that fits over the cylinder can be sutured to the vulva to secure the intrauterine tandem. Cylinders are available in various diameters (1–5 cm) and lengths to fit any vaginal width and length. Some cylinders have hollow channels within them that allow for the option of inserting tungsten shields into one or more of the hollow channels to partially shield one or more of the vaginal walls.

Radioisotope. Most LDR intracavitary brachytherapy systems use cesium as the implanted radioisotope. One advantage of cesium-137 over radium-226 is the elimination of radon gas leakage. Another advantage is less required shielding for radiation protection because of the lower energy emitted from the photons, 0.662 MeV versus 0.8 MeV average (2.2 MeV maximum). Cesium may be purchased encapsulated asymmetrically in either platinum or stainless steel. The potential dosimetric consequences of this asymmetry are usually ignored (16). The physical characteristics of one brand may differ somewhat from another. A commonly used cesium source has a physical length of 2 cm, physical width of 0.31 cm, and an active length of 1.4 cm (Figure 21.6).

General Procedure

At the University of Minnesota the insertion of these applicators is usually performed jointly with the gynecologic and radiation oncologist. Although insertion of these appliances is often considered a "minor" surgical procedure, it is advantageous to have an experienced gynecologic oncologist present. Sometimes the tumor has obliterated normal anatomy and finding the uterine canal without creating a false passage or perforating the uterus is difficult.

For insertion of the Fletcher-Suit-Delclos tandem and

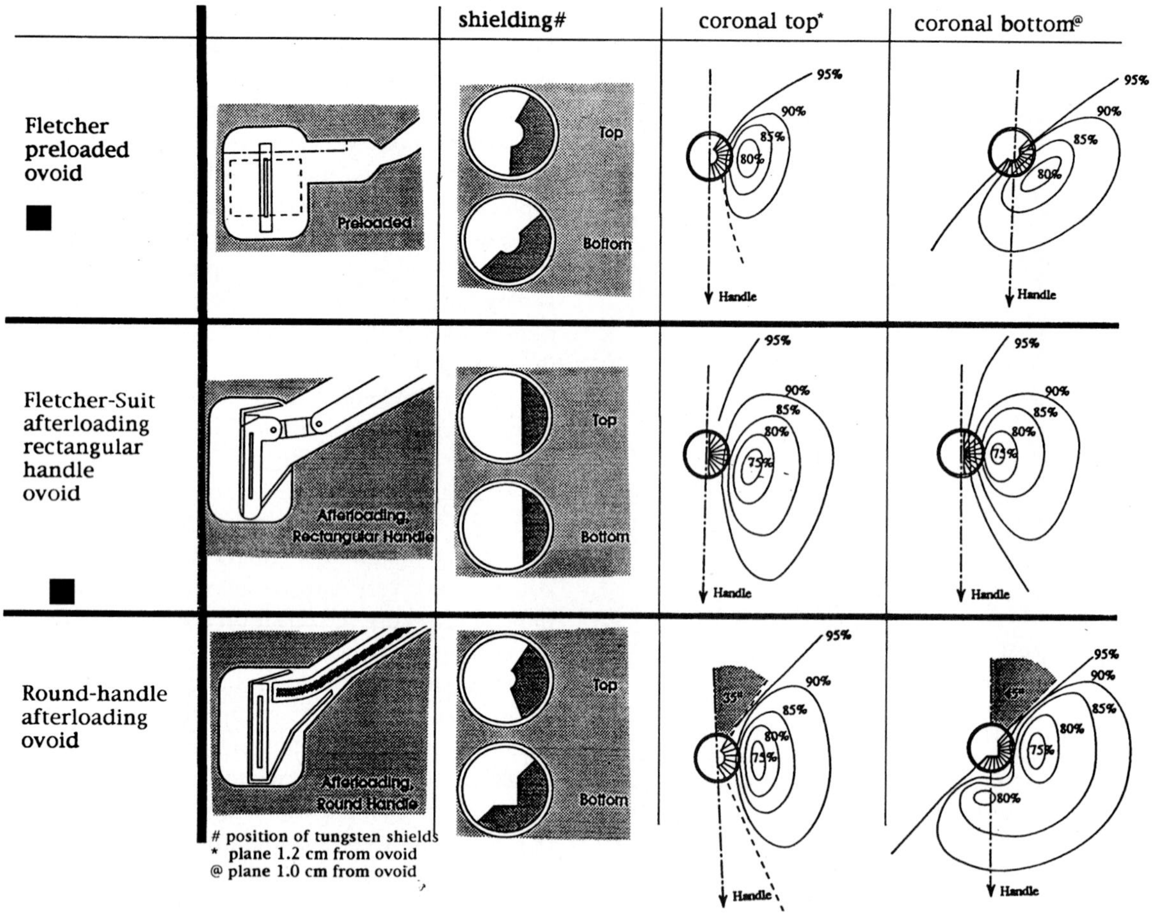

Figure 21.4. Three generations of Fletcher ovoids demonstrating the tungsten shielding design and resultant isodose distributions at 1.2 cm above and 1.0 cm below the ovoids. Modified from Haas et al. [15] and Radium Accessories Services, Inc, Marathon, Fl; both used with permission.

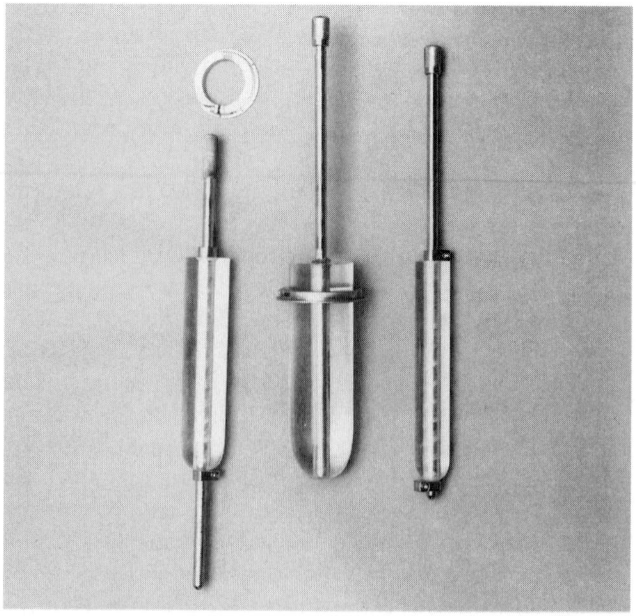

Figure 21.5. Vaginal cylinders are available in a variety of lengths and sizes.

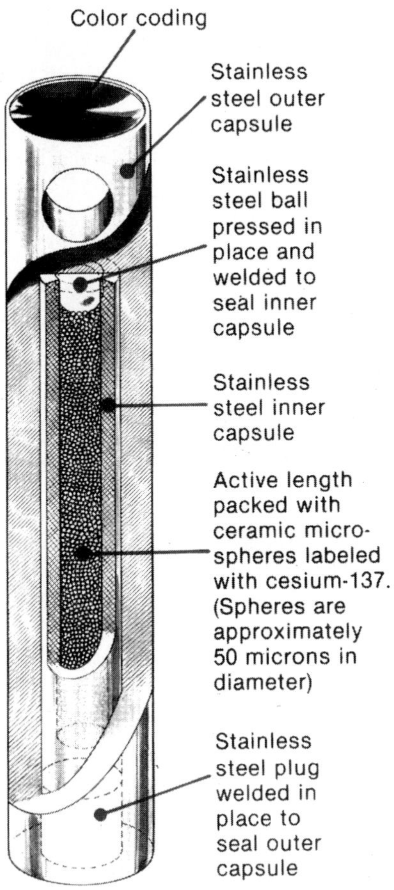

Figure 21.6. Cesium-137 tubes consist of asymmetrically placed cesium-labeled ceramic microspheres packed within a stainless steel or platinum casing. The eyelet is usually color-coded to correspond to the nominal strength of the cesium. (From Medical Products Division/ 3M. St. Paul, MN 55144. Used with permission.)

ovoids, the patient can choose either spinal or general anesthesia. Spinal anesthesia has the advantage that it wears off slowly, usually not until after completion of the simulation and after the patient has been transported to her room. By then other analgesics are available allowing for a smooth transition to either oral or parenteral pain control. Since the patient will be confined to bed rest for up to 3 days, preventing the development of a deep venous thrombosis is important. At the University of Minnesota, we use sequential pneumatic devices (pneumoboots) and low-dose (5000 units twice daily) subcutaneous heparin. Antibiotics are not prescribed unless the cervix is extremely necrotic or we suspect that the uterine wall was inadvertently perforated or a false passage created during the insertion.

Insertion of the Fletcher-Suit Tandem and Ovoids. In addition to the brachytherapy equipment, additional surgical equipment (usually found in a standard dilatation and curettage tray) is necessary for insertion of the tandem and ovoids (Figure 21.7). The patient is placed in the dorsal lithotomy position and examined. The extent of disease is delineated and compared to the preradiation therapy examination. It is particularly important to feel the position of the uterus. In most, but not all, patients the uterus is slightly anteverted. Knowing the uterine position will help guide the sounding of the uterine canal. The perineum and vagina are then prepped with an antiseptic solution. The field is draped with sterile towels. A Foley catheter is placed into the bladder and the balloon filled with 7 cc of radiopaque contrast material (diatrizoate meglumine Hypaque®, Sandi Winthrop Pharmaceuticals, NY). A weighted speculum is placed in the vagina. The anterior cervical lip is grasped with a single tooth tenaculum or Allis clamp. The uterine canal is sounded with a uterine sound and its length noted. Care is taken to not perforate through the uterine wall. If the uterine canal is difficult to find, ultrasound guidance can provide assistance (Figure 21.8a-c). Serial dilatation of the cervical os is performed. A size of #7 Hegar (or #16 Hanks) is usually adequate to inert the tandem.

The collar on the tandem is placed at the mark on the tandem corresponding to the length of the uterine canal. Cesium sources are generally 2 cm in length, and since the aim is to have the lowest cesium source in the tandem at the level of the cervix, it is convenient if the uterus sounds to an even length (i.e., 6 or 8 cm). The collar then can be set at the 6 or 8 cm mark (Figure 21.9). If the uterus sounds to an odd length (i.e., 5 or 7 cm) the mark closest (but shorter) than the sounded length should be used. If the

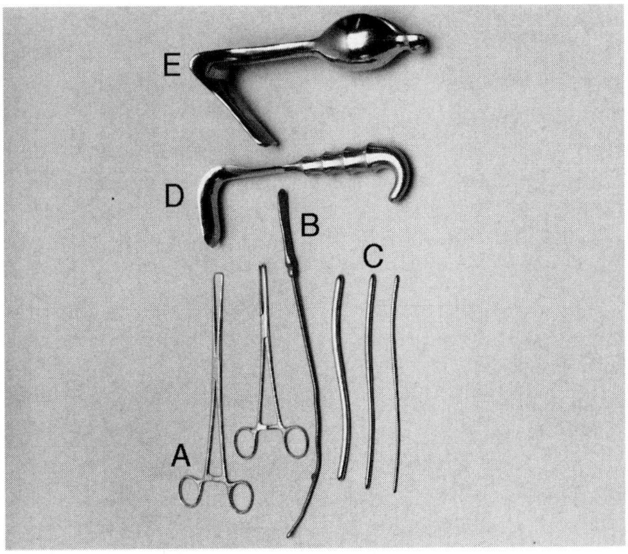

Figure 21.7. A dilatation and curettage tray usually has the major surgical equipment necessary for a tandem and ovoid application including an Allis clamp or single tooth tenaculum to grasp the cervical lip (A), a uterine sound (B), Hegar dilators to dilate the uterine canal (C), and a retractor and weighted speculum to help visualize the cervix (D).

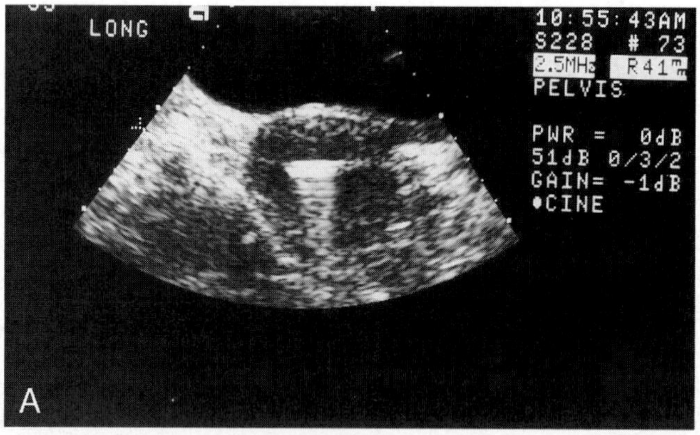

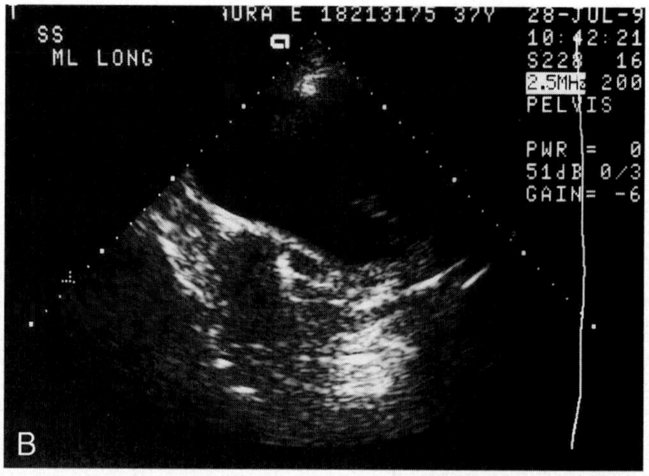

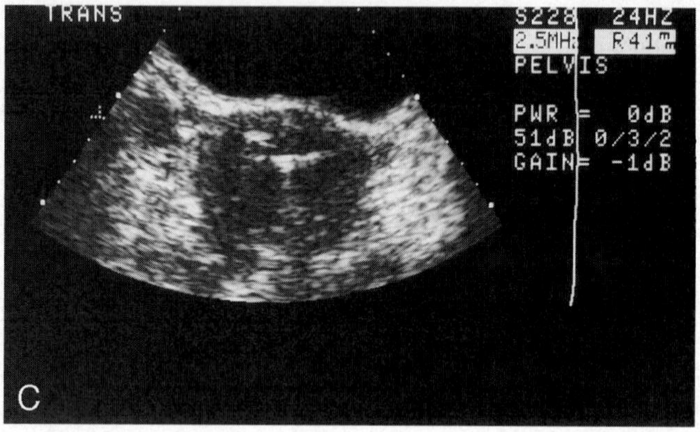

Figure 21.8. A. Longitudinal ultrasound image through the uterus demonstrating bladder, myometrium, and correct position of tandem within the uterine cavity. B. Longitudinal ultrasound image showing two echogenic stripes consisting of the tandem in a false passage and endometrial stripe where tandem should be. C. Transverse ultrasound image through the uterus demonstrating a false passage that was inadvertently created and the true uterine canal.

uterine canal sounds to a length of greater than 8 cm, we generally set the cervical collar at the 8 cm mark.

At the University of Minnesota, we routinely suture the collar to the cervix using nonabsorbable suture material to ensure that the tandem will not dislodge. The suture is either run through the small tunnel at the collar and tied at the cervix, or a second collar is placed more distally (Figure 21.10) and the suture is run through both collars and tied at the distal collar. The knot is cut long to facilitate removal.

One of the advantages of the Fletcher-Suit tandem and ovoid applicators is that the tandem is inserted separately from the ovoids. By using various size caps and angles on the ovoids and curvatures on the tandem, the application can be customized to the patient's tumor and anatomy. The aim is to achieve a high-dose rate within the tumor and a low-dose rate in the critical normal tissues (bladder and rectum). This is usually accomplished by trying to orient the tandem relative to the ovoids so that the resultant isodose distribution around the application bears the typical pear-shaped distribution with the bottom of the pear encompassing the tumor. Achieving this distribution is referred to as "optimizing the geometry" of the application. This idealized geometry does not always correspond to the distribution of the tumor, and what appears to be a less than ideal geometry may actually yield a dose distribution around the tumor that is ideal.

After the tandem is secured, the colpostats are inserted. The size of the vaginal vault dictates which size caps (if any) can be placed on the colpostats. The colpostats should fit snugly against the vaginal fornices. In general, the largest caps that fit and still result in good geometry should be used. This optimizes the depth dose ratio. If the colpostats are too large, they do not fit into the vaginal fornices and are displaced into the distal vagina (caudally). It is sometimes difficult (especially for the novice) to tell if the colpostats are displaced caudally after the tandem and ovoids are in the patient. Therefore, prior to insertion of the tandem into the patient, a useful approach is to put the tandem next to the ovoids and to visualize where the proximal collar should be relative to the ovoids, (Figure 21.11) then set the second collar exactly at the point the ovoid handles come together. This distal collar will then serve as a marker for whether the ovoids are too cranial or too caudal relative to the tandem.

For a narrow vault in which the standard size colpostats will not fit, mini-colpostats can be considered. However, at the University of Minnesota we prefer to use a protruding

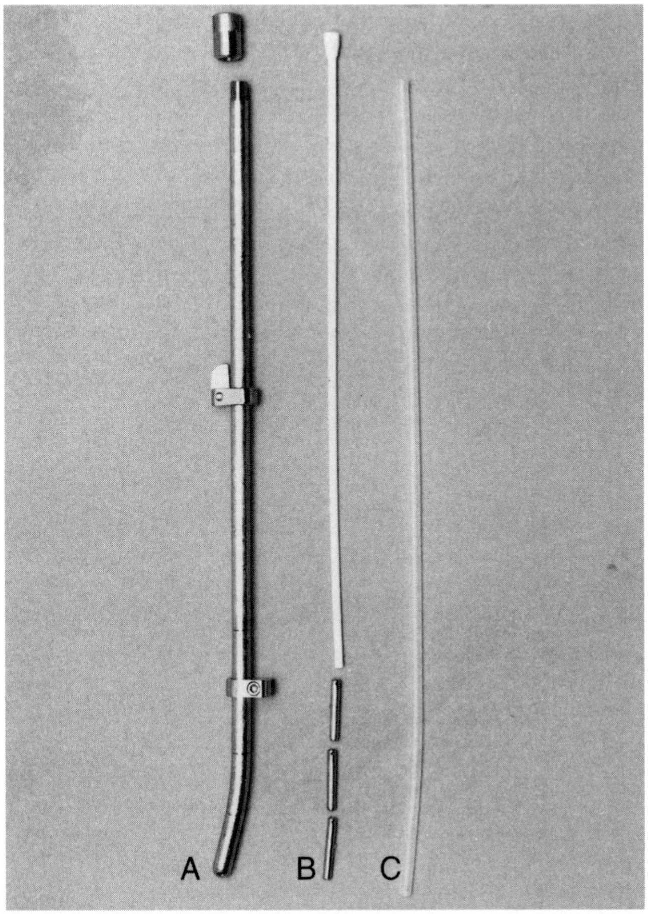

Figure 21.9. A. The proximal collar on the tandem is secured at the appropriate embossed line which will correspond to the eventual position of the cesium within the tandem. B. "Dummies" are oriented eyelet distally. A plunger that keeps the cesium sources at the apex of the tandem. C. The cesium sources are placed in a hollow nylon tube, followed by the plunger.

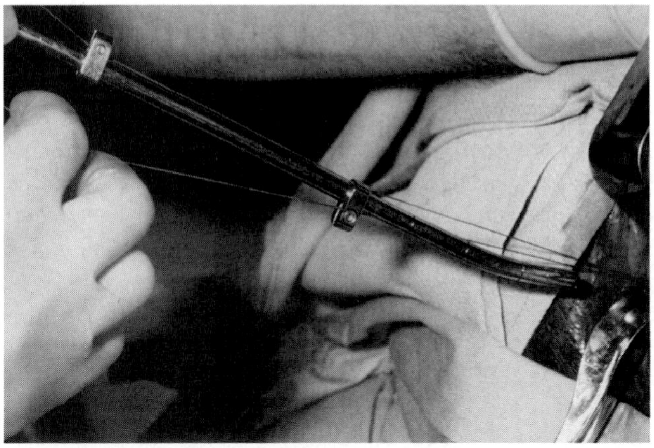

Figure 21.10. To prevent the tandem from dislodging, the proximal collar is sutured to the cervix by placing a suture through the cervix and running the suture through the hollow channel on the collar. Instead of securing the knot at the proximal collar, the suture can be threaded through a second collar placed more distally along the tandem and the knot tied at the distal collar. This facilitates removal of the tandem at the completion of the implant.

vaginal source (also called a hanging tandem) because of a higher incidence of bladder and rectal complications reported with the use of mini-colpostats (17). When the colpostats are in place, the tandem needs to be secured to the ovoids. We use a sterilized rubber band, but umbilical tape also can be used to tie the colpostats to the tandem. Alternatively, some systems have a yoke that secures the tandem to the colpostats and helps align the tandem relative to the colpostats to potentially improve the geometry.

Packing is used to optimize the geometry of the application and to displace the rectum posteriorly and bladder anteriorly away from the colpostats. Rolled gauze soaked in an antibacterial solution (Acriflavine) is used at the University of Minnesota. A metallic ribbon in the gauze helps outline the relative position of the vagina to the bladder and rectum. Because of the weight of the colpostats, there is a tendency for them to displace posteriorly. For that reason, the packing usually begins posteriorly, pushing the

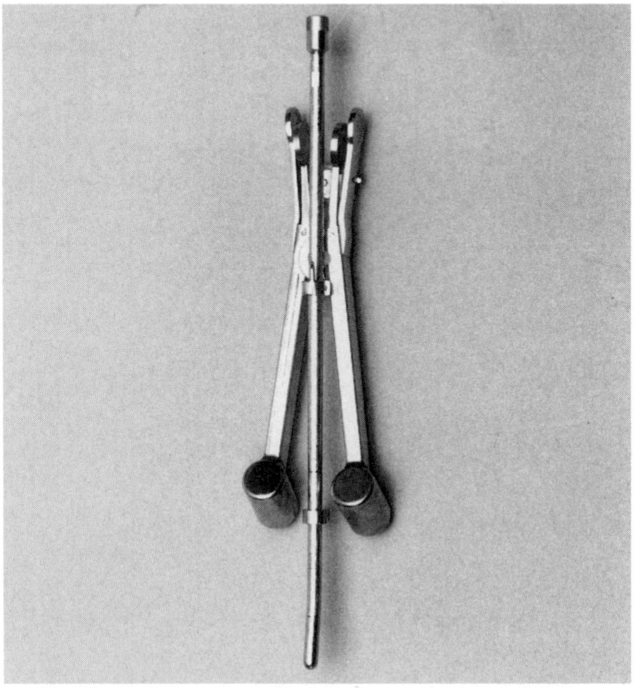

Figure 21.11. Since it is difficult to ascertain whether the ovoids are too proximal or distal relative to the cervix, the tandem and ovoids are placed in their desired orientation and the second collar is conveniently placed at the position where the ovoid handles come together prior to inserting them into the patient. Thus when the tandem and ovoids are in the patient, the distal marker helps determine if the geometry is good.

colpostats anteriorly. Packing anteriorly may be used at the midline to push the bladder anteriorly.

Representations of the desired geometric relationship between the tandem and ovoids are shown in Figure 21.12a-b. An orthogonal pair of radiographs of a Fletcher-Suit tandem and ovoid application with good geometry is shown in Figure 21.13a-b. In general, the aim is to have the tandem bisect the two ovoids. On anterior view, approximately one-third of the ovoid should be superior to the cervical collar and two-thirds should be inferior to the cervical collar. On lateral view, the colpostats should bisect the tandem, although most of the time the ovoids are slightly posterior to the tandem. After the packing is completed, a Foley catheter is placed in the rectum and the balloon filled with contrast material (Hypaque®).

To confirm that a good geometry has been obtained, an anterior and lateral x-ray is taken. This is usually accomplished with a portable x-ray unit. A C-Arm can also be used, but this is not possible with all operating room tables. If the applicator geometry is not "good," the packing is

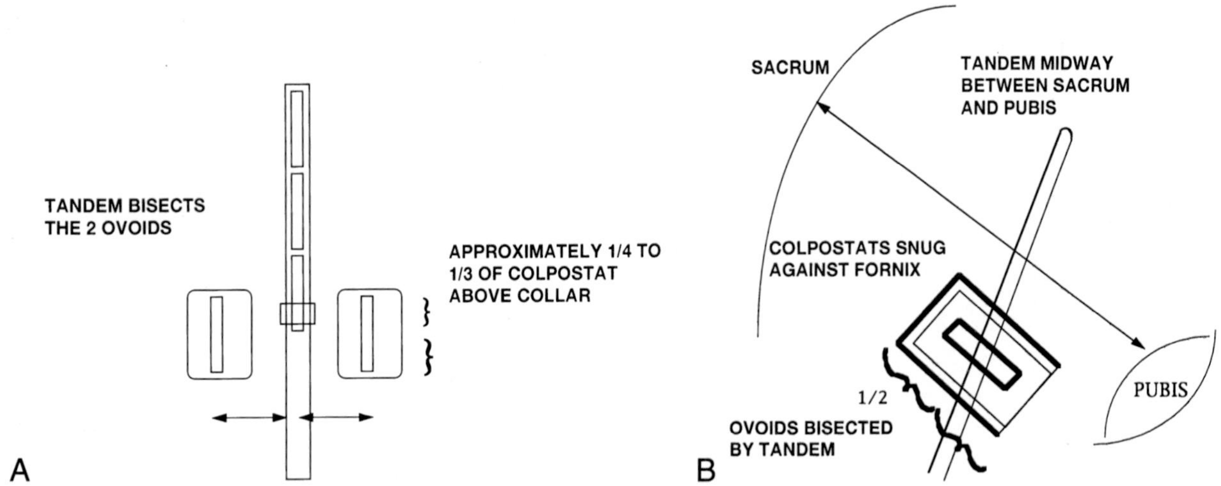

Figure 21.12. A. Diagram illustrating the desired orientation of the tandem relative to the ovoids as seen on an anterior view. B. Diagram illustrating the desired orientation of the tandem relative to the ovoids as seen on a lateral view.

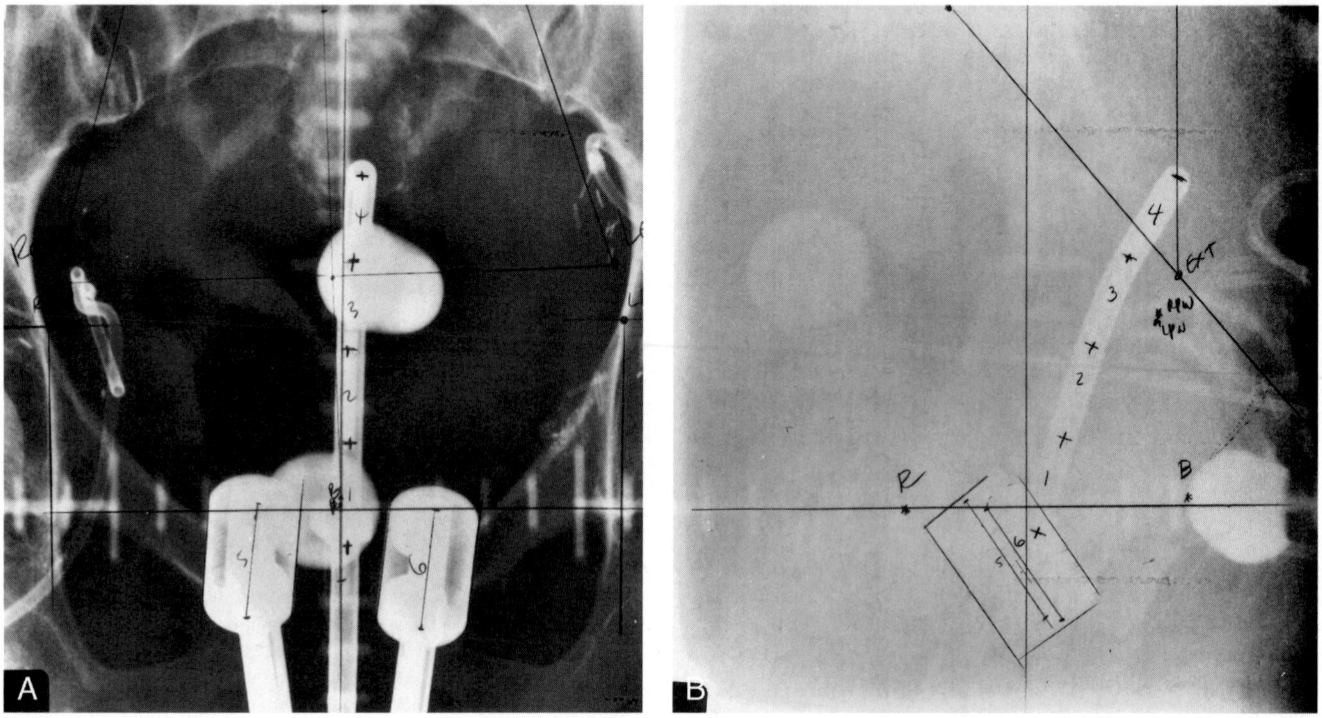

Figure 21.13. Radiographs of desired orientation of the tandem and ovoids. A. Anteroposterior. B. Lateral.

removed and the patient is repacked. The process is repeated as necessary. Examples of poor geometry implants are shown in Figure 21.14A–C. Every attempt should be made to optimize the relationship between the tandem and ovoids. Further repacking is not necessary if after one or two attempts of repacking there is no improvement in geometry either because of the patient's anatomy or tumor extent; at this point, a decision must be made about how to load the tandem and ovoids. In general, if the distorted geometry leads to a higher tumor dose with an acceptable rectal and bladder dose, it is usually loaded with cesium as usual. If this is not the case, alternate loadings, or waiting an additional 1 to 2 weeks for more tumor shrinkage, is advisable.

Occasionally the vault is narrow and although the colpostats (without caps) can be inserted into the vagina, the x-ray may reveal that they are inferior to the cervical collar. Repacking will not be of benefit in this situation because

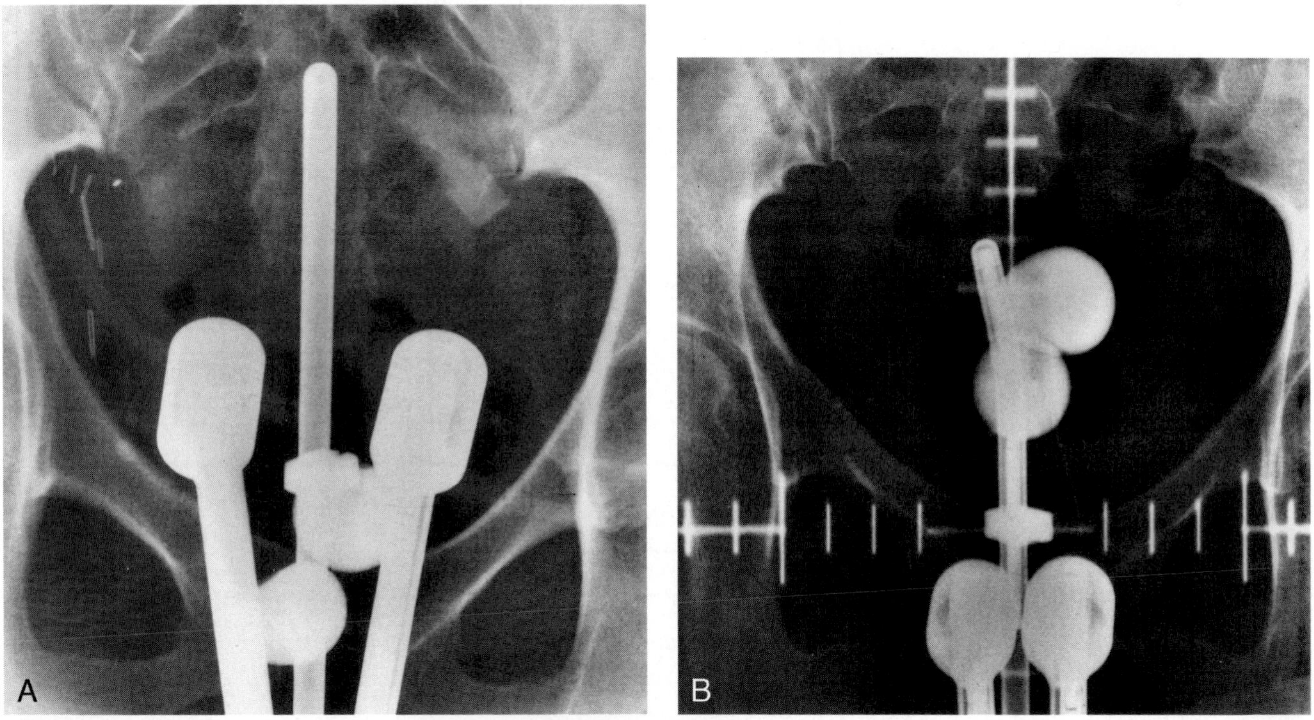

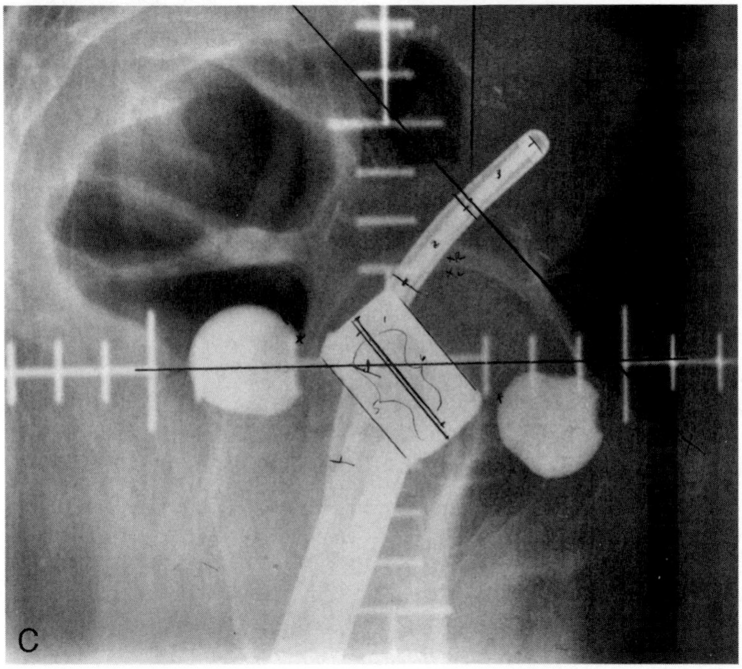

Figure 21.14. Radiographic examples of poor geometry. A. Portable x-ray taken in the operating room demonstrating ovoids that are placed too inferior and posterior relative to the tandem. Repacking is indicated. Note that the ovoids are widely spaced and placing caps on the ovoids may help. B. Radiograph demonstrating ovoids that are too inferior and posterior relative to the tandem. If caps are on the ovoids, removing them might improve the geometry. C. The ovoids are anterior relative to the tandem resulting in a very high bladder dose rate.

Figure 21.15. Prior to placing the cesium in the patient a preliminary written directive must be completed and signed by the radiation oncologist. Prior to the completion of the implant, the final written directive must be completed.

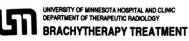

UNIVERSITY OF MINNESOTA HOSPITAL AND CLINIC
DEPARTMENT OF THERAPEUTIC RADIOLOGY
BRACHYTHERAPY TREATMENT

PATIENT IDENTIFICATION PLATE

WRITTEN DIRECTIVE

I. PRIOR TO IMPLANTATION

PATIENT'S NAME		U of M HOSPITAL #
DIAGNOSIS	TREATMENT SITE	
STATION	REFERRING PHYSICIAN	
ISOTOPE USED Cs-137 ☐ Ir-192 ☐ I-125 ☐ Other ☐		BATCH #
APPLICATOR(S) USED		
# Ribbons	#Seeds/Ribbon	Total # seeds
mg. Ra. Equiv. per seed	Total mg. Ra. Equiv.	

DIAGRAM OF APPLICATION	TANDEM? ___YES ___NO	NUMBER OF SOURCES
	COLPOSTATS? ___YES ___NO	DIAMETER OF COLPOSTATS ___ cm
	VAGINAL CYLINDER? ___YES ___NO	DIAMETER OF CYLINDER ___ cm
STAFF SIGNATURE:		

II. PRIOR TO COMPLETION OF IMPLANT

TOTAL HOURS	DOSE [mg. hrs] (1.07 FILTRATION FACTOR INCLUDED)			
DOSE (cGy)	Point A	Point B	BLADDER	RECTUM
	VAGINAL SURFACE			
STAFF SIGNATURE:		PHYSICS SIGNATURE:		

INSERTED	DATE	TIME	BY
REMOVED	DATE	TIME	BY

MR 307, DEC 93 WHITE-MEDICAL RECORD YELLOW AND PINK-THERAPEUTIC RADIOLOGY DEPT.

the problem is not with the alignment of colpostats relative to the tandem, but with the patient's anatomy (narrow vagina). Some authors have advocated mini-colpostats in this situation. Mini-colpostats have a diameter of 16 mm (regular colpostats 20 mm) and a flat inner surface. Early models had no shielding, although newer models are commercially available with tungsten shields. When loaded with 10 mg cesium, mini-colpostats deliver roughly the same vaginal surface dose as the small colpostats. When combined with the tandem, however, the bladder and rectal dose rates may be prohibitive. High bladder and rectal complication rates have been reported with mini-colpostats (17,18). An alternative to mini-colpostats for patients with narrow vaginas is to load the tandem with a source that protrudes below the cervical collar into the upper vagina. This protruding vaginal source increases the dose rate within the cervical tumor without leading to prohibitively high bladder or rectal dose rates. The disadvantages to using the protruding vaginal source are that the distribution of dose near the cervix is not expanded inferiorly as is obtained with the addition of ovoids, that a longer implant duration is required to achieve a certain total point A dose, and that the mg-hr prescription system cannot be used to determine implant duration. Additionally, bowel and bladder complications may be higher than with standard sized ovoids. Alternatively, some institutions use interstitial brachytherapy in these cases.

Insertion of the Intrauterine Tandem and Vaginal Cyl-

inder. The intrauterine tandem is inserted as previously described. The appropriate diameter vaginal cylinder is introduced over the intrauterine tandem and secured with a second collar. A metal ring slides over the cylinder and is tightened just distal to the introitus. The ring has four holes in it to suture the cylinder to the vulva at the corresponding four positions.

Simulation

After insertion of the applicator, "dummy" cesium sources are loaded into the afterloading appliances and an orthogonal pair of radiographs are taken. The isocenter is set at the center of the collar for Fletcher-Suit tandem and ovoid applications. An anterior and lateral pair of orthogonal simulation films are taken. The "dummy" sources and rectal balloon are removed and the patient is transported back to her hospital room.

Applicator Loading Determination

After reviewing the orthogonal films, the "preliminary written directive" for loading the cesium sources is decided upon. It is unusual for the final plan to differ from this preliminary plan, but occasionally this will occur. The Nuclear Regulatory Commission requires that the radiation oncologist provide a "preliminary written directive" that includes the patient's name, identifying information, radioisotope, number of sources, source strength, and date. This must be signed by the authorized user physician before the cesium can be loaded into the patient (Figure 21.15).

The standard loading for a 6-cm intrauterine tandem (from superior to inferior) is 15 mg, 10 mg, 10 mg, and for an 8-cm tandem 15 mg, 10 mg, 10 mg, 10 mg. The standard loading for the vaginal ovoids is 15 mg for 2-cm diameter ovoids (with no caps); 20 mg for 2.5-cm diameter ovoids (with small caps) and 25 mg for 3.0-cm diameter ovoids (with large caps). Exceptions to these guidelines are for patients who have a "barrel-shaped" cervix. These patients have considerable tumor bulk in the expanded lower uterine segment. It is reasonable to put a more active source lower in the tandem for example, 15 mg, 15 mg, 10 mg (or 10 mg, 15 mg, 10 mg) in a 6-cm tandem and 15 mg, 15 mg, 10 mg, 10 mg (or 10 mg, 15 mg, 15 mg, 10 mg) in an 8-cm tandem respectively. A 15 mg source is never placed just above the cervical collar because the contribution of the ovoids to the dose in that area is considerable and the bladder and rectum are close. If ovoids cannot be used because of a narrow vagina, a single protruding vaginal source of 10 mg is added below the collar.

If a vaginal cylinder is used, the activity of the cesium put into the cylinder depends on the cylinder diameter. A computer plan can provide vaginal surface dose rate. However, since the computer plan often takes several hours to complete, and the patients are anxious to complete the implant, it is useful to know the approximate vaginal surface dose rate with a certain diameter cylinder loaded a certain way so that the "preliminary written directive" can be completed and the cesium loaded into the applicator without delay. "Away" tables are useful in this regard (Table 21.3).

Table 21.3. Surface Dose Rates as a Function of Cylinder Diameter and Number of Sources

Diameter of Cylinder (mm)	Source Strength Cesium (mg)	Number of Sources	Effective Length of Vagina Treated (mm)	Lateral Vaginal Surface Dose Rate (cGy/hr)
20	10	1	16	71
"	"	2	34	87
"	"	3	51	108
"	"	4	65	102
26	15	1	19	64
"	"	2	32	91
"	"	3	52	110
"	"	4	62	118
32	20	1	18	57
"	"	2	32	88
"	"	3	48	107
"	"	4	57	116
36	25	1	22	60
"	"	2	33	92
"	"	3	47	115
"	"	4	62	123

Modified from Johnson and Potish used with permission [61].

A 2-cm diameter cylinder with four sources loaded with 10 mg, 10 mg, 10 mg, 10 mg sources will yield a vaginal surface dose rate (at mid-implant) of approximately 100 cGy/hour, and a dose rate at 0.5 cm deep to the surface of 60 cGy/hr. Larger diameter cylinders will give correspondingly lower dose rates. For example, a 3-cm diameter cylinder loaded identically will yield a 60 cGy/hr vaginal surface dose rate. Since the dose falloff is almost linear with distance at very close distances to the brachytherapy applicators, an approximation is possible of the corresponding vaginal surface dose rate. The preliminary written directive can be filled out accordingly, then modified depending on the computer plan.

After the "preliminary written directive" is completed, the cesium can be prepared for transportation to the patient's hospital room. A plastic straw, with a smaller diameter than the tandem, holds the cesium sources in tandem. A plunger keeps the sources at the apex of the straw.

We employ a series of double checks to make sure the correct strength cesium sources are prepared for the patient. The lead pigs that are used to transport the cesium to the patient's room are labeled with the patient's name. A "cesium transport card" accompanies the cesium (Figure

21.16a-b). Before administering the brachytherapy dose, the identity of the patient must be verified by two independent means by checking the name of the patient against the name printed on the written directive. Movable shields are placed on both sides of the patient's bed. After the cesium is placed in the applicator, the date and time of the loading are indicated on the cesium transport card and on the patient's hospital chart, which should also include a diagram of the loading and total source strength.

A survey of the room and surrounding area measure the exposure in mR/hr to assure that exposure rates are within acceptable limits to hospital personnel and patients who might be in adjoining rooms. The exposure rate at the patient's door and at the wall closest to the patient in adjoining rooms must be below 2 mR/hr. If not, additional shielding is placed until these limits are met. Signs on the patient's door alert others to the presence of radioactivity.

Computer Planning: Dose Calculations

For all brachytherapy implants, computerized dosage calculations are performed using the orthogonal film pair to provide the positional data of the sources and the applicators. To accomplish this, a variety of software packages are available. The general procedure includes digitizing the following points on the orthogonal x-rays into the computer planning system:

1. Tips and ends of the cesium sources.
2. Bladder reference point. Foley balloon is filled with 7 cc of radiopaque fluid (Hypaque) and pulled down towards the bladder neck. On the lateral radiograph, the reference point is obtained by drawing a line through the center of the balloon and the posterior surface of the balloon is used as the reference point. On the anterior radiograph, the reference point is

UNIVERSITY OF MINNESOTA HOSPITAL AND CLINIC
DEPARTMENT OF THERAPEUTIC RADIOLOGY–RADIATION ONCOLOGY

ISOTOPE TRANSPORT CARD CESIUM ☐ IRIDIUM ☐ OTHER ☐

PATIENT NAME:	HOSPITAL NO.

APPLICATION NO. ☐ 1 ☐ 2 ☐ 3 ☐ 4 ☐ 5

DIAGRAM OF IMPLANT

APPLICATOR:	mg. RA. EQ.	IF IR-192:
☐ TANDEM	________	Batch #: ________
☐ COLPOSTATS	________	NO. of SEEDS________
☐ CYLINDER	________	mg.Ra.Eq./SEED on________=________ (date)
☐ SIMON'S CAPSULES	________	
☐ NEEDLES	________	Batch #: ________
☐ OTHER: ________	________	NO. of SEEDS________
		mg.Ra.Eq./SEED on________=________ (date)
TOTAL ACTIVITY	________	

	DATE	HOUR	No. of Sources	BY
INSERTED				
REMOVED				

TOTAL HOURS	EQ.MG. HRS.
RADIOISOTOPE CURATOR	STAFF

23424, NOV 93

Figure 21.16. A. Cesium transport card accompanies movement of the cesium outside the radioisotope safe. A convenient place to document some of the quality management program items is on the back of the cesium transport card (B), including the initial room survey (which is done after the cesium is loaded into the patient to assure low exposure rates for nurses and patients in adjoining rooms) and the final room survey (done as a double check to make sure the radioisotope has been removed).

Figure 21.16B. *(continued)*

APPENDIX A-IV
PATIENT ROOM SURVEY FORM
University of Minnesota

Patient identified by two independent means (Yes/No): ________

Diagram of implant, isotope, number of sources, and total activity in hospital chart (Y/N): ______

INITIAL ROOM SURVEY Room Number: ____________
(following insertion of sources)

Instrument used for the survey:
Ionization Survey Meter________________; GM Survey Meter ________________

EXPOSURE RATE: mR/hr

		mR/hr	Less than 2 mR/hr Yes	No
(A)	1 m from patient (unshielded):	______		
(B)	At bedside (behind shield):	______		
(C)	Door to room:	______	______	______
(D)	Wall closest to patient, in adjoining room:	______	* ______	______
(E)	Wall farthest from patient, in adjoining room:	______	* ______	______
(F)	Chair at foot of bed (if applicable):	______	______	______

Patient in adjoining room(s); Room No(s). __________, __________

- If exposure rate for (C) through (E) is greater than 2 mR/hr, reposition the bed and/or shields to reduce the exposure rate to ≤2 mR/hr. If the exposure rate cannot be reduced to ≤2 mR/hr, notify the Therapeutic Radiology physicist on call or a member of the Radiation Protection Staff (see cesium or iridium emergency procedures for contact numbers).

*This need not be done if radioisotopes are present in the adjoining room.

Signature ______________________________ Date/Time ______________

FINAL ROOM SURVEY (following removal of the sources)

Instrument used for the survey:
Ionization Survey Meter________________; GM Survey Meter ________________

EXPOSURE RATE:

Patient __________mR/hr; Room __________mR/hr; Walls __________mR/hr

If exposure rate is greater than 2 mR/hr, indicate the reason: ______________________

- If reason is a dislodged or missing source, immediately contact the physician/resident and Radiation Protection staff member on call (see cesium or iridium emergency procedures for contact numbers).
- If the exposure rate is greater than 2 mR/hr due to a radiation patient in an adjacent room, reposition the bed and/or shields in the adjacent patient's room to reduce the exposure rate to ≤2 mR/hr. If the exposure rate cannot be reduced to ≤2 mR/hr, notify the Therapeutic Radiology physicist on call or a member of the Radiation Protection Staff (see cesium or iridium emergency procedures for contact numbers).

Signature ______________________________ Date/Time ______________

taken at the center of the balloon (Figure 21.17).

3. Rectal reference point. The International Commission of Radiation Units and Measurements (ICRU) rectal reference point is obtained by drawing an anteroposterior line on the lateral radiograph from the lower end of the intrauterine source (or from the middle of the intravaginal sources). The rectal point is taken at a depth of 0.5 cm, posterior to the point where this line traverses the posterior vaginal wall (the vaginal wall is identified by intravaginal radiopaque gauze). The anterior coordinates of the rectal point are at the lower end of the intrauterine source or at the middle of the intravaginal sources at midline (Figure 21.17).

4. The Fletcher Lymphatic Trapezoid Points. A line is drawn from the junction of S1-S2 to the top of the symphysis. Then a line is drawn from the middle of that line to the middle of the anterior aspect of L4. A trapezoid is constructed in a plane passing through the transverse line in the pelvic brim plane and the midpoint of the anterior aspect of the body of L4. A point 6 cm lateral to the midline at the inferior end of this figure is used to give an estimate of the dose rate to the mid-external iliac nodes. At the top of the trapezoid, points 2 cm lateral to the midline at the level of

L4 are used to estimate the dose to the low para-aortic nodes. The midpoint of a line connecting these two points is used to estimate the dose to the low common iliac nodes (Figure 21.18).

5. The Pelvic Wall Points. Pelvic wall reference points can be visualized on an AP and lateral radiograph and related to fixed bony structures. This point is intended to be representative of the absorbed dose at the distal part of the parametrium and at the obturator lymph nodes. On an AP radiograph, the pelvic-wall reference point is intersected by a horizontal line tangential to the highest point of the acetabulum and a vertical line tangential to the inner aspect of the acetabulum. On a lateral radiograph, the highest points of the right and left acetabulum, in the craniocaudal direction, are joined and the lateral projection of the pelvic-wall reference point is located at the mid-distance of these points (Figure 21.19).

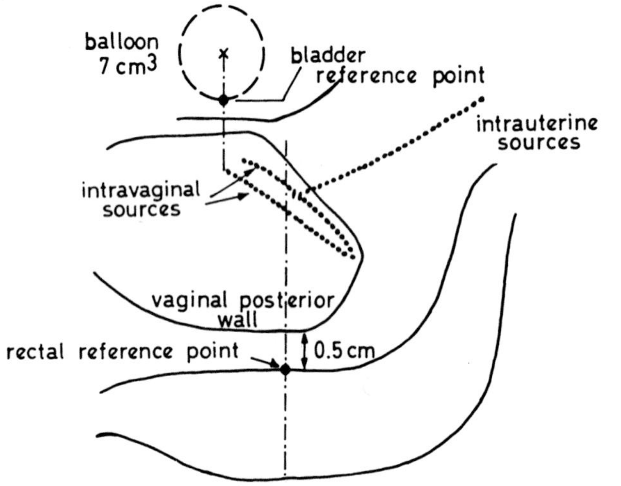

Figure 21.17. Location of bladder and rectum points as specified by the ICRU [33]. (From ICRU Report No. 38. Bethesda, MD: International Commission on Radiation Units and Measurements, 1985. Used with permission.)

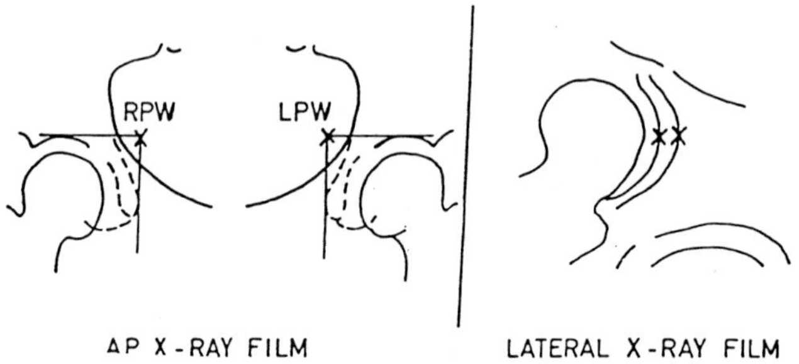

Figure 21.19. Definition of pelvic wall points [33]. Position of right pelvic wall (RPW) and left pelvic wall (LPW) are diagrammed. From ICRU Report No. 38. Bethesda, MD: International Commission on Radiation Units and Measurements, 1985. Used with permission.

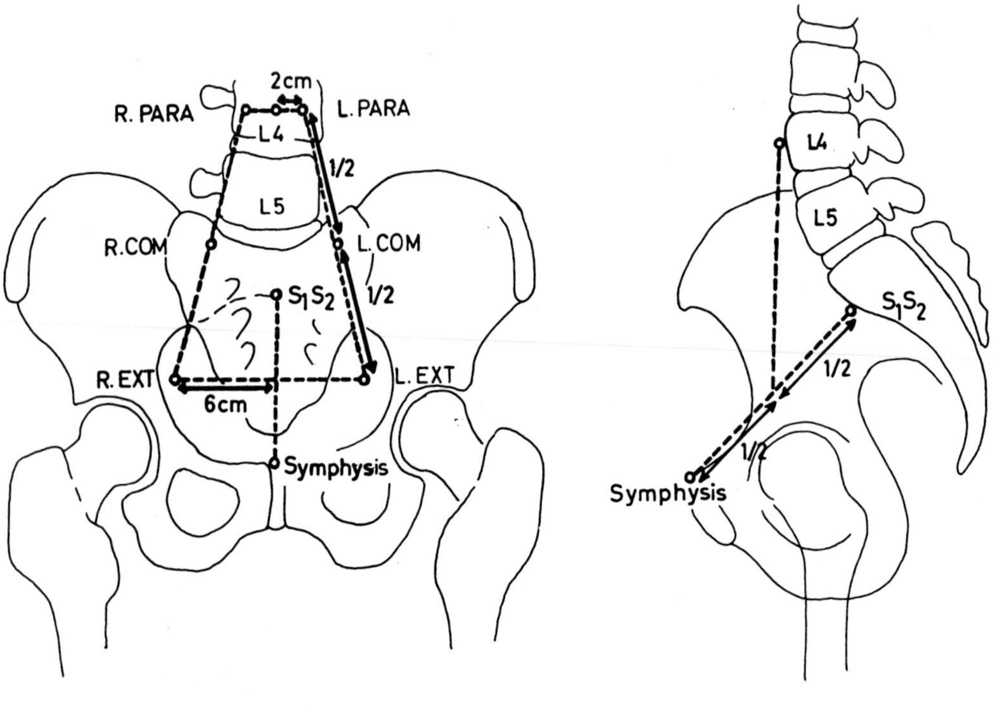

Figure 21.18. Determination of reference points corresponding to the lymphatic trapezoid of Fletcher [33]. (From ICRU Report No. 38. Bethesda, MD: International Commission on Radiation Units and Measurements, 1985. Used with permission.)

Implant Duration

Milligram Hours. When only radium sources were available in the precomputer era, gynecologic brachytherapy applications were specified by the simple mathematical product of the number of milligrams of radium times the duration (in hours) of the implant. Thus an implant with five 10 mg radium sources left in place for 48 hours would yield a dose of 2400 mg-hrs ($10 \times 5 \times 48$). Since its initial use in the early 1900s in Europe, a dose-prescription system evolved and was refined at M.D. Anderson hospital by Dr. Gilbert Fletcher and his colleagues (19). Results obtained at M.D. Anderson are among the best in the world. At the University of Minnesota we depend heavily on the Fletcher mg-hr system to specify dose. A 7% correction factor (8.25/7.71) is used to convert the Fletcher mg-hrs to ICRU mg-hrs, since the mg-hours recommended by Dr. Fletcher are for implants with radium encapsulated in 1 mm platinum (exposure rate constant 7.71 R/cm 2 $h^{-1}mg^{-1}$) and the ICRU specifies that radium sources with 0.5 mm platinum filtration be used as the standard (exposure rate constant 8.25 $R/cm^2\ h^{-1}mg^{-1}$).

Although the mg-hr system is easy to use, this method does not provide information about the dose distribution around that application. The system works because it specifies a particular geometry between the tandem and ovoids and the sources are loaded in a rigidly prescribed manner. It is only applicable when both the tandem and ovoids are implanted. For a tandem loaded with a protruding vaginal source (no ovoids), the mg-hr dose specification is not applicable.

Point A Dose. The second dose prescription system that evolved specifies the dose to four specific points in space around the applicator, Points A, B, Bladder, and Rectum. Originally developed in Manchester, England, this system is often referred to as the Manchester System. Point A was initially defined as the point 2 cm superior to the vaginal fornix and 2 cm lateral to the cervical canal. Point B was 3 cm lateral to point A. Points A and B were said to represent critical anatomic structures, point A representing the site where the uterine vessels crossed the ureter and point B representing the location of the more lateral pelvic nodes.

Although point A is usually described as 2 cm superior and 2 cm lateral to a specified origin, the definition of the point of origin is not standardized. Since the initial description of point A, many different origins have been defined without a clear consensus as to which origin is standard (Figure 21.20a-b) (20). Depending on which origin is chosen, the point A dose can vary widely, especially if the ovoids are displaced either superiorly or inferiorly. A relatively small displacement of the ovoids superiorly results in a large increase in the dose rate to point A. Since dose rates falls off very rapidly with distance from the brachytherapy sources, any point surrounding the applicator will be expected to be in a rapid dose fall off area, another disadvantage of using point A. For small tumors, point A may even lie outside the tumor volume, whereas for larger tumors, the tumor may extend significantly more lateral than point A. Since some definitions of point A are radiographic, point A may end up outside of the cervix all together.

At the University of Minnesota, we specify either point A_v or A_o to attempt to better specify the radiographic location of point A. The subscripts o and v refer to the os and vaginal fornix, respectively. In most situations, point Av is used with the vertical origin determined on lateral radiograph at the point where the colpostat cap crosses the tandem and is 2 cm superior to this point along the axis of the cervical source, then 2 cm lateral. When colpostats are unable to be used (most often due to narrow vaginal vault), A_o cannot be specified (since with the absence of the ovoids, the vaginal fornix is not radiographically outlined), and instead A_o is specified as the vertical origin determined on anterior radiograph at top of cervical collar 2 cm superior to this point along the axis of the cervical source, then 2 cm lateral.

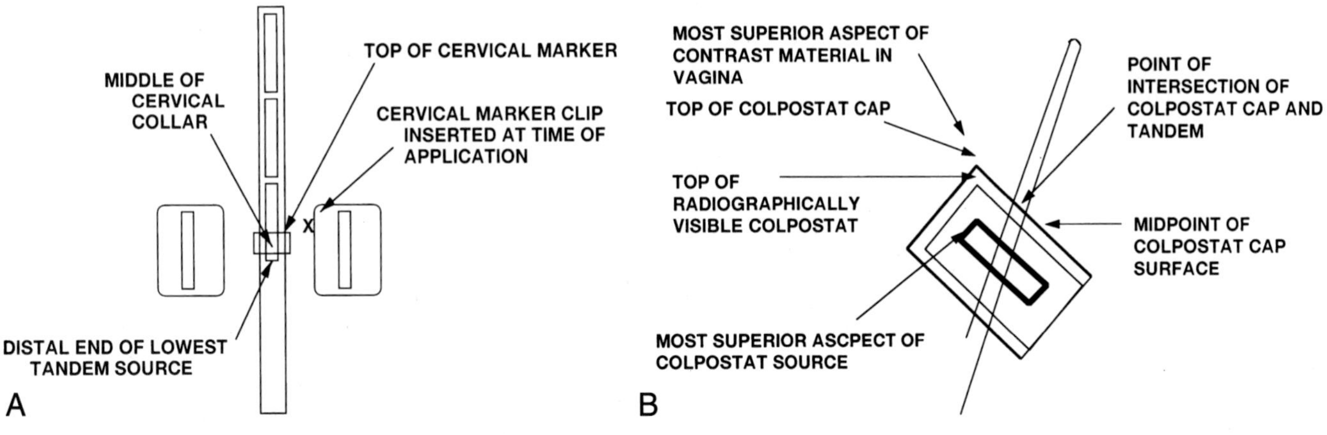

Figure 21.20. A. Possible origins of point A on anterior view. B. Possible origins of point A on lateral view.

Association Between Point A, Point B, and mg-hours. In a perfect Fletcher-Suit implant loaded as described above, point A almost always lies between 50 and 60 cGy/hr. Point B usually lies between 10 and 20 cGy/hr and is largely dependent on the source strength in the ovoids. Because these dose rates for point A and B are usually confined to a narrow range, as are implant durations, it is not surprising that there is an association between these total point doses and milligram-hours (20,21). In an evaluation of almost 100 brachytherapy applications performed at the University of Minnesota, we found a fairly high correlation between milligram-hours of radium and doses at point A and point B (correlation coefficients of 0.73 and 0.89, respectively) (22). However, point A dose was markedly affected by the position of the colpostats relative to the tandem, and considerable inter-patient variability made the routine translation between Fletcher and Manchester systems too unpredictable for clinical use. Despite these limitations, it is useful to roughly translate milligram-hours into point A or point B doses. Bhatnager has suggested a formula that roughly calculates the Point A dose based on the milligrams of radium loaded.

Point A(cGy/hr) = 1.1{(#mg in tandem) + (#mg in ovoids/2)} cGy/hr [26]

Likewise, the following formula roughly converts milligram-hours into the total point B dose:

Point B (total dose in cGy) = (total mg-hrs in 2 implants)/4

International Commission on Radiological Units and Measurements (ICRU). In 1985, the ICRU recommended a system of low-dose-rate brachytherapy dose and volume specifications aimed at redefining and standardizing brachytherapy reporting terminology (23). Three reporting approaches were proposed to specify intracavitary applications (Table 21.4). Since specification of dose in brachytherapy involves complex three-dimensional gradients that do not lend themselves to simple reporting, it was suggested that all three methods be used to complement each other. These methods of dose specification were to report 1) reference air kerma rate, 2) absorbed dose at certain reference points, and 3) isodose reference volume.

The reference air kerma rate was proposed to introduce international units into the brachytherapy reporting. The reference air kerma rate is expressed in mGy/h at 1 meter. The total reference air kerma is therefore the sum of the products of the reference air kerma rate and the duration of the application. The Fletcher mg-hrs can be easily converted into reference air kerma by the following formula (23):

Table 21.4. ICRU Reporting Data

Description of Technique
Source used (radionuclide, reference air kerma rate, shape and size of source, and filtration)
Simulation of linear source for point or moving sources
Applicator geometry (rigidity, tandem curvature, vaginal uterine connection, source geometry, shielding material)
Total Reference Air Kerma
Time Dose Pattern (application duration)
Description of Reference Volume
Reference isodose level
Isodose width, height, and thickness
Dose at Reference Points
Bladder
Rectum
Lymphatic trapezoid (lower periaortic, common iliac, external iliac)
Pelvic wall

ICRU, International Commission on Radiological Units and Measurements.

1 mg hr = 6.5 mGy total reference air kerma (for filtration 1 mm PT)

Total reference air kerma therefore has the same limitations as mg-hr dose specification.

The ICRU also recommended calculating absorbed dose at certain reference points (rectal, bladder, pelvic wall, trapezoid node points), but fell short of trying to standardize definitions for point A or B.

The most radical change proposed by the ICRU report was to specify reporting parameters for the pear shaped reference volume. The report states that "an absorbed dose level of 60 Gy is widely accepted as the appropriate reference level for classical low-dose-rate brachytherapy" and therefore the 60 Gy isodose reference volume was suggested. This reference volume is determined by measuring the width, height, and thickness tissue encompassed by the 60 Gy isodose curves. The method to measure these dimensions are as follows: The height (dh) is the maximum dimension along the intrauterine source and is measured in the frontal plane. The width (dw) is the maximum dimension perpendicular to the intrauterine source measured on the same frontal plane. The thickness (dt) is the maximum dimension perpendicular to the intrauterine source measured in the plane 90° lateral to the frontal plane (sagittal plane).

The height (dh), thickness, (dt) and width (dw) of a 60 Gy isodose reference volume, the product of which is the reference volume. The ICRU chose to subtract any external beam therapy from this 60 Gy reference volume. To choose the relevant isodose surface, the EBRT is subtracted from the 60 Gy volume and the remainder is divided by the implant duration to obtain the isodose surface by which to calculate the reference volume. For instance,

Fairview-University Medical Center
A Division of Fairview

University Campus
420 Delaware Street Southeast
Minneapolis, MN 55455
612-626-3000

Department of Therapeutic Radiology-Radiation Oncology

Conventional LDR Brachytherapy QMP Checklist

Hospital No.: ____________
Patient's Name: ____________
Dates of Implantation: ____________

I. Before Insertion of Radioactive Sources into the Patient

1. Preliminary written directive signed and on file (radioisotope, number of sources, and source strengths). ____________ attending physician (initial and date)
2. Patient positively identified by two independent methods. ____________ resident physician (initial and date)
3. Verification that source preparation is in agreement with signed preliminary written directive. ____________ curator/resident physician (initial and date)
4. Position of sources within patient verified radiographically. ____________ attending physician (initial and date)

II. After Insertion but Prior to Completion of Treatment

5. Recording of actual source loading sequence in patient's chart. ____________ resident physician (initial and date)
6. Final written directive signed and on file (radioisotope, treatments site, total source strength, and exposure time). ____________ attending physician (initial and date)
7. Check of dose calculations, computerized treatment plan, computations in the Daily Dose Record, and the planned implant duration. ____________ physicist (initial and date)
8. Daily physical inspection of implant position. ____________ physician (initial and date) ____________ physician (initial and date) ____________ physician (initial and date)

III. After Source Removal

9. Sources removed at the planned time (temporary implants). ____________ resident physician (initial and date)
10. Check that administered dose agrees with final written directive dose to within ± 10%*. ____________ attending physician (initial and date)

* If delivered dose differs from final written directive by more than ± 10% but less than or equal to ± 20%, this is a recordable event. Notify the physician and physics staff for the required action.

If delivered dose differs from final written directive by more than ± 20%, this is a misadministration. The physician and physics staff need to be notified immediately.

ATTENDING PHYSICIAN ADMINISTERING THERAPY (signature) ____________ DATE ____________

:sah(QMP Brachytherapy Checklist)

Figure 21.21. A checklist of tasks that need to be completed for every patient undergoing a brachytherapy application is a helpful tool to document that these tasks were performed and as a double check to ensure that nothing was overlooked.

if a patient has received 40 Gy external beam therapy and 80 hours of brachytherapy, the 25 cGy/hour isodose surface is chosen to calculate the reference volume:

$$60 \text{ Gy} - 40 \text{ Gy} = 20 \text{ Gy}$$

$$20 \text{ Gy } 80 \text{ hours} = 0.25 \text{ Gy/hr}$$

The 25 cGy/hour isodose surface is chosen.

The ICRU recommendation was an attempt to use the reference volume to further describe the brachytherapy application and shed light on the volume of tissue receiving a particular level of dose. Unfortunately, instead of being a helpful concept, it has only caused confusion and criticism and has been helpful neither for specification nor for reporting (24).

The ICRU report 38 specifies a variety of points and volumes that can be reported but it does not address the question of dose prescription (implant duration). It simply gives recommendations for reporting doses, not prescribing them. The prescription of dose needs to be considered in the framework of the particular implant system being used.

University of Minnesota Dose Specification Guidelines. At the University of Minnesota, we rely heavily on the Fletcher mg-hr dose specification system (Table 21.5) (19). When mg-hrs are inappropriate (protruding vaginal source, vaginal cylinder) point calculations (A_V, or vaginal surface dose) are used. The ICRU points are calculated for all patients, but are not routinely used to specify dose. We find them useful as a double check to assure ourselves that both an adequate tumor dose has been achieved (remembering that point A may have little relationship to the tumor) and that bladder or rectal tolerances have not been exceeded (remembering that a point dose to the rectum

Table 21.5. Treatment of Carcinoma of the Cervix

	Whole Pelvis EBT Dose cGy[a]	Maximum mg/hr in Two Implants[b]	Additional Split Pelvis Radiation
Microinvasive (rarely referred for radiation therapy)	—	10,000	No
Small tumor, no or minimal extracervical extent	2,500–3,500	6,000–7,000	Yes—to bring point "B" up to 5,000–5,500 cGy
Moderate size tumor, definite parametrial extension	3,000–4,000	5,500–6,000	Yes—to bring point "B" up to 6,000 cGy
Large, bulky tumor with or without hydronephrosis	3,500–4,500	5,000–5,500[c]	Yes—to bring point "B" up to 6,000 cGy

[a] Periaortic nodes included if the primary tumor is bulky, or stage II or III, or in surgically staged patients if there is known paraortic spread.
[b] Tandem and ovoid applications 2 weeks apart. Does not take into account 1.07 filtration factor correction factor.
[c] Consider iridium/cesium application if minimal shrinkage at time of first implant.

or bladder provides no information about the dose the rest of the rectum or bladder received).

One of the more difficult aspects of treating cervical cancer is to determine how much pelvic external beam therapy to use relative to brachytherapy. The major advantage of brachytherapy is that a high dose is delivered within a few centimeters of the applicators, and relatively little dose is given a few centimeters away. With brachytherapy the "epicenter" of the cervical tumor receives very high doses, and when possible, the benefit of this high dose should be maximized. However, as the size and extent of a tumor increases, higher doses of whole pelvic EBRT need to be delivered in order to shrink the tumor down in size.

For the rare patient referred to the radiation department with microinvasive disease (FIGO IA), the tumor volume is small, and the risk of pelvic nodal spread is low. These patients can be treated with brachytherapy alone with doses up to 10,000 mg-hr in two applications. For other patients, EBRT is given in conjunction with brachytherapy.

Table 21.5 gives guidelines for external beam and brachytherapy doses. Notice that a range of external beam doses are given for each stage and tumor size. The actual doses are individualized for each patient. A common scenario is to have a patient with a 3-4 cm FIGO Stage IIB cervical tumor extending to the medial parametria. At the University of Minnesota the whole pelvis (and possibly the periaortic nodes, depending on the results of the surgical staging) would be treated to a dose of approximately 3500 cGy. Two brachytherapy applications would follow, 2 weeks apart for a total dose of up to 6500 mg-hrs. Additional split pelvis EBRT would be given to bring the total "Point B" dose to 6000 cGy.

The amount of split pelvis irradiation given depends on the contribution to "Point B" from the brachytherapy. In general, approximately 1500 cGy is given to Point B in two standard brachytherapy applications totaling 6500 mg-hrs (a rule of thumb is; 6500/4 = 1500). For patients with known positive pelvic lymph nodes or a high estimated risk of pelvic nodal spread (bulky FIGO Stage IB or II disease), split pelvic EBRT is given to bring "Point B" up to a total (EBT and BT) of 6000 cGy.

For tumors with significant vaginal involvement, the implantation volume should include the extent of disease in the vagina. Usually the EBRT leads to shrinkage of the vaginal involvement so that at the time of the first brachytherapy application there is little palpable tumor left. Often the previous tumor is replaced with vague induration. We usually use a vaginal cylinder if this induration is minimal (less than 0.5 cm thick). If there is more tumor than 0.5 cm of induration remaining, implanting the vaginal component of the tumor with iridium should be considered. Tolerance of the vaginal wall to high doses of radiation probably depends on the length of vagina treated as well as on the total dose and dose rate. In general, the vaginal apex tolerates more than the distal vagina, with the apex tolerating doses of 10,000 cGy or more. More distal portions of the vagina should probably not receive more than 7,000 to 8,000 cGy.

Many institutions prefer to specify dose to "Point A." Although we usually prescribe by mg-hrs, we also carry the "Point A_v" dose. We use the "Point A_v" dose column primarily to reassure ourselves that neither an excessive nor an inadequate dose to "Point A_v" has been delivered[25,26], keeping in mind that the "Point A_v" dose may have little relationship to the cervical tumor dose. In the setting of a protruding vaginal source (no colpostats), the rules for mg-hrs do not apply. We therefore prescribe to Point A_o in this situation.

For patients who have undergone a hysterectomy, the dose of external beam and brachytherapy needs to be individualized for each patient, type of hysterectomy performed, and the surgical-pathological findings (Table 21.6). If gross disease remains, interstitial therapy is usually given. For microscopic residual, intracavitary therapy is considered. The risk of bowel and bladder complications is high in this setting (27–30), and care must be taken to minimize the risk of a late radiation complication as much as possible.

Dose to Bladder and Rectum. The ICRU suggests a method to choose which point to calculate the rectal and bladder dose. These point doses may have little relationship to the dose received by other parts of the bladder or

Table 21.6. Post-Hysterectomy Dose Guidelines

	Dose (cGy)	
Situation	External Beam Therapy[a]	Brachytherapy
At risk for pelvic recurrence	4,500–5,000	None
At risk for vaginal recurrence	None	8–10,000 VSD (6,500–7,500 to 0.5 cm depth)
At risk for both pelvic and vaginal recurrence	4,500–5,000	4–5,000 VSD (2,500–3,500 to 0.5 cm depth)

[a] 175–200 cGy/day, volume treated individualized to the clinical and histopathological findings at the time of hysterectomy.
VSD, vaginal surface dose.

rectum and may not be the highest dose area. The localization of the bladder and rectum can be achieved by either placing hypaque in a Foley catheter which has been placed in the bladder or rectum, or by the use of rectally inserted ionization chambers. This method, however, is probably no more reliable than the point calculation method.

Generally, the bladder can tolerate more radiation than the rectum. No absolute point dose limit can be set, but it is preferable to keep the bladder point dose below 8,000 cGy and the rectal point dose below 7,000 cGy. Therefore, it is optimal if the rectal dose rate is lower than the bladder dose rate for the brachytherapy application. Additionally, it is also desirable for the dose rate to the bladder point to be 0.8 or less that of the dose rate to point A.

Patient Care During the Implant

At the University of Minnesota, following insertion of the applicator, patients are monitored in the recovery room, then transported to the radiation therapy department where orthogonal pair of simulator films are taken. The patient is then transported to her hospital room. The sources are subsequently loaded either manually or by remote afterloading techniques. Adequate analgesia while the applicator is in place is crucial. We usually order oral narcotics for patients with colpostats or cylinders and parenteral narcotics for patients with intrauterine tandems. Since the prolonged bed rest is stressful, benzodiazepines are given as needed to help sedate patients. The anesthesia sometimes causes nausea postoperatively and antiemetics are routinely prescribed. For the duration of the implant, the subcutaneous heparin is continued and the sequential pneumatic stockings used. Daily inspection of the brachytherapy appliance should be performed to assure that it has not dislodged.

It is important that good nursing care continue despite the presence of the radioactivity. To accomplish this, nurses need to be educated about the level of radiation they are exposed to in the patient's room and how to keep that exposure to within acceptable limits. Patients containing radioactive sources should receive the same medical monitoring as any other hospitalized patients, especially since these patients feel isolated during the brachytherapy application.

Despite careful attention to the care of these patients in the operating room and afterwards while the sources are in place, up to 7% of patients will have life threatening complications (31). In the event of a medical emergency during the implant, emergency care can be administered with the sources in the patient. The emergency care team should follow the proper precautions and maximize their distance from and minimize their time near the patient. At the University of Minnesota, film badges are distributed in a medical emergency to document the exposure to emergency personnel. If CPR is necessary, the person giving chest compressions is alternated at 10-minute intervals. The radiation oncologist should be called immediately and informed of the nature of the emergency, then he or she can decide if it is necessary to remove the radioactive sources. The radiation protection officer for the hospital should also be called.

Implant Removal

Prior to implant removal, patients are premedicated with either oral or parenteral narcotics. We also make use of intravenous short acting benzodiazepines (for example midazolam [Versed; Roche Laboratories, Nutley, NJ]) which are anxiolytic and often cause a retrograde amnesia for the removal.

At the scheduled removal time, the cesium sources are removed, returned to their lead pigs that are put into a lead lined cart, and transported back to the radiation oncology department for storage in the radioisotope safe. After the cesium has been removed, the afterloading appliance may be removed from the patient. For a cylinder, this merely involves cutting the sutures holding the cylinder ring to the perineum and gently pulling the cylinder free. For colpostats, the packing is removed, then the screw holding the colpostats together is removed and each colpostat individually withdrawn from the vagina. For patients with a tandem and ovoid application, the packing and ovoids are removed first, then the suture holding the tandem to the cervix is cut. The tandem then can be slipped out of the intrauterine canal.

Sequelae

Acute sequelae including diarrhea, cystitis, fatigue, and lowered peripheral blood counts are common, but usually resolve within weeks after treatment. Ovarian failure occurs in nearly all patients, unless ovarian transposition outside the pelvis has been performed (32,33). Shrinkage of the vagina can be minimized by daily use of a dilator during and after a course of radiation therapy.

The risk of developing a major complication depends on multiple factors. Patient related factors include the stage and extent of the disease, weight, age (34), smoking history (35), and number of previous abdominal surgical procedures (4,36,37). Treatment related factors include the volume of EBRT field treated, fraction size, the dose of EBRT, the brachytherapy used, and the technique of implantation used (38–44).

The Patterns of Care study reported that from 8 to 15% of patients treated for cervical cancer with definitive irradiation required hospitalization for a complication, half of which required a surgical intervention. Others have reported similar percentages. In a recent review of 1,784 patients treated at M.D. Anderson Hospital with FIGO Stage IB cervix cancer, the risk of a major complication was 9.3% at 5 years and 14.4% at 20 years (45). The most common gastrointestinal complications include proctitis, rectal ulceration, sigmoid stricture, or small bowel obstruction. Urinary complications include cystitis, or ureteral stricture. Rectovaginal or vesicovaginal fistulas are uncommon.

Table 21.7. Five-Year Disease-Free Survival Rates Reported for Carcinoma of the Cervix

Author (reference)	Total Number of Patients	Stage IB	IIA	IIB	III	IVA
Perez (62)	970	85	70	68	45	—
Pettersson (63)	32,428	78	—	—	57	8
Coia (37)	565	74	—	56	33	—
Horiot (51)	1,383	9	85	75	50	20
Montana (56,64)	533	83	76	62	33	—
Potish (65)	153	67	71	70	—	—
Leibel (53)	119	—	—	—	—	—
Gerbaulet (46)	441	89	78	—	—	—
Kramer (66)	48	—	—	—	—	18
Mendenhall (48)	264	70[a]	71	70[a]	—	—
		68[b]	—	43[b]	—	—
Kim (52)	569	82	78	65	48	27
Thoms[c] (67)	371	56[b]	49[b]	53[b]	—	—
Willin (47)	168	88	77	68	—	—

[a] <6 cm.
[b] >6 cm.
[c] 5-year survival.

Table 21.8. Percentage of In-Field Failure Reported for Patients with Carcinoma of the Cervix

Author (reference)	FIGO Stage I	II	III	IV
Coia (37)	12	27	51	
Kim (52)	11.2	8.2 (IIA) 30 (IIB)	52	69
Horiot (51)	8	12 (IIA) 20 (IIB)	37 (IIIA) 43 (IIIB)	82
Montana (56,64)	11	16 (IIA) 34 (IIB)	61 (IIIA) 47 (IIIB)	

Results

The Patterns of Care Study reported 4-year disease-free survivals of 87%, 66%, and 28% for FIGO stage I, II, and III, respectively (37). Results from other individual institutions are shown in Table 21.7. Although results are often reported by FIGO stage, other prognostic factors such as tumor volume or extent of nodal spread may be more important prognosticators of outcome, not currently reflected in the clinical staging system of FIGO. Patients with FIGO Stage IA or small IB disease have an excellent prognosis with 5-year disease-free survival estimates from 80% to 100% (39,46–49). For larger IB lesions, 5-year disease-free survival estimates range from 75 to 90%. Stage IIB disease-free survival results range from 60 to 75 % (50,51) and for IIIB, the 5-year disease-free survival rates drop to 30 to 50% (52,53).

The in-field failure rate increases with increasing initial FIGO stage (Table 21.8). For Stage I patients an in-field recurrence rate of 5 to 9 % has been reported (38,52,54–57). For Stage II patients the in-field recurrences range between 10 to 23%, and for Stage III patients up to a 61% in-field recurrence rate has been reported.

Quality Management Program

A quality management program (QMP) is crucial to the safe functioning of a brachytherapy program (58). This cannot be accomplished without a dedicated physics support. The various components of a QMP may be found in the AAPM Task Group 40 Report (59). However, several issues relative to intracavitary cesium applications deserve emphasis. To assure accurate preparation of the sources that are to be loaded into the patient, a series of double checks should be in place. We use color-coded cesium sources and check each source in a well-ionization chamber. Two people must prepare the sources to double check each other. Sources must be logged in and out of the de-

Table 21.9. Quality Assurance Tests for Intracavitary Brachytherapy Applicators: Frequency of Performance and Acceptable Tolerance Limits

Test	Frequency	Tolerance
Source location	I, Y	D
Coincidence of dummy and active sources	I	1 mm
Location of shields	I, Y[a]	D

I, initial use or following malfunction and repairs; Y, yearly; D, documented and correction applied or noted in report of measurement when appropriate.
[a] Before each use the applicator may be shaken to listen for loose parts [59].

partment (along with a visual count of the remaining sources left in the cesium safe) and all sources leaving the isotope room are always accompanied by a cesium transport card (Figure 21.16a). Regulations mandated by the Nuclear Regulatory Commission are followed. We have found it helpful to have a checklist to ensure compliance with these regulations with every brachytherapy application (Figure 21.21).

Quality assurance (QA) tests for the brachytherapy applicators need to be performed intermittently. A rattling noise when the ovoids are gently shook suggests that the rectal or bladder shields have dislodged and the applicator should be radiographed immediately to verify this. Reports of tandem tips coming off while implanted and remaining within the uterine cavity make it prudent to check the integrity of the tandem tip with each insertion. The AAPM Task Group 40 recommended QA procedures for brachytherapy applicators (59) are outlined in Table 21.9. In addition to these tests, we radiograph the applicators yearly to confirm correct position of the shields.

CONCLUSION

In early stages, cancer of the uterine cervix is highly curable with either surgery or radiation therapy. As the tumor advances, however, the best chance of cure is with aggressive, definitive radiation therapy consisting of a combination of external beam treatments and brachytherapy applications. Both of the components are important, however, it is probably the skilled use of intracavitary brachytherapy that is the most crucial to a successful outcome. This skill is achieved through experience as well as meticulous attention to the details of the treatment outlined here.

References

1. Nag S, Abitbol AA, Anderson LL, et al. Consensus guidelines for high dose rate remote brachytherapy in cervical, endometrial, and endobronchial tumors. Clinical Research Committee, American Endocurietherapy Society. Int J Radiat Oncol Biol Phys 1993;27:1241–1244.
2. Sarkaria JN, Petereit DG, Stitt JA, et al. A comparison of the efficacy and complication rates of low dose-rate versus high dose-rate brachytherapy in the treatment of uterine cervical carcinoma. Int J Radiat Oncol Biol Phys 1994;30:75–82.
3. Brenner DJ, Huang Y, Hall EJ. Fractionated high dose-rate versus low dose-rate regimens for intracavitary brachytherapy of the cervix: equivalent regimens for combined brachytherapy and external irradiation. [Review]. Int J Radiat Oncol Biol Phys 1991;21:1415–1423.
4. LaPolla JP, Schlaerth JB, Gaddis O, et al. The influence of surgical staging on the evaluation and treatment of patients with cervical carcinoma. Gyn Oncol 1986;24:194–206.
5. Heaps JM, Berek JS. Surgical staging of cervical cancer. [Review]. Clin Obstet Gynecol 1990;33:852–862.
6. Paterson R, Russell MH. Clinical trials in malignant disease. VI. Cancer of the cervix uteri: is x-ray therapy more effective given before or after radium? Clin Radiol 1962;13:313–315.
7. Maracial LV, Marcial JM, Krall JM, et al. Comparison of 1 vs 2 or more intracavitary brachytherapy applications in the management of carcinoma of the cervix with irradiation alone. Int J Radiat Oncol Biol Phys 1991;20:81–85.
8. Podczaski E, Stryker JA, Kaminski P, et al. Extended-field radiation therapy for carcinoma of the cervix. Cancer 1990;66:251–258.
9. Potish RA, Twiggs LB, Adcock LL, et al. The utility and limitations of decision theory in the utilization of surgical staging and extended field radiotherapy in cervical cancer. Obstet Gynecol 1984;39: 555–559.
10. Rubin SC, Brookland R, Mikuta JJ, et al. Para-aortic nodal metastases in early cervical carcinoma: long-term survival following extended-field radiotherapy. Gyn Oncol 1984;18:213–217.
11. Nori D, Valentine E, Hilaris BS. The role of paraaortic node irradiation in the treatment of cancer of the cervix. Int J Radiat Oncol Biol Phys 1985;11:1469–1473.
12. Rotman M, Pajak TF, Choi K, et al. Prophylactic extended field irradiation of para-aortic lymph nodes in stages IIB and bulky IB and IIIa cervical carcinomas: ten year treatment results of RTOG 79-20. JAMA 1995;274:387–393.
13. Haie C, Pejovic MJ, Gerbaulet A. Is prophylactic para-aortic irradiation worthwhile in the treatment of advanced cervical carcinoma? Radiother Oncol 1988;11:101–102.
14. Rotman M, Choi K, Guse C, et al. Prophylactic irradiation of the para-aortic lymph node chain in stage IIB and bulky stage IB carcinoma of the cervix, initial treatment results of RTOG 7920 [published erratum appears in Int J Radiat Oncol Biol Phys 1991 Jan;(1):193]. Int J Radiat Oncol Biol Phys 1990;19:513–521.
15. Haas JS, Dean RD, Mansfield CM. Dosimetric comparison of the Fletcher family of gynecologic colpostats 1950–1980. Int J Radiat Oncol Biol Phys 1985;11:1317–1321.
16. Sharma SC, Williamson JF, Khan FM, et al. Dosimetric consequences of asymmetric positioning of active source in Cs 137 and Ra 226 intracavitary tubes. Int J Radiat Oncol Biol Phys 1981;7:555–559.
17. Kuske RR, Perez CA, Jacobs AJ, et al. Mini-colpostats in the treatment of carcinoma of the uterine cervix. Int J Radiat Oncol Biol Phys 1988; 14:899–906.
18. Paris KJ, Spanos WJ, Day TG, et al. Incidence of complications with mini-vaginal colpostats in carcinoma of the uterine cervix. Int J Radiat Oncol Biol Phys 1991;21:911–917.
19. Fletcher GH. Female pelvis: squamous cell carcinoma of the uterine cervix. In: Textbook of Radiotherapy. Saunders: London, 1973.
20. Potish RA, Gerbi BJ. Cervical cancer: intracavitary dose specification and prescription. Radiol 1987;165:555–560.
21. Esche BA, Crook JM, Isturiz J, et al. Reference volume, milligram-hours and external irradiation for the Fletcher applicator. Radiother Oncol 1987;9:255–261.
22. Potish RA, Diebel RC, Khan FM. The relationship between milligram-hours and dose to point A in carcinoma of the cervix. Radiol 1982; 145:479.
23. Wilkinson JM, Ramachandran TP. The ICRU recommendations for reporting intracavitary therapy in gynaecology and the Manchester method of treating cancer of the cervix uteri. Brit J Radiol 1989;62: 362–365.
24. Potish RA, Gerbi B. Role of point A in the era of computerized dosimetry. Radiol 1986;158.
25. Perez CA, Breaux S, Madic-Jones H, et al. Radiation therapy alone

in the treatment of carcinoma of the uterine cervix. Cancer 1983;51: 1393–1402.
26. Lanciano RM, Martz K, Coia LR, Hanks GE. Tumor and treatment factors improving outcome in stage IIIB cervix cancer. Int J Radiat Oncol Biol Phys 1991;20:95–100.
27. Jacobs AJ, Perez CA, Camel HM, et al. Complications in patients receiving both irradiation and radical hysterectomy for carcinoma of the uterine cervix. Gynecol Oncol 1985;22:273–280.
28. Perez CA, Kao MS. Radiation therapy alone or combined with surgery in the treatment of barrel-shaped carcinoma of the uterine cervix (stages IB, IIA, IIB). Int J Radiat Oncol Biol Phys 1985;11:1903–9.
29. Kim RY, Salter MM, Shingleton HM. Adjuvant postoperative radiation therapy following radical hysterectomy in stage IB CA of the cervix—analysis of treatment failure. Int J Radiat Oncol Biol Phys 1988; 14:445–449.
30. Farquharson DI, Shingleton HM, Soong SJ, et al. The adverse effects of cervical cancer treatment on bladder function. Gynecol Oncol 1987;27:15–23.
31. Dusenbery KD, Carson LF, Potish RA. Perioperative morbidity and mortality of gynecologic brachytherapy. Cancer 1991;67:2786–2790.
32. Husseinzadeh N, Nahhas WA, Velkley DE, et al. The preservation of ovarian function in young women undergoing pelvic radiation therapy. Gynecol Oncol 1984;18:373–379.
33. Belinson JL, Doherty M, McDay JB. A new technique for ovarian transposition. Surg Gynecol Obstet 1984;159:157–160.
34. Kucera H, Genger H, Wagner G, et al. Prognosis of primary radiotherapy of cervix cancer in younger females. German. Geburtshilfe und Frauenheilkunde, 1986;46:800–803.
35. Kucera H, Enzelsberger H, Eppel W, et al. The influence of nicotine abuse and diabetes mellitus on the results of primary irradiation in the treatment of carcinoma of the cervix. Cancer 1987;60:1–4.
36. Potish RA, Twiggs LB. An analysis of adjuvant treatment strategies for carcinoma of the cervix. Am J Clin Oncol 1989;12:430–433.
37. Coia L, Won M, Lanciano R, et al. The Patterns of Care Outcome Study for cancer of the uterine cervix. Results of the Second National Practice Survey. Cancer 1990;66:2451–2456.
38. Montana GS, Fowler WC. Carcinoma of the cervix: analysis of bladder and rectal radiation dose and complications. Int J Radiat Oncol Biol Phys 1989;16:95–100.
39. Perez CA, Breaux S, Bedwinek JM, et al: Radiation therapy alone in the treatment of carcinoma of the uterine cervix. II. Analysis of complications. Cancer 1984;54:235–246.
40. Pourquier H, Delard R, Achille E, et al. A quantified approach to the analysis and prevention of urinary complications in radiotherapeutic treatment of cancer of the cervix. Int J Radiat Oncol Biol Phys 1987; 13:1025–1033.
41. Hanks GE, Herring DF, Kramer S. Patterns of care outcome studies. Cancer 1983;51:959–967.
42. Deore SM, Shrivastava K, Viswanthan PS, Dinshaw KA. The severity of late rectal and recto-sigmoid complications related to fraction size in irradiation treatment of carcinoma cervix stage IIIB. Strahlenther Onkol 1991;167:638–642.
43. Unal A, Hamberger A, Seski J, et al. An analysis of the severe complications of irradiation of carcinoma of the uterine cervix: treatment with intracavitary radium and parametrial irradiation. Int J Radiat Oncol Biol Phys 1981;7:999–1004.
44. Crook JM, Esche BA, Chaplain G, et al. Dose-volume analysis and the prevention of radiation sequelae in cervical cancer. Radiother Oncol 1987;8:321–332.
45. Eifel PJ, Levenback C, Wharton T, et al. Time course and incidence of late complications in patients treated with radiation therapy for FIGO Stage IB carcinoma of the uterine cervix. Int J Radiat Oncol Biol Phys 1995;32:1289–1300.
46. Gerbaulet AL, Kunkler IH, Kerr GR, et al. Combined radiotherapy and surgery: local control and complications in early carcinoma of the uterine cervix—the Villejuif experience, 1975-1984. [Review]. Radiother Oncol 1992;23:66–73.
47. Willen H, Eklund G, Johnsson JE, et al. Invasive squamous cell carcinoma of the uterine cervix. VIII. Survival and malignancy grading in patients treated by irradiation in Lund 1969-1970. Acta Radiologica Oncology 1985;24:41–50.
48. Mendenhall WM, Thar TL, Bova FJ, et al. Prognostic and treatment factors affecting pelvic control of Stage IB and IIA-B carcinoma of the intact uterine cervix treated with radiation therapy alone. Cancer 1984;53:2649–2654.
49. Montana GS, Fowler WC, Varia MA, et al. Analysis of results of radiation therapy for stage IB carcinoma of the cervix. Cancer 1987;60: 2195–2200.
50. Montana GS, Fowler WC, Varia MA, et al. Analysis of results of radiation therapy for Stage II carcinoma of the cervix. Cancer 1985;55: 956–962.
51. Horiot JC, Pigneux J, Pourquier H, et al. Radiotherapy alone in carcinoma of the intact uterine cervix according to G. H. Fletcher guidelines: a French cooperative study of 1383 cases. [Review]. Int J Radiat Oncol Biol Phys 1988;14:605–611.
52. Kim RY, Trotti A, Wu CJ, et al. Radiation alone in the treatment of cancer of the uterine cervix: analysis of pelvic failure and dose response relationship. Int J Radiat Oncol Biol Phys 1989;17:973–978.
53. Leibel S, Bauer M, Wasserman T, et al. Radiotherapy with or without misonidazole for patients with stage IIIB or stage IVA squamous cell carcinoma of the uterine cervix: preliminary report of a Radiation Therapy Oncology Group randomized trial. Int J Radiat Oncol Biol Phys 1987;13:541–549.
54. Adcock LL, Potish RA, Julian TM, et al. Carcinoma of the cervix, FIGO Stage IB: treatment failures. Gynecol Oncol 1984;18:218–225.
55. Eifel PJ, Morris M, Oswald MJ, et al. Adenocarcinoma of the uterine cervix. Prognosis and patterns of failure in 367 cases. Cancer 1990; 65:2507–2514.
56. Montana GS, Martz K, Hanks G. Patterns and sites of failure in cervix cancer treated in the USA in 1978. Int J Radiat Oncol Biol Phys 1991; 20:87–93.
57. Sommers GM, Grigsby PW, Perez CA, et al. Outcome of recurrent cervical carcinoma following definitive irradiation. Gynecol Oncol 1989;35:150–155.
58. Dawson J, Roy T, Abrath F, et al. Comprehensive quality management program for radiation oncology. Radiother Oncol 1994;31:187–188.
59. Kutcher GJ, Coia L, Gillin M, et al. Comprehensive QA for radiation oncology: report of AAPM radiation therapy committee task group 40. Medical Physics 1994;21:581–607.
60. Joslin CA. A place for high dose rate brachytherapy in gynaecological oncology: fact or fiction. Activity Selectron Brachytherapy Journal 1991;suppl 2:3–4.
61. Johnson JM, Potish RA. The provision of a uniform vaginal surface dose rate by a novel afterloading vaginal cylinder. Medical Dosimetry 1991;16:193–198.
62. Perez CA, Camel HM, Kuske RR, et al. Radiation therapy alone in the treatment of carcinoma of the uterine cervix: A 20-year experience. Gynec Oncol 1986;23:127–140.
63. Pettersson F, ed. The 19th FIGO Annual Report on the results of treatment in Gynecological Cancer. Stockholm, Sweden: Radiumhemme, 1985, S-10401.
64. Montana GS, Fowler WC, Varia MA, et al. Carcinoma of the cervix stage III: results of radiation therapy. Cancer 1986;1:148–154.
65. Potish RA, Downey GO, Adcock LL, Prem KA, Twiggs LB. The role of surgical debulking in cancer of the uterine cervix. Int J Radiat Oncol Biol Phys 1989;17:979–984.
66. Kramer C, Peschel RE, Goldberg N, et al. Radiation treatment of FIGO stage IVA carcinoma of the cervix. Gynec Oncol 1989;32:323–326.
67. Thoms W, Eifel P, Smith L, et al. Bulky endocervical carcinomas: a 23 year experience. Int J Radiat Oncol Biol Phys 1992;23:491–499.
68. Montana GS, Fowler WC Jr, Varia MA, et al. Carcinoma of the cervix stage IB: Results of treatment with radiation therapy. Int J Radiat Oncol Biol Phys 1983;9:45–49.

Chapter 22

Technical Aspects of Radiation Therapy for Endometrial Carcinoma

Perry W. Grigsby and K. S. Clifford Chao

Carcinoma of the endometrium is currently the most common invasive gynecologic cancer in the United States. More than 30,000 new cases will be diagnosed this year. Appropriate determination of stage or extent of disease at the time of diagnosis is of critical importance in the management of endometrial carcinoma, since both treatment and prognosis are strongly dependent on stage. Staging for endometrial cancer is determined by surgical and pathologic findings. The need for radiotherapy is based on tumor grade, myometrial invasion, and spread of disease beyond the uterus.

After a preoperative workup that usually includes routine blood work, chest x-ray, and EKG, the patient with endometrial cancer undergoes an exploratory laparotomy with hysterectomy and staging to determine the extent of disease. The excised uterus is examined to determine the extent of the tumor. Surgical removal of the lymph nodes may be performed based on the tumor characteristics. In certain circumstances, the lymph node sampling may be omitted based on other medical conditions or undue risk to the patient. These data provide the basis for selection of postoperative radiation therapy.

After surgery, further treatment with radiation may be indicated based on surgical-pathological staging information. The radiotherapy may be given locally in the vagina, to the pelvis, or to the abdomen. Local radiation to the vagina may be performed as an inpatient using a low dose rate delivery system or as an outpatient using a high dose rate delivery system. Pelvic irradiation is given with external beam or vaginal brachytherapy or both. Radiation therapy to the abdomen can be administered with external radiotherapy or with intraperitoneal P-32.

For occasional patients with serious medical conditions, radiation therapy is used as an alternative to surgery. Severe cardiopulmonary disease and morbid obesity are the primary reasons a patient with endometrial carcinoma does not undergo surgery. Patients not undergoing surgery are clinically staged. Radiotherapy may be internal, external, or a combination, depending on tumor characteristics.

Preoperative intracavitary, external irradiation, or both are administered to some patients with high-grade lesions, or advanced stage disease. Radiation therapy is also used in treating patients with recurrent disease after surgery. Palliative radiation therapy is given to relieve symptoms.

The anatomy of the uterus and its draining lymphatics are shown in Figure 22.1. The anatomic distribution of the lymphatics forms the basis for the delivery of irradiation. Lymphatics from the body of the uterus may drain to the pelvic lymph nodes and subsequently to the para-aortic lymph nodes and upper abdomen. These lymphatics may also drain directly to the para-aortic lymph nodes and upper abdomen without coursing through the pelvic lymph nodes. The lymphatics from the lower uterine segment and cervix usually drain to the parametrial tissues and pelvic lymph nodes. Lymphatics from the cervix and upper vagina may also drain to the inguinal lymph nodes. The lymphatics of the distal vagina drain directly to the inguinal lymph nodes.

The purpose of this chapter is to discuss the technical aspects of external radiation therapy and brachytherapy for patients with endometrial cancer. The rationale for patient selection for treatment with these techniques is only discussed in general terms.

PREOPERATIVE IRRADIATION

Low Dose Rate (LDR)

Preoperative irradiation is less common today than in the past. It is still advocated for some patients such as

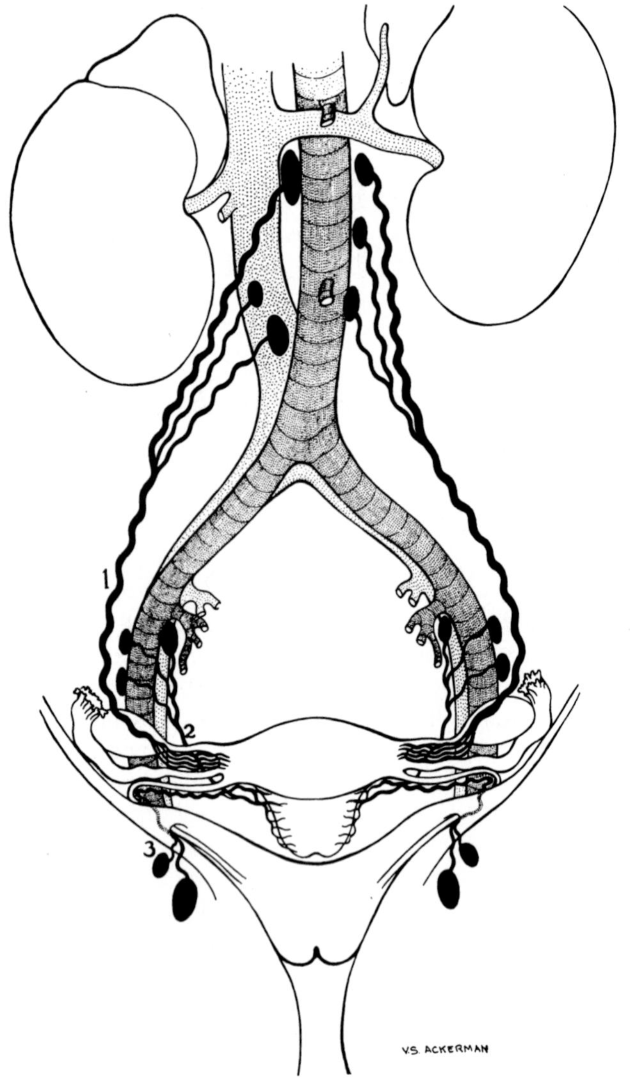

Figure 22.1. Uterine anatomy and lymphatic drainage. (Reprinted with permission from Ackerman LV and del Regato JA: Cancer—Diagnosis, Treatment, and Prognosis, 6th ed. St. Louis: Mosby-Year Book; 1985.)

those with high-grade lesions and Stage II disease. The preoperative implant is performed in the operating room utilizing afterloading applicators consisting of Simon-Heyman uterine capsules and Fletcher-Suit tandem and ovoids (Figure 22.2). Following an examination under anesthesia (EUA), dilation and curettage (D&C), cervical biopsies, and placement of an indwelling bladder catheter with 7cc of contrast material placed into the bulb of the catheter, the implant is placed into the uterus and vagina. Radiopaque markers are placed on the cervix at the 2 and 7 o'clock positions with absorbable suture. The Simon-Heyman capsules have diameters of 6, 8, and 10 mm. The capsules are numbered on their distal end and the order of capsule placement is recorded at the time of placement. Simon-Heyman capsules are placed through the cervical os into the uterine fundus to fill the body of the uterus with these capsules. Small capsules (i.e., 6 mm) are used for a small uterus with a sounding of 6 to 8 cm. Larger capsules (i.e., 8 to 10 mm) are used when the uterus is larger and sounds to 8 to 12 cm. The number of capsules placed into the uterus ranges from 4 to 20, depending upon the size of the uterus. The usual number of capsules that are placed into the fundus is 5 to 7 but in the large uterine cavity there may be as many as 16. The capsules are packed into the uterus in layers. The Fletcher-Suit tandem is then placed into the uterus such that the tip of the tandem abuts the lowest Simon-Heyman capsule. The tandem can be placed in the lower uterine segment to a depth of 4 to 8 cm with an average depth of placement of 6 cm. Fletcher-Suit ovoids are then placed into the vagina, the sizes of the ovoids being the largest that will fill the lateral fornices (usually 2 to 2.5 cm ovoids). The vagina is packed with Iodoform gauze soaked in a dilute solution of Hypaque contrast material (Figure 22.3A and 22.3B). It is usually not necessary to place a suture in the vulva to secure the implant in place since adequate vaginal packing serves this purpose. On occasion a suture is placed in the vulva to hold the implant in place when patients have severe chronic obstructive pulmonary disease (COPD) and cough during their hospitalization or when the patient has a severe cystocele, rectocele, or uterine prolapse.

The implant remains in place about 48 to 72 hours. During the implant, patients are placed on radiation precautions, given mild pain medication, given medication if they have nausea, and are given a low residue diet. Low-dose subcutaneous Heparin is administered for deep vein thrombosis (DVT) prophylaxis. The patient is encouraged to turn from side to side, the head of their bed is elevated as needed, and a footboard is utilized for leg exercises.

When the implant is removed, the patient receives mild pain medication about 30 minutes before removal. The radioactive sources are removed first and placed into storage. The implant removal procedure is performed in the examination room with the assistance of a nurse. Bleeding must be anticipated but rarely occurs. If a labial suture has been placed then it is removed first. The vaginal packing is then removed. This is followed by removal of the vaginal colpostats and intrauterine tandem. The Simon-Heyman capsules obviously need to be removed in reverse order of their placement, hence the importance of the numbering of the capsules at the time of their placement.

The radiation therapy prescription for a typical preoperative implant is shown in Table 22.1. This prescription is empirical and based upon the original method of Heyman with the addition of Fletcher-Suit tandem and ovoids. The Simon-Heyman capsules are loaded with 10 mgRaeq each. The tandem is loaded with three sources; 10 mgRaeq, 20 mgRaeq, and 10 mgRaeq. The purpose of inserting the 20 mgRaeq source in the tandem is to expand the isodose

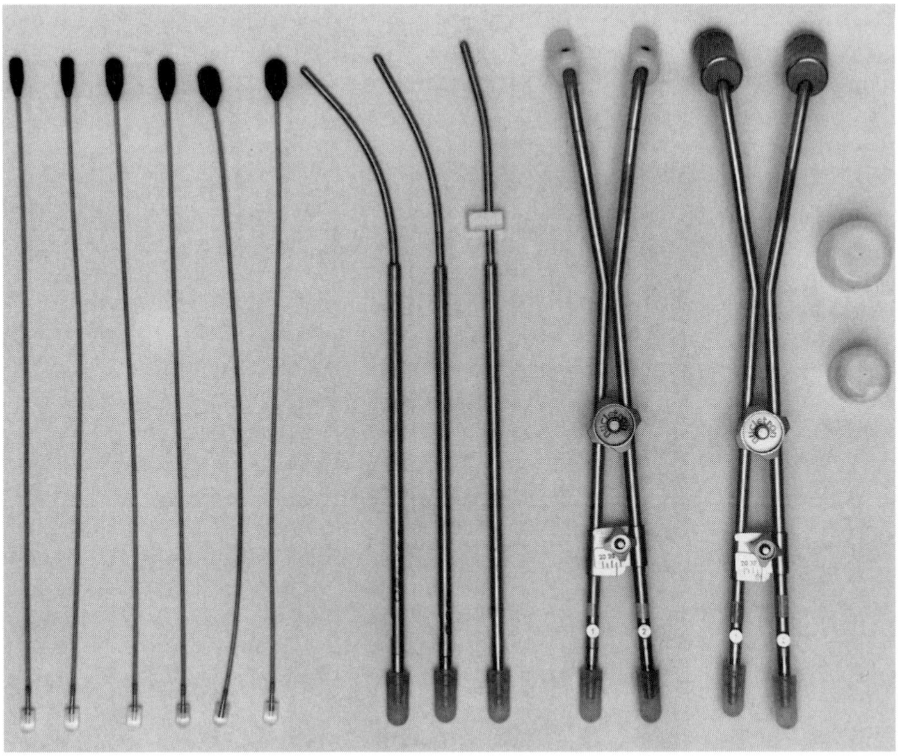

Figure 22.2. Fletcher-Suit afterloading tandems and colpostats and Simon-Heyman afterloading intrauterine capsules.

Table 22.1. Low Dose Rate Preoperative Implant Prescription

([a]6–10) × 10 mg
10 mg
20 mg
10 mg — 3500–4000 mg/hr
20 mg 20 mg — 6500 cGy SD

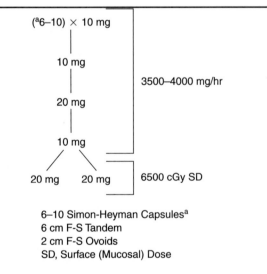

6–10 Simon-Heyman Capsules[a]
6 cm F-S Tandem
2 cm F-S Ovoids
SD, Surface (Mucosal) Dose

curves in the lower uterine segment. This avoids an "hourglass" isodose distribution. The isodose distribution from a preoperative implant is shown in Figures 22.3C and 22.3D. The procedure for calculating the isodose distribution and point doses are similar to that for cervical carcinoma treated with an intrauterine tandem and Fletcher-Suit colpostats. Point A is first located on the lateral radiograph by measuring from the center of the superior surface of the colpostat along the axis of the tandem. On the AP-PA radiograph, point A is 2 cm lateral to the center of the uterine canal that is defined as the center of the intrauterine tandem and the stems of the Simon-Heyman capsules. The center of the canal is the midpoint between the two tandems when two tandems are utilized. Points B and P are 5 and 6 cm lateral, respectively, to the midplane at the level of point A. The bladder reference point is determined as the closest point to the implant on the posterior surface of the urinary catheter balloon. The rectal reference point lays 5 mm posterior to the posterior vaginal wall mucosa at the level of the vaginal colpostats. Adjustments to the loading and prescription are made as a result of uterine and vaginal size, based upon applicator size, number and geometry (Appendix 1).

High Dose Rate (HDR)

The preoperative implant can be performed with HDR brachytherapy rather than LDR brachytherapy. The intrauterine portion of the HDR implant can consist of a tandem and Simon-Heyman capsules (as with LDR brachytherapy) as demonstrated in Figures 22.4A and 22.4B or, two tandems may be placed in the uterus rather than using Simon-Heyman capsules. The HDR preoperative implant is performed in the operating room utilizing the same procedure as for an LDR preoperative implant. The prescription for HDR brachytherapy also follows the same rules for radia-

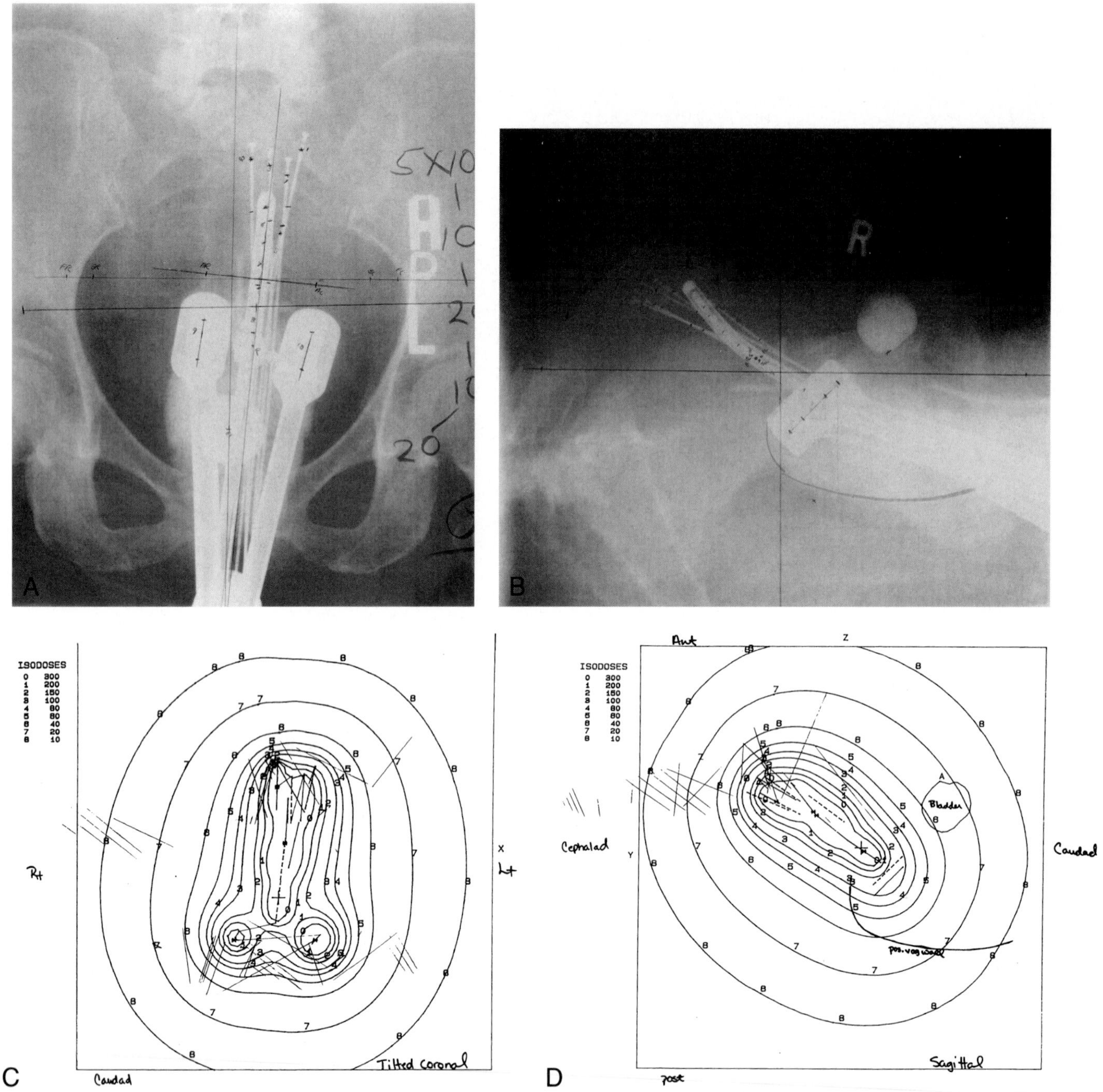

Figure 22.3. Manual afterloading, low dose rate preoperative implant with Simon-Heyman capsules and Fletcher-Suit tandem and ovoids. **A.** AP simulator radiograph; **B.** Lateral simulator radiograph; **C.** AP isodose curves; **D.** Lateral isodose curves.

tion distribution as with LDR brachytherapy. The relative proportions of radiation are maintained in the uterus and vagina. Implants are performed once a week, for 3 consecutive weeks for a total of 3,300 mghr (Table 22.2).

If the only preoperative irradiation that a patient receives is a preoperative implant as specified above, an extrafascial hysterectomy can be performed in 1 to 3 days after completion of the implant. Alternatively, if the extrafascial hysterectomy is not performed within 1 to 3 days, then moderate pelvic inflammation occurs from the irradiation and the hysterectomy must be delayed 4 to 6 weeks when the inflammation from the irradiation has subsided.

Selected patients with Stage I disease and all patients with clinical Stage II disease undergo a preoperative intracavitary implant as described above. Women with Stage II disease with ectocervical involvement also receive preop-

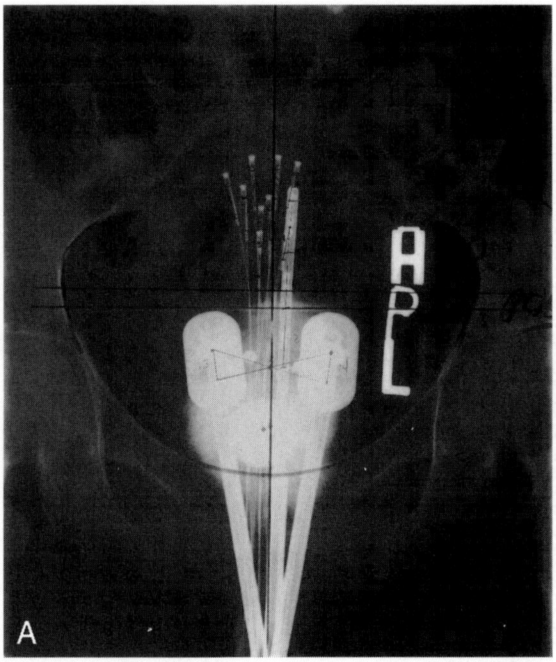

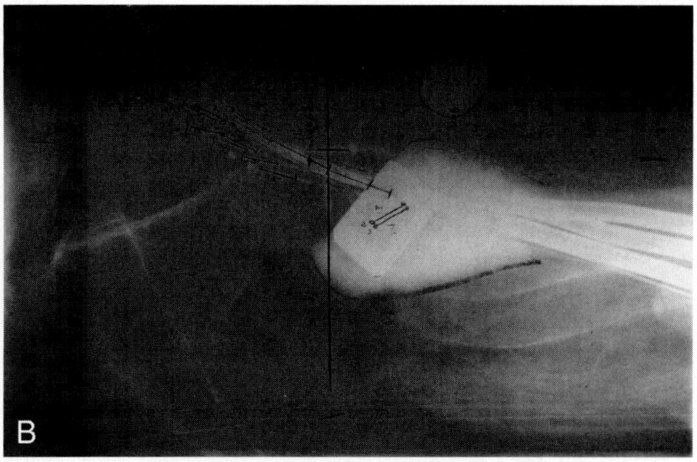

Figure 22.4. Remote afterloading, high dose rate preoperative implant with Simon-Heyman capsules and Fletcher tandem and ovoids. **A.** AP simulator radiograph; **B.** Lateral simulator radiograph.

Table 22.2. High Dose Rate Preoperative Implant Prescription

[a]6 × 10 mg 10 mg 20 mg 10 mg	700 mg/hr
20 mg 20 mg	400 mg/hr

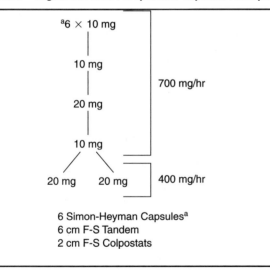

6 Simon-Heyman Capsules[a]
6 cm F-S Tandem
2 cm F-S Colpostats

erative external radiotherapy. Women with suspected or known Stage II disease will undergo an examination under anesthesia, a fractional D&C, cervical biopsies, and a preoperative intracavitary implant. With the results of the D&C and cervical biopsies, and the diagnosis of Stage II disease with ectocervical involvement established, these patients also receive preoperative external irradiation.

External Radiation Therapy

External pelvic irradiation is delivered with AP-PA and sometimes lateral portals and prescribed to the pelvis to a midplane pelvis dose of 50 Gy. Following a single preoperative intracavitary implant, external irradiation is administered with 20 Gy delivered to the whole pelvis (Figure 22.5A and 22.5B) and 30 Gy delivered with a midline step wedge in place to cover the high dose region of the preoperative intracavitary implant. The combined isodose curves from a single preoperative intracavitary implant as outlined in Figures 22.3C and 22.3D is administered in conjunction with postoperative pelvic radiation therapy with 20 Gy whole pelvis and 30 Gy split field is shown in Figure 22.6.

POSTOPERATIVE IRRADIATION

Low Dose Rate (LDR)

The most common application of radiation therapy for patients with endometrial carcinoma is with the use of postoperative irradiation. A postoperative vaginal cuff intracavitary implant is performed for those patients at high risk for failing in the vagina. The postoperative vaginal cuff implant can be performed with either LDR or HDR irradiation. When LDR irradiation is performed, the procedure is performed in the operating room. With the patient under a regional or general anesthetic, a pelvic EUA is performed. Biopsies are performed as indicated. A urinary drainage catheter is placed into the urinary bladder and the bulb of the catheter is filled with 7 cc of Hypaque contrast material. A radio-opaque marker is placed in the center of the suture line of the vaginal cuff with an absorbable suture. Fletcher-Suit afterloading colpostats are placed at the apex with a source-center to source-center separation of about 4 cm. This is most often accomplished

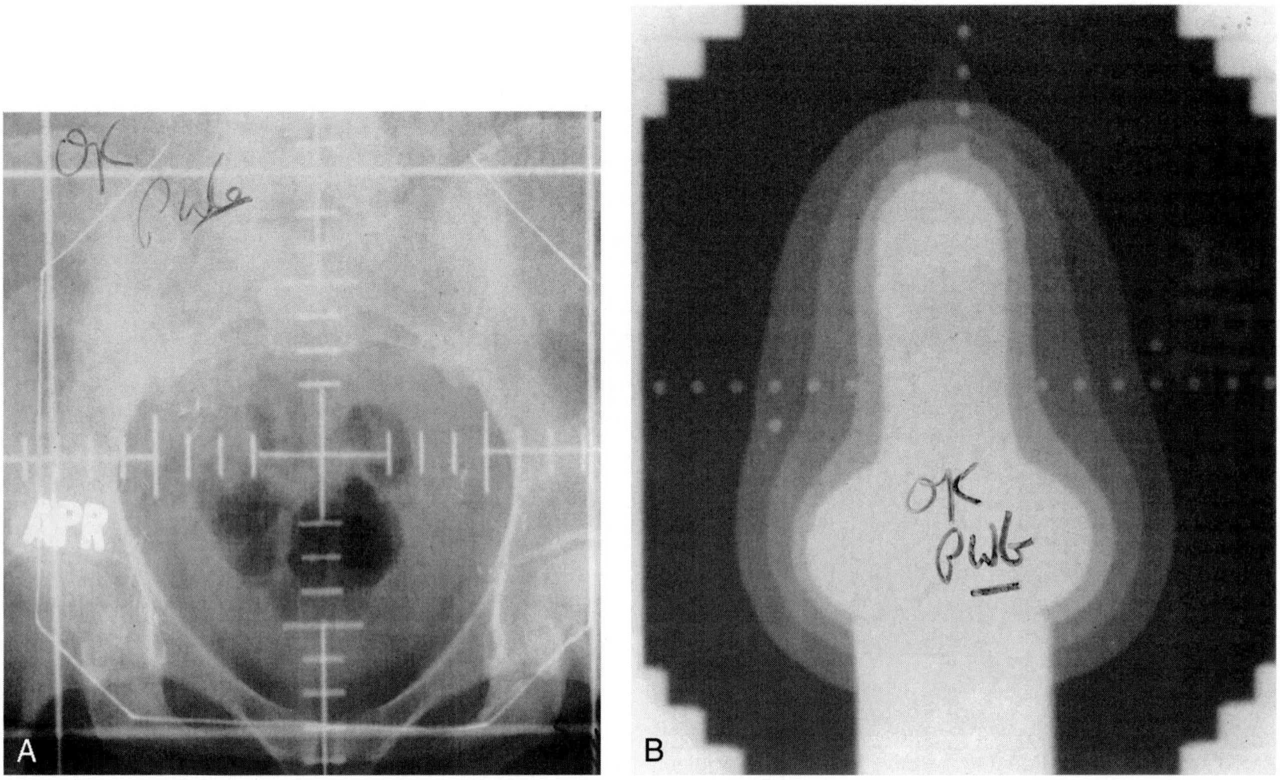

Figure 22.5. **A.** AP simulator radiograph of whole pelvis port; **B.** AP portal of 6A with midline step-wedge.

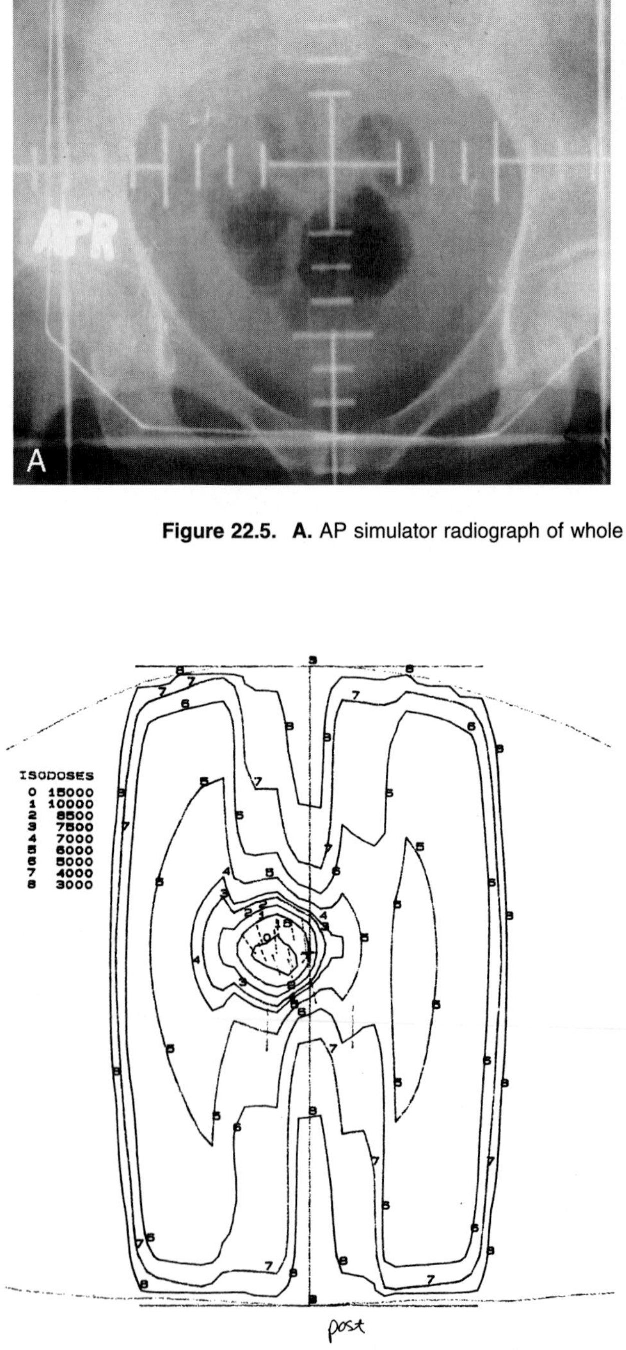

Figure 22.6. Transverse section of combined isodose curves from 20 Gy whole pelvis, 30 Gy split field, and a single preoperative intracavitary implant (5,500 mgh).

with 2 cm colpostats. Larger colpostats are used as indicated. Fletcher-Suit-Delclos mini-ovoids are used for the patient with a small vaginal apex. The vagina is packed with Iodoform gauze soaked in dilute Hypaque contrast material. The vaginal cuff colpostats adequately treat the upper one-third of the vaginal surface. An AP and lateral simulation radiographs of an ovoid cuff implant are shown in Figures 22.7A and 22.7B. Treatment of the entire vaginal length is rarely indicated. When the vaginal cuff is treated with colpostats, the usual prescription is 65 Gy to the surface of the vagina from a single colpostat source. The resultant isodose curves from two 2-cm colpostats are shown in Figures 22.7C and 22.7D. The procedure for calculating the isodose, the dose distributions, and point doses is the same as for the preoperative implant. When 65 Gy is prescribed to the vaginal surface from a single colpostat, the surface dose from the contribution of sources from both colpostats is about 70 Gy and the dose at 0.5 cm depth is about 30 Gy.

High Dose Rate (HDR)

Vaginal cuff implants can also be performed with HDR brachytherapy, which is usually delivered in three procedures at 1- or 2-week intervals. It is our practice to perform the first HDR implant in the operating room with the pa-

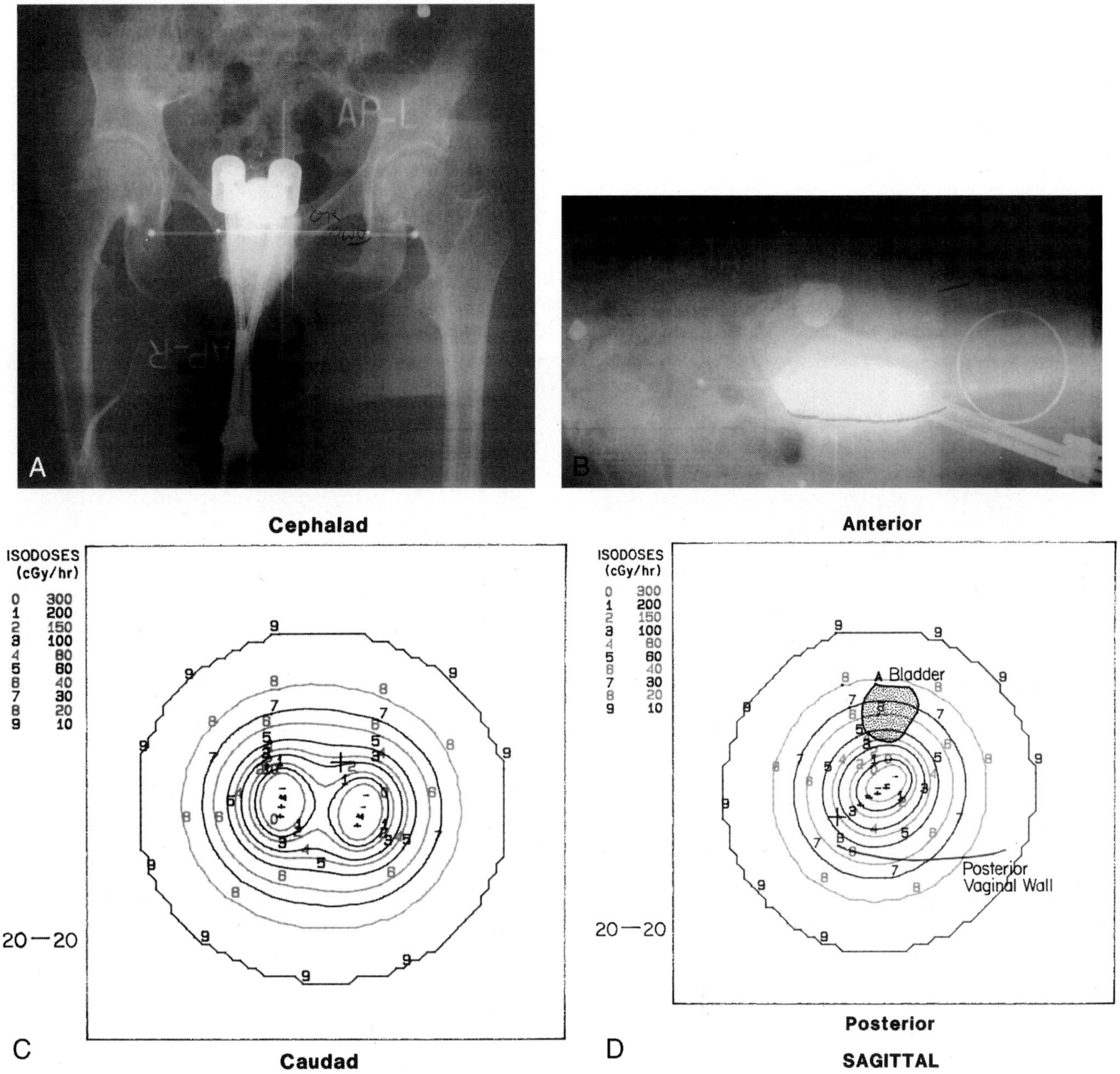

Figure 22.7. Manual afterloading, low dose rate, Fletcher-Suit colpostat vaginal cuff implant. **A.** AP simulator radiograph; **B.** Lateral simulator radiograph; **C.** AP isodose curves; **D.** Lateral isodose curves.

tient receiving regional or general anesthesia. An EUA and biopsies (if indicated) are performed. The vaginal cuff implant is performed with Fletcher-Suit HDR colpostats. The physical characteristics of the intracavitary implant are the same for HDR or LDR brachytherapy. A urinary catheter is placed in the bladder with 7 mL of contrast material placed in the bulb of the catheter. Radiopaque markers are placed at the vaginal apex and radiopaque packing is placed in the vagina. The prescription for HDR brachytherapy is, by convention, defined at a depth of 0.5 cm in tissue from the surface of the vaginal mucosa midway between the two ovoids and the surface dose is also calculated (Figure 22.8). An AP and lateral simulation radiograph of an HDR vaginal cuff implant are shown in Figures 22.9A and 22.9B and the resultant isodose curves are shown in Figures 22.9C and 22.9D. The vaginal packing and applicators are removed from the patient immediately after completion of the treatment.

Both LDR and HDR vaginal cuff brachytherapy can also be performed with standard vaginal cylinders or a domed vaginal cylinder. When a vaginal cylinder is utilized, only the upper one-third of the vagina is treated. The radiation

Figure 22.8. High dose rate prescription point for vaginal cuff colpostats.

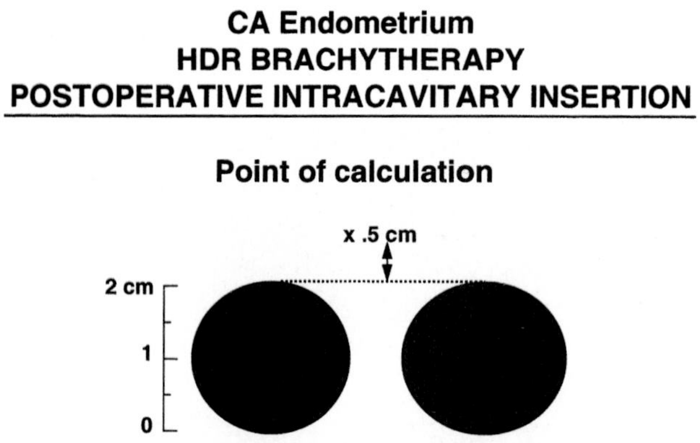

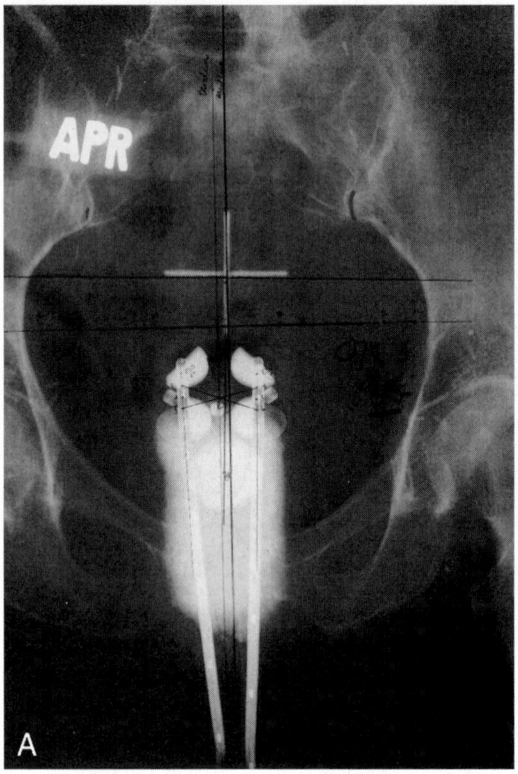

Figure 22.9. Remote afterloading, high dose rate, Fletcher-Suit colpostat vaginal cuff implant. A. AP simulator radiograph; B. Lateral simulator radiograph; C. AP isodose curves; D. Lateral isodose curves.

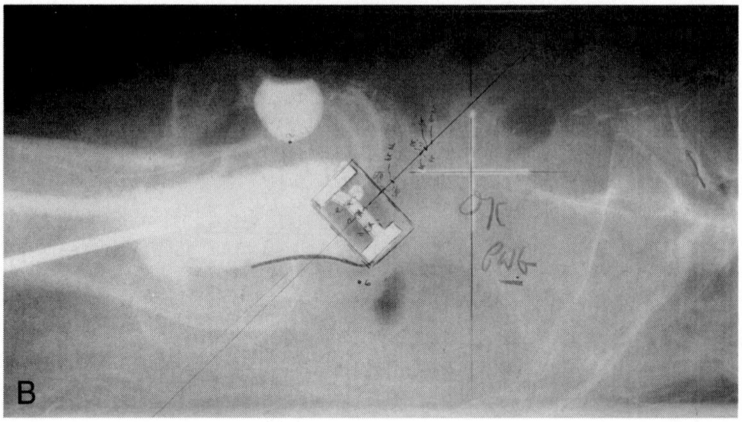

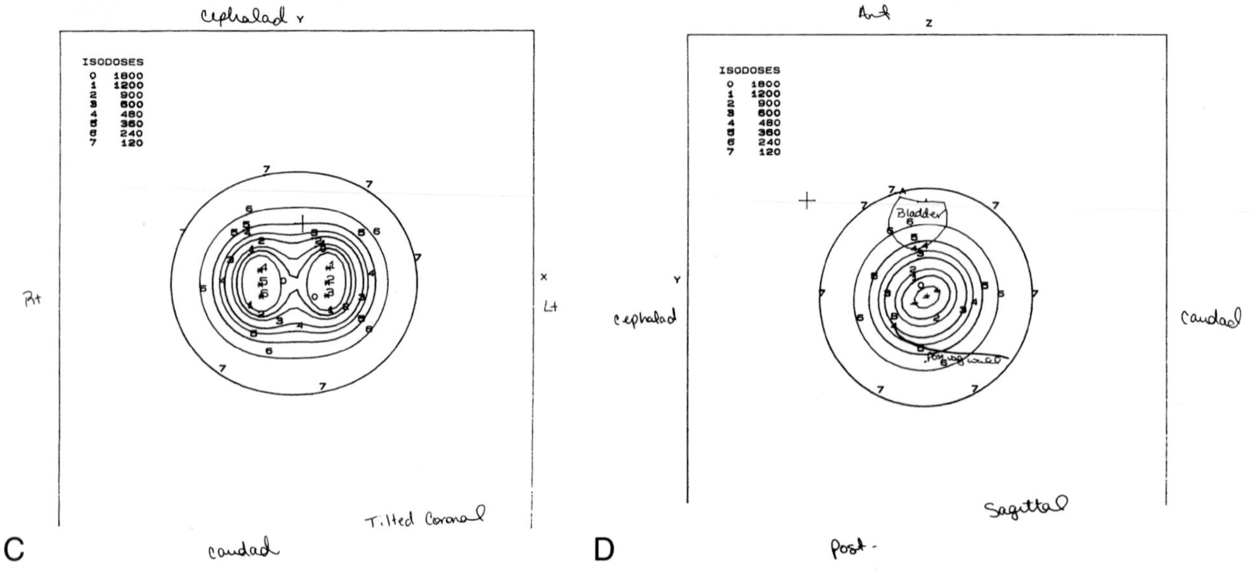

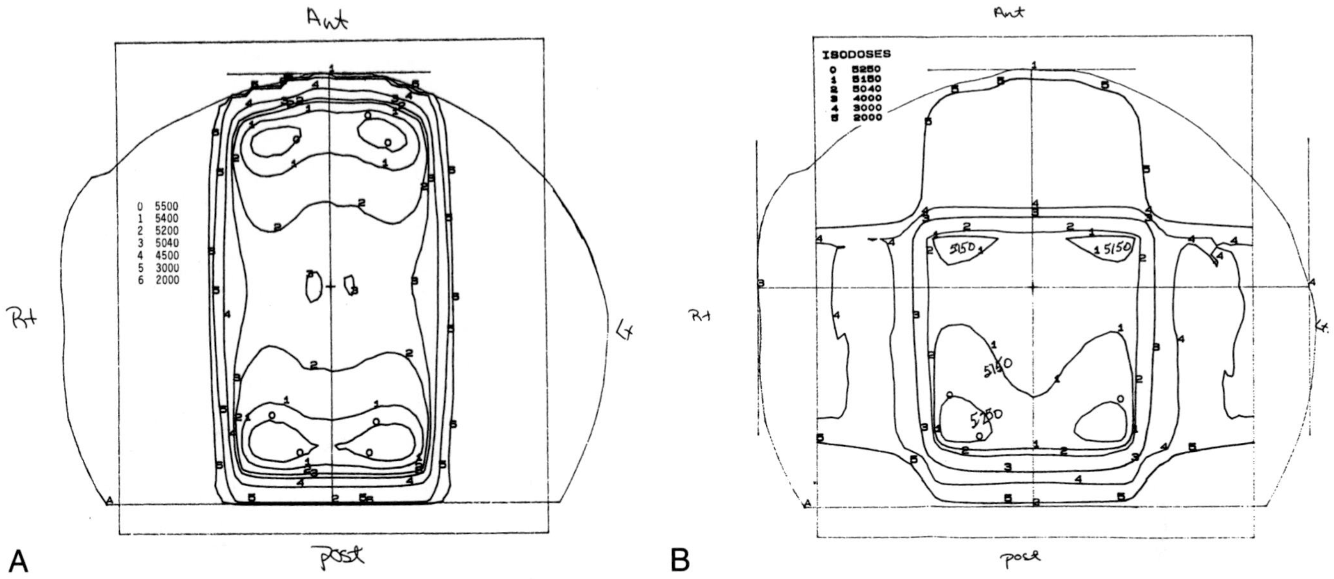

Figure 22.10. **A.** 50 Gy whole pelvis, 18 MV photons, AP-PA ports; **B.** 50 Gy whole pelvis, 18 MV photons, four-field box technique.

therapy prescription can be calculated at the surface of the vaginal cylinder or at a depth of 0.5 cm from the surface of the cylinder.

External Radiation Therapy

Postoperative external irradiation is delivered to selected patients with endometrial carcinoma; at some institutions it is administered without brachytherapy. The prescription for external radiation therapy without brachytherapy is 50 Gy to the whole pelvis. Most patients with endometrial carcinoma are obese; the AP separation tends to be greater than 30 cm. If the AP separation is less than 30 cm then the patient is treated with AP-PA fields with 18 MV photons. Figure 22.10A demonstrates the isodose curves for a prescription of 50 Gy delivered to the pelvis with 18 MV photons using AP-PA fields (Figure 22.5A) for a patient with a separation of 32 cm. The preferred method of treatment for patients with a separation of greater than 30 cm is to use a four-field box technique (Figure 22.10B). The improvement in isodose distribution results in a decreased dose to the rectum and bladder. Figure 22.11 is a simulation radiograph of the lateral field.

If postoperative external radiation therapy is indicated, then it is our practice to administer both external irradiation and an intracavitary cuff implant. The rationale for delivering both types of therapy is to administer a higher radiation dose to the vaginal apex with both treatments than that delivered with 50 Gy whole pelvis external irradiation alone.

Our standard prescription for combined external radiation therapy and brachytherapy for postoperative irradiation for endometrial carcinoma is 20 Gy whole pelvis (Figure 22.5A), 30 Gy split-field with a midline stepwedge (Figure 22.12A), and a vaginal cuff intracavitary implant with either HDR (6 Gy × 3 @ 0.5 cm) or LDR brachytherapy (65 Gy surface dose). The external irradiation is administered with 18 MV photons by AP-PA fields as indicated above. Figure 22.12B demonstrates the combined isodose curves for the prescription 20 Gy whole pelvis, 30 Gy split field and a vaginal cuff implant for 65 Gy. Patients who have positive or close vaginal margins may receive 45 Gy whole pelvis irradiation and the irradiation dose from the vaginal cuff implant is subsequently modified (Appendix 2).

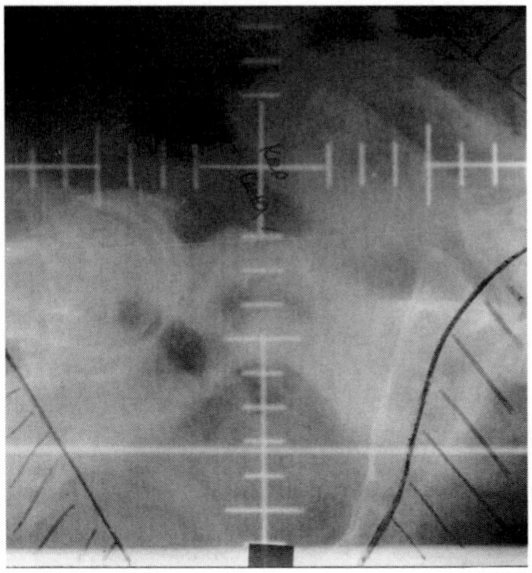

Figure 22.11. Lateral simulator radiograph of the whole pelvic port.

If the para-aortic lymph nodes are found to be positive, the entire para-aortic region is treated to 45 Gy up to the

Figure 22.12. A. Postoperative AP port with colpostat step-wedge; **B.** 20 Gy whole pelvis, 30 Gy split field, 65 Gy surface dose, low dose rate.

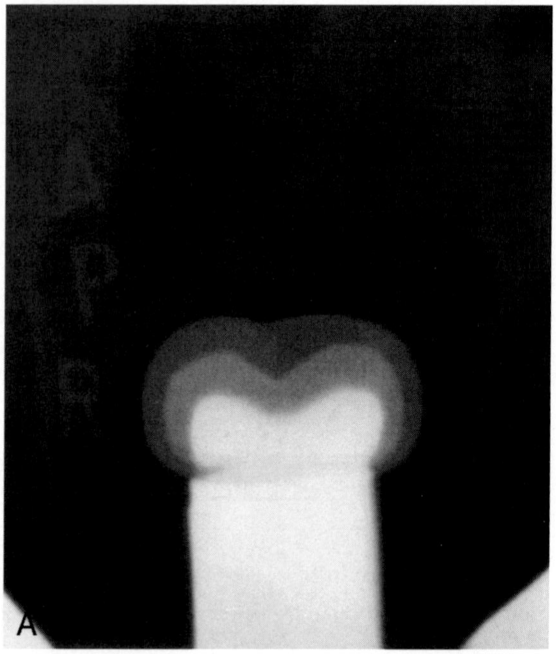

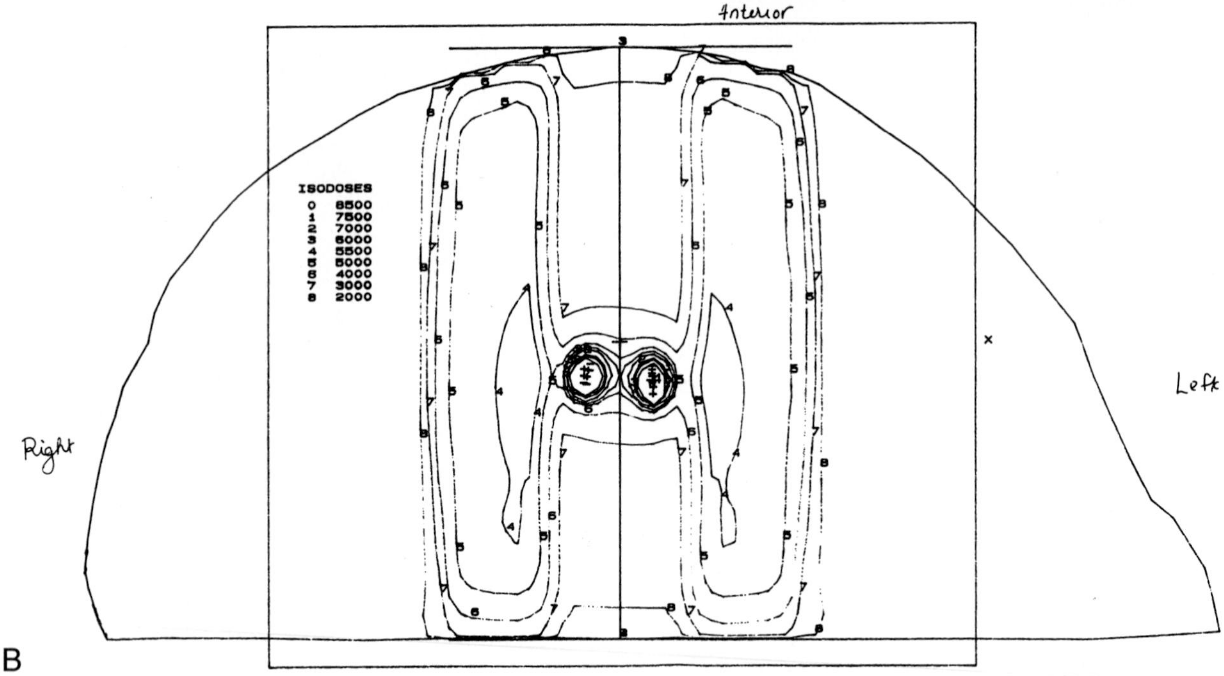

level of the T12-L1 interspace. An additional 500 cGy boost is delivered to a small field encompassing the area of the positive lymph nodes. In postoperative patients these sites are usually well delineated by surgical clips.

RADIATION THERAPY ALONE

Medically inoperable patients with endometrial carcinoma and patients with Stage III or IV disease are treated with irradiation alone. Patients with clinical Stage I disease who are at low risk for having pelvic lymph node metastasis are treated with brachytherapy without external radiotherapy. The prescription for patients treated with brachytherapy is to administer 8,000 mghr utilizing Simon-Heyman capsules, Fletcher-Suit tandem and colpostats in two intracavitary procedures, separated by 2 weeks. The radiation exposure is divided as demonstrated in Table 22.3. As outlined in the section on the use of the preopera-

Table 22.3. Low Dose Rate Brachytherapy Alone Prescription

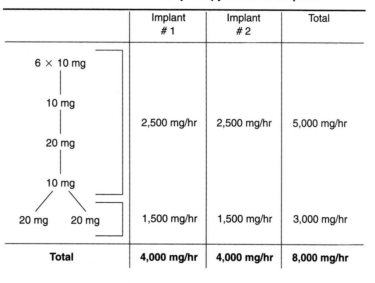

	Implant # 1	Implant # 2	Total
6 × 10 mg — 10 mg — 20 mg — 10 mg	2,500 mg/hr	2,500 mg/hr	5,000 mg/hr
20 mg, 20 mg	1,500 mg/hr	1,500 mg/hr	3,000 mg/hr
Total	**4,000 mg/hr**	**4,000 mg/hr**	**8,000 mg/hr**

tive implant, the fundus of the uterus is packed with Simon-Heyman capsules and a Fletcher tandem. Colpostats are placed in the vagina. Two LDR intracavitary implants are performed and are separated by 2 weeks.

Patients with clinical Stage I disease who are at risk for having positive pelvic lymph nodes, patients with medically inoperable Stage II disease, and patients with clinical Stages III and IV disease receive external radiation therapy plus intracavitary brachytherapy. External radiotherapy is prescribed as 20 Gy whole pelvis and 30 Gy split field and is administered with AP-PA fields or a four-field box technique as described for postoperative pelvic irradiation. Typically, an intracavitary implant with Fletcher tandem and ovoids and Simon-Heyman capsules is performed. External radiotherapy is administered for 2 weeks and the second intracavitary implant is performed. This is followed by an additional 4 weeks of external radiotherapy. If the para-aortic lymph nodes are positive, 45 Gy is prescribed to the para-aortic region up to the T12-L1 interspace and an additional 500 cGy boost is delivered to a small field encompassing the positive lymph nodes.

If HDR brachytherapy is used rather than LDR brachytherapy the implant procedure is performed as discussed in the section on preoperative brachytherapy, with two intrauterine tandems and vaginal colpostats or with an intrauterine tandem, intrauterine Simon-Heyman capsules and vaginal colpostats. A total of six HDR implants are performed at weekly intervals during the course of external radiotherapy. The prescription for the high dose rate implant is shown in Table 22.4. A total of 500 mg/hr is delivered to the uterus and 300 mg/hr is delivered to the vagina for each implant for a total of 4,800 mg/hour delivered in six weekly implant procedures.

Table 22.4. High Dose Rate Brachytherapy Alone Prescription

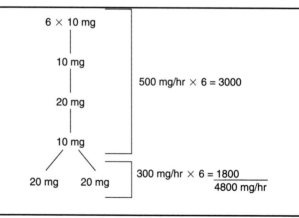

6 × 10 mg — 10 mg — 20 mg — 10 mg	500 mg/hr × 6 = 3000
20 mg, 20 mg	300 mg/hr × 6 = 1800
	4800 mg/hr

RECURRENT ENDOMETRIAL CANCER

Locally recurrent endometrial cancer after surgery is treated with radiotherapy. The location of the pelvic recurrence is usually on the pelvic sidewall or is isolated in the vagina. Vaginal recurrences are usually at the vaginal apex or in the suburethral region.

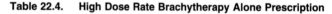

Patients with pelvic sidewall recurrences from endometrial cancer are rarely cured of their disease. Therefore, the intent of therapy (i.e., palliation or cure) should be determined. If the goal of therapy is to cure the patient of their disease, then whole pelvis irradiation to 50 Gy is administered via AP-PA portals, or with a four-field box technique. A pelvic sidewall boost with 1 to 2 cm margins to cover the residual disease is performed to deliver an additional 10 to 16 Gy with AP-PA portals. An intraoperative I-125 seed implant may be performed in selected patients.

Patients with recurrences at the vaginal apex receive 50 Gy to the pelvis with AP-PA ports or with a four-field box technique. Near the completion of their external radiation therapy, patients undergo one or two intracavitary and/or interstitial brachytherapy procedures depending upon tumor size and the total tumor dose. The implant is performed with the patient subjected to regional or general anesthesia. Examination under anesthesia, performed during the last 1 to 2 weeks of external irradiation to the pelvis will often reveal a mobile or tethered mass. Interstitial Flexiguide afterloading catheters are placed through the vagina into the tumor mass and surrounding marginal tissues in a 1 × 1 cm matrix. It is often possible to palpate the superior extent of the vaginal apex tumor mass on rectal examination. Therefore, when interstitial catheters are placed into and through the tumor mass, a finger in the rectum (palpating the cephalad extent of the tumor) is able to detect when the interstitial catheters have passed through the tumor mass with a 1 cm margin). The interstitial catheters are placed without the aide of a template because of the logistical problem of placing a template at the vaginal apex. The use of the Syed template does not allow direct palpation of the tumor mass during catheter placement and is not utilized. We do utilize a template on the perineum to secure the placement of the individual interstitial catheters. The catheters are fixed to the template with SuperGlue after the catheters have been placed into the tumor. The template is then secured to the perineum with prolene sutures. These implants are performed with flexible catheters and usually only oral pain medications are required during the patient's 48- to 72-hour hospital admission. Following the completion of the implant and the removal and storage of the iridium sources, the prolene sutures are removed and the template and its attached Flexiguide catheters are removed as a single unit. Removal of the implant is performed in the exam room with the assistance of a nurse. Bleeding must be anticipated, but rarely occurs. Patients are administered pain medication prior to the removal of the implant.

The interstitial catheters are placed in a 1 × 1 cm matrix. The general rules for a volume implant with a tumor margin are followed. The cephalad and caudad extent of the interstitial catheters extend in length 1 to 2 cm beyond the tumor margin. This allows sufficient coverage of the tumor in these two dimensions. The minimal tumor dose rate is calculated to be 40 cGy/hour. This often results in a maximum tumor dose rate of about 60 cGy/hour. Prescriptions for interstitial therapy are dependent on tumor size. Combined total tumor doses from both external radiotherapy and interstitial and brachytherapy range from about 70 Gy to 85 Gy. One or two interstitial implants are performed. One interstitial implant is performed if the total interstitial dose is to be limited to 2000 cGy. If the total interstitial dose is increased to 30 to 35 Gy, then two implants are performed, each of equal doses, at a 2-week interval.

Vaginal recurrences in the suburethral region are treated in a manner similar to that for patients with urethral carcinoma. External radiation therapy is delivered to the pelvis at a dose of 50 Gy. The groins are included in the AP-PA pelvic ports and the dose to the lymph nodes is 66 Gy. A separate groin boost is delivered if the pelvis is treated with a four-field box technique or if there are positive lymph nodes in the groin. As with lesions in the vaginal apex, interstitial therapy is a reflection of tumor location and size. At our institution, a specially designed interstitial and intracavitary template is used for patients with urethral carcinoma, vaginal carcinoma, or suburethral metastasis from endometrial carcinoma. A complete series of Delclos vaginal cylinders with diameters of 2.0, 2.5, and 3.0 cm has been modified by drilling a series of holes in the long axis of the cylinder segments near the surface to allow the placement of flexible interstitial needles into the cylinder. Surrounding the vaginal cylinder is a circular template that allows for the interstitial placement of flexible needles in the peri-urethral tissues in a single, double, or triple curved plane configuration that is performed depending on the size of the tumor mass to be implanted. The use of the vaginal cylinder allows the posterior vaginal mucosa and the anterior rectal wall to be displaced posteriorly to decrease the radiation dose to those structures. Irradiation dose rates are calculated to be approximately 40 to 50 cGy/hour to surround the intended treatment volume. The tumor size and the use of combined treatment with external radiotherapy determine the total irradiation dose from the implant. One or two interstitial implants may be utilized during the course of treatment.

Whole Abdominal Irradiation

Whole abdominal irradiation is administered to patients at high risk for failing in the upper abdomen. The usual prescription for whole abdominal therapy is 30 Gy to the whole abdomen, 45 Gy to the para-aortic region for positive para-aortic lymph nodes, and 50 Gy to the pelvis and vaginal cuff brachytherapy with LDR or HDR brachytherapy. The kidneys are shielded to keep the dose below 18 Gy; this is accomplished with 5 HVL blocks placed on the PA portals. The liver should not receive doses higher than 30 Gy. If conventional simulation is performed, intravenous contrast with films obtained during the nephrogram phase are obtained so that the kidneys can be localized for placement of the kidney blocks. It is our policy to perform computer tomography (CT) simulation for these patients; intravenous contrast is not necessary and the kidneys and other normal organs and structures can be contoured. It is our clinical impression that CT simulation provides more accurate localization of the kidneys and the

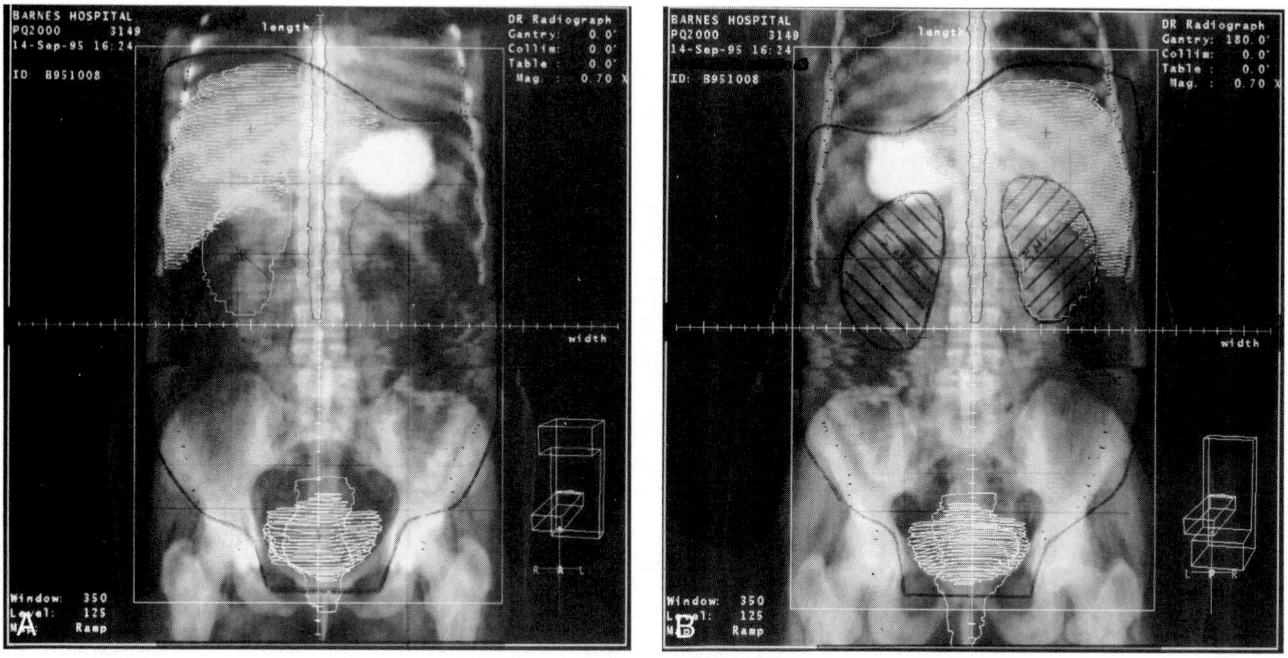

Figure 22.13. (**A**) AP, and (**B**) PA CT simulator radiograph of whole abdomen port.

diaphragm. Simulation is performed with the patient supine in the treatment position at 100 cm SAD. Full inspiration is maintained during CT scanning of the upper abdomen. The upper border of the whole abdominal port is 1 cm cephalad to the diaphragm. The lateral borders of the field extend laterally so that the entire peritoneal surface is covered with margin. Falloff laterally may or may not occur but has no clinical relevance since the whole abdominal dose is limited to 30 Gy. Inferiorly, the port covers the pelvis in the routine and standard fashion. CT simulation films for the whole abdominal ports are shown in Figures 22.13A and 22.13B. The whole abdomen is treated with 150 cGy daily fractions to 30 Gy. If the para-aortics are to be treated, then the para-aortics and pelvis are treated with 150 cGy daily fractions to a total dose of 45 Gy and then the pelvis only is treated to a total of 50 Gy with placement of a mid-line stepwedge. Low dose rate or high dose rate vaginal cuff brachytherapy is temporally integrated during the course of external radiotherapy.

Intraperitoneal P-32

Intraperitoneal P-32 is administered to those patients who are at low risk of failure in the pelvis but are found to have a positive peritoneal cytology at the time of hysterectomy. Patients receiving intraperitoneal P-32 should not receive simultaneous or immediate sequential external radiotherapy to the pelvis because the complication rate from this combined therapy is unacceptably high. Patients who have received P-32 and develop recurrent disease months to years later may subsequently be treated with limited field palliative external radiotherapy to the pelvis or abdomen without overdue concern for complications from combined P-32 and external radiotherapy.

Ideally, patients who are going to receive intraperitoneal P-32 should have their intraperitoneal catheter placed at the time of surgery. However, as a practical matter for patients with endometrial carcinoma, this does not occur. Rather, once the pathologic evaluation of the uterine specimen, lymph nodes, and peritoneal cytology is completed, then a few days have lapsed since the surgery. It is at this time that the decision to administer P-32 is made. An intraperitoneal catheter is placed. The typical prescribed activity for intraperitoneal P-32 is 15 mCi. The procedure for administration is as follows: normal saline (about 100 ml) is instilled into the peritoneal cavity. Tc-99-m sulfur colloid (2 mCi) is also instilled into the peritoneal cavity. The patient is instructed to roll from side to side, lie on her back, and then lie on her abdomen in order to distribute the isotope. An AP and lateral Tc-99m scan of the abdomen is obtained. If the isotope distribution indicates loculation (Figure 22.14A), then the procedure is terminated and external whole abdominal irradiation is delivered. If the isotope distribution throughout the abdomen is adequate (Figure 22.14B and 22.14C), then P-32 administration is performed. The P-32 is instilled into the peritoneal cavity with an additional 100 to 200 ml of normal saline. The patient is instructed to roll from side to side, on her back, and on her abdomen for 30 to 45 minutes to distribute the therapeutic isotope. The intraperitoneal catheter is removed and the puncture site is closed with a purse string

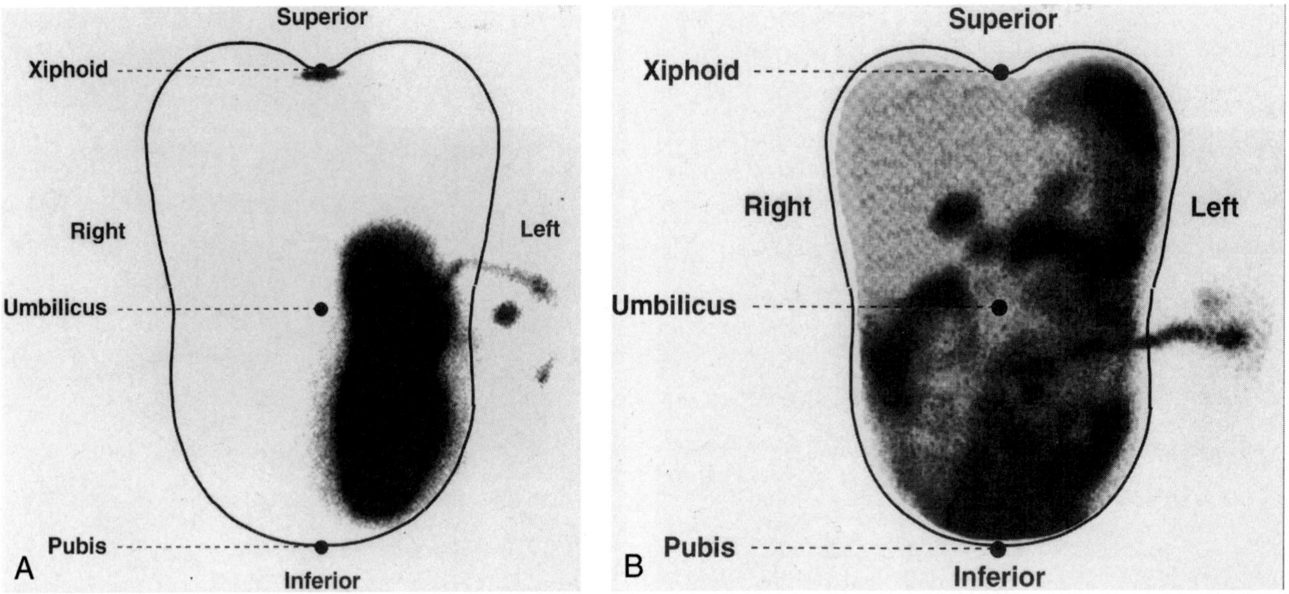

Figure 22.14. **A.** AP Tc-99m peritoneal scan demonstrating loculation of the radioisotope; **B.** AP Tc-99m peritoneal scan demonstrating adequate intraperitoneal distribution; **C.** Lateral scan of **B.**

suture. The patient is usually observed for 24 hours and then discharged from the hospital.

Palliative Irradiation

Patients with locally advanced or metastatic endometrial cancer who have symptoms of pain and bleeding may receive external radiotherapy to the pelvis to relieve these symptoms. When palliation is the goal of therapy for this patient population, it is important to fully evaluate the patient's medical status. Patients requiring palliation but who have an expected survival of greater than 1 year are treated with external therapy to the pelvis to 50 Gy with 180 to 200 cGy daily fractions. Patients with a life expectancy of less than 1 year and those with other severe medical conditions causing disability are treated with 370 cGy twice daily for 2 consecutive days, given a 2-week break, and then treated with radiotherapy twice daily for 2 more days. Then they are given another 2-week break and 2 more days of twice daily therapy is administered. The total dose to the pelvis following this regime of twice daily radiotherapy is 44.4 Gy.

Palliative irradiation may also be administered with an intracavitary implant. Patients with a large volume of disease in the pelvis usually have bleeding and pain. If there is a large volume of disease then external radiotherapy is the treatment of choice. If the patient has a small volume of disease and bleeding is the primary symptom, then an intracavitary implant with Simon-Heyman capsules,

Appendix 22.2 High Dose Rate and External Radiotherapy Prescriptions

Postoperative Cuff Brachytherapy
Mallinckrodt Institute of Radiology
HDR Policy

External		Implant
Whole Pelvis	*Split Field*	*@ ½ cm*
- 0 -	- 0 -	700 cGy × 3
2000	3000	600 cGy × 3
4000	1000	500 cGy × 3

Appendix 22.1. Intracavitary Prescription Modifications Based On Applicator Size

Implants: Preoperative or Radiation Therapy Only

Simon-Heyman capsules are placed in the uterine cavity. Either 10, 8, or 6 mm capsules are used depending on the size of the uterus. But, in general, the cavity is filled with as many sources as possible. If only one to two capsules can be inserted, use the tandem alone.

Standard uterine dose (capsules and tandem): 3500 mg/h

Increase to 3500–4000 mg/h for G3 or sounding ~ 10 cm

Increase to 4000–4500 mg/h for G3 sounding > 12 cm

The standard ovoids (2.0 cm Fletcher-Suit) are used to deliver 6500 RSD. If 2.5 cm caps are used, the dose is decreased to 6000–6500 RSD. If mini-ovoids (1.6 cm diameter) are used, the dose is increased to 6500–7000 RSD.

Fletcher-Suit tandem, and ovoids is performed for a prescribed 4000 mghr. If the bleeding does not resolve, then a second intracavitary implant is performed in 2 to 3 weeks. If the bleeding does resolve, then a second implant is not performed. A second implant could be performed if the bleeding does recur. Palliative implants can also be performed with HDR brachytherapy.

SUMMARY

Radiation therapy is administered to patients with endometrial carcinoma in many clinical situations. Many physicians and physicists at the Mallinckrodt Institute of Radiology have developed over the years the techniques described in this chapter.

Chapter 23

Carcinoma of the Vulva

Ellen Bellairs and Roger A. Potish

INTRODUCTION

Radiation therapy for cancer of the vulva is becoming increasingly important in view of the aging of the population and the diminishing role of surgery. As demonstrated for squamous cell carcinoma of the anus, vulvar cancer may be radiosensitive and chemosensitive enough, such that surgery and its attendant physical and psychological morbidity can frequently be minimized or avoided altogether (1–4). This chapter addresses the practical aspects of radiation treatment for vulvar cancer.

Anatomy

The terms vulva, pudendum, and female external genital organs are synonymous (5). The perineum consists of the otherwise unnamed region between the posterior frenulum (described below) and the anus. The named structures of the vulva are divided into several superficial regions (Figure 23.1). Serving as a reference point for anatomic delineation of vulvar structures, the mons pubis is the rounded mound of adipose tissue anterior to the pubic symphysis. The labia majora are bilateral elongated prominent longitudinal skin folds originating at the mons pubis where they merge to form the anterior commissure. The labia majora extend posteriorly and merge again to form the posterior commissure, located 2.5 cm to 3 cm in front of the anus. The anterior portion of each labium majus receives the fibrous end of the round ligament as it leaves the superficial inguinal ring (1,5).

The labia minora are 4-cm-long skin folds that are free of hair follicles and extend posteriorly from the clitoris and medially from the labia majora. Anteriorly and posteriorly the labia minora merge to form the respective anterior and posterior frenulum. Situated between the labia minora, the vestibule contains the vaginal and urethral orifices as well as many glandular openings. The external urethral orifice or urinary meatus is 2.5 cm posterior and inferior to the clitoris. The introitus, also known as the vaginal orifice, is posterior and inferior to the urethral orifice. Deeper vulvar structures include the vestibular bulbs and Skene glands, which open into the vestibule (1,5).

The vulva is drained by a complicated network of lymphatic anastomoses with frequent extension across the midline. The superficial external pudendal nodes drain the vulva, the distal third of the vagina, the perineum, and the perianal region. Lymphatic vessels of the labia initially drain anteriomedially toward the pubis but then turn laterally and penetrate the cribriform fascia to the superficial inguinal and femoral lymph nodes. Approximately ten superficial inguinal lymph nodes lie along the saphenous vein and its branches between Camper's fascia and the cribriform fascia overlying the femoral vessels. The superficial nodes are located within the triangle formed by the inguinal ligament superiorly, the border of the sartorius muscle laterally, and the border of the adductor longus muscle medially. The superficial inguinal nodes drain to the deep inguinal nodes and then to the external iliac lymph nodes. There are usually three to five deep inguinal nodes, the most superior of which, located under the inguinal ligament, is known as Cloquet's node (Figure 23.2) (5–7).

Due to frequent anastomoses across midline, the lymphatics of the labia minora and other central or medial structures do not always follow predictable patterns of spread. Lymphatics of medial structures often drain bilaterally or directly to the deeper femoral nodes bypassing more superficial inguinal lymph nodes. Clitoral and other central tumors can bypass both the superficial and deep femoral nodes and drain directly to urethral or external iliac and obturator nodes. Although lateral vulvar lesions usually spread predictably, the possibility of bilateral groin involvement must be kept in mind. If there are extensive lymphatic metastases, retrograde spread can involve the lymphatics of the vulva, lower abdominal wall, buttocks, thigh, and contralateral inguinal area (1,5,8,9).

Detection and Evaluation

A disease of older women with a peak incidence in the sixth and seventh decades and a mean age of 63 years at diagnosis, vulvar cancer accounts for 3 to 5% of gynecologic cancers and 0.3% of all cancers (10). Risk factors include hypertension, obesity, smoking, low parity, prior leukoplakia or vulvar inflammation, as well as viral infection (11). Condyloma acuminata is noted in 5 to 10% of patients (12). Vulvar Intraepithelial Neoplasia (VIN) occurs at a median age of 45 and progresses to invasive cancer in approximately 10% of women, with a higher risk of progression in older individuals (13).

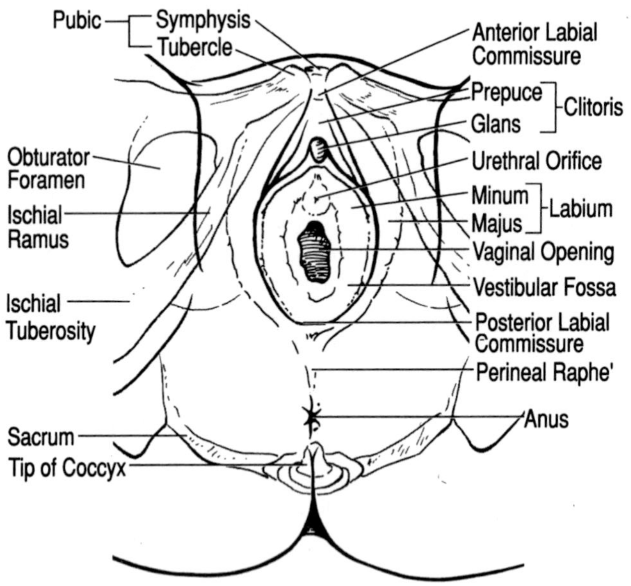

Figure 23.1. Vulvar anatomy in relation to the bony pelvis.

As many as half of the patients present with advanced disease; of these, 5 to 10% have multifocal disease (1,11,14–16). Vulvar, pelvic, and rectal examinations are the best means to assess the characteristics and local extension of vulvar tumors and to rule out concurrent invasive or preinvasive lesions. Of equal importance, but quite variable in both sensitivity and specificity, is the clinical examination of both groins. Although computed tomography (CT) is useful to evaluate lymph nodes, it leads to a 30 to 40% false positive rate upon pathologic examination of suspicious groin adenopathy (8,17,18). Also noteworthy is the 15 to 20% false negative rate for inguinal node metastasis (18,19). Fine needle aspiration of groin nodes may help to prove nodal metastases. Despite its low yield, chest radiography is generally performed as part of the overall evaluation. Other studies such as cystourethroscopy and proctoscopy are useful if tumor is in close proximity to the urinary or anal orifices. Bone imaging is beneficial if tumor fixation or skeletal metastases are suspected, as this can occur from local tumor extension, particularly in the pubic region (1,8).

Figure 23.2. Surgical anatomy of the inguinal lymph nodes. Note the primary relationship to the tributaries of the external iliac chain. (Reprinted with permission from Hacker NF, ed. Essentials of obstetrics and gynecology. WB Saunders: Philadelphia, 1992.)

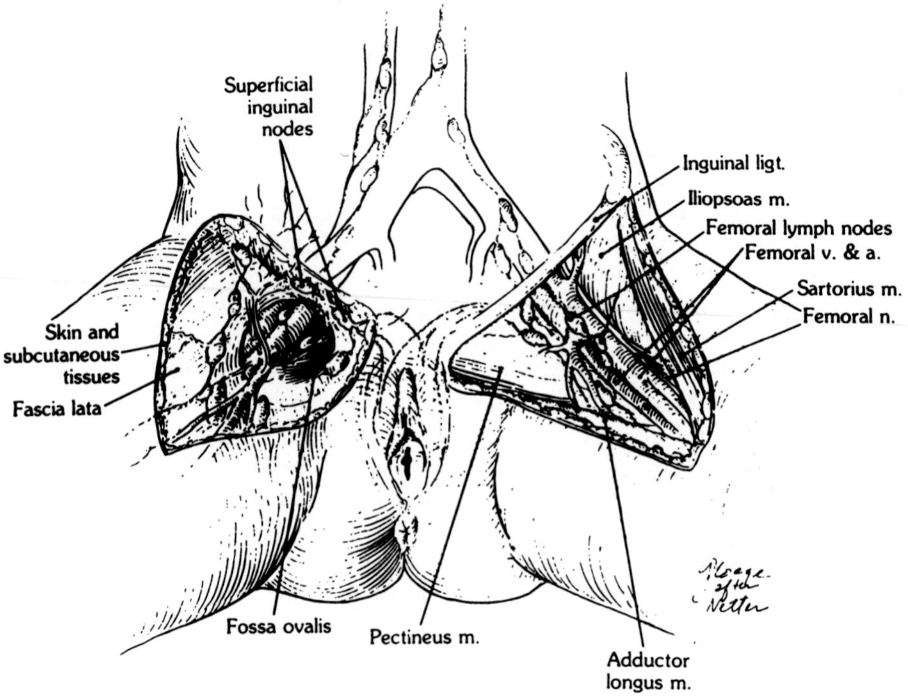

Patterns of Spread, Prognosis, and Staging

Vulvar neoplasms originate in the cutaneous epithelium or in a small region of mucous membrane adjacent to the vagina. Of the 70% of vulvar cancers that arise in the labia, three-quarters occur in the labia majora and one-quarter in the labia minora. An additional 15% occur on the clitoris, with the remainder scattered elsewhere. The majority of lesions are epithelial in origin (8,11,12).

Tumors grow in a variety of patterns. Combinations of exophytic, ulcerative, or infiltrative lesions are common. Vulvar neoplasms spread by local extension and by regional lymphatics. Local extension may involve the adjacent vulvar and perianal regions as well as the vagina, urethra, bladder, anus, rectum, and pubis. Lateral growth can be considerable, even extending to the leg. Hematogenous spread is rare but can include the liver, lungs, or bone (11,12).

Inguinal node metastases are the most common site of spread (17–19). At diagnosis, 30 to 40% of patients have positive groin nodes; of these, 20% have pelvic node metastasis (9,19,20). The incidence of positive nodes is related to tumor size, depth, and stage. Even within clinical Stage I tumors, the incidence of nodal metastasis varies considerably and is primarily related to the depth of tumor invasion (20–22). Tumors from 1 to 2 mm in depth have a 6% incidence of positive lymph node findings while those measuring from 4 to 5 mm are associated with a 25% rate of positive nodes (17,21,23).

Nodal involvement is the most significant prognostic factor in vulvar tumors (9,18,20). Nodal spread cuts survival in half. When more than three groin nodes are involved, 5-year survival ranges from 0 to 20% (8,18,19). At 5 years, less than 10% of patients with positive pelvic nodes are alive. As reflected in the staging rules, nodal involvement is classified as Stage III or IV disease, regardless of the size of the primary lesion (19,24). Factors leading to an increased risk of groin recurrence are fixed or ulcerated nodes and multiple positive nodes. Nodal metastases increase the risk of inguinal and pelvic relapse but do not influence the probability of vulvar relapse (13,18,19,23,25).

Unfavorable pathologic factors prognostic for central recurrence include depth of stromal invasion, histology, lymph vascular invasion, and perineural involvement (1,13,16). Central recurrence is closely related to the adequacy of surgical margins. The margin of clearance of the tumor is the best predictor of local recurrence. In a surgical study every recurrence was noted in specimens from patients with tumor less than 8 mm from the surgical margin (26). Other features prognostic for vulvar recurrence are tumor size greater than 4 cm and capillary lymphatic space involvement (13,19,25). When neither is present, risk of central recurrence is 9.2% compared to 20% when one of these two factors is noted. Hematogenous metastases are rare but confer a bleak prognosis (1,19).

Staging of vulvar cancer was based exclusively on physical examination before 1989 (24). Subsequently, surgical staging was instituted because of the prognostic value of pathologically positive nodes and the limited accuracy of clinical examination of groin nodes (9,26). Stage I and II vulvar cancers are both confined to the vulva, with Stage II disease distinguished by a tumor diameter of more than 2 cm (Table 23.1) (1,27). Because of the minimal risk of nodal involvement in some Stage I patients, a subgroup of Stage I, Stage Ia, has been proposed for solitary lesions less than 2 cm in diameter with clinically negative nodes and a depth of less than 1 mm of stromal invasion (27,28). Stage III tumors have either unilateral inguinal lymph node metastases or regional spread to the adjacent lower urethra, vagina, or anus. Stage IVa disease includes either bilateral inguinal lymph node metastases or more extensive regional spread to the upper urethra, bladder or rectal mucosa, or pelvic bone. Stage IVb tumors are defined by either pelvic lymph node metastases or more distant spread, such as to periaortic nodes, lung, or liver (19,24,27).

The numeric FIGO staging criteria do not always allow for clear separation of early and advanced vulvar cancer, which is useful for prognosis and definition of treatment based on disease extent (Table 23.2). The American Joint

Table 23.1. 1995 FIGO Staging of Vulvar Carcinoma

Stage	Clinical Findings
Stage 0	Carcinoma in situ
Stage I	Tumor 2 cm or less, confined to vulva or perineum
Stage 1a	Stromal invasion 1.0 mm or less
Stage 1b	Stromal invasion > 1.0 mm
Stage II	Tumor > 2 cm, confined to vulva or perineum
Stage III	Any size tumor with adjacent spread to urethra, vagina or anus, or unilateral groin node metastasis with any size tumor
Stage IVa	Any size tumor invading upper urethra, bladder mucosa, rectal mucosa, or pelvic bone or bilateral groin node metastases
Stage IVb	Any distant metastasis including pelvic lymph nodes

Table 23.2. Advanced and Early Vulvar Cancer as Characterized by Primary and Nodal Features

Primary and Nodal Features	Disease Stage	
	Early	Advanced
T	T1B	T2 (>4 cm)
	T2 (<4 cm)	T3, T4
N	N0	N1 Fixed
	N1 Not fixed	Ulcerated
	Not ulcerated	Multiple
	Not multiple	N2

Committee on Cancer (AJCC) categories of T3 (spread to adjacent lower urethra, vagina, or anus) and T4 (further involvement or spread to upper urethra, bladder or rectal mucosa or pelvic bone) signify advanced disease (29). Size is also an important indicator of early and advanced disease with 4 cm generally regarded as the discriminator for bulk of primary involvement. Early nodal disease is defined as absent or solitary adenopathy. In the AJCC classification, N1 is unilateral adenopathy while N2 is bilateral or pelvic and inguinal involvement. However, any nodal spread that is multiple, fixed, or ulcerated is indicative of late nodal disease but not accounted for in either the FIGO or AJCC staging system (27,29). Collectively, these factors are accounted for in patient management decisions (Figure 23.3) (13,30).

Treatment Modalities

Several advances have been made in the treatment strategy of vulvar cancer in the last two decades resulting from a better understanding of the natural history of the disease and from efforts to incorporate less radical surgery. This has allowed the role of radiation therapy and chemotherapy to expand so that individual therapy can be more fully optimized (1,8,30,31). A brief discussion of the major refinements involving the role of surgery, radiation, and chemotherapy in treatment of vulvar cancer follows.

Surgery

Radical vulvectomy and bilateral inguinal lymphadenectomy with pelvic lymph node dissection has achieved

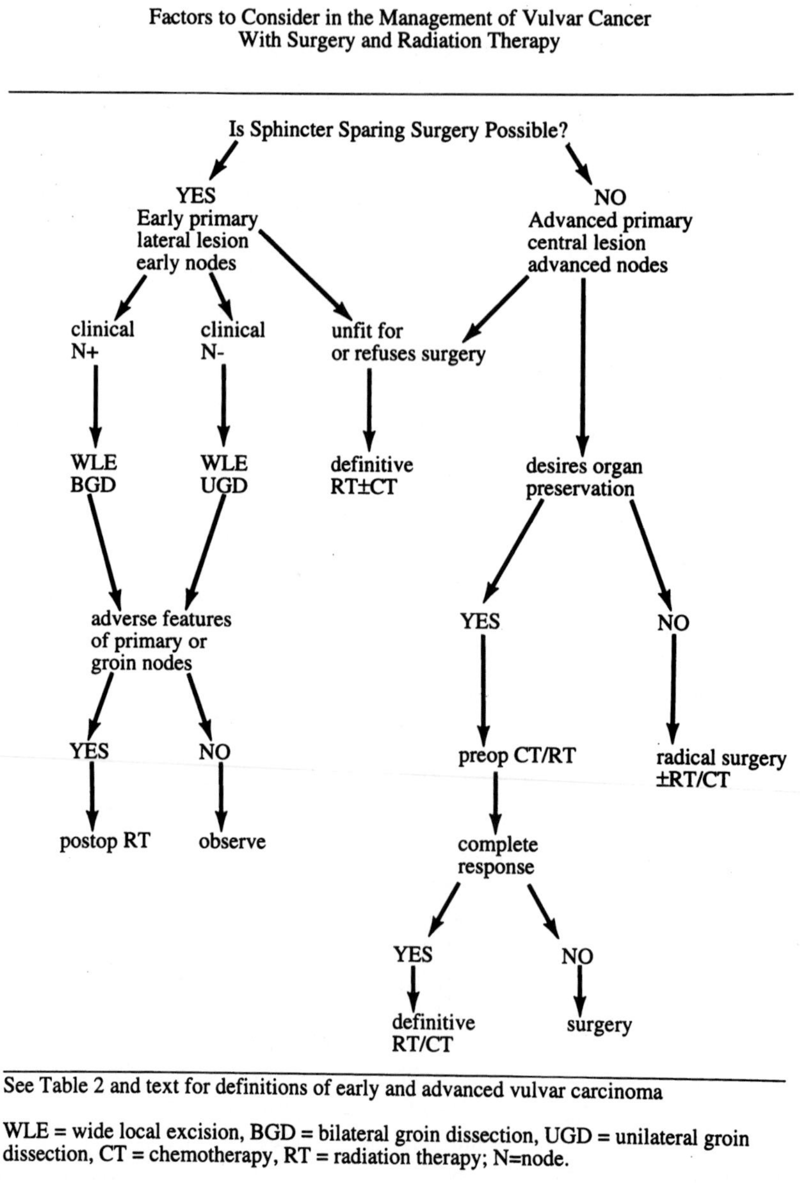

Figure 23.3. Algorithm for the treatment of vulvar cancer. RV, radical vulvectomy; BLGD, bilateral lymph groin dissection; CLS, capillary lymphatic space involvement; RT, radiation therapy; ULGD, unilateral lymph groin dissection.

overall 5-year survival rates of 50 to 75%, with disease-free survival 10 to 20% higher (32,33). This standard surgical approach is not without major complications as wound breakdown can occur in up to 85% of patients, and 30 to 70% of patients experience chronic leg edema (34). Up to 15% of patients require reoperation for surgical complications (8,32,33,35).

In view of this morbidity, less radical surgery is now considered (36,37). For example, patients with lateralized tumors less than 2 cm in diameter treated with radical local excision have a central recurrence rate of 7%, virtually identical to the 6% rate of central recurrence in patients treated with radical vulvectomy (38,39). Surgical margins include 2 cm of normal tissue around the tumor with the depth of resection extending to the inferior fascia of the urogenital diaphragm (18,19,31).

Attempts to diminish the extent of the groin lymphadenectomy have not been as successful (40). The classic inguinofemoral node dissection involves removal of the superficial and deep nodes to the cribriform fascia, thus fully exposing the femoral vessels (18,31). The need for routine dissection of the deeper femoral lymphatics remains controversial (18,25,31,40). However, routine pelvic lymphadenectomy and contralateral groin dissection has been discontinued as routine procedures (Figure 23.4) (18,25,38).

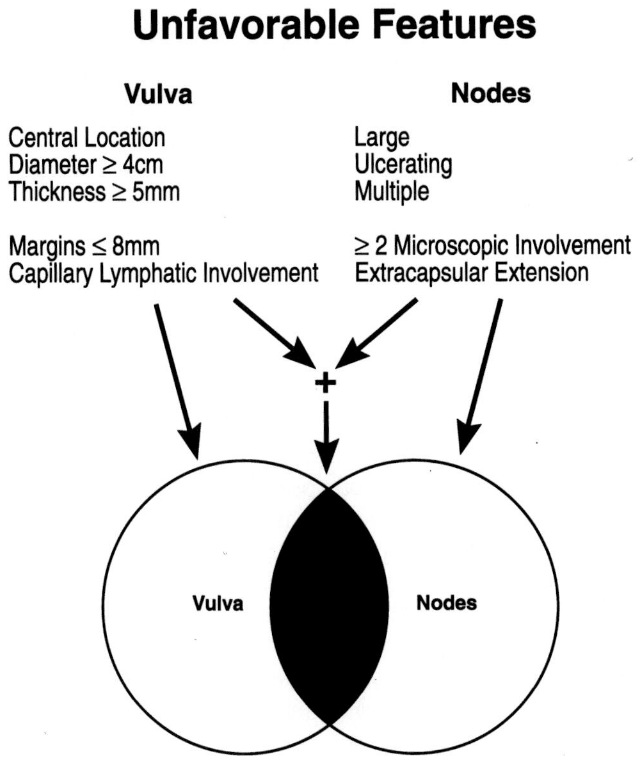

Figure 23.4. Unfavorable prognostic features for vulvar cancer.

Radiation Therapy and Chemotherapy

The most definitive data supporting the efficacy of radiation therapy for treatment of vulvar cancer are derived from a randomized trial for management of the regional lymphatics in which patients with positive groin nodes at radical vulvectomy and bilateral groin dissection were randomized to receive either surgery to the deep pelvic nodes or postoperative radiation therapy to the groin and pelvic nodal regions. When more than one node was positive, postoperative irradiation to the pelvic and groin nodes improved survival and reduced groin recurrence: 2-year survival was 68% versus 54% and control in the groin was 95% versus 76% with postoperative radiation (39). Others have confirmed these results (17,30,41).

The value of preoperative radiation therapy for advanced vulvar cancer is well documented in its capacity to make a once inoperable lesion operable (1,31,42). Further experience using 50 Gy to the whole pelvis, vulva, and groins preoperatively achieved 5-year survival rates of 76% for primary tumors and 63% for recurrent vulvar cancer (43). In another series, 44 to 55 Gy was given preoperatively to patients who would have otherwise required exenteration; half had no pathologic evidence of tumor, and local control was obtained in three-quarters, with avoidance of exenteration in all patients (44). Subsequently, investigators have confirmed the efficacy of preoperative radiation therapy for organ preservation and minimization of surgical resection (45,46).

The medical literature concerning definitive radiation therapy for vulvar cancer is difficult to apply to individual patient management. The role of radiation therapy has not been delineated in a systematic fashion with randomized clinical trials. There are no randomized studies comparing primary surgery to definitive radiation therapy (6,25). Earlier reports of radiation therapy in the treatment of carcinoma of the vulva are difficult to apply since much of the data is derived from small numbers of patients treated by radiation therapy alone either because of unfitness for or refusal of surgery (45,47–50). Also, some early series used outmoded equipment and variable techniques. Although scattered reports of subsequent radionecrosis, femoral neck fractures, and integumentary morbidity helped to discredit radiation therapy (51–55), improvements have occurred with modern equipment and doses (1,55). Although radiation therapy can cause morbidity, 5-year survivals of 40 to 50% have been reported for primary vulvar cancers, with local control rates of 15 to 20% higher (45,47). Rates of cure and local control range from 25 to 75% when radiation therapy is administered for recurrent disease (52,56,57). Collectively, these data support the curative ability of radiation therapy for squamous cell carcinoma of the vulva (1,29).

The success of postoperative radiation therapy in treatment of patients with positive groin nodes led to investigation of the possibility of replacing groin dissection with groin irradiation in patients with a clinically negative groin exam (41,58). This question was studied in a GOG randomized clinical trial with disappointing results (25,59). Groin irradiation led to increased groin failure and a subsequent decrease in survival compared to groin dissection with adjuvant irradiation for positive nodes. Unfortunately, because of the failure to deliver a tumoricidal dose to the actual target depth, the question of whether elective nodal irradiation has a similar or better outcome compared to groin dissection was not adequately answered by this study (59,60). The consequences resulting from failure to account for adequate target coverage should serve as an important lesson for radiotherapists in treatment of inguinal targets (61,62). A subsequent retrospective study with superior irradiation techniques has shown no significant survival advantage to groin dissection over groin irradiation, as well as less morbidity with radiation therapy compared to surgery (63). For patients with clinically negative groin nodes who refuse or are medically unfit to withstand groin surgery, groin irradiation is currently an acceptable alternative, but needs further prospective randomized study (30,62–65).

Chemotherapy, particularly with concurrent 5-fluorouracil (5FU) may act as a radiation sensitizer and enhance tumor cell kill (66,67). In an adjacent tumor site, the use of concurrent 5FU and radiation in squamous cell carcinoma of the anal canal has produced local control rates of 90 to 95% and greatly reduced the necessity of abdominal perineal resection (4,68). In vulvar cancer, complete responses occur in half of patients treated with radiation therapy, mitomycin C, and 5FU (69). In patients with locoregionally advanced disease treated with 40 Gy irradiation and weekly cisplatin and 5FU, half of the patients who had vulvar resection after chemoradiation have no residual disease in the pathologic specimen and remain disease free (70). Toxicity is not excessive and does not result in increased surgical complications (69,70). Short-term disease-free survival rates of 45 to 85% have been achieved (71–73). Neoadjuvant chemoradiation continues to be investigated (72,74–78).

Treatment Choices

Early vulvar cancer is defined by the extent and location of the primary tumor such that a curative excision can be accomplished without sacrifice of the ureteral or anal sphincters (30). Early vulvar lesions are small (less than 4 cm) and well lateralized (29). The treatment of choice for early disease is surgery (18,31). Microinvasive lesions can be managed with wide local excision alone (9,18,28). All other patients with early disease are treated with wide or radical local excision and groin dissection (Figure 23.3). For patients unfit for or refusing surgery, definitive radiation is an option. Radiotherapy to the tumor bed improves local control when tumor is within 8 mm of the surgical margin, when tumor thickness is over 5 mm, or when tumor is found in the capillary lymphatic space (18,23,26).

Women with negative inguinal exams constitute the majority of patients with early disease (30). When clinical examination reveals solitary adenopathy, without fixed or ulcerated nodes, the disease is still considered early (18). If a unilateral lymph node dissection has been performed for lateralized disease and one lymph node is found to be positive, then the contralateral inguinal area is dissected. If no additional nodes contain metastases, the cancer is still considered early, and adjuvant treatment is not necessary (35,39,79). There is a survival benefit for postoperative radiotherapy when more than one node has microscopic invasion, if macroscopic involvement is found, or if disease penetrates through the nodal capsule (18,23,37,39).

Advanced disease is characterized by palpable inguinal disease or the necessity of sphincter sacrifice or exenteration to adequately remove the primary tumor (Table 23.2 and Figure 23.3). Features of the primary lesion that classify tumors as advanced include multifocal lesions and centrally located tumors involving the clitoris, urethra, vagina, or anus such that any adequate surgical procedure would not allow organ preservation (18,30,31,44). Unfavorable or advanced nodal involvement occurs when fixed, ulcerated, or multiple nodes are found on exam (19,23).

Treatment options for women with advanced central or inguinal disease have traditionally involved radical or exenterative surgery (32). Chemoradiation may obviate the need for extensive surgery in some of these women. When locally advanced vulvar lesions and/or fixed or ulcerated inguinal lymph nodes are present, chemoradiotherapy can be given preoperatively or definitively (68,69). Several trials of concurrent chemoradiation using fluorouracil with or without cisplatin resulted in complete response rates of 50 to 90% for primary unresectable disease or for patients who would have otherwise required exenterative surgery (69,72,74,77,78).

Radiation Techniques

Radiation Volume

Radiation doses and volumes are dependent on the extent and location of both primary and nodal disease. Three main situations are encountered: treatment of the vulva and regional lymphatics together, the regional lymphatics alone, or the vulva alone. The indications for choosing among these three different volumes and consequent treatment portals are delineated below and in Figures 23.3 and Table 23.2. Regardless of target volume, techniques are similar for the definitive, preoperative, or postoperative setting (1,20).

A variety of situations is encountered that leads to radiation fields confined to the vulva or its postoperative tumor bed. Only the vulva needs to be treated in patients with Stage Ia carcinomas if they decline or are unfit to undergo surgery. Patients with lateralized disease need postoperative radiation to the resected vulvar tumor bed when pathologic examination reveals close or positive margins, a tumor depth greater than 5 mm, or capillary lymphatic space involvement (9,25,26,30,65).

Treatment of vulvar lymphatics without including central vulvar structures occurs in the absence of pathologic risk factors for central recurrence combined with the presence of risk factors for nodal failure. The latter include microscopic involvement of multiple nodes, gross involvement of one or more nodes, extracapsular extension, or bulky or ulcerated nodes (Figure 23.4) (20,23,25). Preoperative nodal radiation may be useful in patients with fixed, large, or ulcerating groin nodes with subsequent surgical management of the primary. A role for definitive groin and pelvic nodal irradiation as a replacement for lymphadenectomy, in patients with N0 and N1 clinical disease, is emerging but is not yet standard (50,59,63,65,80).

Both the regional nodes and vulva are irradiated in patients with advanced lesions that would otherwise require a more radical surgical procedure or exenteration if the patient were to be offered surgery for cure (3,18). Chemotherapy is often added in the preoperative setting while radiation without chemotherapy is more common postoperatively. In the latter setting, risk factors for local recurrence are noted upon pathologic examination of both the primary and nodal specimens (Table 23.2) (18,26). Definitive radiation therapy can be given without chemotherapy for earlier lesions and with chemotherapy for more advanced situations with the option of surgical salvage if indicated (1,60,73,74,78).

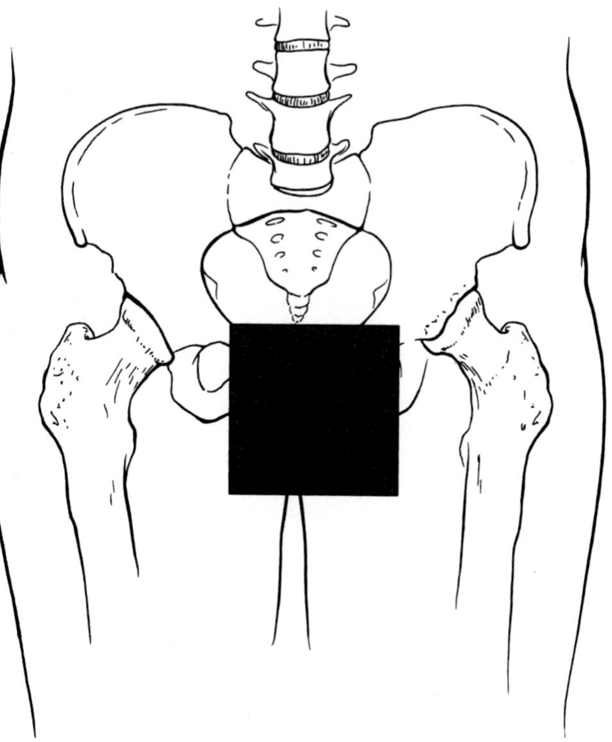

Figure 23.5. Anterior and posterior portals for photon treatment of the vulva alone. Field margins are determined by the characteristics and location of the primary lesion. The superior border is placed above the pubis, and there is falloff on the inferior margin. Lateral field margins include at least 3 cm of normal tissue on either side of the lesion.

Portal Design

Vulva Alone. There is a dearth of published guidelines or recommendations to assist the radiation oncologist in designing vulvar portals. The target for definitive radiation therapy for early lateral Stage Ib and Stage Ia lesions includes only the vulva, with the depth of coverage extending to the level of the urogenital diaphragm. Recommendations for target coverage are based on experience with surgical margins, tumor characteristics, daily setup parameters, and characteristics of the radiation beam (31,35,38). Target coverage should extend to the depth of the urogenital diaphragm. The rationale is to deliver a tumoricidal dose to the area which would have been otherwise surgically resected. Three centimeters around the gross tumor to the beam edge provide for 2 cm around the clinical target volume and also account for 1 cm of daily setup variation within the planning treatment volume. Similar treatment volumes are applicable for postoperative radiation therapy with 2-cm margin surrounding the tumor bed (7,31,38). The adequacy of target coverage is ideally assessed by CT, physical examination, and computerized treatment planning since the depth of the pelvic floor can be quite variable (31,61,81). Regardless of portal orientation, field borders for exclusive vulvar radiation are determined by target coverage, with the objective of providing a 3-cm margin from the lesion (i.e., the gross tumor volume) or tumor bed to the geometric field edge (Figures 23.5 and 23.6) (1,82).

Whenever the vulva is treated, all visible lesions and incisions should be delineated at simulation with radiopaque markers including lead wire, surgical clips, or gold seeds. Lugol's iodine or acetic acid may help delineate the extent of tumor if multifocal disease is suspected or the lesion is difficult to visualize. If the vagina or anus are involved with tumor, they should be identified with radiopaque markers. The sloping skin surface can be seen radiographically by placement of a radiopaque wire or a chain for visualization on the lateral orthogonal simulation film. Customized blocking is mandatory to spare as much normal tissue as possible (82).

Anterior and posterior parallel opposed photon pelvic portals are one option for vulvar radiation (Figure 23.5). Field size is determined by the extent and location of the primary lesion. The vulvar target is covered to the depth

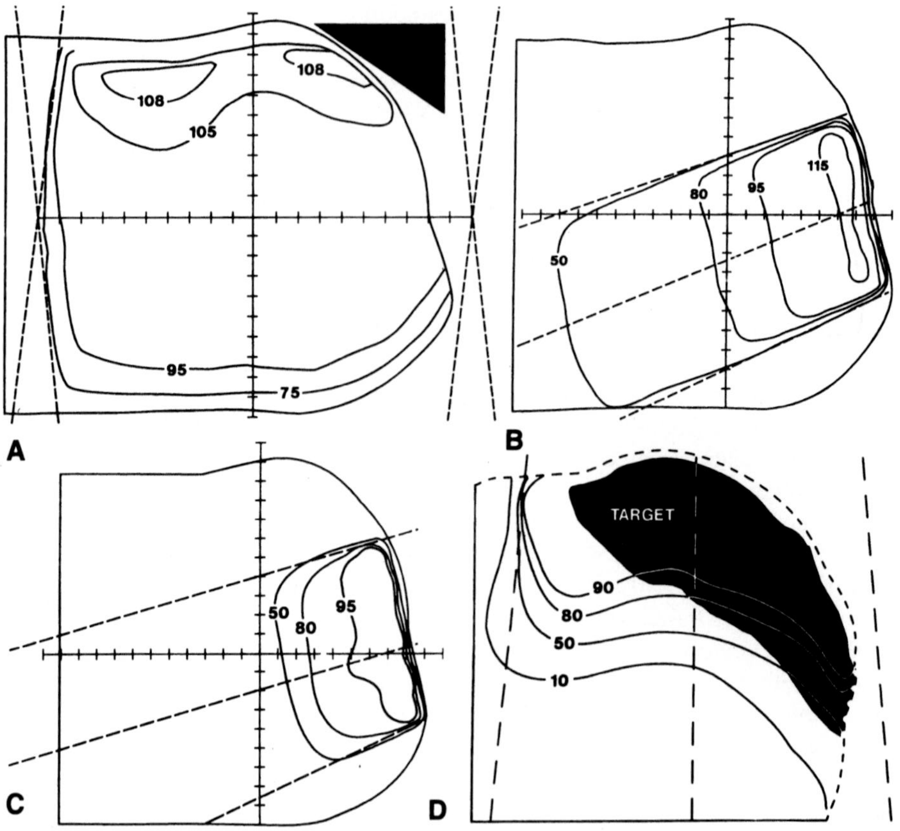

Figure 23.6. Multiple options for perineal treatments. A. Anterior 6-MV and posterior 18-MV parallel opposed beams enter a sagittal contour of the pelvis and vulva with an anterior tissue compensator. Although the compensator does not abolish tangential dose effects, it reduces vulvar dose by 15%. B. A 6-MV perineal photon beam enters the same contour. Bolus is necessary over the vulvar lesion to assure dose buildup. C. An 18-MeV perineal electron beam enters the same contour. Penetration is not as deep, and very little skin sparing occurs. D. An 18-MeV electron beam does not adequately cover the target if it is not oriented properly. (Reprinted with permission from Potish RA. Elements of radiation therapy for the gynecological oncologist. In: Greer BJ, Berek JS, eds. Gynecologic oncology: treatment rationale and techniques. New York: Elsevier, 1991;87–116.)

of the pelvic floor. The superior margin of the field extends 1 or 2 cm above the pubic symphysis. Lateral margins include 3 cm of tissue on either side of the lesion and the field extends beyond the vulvar skin inferiorly.

The three dimensions of treatment planning are particularly important in view of the irregular topography of the vulva and perineum as well as the tangential incidence of the beam. Individualized compensation is critical to minimize skin reaction and to avoid overdose and added perineal discomfort (Figure 23.6A). Treatments are given in the supine position with slight to moderate separation of the legs to minimize skin fold overlap. Other normal tissues, such as a pannus extending into the fields, can be separated or taped (82,83).

Perineal electrons or photons provide another technique to treat the vulva, either primarily or as a boost (Figures 23.6B and 23.6C) (82,83). In order to use a perineal field the patient needs to attain a stable setup in a supine position with adequate support for the separated legs. Although perineal fields include structures from the mons pubis to the anus, target coverage and blocking depends upon the extent and location of the lesion (Figure 23.7). Electron fields need to be slightly larger than photon fields to account for a broader penumbra (82,84). The electron energy is chosen to deliver 90% of the dose to the depth of the urogenital diaphragm. Electron beams are oriented perpendicular to the surface so as to avoid underdosage due to the rapid falloff of electrons in tissue (Figure 23.6D) (84). In selected cases an electron cone can be used for the boost, particularly if a periscope is available for daily setup verification. Applied flush to the vulva, the cone aids in separating the labia to boost central lesions.

Generally, 5 to 10 mm of bolus is placed on the entire field on a daily basis, as tolerated by the skin. The need for bolus on the vulva or perineum is a controversial issue that is determined on an individualized basis. In patients treated with definitive radiation therapy, vulvar bolus was correlated with a nonsignificant trend toward improved local tumor control: 72% with bolus compared to 69% without (57,85). Bolus may not be necessary over the tumor bed when the surgical margins are negative. When the area at risk is encompassed by tangential photons, the skin sparing effect of the beam is lost and diminishes the need for bolus. If the labia are not separable because of tumor or anatomic constraints, they may provide self bolus. Thermoluminescent dosimetry assists to determine the extent of bolus necessary to achieve a surface dose of at least 90% (84).

Brachytherapy. Limited published data exist to provide explicit guidelines for the use of brachytherapy for vulvar tumors (57,86). Superficial lesions can be treated with single plane interstitial implants. Deeper lesions require dou-

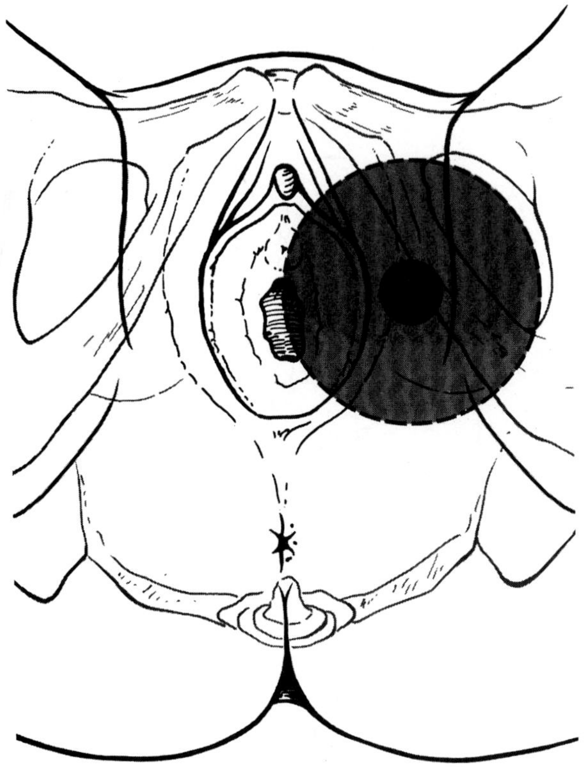

Figure 23.7. Perineal portal for photon or electron treatment of the vulva. The field is determined by the location and size of the primary lesion and includes 3-cm margin of normal tissue in all directions around the area of gross tumor volume (GTV).

ble plane or other volume implants. A vaginal cylinder or interstitial implant lends itself to treatment of vaginal extension of a primary vulvar tumor (87). In one recent brachytherapy series, tumor control was 100% for primary tumors and 50% for recurrent disease (88). A study using iridium-192 with the Paris system that delivered a median dose of 60 Gy to treat both recurrent and primary vulvar lesions reported 5-year local control rates of 23 to 73% (88). A number of investigators have obtained local tumor control rates from 40 to 80% (1,56,89).

Regional Nodal Irradiation. Treatment of vulvar lymphatics without including central vulvar structures is indicated when only risk factors for groin failure are found at pathologic examination (Figures 23.4 and 23.8). The nodal targets (i.e., the clinical target volume) include both the superficial and deeper inguinal groups and the external iliac chain and a variable portion of the internal iliacs. When both the pelvic and inguinal nodes are treated, dose is prescribed to each target separately. Coverage of all nodal targets must be assessed by CT in view of the widely variable location of the femoral vessels and their associated lymphatics (6,61). Surgery and CT confirmed that the groin nodes are frequently much deeper than 3 cm (6, 61, 81). The actual inguinal node depth has a mean value of 6.1 cm and ranges from 2 cm to 18.5 cm (62,76,81). The depth of the groin target is a critical aspect of planning for both the target volume and consequent treatment portals when inguinal nodes are irradiated (62,81).

A parallel opposed rectangular photon field is recommended for treatment of the regional inguinopelvic lymphatics (1,90) (Figure 23.8). Treatment portal borders may be based on bony landmarks. The superior border of the photon field is the most variable and depends upon the extent of iliac nodes at risk for recurrence. Common iliac coverage requires an upper border at L4, with the lower borders designed to cover the external iliac and inguinal nodes. The lateral border extends to the anterosuperior iliac spine or 1 cm lateral to the femoral head. The inferior border extends 3 cm below the pubis or 2 cm below the bottom of the ischial tuberosities. The midline block or medial border is 5 to 6 cm wide and extends from 2 cm above the pubis to the bottom of the field.

If CT proves that both superficial and deep inguinal nodes are close to the surface and if the contour is flat, electrons may be considered when the target does not include the deep pelvic nodes (6,82). Electron fields typically have a superior-lateral border just above the anterosuperior iliac spine, a medial border 2 cm to 3 cm lateral to

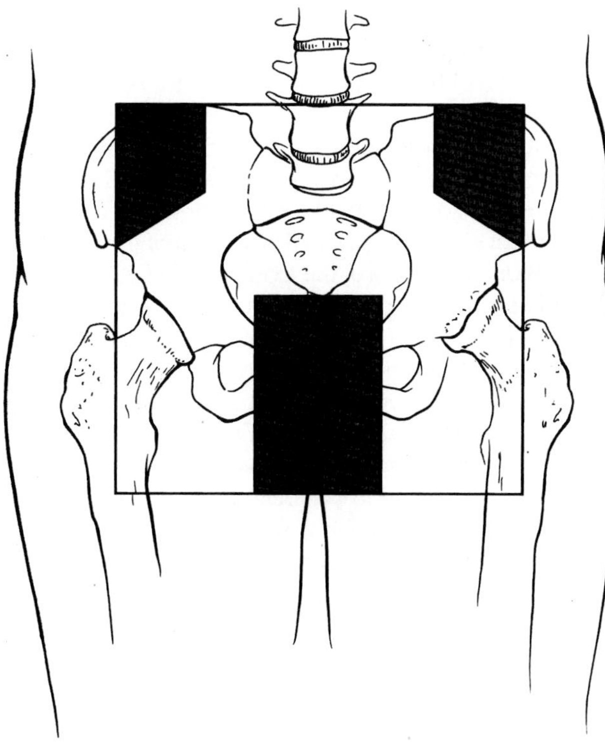

Figure 23.8. Photon portals for treating inguinal and external, internal, and common iliac nodes for patients with vulvar cancer. The superior border is placed at L4 with blocking of midline structures up to the coccyx. The lateral borders extend 1 cm beyond the lateral aspect of the femoral heads or to the anterior superior iliac spine with the bottom of the field placed about 3 cm below the bottom of ischial tuberosities.

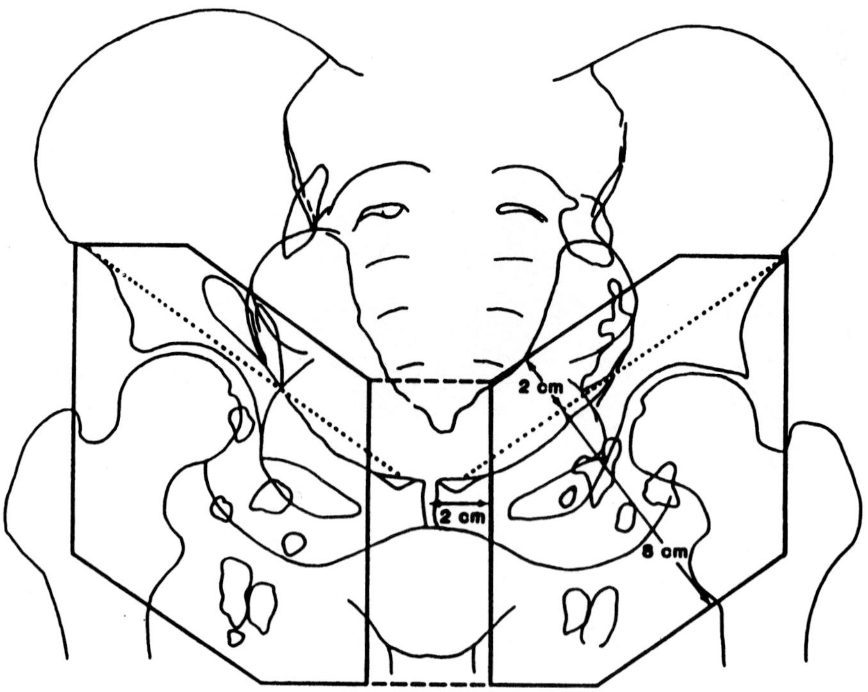

Figure 23.9. Electron portal for treating the inguinal nodes recommended in Gynecologic Oncology Group (GOG). Protocol #88. (Reprinted with permission from Stehman FB et al. Groin dissection versus groin radiation in carcinoma of the vulva: a Gynecologic Oncology Group study. Int J Radiat Oncol Biol Phys 1992,24:389–396).

midline at the level of the pubis, and an inferior border 3 to 4 cm below the pubis thereby including the entirety of the femoral head and a majority of the inguinal ligament (Figure 23.9) (59,91).

Regardless of whether photons or electrons are chosen for treatment, simulation and treatment are performed in the supine position. Slight separation of the legs may minimize skin folds, the judicious use of tape can flatten out areas of redundant skin. Bladder distention may aid in the displacement of part of the small bowel out of the radiation fields (1,82). Orthogonal simulation films and CT are helpful in delineating pelvic and inguinal nodal targets. Surgical scars or palpable adenopathy are delineated with lead wire or radiopaque markers. Contour asymmetry can be quite variable in the inguinopelvic region as well and should be taken into account by tissue compensation and individualized treatment planning. When photons are chosen, bolus is placed over scars and protuberant nodes. The amount of bolus needed to provide a surface dose of 90% with either electrons or photons can be verified with thermoluminescent dosimetry (82,84).

Vulva and Regional Lymphatics. The complexity of treating advanced vulvar cancer with radiation therapy is a consequence of having a superficial yet midline vulvar target, an anterolateral inguinal node target, and a deep pelvic node target. The varied locations of these three targets must be kept in mind with respect to their three-dimensional orientation when determining radiation fields (62,92).

The most common and least complicated technique for coverage of these targets is a pair of parallel opposed anteroposterior inguinopelvic photon fields (Figure 23.10). Simulation and treatment are performed with a combination of the opposed photon vulvar and regional nodal fields described above so as to simply omit the midline block from the latter (93,94). The standard superior border for the anteroposterior and posteroanterior inguinopelvic field is placed at L4 with the bottom of the field extending below the vulva. The lateral field margins are defined by the inguinal nodes that follow the inguinal ligament to the anterosuperior iliac spines (Figure 23.10) (82). Depending on the clinical or pathologic situation and the extent of iliac nodes at risk for recurrence, the upper border may be modified. Treatment is initiated with the superior border at L4 to include the entirety of the common external and internal iliacs. If periaortic node metastases are treated, the superior border is raised accordingly (1,82).

Another combination of portals used for treatment of the vulva and regional nodes consists of a similar large anteroposterior photon field encompassing the vulvar, pelvic, and inguinal targets. The narrower posteroanterior field includes only the central pelvic and vulvar target. Additional dose to the inguinal nodes at depth may be added with an electron field to minimize dose to the femoral heads. The electron contribution and energy is calculated from the CT-determined depth of the deep femoral vessels. This technique, shown in Figure 23.11, is fraught with setup and dosimetric difficulty (1,6,16,71).

Beam weighting with photons is adjusted to maximize dose uniformity across the target and to minimize dose to normal structures such as the small bowel and femoral heads. The combination of lower energy photons (4- or

6-MV) anteriorly and higher energy photons (10 or 24 MV) posteriorly results in favorable dose distribution (Figures 23.6a and Figures 23.11) (82). Care must be taken to prevent overdosing the thinner and sensitive central vulvar area. This can be managed with an anterior compensator or a partial transmission block (93,94). Contour asymmetry can be substantial in the inguinopelvic region as well and usually requires tissue compensation. It is important to verify and document the dose to the midpelvic, vulvar, and inguinofemoral targets (62,82,93). The role of bolus is determined on an individualized basis, according to the characteristics of the primary lesion noted above.

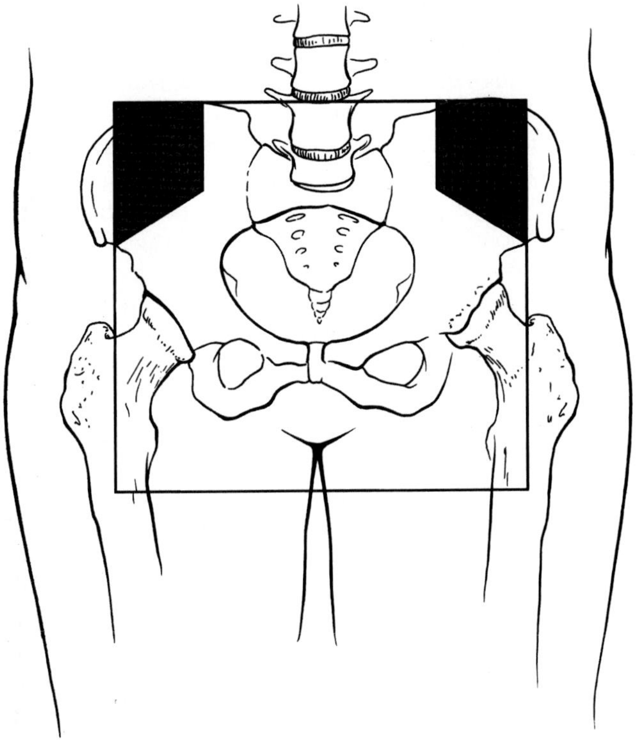

Figure 23.10. Photon portal for treating vulvar, pelvis, and regional nodes.

Radiation Dose and Fractionation

Dose recommendations for definitive vulvar radiation are related to tumor characteristics and stage. External beam irradiation to the vulva alone for minimally invasive early T1a disease entails total doses of 60 to 65 Gy (1). After an initial 40 to 45 Gy is delivered with vulvar portals, the remaining 15 to 20 Gy is administered to a reduced boost field using either electrons, photons, or an implant. With more advanced and larger lateralized Stage Ib and II tumors the vulva and regional lymphatics receive 45 to 50 Gy with vulvoinguinal portals. A boost of 15 to 25 Gy follows to achieve a dose of 65 to 70 Gy to the gross tumor volume. Final dose depends upon initial tumor size, tumor response, and skin tolerance (1,30,82,85).

Treatment of more advanced tumors usually entails a combination of radiation therapy and chemotherapy. As a rough "rule of thumb," when radiation is offered with chemotherapy the total dose of radiation is reduced by 10 Gy. Chemoradiation, in either the preoperative or definitive setting, provides for 45 to 50 Gy to an inguinopelvic field. The upper limit of 55 to 60 Gy is advocated only when a vulvar boost for gross disease is necessary (1,30,85). Lower doses (45 to 50 Gy) are also preferred for preoperative chemoradiation (70,74). An ongoing GOG clinical trial recommends radiation therapy doses of 55 Gy with concomitant fluorouracil and cisplatin (25).

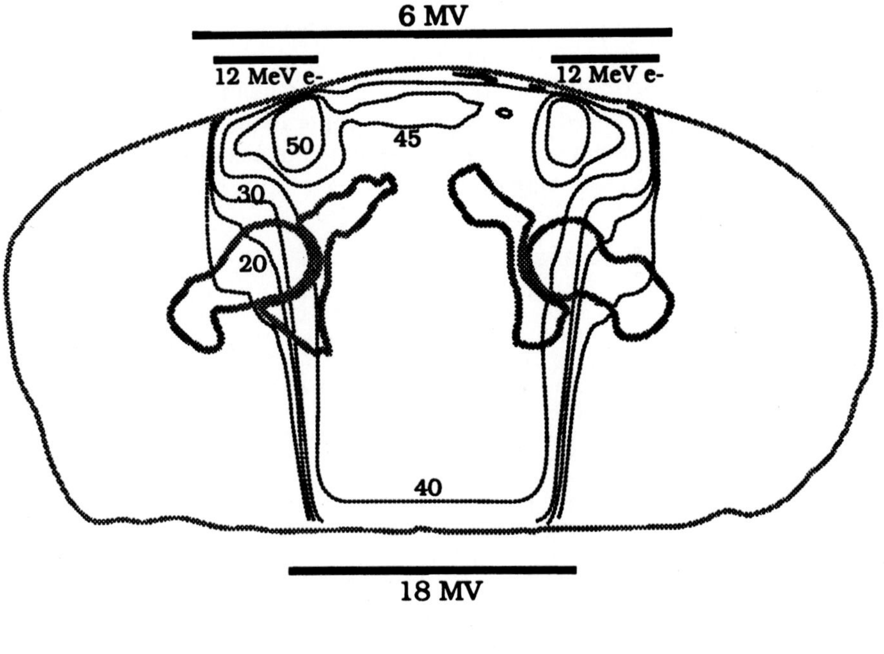

Figure 23.11. Typical isodose distribution for treatment of the lower pelvis and inguinal nodes using a combination of 6- and 18-MV photons and 12 MeV electrons to boost the lateral inguinal regions that are excluded from the posterior photon field. (Reprinted with permission from Eifel PJ. Vulvar carcinoma: radiation therapy or surgery for lymphatics? Front Radiat Ther Oncol 1994; 28:218–225).

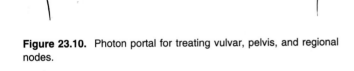

Dose for adjuvant radiation is individualized as well. In either the preoperative or postoperative setting, 45 to 50 Gy is frequently used with an added boost of 10 to 15 Gy for positive margins or gross disease. Similar doses are recommended for adjuvant nodal radiation. The lymphatics at risk are given 50 Gy, with 40 to 45 Gy delivered to the next nodal echelon. This is also customary for definitive nodal radiation in N0 disease (63). A boost of 10 to 20 Gy, to a reduced field is added for N1 disease treated with radiation alone. Advanced nodal disease including protuberant or ulcerating nodes are treated to a total dose of 60 to 70 Gy, with the lower limit used when surgical resection for residual disease is considered (1).

Fraction sizes between 1.7 to 2.0 Gy are standard for daily inguinopelvic photon treatments, with adjustment for concurrent chemotherapy. Five fractions are given weekly with all fields treated daily. When a lower fraction size is chosen, late vulvar fibrosis, atrophy, telangiectasia and necrosis are less likely (30). When fields extend more superiorly or if chemotherapy is administered, a photon fraction size of 1.7 to 1.8 Gy results in less late morbidity (1,30). Daily fraction sizes of 2.0 Gy are generally tolerated for electron boost (82,84). Electron fraction sizes over 3.0 Gy result in undesirable late skin effects (47).

Timing or sequencing considerations are of concern with combined modality treatment. Postoperative treatment begins 6 weeks after surgery or when wound healing permits. With less radical surgery, and if the groins are not to be treated, radiation therapy may begin 2 to 3 weeks after surgery. In the definitive or preoperative setting, treatment should begin without delay, once staging studies are complete.

Treatment interruptions may be anticipated, especially when chemotherapy is added. Moist desquamation is expected after 30 Gy. Some investigators plan for a 1- to 2-week treatment break after the third or fourth week of treatment, while others closely monitor skin tolerance and make individualized decisions as to the need for treatment interruptions. The radiobiological consequences of prolonged treatment times in vulvar tumors are unknown but extrapolating from other related tumor sites, greatly protracted courses should be avoided when possible (1,85,95).

Adverse Effects

The radiosensitivity of structures within traditional inguinopelvic portals is quite variable both among structures irradiated and among different individuals. Of primary concern in treatment of vulvar cancer is the skin tolerance. Skin necrosis is the dose limiting complication for vulvar irradiation in both the short and long term. Diarrhea is a common acute side effect with any pelvic portal but is generally well controlled with medication and dietary changes. A variety of constitutional symptoms occur, such as anorexia and fatigue, which are managed conservatively. Most acute effects are related to the fraction size, treatment volume, and use of concurrent chemotherapy but resolve with conservative management after treatments end (30,82,96).

The late complications of integumentary fibrosis, atrophy, telangiectasis and necrosis are minimized if the radiation fraction size is less than or equal to 1.8 Gy, provided excessive total doses are not used. For definitive radical radiation therapy, the dose limiting integumentary toxicity may be as high as 70 Gy without chemotherapy (30,96). Vaginal ulceration may not occur even with doses in excess of 100 Gy to the vaginal surface, but vaginal dryness and stenosis are commonly seen with standard pelvic doses (1). The latter may be minimized in part if the patient is able to comply with routine use of a vaginal dilator. Sexual dysfunction is multifactorial, with vaginal function playing only a limited overall role in treatment of vulvar structures. The psychosexual consequences from a radical surgical procedure can be considerable (34). In most instances dose will exceed 24 Gy or the dose at which ovarian ablation is inevitable (1,84).

Chronic tolerance of the internal pelvic structures varies as well (1,82,95). Small bowel tolerance limits the total doses of radiation delivered to the pelvis. The incidence of late bowel complications increases considerably at doses above 50 Gy and is also a function of volume, constitution, and fraction size (1,51,96). Adverse effects can include intestinal obstruction, fistula formation, malabsorption, and proctitis or rectal bleeding. There is a 5% actuarial 5-year incidence of femoral fractures in patients receiving doses of 50 Gy or more to the femoral heads (51).

In conclusion, treatment of vulvar cancer has improved over the past 2 decades because of a better understanding of the natural history of the disease as well as from efforts to use less radical surgery. This has allowed the role of radiation therapy and chemotherapy to expand so that individual therapy can be more fully optimized. A natural consequence of the success of multimodal treatments has led to their ever growing application, not only in the preoperative or adjuvant setting, but also for primary definitive therapy of vulvar cancers.

References

1. Perez C, Grigsby PW, Chao KSE, Garipagaoglu M. Vulva. In: Perez C, Brady L, eds. Principles and practice of radiation oncology. Philadelphia: Lippincott-Raven, 1997:1915–1942.
2. Merrow CP, Curtin JP, Townsend DE. Synopsis of gynecologic oncology, 4th ed. New York: Churchill Livingston, 1993:215–310.
3. Russell AH, Mesic JB, Scudder SA, Rosenberg PJ, Smith LH, Kinney WK. Synchronous radiation and cytotoxic chemotherapy for locally advanced or recurrent squamous cancer of the vulva. Gynecol Oncol 1992;47:14–20.
4. Cummings BJ, Keane TJ, O'Sullivan B, Wong CS, Catton CN. Epidermoid anal cancer: treatment by radiation alone or by radiation and 5-fluorouracil with and without mitomycin C. Int J Radiat Oncol Biol Phys 1991;21:1115.

5. Grey H. Grey's anatomy: the anatomical basis of medicine and surgery, 38th ed. New York: Churchill Livingstone, 1993:1861–1880.
6. Eifel PJ. Vulvar carcinoma: radiotherapy or surgery for the lymphatics. Front Radiat Ther Oncol 1994;28:218–225.
7. Hacker NF, ed. Essentials of obstetrics and gynecology. Philadelphia: WB Saunders, 1992.
8. Burke TW, Eifel P, McGuire W. Vulva. In: Hoskind WJ, Perez CA, Young RC, eds. Principles and practice of gynecologic oncology, 2nd ed. Philadelphia: Lippincott-Raven, 1996.
9. Homesley HD, Bundy BN, Sedlis A, Yordan E, Berek JS, Jahshan A. Prognostic factors for groin node metastasis in squamous cell carcinoma of the vulva (a gynecologic oncology group study). Gynecol Oncol 1993;49:279–283.
10. Boring CC, Squires T, Tong T. Cancer Statistics, 1997. CA Cancer J Clin 1997;47:1–20.
11. Lininger RA, Tavassoli FA. The pathology of vulvar neoplasia. Curr Opin Obstet Gynecol 1996;8:63–68.
12. van der Velden J, Hacker NF. Prognostic factors in squamous cell cancer of the vulva and the implications for treatment. Curr Opin Obstet Gynecol 1996;8:3–7.
13. Rutledge F, Mitchell M, Munsell M. Prognostic indicators for invasive carcinoma of the vulva. Gynecol Oncol 1991;42:239–244.
14. Franklin E, Rutledge F. Prognostic factors in epidermoid carcinoma of the vulva. Obstet Gynecol 1971;39:892–901.
15. Rutledge F, Smith JP, Franklin E. Carcinoma of the vulva. Am J Obstet Gynecol 1970;106:1117–1121.
16. Donaldson E, Powell D, Hanson M. Prognostic parameters in invasive vulvar cancer. Gynecol Oncol 1981;11:184–190.
17. Homesley H. Lymph node findings and outcome in squamous cell carcinoma of the vulva. Cancer 1994;74:2399–2402.
18. Homesley HD. Management of vulvar cancer. Cancer 1995;76: 2159–2170.
19. Homesley HD, Bundy BN, Sedlis A, Yordan E, et al. Assessment of current International Federation of Gynecology and Obstetrics staging of vulvar carcinoma relative to prognostic factors for survival: A Gynecologic Oncology Group study. Am J Obstet Gynecol 1991;164: 997–1004.
20. Hacker NF, Berek JS, Lagasse LD, Leuchter RS, Moore JG. Management of regional lymph nodes and their prognostic influence in vulvar cancer. Obstet Gynecol 1983;61:408–412.
21. Sedlis A, Homesley H, Bundy B. Positive groin lymph nodes in superficial squamous cell vulvar cancer. Am J Obstet Gynecol 1987;156: 1159–1164.
22. Collins C, Lee F, Lopez J. Invasive carcinoma of the vulva with lymph node metastases. Am J Obstet Gynecol 1971;109:446–452.
23. Paladini D, Cross P, Lopes A, Monaghan JM. Prognostic significance of lymph node variables in squamous cell carcinoma of the vulva. Cancer 1994;74:2491–2496.
24. Shepherd J. Revised FIGO staging for gynecologic cancer. Br J Obstet Gynaecol 1989;96:889–892.
25. Keys H. Gynecologic oncology group randomized trials of combined technique therapy for vulvar cancer. Cancer 1993;71(suppl): 1691–1696.
26. Heaps JM, Fu YS, Montz FJ, Hacker NF, Berek JS. Surgical-pathologic variables predictive of local recurrence in squamous cell carcinoma of the vulva. Gynecol Oncol 1990;54:309–314.
27. Pettersson F. Annual reports on results on treatment in gynecologic cancer, vol. 22. Stockholm: International Federation of Gynecologic Oncology, 1995;103–110.
28. Kelly JL, Stringer CA, Gerhenson DM, et al. Minimally invasive vulvar carcinoma: an indication for conservative surgical therapy. Gynecol Oncol 1992;44:240.
29. American Joint Committee on Cancer. Cancer staging manual. 5th ed. Philadelphia: Lippincott-Raven, 1997;81–84.
30. Thomas GM et al. Changing concepts in the management of vulvar cancer. Gynecol Oncol 1991;42:9–21.
31. Cavanagh D, Hoffman MS. Controversies in the management of vulvar carcinoma. Br J Obstet Gynaecol 1996;103:293–300.
32. Boutselis J. Radical vulvectomy for invasive squamous cell carcinoma of the vulva. Obstet Gynecol 1972;39:827–836.
33. Benedet J, Turko M, Fairey R. Squamous carcinoma of the vulva. Results of treatment, 1938–1976. Am J Obstet Gynecol 1979;134: 201–207.
34. Lin JY, Dubeshter B, Angel C, Dvoretsky PM. Morbidity and recurrence with modifications of radical vulvectomy and groin dissection. Gynecol Oncol 1992;47:80–86.
35. Sutton GP, Miser MR, Stehman FB, Look KY, Ehrlidi CE. Trends in the operative management of invasive squamous carcinoma of the vulva at Indiana University, 1974 to 1988. Am J Obstet Gynecol 1991; 164(6 Pt 1):1472–1478; discussion 1478–1481.
36. Hacker N, Leuchter RS, Berek JS, Castaldo TW, Lagasse LO. Radical vulvectomy and bilateral inguinal lymphadenectomy through separate groin incisions. Obstet Gynecol 1981;58:574–581.
37. Burke TW, Stringer A, Gershenson DM, Edwards CL, Morris M, Wharton JT. Radical wide excision and selective inguinal node dissection for squamous cell carcinoma of the vulva. Gynecol Oncol 1990;38: 328–332.
38. Hacker NF, van der Velden J. Conservative management of early vulvar cancer. Cancer 1993;71:1673–1677.
39. Homesley HD, Bundy BN, Sedlis A, Adcock L. Radiation therapy versus pelvic node resection for carcinoma of the vulva with positive groin nodes. Obstet Gynecol 1986;68(6):733–740.
40. Stehman FB, Bundy BN, Dvoretsky PM, Creasman WT. Early Stage I carcinoma of the vulva treated with ipsilateral superficial inguinal lymphadenectomy and modified radical hemivulvectomy: a prospective Gynecology Oncology Group Report. Obstet Gynecol 1992;79: 490–497.
41. Lanza A, Valli M, Caldarola B, D'Addato F, Re A, Boidi Trotti A. Radical vulvectomy and inguinal lymphadenectomy versus inguino-pelvic lymphadenectomy combined with radical vulvectomy and the role of radiotherapy. Eur J Gynaecol Oncol 1988;9(1):67–73.
42. Boronow R. Combined therapy as an alternative to exenteration for locally advanced vulvovaginal cancer. Cancer 1982;49:1085–1091.
43. Boronow RC, Hickman BT. Combined therapy as an alternative to exenteration for locally advanced vulvovaginal cancer. Am J Clin Oncol 1987;10(2):171–181.
44. Hacker N, Berek JS, Julliard GJ, Lagasset D. Preoperative radiation therapy for locally advanced vulvar cancer. Cancer 1984;54: 2056–2061.
45. Acosta A, Given F, Frazier A. Preoperative radiation therapy in the management of squamous cell carcinoma of the vulva: preliminary report. Am J Obstet Gynecol 1978;132:198–205.
46. Atlante G, Lombardi A, Mariani L, Vincenzoni C. Carcinoma of the vulva (1981–1985): analysis of a radio-surgical approach. Eur J Gynaecol Oncol 1989;10(5):341–348.
47. Frischbier H, Thomsen K. Treatment of cancer of the vulva with high energy electrons. Am J Obstet Gynecol 1971;111:431–435.
48. Frankendal B, Larson L, Westling P. Carcinoma of the vulva. Acta Radiologica 1973;12:165–174.
49. Ellis F. Cancer of the vulva treated by radiation. Br J Radiol 1949;22: 513–520.
50. Daly J, Million R. Radical vulvectomy combined with elective node irradiation for TxNO squamous carcinoma of the vulva. Cancer 1974; 34:161–165.
51. Grigsby P, Roberts H, Perez C. Femoral neck fracture following groin irradiation. Int J Radiat Oncol Biol Phys 1995;32:63–67.
52. Prempree T, Amormorn R. Radiation treatment of recurrent carcinoma of the vulva. Cancer 1984;54:1943–1949.
53. Helgason N, Hass A, Latourette H. Radiation therapy in carcinoma of the vulva. Cancer 1972;30:997–1000.
54. Slevin NJ, Pointon RC. Radiation radiotherapy for carcinoma of the vulva. Br J Radiol 1989;62:145–147.
55. Anderson JA, Cassady R, Shimm DS, Stea B. Vulvar Carcinoma. Int J Radiat Oncol Biol Phys 1995;32(5):1351–1357.
56. Pao WM, Perez CA, Kuske RR, Sommers GM, Camel HM, Galakatos AE. Radiation therapy and conservation surgery for primary and recurrent carcinoma of the vulva: report of 40 patients and a review of the literature. Int J Radiat Oncol Biol Phys 1988;14(6):1123–1132.
57. Perez CA. Management of vulvar cancer. Front Radiat Ther Oncol 1991;25:183–186, discussion, 207–208.
58. Randall ME, Evans L. Issues in gynecologic radiation oncology. Curr Opin Oncol 1991;3:920–929.
59. Stehman FB, Bundy BW, Thomas G, Varia M, Okagaki T, Roberts J. Groin dissection versus groin radiation in carcinoma of the vulva: a Gynecologic Oncology Group study. Int J Radiat Oncol Biol Phys 1992;24(2):389–396.

60. Koh WJ, Chiu M, Stelzer KJ, Greer BE, Mastras D, Comsia N. Femoral vessel depth and the implications for groin node radiation. Int J Radiat Oncol Biol Phys 1993;27:969–974.
61. Kalidas H. Influence of inguinal node anatomy on radiation therapy techniques. Med Dosimetry 1995;20(4):295–300.
62 Lanciano RM, Corn BW. Groin node irradiation for vulvar cancer: treatment planning must do more than scratch the surface. Int J Radiat Oncol Biol Phys 1993;27(4):987–989; discussion 991.
63. Petereit DG, Mehta MP, Buchler DA, Kinsella TJ. A retrospective review of nodal treatment for vulvar cancer. Am J Clin Oncol 1993; 16(1):38–42.
64. Petereit DG, Mehta MP, Buchler DA, Kinsella TJ. Inguinofemoral radiation of N0,N1 vulvar cancer may be equivalent to lymphadenectomy if proper radiation technique is used. Int J Radiat Oncol Biol Phys 1993;27(4):963–967.
65. Kucera H, Weghaupt K. The electrosurgical operation of vulvar carcinoma with postoperative irradiation of inguinal lymph nodes. Gynecol Oncol 1988;29(2):158–167.
66. Jaakkola M, Rantanen V, Greman S, Kulmala J, Grenman R. In vitro concurrent paclitaxel and radiation of four vulvar squamous cell carcinoma cell lines. Cancer 1996;77:1940–1946.
67. Pekkola-Heino K, Kumala J, Grenman S, Carey TE, Grenman R. Radiation response of vulvar squamous cell carcinoma (UM-SCV-1A, UM-SCV-1B, UM-SCV-2, and A-431) cells in vitro. Cancer Res 1989;49(17): 4876–4878.
68. Evans LS, Kersh CR, Constable WC, Taylor PT. Concomitant 5-fluorouracil, mitomycin-C, and radiotherapy for advanced gynecologic malignancies. Int J Radiat Oncol Biol Phys 1988;15(4):901–906.
69. Thomas G, Dembo A, DePetrillo A, Pringle J, Ackerman I, Bryson P. Concurrent radiation and chemotherapy in vulvar carcinoma. Gynecol Oncol 1989;34(3):263–7.91.
70. Eifel PJ, Morris M, Burke TW, Levenback C, Gershenson DM. Prolonged continuous infusion cisplatin and 5-fluorouracil with radiation for locally advanced carcinoma of the vulva. Gynecol Oncol 1995; 59(1):51–56.
71. Eifel PJ. Radiotherapy versus radical surgery for gynecologic neoplasms: carcinomas of the cervix and vulva. Front Radiat Ther Oncol 1993;27:130–142.
72. Lupi G, Raspagliesi F, Zucali R, Fontanelli R, Paladini D, Kenda R. Combined preoperative chemoradiation followed by radical surgery in locally advanced vulvar carcinoma. A pilot study. Cancer 1996; 77(8):1472–1478
73. Berek JS, Heaps JM, Fu YS, Julliard GJ, Hacker NF. Concurrent cisplatin and 5-fluorouracil chemotherapy and radiation therapy for advanced-stage squamous carcinoma of the vulva. Gynecol Oncol 1991; 42(3):197–201.
74. Landoni F, Maneo A, Zanetta G, Colomb A, Nava S, Placa F. Concurrent preoperative chemotherapy with 5-fluorouracil and mitomycin C and radiotherapy (FUMIR) followed by limited surgery in locally advanced and recurrent vulvar carcinoma. Gynecol Oncol 1996; 61(3):321–327.
75. Wahlen SA, Slater JD, Wagner RJ, Wang WA, Keeney ED, Hocko JM. Concurrent radiation therapy and chemotherapy in the treatment of primary squamous cell carcinoma of the vulva. Cancer 1995;75: 2289–2294.
76. Koh WJ, Wallace HJ III, Greer BE, Cain J, Stelzer KJ, Russell KJ. Combined radiotherapy and chemotherapy in the management of local-regionally advanced vulvar cancer. Int J Radiat Oncol Biol Phys 1993; 26(5):809–816.
77. Roberts WS, Kavanaugh JJ, Greenberg H, Bryson SC, La Polla JP, Townsend PA. Concomitant radiation therapy and chemotherapy in the treatment of advanced squamous carcinoma of the lower female genital tract. Gynecol Oncol 1989;34:183–186.
78. Roberts WS, Hoffman MS, Kavanaugh JJ, Fiorica JV, Greenberg H, Finan MA. Further experience with radiation therapy and concomitant intravenous chemotherapy in advanced carcinoma of the lower female genital tract. Gynecol Oncol 1991;43(3):233–236.
79. Hoffman MS, Roberts WS, La Polla JP, Cavanaugh D. Recent modifications in the treatment of invasive squamous cell carcinoma of the vulva. Obstet Gynecol Survey 1989;44(4):227–233.
80. Manavi M, Gerger A, Jucera E, Vavra N, Kucera H. Does T1, NO-1 vulvar cancer treated by vulvectomy but not lymphadenectomy need inguinofemoral radiation? Int J Radiat Oncol Biol Phys 1997;38(4): 749–753.
81. McCall AR, Olson MC, Potkul RK. The variation of inguinal lymph node depth in adult women and its importance in planning elective irradiation for vulvar cancer. Cancer 1995;75(9):2286–2288.
82. Potish RA. The gynecologic malignancies. In: Khan FM, Potish RA, eds. Treatment planning in radiation oncology. Baltimore: Williams & Wilkins, 1998;354–368.
83. Nobler M. Efficacy of a perineal teletherapy portal in the management of vulvar and vaginal cancer. Radiology 1972;103:393–397.
84. Khan FM. The physics of radiation therapy. 2nd ed. Baltimore: Williams & Wilkins, 1994.
85. Perez CA, Grigsby PW, Galakatos A, Swanson R, Camel HM, Kao MS. Radiation therapy in management of carcinoma of the vulva with emphasis on conservation therapy. Cancer 1993;71(11):3707–3716.
86. Tod M. Radium implantation treatment of carcinoma of the vulva. Br J Radiol 1949;22:508–512.
87. Hoffman M, Greenberg S, Greenberg H, Fiorica JV, Roberts WS, La Polla JP. Interstitial radiotherapy for the treatment of advanced or recurrent vulvar and distal vaginal malignancy. Am J Obstet Gynecol 1990;162(5):1278–1289.
88. Pohar S, Hoffstetter S, Peiffert D, Luporsi E, Pernot M. Effectiveness of brachytherapy in treating carcinoma of the vulva. Int J Radiat Oncol Biol Phys 1995;32(5):1455–1460.
89. Jafari K, Magalotti M. Radiation therapy in carcinoma of the vulva. Cancer 1981;47:686–672.
90. Wang C, Chin YY, Leung S, Chen HC, Sun LM, Fang FM. Topographic distribution of inguinal lymph nodes metastasis: significance in determination of treatment margin for elective inguinal lymph nodes irradiation of low pelvic tumors. Int J Radiat Oncol Biol Phys 1996;35: 133–136.
91. Eifel PJ. Radiotherapy versus radical surgery for gynecologic neoplasms: carcinomas of the cervix and vulva. Front Radiat Ther Oncol 1993;27:130–142.
92. Burke TW, Stringer CA, Gershenson DM, Edwards CL, Morris M, Wharton JT. Radical wide excision and selective inguinal node dissection for squamous cell carcinoma of the vulva. Gynecol Oncol 1990; (38)328–332.
93. Dusenbery KE, Carlson JW, LaPorte RM, Unger JA, Goswitz JJ, Roback DM. Radical vulvectomy with postoperative irradiation for vulvar cancer: therapeutic implications of a central block. Int J Radiat Oncol Biol Phys 1994;29(5):989–998.
94. King GC, Sonnik DA, Kalend AM, Wu A, Kalnicki S. Transmission block technique for the treatment of the pelvis and perineum including the inguinal lymph nodes: dosimetric considerations. Med Dosimetry 1993;18(1):7–12.
95. Hall E. Radiobiology for the radiologist. 4th ed. Philadelphia: JB Lippincott, 1994.
96. Snijders-Keilholz T, Trimbos JB, Hermans J, Leer JW. Management of vulvar carcinoma radiation toxicity, results and failure analysis in 44 patients (1980–1989). Acta Obstetricia et Gynecologica Scandinavica 1993;72(8):668–673.

Chapter 24

Carcinoma of the Vagina

Carlos A. Perez

ANATOMY

The vagina is a muscular, dilatable tube, approximately 7.5 cm in length, located posterior to the base of the bladder and urethra and anterior to the rectum. The upper fourth of the posterior wall is separated from the rectum by a reflection of peritoneum called the pouch of Douglas. At its uppermost extent the vaginal wall merges with the uterine cervix, attaching at a higher point on the posterior wall than on the anterior wall, which constitutes the vaginal fornices. The vaginal wall is composed of three layers: the mucosa, the muscularis, and the adventitia. The inner mucosal layer is formed by a thick, nonkeratinizing, stratified, squamous epithelium overlying a basement membrane containing many papillae. The epithelium normally contains no glands but is lubricated by mucous secretions originating in the cervix. The muscularis layer is composed of smooth muscle fibers arranged circularly on the inner portion and longitudinally on the thicker outer portion. A vaginal sphincter is formed by skeletal muscle at the introitus. The adventitia is a thin, outer connective tissue layer that merges with that of adjacent organs.

The lymphatics in the upper portion of the vagina drain primarily via the lymphatics of the cervix, whereas those in the lowest portion of the vagina drain either cephalad to cervical lymphatics or follow drainage patterns of the vulva into femoral and inguinal nodes. The anterior vaginal wall usually drains into the deep pelvic nodes, including the interiliac and parametrial nodes.

NATURAL HISTORY AND PATTERNS OF FAILURE

Vaginal cancers occur most commonly on the posterior wall of the upper third of the vagina. In an extensive review of the literature, Plentl and Friedman (1) found that 51.7% of primary vaginal cancers occurred in the upper third of the vagina and 57.6% on the posterior wall.

Tumors originating in the vagina may spread along the vaginal wall to involve the cervix or vulva. It is noteworthy that, if biopsies of the cervix or the vulva are positive at the time of initial diagnosis, the tumor cannot be considered a primary vaginal lesion.

Because of the absence of anatomic barriers, vaginal tumors readily extend into surrounding tissues. Lesions on the anterior vaginal wall may penetrate the vesicovaginal septum; those on the posterior wall may eventually invade the rectovaginal septum. Vaginal cancer may invade the paracolpal and parametrial tissues, extending into the obturator fossa, cardinal ligaments, lateral pelvic walls, and uterosacral ligaments.

The incidence of positive pelvic nodes at diagnosis varies with stage and location of the primary tumor. Because the lymphatic system of the vagina is so complex, any nodal group may be involved, regardless of the location of the lesion (1). Involvement of inguinal nodes is most common when the lesion is located in the lower third of the vagina (2). Chyle et al (3), in an update of the M.D. Anderson Cancer Center series (301 patients), noted a 10-year actuarial pelvic nodal failure rate of 28% and an inguinal failure rate of 16% in patients who developed local recurrence in contrast to 4% and 2%, respectively, in the group without local recurrence ($P < 0.001$).

Because of the multicentricity of the disease, a few local failures (5 to 10%) have been noted in patients with stage 0 disease, but pelvic recurrences or distant metastases have not been reported. In patients with stage I disease, the frequency of pelvic recurrence is 10 to 20%. Comparable figures are reported for distant metastases. In patients with stage II disease, in which there is more paravaginal or parametrial infiltration, the incidence of pelvic recurrence increases to 35%, and distant metastases are more common (20 to 25%). In patients with stage III disease, the incidence of local recurrence varies between 25 and 37%, and the distant metastasis rate is 50%. Patients with stage IV disease have a high incidence of pelvic failure (58%) and distant metastases (about 50%).

PROGNOSTIC FACTORS

The most significant factor influencing prognosis is clinical stage of the tumor, which reflects size and depth of penetration into the vaginal wall or surrounding tissues (3,4). Patient age, extent of mucosal involvement, gross appearance of the lesion, and degree of differentiation and keratinization do not appear to be significant factors (4,5). In patients with adenocarcinoma of the vagina, Chyle et al (3) noted a higher incidence of local recurrence compared with squamous cell carcinoma (52% and 20%, respectively, at 10 years), higher distant metastasis rate (48% and 10%, respectively), and lower 10-year survival (20% versus 50%).

Patients with nonepithelial tumors (sarcoma, melanoma) have a poor prognosis with a high incidence of local failure and distant metastasis.

Livingstone (6) reported that lesions located in the upper vagina have a better prognosis. Chyle et al (3) observed 17% pelvic relapse in patients with upper vagina tumors, 36% with mid- or lower vagina tumors, and 42% with whole-vaginal involvement. Local relapse for tumors in the posterior wall was 38% compared with 22% for other locations. However, other authors have found no correlation between location of the primary tumor and treatment results (4,7–9).

Overexpression of HER-2/neu oncogenes in squamous cancer of the lower genital tract is a rare event that may be associated with aggressive biologic behavior (10).

GENERAL MANAGEMENT

Some authors advocate a surgical approach (11), but operations are generally discouraged because of the excellent tumor control and good functional results obtained with adequate radiation therapy. Surgery may be appropriate treatment, particularly in patients with localized intraepithelial disease, in young patients in whom there is a desire to preserve ovarian function, and in patients with verrucous carcinoma (12). Surgery may be reserved for the treatment of irradiation failures, for nonepithelial tumors, and for stage I clear cell adenocarcinomas in young women (13).

Radiation therapy is the preferred treatment for most carcinomas of the vagina. Paravaginal or parametrial interstitial implants or both should be considered if residual tumor is present after the planned external and intracavitary therapy is completed. Additional doses of 20 to 25 Gy to a limited volume are usually well tolerated (14–16).

For locally extensive tumors, a combination of irradiation and surgery has been suggested to improve therapeutic results (17), although more complications may occur with combined therapy.

Carcinoma in Situ

An intracavitary low dose rate (LDR) application delivering 65 to 80 Gy to the involved vaginal mucosa is usually sufficient to control in situ lesions, which do not extend beyond the basement membrane of the squamous epithelium. Higher doses may cause significant vaginal fibrosis and stenosis. Because vaginal carcinoma tends to be multicentric, the entire vaginal mucosa should be treated to a dose of 50 to 60 Gy.

Stage I

These invasive lesions are usually 0.5 to 1 cm thick and may involve one or more vaginal walls. Superficial tumors may be treated with only an intracavitary cylinder covering the entire vagina (60 Gy LDR mucosal dose) and an additional 20 to 30 Gy mucosal dose to the tumor area.

If the lesion is thicker and localized to one wall, a single-plane implant may be used with an intracavitary cylinder to increase the depth dose and limit excessive irradiation to the vaginal mucosa. A dose of 60 to 65 Gy is delivered to the entire vaginal mucosa with the cylinder and an additional 15 to 20 Gy to the gross tumor, calculated 0.5 cm beyond the interstitial implant plane, with the involved vaginal mucosa receiving an estimated 80 to 100 Gy (Figure 24.1) (18).

Use of external-beam irradiation for stage I disease should be reserved for aggressive lesions (more invasive, infiltrating, or poorly differentiated) to supplement intracavitary and interstitial therapy. The whole pelvis is treated with 10 or 20 Gy; additional parametrial dose should be delivered with a midline 5 half-value layer (HVL) block shielding the brachytherapy-treated volume to give a total of 45 to 50 Gy to the parametria.

Stage IIA

Patients with stage IIA tumors have more advanced paravaginal disease without extensive parametrial infiltration. They should be treated with a greater external irradiation dose: 20 Gy to the whole pelvis and additional parametrial dose with a midline block (5 HVL) for a total of 45 to 50 Gy. A combination of interstitial and intracavitary therapy may also be used to deliver a minimum of 45 to 55 Gy 0.5 cm beyond the deep margin of the tumor (in addition to the whole-pelvis dose). Double-plane implants may be necessary because of extensive tumor volume (Figure 24.2).

Stage IIB, Stage III, and Stage IV

For advanced tumors 40 Gy whole pelvis and 55 to 60 Gy total parametrial dose (with midline shielding) have

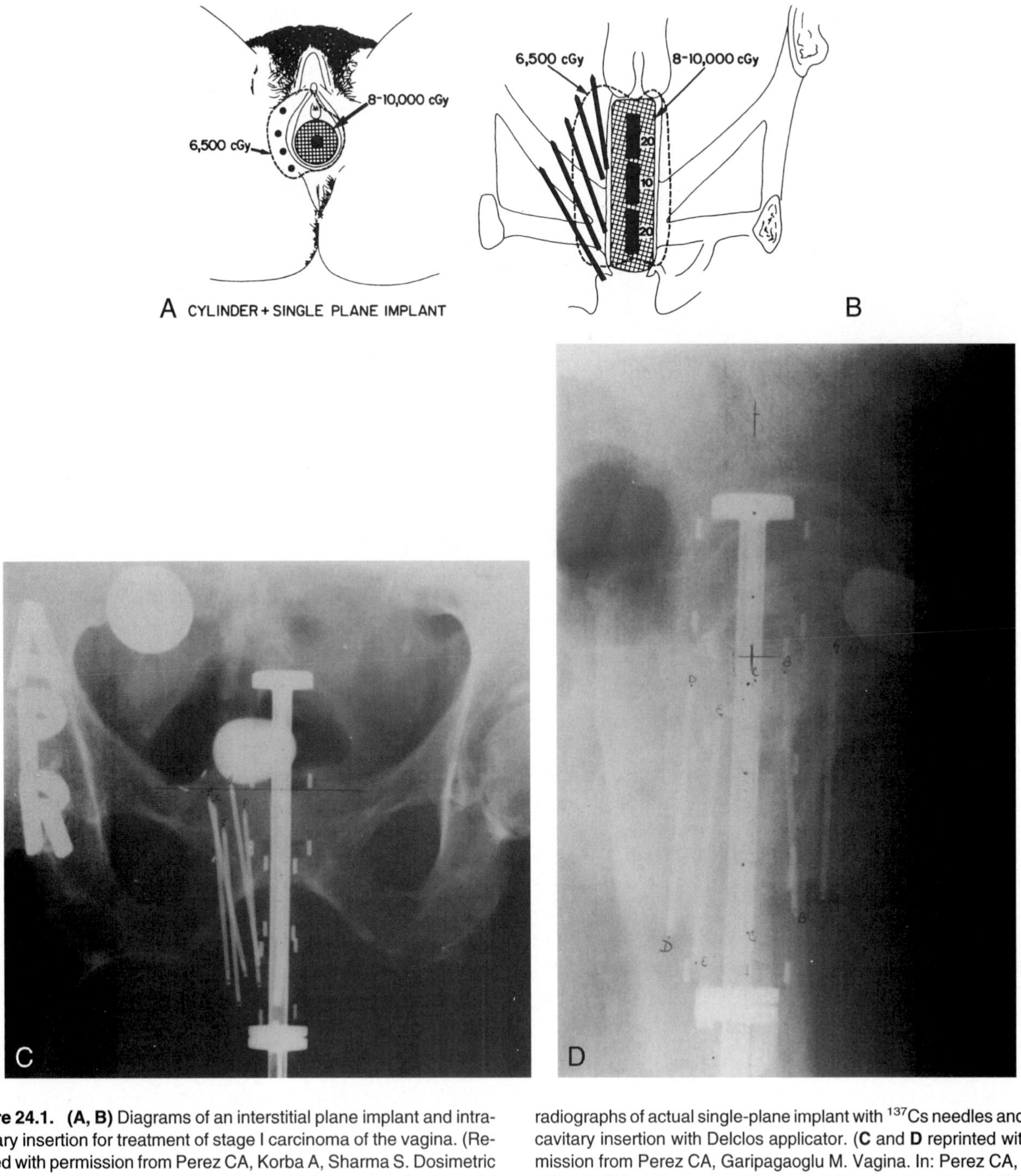

Figure 24.1. (A, B) Diagrams of an interstitial plane implant and intracavitary insertion for treatment of stage I carcinoma of the vagina. (Reprinted with permission from Perez CA, Korba A, Sharma S. Dosimetric considerations in irradiation of carcinoma of the vagina. Int J Radiat Oncol Biol Phys 1977;2:639–649.) Anteroposterior **(C)** and lateral **(D)** radiographs of actual single-plane implant with ^{137}Cs needles and intracavitary insertion with Delclos applicator. (**C** and **D** reprinted with permission from Perez CA, Garipagaoglu M. Vagina. In: Perez CA, Brady LW, eds. Principles and practice of radiation oncology. 3rd ed. Philadelphia: Lippincott-Raven; 1998.)

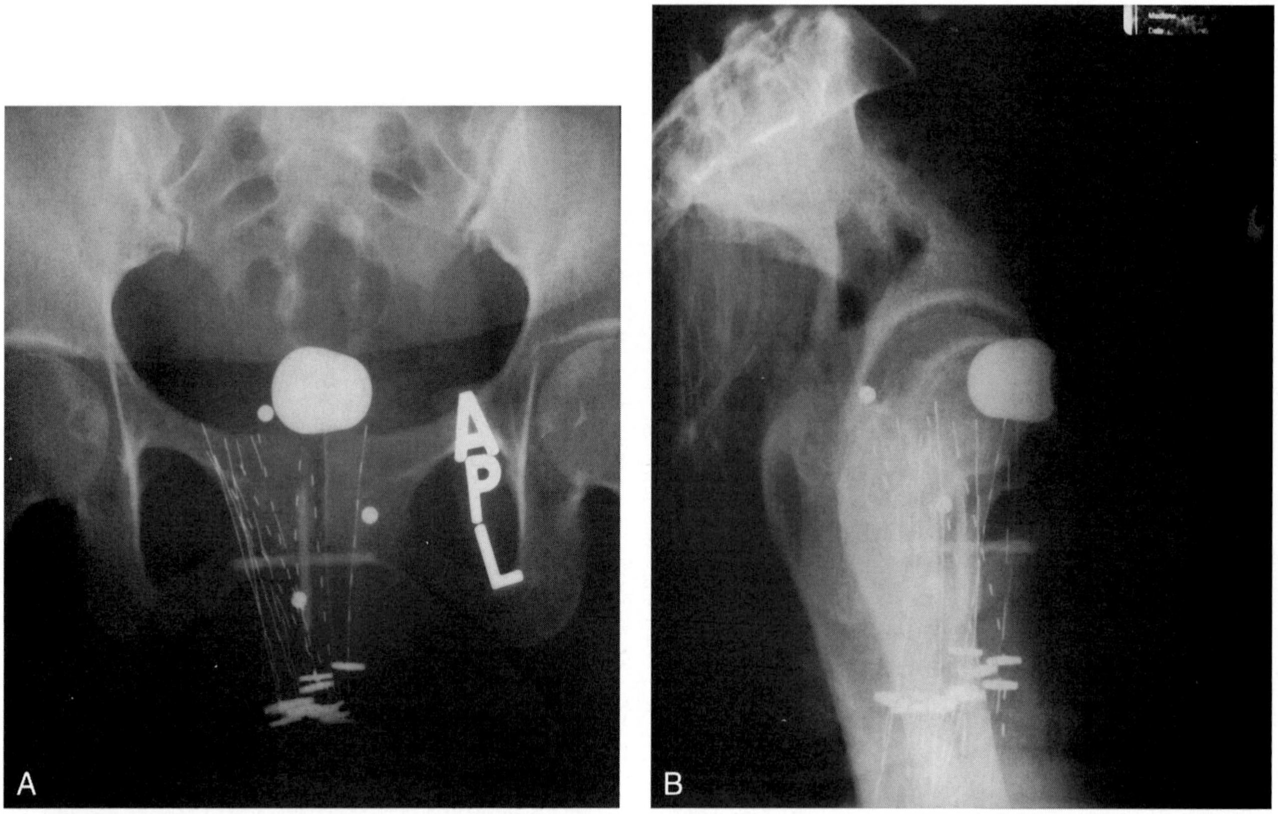

Figure 24.2. Anteroposterior **(A)** and lateral **(B)** radiographs of intracavitary/interstitial implant in patient with stage II carcinoma of the vagina. (Reprinted with permission from Perez CA, Garipagaoglu M. Vagina. In: Perez CA, Brady LW, eds. Principles and practice of radiation oncology. 3rd ed. Philadelphia: Lippincott-Raven; 1998.)

been given in combination with intracavitary insertions and interstitial implants to deliver a total tumor dose of 75 to 80 Gy to the vaginal tumor and 65 Gy to parametrial and paravaginal extensions. The interstitial implant boost dose sometimes given to patients with extensive parametrial infiltration is 20 to 25 Gy (Figures 24.2 and 24.3).

Boronow et al (17) proposed an alternative to exenterative procedures for locally advanced vulvovaginal carcinoma, using radiation therapy to treat the pelvic (internal genital) disease and a radical vulvectomy with bilateral inguinal node dissection to treat the external genital tumor. External irradiation to the pelvis and inguinal nodes consists of 45 to 50 Gy. When combined with intracavitary insertions, maximum doses of 80 to 85 Gy are delivered to the vaginal mucosa with both modalities.

Radiation therapy guidelines for vaginal carcinoma are outlined in Table 24.1.

RADIATION THERAPY TECHNIQUES

External Irradiation

The technical approach to vaginal carcinoma is similar to that for carcinoma of the uterine cervix. External irradiation should be administered using anteroposterior (AP-PA) pelvic portals that encompass the entire vagina down to the introitus and the pelvic lymph nodes to the upper portion of the common iliac chain. Portals of 15 × 15 cm or 15 × 18 cm at the skin (16.5 cm^2 or 16.5 × 20.5 cm at isocenter) are usually adequate. The distal margin of the tumor should be identified with a radiopaque marker or bead when simulation radiographs are taken. In tumors involving the middle or lower third of the vagina, the inguinal and adjacent femoral lymph nodes should be electively treated (45 to 50 Gy), which requires a modification of the standard portals (Figure 24.4A). For patients with clinically palpable nodes, additional doses of 15 Gy (calculated at 4 to 5 cm) are necessary with reducing portals (Figure 24.4B). These doses can be achieved by using unequal loadings (2AP to 1PA) with 10 to 18 MV photons, in which case a 2-cm bolus should be used when palpable lymph nodes are present. Alternatively, equal loading with photons may be used to deliver 45 to 50 Gy to the pelvic and inguinal nodes. If necessary, reduced AP portals are used to deliver a boost dose to the inguinal nodes with Cobalt-60 (^{60}Co) or electrons (12 to 16 MeV). Special attention is needed to avoid areas of overlap (Figure 24.4B). A combination of 6 MV x-rays on the AP portal and 18 MV photons

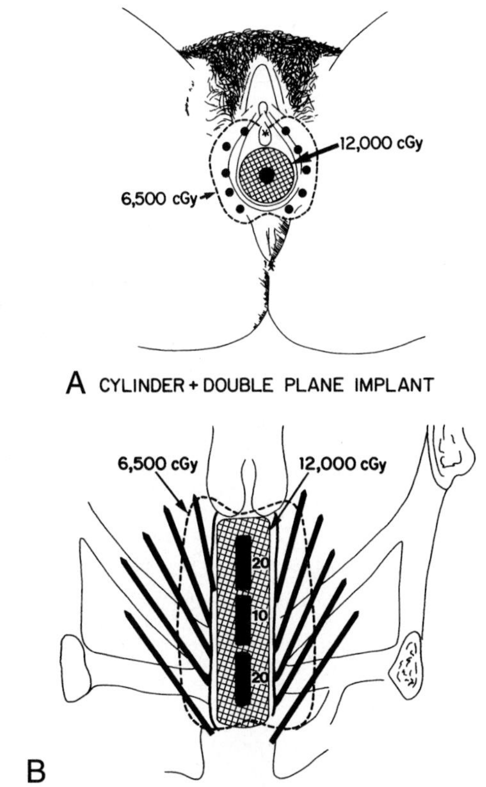

Figure 24.3. A. Cross-section (perineal) view of source arrangement for interstitial and intracavitary implant in a patient with involvement of the right and left lateral vaginal walls and paravaginal tissues. **B.** Coronal illustration of interstitial and intracavitary implant for same patient. (Reprinted with permission from Perez CA, Grigsby PW, Williamson JF. Clinical applications of brachytherapy I. Low-dose-rate. In: Perez CA, Brady LW, eds. Principles and practice of radiation oncology. 3rd ed. Philadelphia: Lippincott-Raven; 1998.)

on the PA portal will yield a higher dose to the inguinal nodes in relation to the midplane tumor dose. After a specified tumor dose is delivered to the whole pelvis (20 to 40 Gy, depending on extent of tumor), a midline rectangular or wedge block is interposed (Figure 24.4C), and additional irradiation is given to the parametrial tissues.

Low Dose Rate Brachytherapy

Intracavitary Applicators

Intracavitary therapy is carried out using vaginal cylinders such as the Burnett, Bloedorn, Delclos, or MIRALVA applicator. The largest possible diameter should be used to improve the ratio of mucosa to tumor dose. Afterloading vaginal cylinders have been designed using a central hollow metallic cylinder, in which the sources are placed, and plastic "jackets" of varying diameter and 2.5 cm in length, which are inserted over the cylinder.

When indicated, domed cylinders are used for homogeneous irradiation of the vaginal cuff. Delclos (19) recommends that a short cesium source be used at the top to obtain a uniform dose around the dome, since a lower dose is noted at the end of the linear cesium sources. Sharma and Bhandare (20) described an ellipsoid design for the dome of Delclos applicators to obtain a more homogeneous dose. The Bloedorn applicator consisted of a device incorporating the configuration of vaginal colpostats and a vaginal cylinder. Although extensively used, it was never described in detail (19).

When the lesion is in the upper third, the upper vagina can be treated with the same intracavitary arrangement used for carcinoma of the uterine cervix, including an intra-

Table 24.1. Carcinoma of Vagina: Treatment Guidelines at Mallinckrodt Institute of Radiology

	External Radiation Therapy (Gy)			
FIGO Stage	Whole Pelvis	Parametrial (midline block)	Brachytherapy (Gy)	Total Tumor Dose (Gy)
0	—	—	Intracavitary: 65–80 SD to tumor, 60 to entire vagina	65–80
I Superficial	—	—	Intracavitary: 65–80 SD to entire vagina	65–80
0.5 cm thick	—	—	Intracavitary/interstitial: 65–70 at 0.5 cm (mucosa, 100)	65–70
IIA	20	30	Intracavitary/interstitial: 60–65 TD	70–75
IIB	20	30	Intracavitary/interstitial: 65–70 TD	75
III, IV	40	10[a]	Intracavitary: 50–60 Interstitial: 20–30 boost to parametrium	80

Distal vagina lesions: inguinal lymph nodes receive 50 Gy (at 3 cm). Interstitial doses are usually calculated 0.5 cm from plane of implant.
SD, surface dose; TD, tumor dose.
[a] Additional 10 Gy boost to parametrium.
(Reprinted with permission from Perez CA, Garipagaoglu M. Vagina. In: Perez CA, Brady LW, eds. Principles and practice of radiation oncology. 3rd ed. Philadelphia: Lippincott–Raven, 1998)

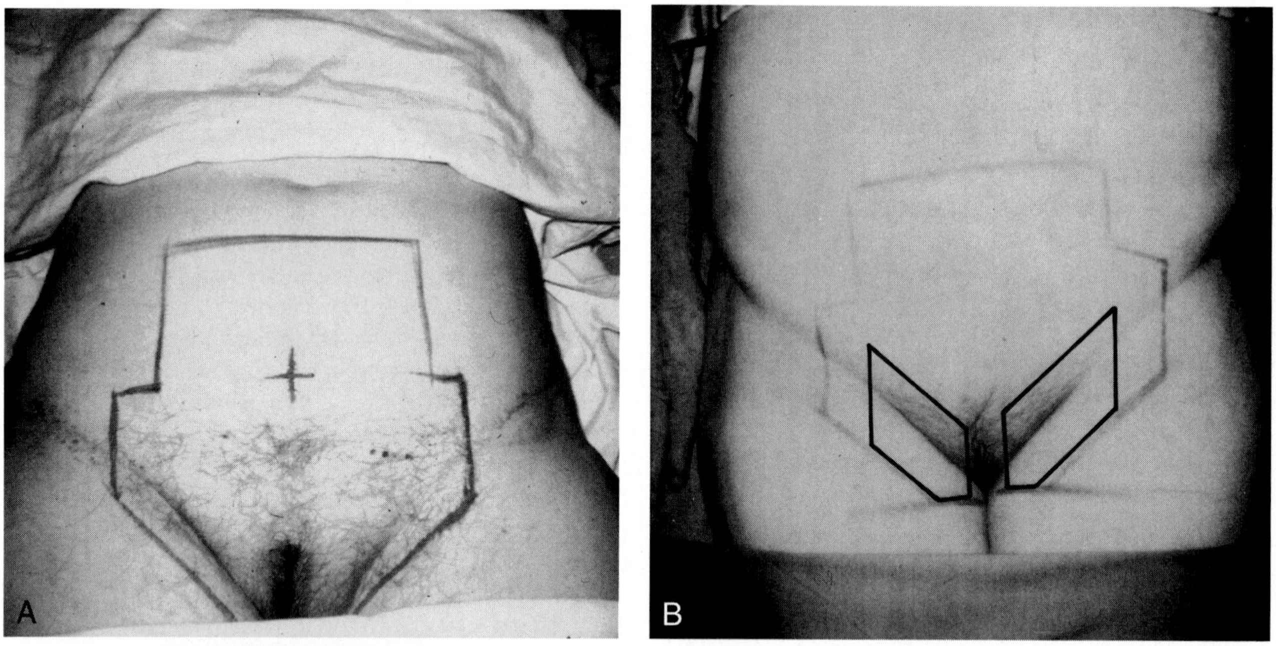

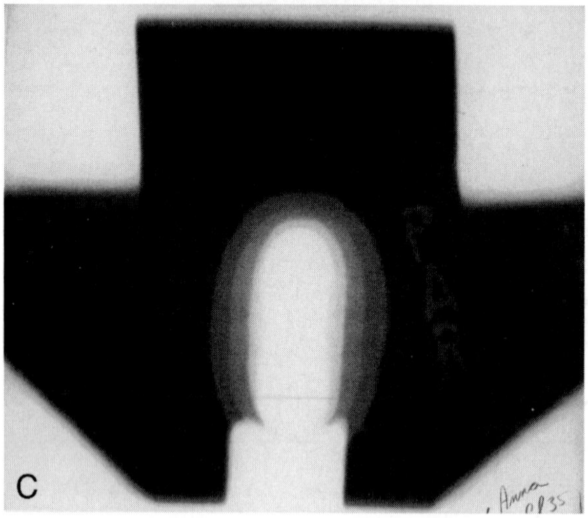

Figure 24.4. A. Example of portal used to treat the whole pelvis and inguinal lymph nodes in carcinoma of the vagina. **B.** Variation of treatment portals, with small fields to boost the inguinal lymph node dose with ^{60}Co or electrons (12 to 16 MeV). Overlap of this field should be carefully avoided. **C.** A step-wedged midline block is used to shield the area treated with higher intracavitary doses (for a portion of the treatment). (Reprinted with permission from Perez CA, Garipagaoglu M. Vagina. In: Perez CA, Brady LW, eds. Principles and practice of radiation oncology. 3rd ed. Philadelphia: Lippincott-Raven; 1998.)

uterine tandem and vaginal colpostats. The middle and distal vagina are treated with a subsequent insertion of a vaginal cylinder. If the entire dose has been delivered to the upper vagina, a blank source should be used in the cylinder. Otherwise, a lower intensity source can be inserted to deliver the desired dose. Alternatively, the insertion can be condensed in one procedure using the MIRALVA (afterloading vaginal applicator) designed by Perez et al (21), which incorporates two ovoid sources and a central tandem that can be used to treat the entire vagina (alone or in combination with the uterine cervix).

Vaginal molds for individualized intracavitary applications have been used (22). When any type of vaginal applicator is used, it is important to determine the surface dose in addition to the tumor dose. Tables have been generated for ^{137}Cs sources (23,24).

Muench and Nath (25) described a shielded vaginal applicator used with encapsulated Americium (^{241}Am) and published dosimetry studies. A few patients with recurrent pelvic, including vaginal, tumors have been treated with this applicator with significant reduction of bladder and rectal doses because of the profound effect of the shielding on the 16 keV photons emitted by the isotope.

Interstitial therapy with ^{137}Cs, ^{226}Ra needles, or afterloading Iridium-192 (^{192}Ir) needles has been used. Depending on the extent and thickness of the tumor, single-plane, double-plane, or volume implants should be planned. ^{252}Cf has been used in a few patients (26). In general, the vulva is sutured with silk or chromic catgut for the duration of the cylinder implant.

A description of the most frequently used applicators follows.

Vaginal Cylinders Afterloading vaginal cylinders were designed in the mid-1960s (27) to irradiate the vagina when disease extends from the uterine cervix along the vaginal walls; they are also used to hold a vaginal source when the vaginal anatomy is compromised (too narrow for ovoids) and to irradiate some vaginal tumors.

Cylinders are available in various diameters (2 to 5 cm) to fit any vaginal diameter (Figure 24.5) (28). They can be used in the same diameter or combined in different

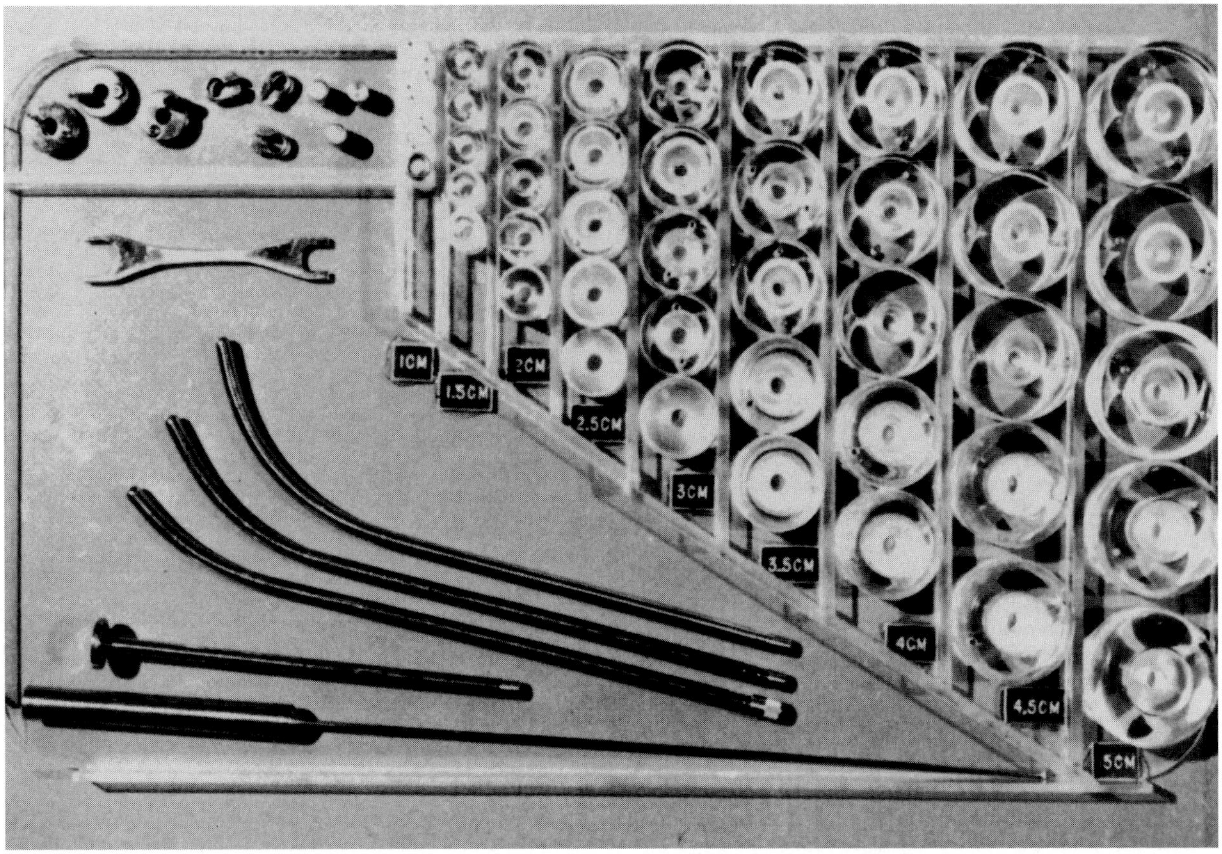

Figure 24.5. Tray with afterloadable tandems and vaginal cylinders. Cylinders are 2.5 cm in height each and are available from 1 to 5 cm in diameter to fit any vaginal diameter. As many cylinders as needed are mounted on vaginal component of intrauterine tube. Lead markers inserted at top and bottom identify cylinder and relationship to uterine cervix or to extension of tumor along vagina. (Reprinted with permission from Delclos L, Fletcher GH, Moore EB, et al. Minicolpostats, dome cylinders, other additions and improvements of the Fletcher-Suit afterloadable system: indications and limitations of their use. Int J Radiat Oncol Biol Phys 1980;6:1195–1206.)

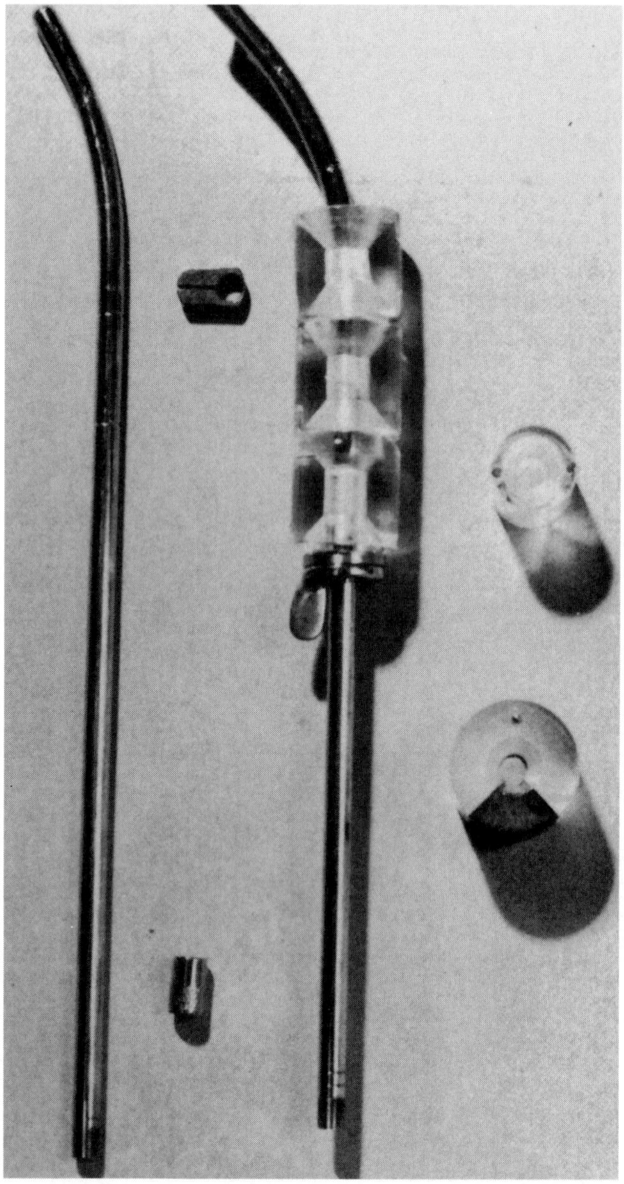

Figure 24.6. From left to right: intrauterine tandem, flange without keel, sample of three vaginal cylinders mounted on vaginal component of intrauterine afterloading tandem, keeled flange, and top view of two cylinders, one with and one without lead shielding. (Reprinted with permission from Delclos L, Fletcher GH, Suite HD, et al. Afterloading vaginal irradiators. Radiology 1970;96:666–667.)

diameters to fit conical vaginas. Cylinders are provided with or without added lead shielding to protect selected vaginal areas, the bladder, or the rectum (Figure 24.6) (29). The cylinders can be mounted in the vaginal component of an intrauterine tandem, or along the stem of a dome cylinder (Figure 24.7) (30). Before the cylinders are mounted into the vaginal component of an intrauterine tandem, the tandem is inserted into the uterus (when this organ has not been removed), and the cylinders are fitted along the protruding tandem. The cylinders have an inside groove on the distal side (28). With the proper hook, the cylinders can be removed one by one if at the time of removal the system is too tight, decreasing the possibility of vaginal tears.

To minimize the rotation of the intrauterine tandem when the cylinders are used in combination with a tandem, a flat, round flange with keel is placed below the last cylinder and is kept in position with some packing (31). The labia are sutured with proline or silk to prevent the system from slipping out and causing a severe vulvar reaction. Figure 24.8 shows examples of the use of the intrauterine tandem and vaginal cylinders. Tables are available with source placement and Ra eq dose rates for ^{137}Cs sources in remote afterloading devices (Tables 24.2 and 24.3) (32,33).

Dome Cylinders Dome cylinders (Figure 24.7) (28) were designed as a substitute for the Bloedorn applicators in irradiating the vaginal cuff alone, or the whole vaginal surface, in patients who have had a hysterectomy. To obtain a uniform isodose around the dome, a minicesium source must be used at the top (28); cesium linear sources are too long (1.5 to 2 cm) for a hemispheric dose distribution.

Radioactive Source Carrier The radioactive sources can be afterloaded into the applicators in the patient's room manually or by remote control. For manual afterloading, the sources are mounted in the laboratory in a Teflon tube of a smaller diameter than the stainless steel tandem or in small carriers to be inserted in ovoids (Figure 24.9) (34).

MIRALVA Perez et al (22) designed a vaginal applicator that incorporates two ovoid sources and a central tandem than can be used to treat the entire vagina (alone or in combination with the uterine cervix). The applicator has vaginal apex caps and additional cylinder sleeves that allow for increased dimensions (Figure 24.10) (35). The dosimetry and dose specifications for this applicator have been published (36), showing that the applicator delivers 1.1 to 1.2 Gy/hour to the vaginal apex and 0.95 to 1 Gy/hour to the distal vaginal surface when loaded with 20 mg Ra eq ^{137}Cs tubes in each ovoid and 10, 10, and 20 mg Ra eq tubes in the vaginal cylinder (Figure 24.11). The tandem in the uterus can be used when clinically indicated with standard loadings, depending on the depth of the uterus (20-10-10 or 20-10 mg Ra eq). When the tandem and vaginal cylinder are used, the strength of the sources in the ovoids should always be 15 mg Ra eq. The vaginal cylinder or uterine tandem never carries an active source at the level of the ovoids.

Special Vaginal Surface Applicators In certain situations, it is necessary to treat selected areas of the vagina while minimizing irradiation to the opposite side (i.e., when the patient has had previous irradiation). Customized cylinders are manufactured that keep the radioactive

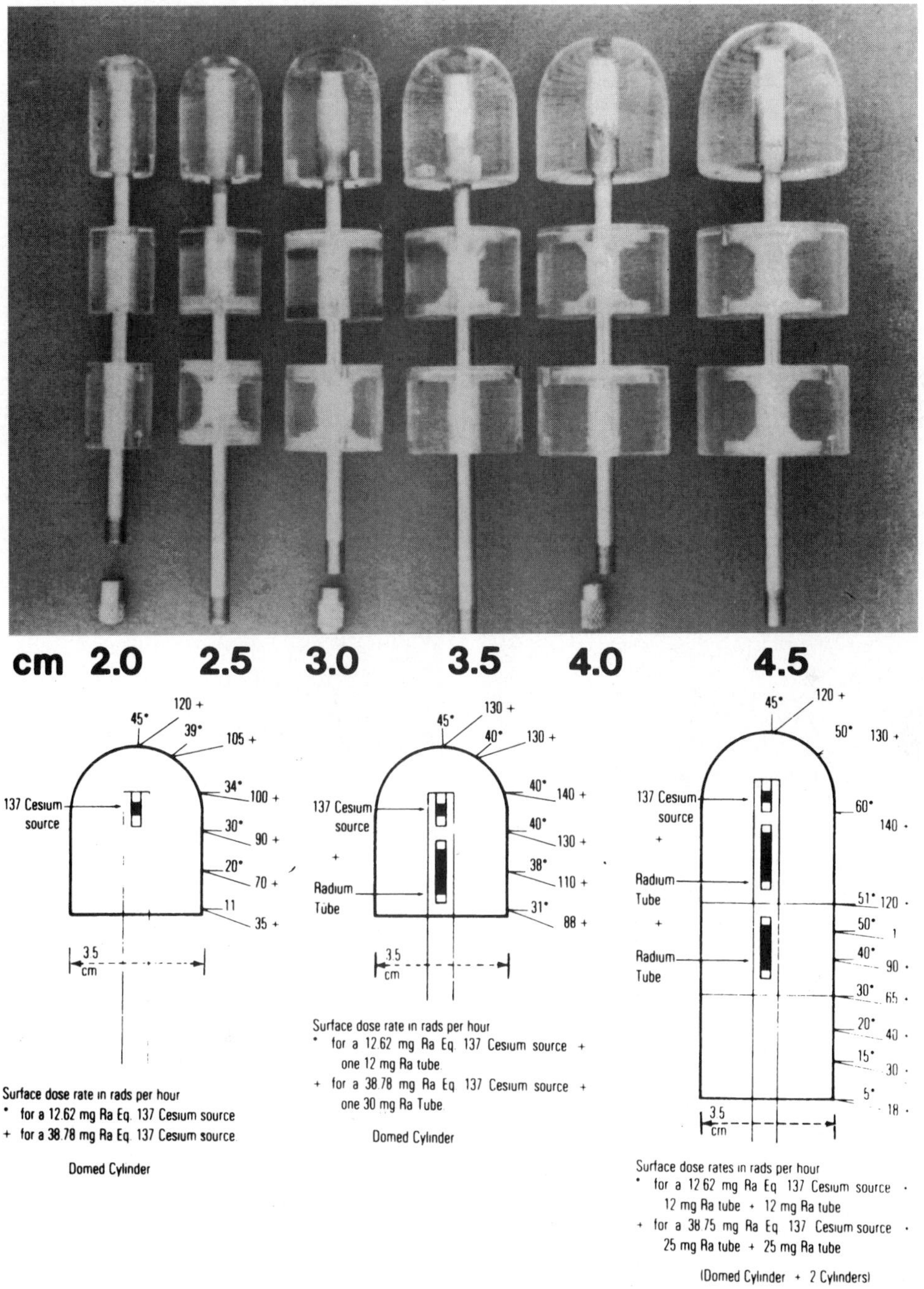

Figure 24.7. Domed colpostats made to treat vaginal cuff alone or vaginal cuff and any selected vaginal length in patient after hysterectomy. Curvature of each done cylinder follows isodose of ^{137}Cs minisource placed at adequate distance from dome in afterloading stem. Previously described vaginal cylinders can be added as shown. Any length of vaginal surface can be treated by combining ^{137}Cs minisource with other cesium sources. (Reprinted with permission from Delclos L, Wharton JT, Rutledge FN. Tumors of the vagina and female urethra. In: Fletcher GH, ed. Textbook of radiotherapy. 3rd ed. Philadelphia: Lea & Febiger; 1980.)

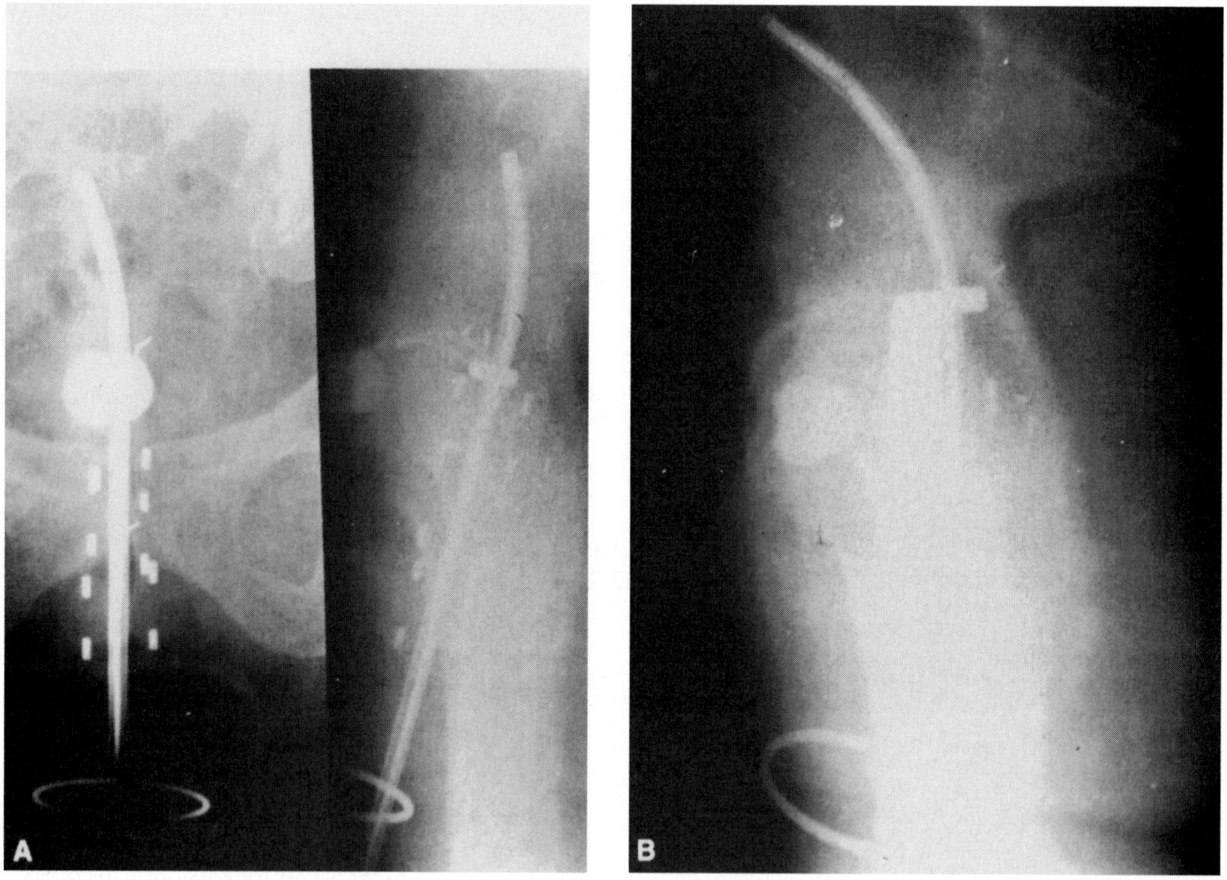

Figure 24.8. A. Intrauterine tandem with three vaginal cylinders along vaginal component of tandem. Note two silver seeds in anterior cervical lip, one in posterior lip, and two in posterior vaginal wall, marking lower extent of vaginal tumor extension. Position of cylinders and dummy sources in relation to tumor is identified easily, allowing proper placement of radioactive sources. **B.** Same system with leaded set of cylinders that reduces dose to bladder and urethra. (Reprinted with permission from Delclos L, Fletcher GH, Moore EB, et al. Minicolpostats, dome cylinders, other additions and improvements of the Fletcher-Suit afterloadable system: indications and limitations of their use. Int J Radiat Oncol Biol Phys 1980;6:1195–1206.)

Table 24.2. Ovoid Surface Dose Rates for Clinical Loadings

Corresponding mg Ra eq 3M tube strength[a]	10	20	25	30
Ovoid diameter	1.6	2.0	2.5	3.0
Source configuration	x2xx5x	1x34x6	123x56	123456
Ovoid surface dose rate[b] (cGy/mg/hr)				
Radial surface	10.24	6.40	4.25	3.09
Bladder	4.28	4.57	4.47	4.39
Rectum	4.28	4.57	3.14	2.16

[a] Assuming 5 mg Ra eq nominal strength/pellet.
[a] Per total mgh in the ovoid.
(Reprinted with permission from Grigsby PW, Williamson JF, Perez CA. Source configuration and dose rates for the Selectron afterloading equipment for gynecologic applicators. Int J Radiat Oncol Biol Phys 1992;24:321–327.)

Table 24.3. Surface Dose for Vaginal Cylinders

Cylinder Diameter (cm)	Cylinder Length (cm)	cGy/hr Constant Factor[a]	Active Pellet Position
2.0	2.5	26.4	1-3-5-8-10
	5.0	21.1	1-2-6-10-14-19-20
	7.5	23	1-2-6-10-14-18-22-26-29-30
	10.0	22.1	1-2-6-10-14-18-22-26-30-34-39-40
2.5	2.5	20.6	1-2-3-8-9-10
	5.0	20.8	1-2-3-7-11-15-18-19-20
	7.5	23	1-2-3-6-9-12-15-18-21-24-28-29-30
	10.0	22.9	1-2-3-6-9-12-15-18-21-24-27-30-34-38-39-40
3.0	2.5	22.5	1-2-3-4-7-8-9-10
	5.0	24.7	1-2-3-4-5-8-11-14-16-17-18-19-20
	7.5	22.6	1-2-3-4-5-10-11-15-16-20-21-26-27-28-29-30
	10.0	24.2	1-2-3-4-5-9-10-14-15-19-20-23-26-27-31-32-36-37-38-39-40
3.5	2.5	22.6	1-2-3-4-5-6-7-8-9-10
	5.0	21.3	1-2-3-4-5-6-9-12-15-16-17-18-19-20
	7.5	23.5	1-2-3-4-5-6-7-11-12-15-16-19-20-24-25-26-27-28-29-30
	10.0	22.8	1-2-3-4-5-6-7-11-12-17-20-21-24-25-29-30-34-35-36-37-38-39-40

[a] The constant is multiplied times the mg Ra eq of the ^{137}Cs pellet.
(Reprinted with permission from Grigsby PW, Williamson JF, Perez CA. Source configuration and dose rates for the Selectron afterloading equipment for gynecologic applicators. Int J Radiat Oncol Biol Phys 1992;24:321–327.)

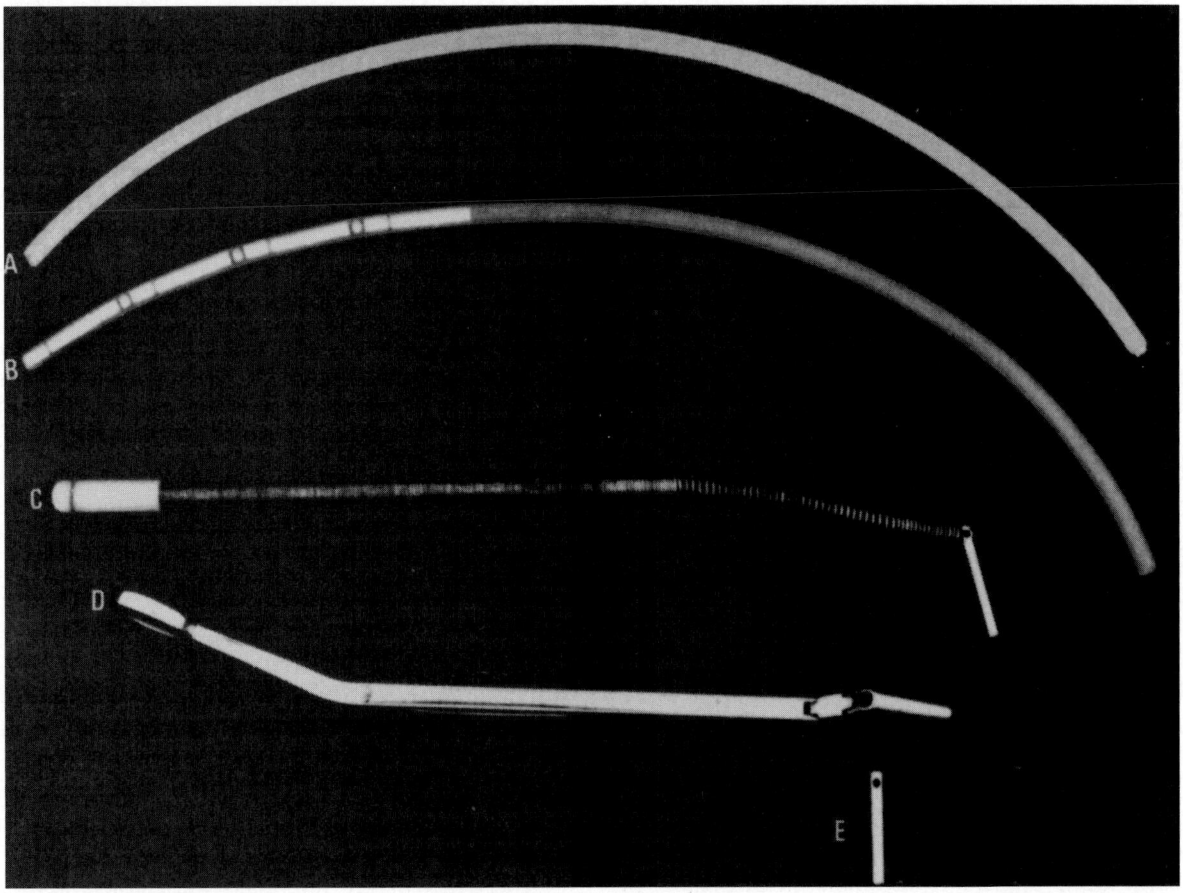

Figure 24.9. A. Empty Teflon tube narrowed at one end. **B.** Three radium or cesium dummies with spaces in Teflon tube carrier. **C.** Dummy source attached at end of spring for afterloading of roundhandle ovoids. **D.** Source carrier for Fletcher-Suit rectangular-handle ovoid. **E.** Dummy radium source with eyelet. (Reprinted with permission from Roosenbeek EV, et al. The radioactive patient: care, precautions, procedures in diagnosis and therapy. Flushing, NY: Medical Examination Publishing; 1975.)

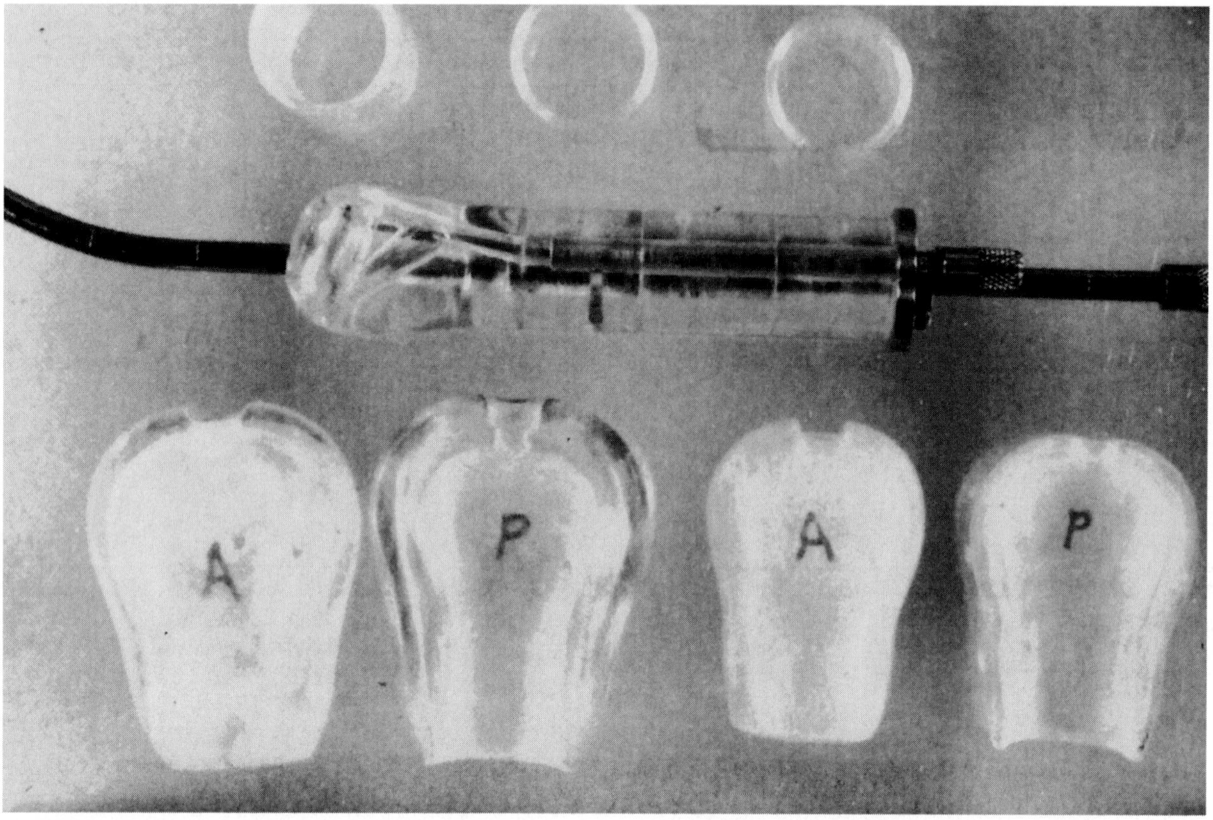

Figure 24.10. MIRALVA applicator with plastic sleeves to increase diameter of vaginal cylinder, afterloading tandem, and plastic caps (A-P) of different sizes to increase diameter of vaginal cuff portion of applicator. (Reprinted with permission from Perez CA, Grigsby PW, Williamson J. Clinical applications of brachytherapy: I, LDR. In: Perez CA, Brady LW, eds. Principles and practice of radiation oncology. 3rd ed. Philadelphia: Lippincott-Raven; 1998.)

sources at a short treating distance from the selected surface and add shielding to protect the opposite side (Figure 24.12) (37). This customized cylinder can be mounted along the vaginal component of an intrauterine tandem if the uterus is present or along the stem of the dome cylinder if there is no uterus.

A tray should be arranged, as shown in Figure 24.13, with instruments for the insertion of intrauterine tandems, colpostats, capsules, dilators, and inserters.

Interstitial Implants

Indications for and techniques of interstitial therapy for carcinoma of the vagina have been described (7,19,38). Rigid metallic or preferably flexible Teflon guides are inserted into the vaginal tissues, using a single, double-plane, or volume implant arrangement. With manual or remote afterloading, radioactive sources of the appropriate activity are inserted in the guides. The ideal LDR is about 0.45 Gy/hour, to deliver approximately 10 Gy per day.

Templates In an attempt to make the insertion of interstitial guides easier and to improve their spatial placement, Aristizabal et al (39), Martinez et al (40), and Syed et al (41) have popularized the use of interstitial implants using perineal templates for guidance of spacing and alignment, with introduction of long metallic guides through the perineum into the parametrial tissues. Also, individually designed acrylic templates can be constructed to accommodate specific tumor geometries (Figure 24.14). Iridium-192 seeds or ^{137}Cs microspheres in nylon tubes are inserted in an afterloading fashion after x-ray films are obtained with dummy sources for dosimetry computations. Aristizabal et al (39) modified their technique by deleting three anteriorly and three posteriorly placed needles in the central row; the central tandem was also omitted in an effort to decrease an initial high incidence of vesicovaginal or rectovaginal fistula.

These patients are potentially vulnerable to severe complications because of the reported lower tolerance of the distal vagina to irradiation and because of the thin rectovaginal septum and proximity of the rectum; therefore it is im-

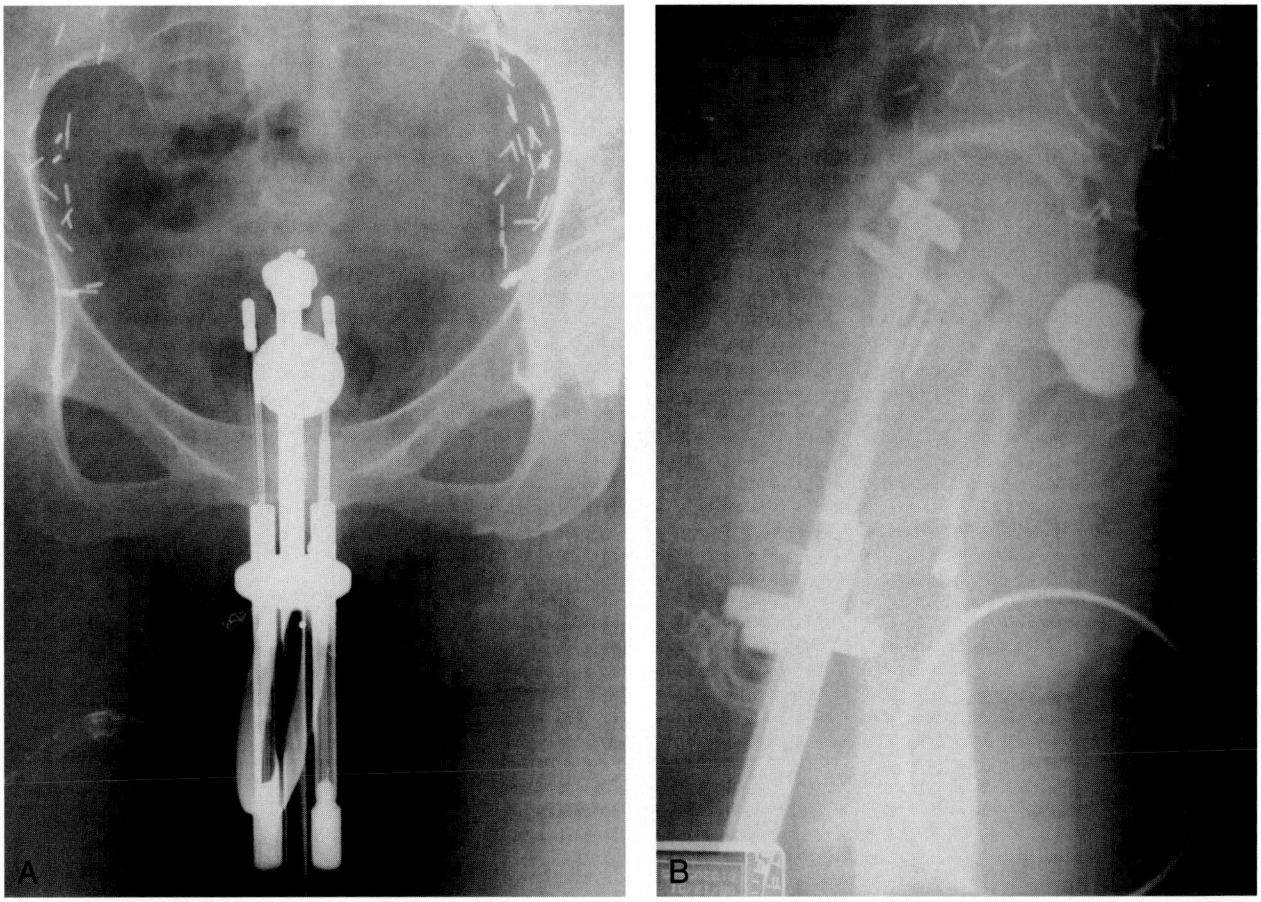

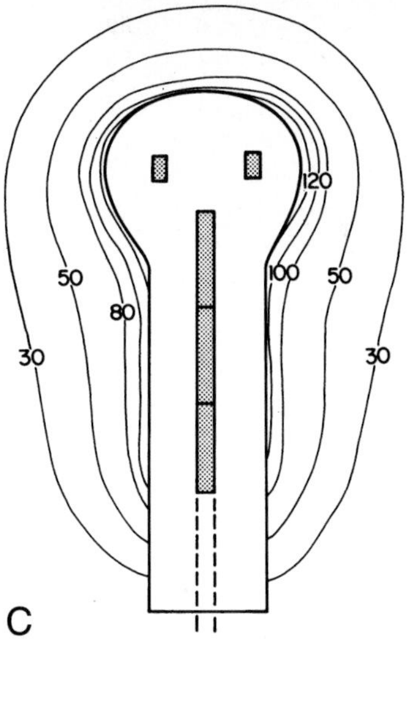

C

Figure 24.11. Anteroposterior **(A)** and lateral **(B)** radiographs depicting position of MIRALVA applicator for treatment of patient with vaginal recurrence of carcinoma of uterine cervix previously treated with a radical hysterectomy. **(C)** Isodose curves of the MIRALVA applicator. (Reprinted with permission from Perez CA, Grigsby PW, Williamson J. Clinical applications of brachytherapy. I. LDR. In: Perez CA, Brady LW, eds. Principles and practice of radiation oncology. 3rd ed. Philadelphia: Lippincott-Raven; 1998.)

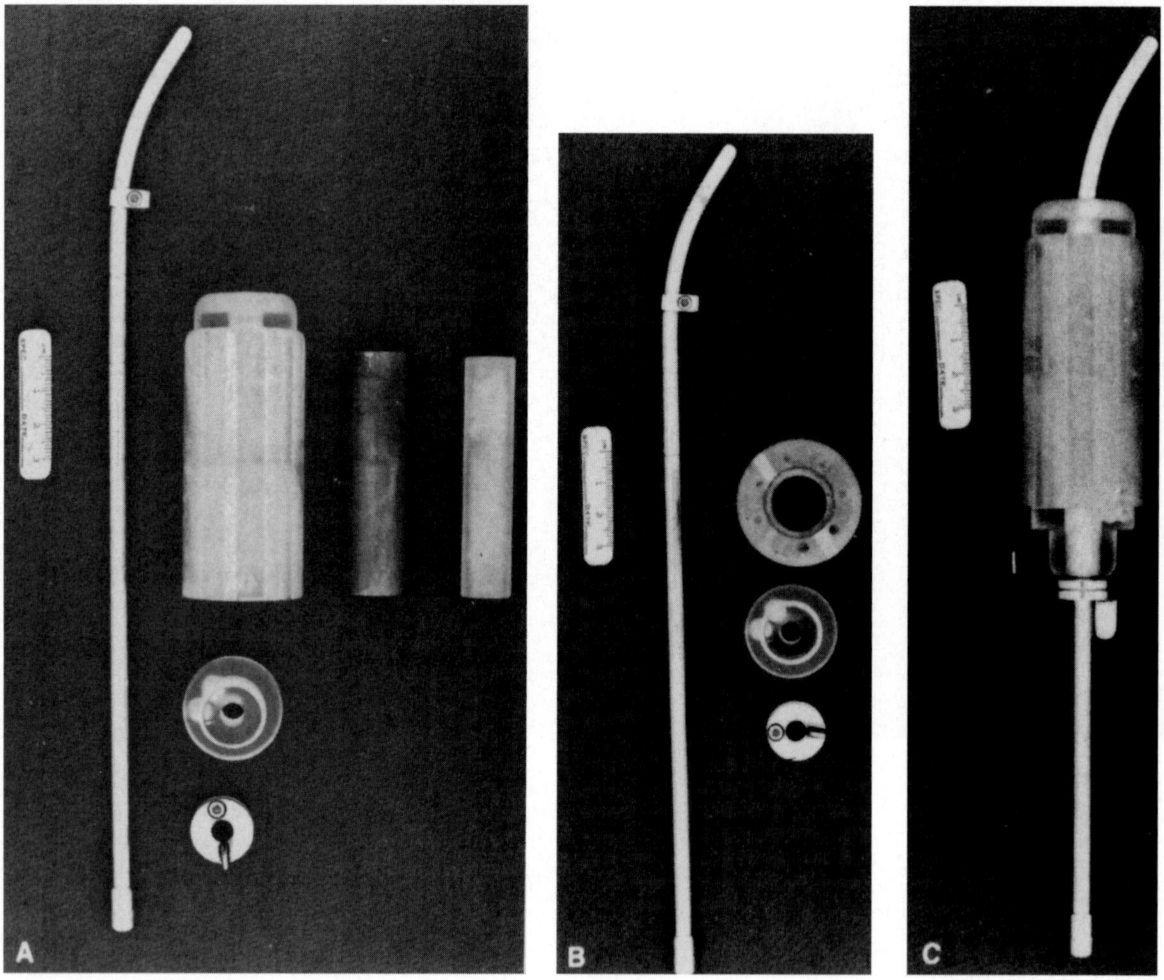

Figure 24.12. **(A)** and **(B)** Dismantled, afterloading short-distance surface cylinder. Note holes in cylinder periphery that accommodate radioactive sources (radium, cesium needles, or iridium wires) and central lead core that shields opposite side. **(C)** Cylinder mounted on vaginal component of intrauterine tandem. (Reprinted with permission from Delclos L, Fletcher GH. Gynecologic Cancers. In: Levitt SH, Tapley N, eds. Technological basis of radiation therapy: practical clinical applications, 2nd ed. Philadelphia: Lea & Febiger; 1992:263–288.)

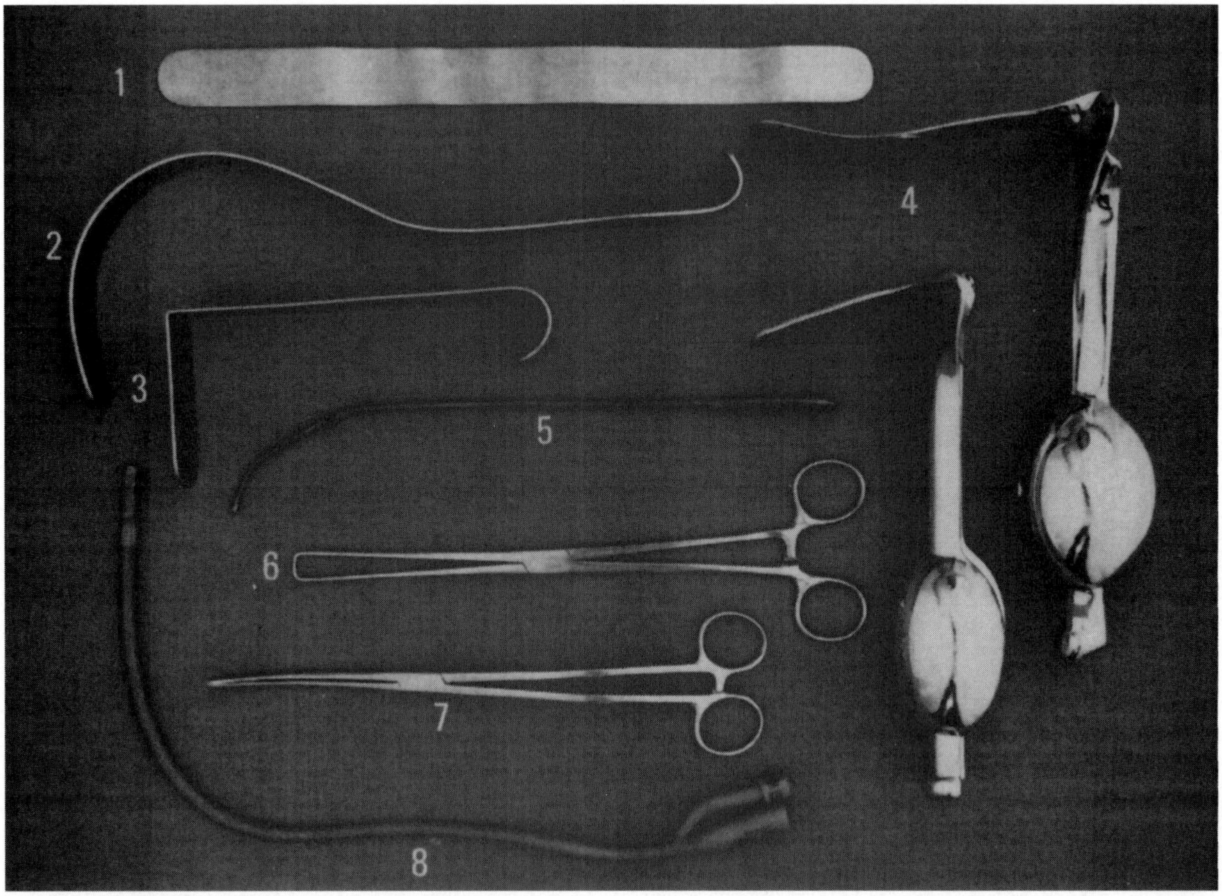

Figure 24.13. Instruments for inserting afterloadable intrauterine tandems and colpostats. 1) Flexsteel ribbon retractor, available in 1-, 1½-, and 2-inch widths. 2) Deaver retractor, available in 1-, 1½-, and 2-inch widths (two of each). 3) Heaney or Kristeller retractors, available in 1-, 1½-, and 2-inch widths (two of each). 4) Auvard weighted retractors, 3, 4, and 5 inches in length (one of each). 5) Malleable hysterometer (one). 6) Braun or Duplay uterine tenaculum (two). 7) Boseman or De Lee uterine packing forceps (two). 8) No. 16 to 18 Foley catheter with 5 ml balloon. (Reprinted with permission from Delclos L, Fletcher GH. Gynecologic cancers. In: Levitt SH, Tapley N, eds. Technological basis of radiation therapy: practical clinical applications. 2nd ed. Philadelphia: Lea & Febiger; 1992:263–288.)

portant to minimize irradiation to the surrounding normal areas. Maximum mucosal dose tolerated by the proximal vagina is 140 Gy and by the distal vagina 98 Gy (42).

Use of interstitial implants ideally should be limited to a volume encompassing 75% or less of the circumference of the vagina, particularly when the lesion involves the posterior wall and rectovaginal septum. Special attention should be paid not to have any guides or radioactive sources in direct contact with the vaginal mucosa (they should be at 0.5 cm depth) or crossing the urethral lumen. At the completion of the procedure it is important to gently perform a rectal examination to ascertain that no guides or radioactive sources are in direct contact with the rectal mucosa. The remaining normal tissues should be kept away from the implanted area as much as possible, with the judicious use of gauze packing, cylinders, or templates. Two rolls of gauze are placed on top of and between the thighs, so that when the legs are brought down from the lithotomy position (in which the implant is done), the inside surfaces of the thighs are separated as much as possible from the vaginal radioactive sources.

High Dose Rate Brachytherapy

High dose rate (HDR) remote afterloading applicators are increasingly used in the treatment of cancer, particularly in gynecologic malignancies. With HDR there is a need to adjust the total dose and additional fractionation is necessary, compared with LDR brachytherapy, because of biologically equivalent dose considerations. In carcinoma of the cervix, Orton et al (43) showed that the ratio of HDR/LDR dose is 0.5 to 0.6; we assume that a similar principle applies to vaginal carcinoma.

Nanavati et al (44) reported on 13 patients with primary vaginal carcinoma (5 stage I tumors, 4 stage IIA, and 4 stage IIB) treated with this modality in combination with

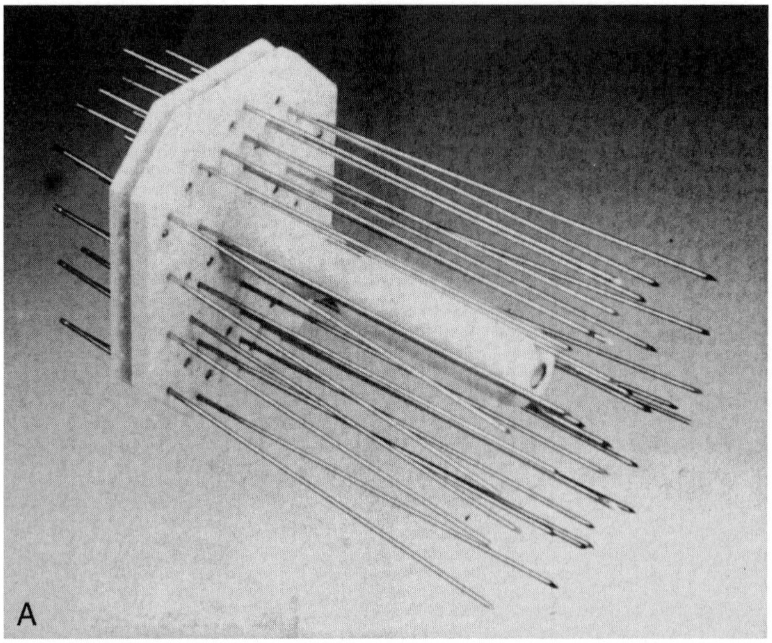

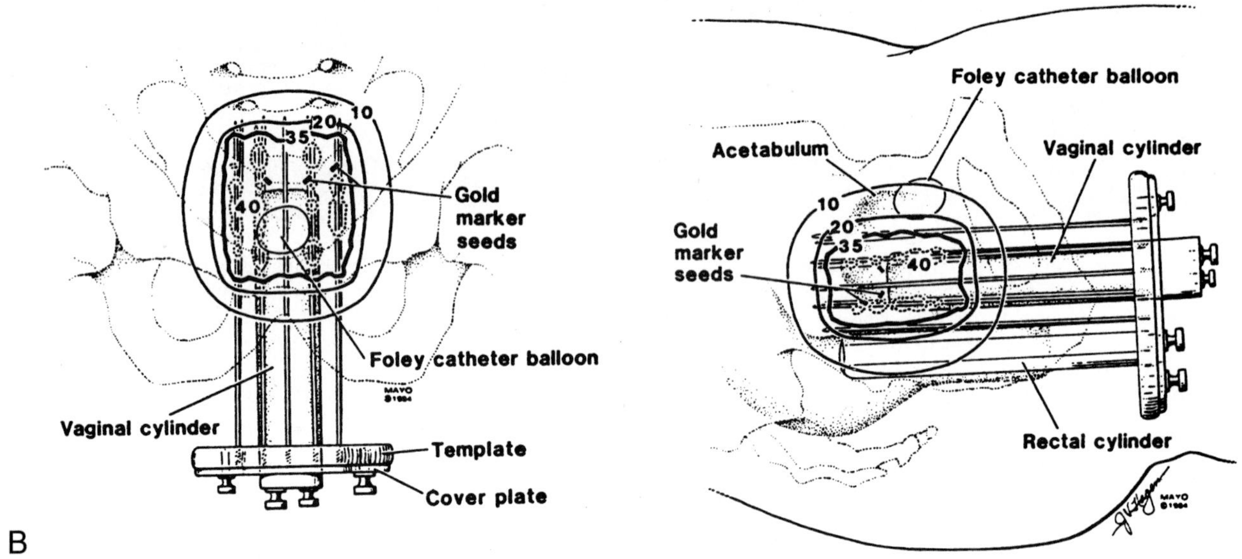

Figure 24.14. **A.** Martinez Universal Perineal Interstitial Template. (Courtesy of Dr. Alvaro Martinez, William Beaumont Hospital, Detroit, MI). **B.** Diagrammatic presentation in coronal and sagittal plane of the same template. (Reprinted with permission from Martinez A, Edmundson GK, Cox RS, et al. Combination of external beam irradiation and multiple-site perineal applicator (MUPIT) for treatment of locally advanced or recurrent prostatic, anorectal, and gynecologic malignancies. Int J Radiat Oncol Biol Phys 1985;11:391–398.)

external irradiation (45 Gy to the pelvis in 1.8 Gy daily fractions, AP-PA and lateral opposed fields, using 10 or 18 MV photons). Brachytherapy was administered with a Microselectron HDR unit, 10 Ci ^{192}Ir source, and a 3-cm diameter vaginal applicator (including intrauterine tandem when an intact uterus was present). Initially doses ranged from 20 to 28 Gy in three or four weekly fractions of 7 Gy. Because of fewer complications with increased fractionation, the dose prescription was changed to 20 Gy in four 5 Gy fractions. There was no significant acute or chronic intestinal or urinary tract grade 3 or 4 toxicity; moderate-to-severe vaginal stenosis occurred in six patients (46%).

Stock et al (45) described results in 15 patients with carcinoma of the vagina treated with HDR brachytherapy; dose per treatment ranged from 3 to 8 Gy, with a median dose of 7 Gy, for a total dose of 21 Gy; median interval between fractions was 2 weeks. Brachytherapy was combined with external irradiation (30 to 63 Gy with a median dose of 42 Gy, 1.8 to 2.92 Gy per fraction). The median total tumor dose from both components was 63 Gy.

References

1. Plentl AA, Friedman EA. Lymphatic system of the female genitalia: the morphologic basis of oncologic diagnosis and therapy. Philadelphia: W.B. Saunders; 1971:51–74.
2. Perez CA, Garipagaoglu M. Vagina. In: Perez CA, Brady LW, eds. Principles and practice of radiation oncology. 3rd ed. Philadelphia: Lippincott-Raven; 1998:1891–1914.
3. Chyle V, Zagars GK, Wheeler JA, et al. Definitive radiotherapy for carcinoma of the vagina: outcome and prognostic factors. Int J Radiat Oncol Biol Phys 1996;35:891–905.
4. Perez CA, Bedwinek JM, Breaux SR. Patterns of failure after treatment of gynecologic tumors. Cancer Treat Symp 1983;2:217–231.
5. Perez CA, Arneson ANA, Dehner LP, et al. Radiation therapy in carcinoma of the vagina. Obstet Gynecol 1974;44:862–872.
6. Livingstone RC. Primary carcinoma of the vagina. Springfield, IL: Charles C Thomas; 1950.
7. Perez CA, Camel HM, Galakatos AE, et al. Definitive irradiation in carcinoma of the vagina: long-term evaluation of results. Int J Radiat Oncol Biol Phys 1988;15:1283–1290.
8. Rutledge F. Cancer of the vagina. Am J Obstet Gynecol 1967;97: 635–655.
9. Whelton J, Kottmeier HL. Primary carcinoma of the vagina: a study of a Radiumhemmet series of 145 cases. Acta Obstet Gynecol Scand 1962;41:22–40.
10. Berchuck A, Rodriguez G, Kamel A, et al. Expression of epidermal growth factor receptor and HER-2/neu in normal and neoplastic cervix, vulva, and vagina. Obstet Gynecol 1990;76:381–387.
11. Underwood RB, Smith RT. Carcinoma of the vagina. JAMA 1971;217: 46–52.
12. Powell JL, Franklin EW III, Nickerson JF, et al. Verrucous carcinoma of the female genital tract. Gynecol Oncol 1978;6:565–573.
13. Wharton JT, Rutledge FN, Gallagher HS, et al. Treatment of clear cell adenocarcinoma in young females. Obstet Gynecol 1975;43:365–368.
14. Laufe LE, Bernstein ED. Primary malignant melanoma of the vagina. Obstet Gynecol 1971;37:148–154.
15. MacNaught R, Symmonds RP, Hole D, et al. Improved control of primary vaginal tumors by combined external beam and interstitial radiotherapy. Clin Radiol 1986;37:29–32.
16. Puthawala A, Syed AMN, Nalick R, et al. Integrated external and interstitial radiation therapy for primary carcinoma of the vagina. Obstet Gynecol 1983;62:367–372.
17. Boronow RC, Hickman BT, Reagan MT, et al. Combined therapy as an alternative to exenteration for locally advanced vulvovaginal cancer: II, Results, complications, and dosimetric and surgical considerations. Am J Clin Oncol 1987;10:171–181.
18. Perez CA, Korba A, Sharma S. Dosimetric considerations in irradiation of carcinoma of the vagina. Int J Radiat Oncol Biol Phys 1977;2: 639–649.
19. Delclos L. Gynecologic cancers: pelvic examination and treatment planning. In: Levitt SH, Tapley N, eds. Technological basis of radiation therapy: practical clinical applications. Philadelphia: Lea & Febiger; 1984:193–227.
20. Sharma SC, Bhandare N. A new design of Delclos dome cylinders using standard Cs-137 sources. Int J Radiat Oncol Biol Phys 1991;21: 511–514.
21. Perez CA, Slessinger E, Grigsby PW. Design of an afterloading vaginal applicator (MIRALVA). Int J Radiat Oncol Biol Phys 1990;18: 1503–1508.
22. Bertoni F, Bertoni G, Bignardi M. Vaginal molds for intracavitary curietherapy: a new method of preparation. Int J Radiat Oncol Biol Phys 1983;9:1579–1582.
23. Fletcher GH. Squamous cell carcinoma of the uterine cervix. In: Fletcher GH, ed. Textbook of radiotherapy. 3rd ed. Philadelphia: Lea & Febiger; 1980:720–773.
24. Sharma SC, Gerbi B, Madoc-Jones H. Dose rates for brachytherapy applicators using ^{137}Cs sources. Int J Radiat Oncol Biol Phys 1979;5: 1893–1897.
25. Muench PJ, Nath R. Dose distributions produced by shielded applicators using ^{241}Am for intracavitary irradiation of tumors in the vagina. Med Phys 1992;19:1299–1306.
26. Shpikalov VL, Atkochyus VB. Interstitial radiotherapy of malignant tumors of the vagina. Neoplasma 1989;36:729–737.
27. Suit HD, Moore EB, Fletcher GH, et al. Modification of Fletcher ovoid system for afterloading using standard sized radium tubes (milligram and microgram). Radiology 1963;81:126.
28. Delclos L, Fletcher GH, Moore EB, et al. Minicolpostats, dome cylinders, other additions and improvements of the Fletcher-Suit afterloadable system: Indications and limitations of their use. Int J Radiat Oncol Biol Phys 1980;6:1195–1206.
29. Delclos L, Fletcher GH, Suite HD, et al. Afterloading vaginal irradiators. Radiology 1970;96:666–667.
30. Delclos L, Wharton JT, Rutledge FN. Tumors of the vagina and female urethra. In: Fletcher GH, ed. Textbook of radiotherapy. 3rd ed. Philadelphia: Lea & Febiger; 1980.
31. Hammoudah MM, Henschke UK. Supervoltage beam films. Int J Radiat Oncol Biol Phys 1977;2:571–577.
32. Wall JA, Arnold H. Preliminary observations on retroperitoneal lymphadenectomies. Tex Med 1953;49:93.
33. Grigsby PW, Williamson JF, Perez CA. Source configuration and dose rates for the Selectron afterloading equipment for gynecologic applicators. Int J Radiat Oncol Biol Phys 1992;24:321–327.
34. Roosenbeek EV, et al. The radioactive patient: care, precautions, procedures in diagnosis and therapy. Flushing, NY: Medical Examination Publishing; 1975.
35. Perez CA, Grigsby PW, Williamson J. Clinical applications of brachytherapy, I: LDR. In: Perez CA, Brady LW, eds. Principles and practice of radiation oncology. 3rd ed. Philadelphia: Lippincott-Raven; 1998: 487–560.
36. Slessinger ED, Perez CA, Grigsby PW, et al. Dosimetry and dose specification for a new gynecological brachytherapy applicator. Int J Radiat Oncol Biol Phys 1992;22:1117–1124.
37. Delclos L, Fletcher GH. Gynecologic cancers. In: Levitt SH, Tapley N, eds. Technological basis of radiation therapy: practical clinical applications. 2nd ed. Philadelphia: Lea & Febiger; 1992:263–288.
38. Perez CA, Kuske R, Glasgow GP. Review of brachytherapy for gynecologic tumors. Endocurie Hypertherm Oncol 1985;1:153–175.
39. Aristizabal SA, Valencia A, Ocampo G, et al. Interstitial parametrial irradiation in cancer of the cervix stage IIB-IIB: An analysis of pelvic control and complications. Endocurie Hypertherm Oncol 1985;1: 41–48.
40. Martinez A, Edmundson GK, Cox RS, et al. Combination of external beam irradiation and multiple-site perineal applicator (MUPIT) for treatment of locally advanced or recurrent prostatic, anorectal, and gynecologic malignancies. Int J Radiat Oncol Biol Phys 1985;11: 391–398.
41. Syed AMN, Puthawala AA, Tansey LA, et al. Temporary ^{192}Ir implantation in the management of carcinoma of the prostate. In: Hilaris BS, Batata MS, eds. Brachytherapy oncology—1983. NY: Memorial Sloan-Kettering Cancer Center; 1983:83–91.
42. Hintz GL, Kagan AR, Chan P, et al. Radiation tolerance of the vaginal mucosa. Int J Radiat Oncol Biol Phys 1980;6:711–716.
43. Orton CG, Seyedsadr M, Somnay A. Comparison of high and low dose rate remote afterloading for cervix cancer and the importance of fractionation. Int J Radiat Oncol Biol Phys 1991;21:1425–1434.
44. Nanavati PJ, Fanning J, Hilgers RD, et al. High-dose-rate brachytherapy in primary stage I and II vaginal cancer. Gynecol Oncol 1993; 51:67–71.
45. Stock RG, Mychalczak B, Armstrong JG, et al. The importance of brachytherapy technique in the management of primary carcinoma of the vagina. Int J Radiat Oncol Biol Phys 1992;24:747–753.

Chapter 25

Prostate

Carlos A. Perez, Jeff M. Michalski, and Alvaro A. Martinez

ANATOMY

The prostate gland is a walnut-shaped solid organ that surrounds the male urethra between the base of the bladder and the urogenital diaphragm and weighs about 20 g. The prostate is attached anteriorly to the pubic symphysis by the puboprostatic ligament. It is separated from the rectum posteriorly by Denovilliers' fascia (retrovesical septum), which attaches above to the peritoneum and below to the urogenital diaphragm. The seminal vesicles and the vas deferens pierce the posterosuperior aspect of the gland and enter the urethra at the verumontanum (Figure 25.1). The lateral margins of the prostate, usually delineated against the levator ani muscles, form the lateral prostatic sulci.

The prostate is divided into five histologically distinct lobes: anterior, posterior, median, and two lateral lobes. It is the posterior lobe, extending across the entire posterior surface of the gland, that is felt on rectal examination.

Myers et al (3), in a study of 64 gross prostatectomy specimens, noted variations in the shape and exact location of the prostatic apex, and pointed out that the configuration of the external striated urethral sphincter was related to the shape of the prostatic apex. Two basic prostatic shapes were recognized, distinguished by the presence or absence of an anterior apical notch, depending on the degree of lateral lobe development and the position of its anterior commissure. Observations by these authors that the urethral sphincter is a striated muscle in contact with the urethra from the base of the bladder to the perineal membrane corroborates the previous description by Oelrich (4), who pointed out that there is no distinct superior fascia of the so-called urogenital diaphragm separating the sphincter muscle from the prostate. The anatomy of the male pelvis at right angles to the perineal membrane, through the membranous urethra, is illustrated in Figure 25.2.

NATURAL HISTORY

Local Growth Patterns

Almost all prostatic carcinomas develop in the peripheral glands of the prostate, whereas benign prostatic hyperplasia arises from the central (periurethral) portions (5). In recent years, more attention is being paid to tumors arising in the transitional zone.

Breslow et al. (6) found that 64% of 350 carcinomas were present in a slice taken 5 mm from the distal end of the prostate. Therefore, the urethra must be transected distal to the prostate to avoid leaving prostatic cancer behind (5,7). This is an important detail in the design of external irradiation portals or in brachytherapy of prostate cancer.

Jewett (8) reported that multiple foci of tumor were found throughout the prostate in 77% of prostatectomy specimens. Andriole et al. (9) described bilateral lobe pathologic involvement in 13 of 15 patients (87%) with clinical stage A1 (T1a) cancer. Therefore, the entire gland (with a margin) must be treated.

As the tumor grows, it may extend into and through the capsule of the gland, invade seminal vesicles and periprostatic tissues, and later involve the bladder neck or the rectum. Tumor may invade the perineural spaces, the lymphatics, and the blood vessels, producing lymphatic or distant metastases. The incidence of microscopic tumor extension beyond the capsule of the gland (at time of radical prostatectomy) in patients with clinical stage A2 or B ranges from 18 to 57% (10,11).

Oesterling et al. (12), in an analysis of patients with stage T1c disease treated with radical prostatectomy, noted that 53% had pathologically organ-confined tumors, 35% had extracapsular extension, and 9% had seminal vesicle invasion. In the last group, 66% of patients had positive surgical margins, an incidence comparable to clinical stage T2 tumors. In a similar group of patients with T1c tumors,

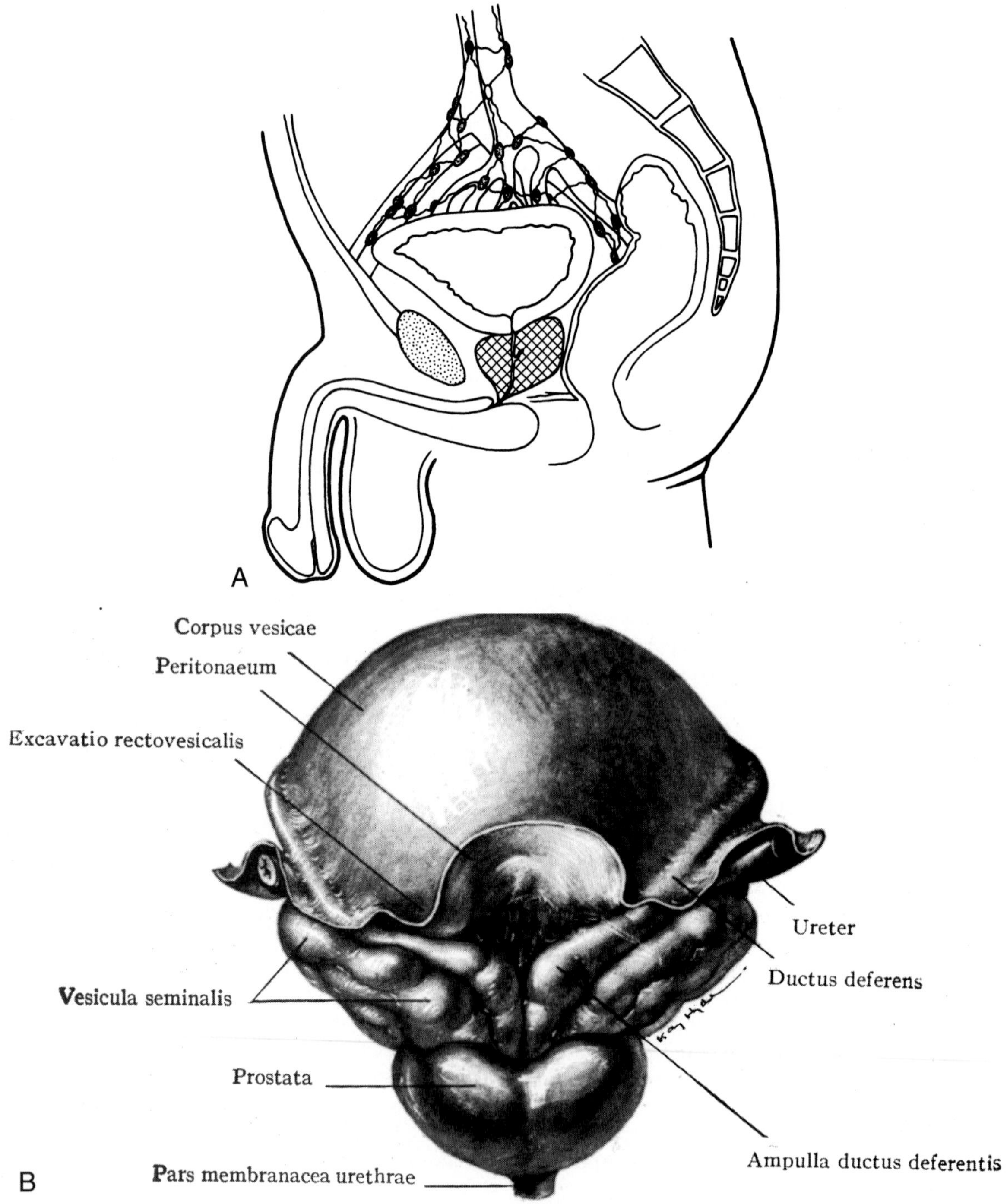

Figure 25.1. **A.** Sagittal diagram of pelvis illustrating anatomic relationships of the prostate. (Perez CA. Prostate. In: Perez CA, Brady LW, eds. Principles and practice of radiation oncology. 3rd ed. Philadelphia: Lippincott-Raven, 1998.) (1). **B.** View of posterior urinary bladder, illustrating close relationship of prostate and seminal vesicles. (Anson BJ, McVay CB. Surgical Anatomy. 5th ed. Philadelphia: WB Saunders, 1971;2:771.) (2)

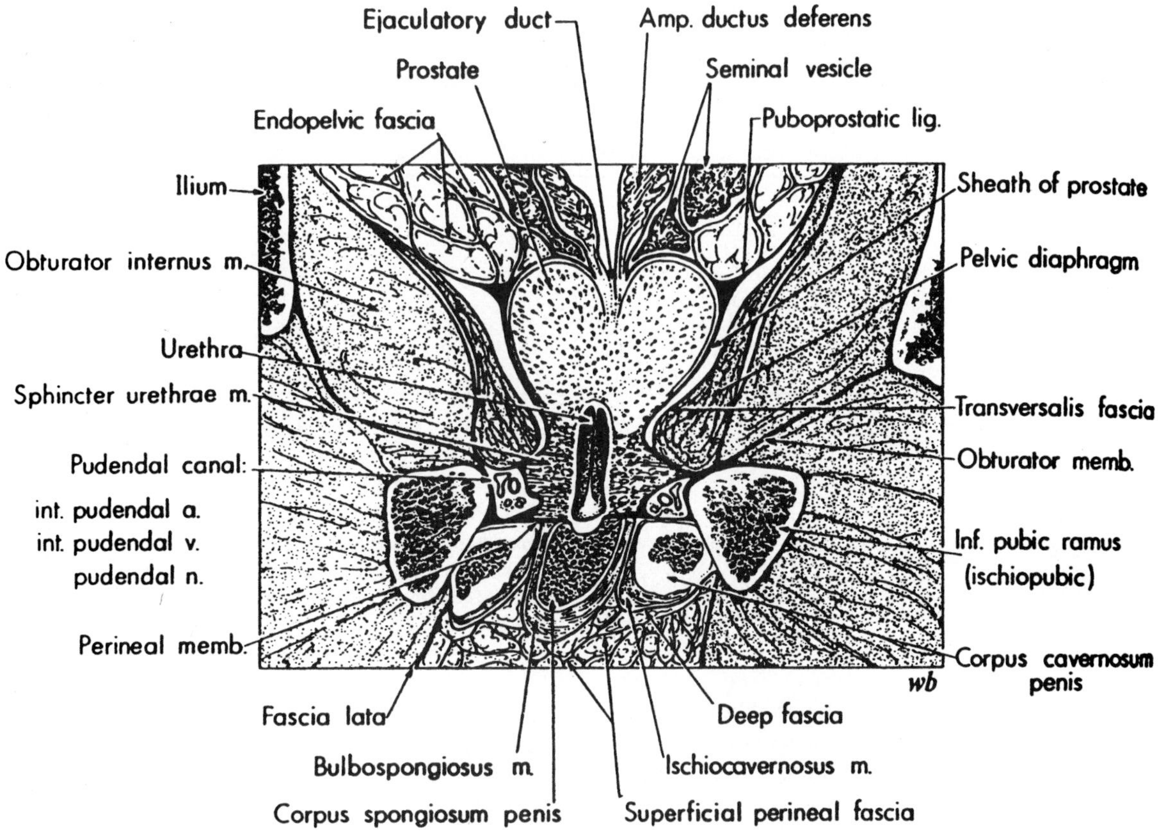

Figure 25.2. Frontal section of male pelvis at right angles to perineal membrane. (Oelrich TM. The urethral sphincter muscle in the male. Am J Anat 1980;158:229–246.) (4)

Epstein et al. (13) found that 34% had established extracapsular extension, 6% seminal vesicle invasion, and 17% positive surgical margins.

Stone et al. (14) reported none of 13 patients with prostate-specific antigen (PSA) less than 4 ng/ml, 11 of 99 patients (11%) with PSA of 4.1 to 20 ng/ml, and 12 of 45 patients (27%) with PSA greater than 20 ng/ml having positive seminal vesicle biopsy. None of the patients with stage T1a, T1b, or T1c had positive seminal vesicle biopsies, compared with 2 of 33 (6%) with T2a, 14 of 80 (17.5%) with T2b, and 7 of 23 (30%) with T2c tumors. Seminal vesicle involvement has been observed in 10% of patients with A2 tumors to 30% of the patients with B2 lesions (15).

Stock et al. (16), in 120 patients with clinical stage T1b to T2c carcinoma of the prostate on whom transrectal ultrasound-guided needle biopsies of the seminal vesicles were performed, reported on 99 who also underwent laparoscopic lymph node dissection. The incidence of seminal vesicle involvement was correlated with PSA level, Gleason score, and clinical stage (Table 25.1). When PSA level and Gleason score were correlated, none of the patients with Gleason scores of 4 or lower showed seminal vesicle involvement, regardless of PSA level. Patients with Gleason scores of 5 and 6 and PSA of 4 to 20 ng/ml had 10 to

Table 25.1. Correlation of Prostate-Specific Antigen Levels, Gleason Score, and Clinical Stage with Positive Seminal Vesicle Biopsy Specimen

	Number of Positive Seminal Vesicle Biopsy Specimens (%)	*P* Value
PSA ≤10	3 (6)	
PSA >10	15 (21)	0.02
PSA ≤20	8 (9)	
PSA >20	10 (37.5)	0.005
Grade <7	6 (7)	
Grade ≥7	12 (37.5)	<0.0001
T1a–T2a	2 (5)	
T2b–T2c	16 (20)	0.03

(Reprinted with permission from Stock RG, Stone NN, Ianuzzi C, et al. Seminal vesicle biopsy and laparoscopic pelvic lymph node dissection: implications for patient selection in the radiotherapeutic management of prostate cancer. Int J Radiat Oncol Biol Phys 1995;33:815–821) (16).

Table 25.2. Incidence of Pelvic Lymph Node Metastasis Correlated with Clinical Stage and Histologic Grade

	Grade							
	Well Differentiated		Moderately Differentiated		Poorly Differentiated		Total	
Stage	No./Total	Percent	No./Total	Percent	No./Total	Percent	No.	Percent
A1	0/28		0/12		0/1		0/41	
A2	0/7		5/19	26	3/7	43	8/33	24
B1	2/53	4	13/94	14	3/9	33	18/156	12
B2	5/27	19	29/106	27	9/21	43	43/154	28
C	5/10	50	18/44	41	13/14	93	36/68	53
Total	12/125	10	65/275	24	28/52	54	105/452	23

(Reprinted with permission from Middleton RG. Value of and indications for pelvic lymph node dissection in the staging of prostate cancer. NCI Monogr 1988;7:41–43). (20).

11% and those with PSA greater than 20 ng/ml had 14% positive seminal vesicle biopsy. With Gleason scores of 7 or higher, 25% of patients with PSA of 4 to 20 ng/ml and 53% of those with PSA greater than 20 ng/ml had seminal vesicle involvement.

D'Amico et al. (17), in a pathologic evaluation of 347 radical prostatectomy specimens, reported none of 38 patients with PSA of 4 ng/ml or less having seminal vesicle involvement in contrast to 6% of 144 patients with PSA of 4 to 10 ng/ml, 11% of 101 with PSA of 10 to 20 ng/ml, 36% of 45 with PSA of 20 to 40 ng/ml, and 42% of 19 with PSA greater than 40 ng/ml. The incidence of positive surgical margins was 11%, 20%, 33%, 56%, and 63%, respectively.

Roach (18) proposed a formula based on analysis of radical prostatectomy specimens to estimate the probability of seminal vesicle involvement:

$$SV+ = PSA + (\text{Gleason score} - 6) \times 10$$

Regional Lymph Node Involvement

Tumor size and degree of differentiation affect the tendency of prostatic carcinoma to metastasize to regional lymphatics (19). The relationship between clinical stage, histologic differentiation, and pelvic nodal metastases in the pre-PSA era is shown in Table 25.2 (20).

Ohori et al. (21), in 478 patients treated with radical prostatectomy, reported no pelvic lymph node metastases in 70 patients with stage T1a,b, 1 of 43 (2%) in patients with stage T1c, 5 of 96 (5%) with stage T2a, and 19 of 269 (7%) with stage T2b,c. The incidence of seminal vesicle invasion was 6%, 11%, 5%, and 17%, respectively.

In a review of 2439 patients treated with radical prostatectomy, Pisansky et al. (22) reported positive pelvic nodes in 12 of 457 (2.6%) with stage T1a–c, 15 of 456 (3.3%) with stage T2a, 130 of 1206 (10.8%) with stage T2b,c, and 81 of 320 (25%) with stage T3 tumors.

Table 25.3. Correlation of Prostate-Specific Antigen Level, Gleason Score, Clinical Stage, and Status of Seminal Vesicle Biopsy Specimen with Incidence of Positive Pelvic Lymph Nodes

	Number with Positive Pelvic Lymph Nodes (%)	*P* Value
PSA ≤10	2 (6)	
PSA >10	7 (15)	0.3
PSA ≤20	2 (3)	
PSA >20	7 (24)	0.003
Grade <7	1 (2)	
Grade ≥7	8 (35)	<0.0001
T1a–T2a	0 (0)	
T2b–T2c	9 (18)	0.03
Positive seminal vesicle biopsy specimen	9 (50)	
Negative seminal vesicle biopsy specimen	0 (0)	<0.0001

(Reprinted with permission from Stock RG, Stone NN, Ianuzzi C, et al. Seminal vesicle biopsy and laparoscopic pelvic lymph node dissection: implications for patient selection in the radiotherapeutic management of prostate cancer. Int J Radiat Oncol Biol Phys 1995;33: 815–821.) (16)

Stock et al. (16), in 99 patients who underwent laparoscopic lymph node dissection, correlated incidence of positive nodes with PSA, Gleason score, stage, and involvement of seminal vesicles (Table 25.3). None of the patients with a Gleason score of 4 or lower, even with PSA greater than 20 ng/ml, had positive pelvic lymph nodes, and 8% in the group with Gleason scores of 5 or 6 and PSA levels of 4 to 10 ng/ml had positive nodes. However, the incidence of positive lymph nodes increased significantly (24%) in patients with PSA greater than 20 ng/ml.

Bluestein et al. (23), Narayan et al. (24), Partin et al. (25), and Spevack et al. (26) have offered comparable models based on pathologic data that may predict risk for lymph node metastases, to decide whether the patient should be subjected to a staging lymphadenectomy (including laparoscopic technique) or considered for irradiation of the pelvic lymph nodes.

Stone et al. (14) reported that none of 11 patients with PSA less than 4 ng/ml, 4 of 77 (9%) with PSA of 4 to 20 ng/ml, and 10 of 42 (24%) with PSA greater than 20 ng/ml had positive nodes. When correlated with clinical stage, none of the patients with stage T1b,c or T2a had positive nodes compared with 10 of 69 (15%) with T2b and 4 of 17 (24%) with T2c tumors. Eleven of 23 patients (48%) with positive seminal vesicles also had positive nodes compared with 3 of 107 (3%) with negative seminal vesicle biopsy.

Roach (18) suggested a revised formula based on pathologic findings in prostatectomy specimens incorporating clinical stage, to estimate the incidence of metastatic pelvic lymph nodes:

$$\text{Risk of N+} = 2/3\ \text{PSA} + [(\text{GS}-6) + \text{TG} - 1.5)] \times 10 \qquad (1)$$

where GS is Gleason score, and TG is clinical tumor group. TG is as follows: TG 1 (stages T1c and T2a) is assigned a value of 1; TG 2 (T1b and T2b) is given a value of 2; and TG 3 (T2c and T3) is assigned a value of 3.

Periprostatic and obturator nodes are involved first, followed by external iliac, hypogastric, common iliac, and periaortic nodes (Table 25.4) (27). Approximately 7% of patients have involvement of the presacral and presciatic lymph nodes (including promontorial and middle hemorrhoidal group) without evidence of metastases in the external iliac or hypogastric lymph nodes (27).

McLaughlin et al. (28) point out that multiple lymph nodes are frequently found in patients with well-differentiated tumors as well as those with poorly differentiated lesions.

Table 25.4. Lymph Node Involvement in Adenocarcinoma of the Prostate (93 Patients)

Lymph Node Group	Number of Patients Undergoing Biopsy	Patients With Tumor	Percent Opacified*
Paraaortic	74	13 (18%)	93
Common iliac	76	13 (17%)	95
External iliac	74	16 (22%)	94
Internal iliac	63	16 (24%)	87
Obturator	51	16 (31%)	94

* Refers to histologic evidence of retained contrast material within the lymph node specimen.

(Reprinted with permission from Pistenma DA, Bagshaw MA, Feiha FS. Extended-field radiation therapy for prostatic adenocarcinoma: status report of a limited prospective trial. In: Johnson DE, Samuels ML, eds. Cancer of the genitourinary tract. New York, NY: Raven Press, 1979.) (27)

Prognosis is closely related to the presence of regional lymph node metastases; patients with positive pelvic lymph node metastasis have a significantly greater probability (over 85% at 10 years) of developing distant metastasis than those with negative nodes (less than 20%) (29).

Gervasi et al. (29) reported that the risk of metastatic disease at 10 years was 31% for patients with negative lymph nodes compared with 83% for those with positive nodes. The risk of dying of prostate cancer was 17% and 57%, respectively.

Rukstalis et al. (30) compiled data from the literature that documented the strong prognostic implications of the number of involved lymph nodes; in general, patients with a single metastatic lymph node have a 5-year survival rate ranging from 60 to 80%, whereas in those with more involved lymph nodes, the 5-year survival rate is 20 to 54%.

Metastases to the periaortic nodes are seen in 5 to 25% of patients, depending on tumor stage and histologic differentiation (27); they are associated with a higher incidence of distant metastases and lower survival (31).

Distant Metastases

Prostatic carcinoma metastasizes to the skeleton, liver, lungs, and occasionally to the brain or other sites. Perez et al. (32) reported an overall incidence of distant metastases of 20% in stage B, 40% in stage C, and 65% in stage D1.

PROGNOSTIC FACTORS

Intrinsic (Tumor Related)

Tumor Stage, Pretreatment PSA, and Histologic Features

The strongest prognostic indicators in carcinoma of the prostate are clinical stage, pretreatment PSA level, and pathologic tumor differentiation (1). This is a consequence of the more aggressive behavior and greater incidence of lymphatic and distant metastases in the larger and less differentiated tumors. Bastacky et al. (33) noted that perineural invasion on prostate biopsies is correlated with a higher probability of capsular penetration, and Bonin et al. (34) reported a lower 5-year biochemical failure-free survival rate in the presence of perineural invasion (39 versus 65%, $P = .0009$) in patients with PSA less than 20 ng/ml treated with three-dimensional conformal radiation therapy (3-D CRT).

Several reports strongly suggest a close correlation of pretreatment or posttreatment follow-up PSA levels with incidence of failures and survival (35,36).

Rising PSA values after radical prostatectomy or 6 to 12 months after definitive irradiation are sensitive indicators of persistent disease.

DNA Index

Combined with histologic grade, PSA, and pathologic stage, DNA ploidy provides a highly sensitive prognostic indicator. Aneuploidy has usually been associated with more aggressive tumors in comparison with diploid lesions (37,38).

Song et al. (39) showed that DNA ploidy is a strong independent marker of tumor aggressiveness in patients with carcinoma of the prostate treated with external-beam irradiation. Pollack et al. (40), in a selected group of 76 patients, noted that doubling time of PSA after irradiation probably reflects tumor doubling time and that there is a strong correlation between PSA doubling time and tumor DNA ploidy.

p53

Hall et al. (41) observed a low frequency of p53 mutations (1 in 37, 2.7%) in patients with clinically localized adenocarcinoma of the prostate. Most reports demonstrate that p53 mutations are a late step in the progression of prostate cancer and are associated with advanced disease, dedifferentiation, and acquisition of androgen independence.

Only 20% of 43 patients reported by Prendergast et al. (42) showed p53 alterations. However, they were found more frequently in patients with postirradiation recurrent tumors (13 of 18, 72%) than in those with nonirradiated tumors (5 of 25, 20%). Despite the obvious selection of patients, it is possible that p53 overexpression may be associated with decreased response to irradiation (radioresistance marker).

S-Phase Fraction

S-phase fraction was found to be the better predictor of survival in 57 men with prostate cancer, when compared with DNA ploidy, although it was not an independent prognosticator in patients with locally advanced or metastatic prostate cancer (43). Median survival was 5.9 years with S-phase fraction less than 8% compared with only 1.3 years with higher than 8%.

Extrinsic (Host Related)

Age

A higher locoregional failure rate and decreased survival in patients younger than 50 years of age has been reported (44). In the patients with stage B disease treated at Washington University, there was no difference in survival for the various age groups; stage C patients younger than 60 had lower 10-year survival (25%) than those older than 60 years (40 to 55%) (45).

Race

Several authors have observed lower survival rates for a given stage of the disease in black men when compared with white patients (46,47), although this observation is not consistent.

Moul et al. (48), in 366 white and 107 black patients treated with radical prostatectomy, observed 5-year disease-free survival rates of 60 and 38%, respectively ($P = 0.018$). Pathologic tumor characteristics in both groups were comparable. On multivariate analysis, race was a significant prognostic factor.

This difference may be related to a lower immune competence, more biologically aggressive tumors, testosterone levels, environmental or socioeconomic conditions, and genetic or other unknown factors (46,49). In 117 patients reported by Aziz et al. (46) with various clinical stages, a greater percentage of black patients presented with high Gleason scores compared with whites (43% and 27%, respectively).

Kim et al. (50), in a review of 489 white and 157 black men treated with irradiation for localized carcinoma of the prostate, noted that black men had more aggressive tumors with a higher incidence of distant metastases and lower survival than white men. This was particularly true in patients with stage C tumors (10-year survival of 58 versus 28%). However, in patients with stage A2 and B tumors, there was no significant difference in survival between black and white patients, similar to our experience (51).

In contrast, in an analysis of 1606 patients (92.5% white, 7.5% black) diagnosed with prostate cancer at military facilities, no significant difference in survival was noted (52). Also, a Veterans Administration Hospital Report failed to correlate financial access to health care with the higher incidence of distant disease and poorer survival of black patients with prostate cancer compared with whites (53).

Moreover, Fowler et al. (54), in 190 black and 167 white men with stage T1b or T2 disease treated with surgery or radiation therapy and 39 black and 42 white men with stage T3 and T4 tumors treated with irradiation, noted that race had no significant impact on stage-specific survival.

RADIATION THERAPY TECHNIQUES

External Irradiation

With the advent of megavoltage equipment, an increase in the use of external irradiation rapidly emerged for the treatment of patients with carcinoma of the prostate (55). Various techniques have been used, ranging from parallel anteroposterior (AP) portals with a perineal appositional field to lateral portals (box technique) or rotational fields to supplement the dose to the prostate (55–57). In recent years, 3-D conformal techniques have been increasingly used (58–60).

In patients on whom transurethral resection of prostate (TURP) has been carried out for relief of obstructive lower urinary tract symptoms, 4 weeks should elapse before radiation therapy begins in order to decrease sequelae (urinary incontinence, urethral strictures) (1).

Volume Treated

When the pelvic lymph nodes are treated, as is occasionally done at Washington University, the field size is 15 × 15 cm at the patient surface (16.5 cm at isocenter). Patients younger than 71 years of age with clinical stage A2, B (T1c, T2a) and Gleason score of 6 or greater, or PSA of 20 ng/ml or greater or with stage B2 (T2b,c) and all patients with stage C (T3) lesions are treated to the whole pelvis with four fields (45 Gy) and additional dose to complete 70 Gy or higher to the prostate, as indicated per protocol, with seven-field 3-D conformal techniques. For stage D1 tumors, the field size is increased to 15 × 18 cm at the patient surface (16.5 × 20.5 cm at isocenter) to cover the common iliac lymph nodes. The inferior margin of the field should be determined using an urethrogram with 25% radiopaque iodinated contrast material. The margin usually is 1.5 to 2 cm distal to the junction of the prostatic and membranous urethra (usually at or caudad to the bottom of the ischial tuberosities). The lateral margins should be about 1 to 2 cm from the lateral bony pelvis (Figure 25.3A).

With lateral portals, which are used with the box technique (including the lymph nodes) or to irradiate the prostate with two-dimensional (2-D) stationary fields or rotational techniques, it is important to delineate anatomic structures of the pelvis and the location of the prostate in relation to the bladder, rectum, and bony structures with computed tomography (CT) scan or magnetic resonance imaging (MRI).

The initial lateral fields encompass a volume similar to that treated with AP-posteroanterior (PA) portals. The anterior margins should be 1.5 cm posterior to the projection of the anterior cortex of the pubic symphysis (Figure 25.3B). Some of the small bowel may be spared anteriorly, keeping in mind the anatomic location of the external iliac lymph nodes. Posteriorly, the portals include the pelvic and presacral lymph nodes above the S3 segment, which allows for some sparing of the posterior rectal wall distal to this level.

Figure 25.4 shows examples of standard simulation films outlining the AP and lateral portals used for the box technique. For the boost with 2-D treatment planning, the upper margin is 3 to 5 cm above the pubic bone or acetabulum, depending on extent of disease and volume to be covered (i.e., prostate or seminal vesicles). The anterior margin is 1.5 cm posterior to the anterior cortex of the pubic bone; the inferior margin is 1.5 cm inferior to the genitourinary diaphragm as demonstrated by urethrogram. The posterior margin is 2 cm behind the marker rod in the rectum. Figure 25.5 illustrates the reduced volume for the prostate boost when the seminal vesicles should be irradiated.

The reduced fields for treatment of the prostatic volume can be about 8 ∞ 10 cm at isocenter for stages A2 or B (T1,2) to 10 × 12 or 12 ∞ 14 cm for stages C (T3) or D1 (T4) (Figure 25.3C) or ideally are anatomically shaped fields, using CT scans or MRI volume reconstructions of the prostate and seminal vesicles. In a study of nine patients implanted with Iodine-125 (^{125}I) seeds undergoing simulation for external-beam radiation therapy, the pelvic bony anatomy reflected fairly well the position of the prostate and its variations in position. Average variations in position of the prostate relative to bony anatomy were 1.7 mm in the craniocaudal, 1.5 mm in the ventrodorsal, and 0.8 mm in the lateral axis (61).

The seminal vesicles are located high in the pelvis and posterior to the bladder (Figure 25.6), which is particularly critical when reduced fields are designed in patients with clinical or surgical stage C2 (T3b) tumors. Perez et al. (62) demonstrated a correlation between size of the reduced portal and probability of pelvic tumor control.

The boost portal configuration and size should be individually determined for each patient, depending on clinical and radiographic assessment of tumor extent.

After the appropriate portals have been determined, the central axis and some corners of the reduced portals for both portals are tattooed on the patient with India ink.

To simulate these portals with the patient in the supine position, a small plastic rod with radiopaque markers 1 cm apart is inserted in the rectum to localize the anterior rectal wall. After thorough cleansing of the penis and surrounding areas with Betadine, using sterile technique, 25 to 40% iodinated contrast material is injected in the urethra until the patient complains of mild discomfort. AP and lateral radiographs are taken after the position of the small portals is determined under fluoroscopic examination; for 3-D CRT a topogram and a CT scan of the pelvis are performed. The urethrogram documents the junction of the prostatic and bulbous urethra and accurately localizes (within 1 cm) the apex of the prostate, which may be difficult to identify on CT or MRI scans without contrast.

A great deal of controversy has developed in reference to the most accurate anatomic location of the prostate apex. In a study of 115 patients, none of the urethrograms showed the urethral sphincter to be caudal to the ischial tuberosities; 10% were located less than 1 cm cephalad to a line joining the ischial tuberosities. If 2 cm or more are arbitrarily considered, 42.5% of patients would have received unnecessary irradiation to small volumes of normal tissues (63).

Cox et al. (64) evaluated urethrogram and CT scans of the pelvis for treatment planning in prostate cancer. Interobserver identification of the prostatic apex varied in 70% of cases. This variability resulted in an inadequate margin (less than 1 cm) beneath the urogenital diaphragm in 5% of patients. In contrast, placing the inferior border of the portal at the ischial tuberosities or the base of the

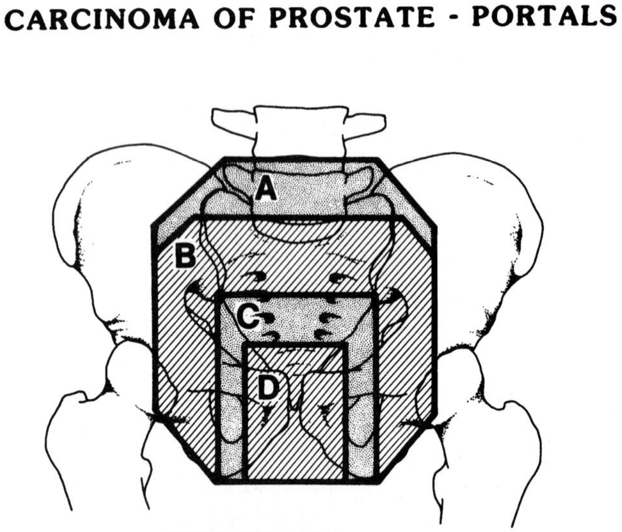

A

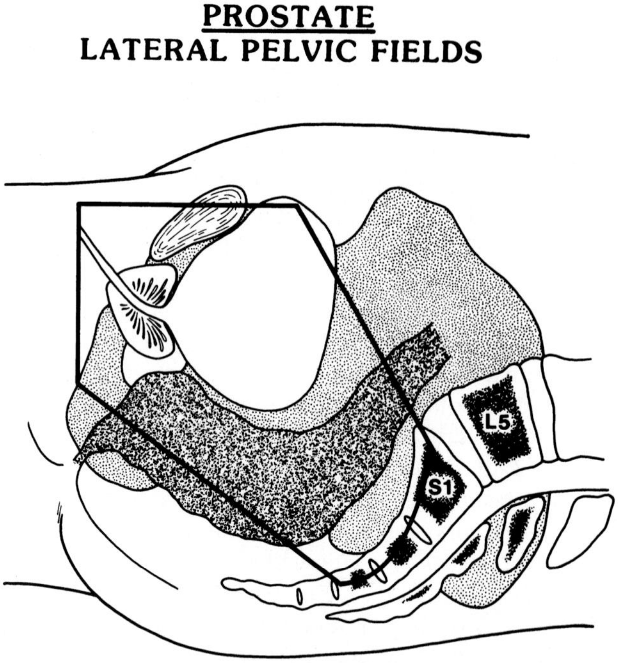

B

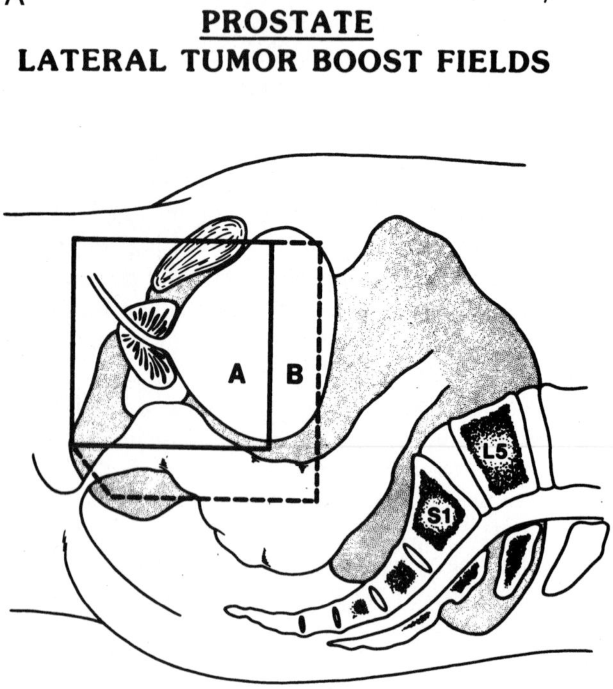

Figure 25.3. A. Diagrams of the pelvis showing volumes used to irradiate the pelvic lymph nodes, when indicated, and the prostate. Lower margin is at or even 1 cm below ischial tuberosities. At the Mallinckrodt Institute of Radiology, 15 × 15 cm portals at source-to-skin distance are used for selected stage A2, B, and all stage C disease and for high-risk postoperative patients, whereas for stage D1 disease, 18 × 15 cm portals are used when necessary to cover all lymph nodes up to the bifurcation of the common iliac vessels. Sizes of reduced fields are larger (up to 12 × 14 cm) when seminal vesicles and/or periprostatic tumor is irradiated compared with prostate boost only (up to 8 × 10 cm) or larger for patients with stage C tumors. **B.** Lateral portal used in box technique to irradiate pelvic tissues and prostate. The anterior margin is 1 cm posterior to projected cortex of pubic symphysis. Presacral lymph nodes are included down to S3; inferiorly the posterior wall of rectum is spared. C) Boost fields, lateral projection, used to irradiate the prostate. (Perez CA. Prostate. In: Perez CA, Brady LW, eds: Principles and practice of radiation oncology. 3rd ed. Philadelphia: Lippincott-Raven, 1998.) (1)

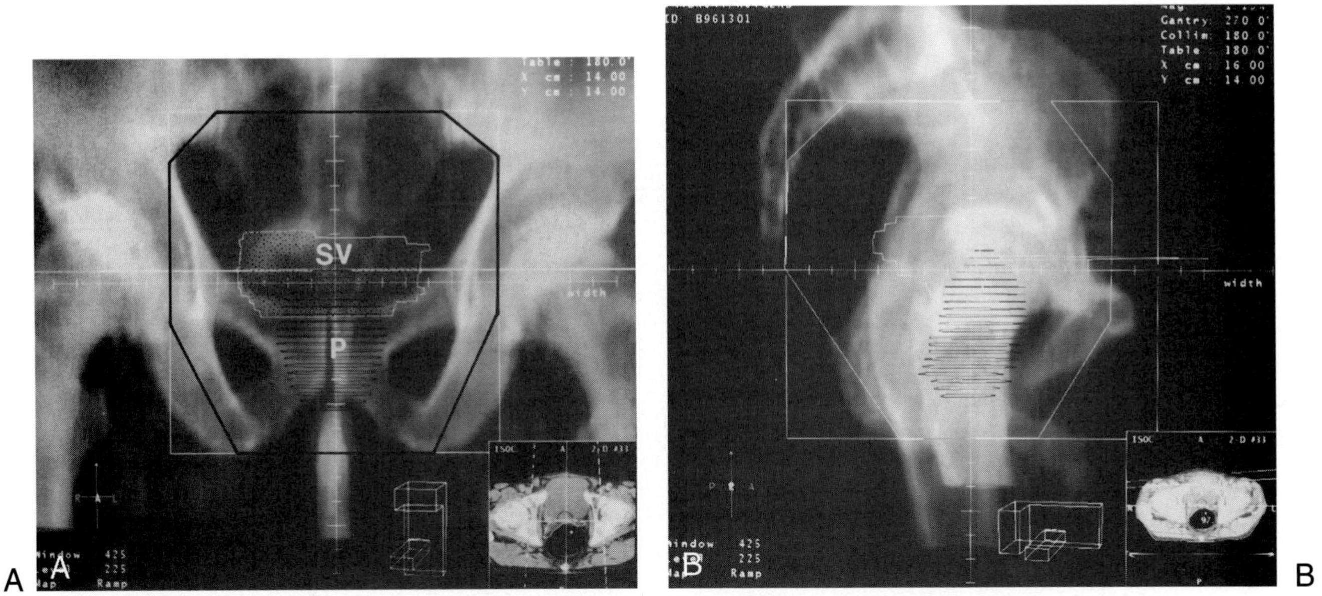

Figure 25.4. Anteroposterior A) and lateral B) 3-D volume reconstructions and portals for carcinoma of the prostate. The junction of the prostatic and bulbous urethra (distal margin of prostate) is identified by ureterogram. Note the relationship of the portals to the roof of the acetabulum, the pubic symphysis anteriorly, and the ischial tuberosities posteriorly. Note the position of the seminal vesicles (SV) above and posterior to the prostate (P). (Perez CA. Prostate. In: Perez CA, Brady LW, eds: Principles and practice of radiation oncology, 3rd ed. Philadelphia: Lippincott-Raven, 1998.) (1)

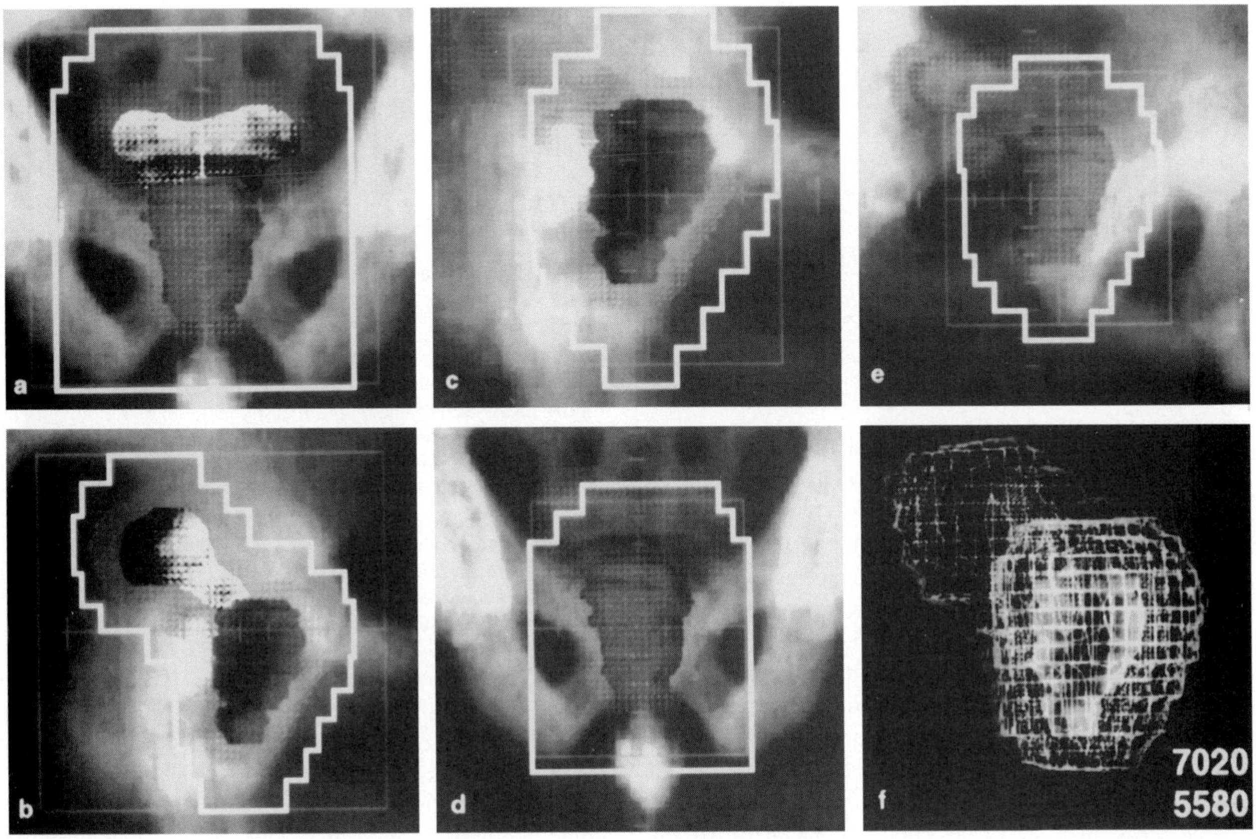

Figure 25.5. Three-dimensional volume reconstruction and portals for patient with seminal vesicle irradiation (dose 55.8 Gy) and prostate boost to 70.2 Gy. **A** and **B.** Larger portals for both seminal vesicles and prostate. **C** to **E.** Prostate-only portals. **F.** Volume isodose display. (Perez CA. Prostate. In: Perez CA, Brady LW, eds. Principles and practice of radiation oncology, 3rd ed. Philadelphia: Lippincott-Raven, 1998.) (1)

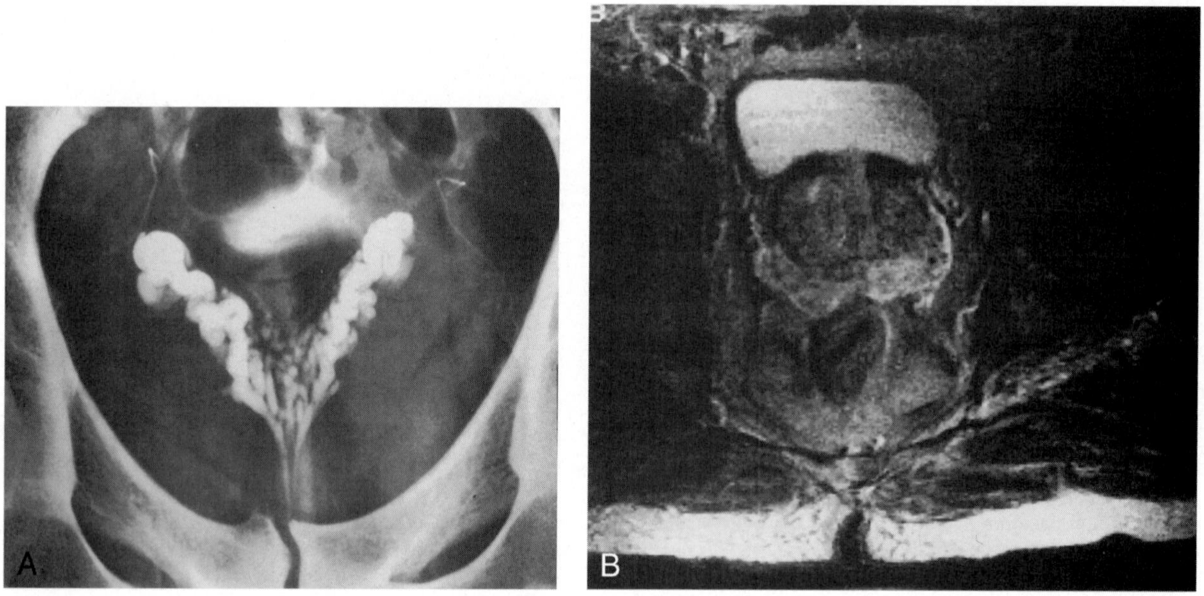

Figure 25.6. **A.** Anteroposterior radiograph of seminal vesicles with contrast material showing their high location. **B.** Cross-section of MRI scan of the pelvis illustrating position of enlarged seminal vesicle. This anatomic location must be kept in mind in patients with seminal vesicle extension, in whom the portals must be enlarged accordingly. (Perez CA. Prostate. In: Perez CA, Brady LW, eds. Principles and practice of radiation oncology, 3rd ed. Philadelphia: Lippincott-Raven, 1998.) (1)

penis, as seen on CT scans, ensured an adequate margin for all patients. They concluded that urethrography is more accurate than CT scanning in determining the inferior extent of the urogenital diaphragm.

Wilson et al. (65) determined the anatomic location of the apex of the prostate in 153 patients undergoing ^{125}I implants by direct surgical exposure (133 patients) or transrectal ultrasound (TRUS) (20 patients). There was excellent agreement in the estimate of location of the prostatic apex between the two methods. It was located 1.5 cm or more above the ischial tuberosities in approximately 95% of patients and within 1 cm in 98% (150 of 153) (Figure 25.7).

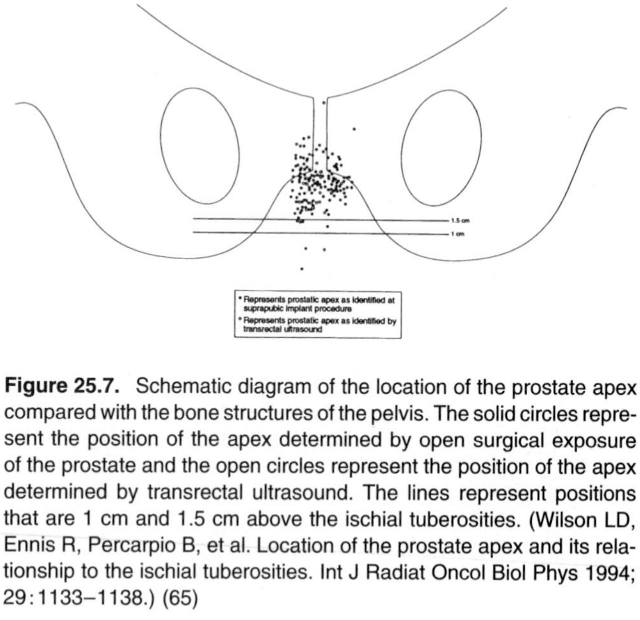

Figure 25.7. Schematic diagram of the location of the prostate apex compared with the bone structures of the pelvis. The solid circles represent the position of the apex determined by open surgical exposure of the prostate and the open circles represent the position of the apex determined by transrectal ultrasound. The lines represent positions that are 1 cm and 1.5 cm above the ischial tuberosities. (Wilson LD, Ennis R, Percarpio B, et al. Location of the prostate apex and its relationship to the ischial tuberosities. Int J Radiat Oncol Biol Phys 1994; 29:1133–1138.) (65)

Algan et al. (66) reviewed the location of the prostatic apex in 17 patients on whom an MRI scan was obtained in addition to retrograde urethrogram and CT scan of pelvis for 3-D treatment planning. The location of the prostatic apex as determined by the urethrogram alone was, on average, 5.8 mm caudad to the location on the MRI, while the location of the prostatic apex as determined by CT/urethrogram was 3.1 mm caudad to that on MRI. If the prostatic apex is defined as 12 mm instead of 10 mm above the urethrogram tip (junction of membranous and prostatic urethra), the difference between the urethrogram and MRI locations of the prostatic apex is no longer present.

Crook et al. (67), in 55 patients with localized carcinoma of the prostate, placed one gold seed under TRUS at the base of the prostate near the seminal vesicles, at the posterior aspect, and the apex of the prostate. At the time of first simulation a urethrogram was performed, and the rectum was opacified with 10 to 15 cc of barium. The tip of the urethrogram cone varied in position from 0 to 2.8 cm above the most inferior aspect of the ischial tuberosities. At initial simulation the apex of the prostate was less than 2 cm above the ischial tuberosities in 42% of patients, less than 1.5 cm in 19%, and less than 1 cm in 8%. Because of variability in the thickness of the urogenital diaphragm, only 12 of 22 (55%) of these low-lying prostates would have been detected by urethrogram.

Periaortic Lymph Node Irradiation

The periaortic lymph nodes can be treated through an extended AP-PA portal that includes both the pelvic and periaortic lymph nodes (Figure 25.8A), if large-field linear accelerator beams are available. Otherwise, a separate periaortic portal is placed above the pelvic fields, in which case calculations for an appropriate gap (usually about 3 cm) should be carried out (Figure 25.8B). To cover all of the periaortic lymph nodes, the portal's superior margin should be at the T12-L1 vertebral interspace. The width, which usually is about 10 cm, can be determined with the aid of a lymphangiogram or CT scans. If these studies are not available, the intravenous pyelogram indicates the trajectory of the ureters, which may be used as landmarks, although not 100% accurate. The dose to the distal spinal cord should be limited to 45 Gy with a 2 cm wide posterior 5 half-value layer block above the L2-3 interspace.

Beam Energy and Dose Distribution

Ideally, high-energy photon beams (>10 MV) should be used to treat these patients, which simplify techniques and decrease morbidity.

With photon beam energies below 18 MV, lateral portals are always necessary to deliver part of the dose in addition to the AP-PA portals (box technique). With photon energies above 18 MV, the lateral portals are not strictly necessary to deliver up to 45 Gy, except in patients with an AP diameter over 20 cm, because the improvement in the dose distribution is marginal. In our experience, the main advantage of using the box technique is a decrease in erythema and skin desquamation in the intergluteal fold, which occurs more frequently with the AP-PA portals. The additional prostate dose is administered with anatomically shaped lateral and oblique or rotational portals.

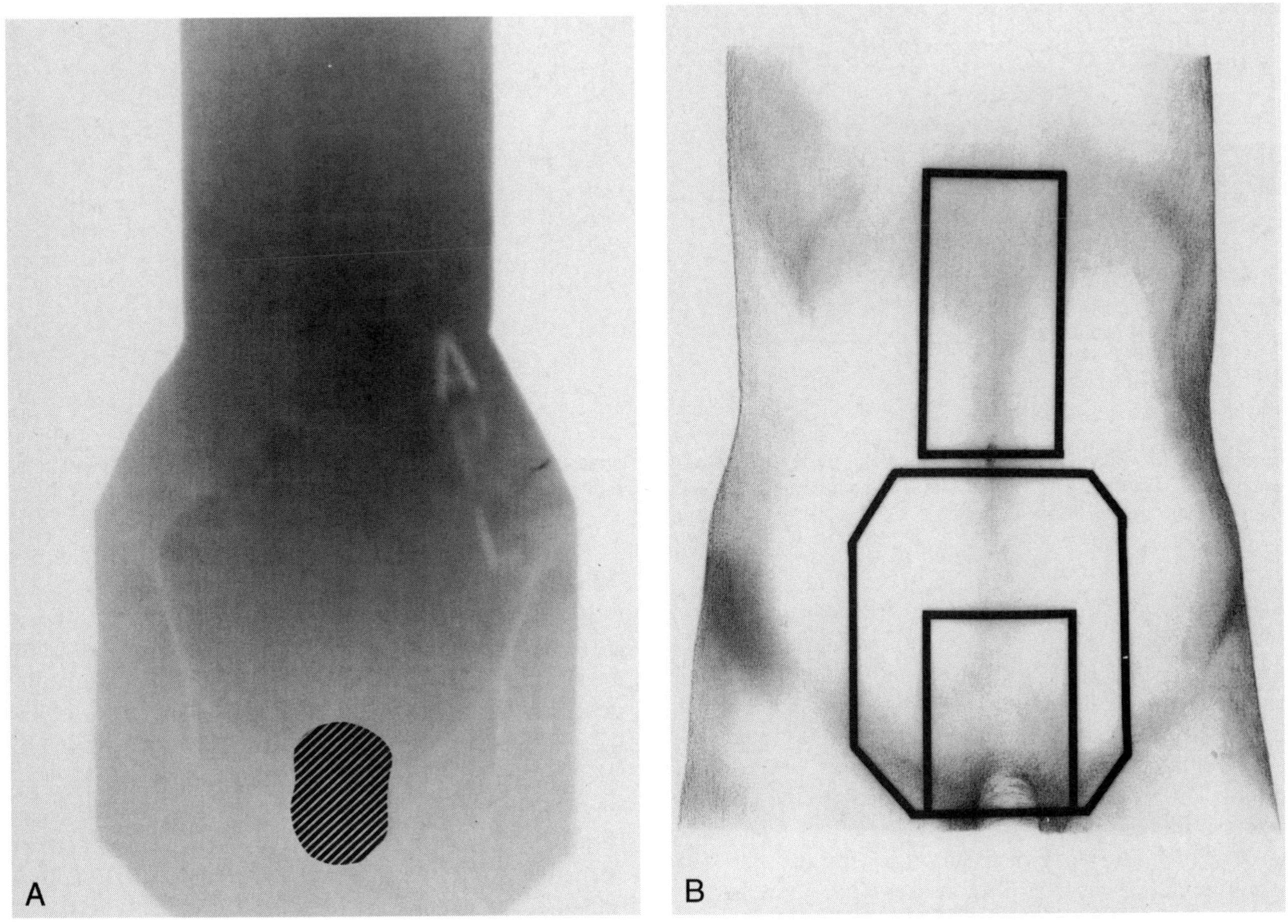

Figure 25.8. A. Localization film showing an extended portal for irradiation of the periaortic and pelvic lymph nodes in carcinoma of the prostate. **B.** Separate portals used for irradiation of the periaortic lymph nodes when large fields are not available. Gap separation must be calculated for each individual patient. (Perez CA. Prostate. In: Perez CA, Brady LW, eds. Principles and practice of radiation oncology. 3rd ed. Philadelphia: Lippincott-Raven, 1998.) (1)

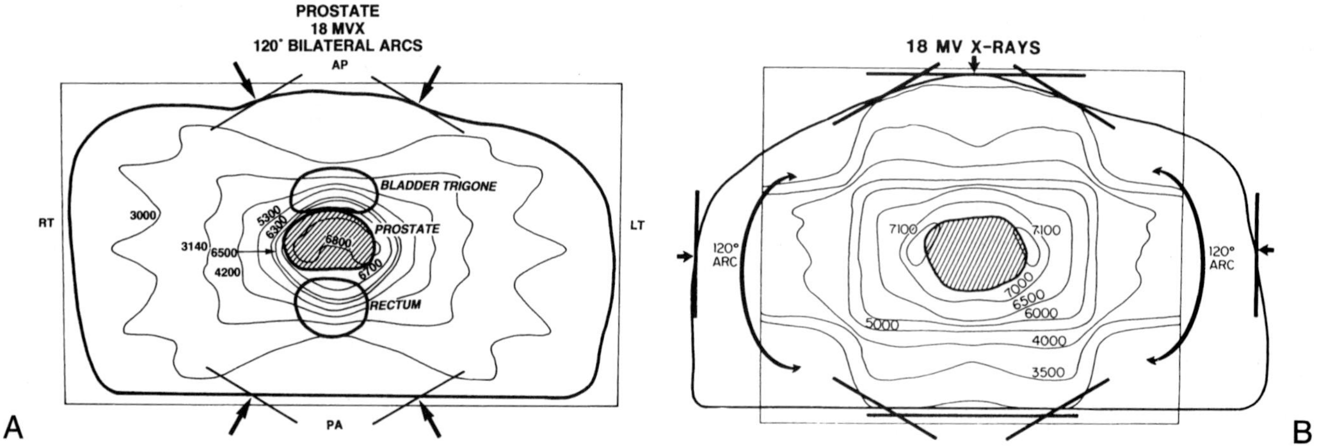

Figure 25.9. A. Isodose curves to deliver 68 Gy to the prostate with 18-MV photons, bilateral 120-degree arcs, skipping 60-degree anterior and posterior vectors. **B.** Isodose curves for irradiation of pelvic lymph nodes and prostatic volume using AP-PA and lateral fields to deliver 45 Gy to the pelvis and 26 Gy to prostate with reduced fields, bilateral 120-degree arcs. (Perez CA. Prostate. In: Perez CA, Brady LW, eds. Principles and practice of radiation oncology, 3rd ed. Philadelphia: Lippincott-Raven, 1998.) (1)

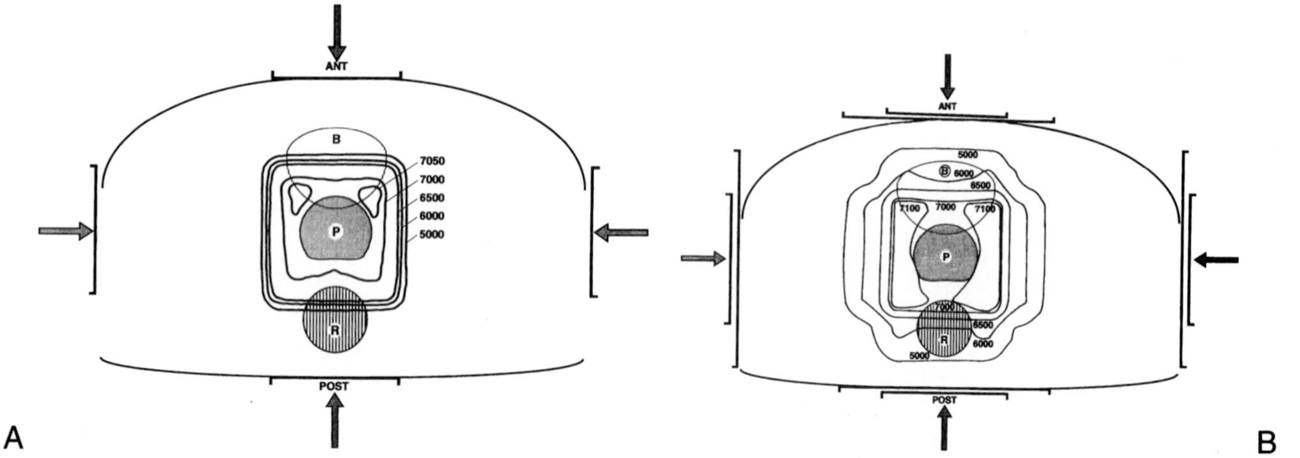

Figure 25.10. A. Dose distribution for box technique for AP/PA and lateral portals encompassing the prostate with a small margin. **B.** Box technique for pelvic fields to deliver 45 Gy to pelvic lymph nodes and additional dose for a total of 71 Gy to the prostate with reduced portals.

For the reduced volume, a reasonable dose distribution is obtained with bilateral 120° arc rotation, skipping the midline anteriorly and posteriorly (60° vectors). Figure 25.9A illustrates the dose distribution for 8 × 10 cm bilateral 120-degree arcs. The composite isodose of AP-PA portals with lateral portals to deliver 45 Gy to the pelvic lymph nodes with the addition of a boost of 24 to 26 Gy to the prostate and surrounding tissues with 120° bilateral arcs is shown in Figure 25.9B. The dose distribution for the prostate box technique portals alone is illustrated in Figure 25.10.

Standard Tumor Doses

A frequently used minimum tumor dose to the prostate is 64 to 66 Gy for stage A1 (T1a) when these patients are irradiated, 68 to 72 Gy for stage A and B (T1b,c) tumors, and approximately 72 Gy for stage C. For stage D1 lesions, treatment is usually palliative, and the minimum tumor dose can be held at 60 to 65 Gy to decrease morbidity. Most institutions treat with daily fractions of 1.8 to 2 Gy, five fractions per week (68,69). Treatment guidelines at Washington University are summarized in Table 25.5. Occasionally four weekly fractions of 2.25 Gy have been used (70). At least two portals should be treated daily to improve tolerance to irradiation.

Biggs and Russell (71) described an average dose decrease of approximately 2% for patients with metallic hip prostheses who were treated with lateral portals, and an average increase of 2% for 10-MV x-rays and 5% for ^{60}Co.

Table 25.5. Summary of Treatment Guidelines for Adenocarcinoma of Prostate Using High-Energy Photon Conventional Techniques

	Portal Size (cm at isocenter)		Tumor Doses[a] (Gy)	
Stage	Pelvic	Prostate	Pelvic Lymph Nodes	Boost
A1 (less than well differentiated)		8 × 10	0	64/6.5 wk
A2, B—Staging lymphadenectomy, negative pelvic lymph nodes		8 × 10 or 10 × 12	0	68–72/7 wk
A2–B1—No staging		10 × 12	0	68–72/7 wk
B2—No lymphadenectomy	16.5 × 16.5	8 × 10	45/5 wk	24/2 wk
A2, B—Any histology, older than 71 years		8 × 10 or 10 × 12	0	68–70/7 wk
A2, B—Positive common iliac nodes (plus 45 Gy to periaortic nodes)[b]	16.5 × 21	8 × 10	45/5 wk	24/2 wk
C—Negative lymphadenectomy	16.5 × 16.5	12 × 12 or 12 × 14	45/5 wk	26/2.5 wk
C—Positive external iliac or hypogastric nodes by any evaluation	16.5 × 21	10 × 12 or 12 × 14	45/5 wk	26/2.5 wk
C—Positive common iliac or periaortic nodes (plus 45 Gy to periaortic nodes)[b]	16.5 × 21	8 × 10 or 10 × 12	45/5 wk	26/2.5 wk
D1	16.5 × 21	10 × 12 or 12 × 14	45/5 wk	20/2 wk

[a] Daily dose: Large pelvis fields, 1.8 Gy; boost prostate portals, 2 Gy.
[b] In case of "grossly positive" periaortic nodes, add 5 to 10 Gy with reduced portals. In stage C, if seminal vesicles are involved (C2), boost portal may be 12 × 14 cm.
(Reprinted with permission from Perez CA. Prostate. In Perez CA, Brady LW, eds. Principles and practice of radiation oncology. 3rd ed. Philadelphia: Lippincott-Raven, 1998.) (1)

The usual dose for the pelvic and periaortic lymph nodes (when the latter are to be irradiated) is 45 Gy, with a boost (24 to 26 Gy) to the prostate or enlarged periaortic lymph nodes (5 Gy) through reduced fields (1).

Treatment Planning for Three-Dimensional Conformal Radiation Therapy

The theoretic basis and process of this approach are described in Chapter 9. For 3-D CRT of prostate cancer, four anterior and posterior oblique fields, an anterior, and two lateral fields are used to irradiate the prostate and, when indicated, the seminal vesicles (Figure 25.11). Following International Commission on Radiation Units (ICRU) Bulletin No. 50 (72) guidelines as determined on serial CT scans of the pelvis, gross tumor volume (GTV) for stages A2 and B (T1 and T2) is the prostate. The clinical target volume (CTV) is arbitrarily set as 0.5 cm around the prostate for stage A2 (T1c) and B1 (T2c) tumors and 0.8 cm around the prostate and seminal vesicles for stage B2 (T2b,c) or periprostatic tumor.

The planning target volume (PTV) has been reduced to 0.5 to 0.8 cm. The dose calculation algorithm used in our 3-D treatment planning system requires that an additional 0.7 cm margin from the PTV to the block edge be added to account for penumbra (73) (Table 25.6).

Pickett et al. (74) documented the value of nonuniform margins in 3-D CRT; 1.5 and 2 cm uniform margins adequately covered the CTV, but significantly higher doses were delivered to the bladder and rectum. Therefore, as we recommend, nonuniform margins to outline the CTV and PTV should be used in planning 3-D CRT in these patients (0.5 cm or even less after 70 Gy posteriorly along the anterior rectal wall).

When pathologic data from Bluestein et al (23) and Partin et al (25) and the formula proposed by Roach et al (75) are used, in patients with 15% or greater probability of seminal vesicle involvement, this volume is incorporated into the CTV (0.8 cm margin for PTV) to electively deliver 55.8 Gy. If the seminal vesicles are grossly involved, higher doses (64 Gy) are necessary. Thereafter, the prostate volume only is taken to the prescribed total dose.

Diaz et al. (76), using an empirical equation (75,77) in 188 patients treated with radical prostatectomy, noted that 20% of the rectal volume received an average above 86% of the total prostate dose in five plans that included the seminal vesicles compared with 68% volume for five plans excluding the seminal vesicles. The doses administered to 40% of the rectal volume were 64% and 37% of the tumor dose if the seminal vesicles were included or excluded, respectively. Dose to the bladder and femoral heads was also decreased but to a lesser extent when the seminal

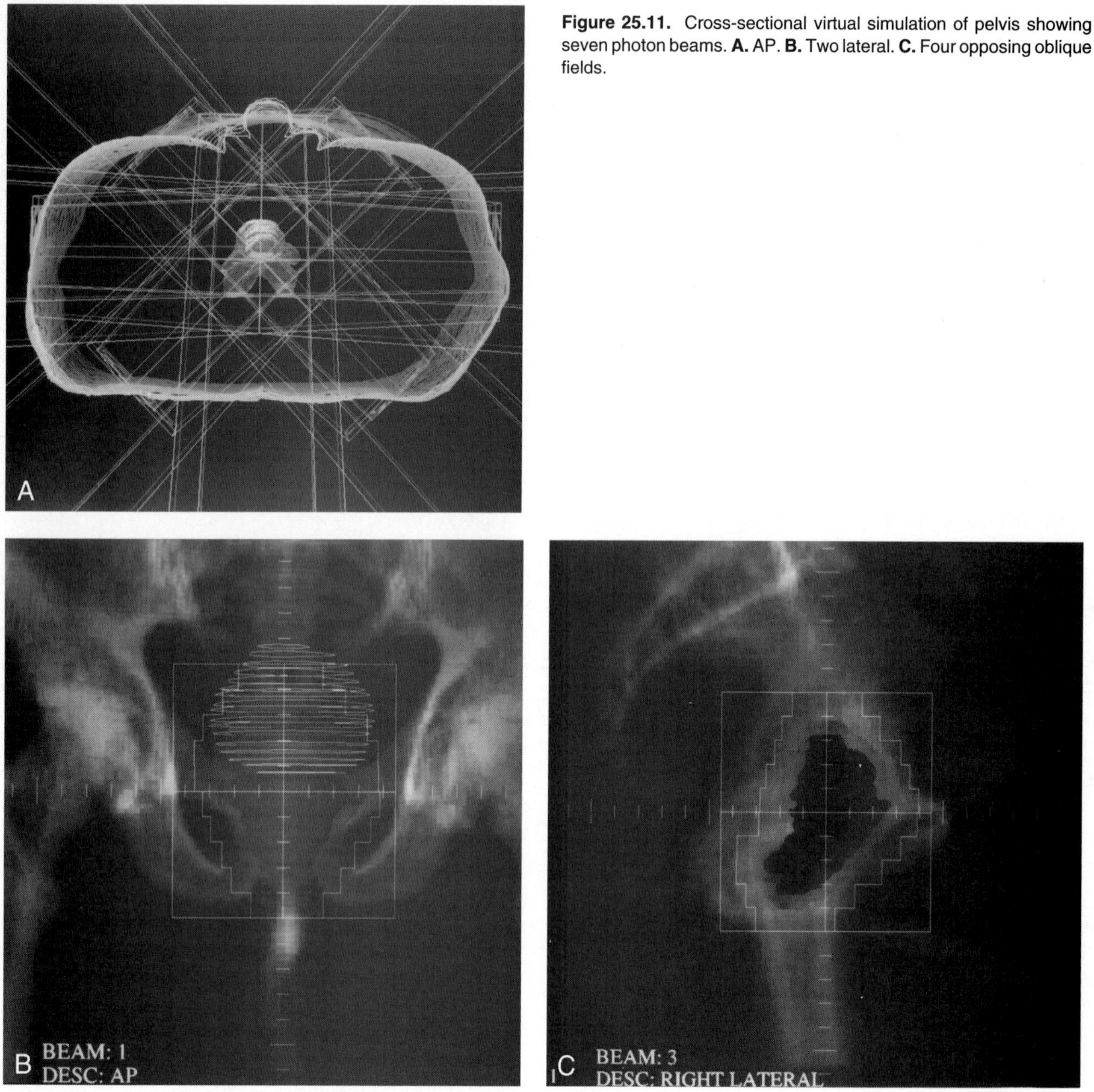

Figure 25.11. Cross-sectional virtual simulation of pelvis showing seven photon beams. **A.** AP. **B.** Two lateral. **C.** Four opposing oblique fields.

Table 25.6. Conformal Radiation Therapy Prostate Target Volumes

Stage	Gross Target Volume	Clinical Target Volume Equals Gross Target Volume Plus	Planning Target Volume Equals Clinical Target Volume Plus
A1	Prostate	0.0 cm margin	0.5 cm
A2	Prostate	0.5 cm margin	0.8 cm
B1	Prostate	0.5 cm margin	0.8 cm
B2	Prostate and seminal vesicles	0.8 cm margin; 0.5 cm posterior	0.8 cm
C1/C2	Prostate, seminal vesicles, and periprostatic extension	0.7 cm margin	0.8 cm

Note: Treatment of pelvic nodes is not part of 3-D treatment planning and is the decision of the radiation oncologist. Use AP-PA and right and left lateral portals.

(Reprinted with permission from Perez CA. Prostate. In Perez CA, Brady LW, eds. Principles and practice of radiation oncology. 3rd ed. Philadelphia: Lippincott-Raven, 1998.) (1)

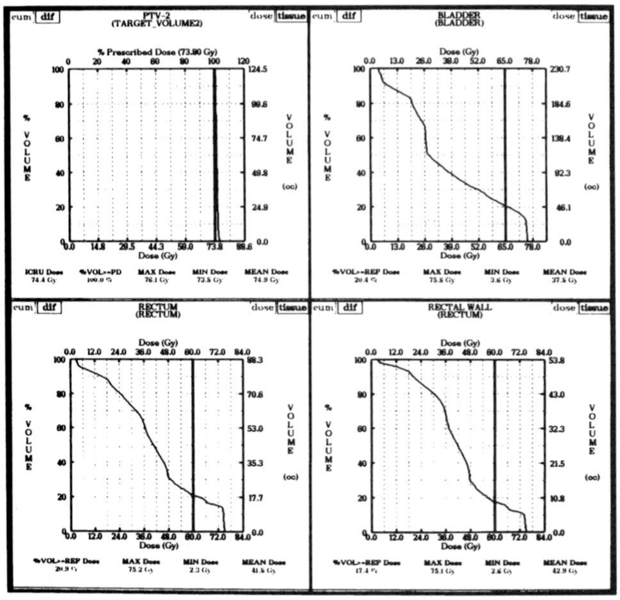

Figure 25.12. Dose-volume histograms for bilateral-arc rotation and seven-field 3-D conformal irradiation for planning target volume, bladder, rectum, and rectal wall.

vesicles are not irradiated. Thus, it is extremely important to identify patients at risk for seminal vesicle involvement and select the appropriate volumes for high-dose irradiation.

With virtual simulation, the outline of the portals is designed following 3-D volumetric reconstruction of the prostate and seminal vesicles and a margin. Three-dimensional planning is carried out in all patients, volumetric dose displays are generated, and percent of target volume receiving maximum, mean, and minimum tumor dose is determined (Figure 25.5F). Dose-volume histograms are routinely calculated for GTV, PTV, bladder, rectum, and femora (Figure 25.12) (60).

Neal et al. (78), in twelve patients with early prostate cancer treated with isocentric coplanar beams with three, four, six, or eight portals and optimized beam weights using dose-volume histograms, determined that six and eight fields had an advantage compared with three or four fields in respect to the percent of volume of femoral head receiving greater than 50% of the prescribed dose. The four-field plan was the best in reducing rectal irradiation (although this is not our experience), and the six-field plan provided more sparing of the bladder. The selection of optimal plans must be determined by the limits of radiation tolerance, expected toxicity in various structures within the irradiated volume, and complexity of delivery with more portals.

Roach et al. (79), based on dose-volume histograms, concluded that bilateral 120° arc rotation techniques or four-field conformal techniques would not allow significant dose escalation without increasing the risk of complications in comparison with six-field conformal techniques.

Motion of internal organs has been a source of concern when 3-D CRT is used. Beard et al. (80) evaluated prostate and seminal vesicle position changes between treatment planning and delivery in 30 patients. Although maximum target displacement of 1.3 to 2.2 cm did occur, the majority of the prostate and seminal vesicle median motion was between 0.1 and 0.3 cm in the various directions. Only about 20% of the patients had motion greater than 0.5 cm in the anterior and posterior directions, none in the right and left directions, and 7% and 23%, respectively, in the superior direction. Motion greater than 1 cm occurred in only 3% of patients in the posterior direction. Both rectum volume and diameter changes correlated with target motion for both the prostate and the seminal vesicles.

Rudat et al. (81) assessed patient positioning variability on 125 portal films (27 patients) compared with orthogonal simulator films and prostate motion on 107 CT scans of the pelvis (28 patients). They reported that the standard deviation (SD) of patient positioning error ranged from 3.1 to 5.4 mm. The prostate motion was significantly greater in the anteroposterior direction (1 SD = 2.8 mm) than in the mediolateral direction (1 SD = 1.4 mm). The 1 SD of the estimated combined error in the anteroposterior direction was 6.1 mm and in the mediolateral direction, 3.6 mm.

In a study by Crook et al. (67), there was minimal prostate motion in the lateral directions (0.1 to 0.5 cm). Movement in the craniocaudal axis was usually in the caudal direction (about 0.5 cm on average); 43% of patients showed more than 0.5 cm inferior displacement of the prostate and 11%, more than 1 cm. Average displacement in the posterior or dorsal direction was 0.72, 0.62, and 0.46 cm for seeds placed at the seminal vesicles, posterior aspect of the prostate, or apex of the gland, respectively; 60% of patients showed more than 0.5 cm posterior displacement of the prostate base and 30%, more than 1 cm. Roeske et al. (82) evaluated 10 patients on whom 42 CT scans of the pelvis were performed. Average motion was 6 mm for left to right, 6 mm in the anteroposterior direction, and 5 mm in the superior-inferior direction. Prostate motion in the anteroposterior direction was a strong factor in increasing rectal volume irradiated over the length of the prostate. Variations in the anteroposterior motion of the seminal vesicles also had a strong influence on changing rectal volume. However, there were no significant changes in the bladder volume with anteroposterior or superior-inferior motion of the prostate.

Published data suggest mean internal organ motion for the prostate of 5 to 10 mm in the anteroposterior direction, 1 to 2 mm in the lateral, and about 10 mm in the cephalad-caudal direction (60) (Table 25.7). For the seminal vesicles, motion may be greater (10 to 20 mm), particularly in the anteroposterior direction. This motion is primarily related to the contents (filling) of the bladder and the rectum.

Table 25.7. Prostate Internal Motion

Series	Anatomy	Range (mm)	Mean (mm)	Comments
Balter et al. (84)	Total (seeds)	0–7.5	"Typical" <4	Maximum expected: AP < 4.5, LR < 1.7, IS < 3.7
Beard et al. (80)	CT prostate anterior	0–10	4	CT study
	CT prostate lateral	0–3	1	
	CT seminal vesicles posterior	0–16	4.5	
Forman et al. (84)	CT prostate and seminal vesicles	0–37	12	Serial CTs
Melian et al. (85)	CT "target" anterior/posterior	0–30	Not stated	CT study
	CT "target" lateral	0–15	Not stated	
Schild et al. (86)	Prostate posterior (CT)	0–9	1	CT study
	Prostate anterior (CT)	0–8	2	
	Seminal vesicles (posterior/border)	0–10	2	
	Seminal vesicles (anterior/border)	0–17	1	
Ten Haken et al. (87)	Total (seeds)	0–20	5	Test in simulator with contrast
	Total (CT)	0–8	Not stated	
van Herk et al. (88)	Prostate (CT)		2.7 (SD)	4-degree rotation

AP, Anterior-posterior; LR, left-right; IS, inferior-superior; CT, computed tomography.
(Reprinted with permission from Perez CA, Michalski J, Drzymala R, et al. Three-dimensional conformal therapy (3-D CRT) and potential for intensity-modulated radiation therapy in localized carcinoma of prostate. In: Sternick ES, ed. The theory and practice of intensity modulated radiation therapy. Madison, WI: Advanced Medical Publishing, 1997:199–217.) (60)

In the technical implementation of 3-D CRT or intensity-modulated radiation therapy for treatment of prostate cancer, a critical parameter to be determined is the PTV (margins around the tumor volume). Allowance must be made in treatment planning for average organ motion to avoid systematic marginal misses that may compromise tumor control.

Diminishing the variability of patient positioning with 3-D CRT has been emphasized, and several methods have been described. In a prospective study of 90 patients receiving pelvic irradiation, Huddart et al. (89) observed mean portal placement errors of 0.25 to 0.42 cm. On each treatment day, 29% of anterior films and 45% of lateral films had at least one 0.5 cm error (9% of all portals had 1 cm error). This study showed that without customized immobilization devices to cover 95% of random and systematic errors, margins of 0.9 cm in the anteroposterior direction and 0.6 cm in the right-left lateral direction should be allowed between CTV and PTV.

Lebesque et al. (90) described their preliminary experience with 3-D treatment planning and conformal therapy in patients with T3 carcinoma of the prostate and pointed out significant variations in the high-dose rectum wall volume. They concluded that planning CT scan overestimates rectum and bladder filling during treatment and that only the wall structures have relatively constant volume during fractionated treatment. Along the same lines, Lu et al. (91) described a method of analyzing rectal surface area irradiated with conformal therapy by means of dose-surface histograms, which exclude the contents of a hollow organ that are irrelevant to biologic response of the organ. The wall volume of the whole organ is delineated easily and accurately on CT imaging. Dose-surface histograms are computed in a similar fashion as a dose-volume histogram, and normal tissue complication probability can be defined as a function of the dose-surface histogram.

Lee et al. (92) reported on 257 patients with localized prostate cancer treated with 3-D CRT to doses of 71 to 79 Gy. A small rectal block was added to the lateral boost fields for the last 10 Gy in 88 patients to reduce the dose to the anterior rectal wall. The posterior margin from CTV to PTV was reduced from 10 mm to 0 mm, and only 5 mm margin around the posterior edge of the prostate to the block edge was allowed for adequate buildup. There was a reduction by a factor of two in the incidence of grade 2 and 3 rectal morbidity in comparison with patients without use of a rectal block (Table 25.8). No data were provided on tumor control or chemical disease-free survival, which will be critical to obtain, because of the small margins and possible geographic misses.

Song et al. (93), in 62 patients treated with a four-field pelvic technique, compared no immobilization with three types of immobilization using Alpha cradle, Styrofoam leg immobilizer, or Aquaplast cast. The maximum variation in position was 2 cm, and the median was 1.2 cm. There was no significant difference in overall movement with any of the immobilization devices compared with no immobilization, but there was less vertical (9% versus 18%) ($P = .03$) and anteroposterior (6 versus 15%) ($P = .14$) movement with the Aquaplast than with any other device. However, in the lateral direction the Aquaplast had significantly more movement (32 versus 9%) ($p < 0.001$) than other devices.

Hanley et al. (94) described the value of on-line portal imaging in detecting errors in daily treatment setup in com-

Table 25.8. Crude and Actuarial Rate of Grade 2 and 3 Rectal Morbidity Correlated with Use of a Rectal Block

	With Rectal Block		No Rectal Block	
Central Axis Dose (Gy)	No. of Complications/No. of Patients (%)	Actuarial Rate[a] (%)	No. of Complications/No. of Patients (%)	Actuarial Rate[a] (%)
<74	0/3	0	1/16 (6)	8
74–76	6/85 (7)	10	29/121 (24)	19
Total	6/88 (7)	9	30/137 (22)[b]	18

[a] Actuarial rate at 18 months.
[b] $P = 0.003$.
(Reprinted with permission from Lee WR, Hanks GE, Hanlon AL, et al. Lateral rectal shielding reduces late rectal morbidity following high dose three-dimensional conformal radiation therapy for clinically localized prostate cancer: further evidence for a significant dose effect. Int J Radiat Oncol Biol Phys 1996;35:251–257.) (92)

parison with simulation films. Using 2-D representation of the patient's anatomy on the portal images could not account for patient rotations out of the image plane and, therefore, would result in erroneous correction of patient position as well as changes in the dose distribution calculated with 3-D dosimetry. The errors introduced in patient position by 2-D images were less than 1 mm and 1° when no out-of-plane rotations were present, and these errors caused insignificant effect on the 3-D dose distribution of the prescribed dose.

Brachytherapy

Permanent Interstitial Implants

Nearly abandoned as a method to treat early prostate cancer in the 1980s, prostate brachytherapy has regained popularity in the 1990s as a result of several technologic improvements. Brachytherapy offers conceptual advantages in the management of early prostate cancer as radioactive seed implantation delivers a high intraprostatic radiation dose. The isotopes that are commonly used for a permanent implantation, ^{125}I and Palladium-103 (^{103}Pd), have very low energies, and the radiation dose to adjacent organs falls off rapidly. The implant procedure, when done by a transperineal route, is very well tolerated by patients, and the procedure is typically done in 1 to 2 hours on an outpatient basis. Patients frequently resume normal activities within 1 week of the procedure. Patients for whom brachytherapy is appropriate as a sole modality avoid the 7 to 8 weeks of daily visits to the radiation oncology department for external-beam irradiation.

Patient Selection

Successful clinical results with prostate brachytherapy are highly dependent on careful selection of patients for this procedure. The ideal candidate for this procedure should have low-volume cancer with little risk of extraprostatic extension. Tumor stage should be T2b or less (95). Although no absolute limit for PSA or Gleason score has been reported as a contraindication to undergo this procedure, each of these values raises the risk of seminal vesicle invasion, regional lymph node metastases, or distant metastases, making this local therapy inappropriate. Patients with very large glands that exceed 60 cc are inappropriate candidates for prostate brachytherapy for two reasons: with increasing volume of the gland, the number of seeds and total radioactivity increase with a commensurate increased risk of complications, and the lateral aspects of the gland may be difficult to implant because of interference from the arch of the pubic bone, which may obstruct the transperineal placement of implant needles. A patient with a very large gland may be treated with 3 to 4 months of combined neoadjuvant androgen blockade with an luteinizing hormone-releasing hormone agonist and an antiandrogen to downsize the tumor and convert it to an appropriate size for this procedure.

Pubic arch interference can be assessed with a pelvic CT or MRI scan. The borders of the prostate gland can be superimposed on the lymph nodal aspect of the pubic bone as seen on the scan. At Washington University, we have used a digitally reconstructed radiograph with a transperineal projection to determine whether significant pubic arch interference exists (Figure 25.13).

Prostate brachytherapy can be used as the sole modality to treat favorable patients with prostate cancer or used as a boost to the prostate after external-beam irradiation. Appropriate candidates for implant alone include patients with T1a–c, T2a, and small T2b cancers. Patients with initial PSA levels of less than 10 ng/ml and Gleason scores of 6 or less are associated with a low risk of extracapsular extension of prostate cancer (23,74,96). On the other hand, patients with large T2b cancers, PSA level greater than 10 ng/ml, and Gleason score of 7 or higher have significant risk of extracapsular extension or may have larger tumor volume and, therefore, may benefit from a combination of external-beam irradiation and prostate implant (97). Most

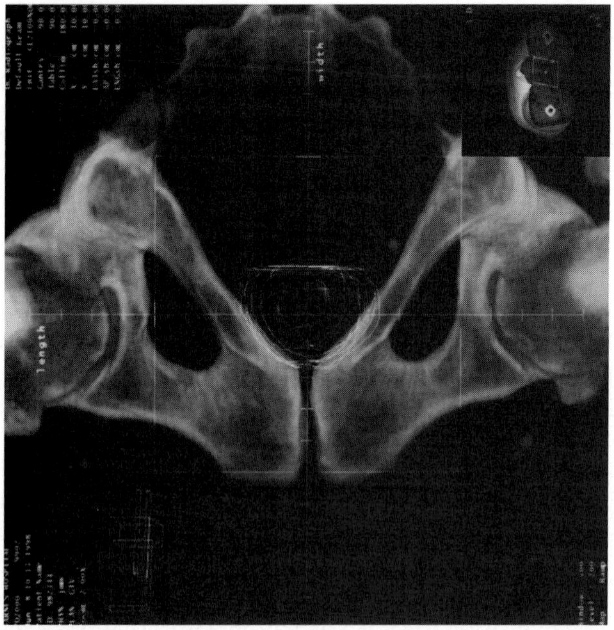

Figure 25.13. Digitally reconstructed radiograph to evaluate pubic arch interference. Contours of the prostate outline are overlaid on the transperineal projection of the pelvis, which illustrates minimal pubic arch interference.

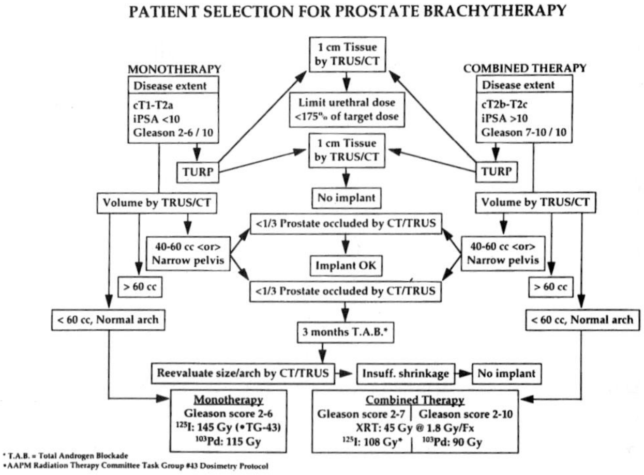

Figure 25.14. Algorithm for patient selection for brachytherapy in carcinoma of the prostate.

Table 25.9. Radionuclides Used in Prostate Brachytherapy

	^{125}I	^{103}Pd	^{192}Ir
Type of implant	Permanent	Permanent	Temporary
Brachytherapy	LDR	LDR	LDR, HDR
Average energy (KeV)	28	21	380
Physical half life (days)	59.6	17	74
Initial dose rate (cGy/hr)	8–10	20–25	Varies
Dose (Gy)			
Implant only dose	145	115	LDR: 65–70
LDR seed strength (mCi)	0.37	1.13	
			HDR: 17–20
Implant and external beam (45 Gy)	108	90	LDR: 30–35
LDR seed strength (mCi)	0.3	1.0	
			HDR: 17–20

LDR, low dose rate; HDR, high dose rate.

centers using the combined radiation therapy program deliver the external-beam therapy first, followed by the implant within 2 to 3 weeks (41.4 to 45 Gy delivered in 1.8 Gy fractions using a four-field pelvic box technique) (97,98). Other centers have used an alternative schedule of implantation followed by external-beam irradiation (99).

Patients who have undergone a prior TURP for benign prostatic enlargement may have an increased risk of urethral complications (100). In the series reported by Blasko et al. (100), 15 of 124 (12%) patients who had prior TURP developed superficial urethral necrosis, whereas only 1 of 262 patients (0.4%) without TURP developed this complication. Wallner et al. (101), on the other hand, described no increased risk of urinary morbidity in patients who underwent a TURP if a peripheral seed loading technique was used. These authors stressed the importance of having at least 1 cm of prostate tissue posterior to the TURP defect in order to maintain an acceptable rectal dose (102).

An algorithm summarizing the above criteria is shown in Figure 25.14.

Isotope Selection

Iodine-125 and ^{103}Pd are currently used for permanent implants (Table 25.9). Each of these seeds has very similar physical dimensions; therefore, techniques used for ^{125}I implantation are applicable to ^{103}Pd. However, ^{103}Pd differs from ^{125}I in possessing a slightly lower energy (21 KeV versus 27 KeV) and a significantly shorter half life (17 days compared with 60 days for ^{125}I). The lower energy of ^{103}Pd results in a minor reduction of tissue penetration when compared with ^{125}I. The dose distribution effect of this difference is insignificant for seed-to-seed distances of 1.7 cm or less and linear planar, biplanar, and cubic configurations are similar for both sources, providing spacing requirements are met (103). Because of the more rapid fall-off of dose beyond 1.7 cm, Blasko and Schumaker (104) strongly recommend a maximum seed spacing of no more than 1 cm seed-to-seed and needle-to-needle with ^{103}Pd to decrease the amount of rectum receiving a high dose (105). Because of the more rapid radial dose fall-off of ^{103}Pd, inexact seed placement or seed migration may compromise the radiation dose distribution with hot or cold spots.

The shorter half-life of ^{103}Pd results in its cumulative total dose being delivered in a substantially shorter time than with ^{125}I. The initial dose rate at the periphery of an implant using ^{103}Pd is typically 21 to 25 cGy per hour compared with about 8 to 10 cGy per hour with ^{125}I. Because of this substantial difference in initial dose rate, the total prescribed dose for ^{103}Pd is reduced to maintain acceptable tolerance of the adjacent critical structures. It has been suggested, yet not clinically proved, that patients with high-grade tumors or more rapid proliferative indices are more sensitive to the higher initial dose rate that accompanies a ^{103}Pd implant than the low dose rate (LDR) that is seen with ^{125}I (106,107). Nag et al. (108), in an experiment with the Dunning R3327 prostate tumor transplanted in the thigh of rats and exposed to interstitial irradiation with equivalent doses of either ^{103}Pd (45.5 Gy in 7 days) or ^{125}I (63.3 Gy in 26 days), observed somewhat greater tumor regrowth delay with ^{103}Pd. In a similar experiment with a poorly differentiated prostate cancer model, tumors treated with ^{103}Pd had a statistically significant improvement in regrowth delay and tumor necrosis compared with the same tumor model treated with ^{125}I (109).

When the brachytherapy literature is reviewed, care should be taken when evaluating prescription and other reported doses with ^{125}I seeds. The American Association of Physicists in Medicine (AAPM) Radiation Therapy Committee Task Group No. 43 (TG-43) published a new dosimetry protocol for LDR interstitial brachytherapy sources (110). Luse et al. (111) described a method for implementing the TG-43 protocol for transperineal implants on commercial planning systems. When the TG-43 formalism is incorporated, the radiation dose that corresponds to the historical 160 Gy prescription is closer to 145 Gy, or 11% lower. If a treatment planning system is used for ^{125}I brachytherapy, the prescribed dose should be adjusted accordingly. When the TG-43 formalism is used, the old 160 Gy prescription dose for ^{125}I prostate brachytherapy is now equivalent to 145 Gy, and the 120 Gy prescription dose is now equivalent to 108 Gy. In this chapter, the ^{125}I doses are assumed to be TG-43 compliant unless stated otherwise.

Brachytherapy Procedures

Retropubic Technique Hilaris and Batata (112) described this implant technique in detail, and at the present time it is only of historical interest. ^{125}I seeds were initially implanted permanently in the prostate through an open retropubic laparotomy incision with the patient in a modified lithotomy position after an extraperitoneal bilateral pelvic lymphadenectomy was performed.

The methods for dose calculation and specification with ^{125}I implants were described by Anderson and Aubrey (113). The matched peripheral dose (MPD) was identified as well as the integral dose within the MPD contour. Although the initial dose rate in the center of the implant could be double this value, the peripheral dose was considered the determining factor. The average MPD was 145 Gy with a standard deviation of 13 Gy.

The retropubic approach to prostate seed implantation has largely been abandoned. Despite early encouraging results at 5 years, late local failures occurred in a large proportion of patients (114,115). It is likely that uneven placement of ^{125}I seeds resulted in underdosed cold spots and eventually local treatment failure.

Transperineal Technique Several authors, including Blasko et al. (116), Holm et al. (117), and Wallner et al. (118), described the technique for ^{125}I implants of the prostate using a transperineal approach under ultrasound or CT-guidance. Following a planning volume study using TRUS (vide infra), a 4 to 7.5 MHZ ultrasound probe is rigidly fixed to the operating room floor or table with a stabilization device. With the patient in the lithotomy position, the scrotum and testis are pulled up anteriorly; after preparation and draping of the perineum and adjacent areas, the ultrasound probe is advanced into the rectum using a precisely calibrated stepping device that moves the probe in 5-mm increments. A template drilled with an array of 17- or 18-gauge holes with 5-mm spacings is attached to the stepping device and placed against the patient's perineum when he is in a dorsolithotomy position (Figure 25.15). The hole positions of the rigid template are displayed on the ultrasound monitor superimposed on the axial ultrasound images of the prostate. This system allows for real-time visualization of needle position within the prostate gland relative to both the hardware template and ultrasound monitor. In addition, fluoroscopic x-ray visualization of needle position can be performed to verify depth of insertion.

Advantages of the transperineal approach over the retropubic approach include avoidance of a major surgical procedure and performance of the procedure in an outpatient setting. One disadvantage of the transperineal approach is the occasional problem with needle insertion in the anterolateral portion of the prostate because of pubic arch interference, which may result in areas of underdosing. This can often be overcome by careful patient selection or, in some patients, preimplant use of neoadjuvant hormone therapy to downsize the prostate gland.

Roy et al. (119) recommend that needles be placed at oblique angles to cover the anterior prostate adequately. However, unless differential loading of source activity is used, it is possible that high doses may be delivered to the central and anterior portions of the gland (120). On the other hand, rapid dose fall-off in the most peripheral portion of the gland may result in underdosing of posterior, peripheral prostate cancer or overdosing of the anterior rectal wall. Roy et al. (121), in an analysis of 10 prostate implants with CT-planned and fluoroscopically guided radioactive ^{125}I seed placement, found that the 150 Gy pre-

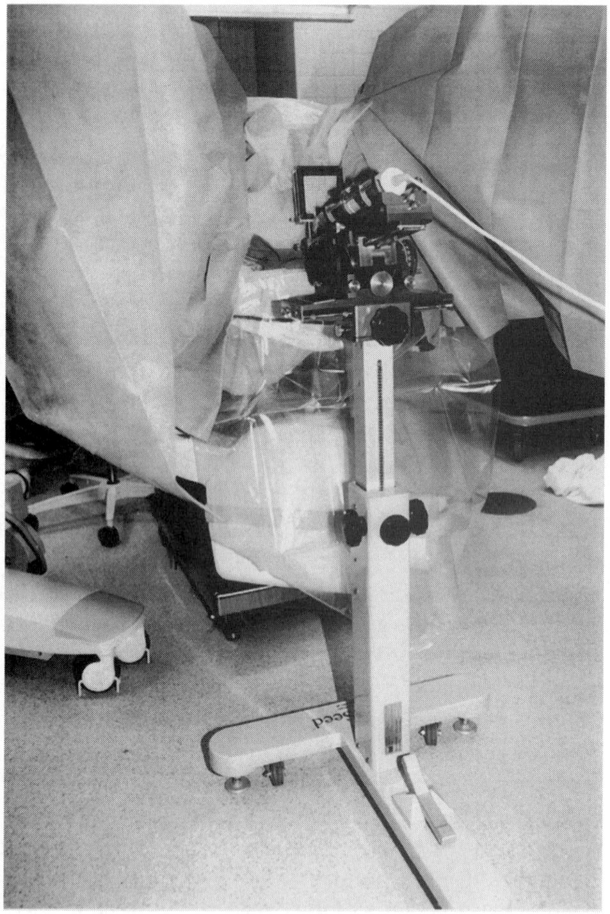

Figure 25.15. Intraoperative photograph of transrectal ultrasound probe in place. Patient is in a dorsolithotomy position. The ultrasound probe is attached to a precision stepping unit with a floor-mounted stabilization device. (Stabilization and stepping units courtesy of Tagman Medical, St. Louis, MO.)

scription isodose line encompassed only 78 to 96% of the total prostate volume.

Preimplant Volume Study and Treatment Planning

In preparation for the actual implant procedure, ultrasound images of the prostate gland are acquired for treatment planning. The patient is placed in a dorsolithotomy position, and a Foley catheter or aerated lubricating jelly is inserted through the penis in order to visualize the prostatic urethra on the ultrasound images. Microbubbles in aerated lubricating jelly serve as an ultrasound contrast agent that shines brightly on the ultrasound images. If a catheter is used to visualize the urethra, care must be taken not to pull the catheter balloon against the prostate base because this may distort the geometry of the gland and compromise the preimplant treatment planning.

Once the prostate is visualized on ultrasound, the prostate base is identified, and its position recorded. The posterior aspect of the prostate is positioned relative to the ultrasound probe so that all parts of the gland are at least 5 mm anterior to the rectal wall and probe surface. The posterior row of needles should be targeted just inside the prostate capsule. Excessive pressure on the prostate from the probe may distort the gland and push the lateral aspects posterior to the implant plane. The prostate images should be centered side-to-side within the implant template. Images of the prostate are acquired in 5-mm increments starting at the base through the apex. On each 5-mm ultrasound slice, the prostate is outlined. Once the ultrasound images have been acquired, additional target and normal tissue contours are added for dosimetry planning. It is our practice to contour the prostatic urethra and anterior rectal wall. A PTV is added around the prostate contours to account for any seed migration, inaccurate placement, intraoperative swelling, or uncertainties in duplicating the prostatic position at the time of the actual procedure. Generally, a 2- to 3-mm margin is added anterolaterally at the midportion of the gland. Superiorly and inferiorly, an additional margin equivalent to a 5-mm ultrasound plane is added to account for 3-D changes in the prostate shape from superior to inferior (Figure 25.16).

Treatment planning is undertaken by a dosimetrist or physicist based on the physician's prescription. When ^{125}I is used as monotherapy, the intent is to deliver 145 Gy to the PTV over the life of the implant. When combined with external-beam irradiation, the prescription is 108 Gy minimum dose to the PTV. Each of these prescription doses reflects the TG-43 changes in ^{125}I dosimetry (114). When ^{103}Pd is used as monotherapy, 115 Gy is prescribed as a minimum to the PTV. When used in combination with external-beam irradiation, a dose of 90 Gy is prescribed to the PTV (100).

Various seed-loading techniques have been described. Blasko et al. (102) described a uniform seed placement technique with 1-cm spacing between needles and each individual seed. For ^{125}I a source strength of 0.37 mCi per seed is used to deliver the 145 Gy prescription. For patients receiving a combination of external-beam irradiation plus an ^{125}I implant, a source activity of 0.30 mCi per seed delivers the prescribed dose of 108 Gy. To deliver 115 Gy with ^{103}Pd, a source strength of 1.3 to 1.5 mCi per seed is required. When combined with external-beam irradiation, a source strength of 1.0 mCi per seed is used to deliver 90 Gy minimum target dose. Uniform seed loading delivers a very high central dose, sometimes exceeding 200% of the prescribed peripheral dose. Because of this high central dose area, efforts have been made to decrease the central loading without compromising the minimum dose to the target volume. Wallner et al. (122) described a technique of using more seeds located peripherally in the prostate gland. Generally, needles are placed within 5 mm of the prostate gland capsule. A source strength of 0.7 mCi per seed has been used to deliver the prescribed dose of

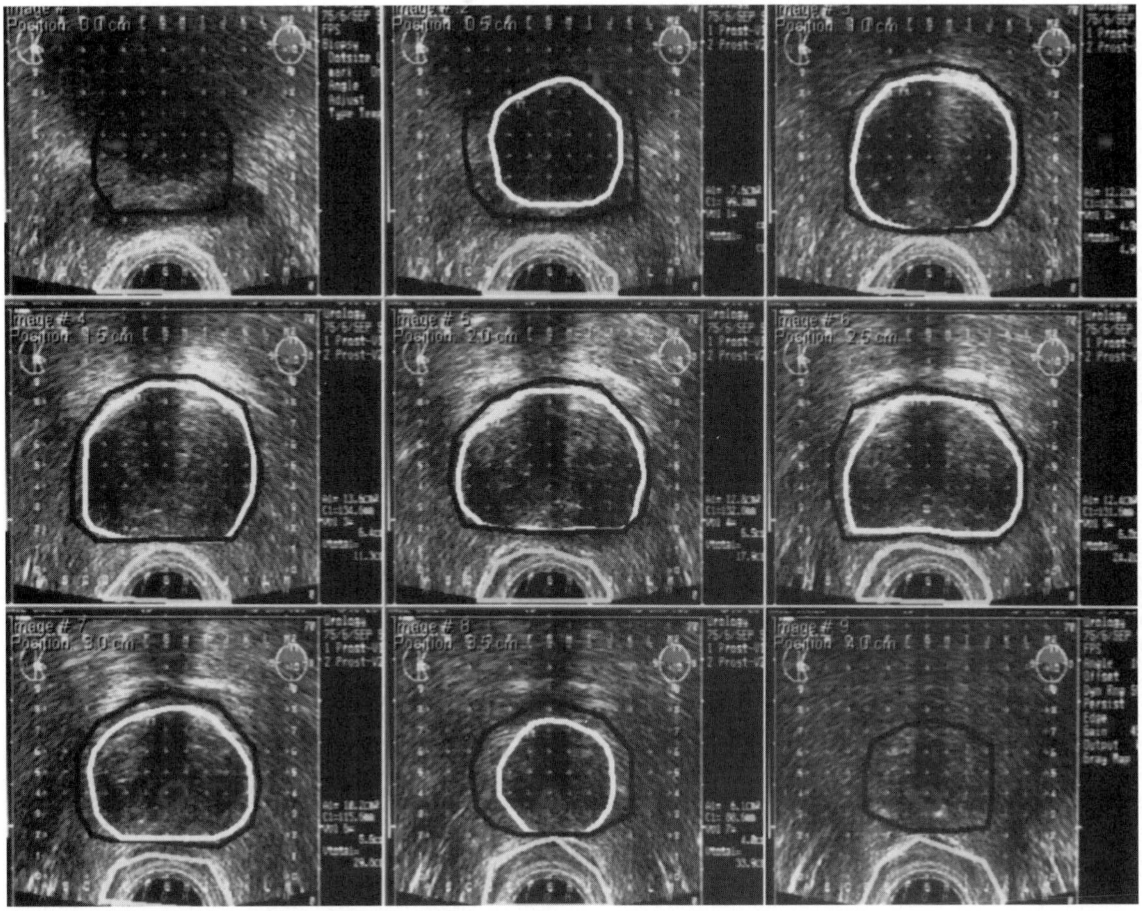

Figure 25.16. Ultrasound volume study for preimplant dosimetry. The prostate is contoured in white and the PTV margin in black. The margin is larger at the prostate base and apex to account for three-dimensional changes in the gland contours. Posteriorly, there is no margin because the ultrasound probe contacts the rectal wall and prostate directly.

145 Gy minimum peripheral dose. This technique results in a lower central dose and, therefore, urethral sparing; however, dose to the rectum may be greater with this method than with the uniform loading method.

A modified loading treatment planning technique has been described by Merrick et al. (123); uniform loading is modified by placing extra needles around the anterior and lateral periphery of the target volume to eliminate cold spots. The seed spacing in these extra needles is kept at 1 cm, but the depth of seed insertion is offset by 5 mm relative to the initially uniformly loaded needles. The central periurethral needles are modified to contain less than one seed per centimeter. These "special" needles may have seeds only at the base and apex with a series of spacers between them to maintain a central urethral dose that does not exceed 150% of the prescription (Figure 25.17).

Wallner et al. (124) suggested dosimetric guidelines that would minimize urethral and rectal morbidity following transperineal ^{125}I prostate brachytherapy. In patients with central urethral doses exceeding 400 Gy (pre-TG-43 value), rectal morbidity was significantly reduced if the rectal surface dose was kept below 100 Gy (pre-TG-43 value). Stone et al. (125) has developed a table to determine the total activity of seeds required to implant a gland of predetermined volume. This look-up table as well as the nomographs described by Anderson et al. (126,127) allow ordering of seeds in advance of the implant without a volume study. This approach requires plan development or modification at the time of the implant procedure.

Implant Procedure

The procedure is performed under either spinal or general anesthesia. The patient is placed into the dorsolithotomy position. Aerated lubricating jelly is instilled into the urethra to allow its visualization on ultrasound. The ultrasound probe is introduced into the rectum, and the prostate is visualized on the ultrasound monitor. Once the prostate position has been duplicated relative to the pretreatment volume study, the ultrasound is secured to the stepping device, and the stepping device is stabilized either to the oper-

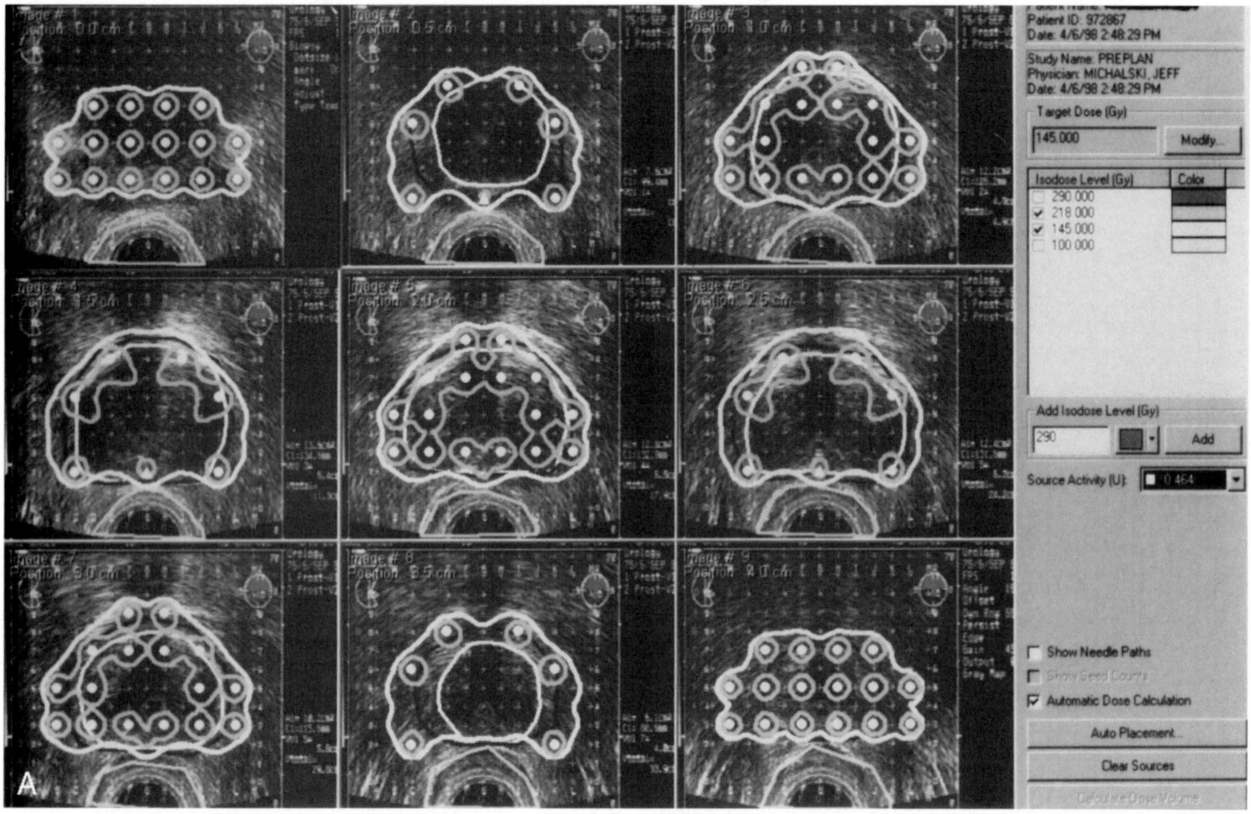

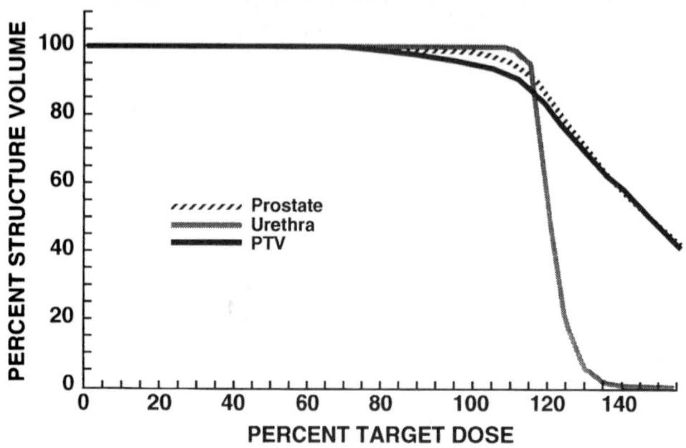

Figure 25.17. A. A preimplant treatment plan using the modified uniform loading technique described by Merrick et al. (123). Isodose curves displayed are 150% and 100%. Source positions are represented by the points on the grid. Alternate slices are loaded heavily or peripherally. The periurethral sources have been removed to decrease the dose to that organ. **B.** A dose-volume histogram of the planned implant for the PTV, urethra, and rectum.

ating room floor or table. The base of the prostate is identified, and its position relative to the stepping unit is recorded. The needle template is then placed against the patient's perineum and needle insertion begins.

Various methods have been described to place needles and seeds into the prostate gland. A Mick applicator inserts sources one at a time as the needle is withdrawn from the patient in 5 or 10 mm increments. Other investigators have used preloaded needles according to the pretreatment volume isodose study plan. Needle tips can be occluded with a small plug of bone wax, and sources are loaded at 1-cm intervals with 5-mm catgut spacers between each source. An alternative to free seed loading is the use of Vicryl suture-encased ^{125}I source arrays. These Vicryl stranded sources can be cut to the desired length with the appropriate number of seeds per strand and loaded directly into an implant needle. Because the Vicryl casing is fragile, these sources may become jammed in the implant needle if it is occluded with a thick plug of bone wax. A technique of plugging the implant needle with melted Anusol-HC suppositories can occlude the needle tip and prevent accidental extrusion of the Vicryl-encased seed array (128). When inserted into the patient, the Anusol-HC melts at body temperature allowing free and easy extrusion of the Vicryl-encased ^{125}I seeds into the targeted position. Care must be given to inserting the Vicryl-encased sources into or around the urethra as this material may trap the source against the sensitive urethral mucosa.

To minimize prostate motion during the implant procedure, stabilization needles may be used. Generally, stabilization needles are placed in the posterolateral aspect of the gland and anterior midline (129,130).

Brachytherapy needle insertion begins in the most anterior aspect of the prostate gland. Depth of insertion is generally measured relative to the prostate base. Under ultrasound visualization, the brachytherapy needles are inserted until the needle tip can be seen as a "star" on the ultrasound monitor. Once position of the needle is visualized on ultrasound, its position can be verified either radiographically using fluoroscopy or manually using a ruler that measures the distance from the needle hub to the template. The radiographic sources are then extruded into the gland by holding the internal trocar steady and withdrawing the implant needle back over the trocar, thereby pushing the seeds into the prostate gland. This procedure is repeated with each needle. The physician works from anterior to posterior in order not to have imaging artifacts from posteriorly placed seeds interfere with anterior needle visualization. Periodically during the procedure, the baseline should be verified because prostate swelling may shift the base plane.

Sagittal ultrasound imaging of the prostate may assist in verifying needle insertion depth and seed placement within the prostate base. At the conclusion of the procedure, cystoscopy is commonly performed to retrieve any seeds that may have been inadvertently placed into the prostatic urethra or beyond the prostate, into the bladder.

Postimplant Dosimetry

Following the implant procedure, a CT scan of the prostate is obtained for postimplant dose calculation. Images are generally obtained in 5-mm slice thickness. Timing of the postimplant CT scan may affect the dosimetry. Within 24 hours of the procedure, prostate edema may make the target volume appear larger than the preimplant volume study, which will make the isodose coverage appear inadequate. In most cases postimplant edema is reduced within 3 weeks (129–131). At some institutions it is not practical to have the patient return 3 to 4 weeks after the procedure, and in those situations the postimplant CT scan is done within 24 hours after the implant procedure. Despite the presence of edema, the early CT scan allows a more rapid evaluation of implant quality. Some investigators have recommended the use of perioperative corticosteroids to minimize this edema (129).

The prostate, rectum, and urethra are outlined on the CT scan for dosimetry calculation. The urethra is identified with the use of a Foley catheter in the patient who has the CT scan done the same day as the procedure (day 0). Because of patient discomfort, a catheter is not commonly placed at 3 weeks after the procedure for CT dosimetry (Figure 25.18).

Quality assessment of postimplant dosimetry is currently under evolution. Stock et al. (132) described a dose-response relationship for patients undergoing prostate brachytherapy with ^{125}I sources. If the D-90 (dose delivered to 90% of the prostate tissue as defined by CT scan) exceeded 140 Gy, the freedom from biochemical failure rate was 92% compared with only 68% in patients who had a D-90 of less than 140 Gy. Another measure of implant quality is the V-100 (percent volume of the prostate covered by 100% of the prescribed dose).

Perioperative Management

Patients frequently have urinary symptoms after transperineal prostate brachytherapy. Prophylactic antibiotics are generally given before and after the implant procedure. Pain from the implant is usually mild and can be managed with nonnarcotic analgesics. Selective alpha blockers such as tamsulosin, prazosin, or terazosin may minimize obstructive urinary symptoms. Nonsteroidal antiinflammatory agents may minimize perioperative edema of the prostate gland and relieve the perineal pain and discomfort associated with the procedure. Some investigators have reported the use of perioperative steroids to minimize prostate edema with reasonably good success (98). Infection should be ruled out in patients with dysuria shortly after the implant procedure. Patients with symptoms of bladder instability with urinary frequency, urgency, and nocturia may benefit from anticholinergics. Phenazopyridine hydrochloride may alleviate mild dysuria in some patients. Patients who are unable to void after the implant may require placement of a Foley catheter. The Foley catheter can be plugged or attached to a leg bag to allow the patient to be discharged. Generally, within 24 to 48 hours most patients can have the catheter removed and can void without further obstructive problems. Occasionally, patients with recurring obstructive symptoms may require intermittent sterile straight catheterization or placement of a suprapubic tube for urinary drainage. Because TURP and transurethral incision of the prostate increase the risk of urinary incontinence, these procedures should be avoided if at all possible.

Removable Interstitial Implants with Iridium 192 Charyulu (133), Syed et al. (134), and Martinez et al. (135) developed interstitial implant techniques using removable ^{192}Ir sources with a transperineal template for the treatment of carcinoma of the prostate.

In Syed's technique, a bilateral pelvic lymphadenectomy is carried out without mobilization of the prostate. With the patient in a semilithotomy position, a bladder catheter with a Foley bag containing 10 ml of Hypaque solution is inserted. The prostate template is placed in the perineum and fixed by 2-0 silk sutures. Metallic guides are inserted transperineally through the prostate and seminal

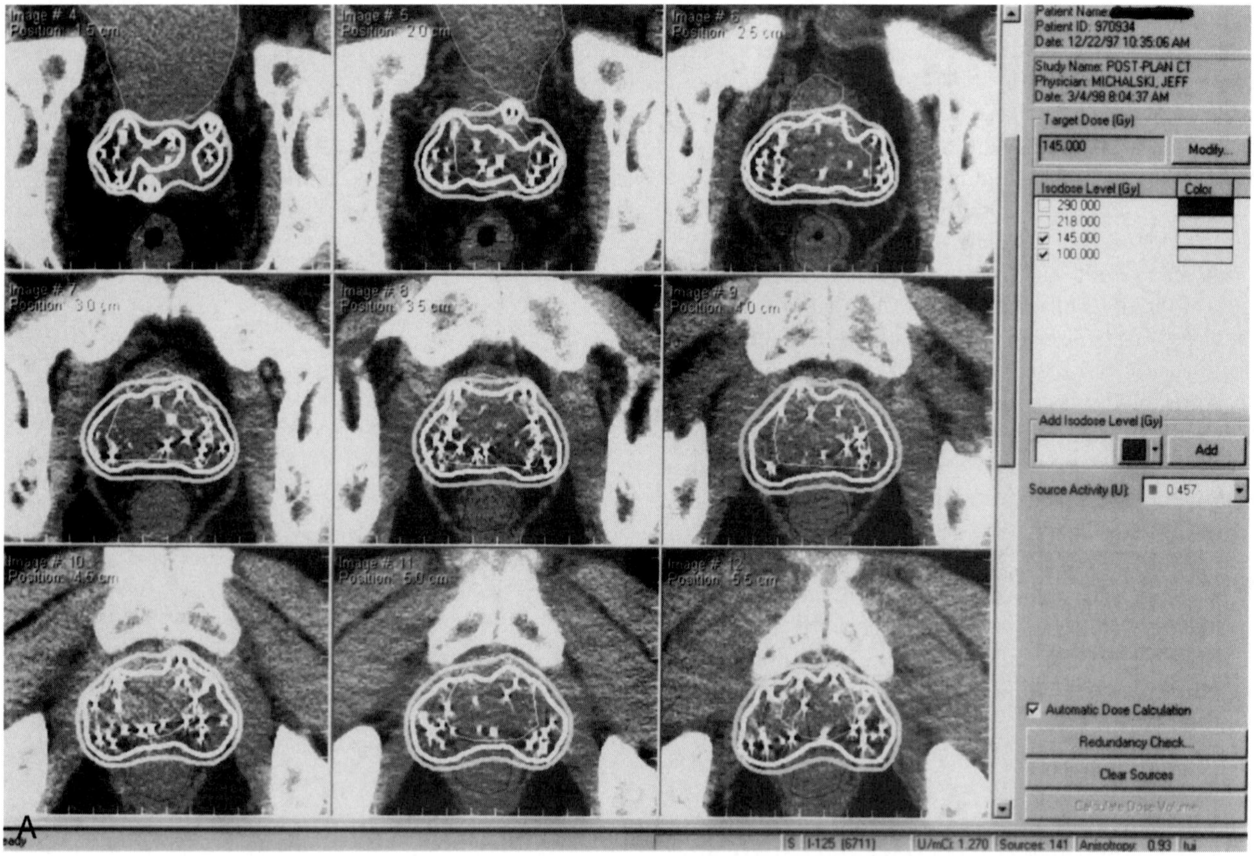

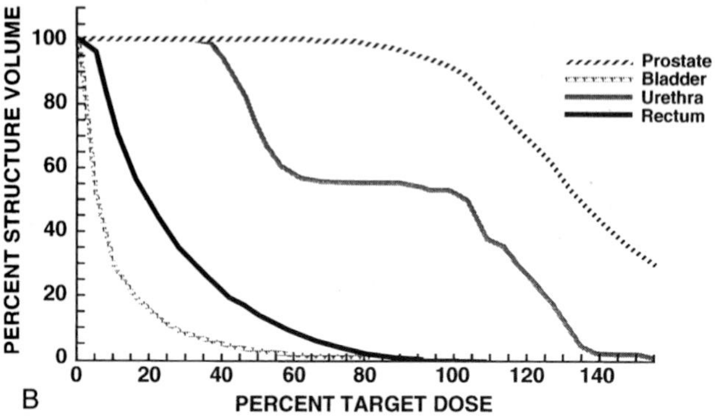

Figure 25.18. A. Postimplant CT scan demonstrating seed placement and 145 Gy and 100 Gy isodose coverage of the prostate. **B.** A dose-volume histogram of the prostate, urethra, bladder, and rectum.

vesicles (if indicated). The tip of the source guides is usually 1 cm above the level of the bladder neck. The hollow guides are loaded with inactive dummy sources for x-ray localization films, which are taken in AP and lateral orthogonal projections. Usually seven seeds of radioactive ^{192}Ir, spaced 1 cm apart, are loaded into each of 18 guides placed through the template. Activity of the iridium sources in the central guides is about 0.25 to 0.3 mg Ra eq and in the outer 12 guides, 0.4 to 0.5 mg Ra eq per seed. Dose rate per hour is 0.7 to 0.9 Gy, with the bladder neck and rectum receiving only 0.3 to 0.4 Gy/hour. The implant is removed after 30 to 35 Gy is delivered (40 to 45 hours). After the interstitial irradiation is completed, the radioactive sources are withdrawn with long forceps, and the template is removed with all guides in place, after the perineal sutures are transected. The Foley catheter is removed 1 day later. This interstitial therapy is combined with 40 Gy of external irradiation to the pelvis. Their results and some modification of technique have been updated by Puthawala et al. (136).

At Washington University we have used another version of this technique with a template directing the insertion of hollow 20-cm 17-gauge metallic guides (Alpha Omega Co.) in the prostate via a perineal route under ultra-

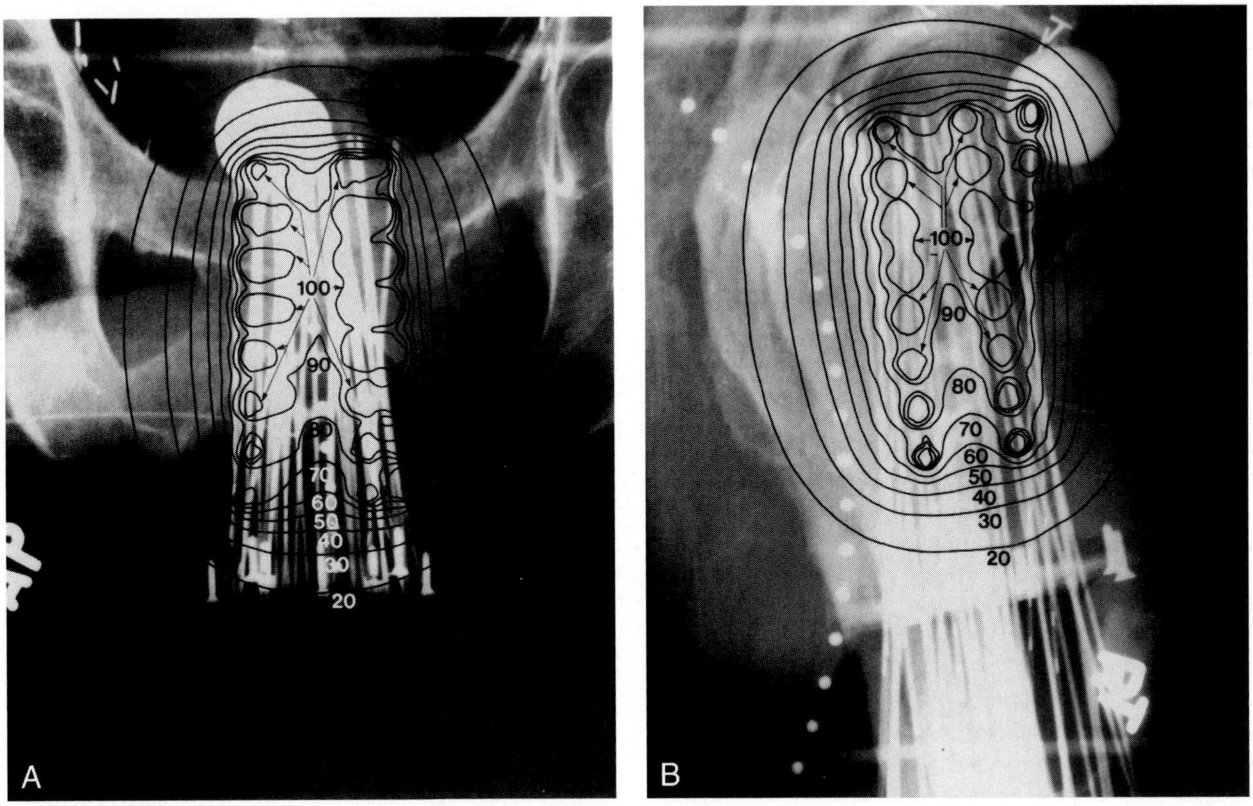

Figure 25.19. Anteroposterior **A)** and lateral **B)** radiographs of pelvis showing position of metallic guides inserted through the perineum under ultrasound control for patient with localized carcinoma of the prostate. Isodose curves are superimposed on films. (Perez CA, Williamson J. Clinical applications of brachytherapy. I. LDR. In: Perez CA, Brady LW, eds. Principles and practice of radiation oncology, 3rd ed. Philadelphia: Lippincott-Raven, 1998.) (137)

sound control. A TRUS scan of the prostate is initially obtained in the transverse and sagittal planes to identify the position and volume of the prostate. The metallic guides are successively inserted under ultrasound visualization (sagittal scanning). After insertion of each guide, a transverse scan is performed to determine the position of the guide being inserted in relation to the others already implanted. The guides are advanced 1 to 1.5 cm beyond the superior aspect of the prostate, avoiding piercing of the bladder or urethra. After all guides are inserted, the template is sutured to the perineal skin.

After the patient has recovered from anesthesia, AP and lateral radiographs of the pelvis are obtained for dose computations (Figure 25.19) (137). Later ^{192}Ir seeds, about eight per ribbon with 0.3 mCi Ra eq, are inserted in the guides (dose rate about 0.7 Gy/hour to periphery of gland). Minimum tumor doses of 30 to 35 Gy are delivered. This is combined with 40 Gy (2 Gy per fraction) to the prostate or the whole pelvis, as required.

Martinez et al. (135) and Brindle et al. (138), in an update of the initial publication, described implantation of the prostate with a perineal template (MUPIT). This technique was developed to replace external-beam boost for patients with stage C disease. A bilateral staging pelvic lymphadenectomy is performed; the length of metallic guides is determined by palpation, and palpable tumor margins are identified with inactive gold seeds. In a modification of the technique, the first needle is placed with the guidance of a finger in the rectum to prevent piercing of that organ. A rectal tube is inserted to help position the template to allow for proper spacing of the rest of the needles. The template is carefully aligned parallel to the floor of the pelvis, not conforming to the perineal slope, to avoid posterior angling of the needles. The needles are differentially loaded with ^{192}Ir seeds on nylon ribbons of varying activity, number of seeds, and the use of ribbon spacers. The posterior needles, in particular, which are primarily directed to the seminal vesicles, are loaded only in the superior half. The implant dose is 33 to 35 Gy, which is combined with external irradiation (5 Gy in one dose before the implant and 30 Gy in 17 fractions after the implant). Stromberg et al. (139) reported their long-term results; local tumor control rates of 100% by clinical examination and 84.5% by biopsy and actuarial disease-free survival of 89% were observed.

Conformal High Dose Rate Interstitial Prostate Brachytherapy

With the advent of TRUS technology, there has been a resurgence of prostate brachytherapy. Currently, there is a consensus among brachytherapists that ultrasound-guided template techniques result in more accurate needle and seed placement (116,140). Based on the linear-quadratic formula, fractionated high dose rate (HDR) schedules have been devised that allow substitution for boost procedures with either LDR ^{192}Ir or external-beam boost (139,141). High dose rate ^{192}Ir, in addition to providing conformal brachytherapy capability, has the appeal of excellent radiation safety and potential for dose optimization (Figure 25.20). The most significant experience with this technique has been accumulated by Bertermann and Brix (142) and Kovacs et al. (143) in Kiel, Germany, Mate et al. (144) in Seattle, Washington, and Martinez et al. (141) at William Beaumont Hospital in Royal Oak, Michigan.

With use of TRUS-guided prostate implantation techniques, HDR remote afterloading, and a specialized planning system, prostate implants are directly performed with the ultrasound images from the volume study concurring with the placement of the needles for radioactive source insertion (Figure 25.21) (145).

Martinez et al. (145) developed a program for intraoperative optimization of needle placement and dwell times for conformal prostate brachytherapy. This planning method can be used in other body sites. The intraoperative optimization of needle placement and dwell times is as follows: The length and cross-section of the target (prostate) and location of urethra and rectum are determined intraoperatively from live ultrasound imaging. The planning program automatically generates a "reference plan" containing needle locations, dwell times, and the resulting isodose distribution. As needles are placed, this information is corrected to account for any deviation of needle placement or movement of the prostate. After all needles are in place, the normalization is adjusted to reconcile remaining hot spots with adequate coverage of the target volume. Optimization is performed in three stages.

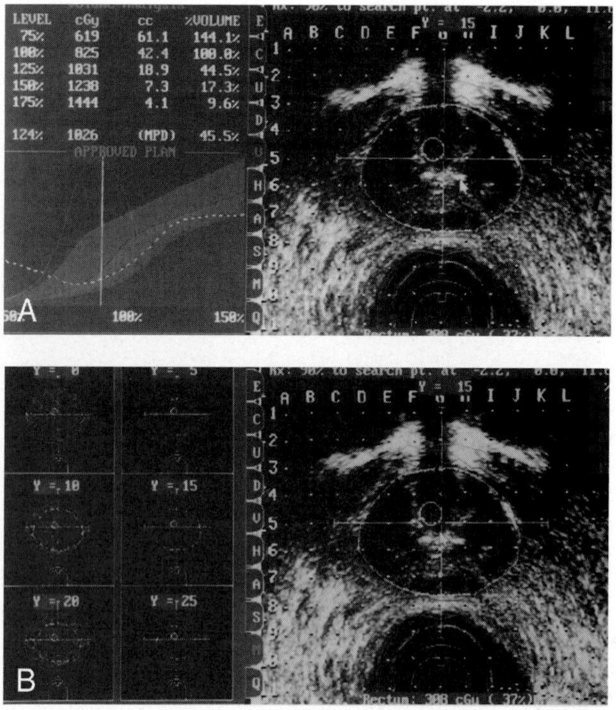

Figure 25.21. **A.** Example of transrectal ultrasound image of prostate and rectum with isodose curves. **B.** Computer-suggested needle coordinates and six concurrent planning levels from the base to the apex of the prostate at 5-mm intervals. (Martinez A: Clinical applications of brachytherapy. II. HDR. In: Perez CA, Brady LW, eds. Principles and practice of radiation oncology. 3rd ed. Philadelphia: Lippincott-Raven, 1998.) (145).

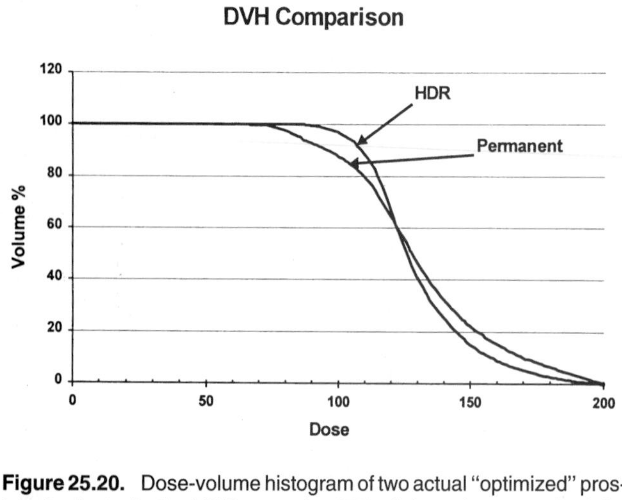

Figure 25.20. Dose-volume histogram of two actual "optimized" prostate implants. In the HDR example, 97% of the volume received the prescribed dose and 88% in the permanent implant. Minimum dose was 90% for HDR versus 72% for permanent implant.

1. *Pattern optimization* attempts to find the most appropriate placement for the needles or catheters and is based on the transverse contour of the target volume. Needles are placed uniformly around the perimeter, and interior needle positions are determined from the cross-sectional area and shape. Critical structures such as the urethra are explicitly avoided. This step provides the overall framework for the implant and is not generally repeated.
2. *Relative dwell time optimization* selects relative dwell times that will give the best uniformity of dose. It works by setting the relative dwell time in each source position inversely proportional to the dose delivered

to that point by the other source positions. It is used in the reference plan and is repeated as each needle is inserted. This provides dosimetric feedback to the physician, who can judge the effect of deviations from the reference plan.

3. *Relative volume optimization* is an interactive method for fine-tuning the normalization, based on volume analysis. The volume analysis is presented in tabular and graphic form, both of which are updated rapidly as the normalization is adjusted. The information is formatted to help the operator judge coverage and uniformity. Special functions are provided that allow the operator to "jump" to special normalization values based on several indices of uniformity or uniformity/coverage. Schedules used in a dose-escalation study are detailed in Tables 25.10 and 25.11

Table 25.10. High Dose Rate Brachytherapy in Localized Prostate Cancer: Biologic Equivalence of Three High Dose Rate Fractions

Pelvis	180 × 28	180 × 12 200 × 12	180 × 12 200 × 12	180 × 12 200 × 12
Prostate	200 × 10	550 × 3	600 × 3	650 × 3
Tumor	7040	6740	7010	7290
Tumor (%)	100	96	100	104
Rectum	7040	5830	6000	6180
Rectum (%)	100	83	854	88

Note: The biologic equivalence shown is based on the biologic effective dose model accounting for different fractionation effects. It assumes an ∂/β ratio of 10 Gy for tumor and 4 Gy for late responding tissues (rectum). The rectal dose from external-beam therapy is 100%; however, for brachytherapy it is assumed to be 60% of the prostate dose due to the loading pattern and dose-specification method. This dose calculation algorithm has been verified extensively with thermoluminescent dosimetry (TLD) measurements. Twenty patients receiving three HDR fractions each had TLD measurements performed during treatment. The calculated and measured rectal dose along 4 cm length of rectum was within ± 6%.

Figure 25.21B depicts not only the computer-suggested needle coordinates but also demonstrates six concurrent planning levels from the base to the apex of the prostate at 5-mm intervals.

For patients with locally advanced disease (stages T2b–T3c), Stromberg et al. (146) recently updated the William Beaumont Hospital experience with conformal HDR boost brachytherapy. While the median pretreatment PSA levels were similar (14 and 14.3 ng/ml), the median Gleason score was 6 for external irradiation patients and 7 for the brachytherapy boost group. The 3-year actuarial biochemical control rates were 85% for the conformal HDR and 52% for conventionally treated patients (P = .001). Table 25.12 shows a comparison of the acute toxicity rates in patients with high-risk localized prostate cancer when treated with three conformal HDR boost implants and external-beam irradiation versus those treated with two HDR implants and external-beam irradiation. Biologic equivalence of the HDR dose schedules was calculated using the linear-quadratic model. Acute toxicity was graded according to the most severe reaction, using a modified Radiation

Table 25.12. High Dose Rate Brachytherapy in Localized Prostate Cancer: Percent of Patients with Modified Radiation Therapy Oncology Group Acute Toxicities

	3 HDR (n = 58)		2 HDR (n = 47)	
	Grade 2	Grade 3	Grade 2	Grade 3
Diarrhea	29.3	1.7	14.9	1.2
Tenesmus	20.7	0	12.8	0
N/V	0	0	0	0
Urinary frequency	32.7	0	19.1	0
Dysuria	46.5	3.4	21.3	0
Incontinence	3.4	0	2.1	0
Retention	13.8	0	6.4	0
Hematuria	41.4	0	17.2	0
Hemospermia	10.3	0	4.1	0
Perineal pain	3.4	0	0	0

Table 25.11. Biologic Equivalence of Two High Dose Rate Fractions

Pelvis	180 × 28	200 × 23	200 × 23	200 × 23	200 × 23
Prostate	200 × 10	825 × 2	875 × 2	950 × 2	1050 × 2
Tumor	7040	7200	7420	7800	8290
Tumor (%)	100	102	105	111	118
Rectum	7040	6320	6370	6600	6930
Rectum (%)	100	88	90	94	98

Note: The biologic equivalence shown is based on the biologic effective dose model accounting for different fractionation effects. It assumes an ∂/β ratio of 10 Gy for tumor and 4 Gy for late responding tissues (rectum). The rectal dose from external-beam therapy is 100%; however, for brachytherapy it is assumed to be 60% of the prostate dose due to the loading pattern and dose-specification method. This dose calculation algorithm has been verified extensively with thermoluminescent dosimetry (TLD) measurements. Twenty patients receiving three HDR fractions each had TLD measurements performed during treatment. The calculated and measured rectal dose along 4 cm length of rectum was within ± 6%.

Therapy Oncology Group grading system. A total of 105 patients were treated in this dose-escalation trial; 58 patients received three HDR fractions of 5.5, 6.0, and 6.5 Gy each and 47 were treated with two HDR fractions of 8.25 and 8.75 Gy each. With mean follow-up of 2.4 years, no increase in acute toxicity was noted with two HDR implants when compared with three implants.

References

1. Perez CA. Prostate. In: Perez CA, Brady LW, eds. Principles and practice of radiation oncology. 3rd ed. Philadelphia: Lippincott-Raven, 1998:1583–1694.
2. Anson BJ, McVay CB. Surgical anatomy. 5th ed, vol 2. Philadelphia: WB Saunders, 1971:771.
3. Myers RP, Goellner JR, Cahill DR. Prostate shape, external striated urethral sphincter and radical prostatectomy: The apical dissection. J Urol 1987;138:543–550.
4. Oelrich TM. The urethral sphincter muscle in the male. Am J Anat 1980;158:229–246.
5. McNeal JE. Origin and development of carcinoma of the prostate. Cancer 1969;23:24.
6. Breslow N, Chan CW, Dhom G, et al. Latent carcinoma of prostate at autopsy in seven areas. Int J Cancer 1977;20:680–688.
7. Blennerhassett JB, Vickery AL. Carcinoma of the prostate gland: an anatomical study of tumor location. Cancer 1966;19:980–984.
8. Jewett HJ. Radical perineal prostatectomy for palpable, clinically localized, nonobstructive cancer: experience at the Johns Hopkins Hospital 1909-1963. J Urol 1980;124:492–494.
9. Andriole GL, Ponas SH, Catalona WJ. The implication of focal well differentiated prostate cancer (CaP) in men with elevated serum PSA and palpably normal prostates. J Urol 1992;147:442A.
10. Catalona WJ, Smith DS. 5-year tumor recurrence rates after anatomical radical retropubic prostatectomy for prostate cancer. J Urol 1994; 152:1837–1842.
11. Villers AA, McNeal JE, Freiha FS, et al. Development of prostatic carcinoma: morphometric and pathologic features of early stages. Acta Oncol 1991;30:145–151.
12. Oesterling JE, Suman VJ, Zincke H, et al. PSA-detected (clinical stage T1c or B1) prostate cancer. Urol Clin North Am 1994;20:293–302.
13. Epstein JI, Walsh PC, Carmichael M, et al. Pathologic and clinical findings to predict tumor extent of nonpalpable (stage T1c) prostate cancer. JAMA 1994;271:368–373.
14. Stone NN, Stock RG, Unger P. Indications for seminal vesicle biopsy and laparoscopic pelvic lymph node dissection in men with localized carcinoma of the prostate. J Urol 1995;154:1392–1396.
15. Catalona WJ, Bigg SW. Nerve-sparing radical prostatectomy: evaluation of results after 250 patients. J Urol 1990;143:538–544.
16. Stock RG, Stone NN, Ianuzzi C, et al. Seminal vesicle biopsy and laparoscopic pelvic lymph node dissection: Implications for patient selection in the radiotherapeutic management of prostate cancer. Int J Radiat Oncol Biol Phys 1995;33:815–821.
17. D'Amico AV, Whittington R, Malkowicz SB, et al. A multivariate analysis of clinical and pathological factors that predict for prostate specific antigen failure after radical prostatectomy for prostate cancer. J Urol 1995;154:131–138.
18. Roach M. Equations for predicting the pathologic stage of men with localized prostate cancer using the preoperative prostate specific antigen. J Urol 1993;150:1923–1924.
19. Fowler JE, Whitmore WF. The incidence and extent of pelvic lymph node metastases in apparently localized prostatic cancer. Cancer 1981;47:1941–1945.
20. Middleton RG. Value of and indications for pelvic lymph node dissection in the staging of prostate cancer. NCI Monogr 1988;7:41–43.
21. Ohori M, Wheeler TM, Kattan MW, et al. Prognostic significance of positive margins in radical prostatectomy specimens. J Urol 1995; 154:1818–1824.
22. Pisansky TM, Zincke H, Suman VJ, et al. Correlation of pretherapy prostate cancer characteristics with histologic findings from pelvic lymphadenectomy specimens. Int J Radiat Oncol Biol Phys 1996; 34:33–39.
23. Bluestein DL, Bostwick DG, Bergstralh EJ, et al. Eliminating the need for bilateral pelvic lymphadenectomy in select patients with prostate cancer. J Urol 1994;151:1315–1320.
24. Narayan P, Fournier G, Gajendran V, et al. Utility of preoperative serum prostate-specific antigen concentration and biopsy Gleason Score in predicting risk of pelvic lymph node metastasis in prostate cancer. Urology 1994;44:519–524.
25. Partin AW, Yoo J, Carter H, et al. The use of prostate specific antigen, clinical stage and Gleason score to predict pathological stage in men with localized prostate cancer. J Urol 1993;150:110–114.
26. Spevack L, Killion LT, West JC Jr, et al. Predicting the patient at low risk for lymph node metastasis with localized prostate cancer: An analysis of four statistical models. Int J Radiat Oncol Biol Phys 1996; 34:543–547.
27. Pistenma DA, Bagshaw MA, Freiha FS. Extended-field radiation therapy for prostatic adenocarcinoma: status report of a limited prospective trial. In: Johnson DE, Samuels ML, eds. Cancer of the genitourinary tract. New York: Raven Press, 1979;229–247.
28. McLaughlin AP, Saltzstein SL, McCullough DL, et al. Prostatic carcinoma: incidence and location of unsuspected lymphatic metastases. J Urol 1976;115:89–94.
29. Gervasi LA, Mata J, Easley JD, et al. Prognostic significance of lymph node metastases in prostate cancer. J Urol 1989;142:332–336.
30. Rukstalis DB, Lawton CA, Brendler CB. Management options for patients with lymph node metastases from prostate cancer. In: Vogelzang NJ, Scardino PT, Shipley WU, et al, eds. Comprehensive textbook of genitourinary oncology. Baltimore: Williams & Wilkins, 1996;838–853.
31. Lawton C, Winter K, Byhardt R, et al. Androgen suppression plus radiation versus radiation alone for patients with D1 (pN +) adenocarcinoma of the prostate (results based on a national prospective randomized trial, RTOG 85-31). Int J Radiat Oncol Biol Phys 1997; 38:931–939.
32. Perez CA, Pilepich MV, Garcia D, et al. Definitive radiation therapy in carcinoma of the prostate localized to the pelvis: experience at the Mallinckrodt Institute of Radiology. NCI Monogr 1988;7:85–94.
33. Bastacky SI, Walsh PC, Epstein JI. Relationship between perineural tumor invasion on needle biopsy and radical prostatectomy capsular penetration in clinical stage B adenocarcinoma of the prostate. Am J Surg Pathol 1993;17:336–341.
34. Bonin SR, Hanlon AL, Lee WR, et al. Evidence of increased failure in the treatment of prostate carcinoma patients who have perineural invasion treated with three-dimensional conformal radiation therapy. Cancer 1997;79:75–80.
35. Ennis RD, Flynn SD, Fischer DB, et al. Preoperative serum prostate-specific antigen and Gleason grade as predictors of pathologic stage in clinically organ confined prostate cancer: implications for the choice of primary treatment. Int J Radiat Oncol Biol Phys 1994;30: 317–322.
36. Stamey TA, Kabalin JN, Ferrari M. Prostate specific antigen in the diagnosis and treatment of adenocarcinoma of the prostate. III. Radiation treated patients. J Urol 1989;141:1084–1087.
37. Benson MC. Application of flow cytometry and automated image analysis to the study of prostate cancer. NCI Monogr 1988;7:25–29.
38. Lieber MM, Murtaugh PA, Farrow GM, et al. DNA ploidy and surgically treated prostate cancer. Cancer 1995;75:1935–1943.
39. Song J, Cheng WS, Cupps RE, et al. Nuclear deoxyribonucleic acid content measured by static cytometry: Important prognostic association for patients with clinically localized prostate carcinoma treated by external beam radiotherapy. J Urol 1992;147:794–797.
40. Pollack A, Zagars GK, El-Naggar AK, et al. Relationship of tumor DNA ploidy to serum prostate-specific antigen doubling time after radiotherapy for prostate cancer. Urology 1994;44:711–719.
41. Hall MC, Navone NM, Troncoso P, et al. Frequency and characterization of p53 mutations in clinically localized prostate cancer. Urology 1995;45:470–475.
42. Prendergast NJ, Atkins MR, Schatte EC, et al. p 53 immunohistochemical and genetic alterations are associated at high incidence with post-irradiated locally persistent prostate carcinoma. J Urol 1996;156:1685–1692.

43. Bratt O, Anderson H, Bak-Jensen E, et al. Metaphase cytogenetics and DNA flow cytometry with analysis of S-phase fraction in prostate cancer: Influence on prognosis. Urology 1996;47:218–224.
44. Johnson DE, Lanieri JP Jr, Ayala G. Prostatic adenocarcinoma occurring in men under 50 years of age. J Surg Oncol 1972;4:207–216.
45. Perez CA, Garcia D, Simpson JR, et al. Factors influencing outcome of definitive radiotherapy for localized carcinoma of the prostate. Radiother Oncol 1989;16:1–21.
46. Aziz H, Rotman M, Thelmo W, et al. Radiation-treated carcinoma of prostate: comparison of survival of black and white patients by Gleason's grading system. Am J Clin Oncol 1988;11:166–171.
47. Pilepich MV, Krall JM, Sause WT, et al. Prognostic factors in carcinoma of the prostate: Analysis of RTOG Study 75-06. Int J Radiat Oncol Biol Phys 1987;13:339–349.
48. Moul JW, Douglas TH, McCarthy WF, et al. Black race is an adverse prognostic factor for prostate cancer recurrence following radical prostatectomy in an equal access health care setting. J Urol 1996; 155:1667–1673.
49. Dayal HH, Polissar L, Dahlberg S. Race, socioeconomic status, and other prognostic factors for survival from prostate cancer. J Natl Cancer Inst 1985;74:1001–1006.
50. Kim JA, Kuban DA, El-Mahdi AM, et al. Carcinoma of the prostate: race as a prognostic indicator in definitive radiation therapy. Radiology 1995;194:545–549.
51. Perez CA, Lockett MA. Localized carcinoma of the prostate: patterns of failure with external beam radiation therapy. In: Petrovich Z, Baert L, Brady LW, eds. Carcinoma of the prostate: innovations in management. Berlin: Springer, 1996:225–241.
52. Optenberg S, Thompson I, Friedrichs P, et al. Race, treatment, and long-term survival from prostate cancer in an equal-access medical delivery system [abstract]. J Urol 1996;155(suppl):486A.
53. Powell IJ, Schwartz K, Hussain M. Removal of the financial barrier to health care: does it impact on prostate cancer at presentation and survival? A comparative study between black and white men in a Veterans Affairs System. Urology 1995;46:825–830.
54. Fowler JE, Terrell F. Survival in blacks and whites after treatment for localized prostate cancer. J Urol 1996;156:133–136.
55. Del Regato JA, Trailings AH, Pittman DD. Twenty years follow-up of patients with inoperable cancer of the prostate (stage C) treated by radiotherapy: Report of a National Cooperative Study. Int J Radiat Oncol Biol Phys 1993;26:197–201.
56. Bagshaw MA, Cox RS, Ray GR. Status of radiation therapy of prostate cancer at Stanford University. NCI Monogr 1988;7:47–60.
57. McGowan DG. The value of extended field radiation therapy in carcinoma of the prostate. Int J Radiat Oncol Biol Phys 1981;7: 1333–1339.
58. Hanks GE, Lee WR, Hanlon AL, et al. Conformal technique dose escalation for prostate cancer: Chemical evidence of improved cancer control with higher doses in patients with pretreatment prostate-specific antigen ≥10 ng/ml. Int J Radiat Oncol Biol Phys 1996;35: 861–868.
59. Leibel SA, Heimann R, Kutcher GJ, et al. Three-dimensional conformal radiation therapy in locally advanced carcinoma of the prostate: preliminary results of a phase I dose-escalation study. Int J Radiat Oncol Biol Phys 1993;28:55–65.
60. Perez CA, Michalski J, Drzymala R, et al. Three-dimensional conformal therapy (3-D CRT) and potential for intensity-modulated radiation therapy in localized carcinoma of prostate. In: Sternick ES, ed. The theory and practice of intensity modulated radiation therapy. Madison, WI: Advanced Medical Publishing, 1997:199–217.
61. Althof VGM, Hoekstra CJM, Te Loo H-J. Variation in prostate position relative to adjacent bony anatomy. Int J Radiat Oncol Biol Phys 1996;34:709–715.
62. Perez CA, Lee HK, Georgiou A, et al. Technical and tumor-related factors affecting outcome of definitive irradiation for localized carcinoma of the prostate. Int J Radiat Oncol Biol Phys 1993;26:565–581.
63. Sadeghi A, Kuisk H, Tran L, et al. Urethrography and ischial intertuberosity line in radiation therapy planning for prostate carcinoma. Radiother Oncol 1996;38:215–222.
64. Cox JA, Zagoria RJ, Raben M. Prostate cancer: Comparison of retrograde urethrography and computed tomography in radiotherapy planning. Int J Radiat Oncol Biol Phys 1994;29:1119–1123.
65. Wilson LD, Ennis R, Percarpio B, et al. Location of the prostatic apex and its relationship to the ischial tuberosities. Int J Radiat Oncol Biol Phys 1994;29:1133–1138.
66. Algan O, Hanks GE, Shaer AH. Localization of the prostatic apex for radiation treatment planning. Int J Radiat Oncol Biol Phys 1995; 33:925–930.
67. Crook JM, Raymond Y, Salhani D, et al. Prostate motion during standard radiotherapy as assessed by fiducial markers. Radiother Oncol 1995;37:35–42.
68. Perez CA. Carcinoma of the prostate: a vexing biological and clinical enigma. Int J Radiat Oncol Biol Phys 1983;9:1427–1438.
69. Taylor WJ, Richardson RG, Hafermann MD. Radiation therapy for localized prostate cancer. Cancer 1979;43:1123–1127.
70. Bagshaw MA, Ray GR, Cox RS. Radiotherapy of prostatic carcinoma: Long- or short-term efficacy (Stanford University experience). Urology 1985;25:17–23.
71. Biggs PJ, Russell MD. Effect of a femoral head prosthesis on megavoltage beam radiotherapy. Int J Radiat Oncol Biol Phys 1988;14: 581–586.
72. International Commission of Radiation Units (ICRU). Bulletin No. 50: Prescribing, Recording, and Reporting Photon Beam Therapy. Washington, DC, ICRU, 1993.
73. Zhu XR, Low DA, Harms WB, et al. A convolution-adapted ratio-TAR algorithm for 3D photon beam treatment planning. Med Phys 1995;22:1315–1327.
74. Pickett B, Roach M III, Verhey L, et al. The value of nonuniform margins for six-field conformal irradiation of localized prostate cancer. Int J Radiat Oncol Biol Phys 1995;32:211–218.
75. Roach M III, Marquez C, Yuo H-S, et al. Predicting the risk of lymph node involvement using the pre-treatment prostate specific antigen and Gleason score in men with clinically localized prostate cancer. Int J Radiat Oncol Biol Phys 1994;28:33–37.
76. Diaz A, Roach M III, Marquez C, et al. Indications for and the significance of seminal vesicle irradiation during 3D conformal radiotherapy for localized prostate cancer. Int J Radiat Oncol Biol Phys 1994; 30:323–329.
77. Roach M. Equations for predicting the pathologic stage of men with localized prostate cancer using the preoperative prostate specific antigen. J Urol 1993;150:1923–1924.
78. Neal AJ, Oldham M, Dearnaley DP. Comparison of treatment techniques for conformal radiotherapy of the prostate using dose-volume histograms and normal tissue complication probabilities. Radiother Oncol 1995;37:29–34.
79. Roach M III, Pickett B, Weil M, et al. The "critical volume tolerance method" for estimating the limits of dose escalation during three-dimensional conformal radiotherapy for prostate cancer. Int J Radiat Oncol Biol Phys 1996;35:1019–1025.
80. Beard CJ, Kijewski P, Bussière M, et al. Analysis of prostate and seminal vesicle motion: implications for treatment planning. Int J Radiat Oncol Biol Phys 1996;34:451–458.
81. Rudat V, Schraube P, Oetzel D, et al. Combined error of patient positioning variability and prostate motion uncertainty in 3D conformal radiotherapy of localized prostate cancer. Int J Radiat Oncol Biol Phys 1996;35:1027–1034.
82. Roeske JC, Forman JD, Mesina CF, et al. Evaluation of changes in the size and location of the prostate, seminal vesicles, bladder, and rectum during a course of external beam radiation therapy. Int J Radiat Oncol Biol Phys 1995;33:1321–1329.
83. Balter J, Sandler H, Lan K, et al. Measurement of prostate motion over the course of radiotherapy. Int J Radiat Oncol Biol Phys 1995; 31:113–118.
84. Forman JD, Mesina CF, He T, et al. Evaluation of changes in the location and shape of the prostate and rectum during a seven week course of conformal radiotherapy. Int J Radiat Oncol Biol Phys 1993; 27(suppl 1):222.
85. Melian E, Kutcher G, Leibel S, et al. Variation in prostate position: quantitation and implication for three-dimensional conformal radiation therapy. Int J Radiat Oncol Biol Phys 1993;27(suppl 1):137.
86. Schild SE, Casale HE, Bellefontaine LP. Movements of the prostate due to rectal and bladder distension: implications for radiotherapy. Med Dosim 1993;18:13–15.
87. Ten Haken RK, Forman JD, Heimburger K, et al. Treatment planning issues related to prostate movement in response to differential filling

of the rectum and bladder. Int J Radiat Oncol Biol Phys 1991;20: 1317–1324.

88. van Herk M, Bruce A, Kroes APG, et al. Quantification of organ motion during conformal radiotherapy of the prostate by three dimensional image registration. Int J Radiat Oncol Biol Phys 1995;33: 1311–1320.
89. Huddart RA, Nahum A, Neal A, et al. Accuracy of pelvic radiotherapy: prospective analysis of 90 patients in a randomized trial of blocked versus standard radiotherapy. Radiother Oncol 1996;39: 19–29.
90. Lebesque JV, Bruce AM, Kroes APG, et al. Variation in volumes, dose-volume histograms, and estimated normal tissue complication probabilities of rectum and bladder during conformal radiotherapy of T3 prostate cancer. Int J Radiat Oncol Biol Phys 1995;33: 1109–1119.
91. Lu Y, Song PY, Li S-D, et al. A method of analyzing rectal surface area irradiated and rectal complications in prostate conformal radiotherapy. Int J Radiat Oncol Biol Phys 1995;33:1121–1125.
92. Lee WR, Hanks GE, Hanlon AL, et al. Lateral rectal shielding reduces late rectal morbidity following high dose three-dimensional conformal radiation therapy for clinically localized prostate cancer: further evidence for a significant dose effect. Int J Radiat Oncol Biol Phys 1996;35:251–257.
93. Song, PY, Washington M, Vaida F, et al. A comparison of four patient immobilization devices in the treatment of prostate cancer patients with three dimensional conformal radiotherapy. Int J Radiat Oncol Biol Phys 1996;34:213–219.
94. Hanley J, Mageras GS, Sun J, et al. The effects of out-of-plane rotations on two-dimensional portal image registration in conformal radiotherapy of the prostate. Int J Radiat Oncol Biol Phys 1995;33: 1331–1343.
95. Fleming ID, Cooper JS, Henson DE, et al., eds. AJCC Cancer Staging Manual, 5th ed. Philadelphia: Lippincott-Raven, 1997.
96. Batata MA, Hilaris BS, Whitmore WF. Factors affecting tumor control. In Hilaris BS, Batata MA, eds. Brachytherapy oncology, 1983: advances in prostate and other cancer. New York: Memorial Sloan-Kettering Cancer Center, 1983;65–73.
97. Grimm PD, Blasko JC, Ragde H. Transperitoneal implantation of I-125 and Pd-103 for the treatment of early stage prostate cancer: technical concepts in planning, operative technique, and evaluation. Atlas Urol Clin N Am 1994:2.
98. Dattoli M, Wallner K, Sorace R, et al. Palladium 103 brachytherapy and external beam irradiation for clinically localized high-risk prostatic carcinoma. Int J Radiat Oncol Biol Phys 1996;35:875–879.
99. Critz FA. Prostate interstitial implantation: half the solution. J Clin Oncol 1996;14:1965.
100. Blasko JC, Grimm PD, Ragde H. Brachytherapy and organ preservation in the management of carcinoma of the prostate. Semin Radiat Oncol 1993;3:240–249.
101. Wallner K, Lee H, Wasserman S, et al. Low risk of urinary incontinence following prostate brachytherapy in patients with a prior transurethral prostate resection. Int J Radiat Oncol Biol Phys 1997; 37:565–569.
102. Blasko JC, Wallner K, Grimm PD, et al. Prostate specific antigen based disease control following ultrasound guided 125 Iodine implantation for stage T1/T2 prostatic carcinoma. J Urol 1995;154: 1096–1099.
103. Nath R, Meigooni AS. Some treatment planning considerations for Palladium-103 and Iodine-125 permanent interstitial implants [abstract]. Endocurie Hypertherm Oncol 1989;5:244.
104. Blasko JC, Schumacher D. Palladium-103 implantation for prostate carcinoma: dose rationale (submitted for publication).
105. Nath R, Meigooni AS, Meillo A. Some treatment planning considerations for 125I and ^{103}Pd permanent interstitial implants. Int J Radiat Oncol Biol Phys 1992;22:1131–1138.
106. Marchese MJ, Hall EJ, Hilaris BS. Encapsulated iodine 125 in radiation oncology: I. Study of the relative biologic effectiveness (RBE) using low dose rate of irradiation of mammalian cell cultures. Am J Clin Oncol 1984;7:607–611.
107. Ling CC. Permanent implants using Au-198, Pd-103, I-125: Radiobiological considerations based on the linear quadratic formula. Int J Radiat Oncol Biol Phys 1982;23:81–87.
108. Nag S, Ribovich M, Cai JZ, et al. Palladium-103 vs Iodine-125 brachytherapy in the Dunning-PAP rat prostate tumor. Endocurie Hypertherm Oncol 1996;12:119–124.
109. Nag S, Sweeney PJ, Wientjes MG. Dose response study of Iodine-125 and Palladium-103 brachytherapy in a rat prostate tumor (Nb A1-1). Endocurie Hypertherm Oncol 1993;9:97–104.
110. Nath R, Anderson LL, Luxton G, et al. Dosimetry of interstitial brachytherapy sources: recommendations of the AAPM Radiation Therapy Committee Task Group #43. Med Phys 1995;22:209–234.
111. Luse RW, Blasko J, Grimm P. A method for implementing the American Association of Physicists in Medicine Task Group 43 dosimetry recommendations for ^{125}I transperineal prostate seed implants on commercial treatment planning systems. Int J Radiat Oncol Biol Phys 1997;37:737–741.
112. Hilaris BS, Batata MA. Brachytherapy techniques. In: Hilaris BS, Batata MA, eds. Brachytherapy oncology—1983. New York: Memorial Sloan-Kettering Cancer Center, 1983:41–56.
113. Anderson LL, Aubrey RF. Computerized dosimetry for ^{125}I prostate implants. In: Hilaris BS, Batata MA, eds. Brachytherapy oncology—1983. New York: Memorial Sloan-Kettering Cancer Center, 1983:41–56.
114. Fuks Z, Liebel SA, Wallner KE, et al. The effect of local control on metastatic dissemination in carcinoma of the prostate: long-term results in patients treated with ^{125}I implantation. Int J Radiat Oncol Biol Phys 1991;21:537–547.
115. Kuban DA, El-Mahdi AM, Schellhammer PF. ^{125}I interstitial implantation for prostate cancer. Cancer 1989;63:2415–2520.
116. Blasko JC, Radge H, Schumacher D. Transperineal percutaneous Iodine-125 implantation for prostatic carcinoma using transrectal ultrasound and template guidance. Endocurie Hypertherm Oncol 1987:3:131–139.
117. Holm HH, Juul N, Pedersen JF, et al. Transperineal ^{125}Iodine seed implantation in prostatic cancer guided by transrectal ultrasonography. J Urol 1983;130:283–286.
118. Wallner KE, Chiu-Tsao S-T, Roy J, et al. An improved method for computerized tomography-planned transperineal ^{125}Iodine prostate implants. J Urol 1991;146:90–95.
119. Roy JN, Wallner KE, Chiu-Tsao S, et al. CT-based optimized planning for transperineal prostate implant with customized template. Int J Radiat Oncol Biol Phys 1991;21:483–489.
120. D'Amico AV, Coleman CN. Role of interstitial radiotherapy in the management of clinically organ-confined prostate cancer: the jury is still out. J Clin Oncol 1996;14:304–315.
121. Roy JN, Wallner KE, Harrington PJ, et al. A CT-based evaluation method for permanent implants: application to prostate. Int J Radiat Oncol Biol Phys 1993:26:163–169.
122. Wallner KE, Roy J, Zelefsky M, et al. Short-term freedom from disease progression after ^{125}I prostate implantation. Int J Radiat Oncol Biol Phys 1994;30:405.
123. Merrick GS, Butler WM, Dorsey AT, et al. Prostatic conformal brachytherapy: ^{125}I/^{103}Pd postoperative dosimetric analysis. Radiat Oncol Invest 1997;5:305–313.
124. Wallner KE, Roy J, Harrison L. Dosimetry guidelines to minimize urethral and rectal morbidity following transperineal ^{125}I prostate brachytherapy. Int J Radiat Oncol Biol Phys 1995;32:465–471.
125. Stone NN, Stock RG, DeWyngaert JK, et al. Prostate brachytherapy: improvements in prostate volume measurements and dose distribution using interactive ultrasound guided implantation and three dimensional dosimetry. Radiat Oncol Invest 1995;3:185–195.
126. Anderson LL, Moni JV, Harrison, LB. A nomograph for permanent implants of Palladium-103 seeds. Int J Radiat Oncol Biol Phys 1993; 27:129–135.
127. Anderson LL. Spacing nomograph for interstitial implants of ^{125}I seeds. Med Phys 1976;3:48–51.
128. Butler WM, Merrick GS. I-125 Rapid Strand™ loading technique. Radiat Oncol Invest 1996;4:48–49.
129. Dattoli M, Wallner KE. A simple method to stabilize the prostate during transperineal prostate brachytherapy. Int J Radiat Oncol Biol Phys 1997;38:341–342.
130. Feygelman V, Friedland JL, Sanders RM, et al. Improvement in dosimetry of ultrasound-guided prostate implants with the use of multiple stabilization needles. Med Dosim 1996;21:109–112.

131. Prestidge BR, Bice WS, Prete JJ, et al. A dose-volume analysis of permanent transperineal prostate brachytherapy. Int J Radiat Oncol Biol Phys 1997;39(suppl):289.
132. Stock RG, Stone NN, Wesson MF, et al. A modified technique allowing interactive ultrasound-guided three-dimensional transperineal prostate implantation. Int J Radiat Oncol Biol Phys 1995;32:219–225.
133. Charyulu KKN. Transperineal interstitial implantation of prostate cancer: a new method. Int J Radiat Oncol Biol Phys 1980;6: 1261–1266.
134. Syed AMN, Puthawala AA, Tansey LA, et al. Temporary iridium-192 implantation in the management of carcinoma of the prostate. In: Hilaris BS, Batata MA, eds. Brachytherapy oncology—1983. New York: Memorial Sloan-Kettering Cancer Center, 1983:83–91.
135. Martinez A, Benson RC, Edmundson GK, et al. Pelvic lymphadenectomy combined with transperineal interstitial implantation of Iridium-192 and external beam radiation for locally advanced prostatic carcinoma: technical description. Int J Radiat Oncol Biol Phys 1985: 11:841–847.
136. Puthawala AA, Syed AM, Tansey LA, et al. Temporary iridium-192 implant in the management of carcinoma of the prostate. Endocurie Hypertherm Oncol 1985:1:25.
137. Perez CA, Grigsby PW, Williamson J. Clinical applications of brachytherapy. I. LDR. In: Perez CA, Brady LW, eds. Principles and practice of radiation oncology. 3rd ed. Philadelphia: Lippincott-Raven, 1998; 487–560.
138. Brindle JS, Martinez A, Schray M, et al. Pelvic lymphadenectomy and transperineal interstitial implantation of ^{192}Ir combined with external beam radiotherapy for bulky stage C prostatic carcinoma. Int J Radiat Oncol Biol Phys 1989;17:1063–1066.
139. Stromberg J, Martinez A, Benson R, et al. Improved local control with survival for surgically staged patients with locally advanced prostate cancer treated with low dose rate iridium-192 prostate implantation and external beam irradiation. Int J Radiat Oncol Biol Phys 1994;28:67–75.
140. Wallner K, Roy J, Zelesky M, et al. PSA response after transperineal I-125 prostate implantation. Int J Radiat Oncol Biol Phys 1993; 27(suppl):228.
141. Martinez A, Gonzalez J, Stromberg J, et al. Conformal prostate brachytherapy: initial experience of a phase I/II dose-escalating trial. Int J Radiat Oncol Biol Phys 1995;33(5):1019–1027.
142. Bertermann H, Brix F. Ultrasonically guided interstitial high dose rate brachytherapy with Ir-192: Technique and preliminary results in locally confined prostate cancer. In: Martinez AA, Orton CF, Mould RF, eds. Brachytherapy HDR and LDR: remote afterloading state of the art. Leersum, The Netherlands: Nucletron International BV, 1990;281–303.
143. Kovacs G, Wirth B, Bertermann R, et al. Prostate preservation by combined external beam and HDR brachytherapy at nodal negative prostate cancer patients: an intermediate analysis after 10 years experience [abstract]. Int J Radiat Oncol Biol Phys 1996;36(suppl 1): 198.
144. Mate TP, Kovacs G, Martinez A. High dose rate brachytherapy of the prostate. In: Nag S, ed. High dose rate brachytherapy: a textbook. New York: Futura, 1994;355–371.
145. Martinez AA, Stitt JA, Speiser BL, Perez CA. Clinical applications of brachytherapy. II. HDR. In: Perez CA, Brady LW, eds. Principles and practice of radiation oncology. 3rd ed. Philadelphia: Lippincott-Raven, 1998;561–582.
146. Stromberg JS, Martinez AA, Horwitz EM, et al. Conformal high dose rate iridium-192 boost brachytherapy in locally advanced prostate cancer: superior prostate-specific antigen response compared with external beam treatment. Cancer J Sci Am 1997;3:346–352.

Chapter 26

Testicular Cancer

David H. Hussey

TESTICULAR CANCER

There have been significant changes in the treatment of cancer of the testis over the last several decades, largely as a result of the development of effective chemotherapy regimens, tumor markers, and new imaging techniques. These advances have made testicular cancer one of the most curable of all cancers, with disease-specific 5-year survival rates in excess of 90% (1).

Radiation therapy still plays a major role in the treatment of patients with pure seminoma, but its place in the management of patients with nonseminomatous testicular cancer has diminished considerably. The objectives of this chapter are to assess the current role of radiation therapy in the management of the primary tumors of the testis and to describe the radiotherapy techniques used in the treatment of pure seminomas.

Incidence

Testicular cancer is a relatively rare tumor, accounting for only about 1% of all cancers in males (58). However, the number of new cases has increased significantly over the last 20 years—from 3.0 cases per 100,000 in 1972 to 4.6 cases per 100,000 in 1992. It is the most common cancer in males between the ages of 15 and 35.

Approximately 10% of testicular cancer patients have a history of cryptorchidism (2,3), and patients with cryptorchidism have about a 35 times greater risk of developing a testicular cancer than patients with normally descended testicles (4). The risk of a cryptorchid testis developing cancer is directly related to the degree of maldescent. Testicular cancer is slightly more common in the right testis than the left, and this correlates with the increased incidence of cryptorchidism in the right testis (5).

A small percentage (1 to 3%) of testicular cancers are bilateral, and over half of the patients with bilateral tumors have a history of cryptorchidism (6). Bilateral testicular cancers may occur synchronously or metachronously, usually within 2 years of each other. However, cancers in the second testis have been noted up to 15 years after the diagnosis of the first cancer.

Pathology

Ninety-five percent of primary cancers of the testis are germ cell tumors. From a treatment standpoint, the germ cell tumors can be divided into seminomas and nonseminomatous tumors. Less than 5% of testicular malignancies originate from the gonadal stroma (e.g., Sertoli cell tumors, Leydig cell tumors, gonadoblastomas). Other tumors that can originate in the testis include lymphomas (usually diffuse large cell lymphomas), melanomas, and rhabdomyosarcomas.

Germ cell tumors of the testis are classified differently in Great Britain and the United States. The British histopathologic classification is based on the theory of the pathogenesis of germ cell tumors proposed by Willis (7). This theory postulates that all nonseminomatous tumors are teratomas which have descended from displaced blastomeres. The United States classification is based entirely on histologic composition. It is similar to the system originally proposed by Friedman and Moore (8), and later modified by Dixon and Moore (9) and Mostofi (10). The United States and British histopathologic classification systems are not easily compared. Seminomas and spermatocytic seminomas are identical in the two classifications, but there is considerable overlap with regard to the various types of nonseminomatous germ cell tumors.

Seminoma (Dixon & Moore Group I)

Seminomas make up ~35% of all germ cell tumors of the testis. They tend to occur in a slightly older age group than nonseminomatous tumors. Three histologic subtypes have been described: classic, anaplastic, and spermatocytic:

Classic Seminomas are comprised of a monotonous sheet of large cells containing a clear cytoplasm and a hyperchromatic nucleus. However, syncytiotrophoblasts may be seen in ~10 to 15% of cases, an incidence that corresponds with the frequency that β-HCG titers are elevated in patients with pure seminoma. Approximately 85% of pure seminomas have a classic pattern.

The diagnosis of *anaplastic Seminoma* is made by finding three or more mitotic figures per high power field. The radiosensitivity of anaplastic seminomas is similar to that of classic seminomas, but patients with anaplastic seminomas usually present with a higher clinical stage (11). Approximately 10 to 12% of seminomas are anaplastic.

Spermatocytic Seminomas contain cells resembling secondary spermatocytes and spermatids. They tend to occur in elderly men, and are characterized by an excellent prognosis. Spermatocytic seminomas account for 4 to 5% of all seminomas.

Embryonal Carcinoma (Dixon & Moore Group II)

Embryonal carcinomas contain cells that resemble malignant epithelial cells. There are two varieties of embryonal carcinoma, an adult type and an infantile type. The infantile variety is known as orchioblastoma, yolk sac tumor, or endodermal sinus tumor. Approximately 20% of germ cell tumors of the testis are embryonal carcinomas. Yolk sac tumors tend to produce alpha feto-protein (AFP), just as the normal yolk sac produces AFP during fetal development.

Teratoma (Dixon & Moore Group III)

Teratomas contain more than one germ cell layer in various stages of maturation. They may contain squamous or neuronal tissue of ectodermal origin, gastrointestinal or respiratory tissue of endodermal origin, and/or cartilage, muscle, or bone of mesodermal origin. Teratomas are benign in infants, but they may metastasize in adults. They account for ~5% of all germ cell tumors.

Choriocarcinoma (Dixon & Moore Group V)

Pure choriocarcinomas are extremely rare (<1%). They are highly malignant and metastasize early in the course of their disease. Choriocarcinomas are composed entirely of syncytiotrophoblasts and cytotrophoblasts, as compared to mixed tumors with foci of choriocarcinoma, which have only scattered syncytiotrophoblasts. Choriocarcinomas produce human chorionic gonadotrophin (HCG) just like the normal placenta does.

Mixed Tumors

Almost 40% of germ cell tumors contain more than one histopathologic type. The most common type of mixed tumor is teratocarcinoma (Dixon & Moore Group IV), which is a combination of teratoma and embryonal carcinoma, with or without seminoma.

Routes of Spread

Local Extension

Testicular cancers may spread locally to the rete testis, epididymis, and spermatic cord. However, this occurs in only 10 to 15% of patients (12). Testis cancer can also extend through the tunica albuginea into the scrotum, but this is even more rare (<5%) because the tunica albuginea forms a natural barrier to direct extension (12,13). This factor is of significance with regard to the design of radiation therapy treatment portals, because in most cases the scrotum does not require treatment.

Lymphatic Metastasis

The primary lymphatic drainage from the testicles follow the internal spermatic vessels to the periaortic area. This is illustrated in Figure 26.1. The major lymphatic channels swing out wide laterally, particularly on the left. However, no attempt is made to include the intervening lymphatic trunks in the treatment portals in patients being managed by radiation therapy (Figure 26.2).

The primary lymphatic drainage from the right and left testis differ. The lymphatics from right testis tend to drain to lymph nodes located along the inferior vena cava from L2 to L5. However, these vessels can cross over directly to terminate in the contralateral left periaortic lymph nodes. The lymphatics from the left testis tend to drain to nodes located just below the renal vein (Figure 26.3). However, they can drain to lymph nodes located elsewhere in the periaortic area. Unlike the lymphatic vessels from the right testis, the vessels from the left testis do not cross over directly to the contralateral side. The lymphatics from either testis can extend to periaortic nodes located above the renal hila or to nodes situated at the level of the aortic bifurcation.

On both sides, some of the lymphatic channels abandon the spermatic vessels after they reach the vesicle peritoneum, ending in nodes lying along the external iliac vein (Figure 26.1). This lymphatic drainage is usually ipsilateral, unless the patient has had groin surgery or retrograde spread due to massive retroperitoneal disease.

Metastases to the lymph nodes above the diaphragm is rare in the absence of involvement of the periaortic lymph nodes. However, supraclavicular metastasis may occur in the absence of mediastinal disease, presumably because

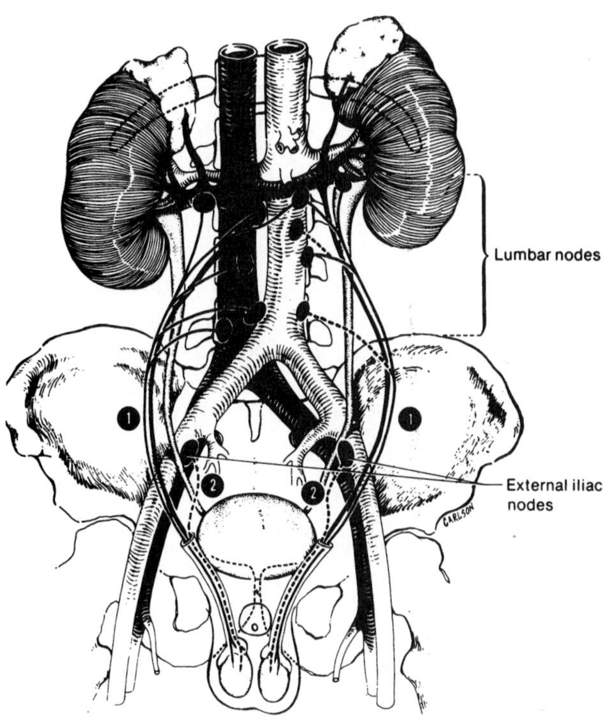

Figure 26.1. Lymphatic drainage system from testis and epididymis. Testicular lymphatics usually drain into ipsilateral para-aortic nodes, although the network of collateral lymphatics is extensive. Nodal connections differ from right and left. On right, most lymphatic channels (1) end in nodes situated between renal vein and aortic bifurcation. On left, most of collecting trunks (1) drain into nodes situated below left renal vein, usually terminating into superior nodes of this group. Lateral nodes at level of renal view may not be visualized by pedal lymphangiography. On both sides, some lymphatic channels (2) abandon spermatic vessels after they reach the vesicle peritoneum, ending in nodes lying along external iliac vein. (Reprinted with permission from Hussey, DH. Radiotherapy in the management of regional lymph node metastases from urologic tumors. In: Weiss L, Gilbert HA, Ballon SC, eds. Lymph Node Metastases. Vol. III. Boston, G.K. Hall Medical, 1980.)

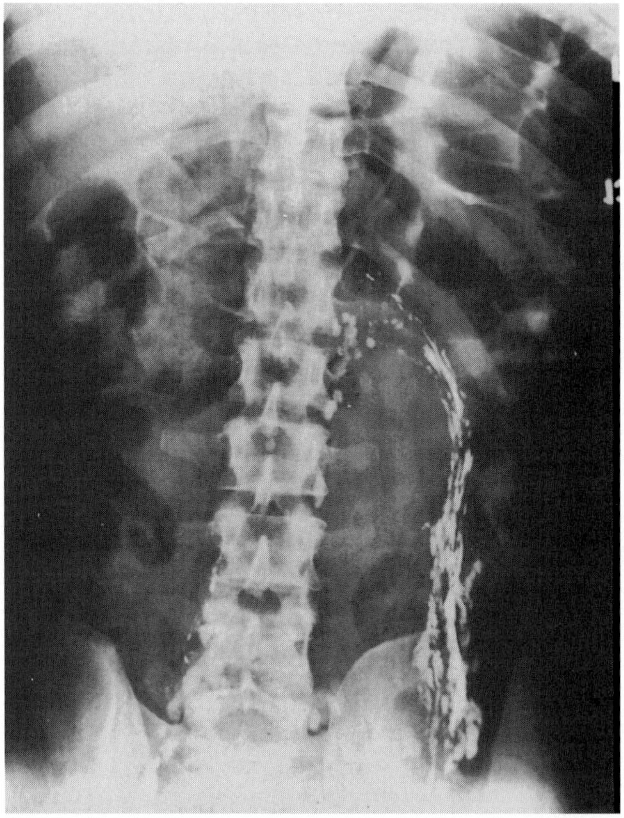

Figure 26.2. Left testicular lymphangiogram. Major lymphatic trunks end in sentinel nodes located near renal hilus. Lymphatic channels follow internal spermatic vessels and lie well lateral to para-aortic nodes.

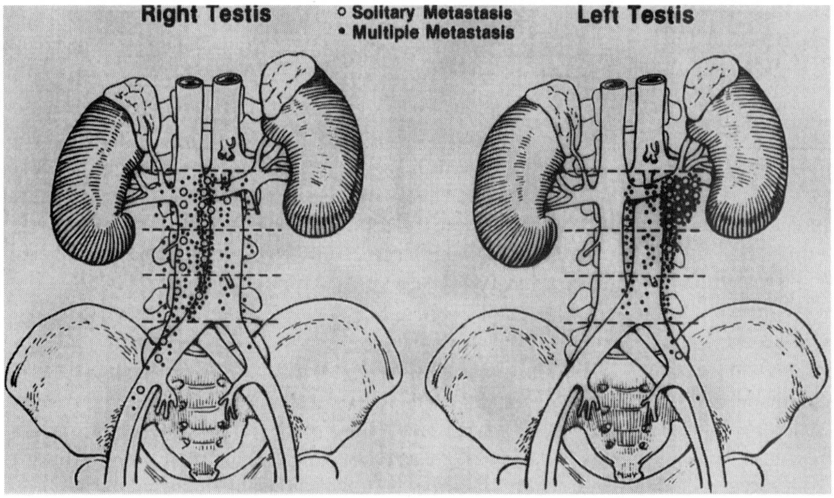

Figure 26.3. Distribution of lymph node metastases found at lymphadenectomy for nonseminomatous tumors. (Drawn from tabular data by Ray B, Hajdu S, Whitmore W. Distribution of retroperitoneal lymph node metastases in testicular germinal tumors. Cancer 33:340, 1974.)

of spread through the thoracic duct. Supraclavicular metastases are usually located on the left side, near the junction of the thoracic duct and the left subclavian vein.

Hematogenous Metastasis

The first site of metastasis from a pure seminoma is almost always the regional lymph nodes, and hematogenous metastasis rarely occurs with this tumor. Embryonal carcinomas and teratocarcinomas also tend to spread to the lymph nodes first, but hematogenous metastasis is not uncommon. On the other hand, choriocarcinomas have usually metastasized hematogenously by the time the diagnosis is established. The lungs are usually the first site of hematogenous spread from a testicular tumor.

Staging

A variety of clinical staging systems have been used for testis cancer. The classification that was used for many years was first proposed by Boden and Gibb (14). A modification of this classification is shown below:

Stage I Tumor clinically limited to the testis and spermatic cord.

Stage II Clinical or radiographic evidence of tumor spread beyond the testis, but limited to the regional nodes below the diaphragm.

Stage IIA Moderate-sized retroperitoneal metastasis.

Stage IIB Massive retroperitoneal metastasis.

Stage III Extension above the diaphragm.

Stage IIIA Extension above the diaphragm, but still confined to the mediastinal or supraclavicular lymphatics.

Stage IIIB Extranodal metastasis.

The two most widely used staging systems today are the AJCC system and the Royal Marsden Hospital system. These are compared in Table 26.1. The AJCC system uses the TNM notation, whereas the Royal Marsden Hospital system closely resembles the original Boden and Gibb classification.

The Royal Marsden classification is used in this chapter whenever possible. This staging system was selected because it subdivides stage II into four subcategories on the basis of the bulk of the retroperitoneal lymph node metastases (<2 cm, 2-5 cm, 5-10 cm, and >10 cm). This makes it easy to convert to other staging systems which may use different cutoffs between moderate and bulky disease. For pure seminomas, 10 cm has usually been used to distinguish between moderately advanced and massive disease, whereas 5 cm has usually been used to differentiate between moderately advanced and massive disease for nonseminomatous testicular cancers (15,16).

Clinical Evaluation

The clinical evaluation of a patient suspected of having a testicular tumor begins with a complete history and physical examination. This includes careful palpation of both testicles and transillumination to differentiate a solid mass from a hydrocele or spermatocele. The abdomen should be examined carefully to evaluate for retroperitoneal lymphadenopathy and/or hepatosplenomegaly. The neck

Table 26.1. Staging Classifications for Germ Cell Tumors of the Testis

AJCC TNM Staging Classification[a]	Royal Marsden Staging System[b]
T–Primary tumor	I Confined to the testis and spermatic cord
pTx Primary tumor cannot be assessed	II Metastasis to lymph nodes below the diaphragm
pTO No evidence of primary tumor	IIA Maximum diameter ≤ 2 cm
pTis Intratubular tumor (CIS)	IIB Maximum diameter 2–5 cm
pT1 Limited to the testis (including rete)	IIC Maximum diameter 5–10 cm
pT2 Extends through the tunica albuginea or to the epididymis	IID Maximum diameter >10 cm
pT3 Involvement of the spermatic cord	III Extension to nodes above the diaphragm (Abdominal status as listed above: A,B,C,D)
pT4 Invades the scrotum	IV Extranodal metastasis
N–Lymph nodes	
Nx Cannot be assessed	
NO No regional lymph node metastasis	
N1 Single lymph node ≤ 2 cm in size	
N2 Single lymph node 2–5 cm in size or multiple lymph nodes	
N3 Metastasis in a lymph node >5 cm in size	
M–Distant sites	
Mx Cannot be assessed	
MO No distant metastasis	
M1 Distant metastasis	

[a] Modified from AJCC Staging, Manual for Staging.

[b] Modified from Thomas GM. Consensus statement on the investigation and management of testicular seminoma. EORTC Genito-Urinary Group, Monograph 7. *In:* Newling DW, Jones WG eds. Prostate Cancer and Testicular Cancer. Wiley-Liss; 1990.

should be palpated because supraclavicular area is the most likely site of lymphatic spread above the diaphragm. The breasts should be evaluated for gynecomastia which is commonly seen with choriocarcinomas.

The initial laboratory studies should include a complete blood count (CBC), urinalysis, liver function studies, and blood urea nitrogen (BUN). If a testis tumor is suspected, testicular ultrasound should be performed and serum markers should be drawn for β-HCG and AFP. Semen analysis and sperm banking should be considered for patients in whom treatment is likely to compromise fertility.

After the initial clinical evaluation, the diagnosis should be established by removal of the primary tumor by a radical orchiectomy through an inguinal incision. Once the diagnosis is confirmed histopathologically, further studies must be performed to accurately stage the extent of the disease. A chest radiograph should be performed to evaluate for pulmonary metastasis and retroperitoneal lymph nodes should be evaluated by pedal lymphangiography and/or abdominopelvic CT scanning.

Abdominal Imaging

Lymphangiography Lymphangiography can detect lymph node metastases as small as 5 to 7 mm. These are usually seen as filling defects beneath the capsule of the node. Other findings suggestive of nodal metastasis include deviation or obstruction of the lymph vessels or nonvisualization of a lymph node group. The accuracy of lymphangiography depends on the experience of the diagnostic radiologist, but it is said to have an overall accuracy of 80% in testicular cancer, with 15 to 20% false negatives and 5 to 10% false positives (17,18). Pedal lymphangiography is useful for detecting regional lymph node metastasis, as an aid to setting up treatment portals, and for following the response to treatment (because the nodes often remain opacified for months after the procedure).

Computed Tomography Computed tomography (CT) is less sensitive than lymphangiography because the nodes must be 1.5 to 2 cm in size or larger to be detected as abnormal. Computed tomography scans have been reported to have an overall accuracy of 76% (19), but the incidence of false negatives is greater with computerized tomography than it is with lymphangiography. Nevertheless, CT scans are useful for evaluating nodes that do not opacify with pedal lymphangiography, such as the sentinel nodes near the renal hila and those located above the renal pedicles.

There is considerable controversy as to whether testicular cancer patients should be staged initially with pedal lymphangiography or with CT. Many oncologists prefer pedal lymphangiography because it is more accurate than CT and has fewer false negatives (20-23). However, others recommend the use of CT scans if the retroperitoneal nodes are to be irradiated anyway. The argument is that any nodal metastasis from seminoma that is not detectable by CT is small enough to be easily controlled with elective doses of radiation therapy (19,24,25). Lymphangiography is not readily available in many institutions, and because of this, most radiation oncologists must rely on CT scans to evaluate patients for retroperitoneal spread.

Tumor Markers

The development of radioimmune assays for β-HCG and alpha feto-protein (AFP) have had a significant effect on the management of testicular cancers. Tumor markers are useful for staging, to monitor the effectiveness of therapy, and to follow patients for the early detection of recurrent cancer.

Tumor markers should be obtained both before and after orchiectomy. However, the postorchiectomy specimen should be obtained after sufficient time has elapsed to allow for metabolism of markers present in the serum at the time of orchiectomy. Human chorionic gonadotropin has a metabolic half-life of 24 hours and AFP has a metabolic half-life of 5 days. If the markers remain elevated after orchiectomy, there is metastatic disease present. However, normal postorchiectomy marker studies are not assurance that metastasis is not present because false negative results occur in 15 to 30% of patients (26).

Human Chorionic Gonadotropin Abnormal β-HCG titers are found in ~40 to 60% of patients with nonseminomatous testicular tumors and in 7 to 10% of patients with pure seminomas (26,27). The elevations seen with pure seminoma are almost always moderate. Human chorionic gonadotropin is not found in normal men or boys. However, it can be elevated with a variety of nontesticular malignancies, e.g., breast, stomach, pancreas, and liver cancer.

Alpha Feto-Protein Elevated AFP concentrations can be detected in newborns, but not in adults. AFP titers may be elevated in patients with hepatomas or other gastrointestinal malignancies, with yolk sac tumors, embryonal carcinomas, or teratocarcinomas of the testis. Elevated AFP values are not found in patients with pure seminomas or choriocarcinomas. Therefore, any patient with a histopathologic diagnosis of pure seminoma and an elevated AFP should be considered to have a mixed tumor.

Tumor markers have improved the accuracy of clinical staging for testis cancer. In a series of 31 patients with nonseminomatous testis cancers initially staged by lymphangiography, Scardino et al (28) found that adding AFP and β-HCG assays to the initial workup reduced the false negative rate from 29% to 13%.

Table 26.2. A Compilation of the Results Achieved with Orchiectomy and Radiation Therapy for Pure Seminoma

	Stage I		Stage II		
Institution	No. of Patients	Results (%)	No. of Patients	Results (%)	Endpoints
Antoni van Leeuwenhoek Hospital (29)	78	95	25	72	3-y RFS
Brooke General Hospital (30)	64	97	—	—	3-y survival
Indiana University (31)	33	94	19	80	2.5-y survival
Johns Hopkins University (21)	42	93	19	89	5-y RFS
Joint Center for Radiation Therapy (32)	79	92	—	—	10-y survival
Institute Gustave Roussy (33)	184	96	—	—	Actuarial 5-y survival
M.D. Anderson Hospital (34)	282	97	68	84	5-y RFS
Massachusetts General Hospital (35)	135	95	25	84	5-y RFS
Norwegian Radium Hospital (36)	329	94	—	—	10-y survival
Princess Margaret Hospital (37)	338	94	86	74	Actuarial 5-y survival
Rotterdam Institute (38)	153	95	74	82	2-y RFS
Royal Marsden Hospital (3)	121	97	54	81	2-y RFS
Stanford University (39)	71	100	27	85	Actuarial 5-y survival
State University of New York (40)	104	94	—	—	5-y survival
U.S. Naval Hospital San Diego (41)	52	94	—	—	3- to 5-y survival
University of Wisconsin (42)	23	96	11	91	3-y survival
Walter Reed General Hospital (43)	284	97	34	76	Actuarial 10-y survival
Washington University (44)	95	100	—	—	5-y survival
Western General Hospital (45)	185	96	53	90	5-y RFS
Yale University (46)	61	98	18	100	5-y disease specific survival
Total	2713	96	513	82	

[a] Whenever possible, the results were reported in terms of 2–5 year relapse-free-survival (RFS) or absolute 5- to 10-year survival rates.

Pure Seminomas

Pure seminomas are set apart from other malignant neoplasms by their remarkable radiosensitivity. Even massive tumors are permanently eradicated by relatively low doses of radiation therapy. Pure seminomas also have an orderly lymphatic spread. They usually metastasize to the retroperitoneal lymph nodes first and then to mediastinal and supraclavicular lymph nodes. Early hematogenous spread is rare. In a review of the literature, the 5-year relapse-free survival rates with orchiectomy and regional lymphatic irradiation are over 95% for stage I and 80% for stage II (Table 26.2).

Although the results achieved with radiation therapy for pure seminoma are excellent, several controversies have arisen in recent years regarding its use in selected clinical situations. These are discussed below.

Surveillance for Stage I Seminoma

Standard treatment for stage I pure seminoma is a radical orchiectomy and elective irradiation of the periaortic and ipsilateral iliac lymph nodes. However, in recent years, a number of investigators have proposed managing these patients with orchiectomy alone and following them closely for disease progression. The arguments for surveillance in stage I seminoma are: 1) that only 15 to 20% of these patients actually have retroperitoneal metastasis, and therefore 80 to 85% are being irradiated needlessly and 2) that most patients who relapse can be salvaged with radiation therapy or chemotherapy when the disease becomes apparent clinically.

Surveillance for stage I pure seminoma has been tested in clinical trials in Denmark, Britain, and Canada (47-50). Each of these studies showed relapse rates in the range of 16 to 20%, which correlates well with the expected incidence of retroperitoneal metastasis in stage I seminoma. Moreover, most of the patients who developed recurrent disease were salvaged with additional therapy, so that the ultimate survival rates were not compromised when the patients were followed closely in a protocol situation.

However, patients undergoing surveillance must be followed much more closely than patients receiving elective irradiation. Furthermore, not all patients are compliant, and a significant number of those who relapse will have bulky disease and require treatment with chemotherapy. In the Royal Marsden Hospital study, for example, two-thirds of those who recurred had either bulky abdominal disease or distant metastasis at relapse, and five of 13 who developed recurrent disease relapsed a second time.

Furthermore, patients undergoing surveillance must be followed for a long period of time because late recurrences are more common with seminomas than they are with nonseminomatous cancers (51). In the Princess Margaret Hospital study, for example, 19% of those who relapsed did so more than 4 years after diagnosis (49). For these reasons, most oncologists today favor elective irradiation for patients with stage I pure seminoma.

Treatment Portals for Stage I-II Seminoma

The standard treatment portals for stage I-II pure seminoma are directed to the periaortic and ipsilateral iliac areas. In the past, these fields have usually included the inguinal orchiectomy scar as well. The hemiscrotum has also been included if the tumor has extended through the tunica albuginea. However, inclusion of the inguinal and scrotal areas results in a significant radiation dose to the contralateral testis, and the risk of tumor seeding in the scrotum and inguinal region is low. Because of this, the International Consensus Conference in Leeds in 1989 recommended that inguinal-scrotal irradiation be omitted, even if the orchiectomy incision extends into the scrotum (15).

Several investigators have proposed treating an even smaller area. These individuals have advocated limiting the irradiation to the periaortic area and omitting treatment of the iliac lymph nodes. (52-54). The principal purpose of limiting the treatment to only the periaortic area is to decrease the risk of second malignancies.

A number of investigators have reported that the incidence of second cancers in patients with seminomas is greater than expected, and some believe that this is due to the irradiation that these patients receive (52,55–58). However, not all of the second cancers reported have been located in or near the radiation therapy treatment portals. Similarly, Kleinerman et al (59) noted a greater-than-expected incidence of second malignancies in patients with testicular cancer who have received no irradiation. Consequently, the high incidence of second cancers may simply represent a predilection for seminoma patients to develop second malignant tumors regardless of the mode of treatment.

Nevertheless, the risk of metastatic disease in the pelvis of patients with clinical stage I seminoma must be quite small. Only 15 to 20% of patients with stage I seminoma have any occult retroperitoneal disease, and this is usually located in the periaortic area (Figure 26.3). Consequently, the risk of occult metastasis within the pelvis is probably only a few percent. This projection correlates well with pelvic failure rates when the iliac lymph nodes have not been irradiated. Van der Maase et al (48), for example, found only a 2% (5/261) incidence of failures in the pelvic nodes in the Danish surveillance study, and Kiricuta et al (60) found only a 2.3% incidence of failure in the inguinal-iliac area in a series of stage I patients treated to only the periaortic region.

Elective Irradiation of the Mediastinal and Supraclavicular Nodes

Before 1985, most patients with stage II pure seminoma received elective irradiation of the mediastinum and supraclavicular areas. The rationale for this policy was that pure seminomas metastasize in a step-wise fashion, first to the retroperitoneal lymph nodes, then to the mediastinum and supraclavicular nodes, and subsequently to distant organs.

Most patients with stage II today do not receive elective irradiation above the diaphragm, largely because of the development of effective chemotherapy for seminoma. The arguments against elective treatment of the mediastinal and supraclavicular nodes are: 1) that the risk of occult disease in these nodes is small if the retroperitoneal disease is limited, 2) that elective irradiation of the mediastinum increases the risk of subsequent coronary artery disease, 3) that irradiation of this area could jeopardize subsequent treatment with chemotherapy which might be needed if the patient were to relapse, and 4) that patients with occult metastasis in this area can be salvaged with additional treatment when the metastases become clinically apparent.

It is generally agreed that elective irradiation to the mediastinum and supraclavicular lymph nodes is not indicated for patients with clinical stage I disease, since only 1 to 2% of stage I patients who receive only irradiation below the diaphragm fail in the mediastinum or supraclavicular area (61). However, there may still be a role for elective irradiation above the diaphragm in selected patients with stage II pure seminoma because a significant number of stage II patients do have occult disease in this area.

Dosmann and Zagars (34), for example, found a 20% actuarial failure rate in the left supraclavicular area in a group of patients with stage IIA-C disease who did not receive elective irradiation in the supraclavicular area. On the other hand, none of those who received elective supraclavicular irradiation failed in this area. Similarly, Thomas et al (62) reported a 22% (10 in 46) relapse rate in the lymphatics above the diaphragm in patients with stage IIB pure seminoma treated to only the retroperitoneal nodes. However, Hermann et al (61) reported only a 4% incidence of mediastinal and supraclavicular failures in patients with stage IIA disease, an observation which suggests that elective irradiation is not necessary if the retroperitoneal disease measures less than 2 cm in size.

Speer et al (63) found that the relapse rate in the mediastinum and supraclavicular area correlated well with the extent of the disease in the periaortic lymph nodes (Table 26.3). In a review of 35 reports involving 389 patients with stage II disease, they found a 9% failure rate in the mediastinum and supraclavicular area in stage IIA, 16% in stage IIB, 23% in stage IIC, and 26% in stage IID (Royal Marsden classification) (63).

Table 26.3. Incidence of Mediastinal and/or Supraclavicular Failure in Stage II Patients Not Receiving Elective Mediastinal and Supraclavicular Irradiation (Review of the Literature)

Royal Marsden Stage	Percent with mediastinal and/or supraclavicular recurrences
IIA (<2 cm)	9 (2/22)
IIB (2–5 cm)	16 (12/76)
IIC (>5 cm or bulky)	23 (38/164)
IID (≥10 cm or "palpable")	26 (33/127)

Modified from Speer TW et al. Testicular seminoma: a failure analysis and literature review. Int J Radiat Oncol Biol Phys 1995;33(1):89–97.

In view of the limited morbidity associated with supraclavicular irradiation, elective irradiation of the supraclavicular area seems to be appropriate for patients with stage IIB-C disease. However, irradiation of the mediastinum is not advocated because of the increased risk of cardiac complications. In Dosmann and Zagars' series (34) most relapses above the diaphragm occurred in the supraclavicular area, indicating that tumor emboli follow normal anatomic channels, bypassing the mediastinum by way of the thoracic duct. If mediastinal irradiation is omitted, the risk of cardiac injury and the compromise of subsequent treatment with chemotherapy should be minimized.

Treatment for Bulky Abdominal Disease

The cure rates with radiation therapy alone for patients with massive retroperitoneal metastasis (Stage IID) is poorer than it is for patients with small-to-moderate sized retroperitoneal disease (stage IIA-C). However, most of the failures following irradiation for bulky retroperitoneal disease are due to distant metastasis. Even massive disease can be eradicated with radiation therapy because seminoma is an exquisitely radiosensitive neoplasm. For example, Anscher et al (64) reported a 38% relapse rate for patients with bulky intraabdominal disease. However, only 15% failed within the treated area (Table 26.4). Zagars and Babaian (16) also reported a significantly greater relapse rate for patients with bulky retroperitoneal metastasis than in those with less extensive disease, but none of the patients in their series developed in-field recurrences.

Today, most patients with bulky retroperitoneal metastasis (stage IID) are treated initially with chemotherapy. These are patients with nodal metastases greater than 10 cm in size. The use of chemotherapy has led to a modest improvement in survival for stage IID patients. Babaian and Zagars (12), for example, reported a 78% disease-free

Table 26.4. Patterns of Relapse After Treatment With Radiation Therapy Alone for Bulky Abdominal Disease

			Sites of Relapse		
Author	No. of Patients	No. of Relapsed	Local Failure Only	Local Failure & Distant Met	Distant Metastases Only
Andrews (2)	4	1	0	0	1
Ball (5)	23	9	2	4	3
Dosoretz (14)	7	4	1	2	1
Epstein (17)	3	1	0	0	1
Gregory & Peckham (21)	14	4	1	2	1
Hunter (27)	3	0	0	0	0
Kellokumpu-Lehtinen (34)	2	0	0	0	0
Lederman (40)	9	6	2	0	4
Lester (41)	4	1	0	0	1
Mason (45)	24	6	0	1	5
Sagerman (54)	11	1	0	0	1
Thomas (65)	26	24	10	0	14
Willan (78)	14	6	0	0	6
Zagars (83)	11	4	2	0	2
Totals	175	67 (38%)	18 (10%)	9 (5%)	40 (23%)

Local Failure Rate = 15%

Distant Metastasis Rate = 28%

Modified from Anscher MS, Marks LB, Shipley WU. The role of radiotherapy in patients with advanced seminomatous germ cell tumors. Oncology 1992;6(8):97–108.

survival rate for patients with stage IID disease after treatment with chemotherapy, compared to 68% for patients treated initially with radiation therapy.

Radiation Therapy Technique

The treatment policy for pure seminoma is outlined in Figures 26.4 and 26.5. The primary tumor in the testis is treated with an inguinal orchiectomy with high ligation of the spermatic cord. The regional lymphatics are treated with radiation therapy. If an incisional biopsy or scrotal orchiectomy has been performed, the spermatic cord is resected before proceeding with treatment of the regional lymphatics. In keeping with the Leeds Consensus Conference (15), the inguinal scar and hemiscrotum are not routinely irradiated in order to limit the dose to the contralateral testicle.

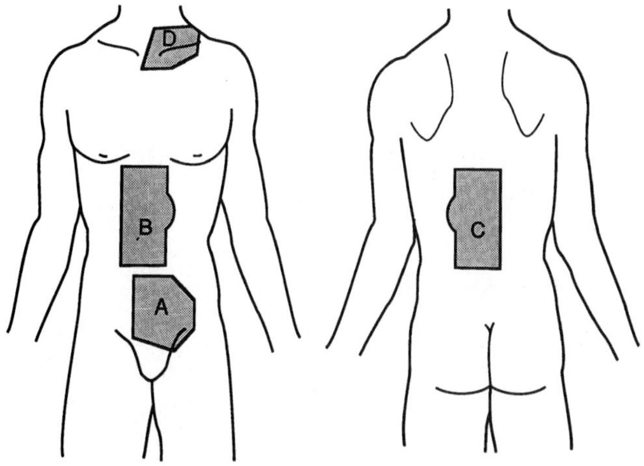

Figure 26.4. Typical field arrangement for treating a seminoma of the left testis using separate periaortic and iliac fields.

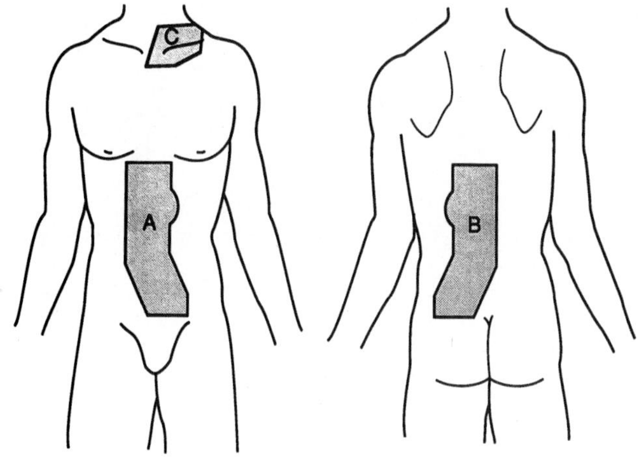

Figure 26.5. Typical field arrangement for treating a seminoma of the left testis using a hockey-stick shaped periaortic/iliac field arrangement.

Stage I

If the seminoma is clinically limited to the testis, the periaortic and ipsilateral iliac areas are irradiated electively because 15 to 20% of these patients will have occult metastasis in the retroperitoneal lymph nodes. Surveillance following orchiectomy may be used in selected patients, but it is not recommended routinely because patients undergoing surveillance must be followed very closely with CT scans and tumor markers for an extended period of time.

A tumor dose of 25 Gy in 15 fractions over 3 weeks is delivered through fields encompassing the periaortic and ipsilateral iliac lymph nodes (Figure 26.4 field A,B,C). The mediastinum and supraclavicular areas are not electively irradiated in stage I because less than 2% of these patients have occult metastasis in this region (61).

Stage IIA

In patients with retroperitoneal metastases measuring less than 2 cm in size, the periaortic and ipsilateral iliac areas are treated through portals similar to those used for stage I. A dose of 25 Gy in 15 fractions over 3 weeks is delivered through these portals (Figure 26.4 fields-A,B,C), followed by an additional 5 to 10 Gy in 2 to 5 fractions through reduced fields encompassing the initially involved areas. Elective irradiation of the mediastinum and supraclavicular area is no longer recommended for stage IIA, because less than 10% of stage IIA patients have occult metastasis in this region (Table 26.3) (63) and most of those who fail in the mediastinal or supraclavicular nodes can be salvaged with radiotherapy or chemotherapy.

Stage IIB-C

In patients with moderate-to-large retroperitoneal metastases, i.e., those measuring 2 to 10 cm in size, the periaortic and ipsilateral iliac lymph nodes are irradiated to a basic dose of 25 Gy in 15 fractions over 3 weeks. However, the total dose delivered to the areas of clinically evident disease may be taken to 35 to 40 Gy using a shrinking field technique (Figure 26.4 fields A,B,C).

Elective irradiation to the left supraclavicular area (Figure 26.4 field D) is recommended for stage IIB-C because approximately 20% of these patients will fail in the supraclavicular nodes if this area is not electively treated (Table 26.3) (34,62,63). The mediastinum is not routinely irradiated because treatment of this area might compromise the subsequent administration of chemotherapy at a later date if it is needed and it may increase the risk of subsequent coronary artery disease. Supraclavicular radiation therapy to a dose of 25 Gy given dose in 3 weeks adds little morbidity, and it can be delivered concurrent with the periaortic and iliac nodal irradiation.

Stage IID

Fifteen years ago, most patients with bulky intraabdominal disease (stage IID) were treated with radiation therapy. Total abdominal irradiation was usually employed, followed by additional treatment through reduced fields. Today, patients with stage IID disease are treated with chemotherapy initially and radiation therapy is reserved for salvage of chemotherapy failures.

Stage III

Patients with stage III pure seminomas are treated initially with chemotherapy, and radiation therapy is used to eradicate residual disease or to palliate local problems. A significant number of patients with stage III disease can be cured with aggressive treatment.

Treatment Portals

The retroperitoneal lymph nodes may be irradiated through either separate periaortic and iliac fields (Figures 26.6 and 26.7) or parallel opposing "hockey-stick" shaped portals (Figure 26.8). The advantages of using separate periaortic and iliac fields are that the blocks are smaller and easier to handle, the dose transmitted to bowel is less, and one can weight the periaortic and iliac fields differently which may be appropriate because the iliac nodes are located more anteriorly than the periaortic nodes. The advantage of using a hockey-stick shaped portal arrangement is that it avoids a field junction between the periaortic and iliac fields.

The periaortic nodes are treated through parallel opposing anterior and posterior portals (Figure 26.6). These fields are weighted equally AP to PA, and the tumor dose is assessed at midplane. The periaortic fields are approximately 10 cm wide and extend from T10 to the L5-S1 junction. The nodes in the renal hila are included, especially on the left where the left spermatic vein joins the left renal vein. The lateral two-thirds of the kidney is excluded whenever possible. The periaortic fields can be extended to include the iliac area in a hockey-stick shaped portal

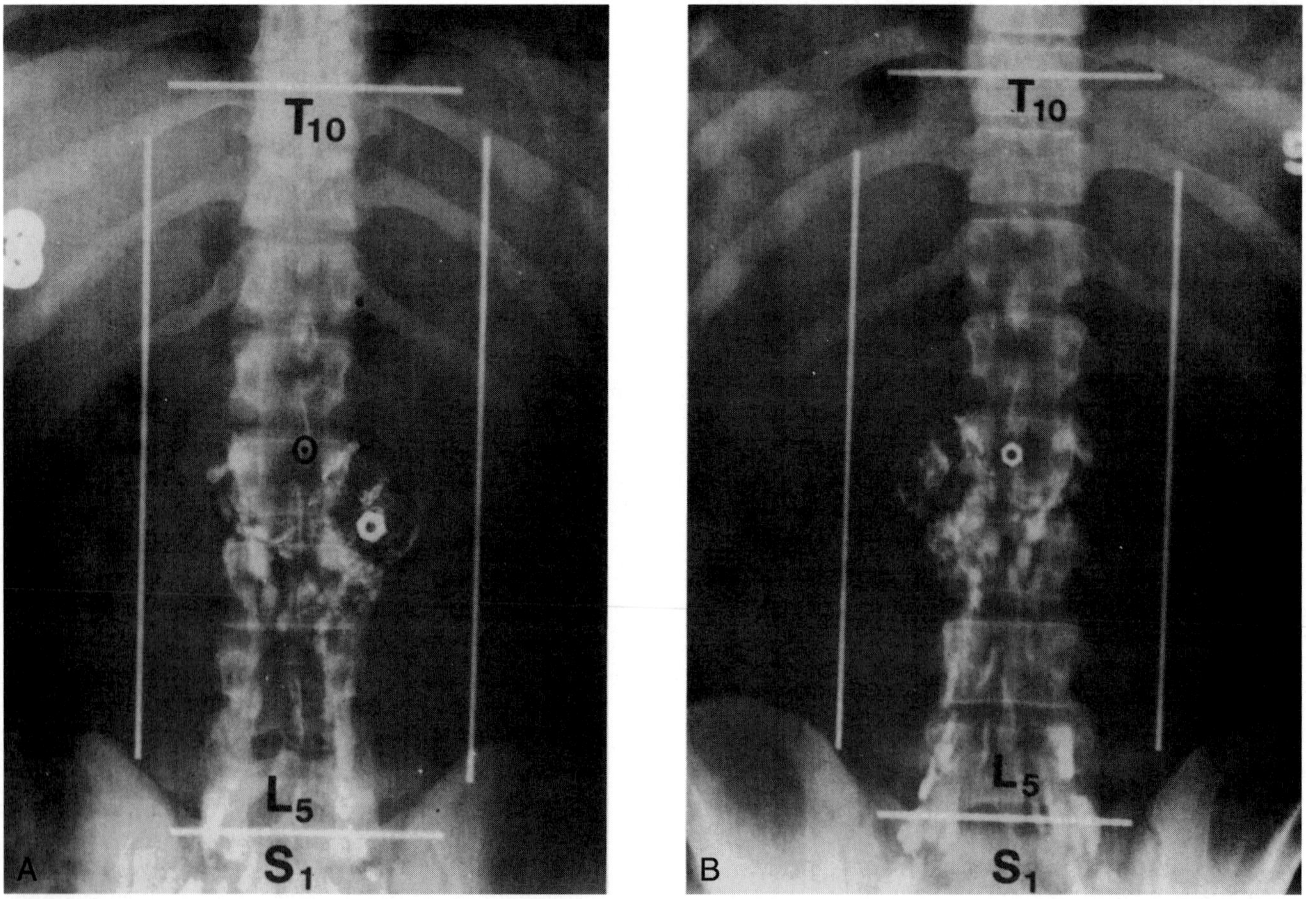

Figure 26.6. Anteroposterior (A) and posteroanterior (B) portal films of para-aortic fields. Fields usually extend from T10 to S1 and are 9 to 10 cm wide. Care is taken to cover "lateral" nodes at renal hila, which may not be filled by pedal lymphangiography. (Reprinted with permission from Fletcher GH. Textbook of radiotherapy. 3rd ed. Philadelphia, Lea & Febiger, 1980.

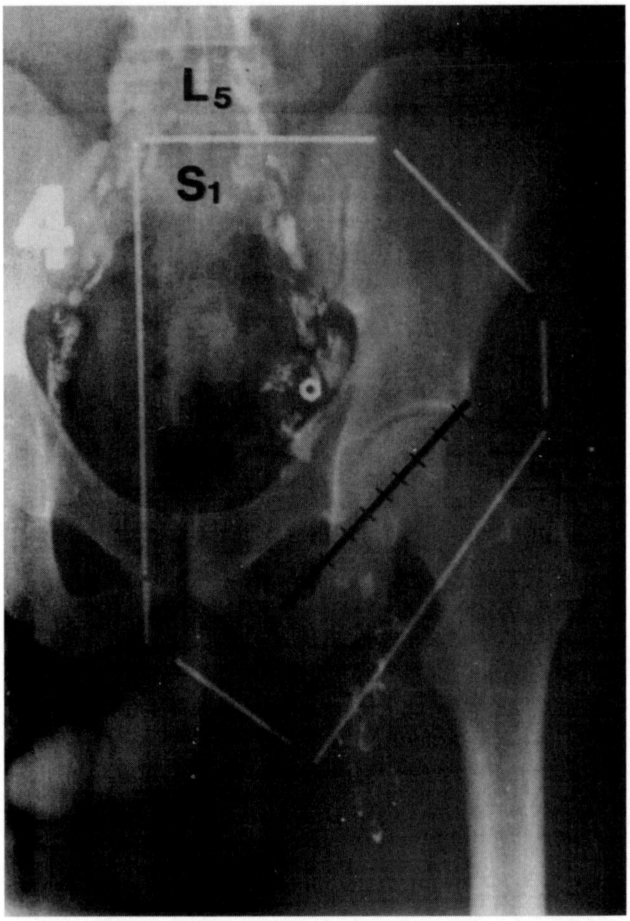

Figure 26.7. Portal film of inguinal-iliac field. Because iliac and inguinal nodes lie anteriorly, only anterior portal is used. Tumor dose is calculated 3 cm anterior to midplane. Superior margin is at L5-S1 level. Medial margin extends 1 cm across midline on skin. Inguinal-iliac areas are treated bilaterally if patient has had herniorrhaphy, orchiopexy, or clinical evidence of inguinal-iliac metastasis. (Reprinted with permission from Fletcher GH. Textbook of radiotherapy. 3rd ed. Philadelphia, Lea & Febiger, 1980.)

(Figure 26.8). In this case, the inferior margin of the field extends to symphysis pubis and the inguinal orchiectomy scar. The iliac crest is shielded, as is the base of the penis.

When the iliac nodes are treated through a separate portal, the superior margin matches the lower border of the periaortic fields at the bottom of the fifth lumbar vertebra. This results in a skin gap of a 2 to 3 cm. These fields should never abut on the skin. Because of the anterior location of the iliac nodes, the iliac treatment is usually delivered through a single anterior field (Figure 26.7). The dose is calculated 3 cm anterior to midplane. The medial margin extends 1 cm across midline on the skin, and the iliac crest is shielded to preserve bone marrow. The inferior and lateral margins are determined by the location of the orchiectomy scar.

The periaortic and iliac fields are usually treated using 4 to 6 MV x-ray beams. However, if the patient has a large AP diameter, 10 to 15 MV x-rays should be employed and the iliac area should be treated with parallel opposing portals to reduce the risk of subcutaneous fibrosis and other late side effects of radiation.

The supraclavicular area is also treated with 4 to 6 MV x-rays (Figure 26.8D). The medial margin of the supraclavicular field includes the sternocleidomastoid muscle with a 1-cm margin, the superior margin is at the cricoid cartilage, and the inferior margin includes the clavicle. The lateral margin usually extends to the junction of the middle and the lateral thirds of the clavicle.

NONSEMINOMATOUS TESTICULAR TUMORS

Chemotherapy was shown to be an effective treatment for nonseminomatous tumors in the early 1980s, and since then radiation therapy has not had a major role in the management of patients with nonseminomas. Nonseminomatous tumors are not as radiosensitive as pure seminomas, and consequently, 45 Gy or more is required to control clinically detectable nonseminomatous testicular cancers. They also have a greater tendency to spread hematogenously, and therefore, they are not as easily cured by any form of locoregional treatment.

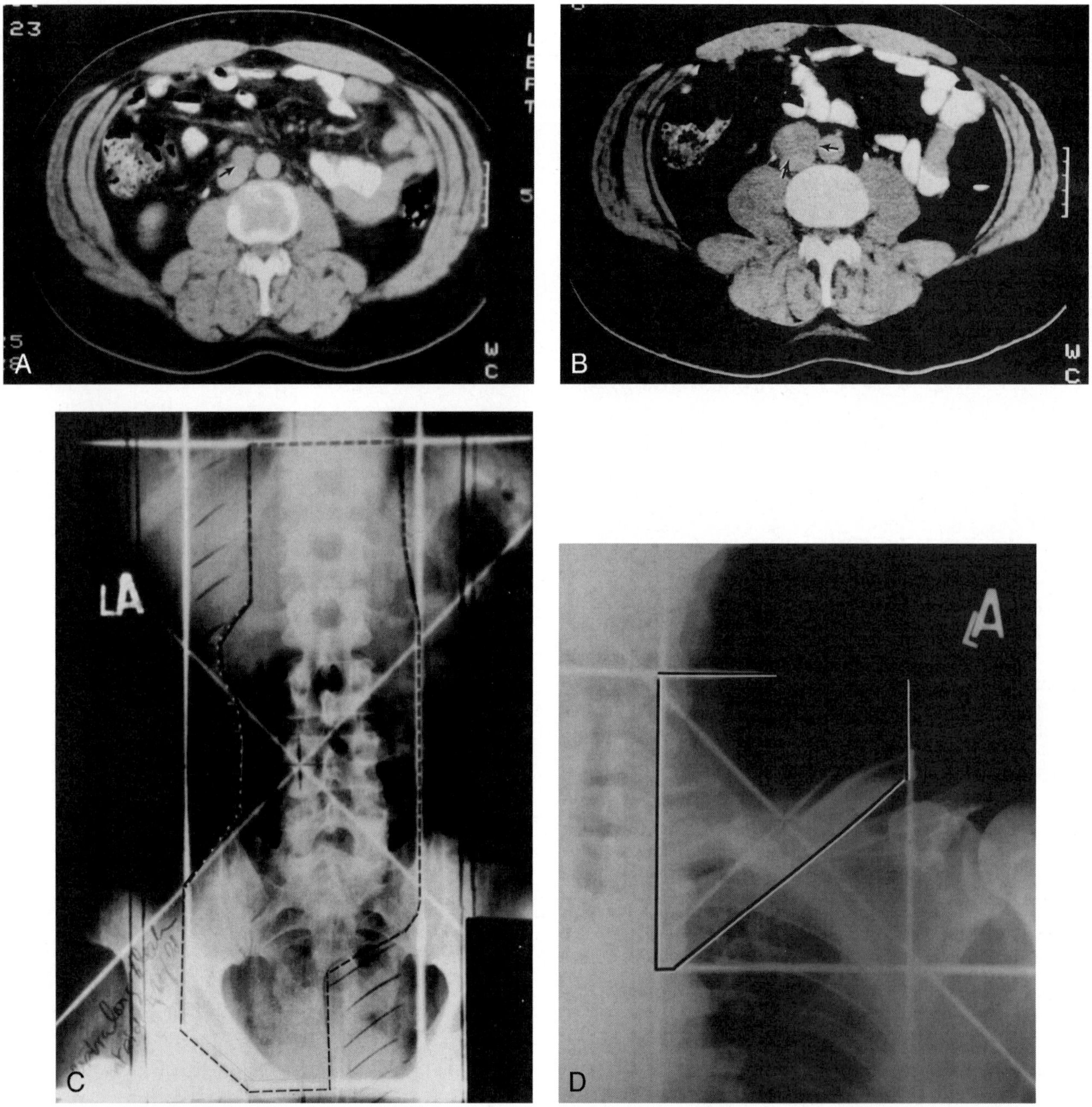

Figure 26.8. (A,B,C,D) Twenty-seven year old man with a 5-week history of progressively enlarging testicular mass. An ultrasound revealed a 2 × 2 cm mass in the upper pole of the right testis. AFP and β-HCG were within normal limits. The patient had a right inguinal orchiectomy which revealed pure seminoma with no extension to the cord or through the tunica albuginea. An abdominopelvic CT scan revealed multiple paracaval nodes measuring 2 to 3 cm in diameter (A and B). The inguinal-iliac and para-aortic area (C) was treated to a dose of 35 Gy in 20 fractions over 28 days, and the supraclavicular area (D) received 25 Gy given dose in 15 fractions through a single anterior field.

References

1. SEER Cancer Statistics Review, 1973-1992 Tables and Graphs. National Cancer Institute NIH Publication #96-2789. Bethesda, MD, 1995
2. Batata MA, Whitmore WF Jr, Chu FC, Hilaris BS, Loh J, Gabstald H, Golbey R. Cryptorchidism and testicular cancer. J Urol 1980;124:382-387.
3. Peckham MJ, McElwain TJ, Hendry WF. Testis and epidydimis. In: Halnan KE, ed. Treatment of Cancer, New York: Igaku-Shoin Medical Publishers, 1982.
4. Peckham MJ. Testicular cancer. Review Oncology 1988;1:439.
5. Presti JC, Herr HW. Genital tumors. 13th ed. Smith's general urology. In: Tanagho MOA, W McAninch, eds. Smith's general urology, 13th ed. Norwalk, CT/ San Mateo, CA: Appleton and Lange, 1992;413.
6. Sokal M, Peckham MJ, Hendry WF. Bilateral germ cell tumours of the testis. Br J Urol 1979;52:158-162.

7. Willis RA. Pathology of tumors. Appleton-Century-Crofts, 1967.
8. Friedman NB, Moore RA. Tumors of the testes. Milit Surg 1946;99: 573-593.
9. Dixon FJ, Moore RA. Tumors of the male sex organs. In Atlas of tumor pathology, Fascicles 31b and 32. Washington, DC: Armed Forces Institute of Pathology, 1952.
10. Mostofi FK. Testicular tumors: epidemiologic, etiologic, and pathologic factors. Cancer 1873;32:1186-1201.
11. Johnson DE, Gomez JJ, Ayala AG. Anaplastic seminoma. J Urol 1975; 114:80.
12. Babaian RJ, Zagars GK. Testicular seminoma: the M.D. Anderson experience. An analysis of pathological and patient characteristics, and treatment recommendations. J Urol 1988;139:311.
13. Sandeman TF, Matthews JP. The staging of testicular tumors. Cancer 1979;43:2514-2524.
14. Boden G, Gibb R. Radiotherapy and testicular neoplasms. Lancet 1951;2:1195-1197.
15. Thomas GM. Consensus statement on the investigation and management of testicular seminoma. EORTC Genito-Urinary Group, Monograph 7. In Newling DW, Jones WG, eds. Prostate cancer and testicular cancer. New York: Wiley-Liss, 1990.
16. Zagars GK, Babaian RJ. The role of radiation in stage II testicular seminoma. Int J Radiat Oncol Biol Phys 1987;13:163-170.
17. Jing BS, Wallace S, Zornoza J. Metastases to retroperitoneal and pelvic lymph nodes: Computed tomography and lymphangiography. Radiol Clin North Am 1981;20:511-530.
18. Maier JG, Schamber DT. The role of lymphangiography in the diagnosis and treatment of malignant testicular tumors. Am J Roentgenol Rad Ther Nucl Med 1972;114:482.
19. Heiken JP, Balfe DM, McClennan BL. Testicular tumors. In: Bragg DG, Rubin P, Youker JE, eds. Oncologic imaging. New York: Pergamon Press, 1985.
20. Cox JD. The testicle. In: Moss WT, Cox JD eds. Radiation oncology rationale, technique, results, 6th ed. St. Louis: The CV Mosby Company, 1989.
21. Epstein BE, Order SE, Zinreich ES. Staging, treatment and results in testicular seminoma: a 12 year report. Cancer 1990;65:405-411.
22. Hussey DH. Testicular cancer. In: Levitt SH, Khan FM, Potish RA, eds. Levitt and Tapley's technological basis of radiation therapy, practical clinical applications, 2nd ed. Philadelphia: Lea & Febiger, 1992.
23. White RL, Maier JG. Testis tumors. In: Perez CA, Brady LW, eds. Principles and practice of radiation oncology. Philadelphia: JB Lippincott, 1987.
24. Marks LB, Anscher MS, Shipley WU. Radiation therapy for testicular seminoma: controversies in the management of early-stage disease. Oncology 1992;6(6):43-48.
25. Zagars G K. Management of stage I seminoma: radiotherapy. In: Horwich A, ed. Testicular cancer. Investigation and management. Baltimore: Williams & Wilkins, 1991.
26. Javadpour N. The role of biologic markers in testicular cancer. Cancer 1980;45:1755.
27. Lange PH, Nochomovitz LE, Rosai J, et al. Serum alpha-fetoprotein and human chorionic gonadotrophin in patients with seminoma. J Urol 1980, 124:472-478.
28. Scardino PT, Cox HD, Waldmann TA, Mcintire KR, Mittenmeyer B, Javadpour N. The value of serum tumor markers in the staging and prognosis of germ cell tumors of the testis. J Urol 1997;118:994-999.
29. Batterman JJ, et al. Testicular tumors, a retrospective study. Arch Chir Neelandicum 1973;XXV-IV:457.
30. Saxena V. Seminoma of the testis. Am J Roentgen 1973;117:643.
31. Lester SG, Morphis JG II, Hornback NB. Testicular seminoma: Analysis of treatment results and failures. Int J Radiat Oncol Biol Phys 1986; 12:353-358.
32. Lederman GS, Herman TS, Jochelson M, et al. Radiation therapy of seminoma: 17 years experience at the Joint Center for Radiation Therapy. Rad Oncol 1989;14:203-208.
33. Giacchetti S, Raoul Y, Wibault P, Droz JP, Court B, Eschwege F. Treatment of stage I testis seminoma by radiotherapy: long-term results—a 30 year experience. Int J Radiat Oncol Biol Phys 1993;27:3-9.
34. Dosmann MA and Zagars GK. Postorchiectomy radiotherapy for stages I and II testicular cancer. Int J Radiat Oncol Biol Phys 1993; 26:381-390.
35. Dosoretz DE, Shipley WU, Blitzer P, et al. Megavoltage irradiation for pure testicular seminoma. Cancer 1981;48:2184-2190.
36. Fossa SD, Aass N, Kaalhus O. Radiotherapy for testicular seminoma stage I: treatment results and long-term post-irradiation morbidity in 365 patients. Int J Radiat Oncol Biol Phys 1989;16:383-388.
37. Thomas GM, Rider WD, Dembo AJ. Seminoma of the testis: results of treatment and patterns of failure after radiation therapy. Int J Radiat Oncol Biol Phys 1982;8:165-174.
38. Van der Werf-Messing B. Radiotherapeutic treatment of testicular tumors. Int J Radiat Oncol Biol Phys 1976;1:235.
39. Earle JD, Bagshaw MA, Kaplan HS. Supervoltage radiation therapy of the testicular tumors. AJR 1973;117:653.
40. van Rooy EM, Sagerman RH. Long-term evaluation of postorchiectomy irradiation for stage I seminomas. Radiology 1994;191:852-861.
41. Kurohara SS, George FW, Dykhuisen RF, Leary KL. Testicular tumors: Analysis of 196 cases treated at the U.S. Naval Hospital in San Diego. Cancer 1967;20:1089.
42. Kademian MT, Bosch A, Caldwell WL. Seminoma: results of treatment with megavoltage irradiation. Int J Radiat Oncol Biol Phys 1976;1: 1075.
43. Maier JG, Van Burskirk KE. Treatment of testicular germ cell malignancies. JAMA 1970;213:97.
44. Lai PP, Bernstein MJ, Kim H, Perez CA, Wasserman TH, Kucik NA. Radiation therapy for stage I and IIA testicular seminoma. Int J Radiat Oncol Biol Phys 1993;28:373-379.
45. Vallis KA, Howard GCW, Duncan W, Cornbleet MA, Keer GR. Radiotherapy for stages I and II testicular seminoma: results and morbidity in 238 patients. Br J Radiol 1995;68:400-405.
46. Hunter M, Peschel RE. Testicular seminoma: results of the Yale University experience, 1964-1984. Cancer 1989;64:1608-1611.
47. Horwich A, Alsanjari N, A'Hern R, Nicholls J, Dearnaley DP, and Fisher C. Surveillance following orchidectomy for stage I testicular seminoma. Br J Cancer 1992;65:775-778.
48. von der Maase H, Specht L, Jacobsen GK, Jakobsen A, Madsen EL, Pedersen M, Roth M, Schultz H. Surveillance following orchiectomy for stage I seminoma of the testis. Eur J Cancer 1993;29(A):1931-1934.
49. Warde P, Gospodarowicz MK, Panzarella T, Catton CN, Sturgeon JFG, Moore M, Goodman P, Jewett MAS. Stage I testicular seminoma: results of adjuvant irradiation and surveillance. J Clin Onc 1995;13(9): 2255-2262.
50. Warde PR, Gospodarowicz MK, Goodman PJ, Sturgeon JF, Jewett MA, Catton CN, Richmond H, Thomas GM, Duncan W, and Munro AJ. Results of a policy of surveillance in stage I testicular seminoma. Int J Radiat Oncol Biol Phys 1993;27:11-15.
51. Whitmore WF. The Marks et al Article Review. Oncology 1992;6(6): 51-52.
52. Hanks GE, Peters T, Owen J. Seminoma of the testis: long term beneficial and deleterious results of radiation. Int J Rad Oncol Biol Phys 1992;24:913-919.
53. Read G, Johnston RJ. Short duration radiotherapy in stage I pure seminoma of the testis: preliminary results of a prospective study. Clin Onc 1993;5:364-366.
54. Willich N, Wendt T, Rohlaff R, Feist H, Meyer-Lenschow T, Lissner J. Radiotherapy of seminoma: small volume irradiation at the stage pT1NoMo—prophylactic irradiation of the mediastinum. Strahlenther Oncol 1986;162:735-741.
55. Hay JH, Duncan W, Kerr GR. Subsequent malignancies in patients irradiated for testicular tumours. Br J Radiol 1984;57:597-602.
56. Møller H, Mellemgaard A, Jacobsen GK, Pedersen D, Storm HH. Incidence of second primary cancer following testicular cancer. Eur J Cancer 1993;29A:672-676.
57. Stein ME, Kessel I, Luberant, and Kuten A. Testicular seminoma stage I: treatment results and long-erm follow-up (1968-1988). J Surg Oncol 1993;53:175-179.
58. van Leeuwen FE, Stiggelbout AM, van den Belt-Dusebout AW, Noyon R, Eliel MR, van Kerkhoff EHM, Delemarre FM, Somers R. Second cancer risk following testicular cancer: a follow-up study of 1,909 patients. J Clin Oncol 1993;11(3):415-424.
59. Kleinerman, RA, Liebermann JV, Li FP. Second cancer following cancer of the male genital system in Connecticut, 1935-82. Natl Cancer Inst Monogr 1985;68:139-147.
60. Kiricuta IC, Sauer J, and Bohndorf W. Omission of the pelvic irradia-

tion in stage I testicular seminoma: A study of postorchiectomy para-aortic radiotherapy. Int J Radiat Oncol Biol Phys 35:293-301, 1996.
61. Herman JG, Sturgeon J, Thomas GM. Mediastinal prophylactic irradiation in seminoma (Abstr). Proc Am Soc Clin Oncol 1983;2:133.
62. Thomas GM. Controversies in the management of testicular seminoma. Cancer 1985;55:2296-2302.
63. Speer TW, Sombeck MD, Parsons JT, Million RR. Testicular seminoma: a failure analysis and literature review. Int J Radiation Oncol Biol Phys 1995;33:89-97.
64. Anscher MS, Marks LB, Shipley WU. The role of radiotherapy in patients with advanced seminomatous germ cell tumors. Oncology 1992;6(8):97-108.

Chapter 27

Extremity Soft Tissue Sarcoma in Adults

Kathryn E. Dusenbery and Roby C. Thompson

BACKGROUND

Although soft tissue sarcomas are uncommon, with an annual incidence of approximately 5000 new cases per year in the United States (1), they are of considerable clinical importance because they are biologically highly aggressive tumors that tend to occur in otherwise young and healthy patients. They pose a particularly complex management problem involving a delicate balance between cure and preservation of function of the affected area of the body. Central to the issue of soft tissue sarcomas is the problem of local recurrence after surgical excision. Simple excision of extremity tumors is followed by a local recurrence rate of 70 to 90%, whereas wide local excision only modestly decreases local recurrence to 30 to 50% (2,3). Only radical excision, defined by Enneking (2) as removal of the entire compartment in which the tumor arises with an uninvolved tissue plane around the compartment, ensures dramatic reduction in local recurrence to as low as 4%. Such extensive surgical procedures frequently necessitate either amputation or significant functional loss—an example is sacrifice of the sciatic nerve in tumors arising in the posterior compartment of the thigh. Moreover, some sarcomas by virtue of size or anatomic location are not suitable for the necessary margin, even with such radical surgery.

In view of the prohibitively high risk of local recurrence with simple excision, and the loss of function and mutilation consequent to amputation with radical surgery, the trend in recent years has been to combine conservative surgery with radiation. Ample evidence has accumulated to suggest that radiotherapy is an effective surgical adjunct (4–8), and, in selected settings, an effective primary treatment for soft tissue sarcomas (9,10). Local control rates comparable to those associated with radical surgery have been reported in several nonrandomized studies using limb-sparing procedures with preoperative or postoperative radiation (Table 27.1) (5,11–25). A randomized trial by the National Cancer Institute (NCI) of 45 patients with high-grade extremity sarcomas assigned to either amputation or limb-sparing surgery with external beam radiation therapy gives further justification for this approach (both groups received postoperative chemotherapy). Although four local recurrences were reported in the limb-sparing group compared to none in the amputation group (P = .004), no differences were noted in either 5-year disease-free (71 and 78%) or overall (83 and 88%) survival rate (26). The NCI published a more recent randomized trial, which again demonstrated the importance of radiation therapy in local control of soft tissue sarcomas (27). In this series of 141 patients, all patients underwent wide local excision. Patients with gross residual tumor after surgery, or multiple positive margins were not included. Patients were then randomized to either no further treatment (all patients with high grade tumors received adjuvant chemotherapy) or postoperative external beam therapy. Overall, local recurrences developed in 17 of the 71 (24%) patients not randomized to radiation therapy compared to only 1 of the 10 (10%) patients receiving adjuvant irradiation (log rank P = .0001). When analyzed by grade, both low and high grade tumors benefited from adjuvant irradiation. Among the low grade tumors, local recurrences developed in 6 out of 19 (31%) of nonirradiated patients compared to 1 out of 22 (5%) in those who did receive radiation therapy (log rank P = .016). Likewise among the high grade tumors, local recurrences developed in 9 out of 49 of the patients who did not receive radiation therapy compared to 0 out of 44 of those who did (log rank P = .03).

MANAGEMENT BY A TEAM OF SPECIALISTS

Patients with soft tissue sarcoma are best managed by a dedicated team of diagnostic radiologists, surgical pa-

Table 27.1. Localized Control Results in Patients Treated by Surgery and Radiation

Reference	No. of Patients	Local Failure (%)
Postoperative		
Suit (11)	176	14
Lindberg (5)	300	22
Abbatucci (12)	89	14
Karakousis (13)	53	14
Potter (14)	128	10
Wilson (15)	23	9
Pao (16)	35	14
Keus (17)	64	8
Fein (18)	67	13
Preoperative		
Mundt (19)	50	24
Suit (11)	181	10
Barkley (20)	110	10
Wilson (15)	39	3
Brant (21)	58	9
Harrison (22)	55	18
Schray (23)	63	8[a]
Chemotherapy and irradiation		
Eilber (24)	371	~10
Wanebo (25)	55	2

[a] Follow-up of 20 months.

thologists, surgeons, medical oncologists, pediatric oncologists, radiation oncologists, and physical therapists whose primary interest and experience is in the treatment of soft tissue neoplasms. The assessment and management plan of an individual patient should be executed only after a coordinated evaluation by the sarcoma team members. As an example, it is critical that the orthopedic surgeon, diagnostic radiologist, and radiation oncologist review the simulation films and ascertain that the desired tissues are included in the treated volume. This level of organization ensures efficient and optimal patient care. Moreover, throughout the treatment and during the subsequent follow-up period, a coordinated effort to attend to the ongoing medical needs and questions of the patient and family members is essential to achieve a successful outcome. At the University of Minnesota, a nurse coordinator helps with these tasks and orchestrates much of the patient education. Weekly tumor conferences and joint follow-up clinics are also used.

CLINICAL DIAGNOSIS AND BIOPSY

Soft tissue sarcomas most frequently manifest as a painless and usually slow growing mass. Asymptomatic patients presenting with a soft tissue mass should be presumed to have a malignant lesion. Appropriate imaging studies to define fully the extent and character of the mass should be performed before biopsy or resection is attempted. A biopsy performed before the appropriate imaging studies are obtained may compromise the chance for future limb preservation (28).

Nonmalignant "tumorous" lesions, such as proliferative fasciitis, myositis ossificans, ganglions, and even soft tissue abscesses, frequently can be diagnosed on the basis of findings of the history, physical examination, and imaging studies. In the absence of a thorough history from the patient, biopsy specimens of many of these reactive soft tissue processes may in fact be mistaken for malignancies.

Sarcomas typically have a characteristic appearance on magnetic resonance (MR) scans (Figure 27.1), with signs of local invasion along nerve fibers, muscle bundles, and fascial planes (29). Intramuscular lipomas also may have a characteristic appearance on computed tomography (CT) or MR scans, and may be observed safely in reliable patients with interval evaluation, unless they are symptomatic. If the diagnosis is uncertain or the mass grows, a biopsy should be performed.

The type and location of the biopsy is determined by the imaging studies. A representative section of the lesion must be obtained. Placement of the biopsy incision should be parallel to the involved muscle bundles and situated so that subsequent surgical resection of the tumor and biopsy scar is possible. In some centers, the preference is needle biopsy either by direct access or CT guidance for diagnosis. The selection of needle versus open biopsy rests primarily on the expertise of the pathologist when making a diagnosis on small fragments of tissue, and on the clinician performing the needle biopsy. When the diagnostic radiologist performs a needle biopsy, consultation with the surgeon should allow placement of the needle tract such that it can be excised easily at the time of definitive resection. When any doubt arises regarding diagnosis, an open biopsy is preferred, with excisional biopsy performed for lesions 3 cm or smaller and incisional biopsy performed for larger lesions. Surgical drains should be avoided because they may tract tumor cells. Meticulous attention to hemostasis is critical; areas of ecchymosis can seed tumor cells and need to be covered by future radiation portals or excised at the time of surgery.

Unfortunately, often little foresight is used when planning such biopsies (30,31), thus some patients are referred to an oncology center with suboptimal pathologic evaluation (Figure 27.2). Mankin et al. demonstrated an 18% incidence of significant problems in patient management resulting from an inappropriate biopsy technique (28); 8% of biopsies produced a significant adverse effect or prognosis, and 5% of biopsies caused or significantly contributed to an otherwise unnecessary amputation. Errors in diagnosis leading to inadequate treatment occurred twice as often when the biopsy was done in a community hospital as opposed to when the biopsy was done after referral to an oncology center. In our experience, local recurrence rates are higher and survival rates are lower in patients

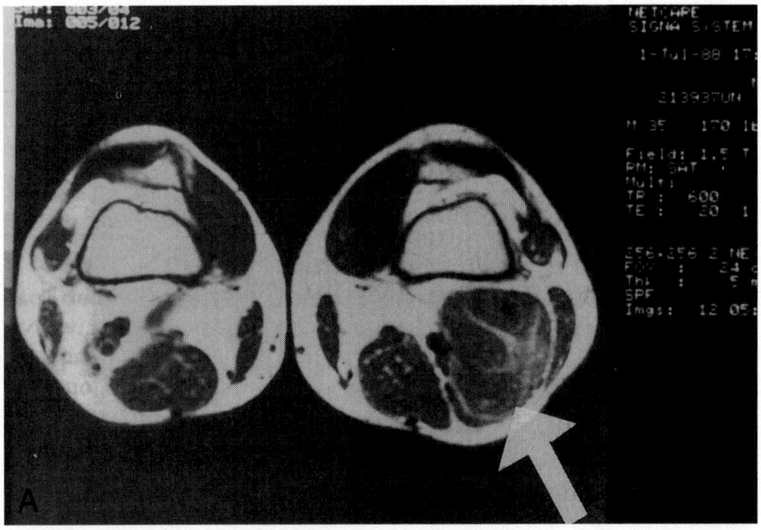

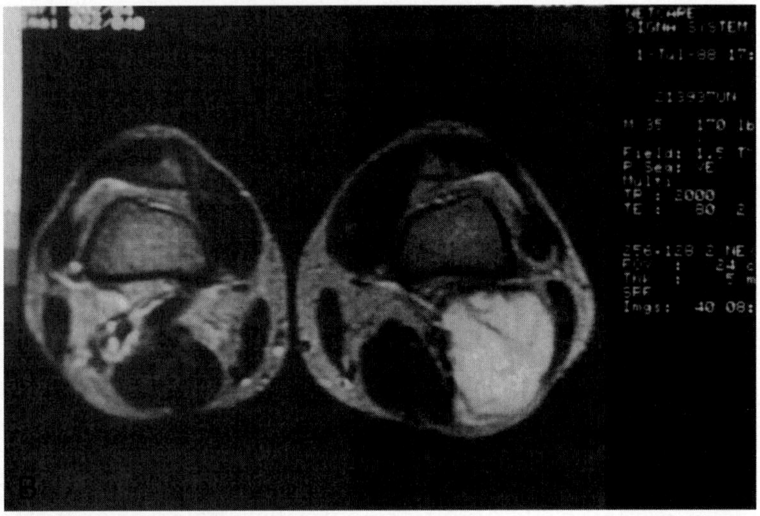

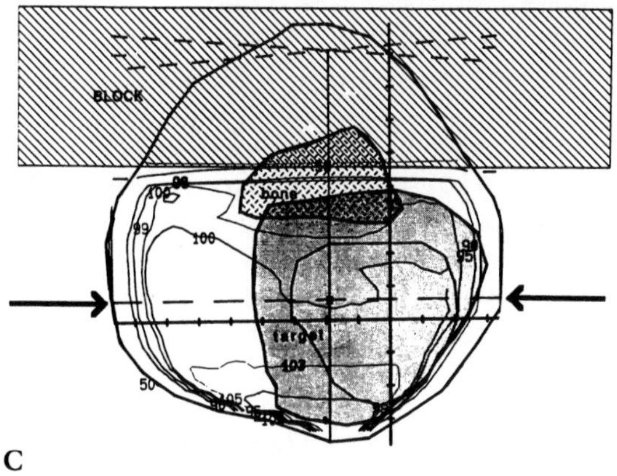

C

Figure 27.1. Magnetic resonance images of asymptomatic soft tissue mass is in 30-year-old man. **A.** T1-weighted image. Signal intensity is similar to that of skeletal muscle (arrow). **B.** T2-weighted image. Signal intensity is greater than that of either skeletal muscle or subcutaneous fat, suggesting tumor. Biopsy confirmed diagnosis of malignant fibrous histiocytoma. **C.** Treatment plan consisted of parallel opposed 6 MV beam arrangement sparing tissue anteriorly.

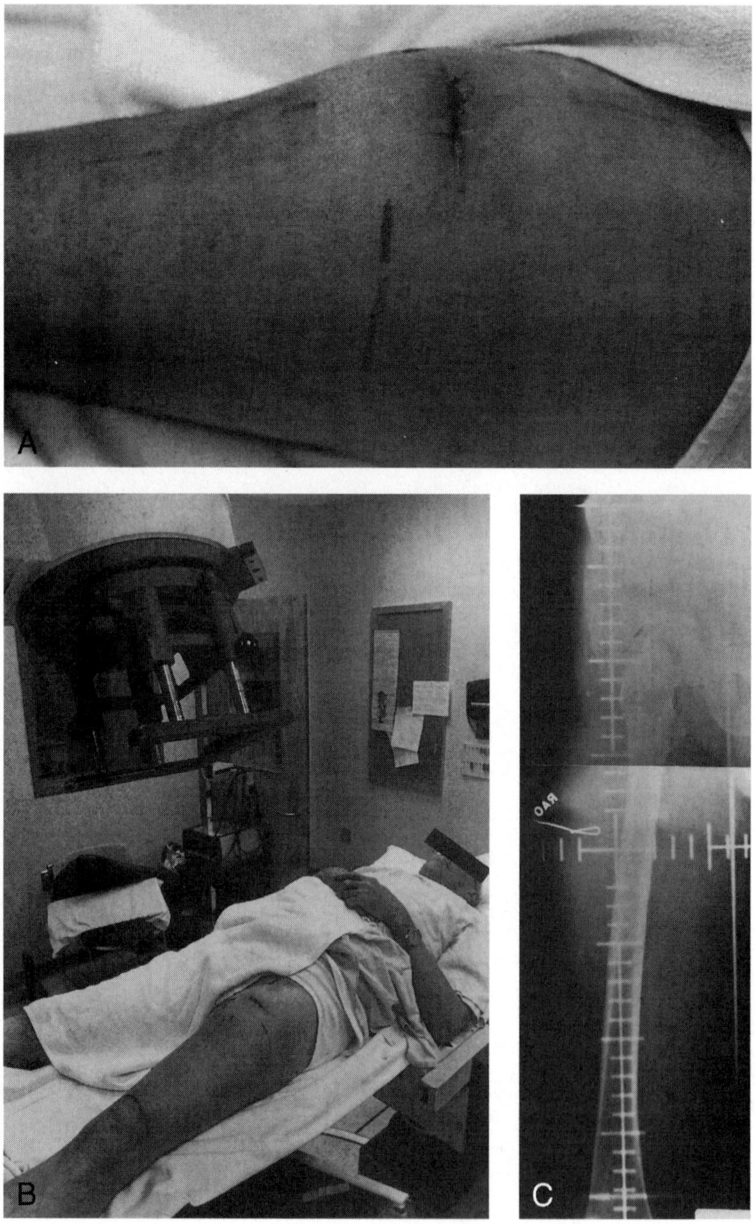

Figure 27.2. Example of inappropriate biopsy technique. **A.** Scar is horizontal, resulting in hemorrhage extending to the knee. Secondary infection delayed initiation of preoperative radiation therapy. **B.** Anterior view of same patient. **C.** Simulation film demonstrates that inferiorly, field edge was extended to include areas involved in post-biopsy hemorrhage, significantly increasing treated volume.

who underwent biopsies at an outside institution (32). Therefore, we recommend referring patients with masses suggestive of sarcoma to an oncology center so that the biopsy can be performed by a surgeon experienced in these details.

HISTOPATHOLOGIC DIAGNOSIS, STAGING, AND PROGNOSIS

The 1998 American Joint Commission on Cancer (AJCC) staging protocol of sarcoma of soft tissue is based on a grade (G), Tumor (T), node (N), and metastasis (M) system and is outlined in Table 27.2. Stage depends primarily on grade, size, and depth of the tumor. The previous AJCC staging system relied on grade and size alone. The depth of tumor has been shown to be an independent variable and has been incorporated into the staging system (33). In the 1998 AJCC staging system, superficial tumors are defined as tumors that do not involve the superficial fascia. Deep tumors are either below or invade the superficial (investing) fascia. All intraperitoneal visceral lesions, or lesions with major vessel invasion are considered deep. Depth of the tumor is categorized as a subcategory of tumor size: T1 tumors are less than 5 cm in diameter, T1a are superficial tumors, and T1b are deep tumors. Likewise for T2 tumors, T2a are superficial and T2b are deep.

The other system frequently employed is that of the Musculo-Skeletal Tumor Society (Table 27.3) (34). In addi-

Table 27.2. Definition of TNM

Primary tumor (T)	
TX	Primary tumor cannot be treated
TO	No evidence of primary tumor
T1	Tumor 5 cm or less in dimension
	T1a superficial tumor
	T1b deep tumor
T2	Tumor more than 5 cm in greatest dimension
	T2a superficial tumor
	T2b deep tumor

Note: Superficial tumor is located exclusively above the superficial fascia without invasion of the fascia; deep tumor is located either exclusively beneath the superficial fascia, or superficial to the fascia with invasion of or through the fascia. Retroperitoneal, mediastinal, and pelvic sarcomas are classified as deep tumors.

Regional lymph nodes (N)	
NX	Regional lymph nodes cannot be assessed
NO	No regional lymph node metastasis
NI	Regional lymph node metastasis
Distant metastasis (M)	
MX	Distant metastasis cannot be assessed
MO	No distant metastasis
M1	Distant metastasis
Histopathologic grade	
GX	Grade cannot be assessed
G1	Well differentiated
G2	Moderately differentiated
G3	Poorly differentiated
G4	Undifferentiated

Stage grouping				
Stage I				
A (Low grade, small, superficial and deep)	G1–2,	T1a–1b,	NO,	MO
B (Low grade, large, superficial)	G1–2,	T2a,	NO,	MO
Stage II				
A (Low grade, large, deep)	G1–2,	T2b,	NO,	MO
B (High grade, small, superficial, deep)	G3–4,	T1a–1b,	NO,	MO
C (High grade, large, superficial)	G3–4,	T2a,	NO,	MO
Stage III				
(High grade, large, deep)	G3–4,	T2b,	NO,	MO
Stage IV				
(any metastasis)	any G,	any T,	N1,	MO
	any G,	any T,	NO,	M1

tion to grade, this system separates tumors based on whether they are intracompartmental (A) or have extended into extracompartmental tissues (B) (34). This system does not give weight to the tumor size. Although extracompartmental extension probably increases the risk of local recurrence, in multivariate analysis this factor is not an independent predictive variable for survival. In a report from UCLA, in a series of 99 patients, no relationship was found between intra- or extracompartmental location and survival (27).

The most important prognostic factor for patients with soft tissue sarcomas is histologic grade (35–37). The AJCC on Cancer Soft Tissue Task Force subdivides tumors into low, moderate, and high grade based on cellular and nuclear pleomorphism, presence of mitotic figures, cellularity, differentiation, and necrosis (38). Other prognostic factors include histologic subtype; location (distal versus proximal); invasion of skin, nerve, blood vessel or muscle; presence of necrosis; and possibly gender and age (14,36,39–43). Possible new prognostic indicators under study include markers of cell proliferation and potential for metastasis, such as deoxyribonucleic acid (DNA) ploidy (44), histologic evidence of necrosis after preoperative therapy (45), and presence of oncogenes or certain antigens (46).

Once the diagnosis of sarcoma has been established, a staging evaluation should include a careful physical examination with documentation of the size and location of the tumor. The minimum pretreatment staging should include posteroanterior and lateral chest radiographs and a CT scan of the chest. Routine follow-up studies will require regular chest radiographs and a CT scan if the radiographic findings are suggestive of metastatic disease. The baseline chest radiograph and chest CT scan will be helpful in interpreting future examinations. A CT or MR scan of the involved limb should be performed, which includes the dis-

Table 27.3. Staging System: Musculo-Skeletal Tumor Society

Anatomical compartments	
Intracompartmental (A)	Extracompartmental (B)
Intraosseous	Soft tissue extension
Intraarticular	Soft tissue extension
Superficial to deep fascia	Deep fascial extension
Paraosseous	Intraosseous or extrafascial
Intrafascial compartments	Extrafascial planes of spaces
Ray of hand or foot	Midfoot and hindfoot
Posterior calf	Popliteal space
Anterolateral leg	Groin-femoral triangle
Anterior thigh	Intrapelvic
Medial thigh	Midhand
Posterior thigh	Antecubital fossae
Buttocks	Axilla
Volar forearm	Periclavicular
Dorsal forearm	Paraspinal
Anterior arm	Head and neck
Posterior arm	
Periscapular	

Surgical stages of sarcomas		
Stage	Grade	Site
IA	Low (G1)	Intracompartmental (T1)
IB	Low (G1)	Extracompartmental (T2)
IIA	High (G2)	Intracompartmental (T1)
IIB	High (G2)	Extracompartmental (T2)
III	Any (G)	Any (T)
	Regional or distant metastasis	

(Modified from reference [34]).

tal and proximal extent of the compartment involved and the proximal areas of lymphatic drainage to identify regional node involvement or satellite tumor nodules. Any suspicious lymphadenopathy should be investigated with a biopsy, although it is unusual for sarcomas to spread through the lymphatic system, except for certain histologic subtypes (47).

SELECTION OF LOCAL TREATMENT

Surgical Resection Alone

Surgical resection remains the cornerstone of local treatment for soft tissue sarcomas. As stated earlier, limb-sparing surgery with adjuvant irradiation has become the standard treatment for most patients with extremity soft tissue sarcoma. There are patients for whom surgery alone is sufficient. For patients with small, superficial tumors in whom a wide margin is achieved, the local recurrence after surgery alone is low (48). Rydholm reviewed the results obtained in 123 patients with superficial tumors treated with surgery alone. Among those with negative margins, local control was achieved in 100% of low grade tumors but only 8% of high grade tumors. Local control was worse for patients with marginal resections, with local control of only 67% of the low grade and 33% of the high grade lesions. Thus, for superficial low grade lesions in a location in which re-resection would be feasible, irradiation is possibly not necessary. However, for high grade tumors and for those with less than a wide excision, local recurrence rate is high and irradiation should be given.

Surgery and Radiation Therapy

Virtually every possible sequence of surgery and irradiation has been reported (5,20,49–57). Until randomized trials are available, however, or a particular approach is shown to be superior, the approach to use for a given patient depends mostly on the experience of the involved radiation therapist and surgeon. Additionally, the approach must be individualized, taking into account the size, location, and character of the tumor.

Preoperative Versus Postoperative Radiation Therapy: Potential advantages of postoperative over preoperative radiation are that the entire surgical specimen is available for review for exact histopathologic classification, the extent of microscopic tumor can be assessed directly, and there is no possibility of increased morbidity associated with operating in an irradiated bed. Good results have been achieved, with local failure rates between 8 to 25% and wound complication rates between 6 to 17% (5,11,52,58).

Advantages of preoperative radiation are that it can potentially shrink the tumor and theoretically allow the surgeon to perform a less radical surgical procedure and in some cases may convert a nonresectable tumor into one that may be resected. However, it is theoretically possible that even if the tumor does not appreciably decrease in size during preoperative radiation, the reactive margins around the tumor may regress, making the resection easier, or the tumor may consist of only necrotic debris with little viable tumor at the time of surgery (45,59). Another theoretic benefit of preoperative irradiation is that irradiation may inactivate tumor clonogens, potentially preventing tumor cell seeding at the time of surgical manipulation of the tumor. The major disadvantage to preoperative irradiation is the risk of wound complications. In institutions experienced with preoperative irradiation, the results are also good with local failure rates (9 to 18%) similar to preoperative irradiation (20,25,51,60–64). As might be expected, the rate of wound complications may be higher with preoperative irradiation (60,65,66).

At the University of Minnesota, we generally recommend postoperative shrinking field external beam therapy, but only if the following criteria are met: the tumor must be resectable with acceptable functional deficit and the biopsy must have been performed correctly (needle tract appropriately placed, no postbiopsy hemorrhage or ecchymosis). If the patient has undergone prior excisional biopsy, a magnetic resonance imaging (MRI) or computerized axial tomography (CAT) scan should have been performed prior to the biopsy and the surgeon performing the biopsy must be the surgeon who is performing the definitive wide local excision.

Preoperative radiation therapy is recommended at the University of Minnesota in two situations: 1) for tumors in which extensive amounts of tissue must be removed or amputation is necessary to achieve adequate margins. For these tumors, preoperative radiation may allow the surgeon to decrease the extent of the surgical field and perform a limb-sparing operation; and 2) for patients referred to the university after an excisional biopsy who did not receive imaging studies prior to the biopsy. In this situation, we obtain a postexcisional biopsy MRI, and if the only abnormalities on the MRI are postoperative signal changes, we recommend "preoperative" irradiation followed by a re-excision of the tumor bed and scar. This strategy is based on the rationale that because the surgeon does not have a "road map" of the exact site of the previous tumor, the risk of local recurrence is higher unless radiation therapy is given first to "sterilize" the operative bed. Giuliano and Eilber found that in patients supposedly undergoing a complete surgical excision, 49% had identifiable gross tumor remaining at the time of re-operation (67).

If a definite tumor mass does remain, however, depending on the extent and location of the tumor, a wide local excision is considered and the patient receives postoperative irradiation.

Preoperative Radiation Therapy: Because of concern about subsequent wound healing, preoperative external beam therapy usually is limited to 45 to 50 Gy with 1.8 to

2.0 Gy daily fractions. Resection is carried out 14 to 28 days after completion of the external beam therapy. Clinicians at the M.D. Anderson Hospital reported local failures in only 10% and wound complications in 14% of 110 patients treated preoperatively with 50 Gy (20). No postoperative boost was given. At other institutions, the tumor bed has been boosted postoperatively with additional radiation given by either interstitial brachytherapy, intraoperative electron beam, or postoperative external beam techniques (7). In the series of patients receiving preoperative radiation with a variety of intraoperative and postoperative boost techniques at Massachusetts General Hospital, Suit et al. reported 14% local recurrence and 15% wound complication rates (7,51). Schray et al. reported a 25% wound complication rate with preoperative external beam therapy, followed by surgical excision with a brachytherapy boost (23).

Whether to give a postoperative boost, and whether to give the boost with external beam therapy, brachytherapy, or intraoperative therapy depends on the experience of the involved physicians as well as the size, location, and response of the tumor to the preoperative irradiation. At the University of Minnesota, we generally wait until there is good wound healing and then give an external beam boost of irradiation. The boost dose ranges from 12 to 18 Gy, bringing the final cumulative doses to around 60 Gy (if the margin is negative), or to 62 to 66 Gy (if the margin is "close"). If the margin is "positive" we consider re-resection in order to achieve a "negative " margin. Postoperative Radiation Therapy: Postoperative irradiation is most often given with shrinking field external beam therapy (4,5,7,26). Even with "negative" margins, doses of over 6000 cGy are usually recommended as sarcoma is considered "radio-resistant." Daily doses of 1.8 to 2 Gy are usually recommended. The initial field encompasses the entire tumor, surgical bed, and areas of suspected microscopic disease. After 4500 to 5000 cGy are delivered, the field is reduced to include the previous tumor with a margin. Results with postoperative irradiation have been good, with low rates of severe wound complications (less than 5%) and excellent local control (usually less than 10% local recurrences).

Brachytherapy

Brachytherapy has the potential advantage of the tumor bed being visualized directly at the time of surgical resection. In addition, the highest dose of irradiation can be localized to the region at greatest risk of gross or microscopic disease with relative sparing of normal surrounding tissues. Radiation can be delivered in the immediate postoperative period before scar tissue forms and any residual microscopic disease becomes embedded in hypoxic fibrous tissue. Considerable technical expertise is required to perform brachytherapy, and not all anatomic sites are suitable. Although the local recurrence rate with postoperative brachytherapy alone at Memorial Sloan-Kettering was only 6% at doses of 30 to 50 Gy, major wound complications occurred in 22% of patients and another 22% had moderately severe wound complications (68). In a subsequent series, a delay in loading the radioactivity for 5 to 8 days postoperatively decreased the wound complication rate to a more acceptable rate of 14% (69).

An important finding by the Memorial Sloan Kettering group is that in low grade tumors, postoperative brachytherapy only (without external beam therapy) failed to improve local control over surgery alone (22). In a randomized trial comparing surgery alone to surgery and postoperative brachytherapy, only patients with high grade sarcomas benefited from postoperative brachytherapy with local recurrence rates of 10% in the brachytherapy group versus 35% in the surgery only group.

Schray et al. advocate surgical resection with implantation of brachytherapy catheters followed by a subsequent course of postoperative external beam therapy, and report a wound complication rate of only 5% and excellent local control (8%) with this technique. This method, however, has not been compared directly to either shrinking field postoperative brachytherapy or external beam therapy.

Intraoperative Electron Beam Therapy

In certain locations, such as near major neurovascular structures, brachytherapy is not possible. An alternative local treatment is to boost the involved area with intraoperative electron beam therapy. The Mayo clinic experience with intraoperative electron beam therapy for soft tissue sarcomas has recently been reported with excellent results in carefully chosen patients (70).

ADJUVANT CHEMOTHERAPY

Despite improved control of the primary lesion through advances in surgical and radiotherapeutic techniques, more than one half of patients with high grade tumors will die within 5 years of diagnosis, usually of metastatic disease. Adjuvant chemotherapy has been tested in several prospective trials and its use remains controversial (71–74). Most of the prospective studies involving the use of a variety of chemotherapeutic agents, many of which have included nonextremity sites, have failed to demonstrate a survival advantage to adjuvant chemotherapy (Table 27.4) (26,71,72,74–78). A recent meta-analysis evaluating over 15 randomized trials suggested a small improvement in survival at 5 years (4% advantage), in patients receiving adjuvant chemotherapy (79). The toxicity of these regimens is considerable and the potential small advantage to adjuvant chemotherapy needs to be weighed

Table 27.4. Randomized Adjuvant Trials: Soft Tissue Sarcomas

Center (ref)	CT	Stage	No. of Patients	DFS (%)		Survival (%)	
				Obs	CT	Obs	CT
EORTC (75)	CYVADIC	I-IVA	317	43	56	56	63
MDA (76)	ACVAd	IIB/IIIB	47	83	76	na	na
NCI (26)	ACM	IIA-IVA					
		Extremities	67	28	54	60	54
		Trunk	22	47	77	61	82
		Retroperitoneal	15	49	92	100	47
Mayo Clinic (72)	AVDAd	I-IVB	61	68	65	70	70
Scandinavian (72)	A	III/IVa	139	44	40	55	52
Rizzoli Inst. (77, 78)	A	III/IVA77	77	45	73	70	91
DFCI/MGH (71)	A	IIB-IVA	46	62	67	72	71
ECOG (74)	A	IIV-IVA	36	55	66	52	65

EORTC, European Organization Radiation Therapy Centers; MDA, MD Anderson; NCI, National Cancer Institute; DFCI/MGH, Dana Farber Cancer Institute/Massachusetts General Hospital; ECOG, Eastern Cooperative Oncology Group; A, adriamycin (doxorubicin); C, cyclophosphamide; V, vincristine; E, dacarbazine; Ad, actinomycin D; Obs, observation; CT, chemotherapy; DFS, disease-free survival.

against possible toxicity (especially cardiac toxicity from doxorubicin). Recent studies have shown that the addition of ifosfamide to doxorubicin-based chemotherapy may produce higher response rates. Hopefully in future trials with agents having a higher activity against sarcoma, adjuvant chemotherapy regimens will show a convincing advantage.

INNOVATIVE APPROACHES

Fast neutron beam therapy is a promising approach for locally advanced sarcomas with a variety of treatment schedules with or without photons possible (80–82). With their improved relative biologic effectiveness, fast neutron beams have been used by Catterall, who achieved local control in 21 of 28 patients using 7-MeV neutrons to a dose of 1200 neutron rad in 12 fractions over 4 weeks (80–83). Complications developed, however, in 32% of patients. Hyperthermia in conjunction with chemotherapy or radiation therapy has the theoretic advantage of improving cytotoxicity, especially in hypoxic cells. Findings of preliminary reports suggest improved regression, although this method has not been evaluated prospectively (84–88). Hypofractionation (once weekly doses of 6 cGy) has been attempted with no evidence of an advantage (89). Hyperfractionation of radiation dose in a preliminary trial resulted in increased wound morbidity but it is an interesting avenue of further investigation (90). Neoadjuvant intra-arterial chemotherapy combined with hypofractionated radiation (3.5 Gy × 5 to 10) and subsequent surgery have been studied in a large number of patients (55,91–94). Local failure rates of 5 to 12% were obtained, and complications occurred in between 23 to 43% of patients, depending on the radiation dose.

DESMOID TUMORS

Desmoid tumors (aggressive fibromatosis) are uncommon and may arise at any anatomic site, although they are most common in the torso and lower extremities. By definition they do not metastasize, but have a propensity to spread regionally. Their growth is unpredictable with reports of spontaneous regression as well as apparent growth arrest either spontaneously or after treatment with antiestrogens or nonsteroidal anti-inflammatory agents (indomethacin).

If the diagnosis of aggressive fibromatosis is made, the entire limb involved should be imaged by MRI. If possible, a surgical resection with a relatively wide margin is the treatment of choice. Although histologically "benign," these tumors may destroy normal tissues, causing pain, disability, and rarely, death (95).

For patients in whom a negative margin is achieved, close follow-up surveillance with physical examination and MRI scans are sufficient. For patients with positive margins, a local recurrence is not inevitable. In a series from Goy et al. only 32% of the patients with a positive margin recurred (96). Likewise, in the series from Memorial, actuarial local control at 5 years postsurgery was 74% among the 21 patients with positive margins (97). Because local recurrence is not inevitable, we do not routinely recommend radiation for patients who have had grossly complete resections for a primary desmoid tumor. The exception to this policy is for patients in whom the recurrence would be difficult or impossible to re-resect without severe functional deficit. In that situation adjuvant postoperative irradiation is sometimes recommended after the initial resection.

For patients with recurrent desmoid tumors, re-resection is generally carried out, and once there is secure wound healing, postoperative irradiation is administered. For patients with only microscopic disease, the total dose is between 55 to 60 Gy, given with a shrinking field technique. For patients with gross tumors that are unresectable the dose is 60 Gy or more. As marginal recurrences are the most common site of recurrence after irradiation, the margins are generous.

TECHNIQUE OF RADIATION THERAPY

Design of Target Volume

The most essential step in treatment planning is definition of the target volume. Superior and inferior extent of the tumor need to be carefully ascertained by review of the pertinent MR or CT scans with the diagnostic radiologist. Additional understanding of the areas at risk can be obtained by attending the operative procedure and discussing the precise site of origin with the surgeon. Because sarcomas tend to spread along the muscle or fascial planes, they tend to be confined to the anatomic compartment of origin. Thus, the radiation therapist must understand normal tissue anatomy.

Postoperative radiation fields should cover all tissues suspected of involvement by tumor plus those violated in the surgical procedure. Preoperative radiation fields may be limited to the tumor bed with a margin. Our practice has been to add 5 to 10 cm of margin to the superior and inferior extents of gross tumor. The exact margin added depends on the grade, size, and location. Margins may be more limited perpendicular to the muscle compartment, especially if the fascial planes appear intact on the MR or CT scans.

We attempt to exclude major joints, although if scar crosses a joint, we choose to treat the areas considered at risk, excluding a portion of the joint, if possible, to prevent a frozen joint in the future. Electrons may be useful in this situation, because the depth of penetration can be manipulated by choice of energy.

The optimal portal angles necessary to cover adequately the involved compartment as well as the logical location for the strip of skin that is to be spared direct irradiation may be determined by careful review of these diagnostic studies. Severe fibrosis with pain and permanent massive edema can occur with circumferential irradiation, so careful planning must include exclusion of at least a strip of skin and subcutaneous tissue (Figure 27.3). Ideally, one-third or more of the circumference of the extremity should be spared direct irradiation, but frequently, only a 2- to 3-cm strip is possible. Oblique beams frequently improve the location or amount of skin that can be spared and are well worth the extra planning involved in their setup.

Several specific sites deserve further mention. Irradiation of the hands and feet has been undertaken successfully, although extreme care is necessary to prevent poor functional results (98–101). Because the thickness of the hand or foot may be only several centimeters, sometimes immersion in a water bath or use of three-dimensional compensators is necessary to improve dose homogeneity.

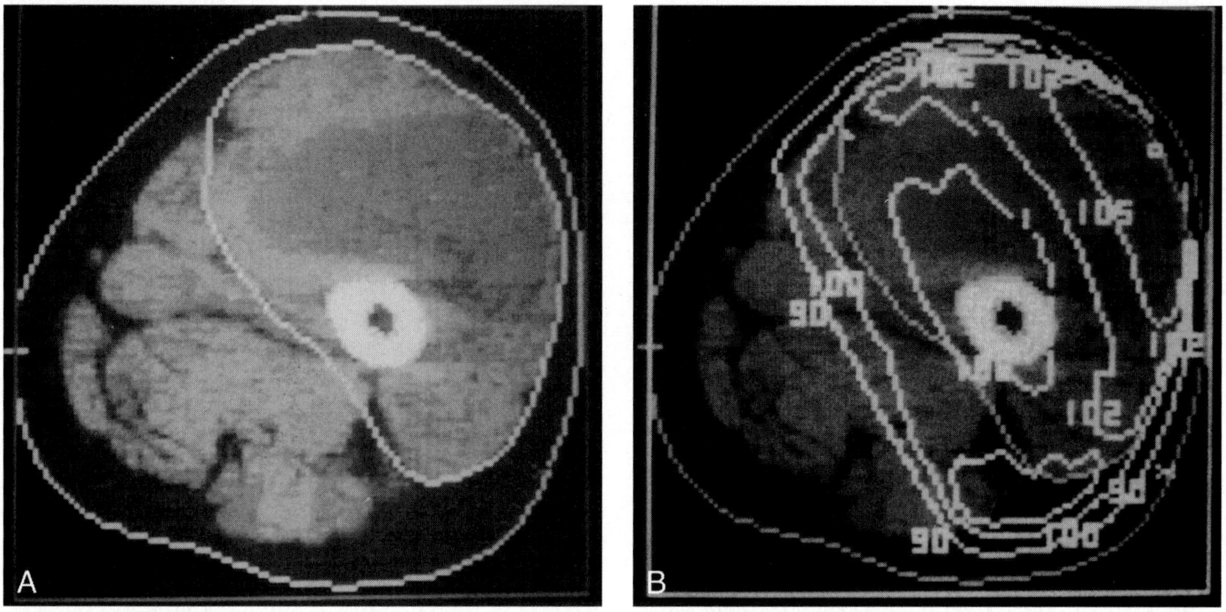

Figure 27.3. A. Delineation of target volume on treatment planning computed tomographic scan in a patient with a large liposarcoma of the thigh. Planning includes sparing a strip of skin from direct irradiation. **B.** Parallel opposed 6 MV beams at oblique angles chosen to give relatively homogeneous dose to the target.

Nail beds should be spared, and care is needed to avoid irradiating the entire sole of the foot (98).

Immobilization

To achieve local tumor control and a good functional result, a reproducible stable daily setup is necessary. A variety of casting materials have been developed that aid in daily repositioning and immobilization. We prefer to use a lightweight, low-density foam casting material (Alpha Cradle Moldmaker Inc., Smithers Medical Products, Hudson, Ohio) which can be mixed at the time of simulation and molded around the area to be immobilized (Figure 27.4). The part of the mold in the treatment field may moderately increase the skin dose in that area, and this fact needs to be considered. For instance, 3 cm of alpha cradle foam will increase the skin dose from approximately 20 to 65% using a 4-MeV beam. (102). If skin sparing is important, an aperture may be cut in the foam. As anatomy changes during treatment because of tumor shrinkage or decreasing edema, the immobilization device may fail to immobilize the extremity appropriately and a second device should be fashioned.

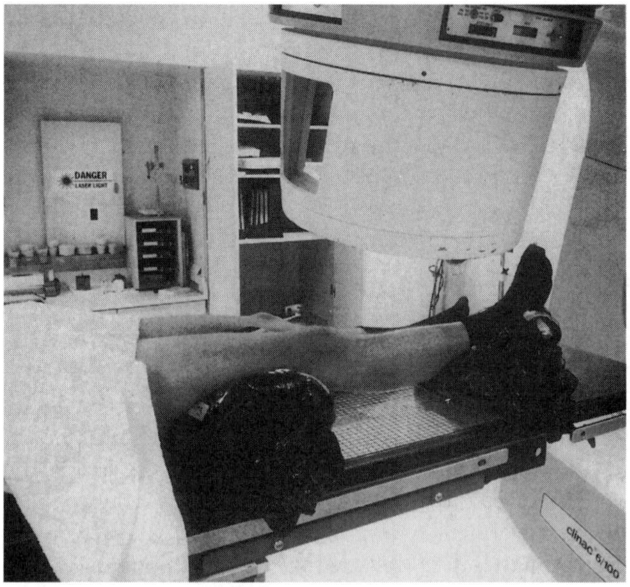

Figure 27.4. Immobilization device (alpha cradle) holds distal extremity in reproducible position for daily treatments. Mold is placed beneath knees and ankle.

Simulation

At simulation, a wire is placed on the scar and/or any palpable tumor. An orthogonal anterior and lateral pair of simulator films is obtained using the previously determined margins. If rotation improves the tumor coverage, radiographs are taken for a more quantitative assessment at the appropriate gantry angle.

With the patient in the treatment position and immobilized appropriately, a treatment planning CT or MRI scan is performed. We place a flat wooden tabletop insert over the curved CT couch and take CT "cuts" at several representative levels. The tumor and target volume can be defined on each CT section throughout the volume of concern. The physicist is able to use this information to generate isodose distribution plans at several levels of interest (Figure 27.5). Various beam weights and energies can be used until the optimal distribution of dose within the defined target is achieved. A three-dimensional planning system, if available, can also be used. In this situation the physician can draw the target volume on multiple scans, usually spaced at less than 0.5-cm intervals. Three-dimensional reconstructions of the limb, target volume, and spared strip of tissue can be visualized on the computer screen and modified quickly (103).

Compensating wedges frequently are useful in improving homogeneity of dose (Figure 27.6). Sagittal planes are helpful in determining whether, because of differences in tissue thickness along the length of the field, acrylic tissue compensation is warranted (Figure 27.7). Generally, a gradient of no more than 10% variation in dose across the target is acceptable.

Field Sizes

Extremely long fields are often necessary to cover the target volume adequately. In this situation, it usually is more satisfactory and easier to treat at extended source-to-skin distances, but field size limits remain. Rather than turning the patient over, because patient rotation may result in overlap, we prefer to treat extremely large fields with two pairs of isocentric fields matching at isocenter. The match line is placed at an area not grossly involved with tumor, and the junction line is moved frequently (every 20 to 30 Gy).

Custom Shaped Fields

Custom blocking is used to shape fields and to shield crucial structures. The tumor or tumor bed is drawn on the simulation films by using MRI and CT scan findings or any other available information; this volume is confirmed by discussion with the radiologist and surgeon. Appropriate margins are added (target volume) and custom blocks are drawn. Points to remember when designing these blocks are day-to-day setup error, as well as falloff of dose to 50% of the central axis dose at the field edge (Figure 27.5). We employ a quality control check on custom blocks to ensure proper mounting and positioning (104). Confirmation port radiographs of planned fields with custom

Vaginal cancer *(Continued)*
lymphatic involvement, 417, 420–*422*
natural history, 417–418
prognostic factors, 418
recurrence patterns, 417–418
stages, 417–418, 421t
treatment guidelines, 418–*420,* 421t
Vaginal cuff irradiation
applicators, 424–*425, 428*
Fletcher-Suit implants, 391, *393–394*
indications, 216–217
postoperative
HDR brachytherapy, 392–*394*
LDR brachytherapy, 391–395
with whole abdominal treatment, 399
Verification techniques
digitally reconstructed radiographs, *116,* 136–*137*
electronic portal imaging, 33–34t, 38, 61, 116
geometric, 38
integration importance, 46
per therapies *(see specific therapy)*
portal films (*see* Portal films)
simulation (*see* Simulation)
VIN (vulvar intraepithelial neoplasia), 404
Vinblastine, 24
Volumes
of interest per ICRU, 36, 53, 108, 110–111
irradiated (*see* Irradiated volume)
reference (*see* Reference volume)
target (*see* Target volumes)
treatment (*see* Treatment volumes)
tumor (*see* Gross tumor volume)
Vulva
anatomy, 403–*404*
neoplasia of, 404
tumors of (*see* Vulvar cancer)
Vulvar cancer
advanced, 405t, 408
chemoirradiation, 408–409, 413–414
detection and evaluation, 404
early, 405t, 408
electron beam therapy, 410–*412,* 414
patterns of spread, 405t–*406*
prognosis, 405, *407*
radiation therapy
adverse effects, 414
brachytherapy, 410–411
dose and fractionation, 412–414, *413*
portal design, *409–413*
postoperative, 407–409
preoperative, 407–409
for regional nodes only, 409, *411–412*
volume factors, 408–409
for vulva alone, *409–410*
for vulva and regional nodes, 412–*413*
recurrence factors, 405, 407, 409
staging, 405t–406
treatment options
algorithm for, *406,* 408
chemotherapy, 408–409, 413–414
radiation therapy, 407–408
surgery, 406–407
Vulvar Intraepithelial Neoplasia, 404

Whole abdominal irradiation, 398–*399*
Whole brain radiation therapy (WBRT), 224, 237–*239*
Whole lung irradiation (WLI), 533
Whole pelvis irradiation, 217, 353–*354,* 364, 391, 395, 420, *422,* 428
World Health Organization (WHO), CNS tumor classification system, 223–224t

X-rays
biologic damage from, 184, 188
linac beams, *65*
in therapy
craniospinal irradiation, 100
electron beam, *72,* 75
with intensity modulated techniques, 142–143

Treatment planning *(Continued)*
techniques, 37–41, 106–116
tumor volume definition, 108–111, *109*
2-D (2-D RTP), limitations, 45, 106, 114
dose focus (*see* Dosimetry)
goals of, 30–31
beam quality, 65, 11238
dose optimization, 38–39, 114–115
per techniques, 38
therapeutic gain ratio, 38–*39*
implementation, 61
importance, 30–31, 41
inverse method, 115, 128–*129,* 143
pencil beam method, 45
per therapies *(see specific therapy)*
per tumor *(see specific anatomical cancer or tumor)*
personnel involved in, 35–36t, 52–53
quality assurance, 46–48, *111*
steps in, 11, *35*–36t, 104–105
beam design and field shaping (*see* Beam design; Field blocks)
dose calculation, 45–46, 112–113
immobilization devices, 54–55, 106–108
relevant normal structure definition, 36–37
repositioning devices, 37–38, 54–55, 106
simulation, 37, 52–62, 108, 111–112
treatment aids evaluation, 37–38
tumor volume definition, *36,* 108–111
techniques
overview, 31–33
per therapy *(see specific therapy)*
Treatment seat, *98*
Treatment stand, *99, 512*
Treatment volumes
defined, *53,* 110
irradiated (*see* Irradiated volume)
per therapies *(see specific disease or therapy)*
standard nomenclature for, *53*
target based (*see* Target volumes)
tumor based (*see* Gross tumor volume)
Trigeminal neuralgia, 152
TRT (*see* Thoracic radiation therapy)
TRUS (*see* Ultrasound, transrectal)
Tumor control probability (TCP)
complications per, 32–*33*
curve evolution, 30–*31*
local *(see specific tumor)*
maximum (*see* Therapeutic gain factor)
per irradiation dose and cancer volume, 9t, *10*–11, 30–32t
special particles for, 45
in treatment planning, 46, 114–115
Tumor staging
per AJCC (*see* American Joint Committee on Cancer)
per cancer *(see specific anatomical cancer or tumor)*
per FIGO (*see* International Federation of Gynecology and Obstetrics)
per Jewett-Strong (*see* Jewett-Strong classification)
per Royal Marsden Hospital (*see* Royal Marsden staging system)
per TNM (*see* TNM classification)
Tumors
classification of (*see* Tumor staging; *specific cancer or tumor)*
control of (*see* Tumor control probability)
growth of
kinetics, 7–*8*
rate considerations, 11
malignant *(see specific anatomy or tumor)*
recurrence of
distant metastases incidence, 41, 43t, *44*
failure factors, 33–35
kinetics of, *8*
locoregional incidence, 41, 43t
treatment planning impact on, 41, 43t
treatment guidelines *(see specific anatomy or tumor)*
volume factors (*see* Gross tumor volume)
TUR (transurethral bladder resection), 349, 352, 356–359
TURP (transurethral resection of prostate), 440–441, 452
Two-D RTP (*see* Treatment planning, 2-D)

Ultrasounds
importance with mastectomy, 303, 305
longitudinal, for tandem placement, *370*
for prostate volume definition, 454–*455*
transrectal (TRUS), 216, 444, 453–*454,* 459–*460*
Upper respiratory tract tumors
recurrence, 8, 10
tumor control probability, 9t
Urethrograms, 444
Urinary bladder
anatomy, 349
reference points, 180, 376–*378*
tumors of (*see* Urinary bladder cancer)
Urinary bladder cancer
brachytherapy, 352
complications, 181–*182,* 210, 218
reference points, 180
chemoirradiation, 22–24, 349, 352, 354, 358t–359
clinical presentation, 350
conformal radiation therapy, 355, *357*
external beam therapy, 352–354, 356, 359
incidence, 349
muscular wall invasion, 349–352
pathology, 351
prognostic factors, 350
radiation therapy
anterior and posterior field design, *353–354*
boost field planning, *355–356*
clinical trials results, 356, 358t
complications, 359
dose factors, *353,* 354, *355–356*
fractionation, 356, 358
indications, 352
lateral fields design, 354
normal tissue tolerance importance, 355
simulation techniques, 352–354
treatment plan, 354–355
whole pelvic fields, *354*
risk factors, 349
staging systems, 350–351t
treatment results per, 356–358
survival rates, 349
transitional cell, 349, 351–352
treatment options, 349, 351–352
chemotherapy/immunotherapy, 352, 356, 358t, 359
irradiation, 352–359
morbidity, 359
surgery, 352, 356–359
workup factors, *350*–351t
Uterine tumors (*see* Endometrial cancer)

Vacuum bags, 54, *96*
Vagina
anatomy, 417
cuff treatment (*see* Vaginal cuff irradiation)
tumors of (*see* Vaginal cancer)
Vaginal cancer
brachytherapy, 421t
cuff focus (*see* Vaginal cuff irradiation)
dosing factors, 423–427t, 428, 432
double-plane, 418, *420,* 423, 428
high dose rate, 431–433
interstitial, 418–421, *419–421,* 428–431
intracavitary, 418–421, *419–421,* 423–428
low dose rate, 418, 421, 423–431
combined radiation therapies, 418, 431–432
external beam therapy
parametrial, 421t
whole pelvis, 418, 420–*422,* 421t

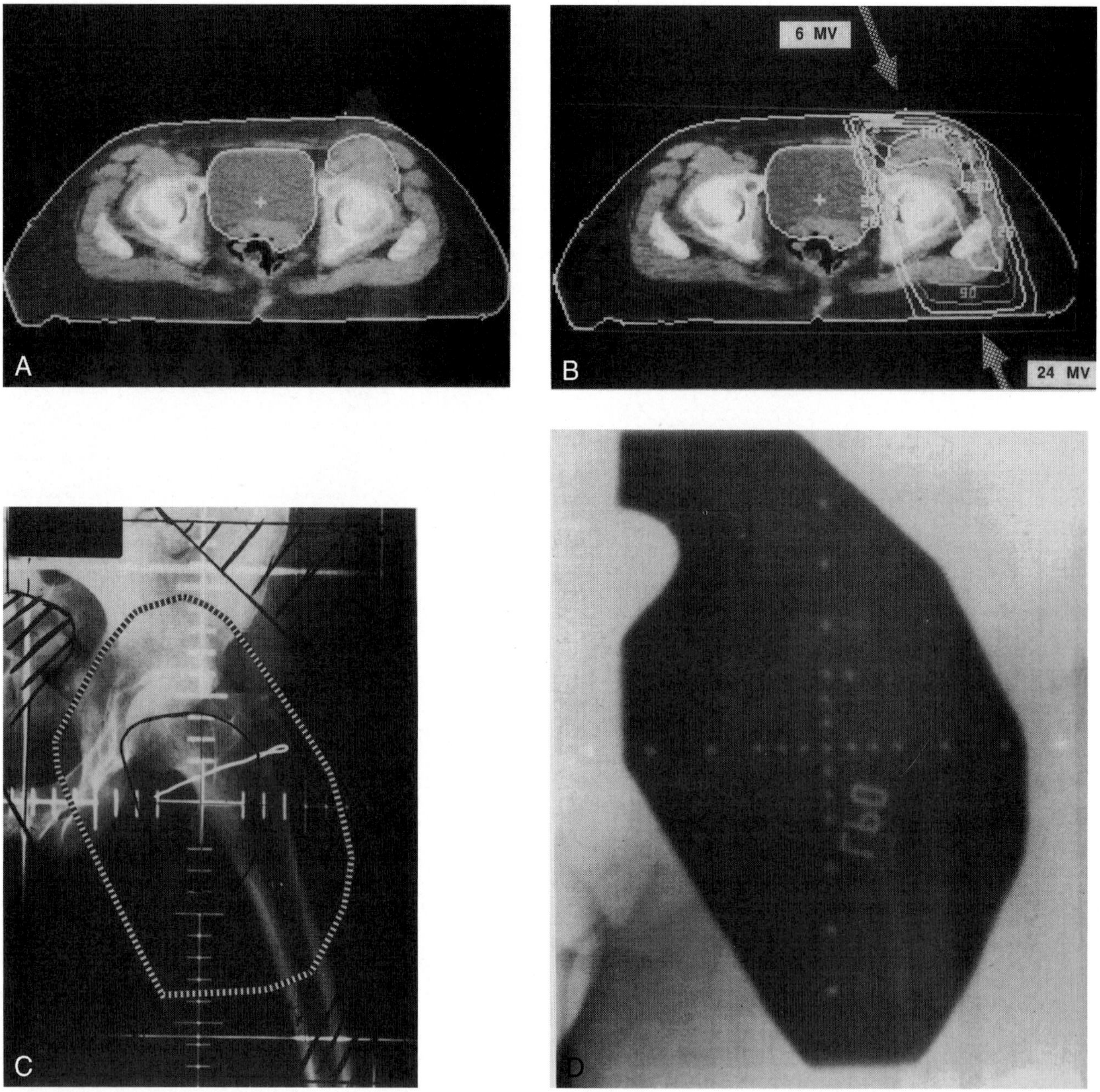

Figure 27.5. A. 50-year-old woman with an incompletely excised hemangiopericytoma of the left femoral artery area was referred for further management. Preoperative radiation therapy with re-excision was planned. Tumor is outlined on treatment planning CT scan. Note flat table top insert on CT couch and markers to delineate central axis points. **B.** Isodoses superimposed on treatment planning CT scan. Mixed 6 MV and 24 MV photon beam arrangement was used to spare tissue posteriorly. Target received 5040 cGy before surgical resection and postoperative boost dose of 1400 cGy with electrons. **C.** Simulation film with tumor (black line) and target volume (dotted line) noted. Custom blocks used to spare as much normal tissue as possible. **D.** Port film confirms correct positioning of patient, blocks, and field.

blocks and the desired gantry angles are obtained at weekly intervals. Circumferential irradiation of an extremity must be prevented with carefully placed blocks, and weekly port films demonstrate preservation of that skin strip. If possible, irradiation of the entire cross-section of an uninvolved bone is prevented to decrease the risk of future pathologic fracture, but this concern is less critical. Areas that may be exposed to repeated trauma such as the skin, Achilles tendon, elbow, and heel should not receive high doses, but it is crucial to remember that the worst complication is a recurrence, which in this situation would probably result in amputation.

Figure 27.6. **A.** Delineation of target volume after resection of synovial sarcoma of lower leg. **B.** and **C.** Isodose distribution of oblique beams without (B) and with (C) 15° compensating wedges. Note compensating wedge improves homogeneity of dose throughout target volume.

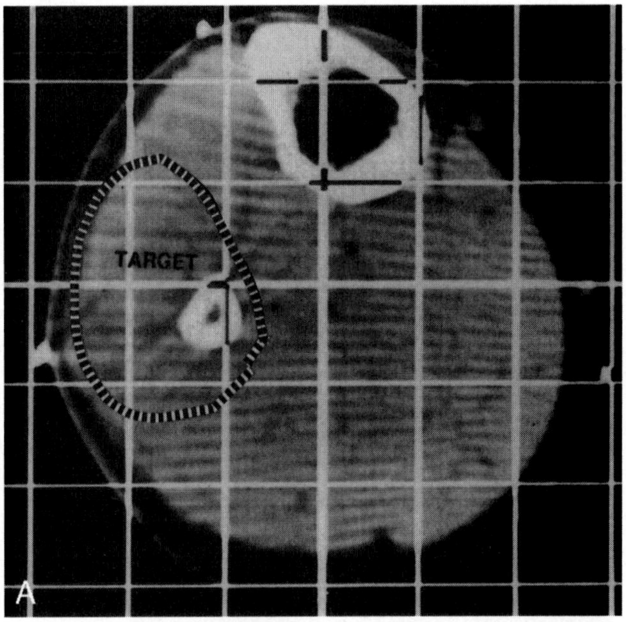

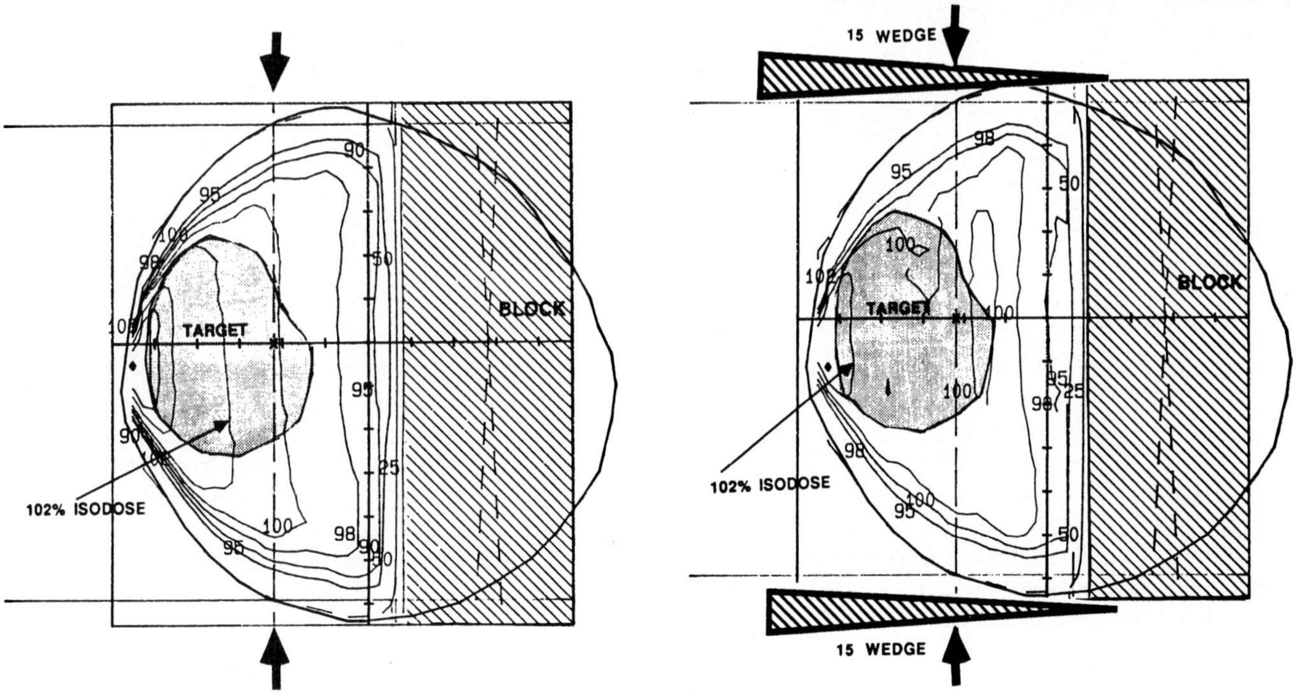

B C

Beam Energy

Because soft tissue sarcomas often involve superficial tissues, using lower energies (i.e. less than 6 MV) generally is better when possible. High energy beams may underdose superficial tissues located in the build-up region. For anteriorly placed lesions, a mixed energy pair of beams may spare posteriorly located tissues without affecting the build-up characteristics anteriorly (Figure 27.5). To assure adequate skin dosage in the area of the surgical scar in postoperatively treated patients, bolus is added to the scar daily. In most preoperatively treated patients, bolus is not used because the biopsy scar and superficial tumor usually are completely resected at the time of surgery.

TIME-DOSE FRACTIONATION

Postoperative Irradiation

Radiation given postoperatively starts 3 to 4 weeks after the surgical procedure to allow for secure wound healing.

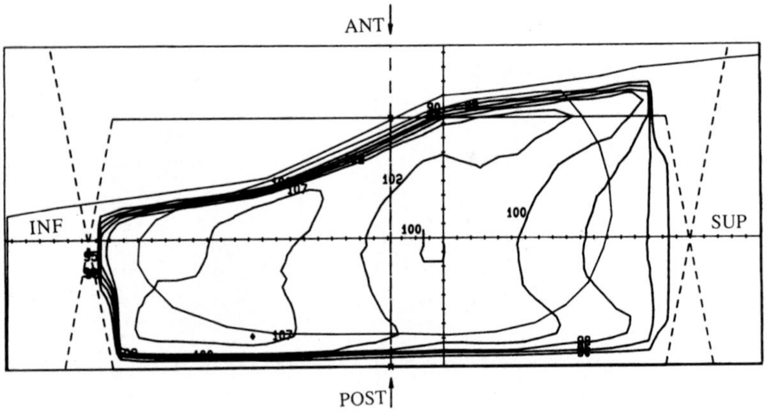

A

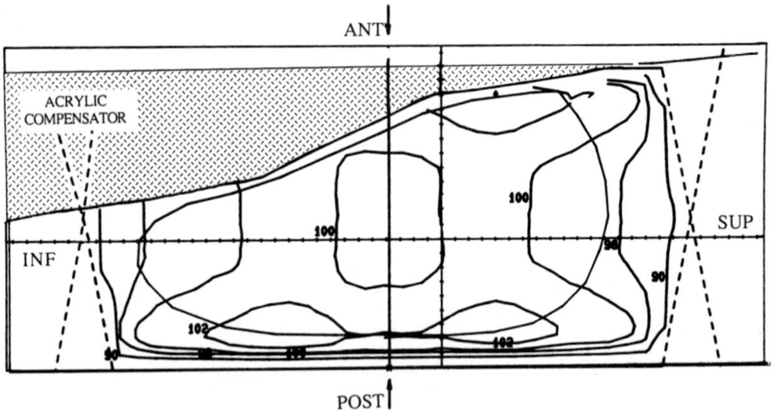

B

Figure 27.7. **A.** Dose distribution in sagittal plane of the thigh. Dose inferiorly is increased because of sloping anterior surface of the thigh. **B.** Effect of acrylic compensator in decreasing area of increased dose inferiorly.

The initial treatment volume is treated to 45 to 50 Gy in 1.8-Gy fractions, and then one or two field reductions follow, to bring the final dose to areas with close margins to 61 Gy. If microscopic residual disease is present, the final dose is 64 to 68 Gy. If gross disease remains after surgical resection, the final dose must be higher, in the range of 70 to 75 Gy. For patients who will receive adjuvant chemotherapy with doxorubicin, these doses usually are decreased empirically by about 10%.

Preoperative Irradiation and Boost

Patients treated preoperatively receive 45 to 50 Gy in 1.8-Gy fractions to the initial volume. From 2 to 4 weeks later, a repeat MR or CT scan of the involved limb is obtained, the response to radiation therapy is assessed, and the surgical procedure is planned. Surgical resection is then carried out, and at the time of the operation, the surgeon and therapeutic radiologist jointly decide if a postoperative boost is necessary based on the operative findings, and whether brachytherapy or external beam is more appropriate. The boost dose ranges from 15 to 20 Gy for a total dose of between 60 and 70 Gy. The postoperative boost is generally given unless there is a wound problem with a prolonged interval between surgery and the postoperative boost, or if there is no tumor left in the operative specimen. In that situation, the boost is omitted only if the functional result would be predicted to be better without the boost (i.e., for an axillary tumor where arm lymphedema is substantially more likely when 60 Gy are given than when only 50 Gy are delivered).

Brachytherapy Boost

Brachytherapy boosts are technically feasible when the tumor does not extend across a joint space and the tumor does not invade deep structures such that visualization of the catheters is not possible. The technique of brachytherapy usually involves placing standard nylon afterloading tubes 1 cm apart into the tumor bed with a 2- to 4-cm margin on the tumor bed (Figure 27.8). Needles are positioned transversely in relation to the extremity, with exit into the skin and subcutaneous tissue outside the tumor bed, and secured with metal buttons. If tumor invades neurovascular structures, the tubes may be placed. After the catheters are positioned, the wound is closed as usual, avoiding staples (to prevent electron scatter once the sources are loaded). Orthogonal films are taken using

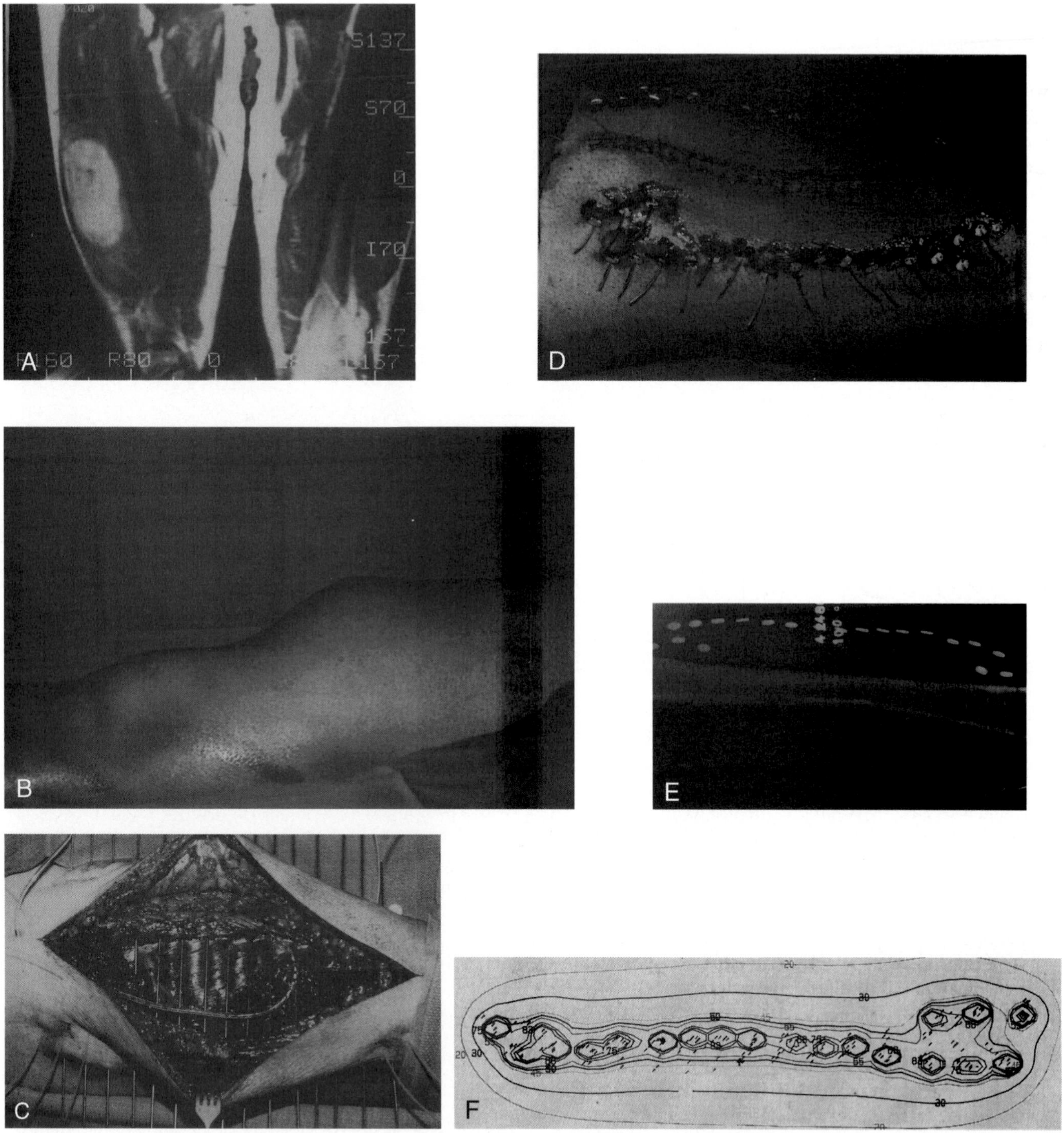

Figure 27.8. Incisional biopsy of an asymptomatic soft tissue mass in the right anterolateral midthigh of a 63-year-old man revealed malignant fibrous histiocytoma. **A.** Magnetic resonance image, coronal plane. Note 10 × 7 × 6 cm mass in deep musculature, not involving bone or major neurovascular structures. **B.** Lateral view. Prominent soft tissue mass proximal to knee. Initial marginal excision was elected. **C.** Transverse needle placement used for implantation of surgical bed (not just tumor bed). At either end, two planes were used through cut muscle bundles. Clip placement defines tumor bed; suction drainage minimized dead space. **D.** Needles were replaced with nylon afterloading tubes, secured with metal buttons. Wound closure was accomplished without metallic staples. Povidone-iodine ointment was placed at tube entry sites. Systemic antibiotics were administered. **E.** Plain film radiograph, 3 days postoperatively, loaded with dummy sources for computerized dosimetry to document 1 cm minimum skin-to-source distance. **F.** Cross-sectional implant dosimetry at center of implantation (expressed in centigrays per hour) with reference isodose of 45 cGy/hour for treatment to 2000 cGy in 44.5 hours. (Reprinted with permission from Schray MF, et al. Soft tissue sarcoma: the integration of brachytherapy, resection, and external irradiation. Cancer 1990;66:451.)

dummy sources on the first or second postoperative day, and computer planning for computerized dosimetry is performed. The iridium sources typically are 1 cm in length with a distance of 1 cm from the center of one source to the center of the next source. Four to 5 days postoperatively, iridium 192 is loaded into the needles such that the sources are at least 1 cm from the skin, and that over the ensuing 24 to 48 hours, a dose of 15 to 20 Gy is given to the tumor bed. The dose usually is calculated at a distance of 0.5 cm from the plane of the implant.

If a brachytherapy boost is not given for technical reasons, an external beam therapy boost is planned. Surgical clips placed at the time of resection are helpful in planning this boost, along with information from the pathologist and surgeon regarding the areas in which margins may be close and sites considered at greater risk for local recurrence. After secure wound healing is well underway (2 to 3 weeks postoperatively), higher risk areas receive an additional 1.4 to 2 Gy, sparing as much of the uninvolved tissues as possible. Electrons of appropriate energy frequently are used because of favorable depth dose characteristics.

PATIENT CARE DURING TREATMENT

We recommend that the patients begin physical therapy as soon after diagnosis as possible and continue physical therapy during and after treatment to maximize the functional result. Skin care includes avoidance of soaps or perfumes and use of a daily moisturizer. The wound is checked daily, with prompt attention paid to any problem. When tumors are located such that the gluteal crease or inguinal fold are in the radiation field, these areas can be taped open to prevent loss of skin sparing and resultant skin reactions.

SEQUELAE

Limb-sparing surgery frequently necessitates extensive resection of muscle and connective tissue, development of large skin flaps, and interruption of vascular and lymphatic channels. Skibber et al. reviewed the experience with limb-sparing surgery for soft tissue sarcomas at the National Cancer Institute, and reported an overall wound complication rate of 34% with serious complications necessitating rehospitalization or reoperation in 10% (105). Adjuvant radiation therapy, either pre- or postoperatively, would be expected to add to wound healing problems, but reported results suggest that with careful attention to the results outlined, the combination of extensive surgery and radiation therapy is well tolerated, and although serious wound complications occur, they are not common.

Lindberg et al. reported a 6.5% incidence of significant complications in 300 patients with extremity lesions treated with conservative surgical excision and postoperative radiation therapy (5). Complications included soft tissue necrosis, fracture, fibrosis, nerve or vascular damage, and edema. Most patients (85%) had a functional limb, and only rare patients eventually went on to amputation.

In patients irradiated preoperatively, the major complication is wound healing delay, which occurred to some extent in 46% of the patients treated by Suit et al. (52). In 20% (10 of 50), the wound problems were severe, necessitating skin grafting (8 patients) or amputation (2 patients). The complications tended to occur in older patients with massive tumors or those sited around major joints. Factors associated with the development of wound complications in these patients included age greater than 59 years, the presence of hypertension, a twice-daily radiation schedule, and a surgical specimen of greater than 205 ml (52).

A common finding in patients who have had large

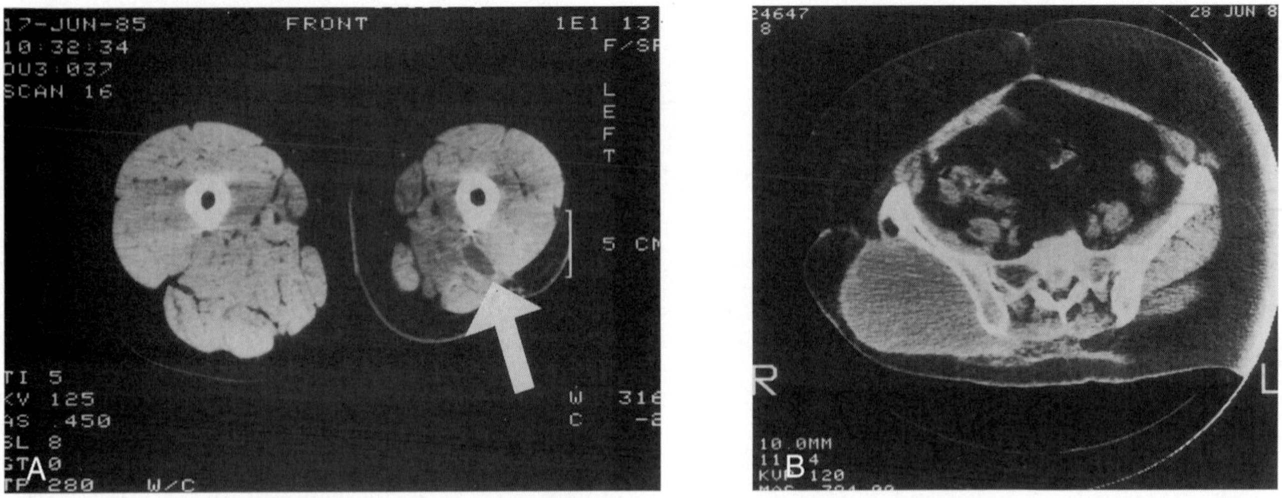

Figure 27.9. A. and **B.** Typical computed tomographic appearance of fluid-filled seromas (arrow) that may develop postoperatively and should not be confused with tumor recurrence.

tumor resection in conjunction with radiation is a fluid-filled defect at the site of the tumor resection that is lined by a fibrotic membrane and shrinks with time. The CT and MR signal in this condition are distinctive (Figure 27.9). Our most troublesome late complication is extremity edema in patients who have required composite resection of major vessels (e.g., the femoral artery and vein with a vascular bypass). Usually, with the use of elastic support stockings, the edema is controlled in 12 to 18 months.

Relatively little attention has been paid to quality of life issues. In a recent report, the authors suggest that a decrease in psychosocial functioning after conservative surgery and chemoradiotherapy may have been underestimated and deserves further study (106). In a randomized trial comparing patients who had surgery alone to those who had surgery and irradiation, there was a significantly worse limb strength, more edema, and a diminished range of motion in patients receiving radiation therapy. These deficits were often transient and had few measurable effects on activities of daily life or global quality of life (106).

SUMMARY

Soft tissue sarcomas are uncommon malignancies that have been the focus of much attention in recent years. Treatment involving a combination of methods has made function-preserving surgery a possibility without jeopardizing the chance for cure. A successful outcome is possible only when the details of diagnosis, staging, and treatment are carefully considered. Cooperation and communication between pathologist, surgeon, and radiation oncologist is critical. For the radiation oncologist, strict attention to the details of treatment is well rewarded with excellent local control and preservation of a functional limb.

References

1. American Cancer Society: Cancer facts and figures—1988. American Cancer Society, 1988.
2. Enneking WF, Spanier SS, Malawer MM. The effect of the anatomic setting on the results of surgical procedures for soft parts sarcoma of the thigh. Cancer 1981;47:1005–1022.
3. Gerner RE, Moore GE, Pickern JW. Soft tissue sarcomas. Ann Surg 1975;181:803–808.
4. Leibel S, et al. Soft tissue sarcomas of the extremities: survival and patterns of failure with conservative surgery and postoperative irradiation compared to surgery alone. Cancer 1982;50:1076–1083.
5. Lindberg R, et al. Conservative surgery and postoperative radiotherapy in 300 adults with soft-tissue sarcomas. Cancer 1981;47: 2391–2397.
6. Mills EED, Hering ER. Management of soft tissue tumors by limited surgery combined with tumor bed irradiation using brachytherapy and supplementary teletherapy. Br J Radiol 1981;54:312.
7. Suit H, et al. Preoperative, intraoperative, and postoperative radiation in the treatment of primary soft tissue sarcoma. Cancer 1985; 55:2659–2667.
8. Tepper JE. Role of radiation therapy in the treatment of sarcoma of soft tissue. Cancer Invest 1985;3:587.
9. Slater JD, McNeese MD, Peters LJ. Radiation therapy for unresectable soft tissue sarcomas. Int J Radiat Oncol Biol Phys 1986;12:1729.
10. Tepper JE, Suit HD. Radiation therapy alone for sarcoma of soft tissue. Cancer 1985;56:475–479.
11. Suit HD. Patterns of failure after treatment of sarcoma of soft tissue by radical surgery or by conservative surgery and radiation. Cancer Treat Symp 1983;2:241.
12. Abbatucci JS, et al. A systematic radio-surgical combination in the treatment of sarcoma of soft tissues in adults. Results in 106 cases at the Centre Francois Baclesse. Ann Radiol (Paris) 1989;32(2): 117–122.
13. Karakousis CP, Proimakis C, Walsh DL. Primary soft tissue sarcoma of the extremities in adults (see comments). Br J Surg 1995;82(9): 1208–1212.
14. Potter DA, et al. Patterns of recurrence in patients with high grade soft-tissue sarcomas. J Clin Oncol 1985;3:353.
15. Wilson A, Davis A, Bell R, et al. Local control of soft tissue sarcoma of the extremity: the experience of a multidisciplinary sarcoma group with definitive surgery and radiotherapy. Eur J Cancer 1994; 30A:746–751.
16. Pao W, Pilepich M. Postoperative radiotherapy in the treatment of extremity soft tissue sarcomas Int J Radiat Oncol Biol Phys 1990;19: 907–911.
17. Keus R, Bartelink H. The role of radiotherapy in the treatment of desmoid tumours. Radiother Oncol 1986;7(1):1–5.
18. Fein D, Lee W, Lanciano R, et al. Management of extremity soft tissue sarcomas with limb-sparing surgery and postoperative irradiation: do total dose, overall treatment time, and the surgery-radiotherapy interval impact on local control? Int J Radiat Oncol Biol Phys 1995;32:969–976.
19. Mundt AJ, et al. Conservative surgery and adjuvant radiation therapy in the management of adult soft tissue sarcoma of the extremities: clinical and radiobiological results. Int J Radiat Oncol Biol Phys 1995;32(4):977–985.
20. Barkley HT, et al. Treatment of soft tissue sarcomas by preoperative irradiation and conservative surgical resection. Int J Radiat Oncol Biol Phys 1988;14:693.
21. Brant TA, et al. Preoperative irradiation for soft tissue sarcomas of the trunk and extremities in adults. Int J Radiat Oncol Biol Phys 1990;19(4):899–906.
22. Harrison LB, et al. Long-term results of a prospective randomized trial of adjuvant brachytherapy in the management of completely resected soft tissue sarcomas of the extremity and superficial trunk. Int J Radiat Oncol Biol Phys 1993;27(2):259–265.
23. Schray M, et al. Soft tissue sarcoma: the integration of brachytherapy, resection, and external irradiation. Cancer 1990;66:451–456.
24. Eilber F, et al. Neoadjuvant chemotherapy and radiotherapy in the multidisciplinary management of soft tissue sarcomas of the extremity. Surg Oncol Clin of North Am 1993;2:611–620.
25. Wanebo H, et al. Preoperative regional therapy for extremity sarcoma. A tricenter update. Cancer 1995;75(9):2299–2306.
26. Rosenberg SA, et al. Prospective randomized evaluation of adjuvant chemotherapy in adults with soft tissue sarcomas of the extremities. Cancer 1983;3:424.
27. Yang JC, et al. Randomized prospective study of the benefit of adjuvant radiation therapy in the treatment of soft tissue sarcomas of the extremity. J Clin Oncol 1998;16(1):197–203.
28. Mankin HJ, Lange TA, Spanier SS. The hazards of biopsy in patients with malignant primary bone and soft-tissue tumors. J Bone Joint Surg 1982;64:1121–1127.
29. Demas BE, et al. Soft tissue sarcomas of the extremities: comparison of MR and CT in determining the extent of disease. AJR 1988;150: 615.
30. Enneking W, Jewitt E. The issue of the biopsy. J Bone Joint Surg Am 1982;64:1119–1120.
31. Simon MA. Current concepts review: biopsy of musculoskeletal tumors. J Bone Joint Surg Am 1982;64:1253–1257.
32. Thompson RC, et al. Local recurrence and survival in soft tissue sarcomas: the relation of biopsy location to local recurrence. (Submitted for publication).
33. Gaynor JJ, et al. Refinement of clinicopathologic staging for localized soft tissue sarcoma of the extremity: a study of 423 adults. J Clin Oncol 1992;10(8):1317–1329.
34. Enneking W, Spanier S, Goodman M. The surgical staging of musculoskeletal sarcoma. J Bone Joint Surg Am 1980;62A:1027–1030.

35. Leyvraz S, Costa J. Issues in the pathology of sarcomas of the soft tissue and bone. Semin Oncol 1989;16:273.
36. Markhede G, Angervall L, Stener B. A multivariant analysis of the prognosis after surgical treatment of malignant soft tissue sarcoma tissue tumors of the extremities. Cancer 1987;60:1703.
37. Potter D, et al. High grade soft tissue sarcomas of the extremities. Cancer 1986;58:190–205.
38. Fleming ID, Cooper JS, Henson DE, eds. Soft tissue sarcoma. In: AJCC Cancer Staging Manual. Philadelphia: Lippincott-Raven, 1998: 144–156.
39. Bell RS, et al. The surgical margin in soft tissue sarcoma. J Bone Joint Surg Am 1989;711:3.
40. Collin C, et al. Localized extremity soft tissue sarcoma: an analysis of factors affecting survival. J Clin Oncol 1987;5:601–612.
41. Rooser B, et al. Prognostication in soft tissue sarcoma. Cancer 1988; 61:817–823.
42. Thompson R, et al. Soft tissue sarcomas of the extremity: its prognosis related to local environment? Cancer 1984;54:1726–1730.
43. Torosian MH, et al. Soft-tissue sarcoma: initial characteristics and prognostic factors in patients with and without metastatic disease. Semin Oncol 1988;4:13.
44. Alvegard T, et al. Cellular DNA content and prognosis of high-grade soft tissue sarcoma: the Scandinavian sarcoma group experience. J Clin Oncol 1990;8:538–547.
45. Huth JF, Mirra JJ, Eilber FR. Assessment of in vivo response to preoperative chemotherapy and radiation therapy as a predictor of survival in patients with soft-tissue sarcoma. Am J Clin Oncol 1985;8: 397.
46. Ueda T, et al. Prognostic significance of Ki-67 reactivity in soft tissue sarcomas. Cancer 1989;63:1607–1611.
47. Ariel IM. Incidence of metastasis to lymph nodes from soft tissue sarcomas. Semin Surg Oncol 1988;4:27.
48. Rydholm A. Prognostic factors in soft tissue sarcoma. (Review) (36 refs). Acta Orthopaedica Scandinavica. Supplementum 1997; 273(148):148–155.
49. Collins SE, Paine CH, Ellis F. Treatment of connective tissue sarcomas by local excision followed by radioactive implant. Clin Radiol 1976;27:39.
50. Shiu MH, et al. Surgical treatment of 297 soft tissue sarcomas of the lower extremities. Ann Surg 1975;182:597.
51. Suit H, et al. Preoperative radiation therapy for sarcoma of soft tissue. Cancer 1981;47:2269–2274.
52. Suit HD, et al. Limited surgery and external irradiation in soft tissue sarcomas. In: Ryan JR, Baker LO, eds. Recent concepts in sarcoma treatment. Boston: Kluwer Academic Press, 1988.
53. Tepper J, Rosenberg SA, Glatstein E. Radiation therapy technique in soft tissue sarcomas of the extremity—policies of treatment at the National Cancer Institute. Int J Radiat Oncol Biol Phys 1982;8: 263.
54. Trivette GA, Grayson J, Glatstein EJ. The role of radiation therapy in the treatment of soft tissue tumors. In: Pinedo HM, Verweig J, eds. Clinical management of soft tissue sarcomas. Boston: Martinus Nijhoff, 1986.
55. Weisenberger TH, et al. Multidisciplinary "limb-salvage" treatment of soft tissue and skeletal sarcomas. Int J Radiat Oncol Biol Phys 1981;7:1495.
56. Willett CG, Suit HD. Limited surgery and external beam irradiation in soft tissue sarcoma. Adv Oncol 1989;5:26.
57. Wood WC, et al. Radiation and conservative surgery in the treatment of soft tissue sarcoma. Am J Surg 1984;147:537.
58. Suit HD, Russell WO, Martin RG. Sarcoma of soft tissue: clinical and histopathologic parameters and response to treatment. Cancer 1975; 35:1478.
59. Willett C, et al. The histologic response of soft tissue sarcoma to radiation therapy. Cancer 1987;60:1500–1504.
60. Bujko K, et al. Wound healing after preoperative radiation for sarcoma of surgery, gynecology and obstetrics (Chicago). Ann Surg 1992;216(5):591–595.
61. Cheng EY, et al. Soft tissue sarcomas: preoperative versus postoperative radiotherapy. J Surg Oncol 1996;61(2):90–99.
62. Eilber F, et al. Preoperative therapy for soft tissue sarcoma. (Review) (22 refs). Hematology Oncology Clinics of North America 1995;9(4): 817–823.
63. Suit H, Spiro I. Preoperative radiation therapy for patients with sarcoma of the soft tissues. Cancer Treat Res 1993;67:99–105.
64. Mason M, et al. Preoperative radiotherapy for initially inoperable extremity soft tissue sarcomas. Clin Oncol (R Coll Radiol) 1992;4(1): 36–43.
65. Herbert SH, et al. Severe coronary artery disease after radiation therapy of the chest and mediastinum: clinical presentation and treatment. Br Heart J 1993;69(6):496–500.
66. Bell RS, et al. Wound healing complications in soft tissue sarcoma management: comparison of three treatment protocols. J Surg Oncol 1991;46(3):190–197.
67. Giuliano AE, Eilber FR. The rationale for planned reoperation after unplanned total excision of soft tissue sarcomas. J Clin Oncol 1985; 3:1344–1348.
68. Arbeit JM, Hilaris BS, Brennan MF. Wound complications in the multimodality treatment of extremity and superficial truncal sarcomas. J Clin Oncol 1987;5:480–488.
69. Ormsby MV, et al. Wound complications of adjuvant radiation therapy in patients with soft-tissue sarcomas. Ann Surg 1989;210(1): 93–99.
70. Gunderson LL, et al. External beam and intraoperative electron irradiation for locally advanced soft tissue sarcomas. Arch Surg 1993; 128(4):402–410.
71. Antman K, Suit H, Amato D, et al. Preliminary results of a randomized trial of adjuvant doxorubicin for sarcomas: lack of apparent difference between groups. J Clin Oncol 1984;2:6.
72. Edmonson J, et al. Randomized study of systemic chemotherapy following complete excision of nonosseous sarcomas. J Clin Oncol 1984;2:1390–1396.
73. Eilber FR, et al. A randomized prospective trial using postoperative adjuvant chemotherapy (adriamycin) in high grade extremity soft tissue sarcoma. Am J Clin Oncol 1988;11:39.
74. Lerner HJ, et al. Eastern Cooperative Oncology Group: a comparison of adjuvant doxorubicin and observation for patients with localized soft tissue sarcoma. J Clin Oncol 1987;5:613.
75. Bramwell V, Rouesse J, Steward W, et al. Adjuvant CYVADIC chemotherapy for adult soft tissue sarcoma-reduced local recurrence but no improvement in survival: a study of the European Organization for Research and Treatment of Cancer Soft Tissue and Bone Sarcoma Group. J Clin Oncol 1994;12:1137–1149.
76. Benjamin R, Terjanian T, Fenoglio C, et al. The importance of combination chemotherapy for adjuvant treatment of high-risk patients with soft-tissue sarcomas of the extremities. In: Salmon S, ed. Adjuvant therapy of cancer. Orlando: Grune and Stratton, 1987;735–744.
77. Gherlinzoni F, Bacci G, Picci P, et al. A randomized trial for treatment of high grade soft tissue sarcoma of the extremities: preliminary results. J Clin Oncol 1986;4:552–558.
78. Picci P, Bacci G, Gherlinzoni F, et al. Results of randomized trial for the treatment of localized soft tissue tumors (STS) of the extremities in adult patients. In: Ryan J, Baker L, eds. Recent concepts in sarcoma treatment. Dordrecht: Kluwer Academic Press, 1988; 144–148.
79. Tierney JF, et al. Adjuvant chemotherapy for soft-tissue sarcoma: review and meta-analysis of the published results of randomised clinical trials. Brit J Cancer 1995;72(2):469–475.
80. Laramore GE, et al. Fast neutron radiotherapy for sarcomas of soft tissue, bone, and cartilage. Am J Clin Oncol 1989;12:4.
81. Pikering DG, et al. Fast neutron therapy for soft tissue sarcoma. Int J Radiat Oncol Biol Phys 1987;13:1489.
82. Salinas R, et al. Experience with fast neutron therapy for locally advanced sarcomas. Int J Radiat Oncol Biol Phys 1980;6:267.
83. Catterall M. Fast neutrons in the treatment of Cancer. London: Academic Press, 1979;278–294.
84. Egawa S. Characteristics of the response of soft tissue sarcoma to hyperthermia: the correlation between temperature distribution, radiological examination and histology. Int J Hyperthermia 1989;5:1.
85. Emami B, Perez CA. Combination of surgery, irradiation, and hyperthermia in treatment of recurrences of malignant tumors. Int J Radiat Oncol Biol Phys 1987;13:611.
86. Gerad H, et al. Doxorubicin, cyclophosphamide, and whole body hyperthermia for treatment of advanced soft tissue sarcoma. Cancer 1984;53:2585.
87. Storm FK, et al. Sarcoma: etiology and advances in therapy with immunotherapy, limb salvage surgery, and hyperthermia. Semin Oncol 1981;8:229.
88. Sunao E, et al. Characteristics of the response of soft tissue sarcoma to hyperthermia: the correlation between temperature distribution,

radiological examination, and histology. Int J Hyperthermia 1989; 5:23.
89. Ashby MA, Harmer CL. Hypofractionated radiotherapy for sarcomas. Int J Radiat Oncol Biol Phys 1986;12:13.
90. Bryant M, et al. Soft tissue sarcomas of the extremities: morbidity of combined radiation and limb salvage with special emphasis on twice a day fractionation (abstract). Int J Radiat Oncol Biol Phys 1985;11(Suppl. 1):87.
91. Bramwell VH. Interaarterial chemotherapy of soft-tissue sarcomas. Semin Surg Oncol 1988;4:66.
92. Eilber F, et al. Limb salvage for skeletal and soft tissue sarcomas: multidisciplinary preoperative therapy. Cancer 1984;53:2579–2584.
93. Eilber FR, et al. Neoadjuvant chemotherapy, radiation and limited surgery for high grade soft tissue sarcoma of the extremity. In: Ryan JR, Baker LO, eds. Recent concepts in sarcoma treatments. Boston: Kluwer Academic Press, 1988.
94. Huth JF, Eilber FR. Patterns of metastatic spread following resection of extremity soft-tissue sarcomas and strategies for treatment. Semin Surg Oncol 1988;4:20.
95. Posner MC, Shiu MH. The desmoid tumor: not a benign disease. Am J Surg 1986;151:230–237.
96. Goy BW, et al. The role of adjuvant radiotherapy in the treatment of resectable desmoid tumors. Int J Radiat Oncol Biol Phys 1997; 39(3):659–665.
97. Suit HD. Radiation dose and response of desmoid tumors. Int J Radiat Oncol Biol Phys 1990;19(1):225–227.
98. Kinsella TJ, et al. Extremity preservation by combined modality therapy in sarcomas of the hand and foot: an analysis of local control, disease-free survival and functional result. Int J Radiat Oncol Biol Phys 1983;9:1115.
99. Okunieff P, et al. Extremity preservation by combined modality treatment of sarcomas of the hand and wrist. Int J Radiat Oncol Biol Phys 1986;12:1923.
100. Owens JC, et al. Soft tissue sarcomas of the hand and foot. Cancer 1985;55:2010.
101. Shiu M, et al. Limb preservation and tumor control in the treatment of popliteal and antecubital soft tissue sarcomas. Cancer 1986;57: 1632–1639.
102. Mondalek PM, Orton CG. Transmission and build-up characteristics of polyurethane-foam immobilization devices. Treatment Planning 1982;7:5.
103. Robinson M, et al. High dose hyperfractionated radiotherapy in the treatment of extremity soft tissue sarcomas. Radiother Oncol 1991; 22(2):118–126.
104. Johnson JM, Gerbi BJ. Quality control of custom block making in radiation therapy. Med Dosim 1989;14:199.
105. Skibber JM, et al. Limb-sparing surgery for soft tissue sarcomas: wound-related morbidity in patients undergoing wide local excision. Surgery 1987;102:447.
106. Chang AE, et al. Functional and psychosocial effects of multimodality limb-sparing therapy in patients with soft tissue sarcomas. J Clin Oncol 1989;7:1217.

Chapter 28

Total Body Irradiation in Conditioning Regimens for Bone Marrow Transplantation

Kathryn E. Dusenbery and Bruce J. Gerbi

Since the first successful bone marrow transplantation was performed at the University of Minnesota in 1960 (1), bone marrow transplantation (BMT) has gained prominence as a therapy for a variety of diseases as outlined in Table 28.1. The majority of bone marrow transplants are done in an effort to eradicate malignant disease, but a growing number of patients with autoimmune (2) or genetic disorders are being offered transplantation (3). The rationale for BMT differs depending on the disease treated and the source of bone marrow cells. In both autologous and allogeneic BMT for malignant diseases, the rationale for BMT is to allow chemotherapeutic dose escalation. The BMT "rescues" the patient from what otherwise would be a lethal dose of chemotherapy. In an allogeneic BMT a healthy donor marrow regenerates in its place and the infused donor lymphocytes have a proven antitumor effect (graft versus leukemic effect). Donor lymphocytes can also serve to supply absent enzyme for patients with inborn errors of metabolism (4). In autologous BMT, the infused marrow may be contaminated with malignant cells. Various methods have been used to purge the marrow of residual malignant cells (5,6). As there is no antitumor (graft versus leukemia) effect, various cytokines are being tried in an effort to mimic the graft versus leukemia effect and improve the efficiency of autologous transplantation (7,8). In the future, the autologous cells may be manipulated with genes that confer relative chemotherapeutic resistance, thus allowing for additional post transplantation chemotherapy with little damage to the new bone marrow.

The development of HLA (human lymphocyte antigen) and MLC (mixed lymphocyte culture) assays allowed physicians to determine if potential marrow donors were "histocompatible" (i.e., matched by HLA antigens and nonreactive to MLC cultures) and therefore less likely to develop graft-versus host disease (GVHD) (9). Initially, transplants were only performed between HLA matched related donors, but with the advent of effective therapies directed at decreasing the probability and severity of GVHD, matched unrelated donor transplants have become more common. The National Marrow Donor Program (NMDP) types potential bone marrow donors. More than 4,000 marrow transplants have been performed using unrelated donors provided by the NMDP. With more than 1.9 million donors listed in the registry, over 70% of patients now find an HLA-A, -B, -DR phenotypic match at the initial search (10).

In recent years, in addition to related and unrelated bone marrow donor sources, additional sources of pluripotential stem cells have been investigated including the use of umbilical cord blood, a rich source of stem cells (10–12). A bank of HLA typed umbilical cord blood harvests has also been established (11,12). Another source of pluripotential stem cells are circulating blood stem cells. These cells can be harvested through leukopheresis, frozen for later use, then thawed and reinfused. In addition to sparing the donor the discomfort of a bone marrow harvest, these peripheral stem cell harvests usually result in a more prompt engraftment than occurs with bone marrow infusions (11–16), resulting in a shorter period of pancytopenia and thus less risk of infection.

CONDITIONING REGIMEN

Presumed desired endpoints of pretransplantation conditioning regimen are to eradicate the recipient's native bone marrow, immune suppress the recipient sufficiently to avoid rejection of the donor transplant, and to do this with minimal toxicity to other tissues. In some situations,

Table 28.1. Diseases Treated by Bone Marrow Transplantation

Leukemia	**Congenital/immunodeficiency**
ALL	SCIDS
AML	**Autoimmune diseases**
CML	Rheumatoid Arthritis
CLL	SLE
Myelodysplasia	**Inborn errors of metabolism**
Lymphoma	Hunter's syndrome
NHL	Adrenoleukodystrophy
Hodgkin's disease	Metachromatic leukodystrophy
Multiple myeloma	Globoid cell leukodystrophy
Aplastic anemia	Osteoporosis
Fanconi disease	Mucopolysaccharidoses
Paroxysmal nocturnal hemoglobinuria	**AIDS**
Idiopathic	

Table 28.2. Diseases in Which TBI is Part of the Conditioning Regimen For BMT at the University of Minnesota

Allogeneic
- Acute lymphoblastic leukemia in second or subsequent CR (17)
- Acute lymphoblastic leukemia high risk in first CR
- Chronic myelogenous leukemia (18)
- Acute myeloid leukemia and myelodysplastic syndrome (adults, children beyond first CR) (19)
- Multiple myeloma
- Inborn errors of metabolism (3)
- Unrelated donor marrow transplantation, (20–24)
- T-cell depleted marrow transplant

Autologous
- Acute myeloid leukemia—no other donor available (25,26)
- Acute lymphoblastic leukemia—no other donor available (24)
- Non-Hodgkin's lymphoma (27)
- Neuroblastoma (certain protocols) (28)
- Chronic myelogenous leukemia (29)

CR, complete remission.

these three goals are attainable with a chemotherapy only conditioning regimen; however, multiple variables need to be considered including the age of the patient, the underlying disease, the source of the donor marrow, and whether the donor marrow is manipulated (i.e., T depleted). At the University of Minnesota, total body irradiation (TBI) is generally part of the conditioning regimens for the situations outlined in Table 28.2. These situations include unrelated marrow or cord blood donor transplants, certain underlying malignancies that are considered radiosensitive (acute lymphocytic leukemia [ALL], multiple myeloma), marrow sources that have been T-cell depleted, and for patients where a TBI conditioning regimen has been shown to be superior to a chemotherapy conditioning regimen (acute myeloid leukemia [AML] in second remission) (25,30).

There are theoretical advantages and disadvantages of a TBI-containing preparative regimen. Most often patients undergoing BMT have been exposed to multiple chemotherapeutic regimens; therefore, potential BMT recipients may be relatively chemotherapy "resistant." As most patients undergoing BMT have not been irradiated previously, their malignant cells may be more radiation sensitive than chemotherapy sensitive. Additionally, there are known sanctuary sites where chemotherapy does not penetrate well, such as the central nervous system (CNS) or testicles. There are no sanctuary sites for irradiation and in certain situations, such as relapsed ALL, a TBI-containing regimen may be especially beneficial. Lastly, chemotherapy, usually given intravenously (busulfan is given orally), needs to be metabolized and eliminated from the body. It is known that chemotherapy pharmacokinetics differ among patients and the exposure to the beneficial effects of certain chemotherapeutic agents may vary (31). As it requires the vasculature system to travel through the body, some areas of the body may be exposed to higher or lower concentrations of drug. TBI requires no metabolism or clearance and all areas of the body receive the same dose of irradiation. The theoretical disadvantages of using a TBI regimen are the potential late side effects, such as sterility, cataracts, and growth retardation, as well as the potential neurologic toxicity that may occur with irradiation.

FRACTIONATION AND DOSE RATE

Initial trials with TBI use a single fraction of up to 10 Gy (32). Subsequently, it was suggested that the therapeutic ratio (i.e., increased leukemic cell kill and decreased toxicity of late responding tissues, such as lung, heart, spinal cord, kidney, and CNS) of TBI might be improved by either going to a very low dose rate (not practical since treatment times of up to 24 hours would be required) or using a fractionated schema. This was based on radiobiological data suggesting that leukemic cells (and their normal counterparts, the hematopoietic stem cells) were relatively radiosensitive, with a narrow "shoulder" on the survival curve and with little capacity of sublethal radiation damage repair capacity (33,34). On the other hand, late responding tissues are better able to repair sublethal damage and have a relatively "broad shoulder" on the dose response curve. Formulations based on dose survival models have been proposed to evaluate the biologic equivalence of various doses and fractionation schedules. Assumptions are based on the linear-quadratic model that takes into account the α and β (nonreparable and reparable) components of cell kill. The values for the α and β components of cell kill can be derived experimentally, but are not available for many human tissues. Extrapolating from animal data and cell cultures, it has been found that the ratio of α/β is a useful indicator of the effect of fractionation on cell damage. Tissues with a high α/β include the gastrointestinal tract, skin, bone marrow cells ("early" responding); whereas tissues with a low α/β include tissues

such as spinal cord, kidney, brain, and lung ("late" responding).

Although not completely applicable in the setting of TBI schemes, the biologic effective dose (BED) of one TBI regimen can be compared to another regimen if several estimates are taken into consideration. The units are arbitrary but allow one to compare the theoretic effects of different TBI regimens on different tissues.

$$\text{Biologic effective dose (BED)} = n\,d\,\{1 + d/\alpha/\beta)\}$$

where n = number of fractions
d = dose per fraction
α/β = estimate (10 for early tissues, 3 for late tissues)

In engineering an optimal TBI regimen, the goal is to cause minimal damage to late responding tissues, while having a high probability of damaging the early responding bone marrow cells (and malignant cells). Regimens can be evaluated for their potential effect on late responding tissues or on early responding tissues:

If evaluating for *late* effects of different TBI regimens:

assume an α/β of 3	BED
750 cGy in 1 fraction	26
750 in 3 fractions	14
1200 cGy in 6 fractions	19
13.20 cGy in 8 fractions	20
1395 cGy in 12 fractions	21

One can see that fractionation would be expected to *spare* late effects. One could go to a higher total dose, without increasing the probability of late effects.

If considering the *early* effects of different TBI regimens:

assume an α/β of 10	BED
750 in 1 fraction	13
750 in 3 fractions	9
1200 cGy in 6 fractions	14
1320 cGy in 8 fractions	15
1395 cGy in 12 fractions	16

It becomes apparent that fractionation spares *early* effects. Since bone marrow ablation is desired, the total dose must be increased (greater than or equal to 1200 cGy) to get the same myeloablative effect as a single fraction of 750 cGy.

These theoretical equations are supported by data from reports of bone marrow transplantation regimens (33–36). For example, the risk of a cataract is substantially higher when the TBI is given with a single fraction of TBI (Table 28.3).

Bone marrow graft failure or graft rejection is an uncommon, but life-threatening complication of BMT. It is more common in certain situations, such as with partially mismatched recipients, or when donor marrows are depleted of T cell subpopulations. Certain patients, such as those who have not had previous chemotherapy, may also be at risk. A possible mechanism for graft rejection is that the conditioning regimen incompletely ablates the host bone marrow leaving residual host natural killer cells or possibly other cells that are able to mediate graft rejection. The influence of total body radiation doses and schedules (Table 28.4) suggests that in the setting of T-depletion, fractionated TBI leads to a much higher rate of graft failures than single dose TBI when similar total doses are used. If, however, the total doses are escalated to greater than 13 Gy, the risk of nonengraftment falls (Table 28.5).

Table 28.3. Incidence of Cataracts With Single Fraction Total Body Irradiation Compared to Fractionated Total Body Irradiation

Author (ref)	Single Fraction (%)	Multiple Fraction (%)	*P* Value
Deeg (37)	75	15	
Ozsahin (38)	39	13	0.02

Although no randomized clinical trials exist, the majority of retrospective reviews looking at the rate of interstitial pneumonitis after single fraction TBI compared to multiple fraction TBI strongly suggest an advantage for a fractionated TBI schedule (Table 28.6). One must keep in mind the fact that these trials are nonrandomized and usually compare recently transplanted patients on fractionated schemas with former single fraction patients. Numerous variables are potentially implicated in the development of interstitial pneumonitis (51) including other TBI variables such as dose rate (36), use of lung shielding, and timing of the TBI (before or after chemotherapy).

SEQUENCE

Total body irradiation can either precede or follow the chemotherapy portion of the conditioning regimen. An advantage to delivering the TBI first is that, with the appropriate use of antiemetics, it can be given as an outpatient treatment and thus reduce inpatient costs. Following completion of TBI, patients are then hospitalized for the chemotherapy portion of the conditioning regimen. Clinical data are lacking, however, on whether TBI is less toxic or more effective when given before chemotherapy, although it is theoretically possible that the variety of cytokines released during chemotherapy may influence the incidence of pneumonitis (52).

NORMAL TISSUE SHIELDING

Shielding of normal tissues must be carefully considered in TBI because shielding may potentially reduce the dose to the target volume (bone marrow cells, leukemic

Table 28.4. Graft Failure for Single Fraction TBI Compared to Multiple Fraction TBI in T-Cell Depleted Bone Marrow Transplantation

Author (ref)	Single Fraction	Graft Failure (%)	Multiple Fractions	Graft Failure (%)
Patterson (39)	Single fraction	7% (3/41)	10–12 Gy in multiple fractions	60% (9/15)
Guyotat (40)	10 Gy in single fraction	0% (0/9)	12 Gy in	47% (7/15) 6 fractions

Table 28.5. Comparison of Incidence of Graft Failure Using T-Cell Depleted Bone Marrow as a Function of Total Dose of Fractionated TBI

Author (ref)	Total Dose (Gy)	# FX	Graft Failure (%)	Total Dose (Gy)	# FX	Graft Failure (%)
Martin (41)	12	6	63	15.75	??	11
Champlin (13)	11.25	5	25	13.5	5	11
Burnett (42)	12	6	63	14	7	4
Iriondo (43)	11	3	50	13	3	0

FX, fraction.

Table 28.6. Incidence of Interstitial Pneumonitis Using Single Fraction TBI versus Fractionated TBI

Author (Institution) (ref)	Single Fraction (%)	Multiple Fraction (%)	*P* Value
Pino y Torres (Hopkins) (44)	70	37	0.005
Meyers (Seattle) (45)	13	5	<.001
Shank (MSK) (46)	50	18	
Bluem (47)	28	10	
Unoue (Japan)	65	42	0.0004
Valls (33)	35	25	ns
Cosset (Villejuif) (48)	45	13	0.02
Weiner (36)			ns
Fyles (35)			ns
Kim (Minnesota) (19)	14	10	ns
Socie (France) (49)	33	17	0.02
Vitale (Genova) (50)	58	5	0.002

cells, and circulating stem cells). Despite this concern, there are situations in which partial shielding of critical tissues, including the lungs, kidneys, eyes (lens) and brain, is considered.

Lung Shielding

Because pneumonitis is a leading cause of death after BMT (36,51,53), with total dose of TBI implicated as a potential contributing cause, partial blocking of the lung has been advocated. The dose received by the lungs is influenced by both the irradiation geometry as well as lung density. At the University of Minnesota, when delivering TBI with right and left lateral fields, the arms are placed at the sides; the thickness of the arms is considered in determining if additional compensation is needed to reduce the lung dose to within 10% of the dose received at the prescription point (level of the umbilicus at midplane). Often no additional compensation is needed to achieve this goal, but if needed, tissue compensators are placed to reduce the lung dose to within 10% of the prescription dose.

Using a similar right and left lateral technique, in addition to using the arms to decrease lung dose, some institutions use partial blocks to reduce the lung dose further, usually to an arbitrary amount (for instance 1000 cGy).

For anteroposterior-posteroanterior (AP/PA) fields partial attenuation blocks (80 to 90% transmission) or thicker blocks (usually one half-value layer [HVL]) can be placed in front of the beam to decrease the lung dose to the desired amount. With 1 HVL blocks, the underlying ribs receive approximately half of the prescription dose and electron beams of the appropriate energy can be used to "boost" the underlying ribs. A CT (computed tomography) scan through the lung can be used to determine the appropriate electron energy. This technique was initially reported at Memorial Sloan Kettering Cancer Center, and is used at the University of Minnesota. Some institutions, in an effort to decrease the risk of pneumonitis, omit the electron beam chest wall boost. No increased risk of leukemia relapse has been noted, but a prospective trial is lacking.

Kidney Shielding

The risk of renal injury after BMT is dependent on multiple factors (54–60), including previous chemotherapy, use of nephrotoxic antibiotics, and therapies directed at

the prevention and treatment of GVHD. In a recent review of the incidence of acute renal failure in patients treated at the University of Minnesota BMT program, up to 30% of patients undergoing BMT in 1993 had acute renal failure, defined as a doubling of creatinine over the baseline creatinine. Of these patients, 10% required dialysis.

Late-onset renal failure occurs in up to 20% of survivors of BMT. On the beneficial effect of partial kidney blocking in the setting of T-depleted BMT, Lawton found that the incidence of chronic renal failure was reduced from 26% to 6% when posterior one HVL renal blocks were placed, reducing the estimated kidney dose from 14 to 12 Gy (given at 200 cGy twice a day) (56). In another series of 79 patients transplanted with TBI-containing regimens, Miralbell et al. reported that the 18-month probability of renal dysfunction-free survival decreased from 95% to 74%, to 55% for the patients conditioned with 10, 12, and 13.5 Gy, respectively (61). The other factor that predicted for renal dysfunction was the risk of developing GVHD. Renal dysfunction-free survivals were 93% for patients at lower risk of GVHD and 52% for patients with a high GVHD risk (e.g., unrelated allogeneic BMT, absence of T-cell depletion).

Head Shielding

At the University of Minnesota, we are interested in treating certain inborn errors of metabolism with BMT, such as Hurlers Syndrome, adrenoleukodystrophy, and metachromatic leukodystrophy. Donor lymphocytes have been shown to provide sufficient enzymatic activity to partially reverse the disease process or prevent disease progression (62). For many of these diseases, neurologic deterioration is a hallmark symptom with affected patients showing relentless neurologic decline and an early death. Most patients lack an unaffected HLA matched related donor, therefore matched unrelated donor transplants (MUD) are usually required. Initial experience with MUD transplantation was complicated by severe GVHD. T-cell depleted MUD transplants substantially reduced the incidence of GVHD, but to decrease the risk of graft failure (nonengraftment), a TBI-containing preparative regimen was crucial. Early trials, however, showed a rapid neurologic deterioration soon after BMT in some patients conditioned with a TBI-containing regimen (63). This was especially pronounced for severely symptomatic patients (performance IQ of less than 80) (63). Based on these data, we postulated that irradiation of the brain, even to low doses as with TBI, was detrimental in the context of underlying demyelinating disease. This has been reported in patients with multiple sclerosis, also a demyelinating disease (64).

We therefore initiated a pilot trial to determine whether blocking the brain while giving total body irradiation is feasible. Because as much as 25% of bone marrow is in the skull of a young child, the technique developed uses a combination of electrons and tangential photons to deliver the full dose of TBI to the skull, while sparing the underlying brain. The preliminary results in this pilot study are encouraging. Patients appear to remain neurologically stable, but long-term results are not yet available.

TECHNICAL ASPECTS

Numerous techniques for irradiation of the entire body are described in the literature (46,65–71). At the University of Minnesota, two general TBI techniques are currently in use, with modifications of the techniques for certain situations.

One technique uses right-left lateral photon beams with the patient in a seated position (68), whereas the second technique is an anteroposterior treatment technique patterned after the one developed at Memorial Sloan Kettering (46). For the latter technique, adult patients are treated in a standing position with anterior and posterior beams, while smaller patients are treated in a reclined position if they can fit within the available field size at the floor of the treatment room. The goal of both of these techniques is to deliver a uniform dose to the entire body within ± 10% of the dose at the prescription point.

RIGHT AND LEFT LATERAL TOTAL BODY TECHNIQUE

This technique uses lateral photon beams with the patient in a seated position, as described in the literature (68,72). The treatment is delivered at a source to patient midline distance of 410 cm, which produces a field ~120 cm wide at the 95% isodose line. Aluminum compensators are used to produce a uniform dose through all body regions to within ± 10% of the dose specified at the umbilicus.

Simulation and Patient Measurements

Pretreatment measurements for total body irradiation are performed in the simulator room to accurately reproduce the treatment position within the treatment room and to calculate the size and thickness of the compensating filters. The simulation procedure consists of three steps. In the first step, an anterior chest film is taken to determine the amount of lung traversed by the treatment fields. The radiograph is taken with the patient seated on the simulator couch with his or her back resting against the film cassette holder. The source-skin distance (SSD) to the patient's chest is measured and because the source-film distance (SFD) is known, the magnification factor for the size of the lungs can be determined. Using this information, the thickness of the lung inhomogeneity can be computed. This information is used later when the need for lung compensation is evaluated.

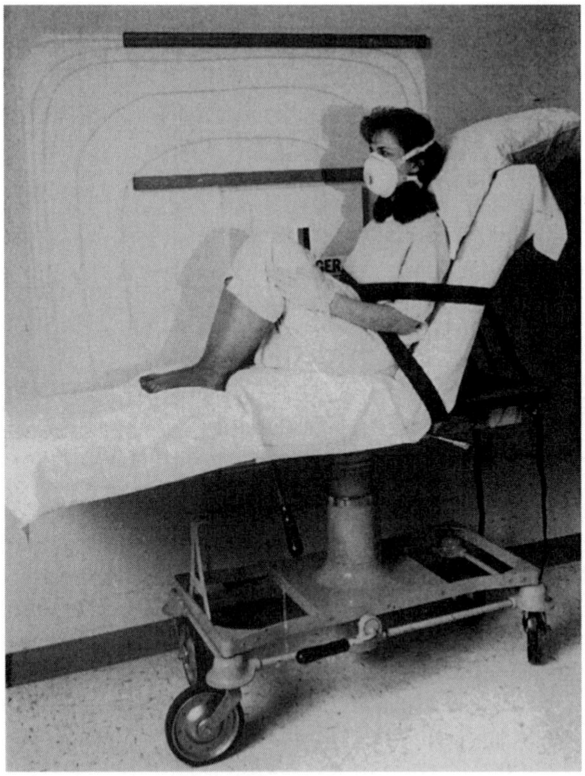

Figure 28.1. For the bilateral technique, the patient is positioned within the homogeneous portion of the beam. The simulation is performed in the simulator room and an overhead projector is used to produce a representation of the treatment field.

The second step is to establish the patient treatment position so that the majority of the body fits within the 98% isodose line. An overhead projector is used to cast an isodose pattern that represents the uniformity of the actual treatment field (Figure 28.1). The head and back of the patient are positioned within the 98% line, while the toes of the feet are within the 95% isodose line of the radiation field. Once this position has been established, setup measurements are recorded on the form as illustrated in Figure 28.2.

To describe the position of the lower extremities, measurements are made from our reference point (the anterosuperior point of the iliac spine [ASIS]) to the knee and to the back of the heel. The length of the feet is also recorded. The distance from the sternal notch to the top of the knee or patella is documented next to describe how compressed the patient is within the field. Finally, with the arms in the treatment position, the distance from the middle of the shoulder to the top of the head is measured. The latter information is used to scale the size of the head compensator. The chin extension, measured from the sternal notch to the point of the chin, is also recorded. Additionally, the need for positional devices, such as pillows for the back of the head, foam sponges underneath the hips, or sandbags under the feet, is recorded on the form. For future reference, the names of the individuals who made and checked the measurements are recorded.

The third step is to measure the right-left lateral thicknesses of the patient at certain anatomic locations. These measurements are recorded on the form shown in Figure 28.3 and constitute the basic data needed to determine the thickness of the compensators at these locations. The key measurement is the width of the patient at the umbilicus, since this is the location where the dose is prescribed. Lateral thicknesses are also measured at the head, neck, shoulders, midmediastinum, pelvis, knees, and the ankles. The midmediastinal thickness is measured midway between the sternal notch and the xiphoid and includes the thickness of the arms.

Once the lateral separations are recorded, the point where the lower extremities compensator is to start must be determined. Since the dose is prescribed for the thickness of the umbilicus, and the pelvis is usually of greater thickness, the compensator must be started at some point below the pelvis. The location where the compensator is to begin is that point on the legs that has the same separa-

LATERAL TOTAL BODY IRRADIATION (TBI) SET-UP DIAGRAM

DIAGNOSIS:
TREATMENT REGIME:
TREATMENT UNITS: Philips 10 MV, Varian 6/2500, or Varian 6/100

NAME: TBI Sample case
UM HOSPITAL #:
DATE:

	Philips 10 MV	Varian 6/2500	Varian 6/100
GANTRY ANGLE:	90°	270°	270°
COLLIMATOR SETTING:	38 x 38 cm²	40 x 40 cm²	40 x 40 cm²
FIELD SIZE @ Rx DISTANCE	156 x 156 cm²	164 x 164 cm²	144 x 144 cm²
TREATMENT SOURCE-AXIS DISTANCE:	410 cm	410 cm	360 cm

OTHER MEASUREMENTS TO BE RECORDED ON THE DIAGRAM:
ANTERIOR CHEST FILM:
SSD = 117 cm
SFD = 140 cm
CHIN EXTENSION = 9 cm

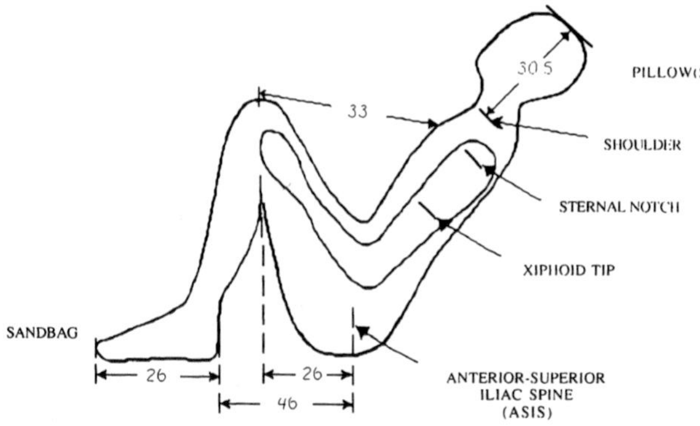

Measurements recorded by:_________ Measurements checked by:________

Figure 28.2. The form used to document the patient treatment position when the bilateral total body technique is used.

CALCULATIONS FOR TBI COMPENSATORS

NAME: TBI Sample case
UM Hospital #:
DATE:

Umbilicus thickness (L_{ref}): 32.5

$$\text{Lateral magnification} = \frac{\text{source-tray distance}}{\text{source-axis distance} - \frac{L_{ref}}{2}} = \frac{72}{410 - \frac{L_{ref}}{2}} = 0.183$$

Compensator material: Aluminum

$$\text{Thickness-ratio correction} = \frac{\tau}{\rho_{comp}} = \frac{0.70}{2.70} = 0.259$$

Site	Lateral thickness (L) (cm)	Lung thickness (cm)	Off-axis ratio (K)[4]	Tissue deficit[2] (g/cm^2)	Compensator thickness (L_c)[3]	Percent Midline Dose
Head	16 cm	0 cm	1.00	16.5	2.1	100%
Neck	12.5 cm	0 cm	1.00	20	20.6	100%
Shoulders	45 cm	0 cm	1.00	-12.5	-1.6	85.6%
Mid-mediastinum	50 cm	27.6 cm[1]	1.00	3.2	0.4	100%
Umbilicus	32.5 **cm**	0 cm	1.00	0	0	100%
Pelvis	39 cm	0 cm	1.00	-6.5	-0.8	92.5%
Knees	25 cm	0 cm	1.00	7.5	1.0	100%
Ankles	14 cm	0 cm	1.00	18.5	2.4	100%

Start Compensator 15 cm below iliac crest

[1]from AP chest film — $\rho_{lung} = 0.25\ g/cm^3$

[2]$TD(g/cm^2) = L_{ref} - L + (1 - \rho_{lung})L_{lung}$ — $\mu_{eff} = 0.024\ cm^2/g$

[3]$L_c = \frac{1}{2}\frac{\tau}{\rho_{comp}} \times TD - \left|\frac{\ln K}{\mu_{eff}} \times \frac{\tau}{\rho_{comp}}\right|$ Calc. by:__________

$= 0.13 \times TD - |10.8 \times \ln K|$ Checked by:__________

[4]normalized to off-axis ratio of 1.0

Figure 28.3. The form used to record the right-left lateral thicknesses of the patient. This information is used to calculate the tissue deficits that exist at various body locations versus the umbilicus thickness. Compensator thicknesses are subsequently calculated from these data. The final column provides a location to document the percent of the prescribed dose delivered to the midline of the indicated regions.

tion as the umbilicus. As final documentation, a photograph is taken of the patient in the treatment position with respect to the radiation field (see Figure 28.1).

Compensators for Total Body Irradiation

Compensator thickness determination. The form shown in Figure 28.3 also serves as the calculation sheet for the determination of compensator thickness at the different locations. The compensators are usually designed in three pieces: one for the lower extremities, one for the head and neck region, and one for the lungs. In most cases, a lung compensator is not required since the effective thickness at the midmediastinum is usually greater than the thickness at the umbilicus. The arms are deliberately positioned in line with the lungs and act to increase the total thickness in this region.

The first step in designing tissue compensators is to determine the tissue deficit (TD), the difference in tissue-equivalent thickness between the prescription point, (which in our case is the umbilicus), and the other locations. The following general equation is used to calculate tissue deficit:

$$TD = L_{ref} - L + (1 - \rho_{lung}) L_{lung} \quad (1)$$

where L_{ref} is the lateral separation at the umbilicus, L is the lateral separation at that particular anatomic location, L_{lung} is the separation of the lung determined from the anterior radiograph, and ρ_{lung} is the density of the lung. For ρ_{lung}, a value of 0.25 g/cm^3 is used as the average lung density for healthy lung tissue (73). Equation 1 is used only for the midmediastinal location where lung tissue is present. At all other locations, L_{lung} is zero and the tissue deficit can be obtained using equation 2:

$$TD = L_{ref} - L \quad (2)$$

L_{lung} is determined using the anterior chest radiograph that was taken in the simulator. The lung thickness is determined at a point midway between the sternal notch and the most superior aspect of the domes of the diaphragms as seen on the radiograph. As shown in Figure 28.4, two lateral measurements are made for both the right and left lobes of the lung: the first measurement, represented by L_{Rt1} and L_{Lt1}, extends from the most lateral aspect of the lung to the most medial portion of the lung. The second measurement, represented by L_{Rt2} and L_{Lt2}, spans from the most lateral extent of the lung to the mediastinum. The lung thickness is calculated using the following equation 3:

$$L_{lung} = \left(\frac{L_{Rt_1} + L_{Rt_2} + L_{Lt_1} + L_{Lt_2}}{2}\right) \times \left(\frac{\frac{1}{2}(SSD + SFD)}{SFD}\right) \quad (3)$$

where SSD is the source-skin distance and SFD is the source-film distance measured when the anterior chest radiograph was obtained during the first step of the simulation. In equation 3, the terms in the second parentheses serve to demagnify the lung dimensions measured on the chest radiograph to life-size at the midplane of the patient.

The compensator thickness, L_c, is determined using the following equation (4) (68):

$$L_c = \frac{1}{2} \times \frac{\tau}{\rho_{comp}} \times TD - \left|\frac{\ln K}{\mu_{eff}} \cdot \frac{\tau}{\rho_{comp}}\right| \quad (4)$$

In this expression, τ is the thickness ratio (74,75). For beam energies from cobalt 60 (Co-60) to 10 MV, a value for τ of 0.70 is a good approximation for compensator dis-

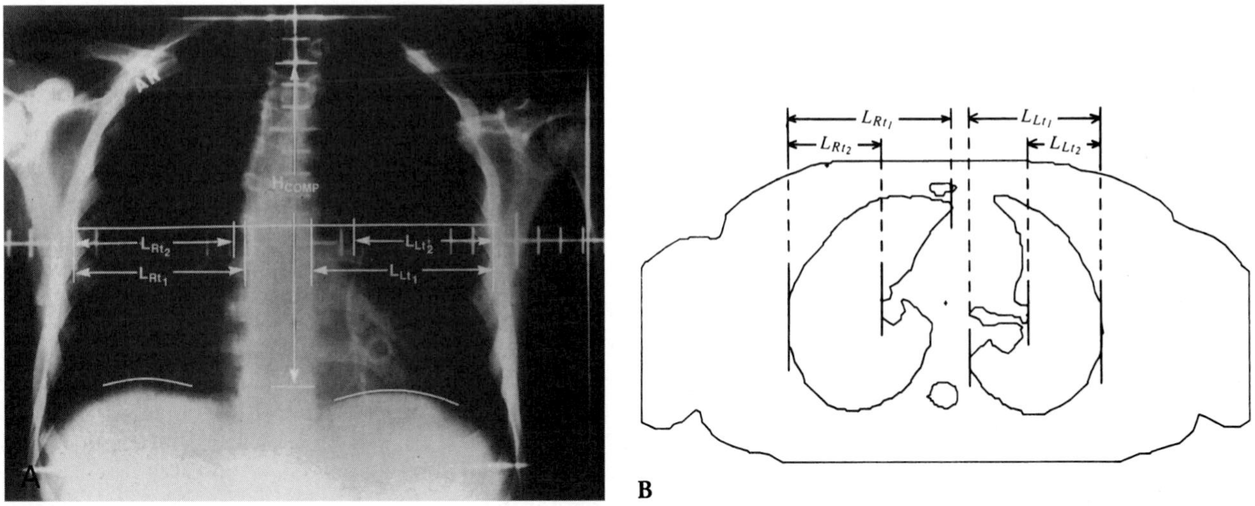

Figure 28.4. A. The anterior chest radiograph obtained during simulation indicating the lateral measurements taken to determine lung thickness, L_{lung}. Also shown is the level where these measurements are taken, the midpoint between the sternal notch and the xiphoid. This dimension, H_{comp}, is also the one used if a lung compensator is required. **B.** The inset, which is a diagrammatic representation of a transverse CT scan through the chest, illustrates the rationale behind these measurements.

tances greater than 20 cm from the surface (68). The density of the compensating material is ρ_{comp} (aluminum in this case), K is the off-axis correction factor that accounts for both the decreases in beam intensity away from the central axis and effective scattering field size for the various locations, and μ_{eff} is the broad-beam linear attenuation coefficient in tissue for this beam energy. The effective field size at various locations can be determined by Clarkson integration (19). The data in Table 28.7 was calculated in this manner for a Rando phantom and represents the equivalent scattering field at various locations of the body as a function of beam energy for an average adult (76). This data can be used to determine accurate values for K in equation 4.

An alternate method to determine compensator thickness for TBI has been suggested by the American Association of Physicists in Medicine (AAPM) (77). Comparisons made between the system of compensator thickness determination described above and that suggested by the AAPM (1986) show that the two systems produce compensators whose thickness varies by less than 1 mm of aluminum.

Finally, the percentage difference in dose between the prescription point and other locations of the body are calculated and recorded in the last column of the form.

Compensator design. The compensators are designed to be located at a distance of 72 cm from the virtual source of the accelerator so that appropriate compensation can be provided without the devices becoming excessively large and difficult to handle. Thus, the measurements recorded on the setup sheet in Figure 28.2 must be demagnified from the treatment distance to the location of their use. Using the information supplied in Figures 28.2 through 28.4, the size of the compensators is determined in the following manner. For the lower extremities compensator, the base length for section A in Figure 28.5 is obtained by taking the ASIS to knee distance, subtracting the distance below the ASIS that the compensator is to start, and multiplying that dimension by the lateral magnification factor:

Table 28.7. The Equivalent Square Field Size For Various Anatomical Locations[a]

	Side of Equivalent Square (cm)				
Photon Energy	Head	Neck	Chest	Umbilicus	Hips
Co-60	17	22	31	30	28
4 MV	16	20	30	29	23
6 MV	18	23	29	27	26
10 MV	17	22	33	27	26
18 MV	>18	>18	>18	>18	>18
Mean	17	22	31	28	26
Lateral dimension	15	12–16	31	27	31
Equivalent length	19	30	31	29	20

[a] Determined at midline in a Rando phantom. The lateral dimensions of the phantom at these locations is also listed in addition to the equivalent lengths required to obtain the calculated field sizes by equivalent square calculation. Reproduced from 76.

$$\text{Lateral Magnification Factor} = \frac{\text{Source-compensator tray distance}}{\left(\text{Source-axis distance} - \frac{L_{ref}}{2}\right)} \quad (5)$$

Section B of the lower extremities compensator is the de-

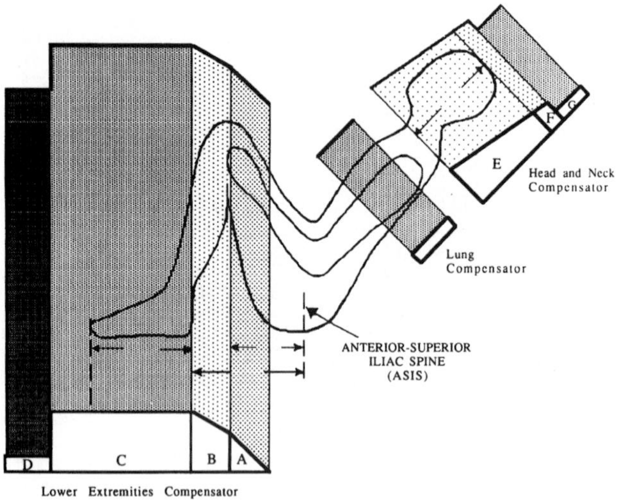

Figure 28.5. A schematic diagram showing the relationship between the compensators used for the bilateral total-body technique and the patient treatment position.

magnified distance from the knee to the back of the heels, while Section C is the demagnified length of the feet plus an additional 2 cm to ensure adequate coverage of the feet. Section D is simply an additional 2 cm of aluminum that is needed to clamp the compensator to the compensator tray during the actual treatment. The thickness of the compensator is obtained from the compensator thickness column as shown on Figure 28.3 for the corresponding anatomic location.

The head and neck compensator is designed in much the same manner. The base length of Section E of this compensator is the demagnified distance from the middle of the shoulder to the top of the head. Section F is an additional 1 cm of material to ensure adequate coverage while Section G is provided for clamping. The thicknesses of the compensator are again obtained from Figure 28.3 for the head and neck regions.

The length of the lung compensator is obtained by demagnifying H_{comp} from the chest radiograph (Figure 28.4) to life size using (1/2) (SSD − SFD) / SFD, then again demagnifying these dimensions to the treatment position of the compensators using Equation 5. The compensator thickness is obtained from Figure 28.3.

The width of the compensators (the dimension of the compensator that is not shown in Figure 28.5) is typically 11 cm for the lower extremities compensator, 6.5 cm for the head and neck compensator, and 7.5 cm for the lung compensator.

Figure 28.6 shows the compensator design form that is sent to the machine shop for fabrication. Figure 28.7A shows the finished aluminum compensators and Figure 28.7B illustrates the compensators in use and how they are attached to the tray using specially designed clamps. The lung compensator, when required, is attached to the tray with double-sided tape.

Machine calibration and treatment calculation. The linear accelerator is calibrated according to the protocol outlined by the AAPM (78). To determine the total number of monitor units (MU) for TBI, the calculation is done as an isocentric treatment at an extended distance. Equation 6 is used in the determination, as follows:

$$MU = \left(\frac{TD \times STF}{k \times S_c(r_o) \times S_p(r_e) \times TMR(d,r_e) \times \left(\frac{f}{f'}\right)^2} \right) \quad (6)$$

In this equation, k is the machine calibration factor equal to 1 cGy per MU in tissue at d_{max} depth at the standard calibration distance, which is f, for the calibration field size of 10 × 10 cm^2; S_c (r_o) represents the collimator scatter correction factor for r_o; the collimator field size, $S_p(r_e)$, is the phantom scatter factor for the effective scattering field, r_e; at the umbilicus, $(f/f')^2$ is the inverse square factor from the calibration distance, f, to the treatment distance, f', set to the midline of the patient; and $TMR(d,r_e)$ is the tissue-maximum ratio for the midline depth, d, for the effective

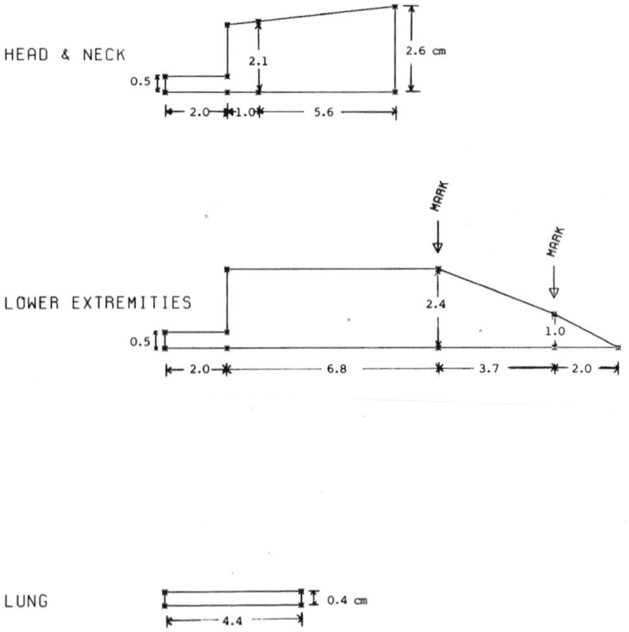

Figure 28.6. The compensator design form showing the information provided to the machine shop for fabrication of the aluminum compensators. For the position on the lower extremities compensator indicated by "Mark," a small peg is inserted into the side of the compensator. This peg aids in aligning the compensator with the knee and the ankle when the patient is in the treatment position.

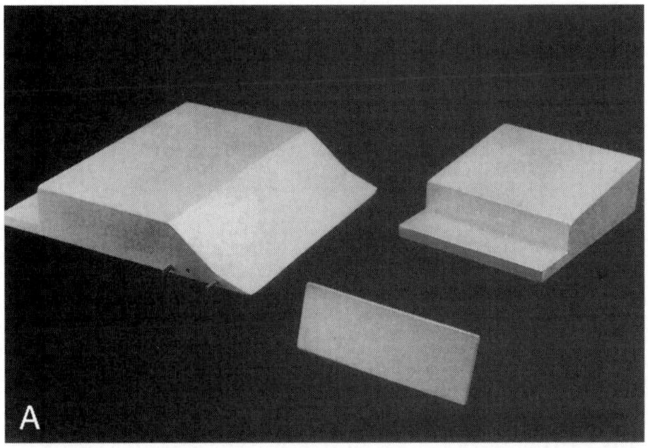

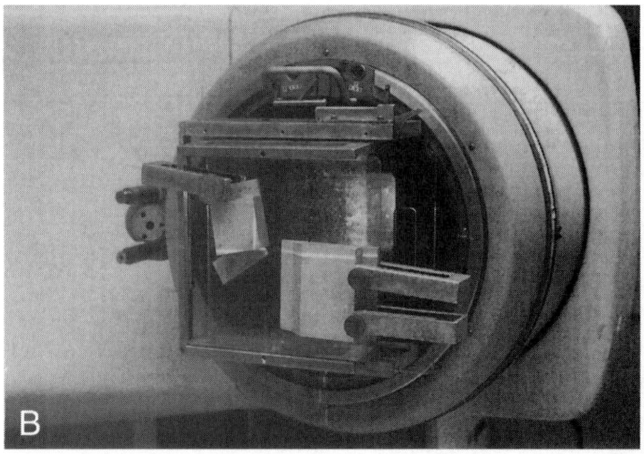

Figure 28.7. The completed aluminum compensators used for the bilateral total body technique. **A.** The aluminum compensators for the lower extremities, lung, and head and neck (from left to right). **B.** An illustration of the aluminum compensators attached to the block tray of the linear accelerator. The head and lower extremities compensators are attached using clamps while the lung compensator is mounted on the tray using double-sided tape.

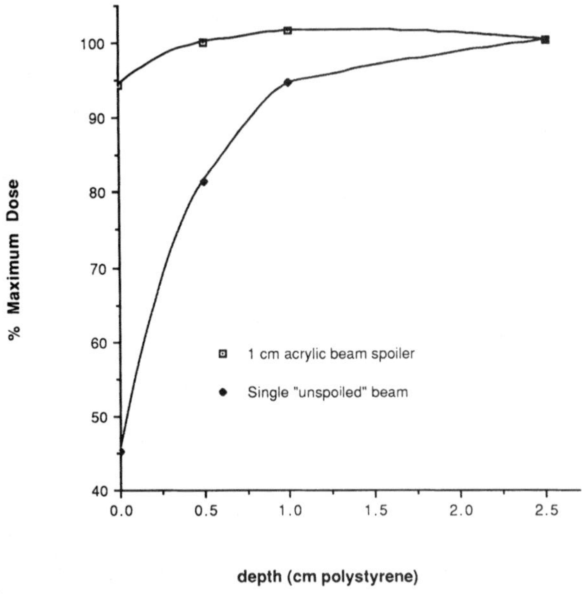

A

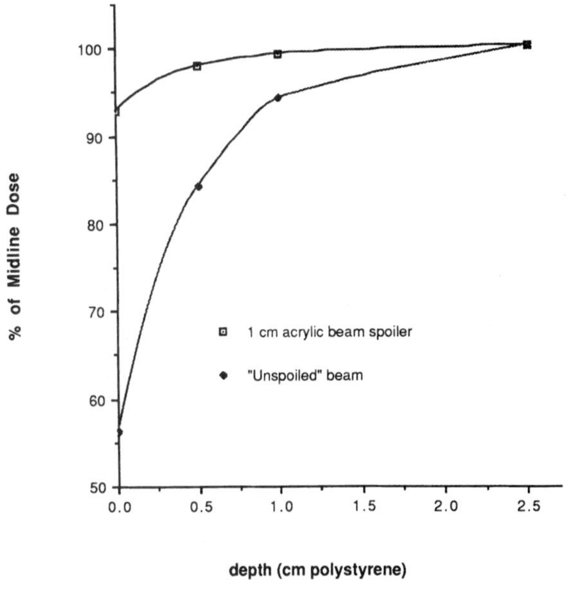

B

Figure 28.8. The buildup characteristics of 10-MV x-rays for **A.** a single incident beam both with and without the beam spoiler in place. The measurements are normalized to d_{max} for the single field in this figure. **B.** This figure shows the percentage surface dose for parallel-opposed 10-MV beams for both open and degraded fields normalized to the dose delivered to the midplane of a 25-cm thick patient.

field size. The accuracy of the TMR values taken at 100-cm source-axis distance has been verified at the extended treatment distance. Finally, a combined spoiler plus tray factor (STF) for both the 1-cm acrylic beam spoiler and the blocking trays that support the compensators, is included.

The beam spoiler or degrader is necessary because of the large degree of skin sparing that is still present for the large field sizes and extended treatment distances employed in TBI. Figure 28.8A illustrates the buildup characteristics of 10-MV x-rays for a single incident beam with and without the beam spoiler in place. The measurements are normalized to d_{max} for the single field in this figure. Figure 28.8B shows the percentage surface dose for parallel-opposed 10-MV beams, for both open and degraded fields, normalized to the dose delivered to the midplane of a 25-cm thick patient. For both data sets, the beam spoiler was placed at a distance of 20 cm from the phantom surface. Without the beam spoiler, the dose delivered to the superficial regions of the patient would be inadequate.

Patient Treatment

To ensure that all the information is accurately transferred to the treatment room, the first setup of every patient is rigorously checked. The treatment position is checked for accuracy versus the data recorded on the setup sheet (Figure 28.2). Next, it is verified that the patient is positioned within the uniformly flat portion of the radiation field. It is verified that the upper arms are properly positioned to provide shielding for the lungs so that they do not receive excessive dose, and that the forearms and hands are in line with the thighs. The fit, size, and positioning of the compensating filters are also checked to ensure that the proper amount of compensation is being applied to each anatomic region. For the lower extremities compensator, positioning is accomplished by aligning the pegs on the side of the compensator (indicated by "Mark" on the compensator design form, Figure 28.6) with the knee and the back of the heel. The head and neck compensator is positioned so that compensation begins at the midshoulder and extends beyond the top of the head. The lung compensator, when required, is placed with the superior border of the compensator at the sternal notch and perpendicular to the back of the treatment couch. The final check before irradiation is to make sure that the beam spoiler is in place and that it is 20 cm or closer to the patient's most proximal surface.

Dose Verification

The dose delivered to the patient during total body irradiation has been verified using both Lithium Fluoride (LiF) thermoluminescent dosimetry (TLD) chips and encapsulated powder. The dosimeters for the head and neck region were taped to the side of these regions and covered by 2.5 cm of wax bolus. The location of the TLDs for the midmediastinal readings was between the upper arm and the chest wall. The TLDs for the lower extremities were all placed between the legs at the indicated locations. The results of these measurements shown in Table 28.8 illustrate that there is fairly good dose uniformity throughout the entire treatment region when using parallel-opposed high energy photon beams.

Dose Prescription

The usual dose prescribed using this technique is 165 cGy twice daily for 4 days for a total of 8 fractions. This results in a cumulative dose of 1320 cGy. Each fraction is separated by at least 6 hours. The dose rate is between 10 and 19 cGy per minute. A summary of the patient treatment schedule is shown in Table 28.9.

ANTEROPOSTERIOR TOTAL BODY IRRADIATION

An anteroposterior total body irradiation technique used at the University of Minnesota is adapted from the one developed at the Memorial Sloan Kettering Hospital in New York (46). The patients are treated in either a standing or reclining position, alternating anterior and posterior surfaces for each fraction. The prescription dose is 1375 cGy to the midplane of the pelvis delivered in eleven 125 cGy fractions using three fractions per day at approxi-

Table 28.8. Lithium Fluoride Thermoluminescent Chip and Disposable Powder Capsule Measurements Showing Percent of Prescribed Dose to Various Anatomic Locations for the Right and Left Lateral TBI Technique

	Anatomic Location							
	Head	Neck	Chest wall	Pelvis	Thigh	Knee	Ankle	Oral cavity
Mean	95.5	99.8	97.8	102.1	97.3	97.2	99.9	109.0
Standard deviation	5.94	7.20	5.76	5.11	6.04	6.54	6.63	10.6
Maximum	110	122	116	111	118	113	116	143
Minimum	84	88	83	90	87	85	88	93
Number	36	35	35	36	36	36	35	20

[a] Aluminum compensators were used to account for differences in thickness. These results are for the 10 MV right-left lateral technique.

Table 28.9. Summary of Patient Treatment Schedule for Right and Left Lateral Total Body Irradiation Treatment

Radiation Therapy BMT Day:	Day 1 −4	Day 2 −3	Day 3 −2	Day 4 −1
	TBI fractions 1, 2: 18 or 25-MV X-rays, 165 cGy/fraction	TBI fractions 3, 4: 18 or 25-MV X-rays, 165 cGy/fraction	TBI fractions 4, 6: 18 or 25-MV X-rays, 165 cGy/fraction	TBI fractions 7, 8: 18 or 25-MV X-rays, 165 cGy/fraction

Table 28.10. Summary of Patient Treatment Schedule for Standing Total Body Technique Showing Timing of Total Body X-Ray and Electron Treatments

TRAD RX.	Day 1	Day 2	Day 3	Day 4
BMT Day:	−7	−6	−5	−4
	TBI fractions 1, 2, 3: 6-MV X-rays, 125 cGy/fraction	TBI fractions 4, 5, 6: 6-MV X-rays, 125 cGy/fraction	TBI fractions 7, 8, 9: 6-MV X-rays, 125 cGy/fraction	TBI fractions 10, 11: 6-MV X-rays, 125 cGy/fraction
	Fraction 1: Testicular electron boost, 400 cGy/fraction		Fraction 7: electron chest wall boost, 300 cGy/fraction	Fraction 10: electron chest wall boost, 300 cGy/fraction

mately a 4½ hour interval. 6-MV x-rays are used at a dose rate of 10 to 19 cGy per minute at the midline of the pelvis, which is the prescription point. For each x-ray treatment, 2.1 cm thick cerrobend lung blocks are used to reduce the dose to the lungs by approximately 50%. The chest wall overlying the lungs, which were shielded by the lung blocks, are given an additional 600 cGy to d_{max} using electron beams of appropriate energy. The electron energy used for these chest wall boost fields is selected to place the 90% isodose line at the lung chest wall interface. In addition, all male patients receive a testicular boost of 400 cGy to d_{max} on day 1. The electron energy for this boost is chosen to set the 90% isodose at the posterior surface of the scrotum. A summary of the patient treatment schedule is shown in Table 28.10.

The workup for the TBI patients consists of a simulation procedure to obtain lung block shape and position during treatment, measurements of patient thickness, and locating the CT scan region that will be used to determine the optimum electron energy for the chest wall boost. Details of the patient workup and treatment procedures are given below.

Simulation and patient measurements. Three steps are associated with the simulation of the patient: 1) fit the patient within the available field size, 2) take both an anterior and a posterior chest radiograph for the location of lung blocks, and 3) measure and record anteroposterior patient thicknesses at specific anatomic sites.

Patient positioning within the treatment field. The simulation of the patient is performed inside the treatment room with the gantry rotated to the lateral treatment position. The gantry is rotated to provide the best coverage of the patient within the visible field. However, the gantry angulation should not deviate by more than 2° from the lateral treatment position so that the proper treatment distance is maintained. The treatment room is preferred over the simulator because fitting the patient within the available field size is a crucial step at our institution. For our treatment distance of 410 cm, the diagonal field size is 170 cm (5'8") inside the 90% isodose line. Patients shorter than 170 cm (5'8") can be easily treated in the standing position. However, it is necessary for taller patients to sit on the seat of the treatment stand in order to fit within the treatment field. Although this is not the optimum treatment position, acceptable dose uniformity can still be achieved.

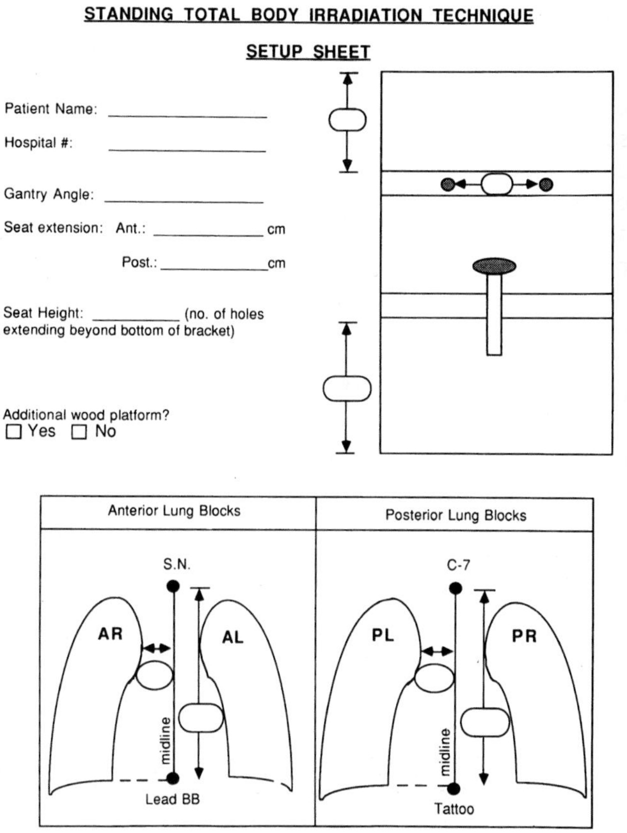

Figure 28.9. The form used to document the patient treatment position when using the standing total body technique.

Films for lung blocks. Once the position of the patient within the treatment field has been determined, chest radiographs are taken. The anterior film is taken with a small BB placed at the tops of the diaphragms. The distance of this BB below the sternal notch is measured and recorded on the form illustrated in Figure 28.9. Additionally, a posterior radiograph is taken with a BB placed at C_7. The location of the BB is indicated on the form and is marked

with a tattoo. Also recorded are the gantry angle of the accelerator, the seat extension and height, the separation of the supports located under the arms, and the position of the hand rests. For shorter patients, an additional wooden platform is placed below their feet to position them more in the center of the beam. The information on this form is later used to duplicate the patient treatment position.

Patient thickness measurements. Following the radiographs, anteroposterior separations are measured at the head, neck, sternal notch, midmediastinum, umbilicus, pelvis, knees, and ankles. The target dose is prescribed at the midplane thickness of the pelvis. The names of the individuals who made and checked the measurements are recorded.

Treatment planning CT scans. The staff physician next outlines the lung blocks on both the anterior and posterior chest radiographs. For adult patients, the blocks are drawn so that there is a 2-cm margin between both the diaphragm and edge of the vertebrae and a 1.5-cm gap between the edge of the block and the rib cage. Once these lung blocks are indicated on the films, the patient is taken for treatment planning CT scans.

The patient is then taken to the diagnostic radiology department for CT scanning through the region of the lung blocks. Treatment planning is performed on the CT scan taken one-third of the way up from the bottom of the lung blocks. Additional scans are taken through the chest region to provide a more complete description of the chest wall thickness under the blocks. Ultrasound scans are occasionally performed instead of CT scans when the chest wall thickness is significantly different with the patient lying supine as compared to the standing position, for instance in women with pendulous breasts.

Once the scanning is completed, computerized treatment planning is performed to determine the appropriate electron beam energy for the electron chest wall boost. This is done by placing the 90% isodose line at the lung-chest wall interface. A typical treatment plan is illustrated in Figure 28.10.

Construction of lung blocks and electron cut-outs. The lung blocks are constructed from the outlines drawn on the anterior and posterior chest films and are held together by a plastic plate that maintains the proper block separation (Figure 28.11). The cerrobend blocks are 2.1 cm thick, which is approximately the half-value thickness, including scatter, for 6-MV photons. The cerrobend cut-out used for the electron chest wall boost fields is an exact negative of the anterior and posterior lung blocks (Figure 28.11B).

Patient Treatment Technique

Total body photon irradiation. The treatment is delivered using 6-MV x-rays with a dose rate between 10 and 19 cGy per minute at the midplane of the pelvis. The patient is treated in the standing position resting against the back plate of the total body treatment stand that was specifically designed for this treatment (Figure 28.12). The treatment distance for this particular setup is 410 cm source-axis distance (SAD) to the midline of the pelvis.

The lungs are shielded with the appropriate lung blocks throughout the total body photon portion of the treatment. The lung blocks are hung by a Lexan™ hook from

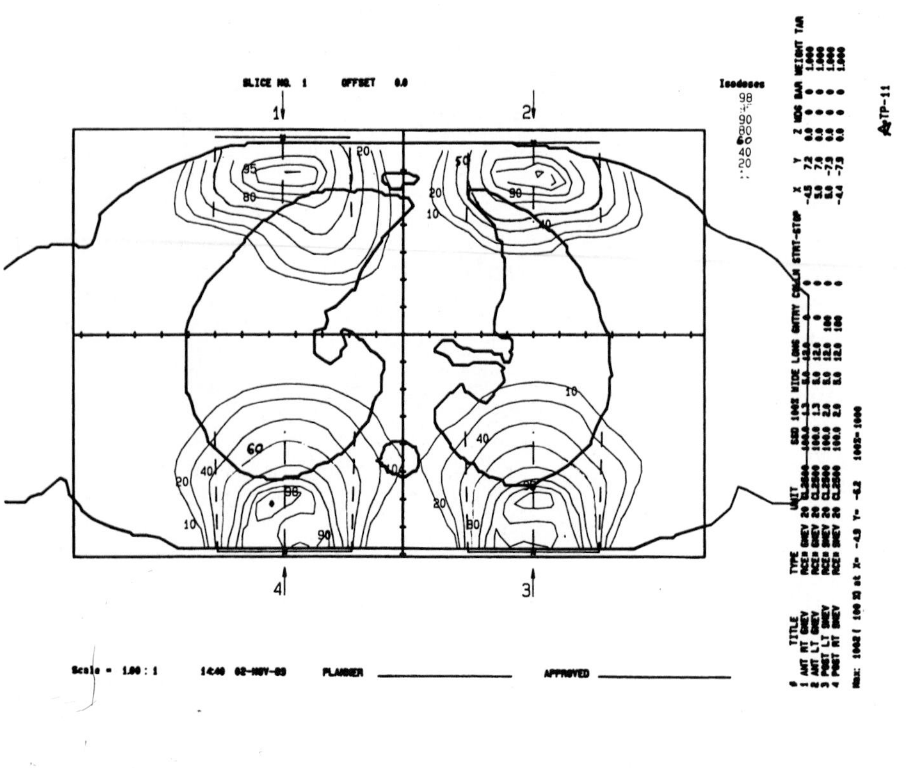

Figure 28.10. A computerized treatment plan done to determine the proper electron energy for the chest wall boost fields. The objective is to place the 90% isodose line at the lung-chest wall interface.

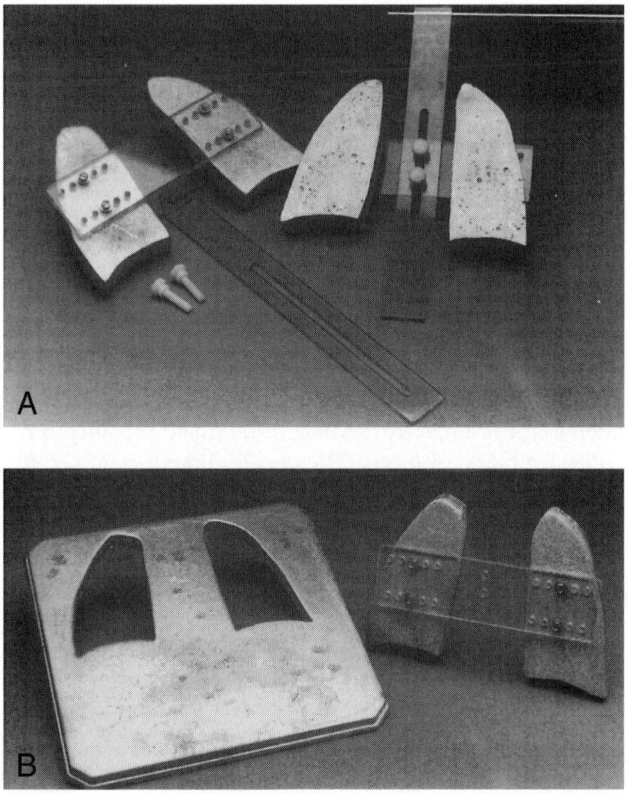

Figure 28.11. The apparatus used to shield the lungs during standing total body irradiation. **A.** The proper separation of the two cerrobend lung blocks is maintained by the acrylic plate. The Lexan™ hook is used to suspend the blocks from the plastic plate that is placed in front of the patient when positioned in the total body treatment stand. This arrangement allows easy adjustment of both the height of the blocks and their right-left placement with respect to the patient. **B.** The cerrobend insert that is used for the chest wall electron boost treatment exactly matches the shape of the cerrobend lung blocks.

the anterior plate of the total body treatment stand. The location of the top of the lung blocks is positioned at the level of the skin tattoos and is verified with measurements from bony landmarks. Verification films confirm the positioning of the blocks during the photon treatments. A 1-cm thick acrylic beam spoiler is placed between the patient and the beam to produce a high dose on the patient's skin surface. The screen is located 20 cm or less from the patient surface. The skin dose with this location of the beam spoiler is approximately 92% of the delivered midline dose for the 6-MV beam.

Electron chest wall boost. For fractions 7 and 10, an electron chest wall boost is given to that portion of the chest wall that was shielded by the lung blocks. A special couch extension has been designed so that both adult and pediatric patients are in the same upright treatment position for the chest wall boost fields as they were for the standing total body treatments (Figure 28.13). The prescribed dose is 600 cGy to d_{max}, delivered in two 300 cGy fractions. The selection of electron energy and the need for bolus is based on the results of computerized treatment planning using the CT scan so that the 90% isodose line is placed at the lung-chest wall interface.

Testicular boost. Male patients are given a testicular electron boost on the first day of treatment. The prescribed dose is 400 cGy to d_{max} in one fraction. The patient is treated in the supine position with a sheet of lead placed under the testes to minimize the dose to the rectal area. A 6-mm thick sheet of wax bolus is placed between the lead and the posterior surface of the scrotum to reduce the amount of backscatter from the lead. The electron energy is based on the thickness of the testes and is chosen so that the 90% isodose line is at the posterior surface of the scrotum.

Infant irradiation. Total body treatments for infants are done with the patient supine on a separate treatment couch positioned on the floor. We have found that these

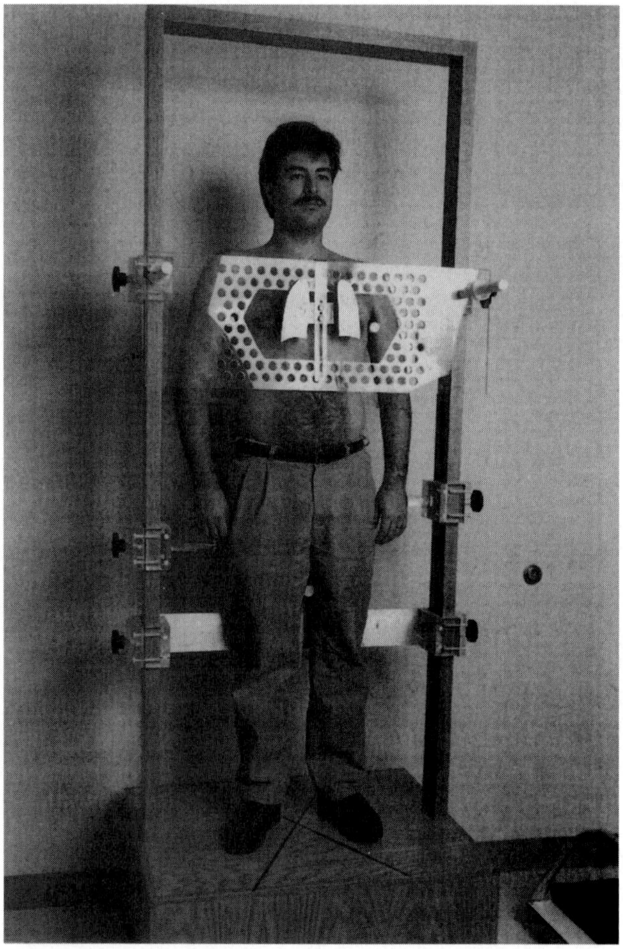

Figure 28.12. The standing total body treatment position with the back of the patient resting against the back plate of the total body treatment stand. The lung blocks are shown, in position, hanging from the front acrylic plate.

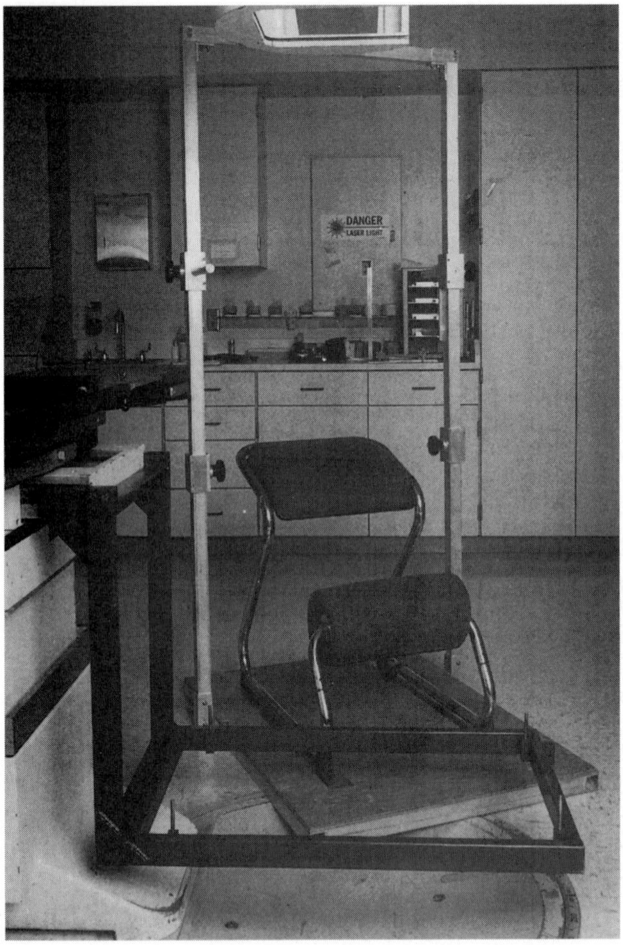

Figure 28.13. A special couch extension designed to reproduce the standing TBI treatment position when treating the electron chest wall boost fields. The device is separated into two pieces for ease of handling and since it is attached directly to the couch, it has the same range of motion as the couch. Patients up to approximately 5 feet tall can be treated in the standing position while taller patients are treated in a seated position. This style of chair keeps the back of the patient in about the same orientation when seated as when they are standing.

treatments are best performed with sedation or anesthesia. The gantry is directed vertically down for these cases and the collimator is rotated 45° to produce the largest available field size. A 1-cm acrylic beam spoiler is positioned approximately 20 cm above the torso of the patient both to provide a high surface dose and to support the lung blocks used for the anterior and posterior x-ray fields. The lower extremities are simply bolused to provide a high skin surface dose (Figure 28.14). The chest wall electron boost is also delivered with the patient in the supine position.

Dose Verification

Lithium fluoride TLD was performed on several patients to establish the homogeneity of dose throughout the treatment field. The TLD chips were covered by approximately 1 cm of bolus to indicate the dose at d_{max} at these locations and were placed at the same locations for both anterior and posterior treatments. The results of the measurements, shown in Table 28.11, indicate an acceptable level of dose homogeneity for this treatment technique.

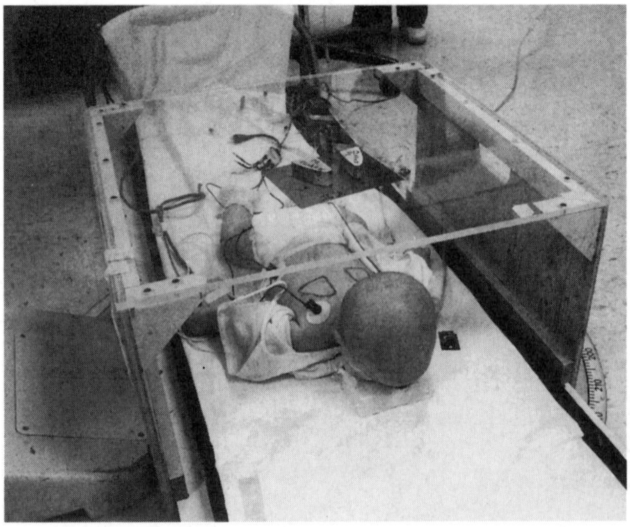

Figure 28.14. An illustration showing the treatment position used for pediatric patients. The lung blocks are placed on top of the acrylic beam spoiler. The lower extremities are bolused to provide a high dose at the surface.

Table 28.11. Lithium Fluoride Thermoluminescent Dosimeters Establish Homogeneity of Dose for Standing TBI Technique[a]

	Pres. Dose (%)				
Anatomical Location	Mean	SD	Highest D	Lowest D	N
Umbilicus	97.4	4.21	104	90	27
Right palm—opposite knuckles	113.9	9.15	134	95	27
Right palm—heel of hand	104.7	8.76	117	90	6
Between breasts	101.0	5.97	118	92	27
Right hip	113.0	9.41	137	98	26
Left inner thigh	107.9	9.59	131	93	25
Perineal	105.2	6.38	120	93	23
Left outer ankle	112.3	11.6	130	103	7
Sternal notch	103.6	6.36	113	85	27
Forehead	97.0	7.44	109	83	26
Left lateral calf	111.7	8.77	128	92	27
Top of head	109.7	11.6	136	96	18
Under lung block	62.5	9.79	86	48	26
Neck-thyroid notch	100.8	6.37	110	92	6

SD, standard deviation; D, deviation.
[a] The TLD chips were covered by approximately 1 cm of bolus to indicate the dose at d_{max} at these locations. The chips were in place during both anterior and posterior treatments.

Brain Sparing Technique

This technique is a variation of the AP/PA technique with the following modifications. A total dose of 1400 cGy in 7 fractions over 3½ days is given. For each fraction of TBI, both the AP and PA fields are treated. Therefore, 100 cGy is given to the prescription point (midpelvis at midplane) for the AP field and 100 cGy is given to the prescription point for the PA field for each fraction of TBI. Additionally, for each fraction of TBI, the brain is blocked with 5 HVL blocks placed on either the beam spoiler (for recumbent patients) or on the front acrylic plate (for standing patients) (Figure 28.15).

The ribs are boosted with electrons (6000 cGy in two fractions) on 2 consecutive days. To properly place the brain blocks, two aquaplast molds are made at the time of simulation, with the patient's head turned as far laterally to the side as possible (Figure 28.16). One mold is made for the AP position and a second mold is made for the PA position. These molds serve both to immobilize the head and to act as a template for later matching of the electron fields. When the patient is treated to the AP photon field, the head is turned to the left (therefore the right side of the skull faces the photon beam), and secured with the aquaplast mold. A simulation film is taken with the patient in this position. When the patient is treated to the PA photon field, the head is also turned to the left. This will result in the opposite (i.e., left side) of the skull to face the photon beam. A second simulation film is taken with the patient in this position. Skull blocks are drawn on these simulation films corresponding to the inner table of the skull. Cerrobend skull blocks (5 HVL thick) are constructed from the outlines drawn on the AP and PA skull radiographs. The cerrobend cut-out used for the electron fields is an exact negative of the AP and PA skull blocks (Figure 28.17).

Prior to the initiation of the first fraction of TBI a port film is taken with the blocks in the approximate position.

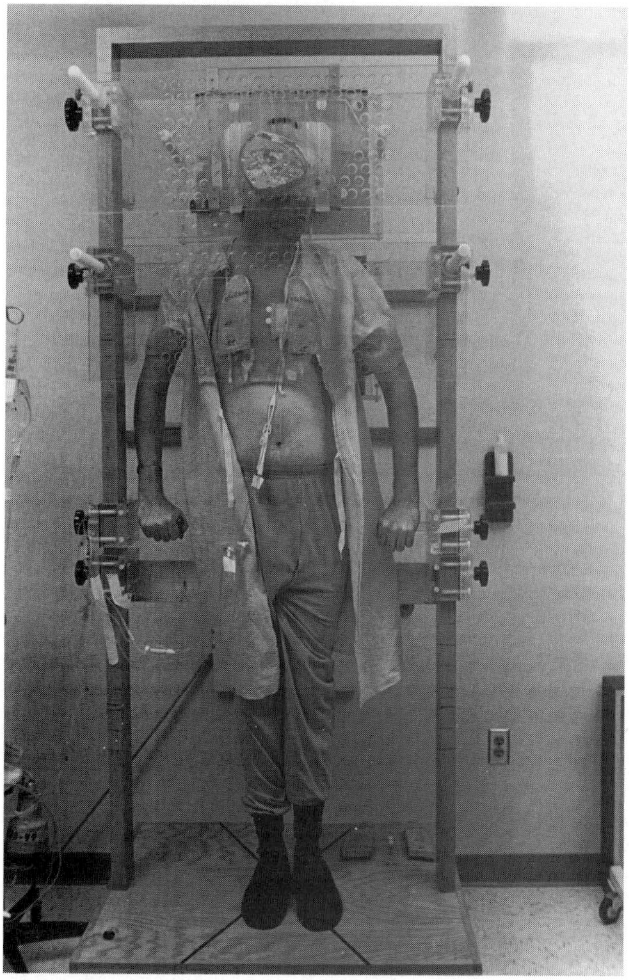

Figure 28.15. Aquaplast head mold is used to secure the head turned position for the "Brain Sparing Technique." With the patient in the standing position, the 5 HVL brain block is fastened to an acrylic plate attached to the TBI stand. With the patient recumbent, the brain block is placed on top of the acrylic beam spoiler. The central portions of the skull are blocked while the outer skull is tangentially included in the TBI photon field.

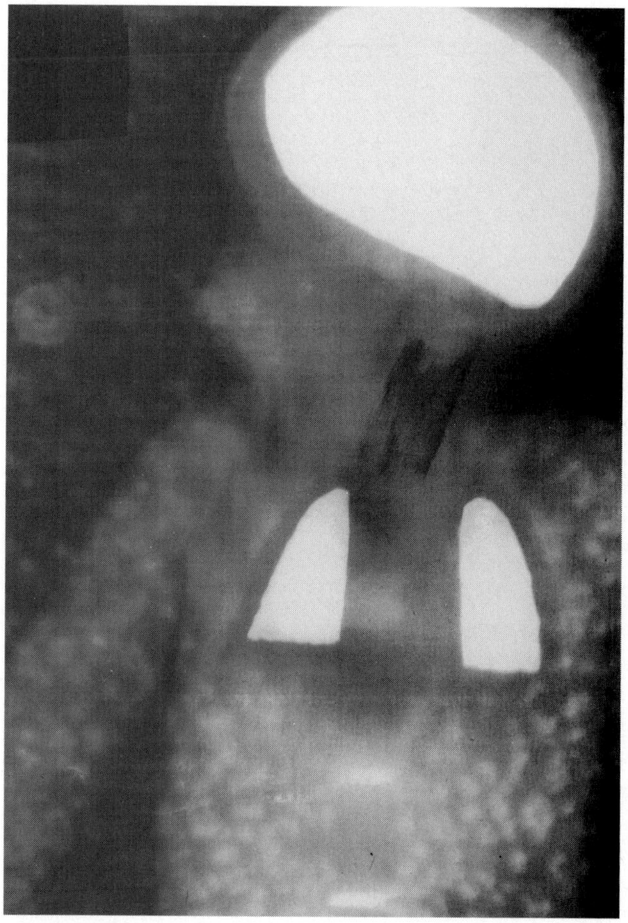

Figure 28.16. Port film demonstrating the placement of the 5 HVL brain block.

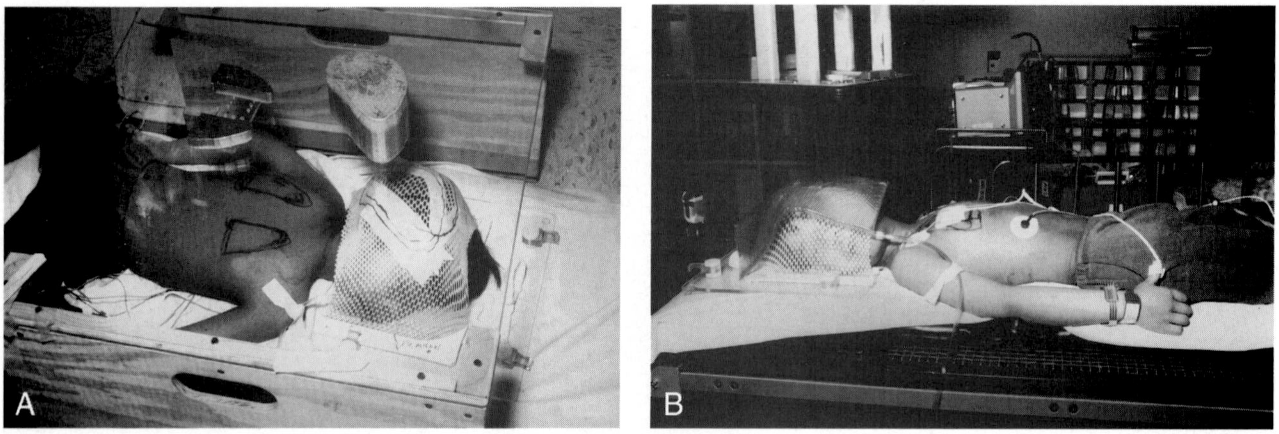

Figure 28.17. **A.** 5 HVL brain block is outlined on the aquaplast mask. **B.** Electron field matches the edge of the photon field, drawn on the aquaplast head mold at the time the photon field was treated.

The edge of the photon field is drawn on the aquaplast mold. The position of the blocks can be modified based on the results of the port film. The modifications are drawn on the aquaplast mold. With the aquaplast mold still in place over the skull, the remainder of the skull is treated with an en face electron beam of appropriate energy. The energy is determined by performing a treatment planning CT scan of the brain (at the same time the chest CT is performed). The electron field abuts the photon field. The fields are matched by aligning the marks drawn on the aquaplast head mold.

The dose schedule for the "Brain Sparing" technique is 200 cGy twice daily for a total of seven fractions. This total dose of 1400 cGy is given over 3 ½ days with a minimum of 6 hours between fractions. As patients treated on this protocol do not have a malignancy, there is no testicular boost.

SPECIAL CONSIDERATIONS FOR TBI IN YOUNG CHILDREN

A fundamental requirement for TBI is immobility during treatment. Whereas many children even as young as 3 years of age are able to cooperate and remain immobile with the encouragement of their parents, many children must be anesthetized. We usually try to determine at the time of simulation whether a patient will require anesthesia. Clues about whether a patient will be cooperative include whether the patient willingly leaves his or her parents for the measurements, whether they listen to the instructions the therapist gives, and how anxious they appear. Additionally, the parents usually have a good indication of how their child has done with other medical procedures. In an effort to avoid needing to use anesthesia, we sometimes arrange for a potential TBI patient come to the department for several consecutive days so he or she can become acquainted with our therapists. The therapist will spend 10 to 15 minutes with the patient in the treatment room practicing for the TBI treatment. As there are intercoms and video monitors, the therapist can place the patient in the treatment position, leave the room, and talk to the patient over the intercom. With practice, even young patients are often able to be spared anesthesia.

Obviously, there are situations where anesthesia is necessary. Anesthesia for TBI presents unique situations not ordinarily encountered by most anesthesiologists. Foremost is the fact that the anesthesiologist cannot be in the treatment room during the TBI. Additionally, for the AP/PA technique the patient is prone, and the airway more difficult to keep patent.

If TBI under general anesthesia is scheduled, the patient fasts for 6 hours before the scheduled procedure. For infants, an interval of 4 hours from intake of formula is sufficient. On arrival to the radiation therapy room, atropine and propofol (79,80) are administered intravenously. Dolasetron is effective at preventing nausea during and after the treatment.

As the patient loses consciousness, a blood pressure cuff is placed around the upper arm and the electrocardiogram (ECG) monitored continuously. Pulse oximetry is used for continuous monitoring of oxygen saturation. Supplemental oxygen is administered with nasal prongs. A continuous drip of propofol is started (79,80). The patient is placed in the treatment position. The child's head is fixed firmly in position by a sponge rubber donut or Styrofoam. Adhesive tape is used to secure the head in the appropriate position so that airway patency and ventilation are secured.

Two closed-circuit television cameras are focused on the patient and on the physiologic monitor console. When the patient is ready for irradiation, all attendant personnel withdraw from the treatment room. During the treatment, airway and respiratory adequacy are observed constantly

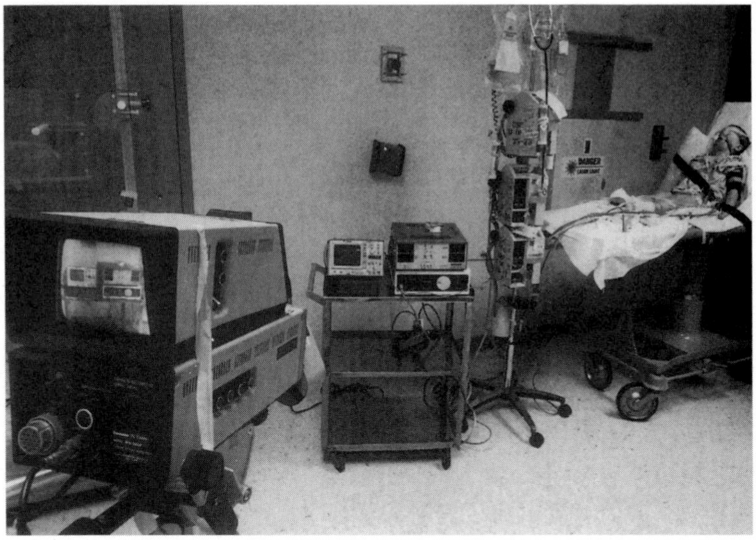

Figure 28.18. Closed circuit television camera is focused on physiologic monitor console. Second camera (not shown) is focused on patient.

with a zoom television monitor system, while blood pressure, ECG, and pulse oximetry are monitored with the second television monitor (Figure 28.18).

After the treatment is complete, the patient is transferred to the postanesthetic recovery room, where surveillance is continued until full arousal occurs. Patients who receive several treatments on consecutive days show increased tolerance to propofol and the dose may need to be increased accordingly.

COMPLICATIONS FOLLOWING PREPARATION WITH TBI

The major causes of morbidity and mortality following a BMT are infectious complications. Additionally, interstitial pneumonitis develops in up to 20% of transplanted patients depending on the source of the marrow and previous therapies received (36,51,53,81–83). Acute side effects of TBI include nausea and vomiting, alopecia, diarrhea, low grade fever, mucositis, and pancytopenia. Intermediate side effects include interstitial pneumonitis, veno-occlusive disease, and nephrotoxicity. Late side effects include restrictive lung disease, possible decreased growth, endocrine abnormalities (especially hypothyroidism) sterility, cataracts, chronic renal failure, and neurologic damage. Sanders (84) reported that boys given single fraction TBI were significantly shorter than boys given fractionated TBI ($P < .03$). Girls showed the same (nonsignificant) trend.

Few studies of neuropsychiatric testing of patients treated after TBI exist. One might expect lower cumulative doses to be associated with less impairment, but data are lacking. In a report from Kaleita et al., four patients, all younger than 2 years of age at the time of TBI, were found to have normal intellectual, language, and perceptual motor development 2 to 6 years later (85). Likewise, Kramer et al., in a series of 15 children (mean age 3 years), found no decrements in psychologic functioning at 1 year follow-up after TBI (86). In a more recent prospective study, 67 children were evaluated at baseline prior to BMT and at 1-year follow-up. Although IQ at 1-year follow-up was significantly lower than baseline, no further changes were evident at the 3 year follow-up evaluation (86). In contrast, Smedler reported a pronounced delay in motor development in the younger TBI patients compared to older patients (86a). In a series of 68 children, McGuire followed IQ and correlated age at irradiation, dose, and years since first irradiation with decreased Wechsler Intelligence Scale (86a).

The incidence of second tumors after BMT is low. Seattle reported 4 in 1800 patients (38). At the University of Minnesota, 53 second malignant neoplasms developed among 2150 patients for an estimated risk of 9.9% at 13 years after transplantation. Second neoplasms were more common in patients likely to have GVHD (88).

References

1. Gatti R, Meuwissen H, Hong R, et al. Immunological reconstitution of sex-linked lymphopenic immunological deficiency. Lancet 1968; 2:1366.
2. Marmont AM. Stem cell transplantation for severe autoimmune disorders, with special reference to rheumatic diseases. Journal of Rheumatology (Suppl) 1997;48:13–18.
3. Krivit W, Lockman LA, Watkins PA, et al. The future for treatment by bone marrow transplantation for adrenoleukodystrophy, metachromatic leukodystrophy, globoid cell leukodystrophy and Hurler syndrome. Journal of Inherited Metabolic Disease 1995;18:398–412.
4. Peters C, Balthazor M, Shapiro EG, et al. Outcome of unrelated donor bone marrow transplantation in 40 children with Hurler syndrome. Blood 1996;87:4894–4902.
5. Fabrega S, Laporte JP, Giarratana MC, et al. Polymerase chain reaction: a method for monitoring cell purge by long-term culture in BCR/ABL positive lymphoblastic leukemia. Bone Marrow Transplant 1993; 11:169–173.

6. Matthay KK, O'Leary MC, Ramsay NK, et al. Role of myeloablative therapy in improved outcome for high risk neuroblastoma: review of recent Children's Cancer Group results. Eur J Cancer 1995;31A(4): 572–575.
7. Katsanis E, Xu Z, Panoskaltsis MA, et al. IL-15 administration following syngeneic bone marrow transplantation prolongs survival of lymphoma bearing mice. Transplantation 1996;62:872–875.
8. Roy J, Blazar BR, Ochs L, et al. The tissue expression of cytokines in human acute cutaneous graft-versus-host disease [published erratum appears in Transplantation 1996 Jan 27;61(2):341]. Transplantation 1995;60:343–348.
9. Hansen JA, Beatty PG, Clift RA. The HLA system in clinical bone marrow transplantation. Advances in immunobiology: blood cell antigens and bone marrow transplantation. McDullough J, Sandler SG, eds. New York: Alan R. Liss, Inc., 1984;299–317.
10. Beatty PG, Kollman C, Howe CW. Unrelated-donor marrow transplants: the experience of the National Marrow Donor Program. Clinical Transplants 1995:271–277.
11. Wagner JE, Kurtzberg J. Cord blood stem cells. Current Opinion in Hematology 1997;4:413–418.
12. Almici C, Carlo SC, Wagner JE, et al. Umbilical cord blood as a source of hematopoietic stem cells: from research to clinical application. Haematologica 1995;80:473–479.
13. Champlin R, Ho WG, Mitsuyasu R, et al. Graft failure and leukemia relapse following T. lymphocyte depleted bone marrow transplantation: effect of intensification of immunosuppressive conditioning. Transplant Proc, 1987;19:2616–2619.
14. Frickhofen N, Korbling M, Fliedner TM. Is blood a better source of allogeneic hematopoietic stem cells for use after radiation accidents? Bone Marrow Transplantation 1996;17:131–135.
15. Ottinger HD, Beelen DW, Scheulen B, et al. Improved immune reconstitution after allotransplantation of peripheral blood stem cells instead of bone marrow. Blood 1996;88:2775–2779.
16. Remes K, Rajamaki A. Autologous stem cell transplantations [editorial]. Ann Med 1996;28:79–81.
17. Weisdorf DJ. Bone marrow transplantation for acute lymphocytic leukemia (ALL). Leukemia 1997;11(Suppl 4):S20–22.
18. Enright H, Daniels K, Arthur DC, et al. Related donor marrow transplant for chronic myeloid leukemia: patient characteristics predictive of outcome. Bone Marrow Transplant 1996;17:537–542.
19. Kim TH, McGlace PB, Ramsay N, et al. Comparison of two total body irradiation regimens in allogeneic bone marrow transplantation for acute non-lymphoblastic leukemia in first remission. Int J Radiat Oncol Biol Phys 1990;9:889–897.
20. Davies SM, Wagner JE, Weisdorf DJ, et al. Unrelated donor bone marrow transplantation for hematological malignancies—current status. Leuk Lymphoma 1996;23:221–226.
21. Davies SM, Ramsay NK, Weisdorf DJ. Feasibility and timing of unrelated donor identification for patients with ALL. Bone Marrow Transplant 1996;17:737–740.
22. Davies SM, Wagner JE, Defor T, et al. Unrelated donor bone marrow transplantation for children and adolescents with aplastic anemia or myelodysplasia. Br J Haematol 1997;96:749–756.
23. Wagner JE, Rosenthal J, Sweetman R, et al. Successful transplantation of HLA-matched and HLA-mismatched umbilical cord blood from unrelated donors: analysis of engraftment and acute graft-versus-host disease. Blood 1996;88:795–802.
24. Weisdorf DJ, Billett AL, Hannan P, et al. Autologous versus unrelated donor allogeneic marrow transplantation for acute lymphoblastic leukemia. Blood 1997;90:2962–2968.
25. Kersey J, Weisdorf D, Nesbit M, et al. Comparison of autologous and allogenic bone marrow transplantation for treatment of high risk refractory ALL. N Engl J Med 1987;317:461.
26. Thomas E, Lochte H, Cannon J. Supralethal whole body irradiation and isologous marrow transplantation in man. J Clin Invest 1959;38: 1709.
27. Weisdorf DJ, Verfaille CM, Miller WJ, et al. Autologous bone marrow versus non-mobilized peripheral blood stem cell transplantation for lymphoid malignancies: a prospective, comparative trial. Am J Hematol 1997;54:202–208.
28. Matthay KK, O'Leary MC, Ramsay NK, et al. Role of myeloablative therapy in improved outcome for high risk neuroblastoma: review of recent Children's Cancer Group results. Eur J Cancer, 1995;31A(4): 572–575.
29. Bhatia R, Verfaillie CM, Miller JS, et al. Autologous transplantation therapy for chronic myelogenous leukemia. Blood 1997;89: 2623–2634.
30. Ringden O, Labopin M, Tura S, et al. A comparison of busulphan versus total body irradiation combined with cyclophosphamide as conditioning for autograft or allograft bone marrow transplantation in patients with acute leukemia. Acute Leukemia Working Party of the European Group for Blood and Marrow Transplantation (EBMT). Br J Hematol 1996;93:637–645.
31. Bostrom B, Blazar B. Role of busulfan pharmacokinetics on outcome after bone marrow transplantation for acute myelogenous leukemia. Blood 1992;80:2947–2948.
32. Thomas E, Lochte H, Lu W, Ferrebee J. Intravenous infusion of bone marrow in patients receiving radiation and chemotherapy. N Engl J Med 1957;257:491.
33. Valls A, Granena A, Carreras E, et al. Total body irradiation in bone marrow transplantation: fractionated vs. single dose. Acute toxicity and preliminary results. Bull Cancer 1989;76:797–804.
34. Cosset JM, Baume D, Pico JL, et al. Single dose vs. hyperfractionated total body irradiation before allogeneic bone marrow transplantation: a nonrandomized comparative study of 54 patients at the Institut Gustave Roussy. Radiother Oncol 1989;15:151–160.
35. Fyles GM, Messner HA, Lockwood G, et al. Long term results of bone marrow transplantation for patients with AML, ALL and CML prepared with single dose total body irradiation of 500 cGy delivered with a high dose rate. Bone Marrow Transplant 1991;8:453–463.
36. Weiner RS, Bortin NM, Gale RP, et al. Interstitial pneumonitis after bone marrow transplantation. Ann Intern Med 1986;104:168–175.
37. Deeg JH, Sullivan KM, Buckner CD, et al. Marrow transplantation for acute non lymphoblastic leukemia in first remission: toxicity and long-term body irradiation. Bone Marrow Transplant 1986;1: 151–157.
38. Ozsahin M, Pene F, Touboul E, et al. Total-body irradiation before bone marrow transplantation. Results of two randomized instantaneous dose rates in 157 patients. Cancer 1992;69:2853–2865.
39. Patterson J, Prentice HG, Brenner MK, et al. Graft rejection following HLA matched T. lymphocyte depleted bone marrow transplantation. Br J Haematol 1986;63:221–230.
40. Guyotat D, Dutou L, Ehrsam A, et al. Graft rejection after T-cell depleted marrow transplantation: role of fractionated irradiation. Br J Haematol 1987;65:499–507.
41. Martin PJ, Hansen JA, Buckner CD, et al. Effects on in vitro depletion of T-cell in HLA identical allogeneic marrow grafts. Blood 1985;66: 664–672.
42. Burnett AK, Hann IM, Robertson RG, et al. Prevention of graft vs. host disease by ex vivo T cell depletion: reduction in graft failure with augmented total body irradiation. Leukemia 1988;2:300–303.
43. Iriondo A, Hermosa V, Richard C, et al. Graft rejection following T lymphocyte depleted bone marrow transplantation with two different TBI regimens. Br J Haematol 1987;65:246–248.
44. Pino y Torres J, Martinez F, Gomez P, et al. Allogeneic bone marrow transplantation versus chemotherapy in the treatment of childhood acute lymphoblastic leukemia in second complete remission. Bone Marrow Transplant 1989;4:609–612.
45. Meyers JD, Flournoy N, Wade JC, et al. Biology of interstitial pneumonia after marrow transplantation. In: Gale R, ed. Recent advances in bone marrow transplantation. New York: Alan R. Liss, 1983;405–423.
46. Shank B, Chu FCH, Dinsmore R, et al. Hyperfractionated total body irradiation for bone marrow transplantation. Results in seventy leukemia patients with allogeneic transplants. Int J Radiat Oncol Biol Phys 1983;9:1607–1611.
47. Bluem KG, Forman SJ, Synder DS, et al. Allogeneic bone marrow transplantation for acute lymphoblastic leukemia during first complete remission. Transplantation 1987;43:389–392.
48. Cosset JM, Socie G, Dubray B, et al. Single dose versus fractionated total body irradiation before bone marrow transplantation: radiobiological and clinical considerations. Int J Radiat Oncol Biol Phys 1994; 30:477–492.
49. Socie G, Devergie A, Girinsky T, et al. Influence of the fractionation of total body irradiation on complications and relapse rate for chronic myelogenous leukemia. The Groupe d'Etude des greffes de moelle osseuse (GEGMO). Int J Radiat Oncol Biol Phys 1991;20:397–404.
50. Vitale V, Bacigalupo A, VanLint MT. Fractionated total body irradiation in marrow transplantation. Br J Hematol 1983;55:547–554.

51. Hartsell WF, Czyzewski EA, Ghalie R, et al. Pulmonary complications of bone marrow transplantation: a comparison of total body irradiation and cyclophosphamide to busulfan and cyclophosphamide. Int J Radiat Oncol Biol Phys 1995;32:69–73.
52. Stewart F, Crittenden R, Lowry P, et al. Long-term engraftment of normal and post-5 fluorouracil murine marrow into normal non-myeloablated mice. Blood 1993;81:2566.
53. Pino y Torres JL, Bross DS, Lam WC, et al. Risk factors in interstitial pneumonitis following allogeneic bone marrow transplantation. Int J Radiat Oncol Biol Phys 1982;8:1301–1307.
54. Cohen EP, Lawton CA, Moulder JE. Bone marrow transplant nephropathy: radiation nephritis revisited. Nephron 1995;70:217–222.
55. Storb R. Graft-versus-host disease and survival in patients with aplastic anemia treated by marrow grafts from HLA-identical siblings. N Engl J Med 1983;308:302.
56. Lawton CA, Barber-Derus SW, Murray KJ, et al. Influence of renal shielding on the incidence of late renal dysfunction associated with T-lymphocyte depleted bone marrow transplantation in adult patients. Int J Radiat Oncol Biol Phys 1992;23:681–686.
57. Kumar M, Kedar A, Neiberger RE. Kidney function in long-term pediatric survivors of acute lymphoblastic leukemia following allogeneic bone marrow transplantation. Pediatr Hematol Oncol 1996;13: 375–379.
58. Leblond V, Sutton L, Jacquiaud C, et al. Evaluation of renal function in 60 long-term survivors of bone marrow transplantation. J Am Soc Nephrol 1995;6:1661–1665.
59. Miralbell R, Bieri S, Mermillod B, et al. Renal toxicity after allogeneic bone marrow transplantation: the combined effects of total-body irradiation and graft-versus-host disease. J Clin Oncol 1996;14:579–585.
60. Patzer L, Hempel L, Ringelmann F, et al. Renal function after conditioning therapy for bone marrow transplantation in childhood. Med Pediatr Oncol 1997;28:274–283.
61. Miralbell R, Chapuis B, Nouet P, et al. Conditioning the leukemic patient before allogeneic value of intensifying immunosuppression in the context different levels of T lymphocyte depletion of the graft. Bone Marrow Transplant 1993;11:447–451.
62. Krivit W, Sung JH, Shapiro EG, et al. Microglia: the effector cell for reconstitution of the central nervous system following bone marrow transplantation for lysosomal and peroxisomal storage diseases. Cell Transplant 1995;4:385–392.
63. Wu D, Keating A. Hematopoietic stem cells engraft in untreated transplant recipients. Exp Hematol 1993;21:251.
64. Quine W. The remedial application of bone marrow. JAMA 1986;26: 1026.
65. Cunningham JR, Wright DJ. A simple facility for whole-body irradiation. Radiol 1962;78:941–949.
66. Davis HP, Revell P, Giangrande P, et al. Safe application of a 13-Gy split dose total body irradiation schedule prior to bone marrow transplantation. Bone Marrow Transplant 1988;3:349.
67. Glasgow GP, Mill WB. Cobalt-60 total body irradiation dosimetry at 220 cm source-axis distance. Int J Radiat Oncol Biol Phys 1980;6: 773–777.
68. Khan FM, Williamson JE, Sewchand W, et al. Basic data for dosage calculation and compensation. Int J Radiat Oncol Biol Phys 1980;6: 745.
69. Pla M, Chenery SG, Podgorsak EB. Total body irradiation with a sweeping beam. Int J Radiat Oncol Biol Phys 1983;9:83–89.
70. Quast U. Physical treatment planning of total body irradiation—patient translation and beam zone method. Med Phys 1985;12:567–573.
71. Sahler OD. Development of a room specifically designed for total body irradiation. Radiology 1959;72:266–267.
72. Khan FM, Kim TH. Total body irradiation. In Syllabus: a categorical course in radiation therapy treatment planning. 72nd Scientific Assembly and Annual Meeting of the Radiological Society of North America.
73. Van Dyk J, Keane TJ, Rider WD. Lung density as measured by computerized tomography: implications for radiotherapy. Int J Radiat Oncol Biol Phys 1982;8:1363.
74. Hall EJ, Oliver R. The use of standard isodose distribution with high energy radiation beams—the accuracy of a compensation technique in correcting for body contours. Br J Radiol 1961;34:43.
75. Khan FM, Moore VC, Burns DJ. The construction of compensators for cobalt teletherapy. Radiology 1970;96:187.
76. Kirby TH, Hanson WF, Cates DA. Verification of total body photon irradiation dosimetry techniques. Med Phys 1988;15:364.
77. American Association of Physicists in Medicine (Task Group 2). The physical aspects of total and half body photon irradiation. AAPM Report No. 17. American Association of Physicists in Medicine, 1986.
78. American Association of Physicists in Medicine (Task Group 2). A protocol for the determination of absorbed dose from high-energy photon and electron beams. American Association of Physicists in Medicine, 1983.
79. McDowall RH, Scher CS, Barst SM. Total intravenous anesthesia for children undergoing brief diagnostic or therapeutic procedures. J Clin Anesthesia 1995;7:273–280.
80. Scheiber G, Ribeiro FC, Karpienski H, et al. Deep sedation with propofol in preschool children undergoing radiation therapy [see comments]. Paediatric Anaesthesia 1996;6:209–213.
81. Kader HA, Khanna S, Hutchinson RM, et al. Pulmonary complications of bone marrow: the impact of variations in total body irradiation parameters. Clin Oncol (R Coll Radiol) 1994;6:96–101.
82. Breuer R, Or R, Lijovetzky G, et al. Interstitial pneumonitis in T cell-depleted bone marrow transplantation. Bone Marrow Transplant 1988;3(6):625–630.
83. Teschler H, Quabeck K, Schafer UW, et al. Pulmonary complications after bone marrow. Pneumologie 1994;48:131–139.
84. Sanders JE, Ritchards S, Mahonet P. Growth and development following marrow transplantation for leukemia. Blood 1986;68:1129–1135.
85. Kaleita TA, Shields W, Tesle RA, et al. Normal neurodevelopment in four young children treated with bone marrow transplantation for acute leukemia or aplastic anemia. Pediatrics 1989;83:753–757.
86. Kramer JH, Crittenden MR, DeSantes K, et al. Cognitive and adaptive behavior 1 and 3 years following bone marrow transplantation. Bone Marrow Transplant 1997;19:607–613.
86a. Smedler AC, Bergman H, Holme P. Neuropsycological functioning in children treated with bone marrow transplantation. J Clin Exp Neuropsycol 1988;325–326. Abstract.
87. McGuire DB, Altomonte V, Peterson DE, et al. Patterns of mucositis and pain in patients receiving preparative chemotherapy and bone marrow transplantation. Oncol Nurs Forum 1993;20:1493–1502.
88. Thomas E. The use and potential of bone marrow allograft and whole-body irradiation in the treatment of leukemia. Cancer 1982; 50:1449.

Chapter 29

Hodgkin's Disease

Chung Kyu Kim Lee

Since 1950, we have witnessed a remarkable expansion in our knowledge of the nature, management, and prognosis of malignant lymphoma. Improved clinical outcome is a direct reflection of our better understanding of the fundamental biologic mechanisms and treatment of the disease. Hodgkin's disease is currently one of the most successfully treated malignancies with survival rates of 80 to 90%. Advances in staging coupled with improved radiation therapy techniques and refinements in combination chemotherapy have played a large role in this success story. This chapter will focus on the role of radiotherapy in the treatment of Hodgkin's disease with emphasis on modern radiation therapy techniques. In recent years, radiotherapy of Hodgkin's disease has become individually tailored to achieve a balance of the best clinical outcomes with the least long-term complications.

DIAGNOSTIC EVALUATION AND STAGING

Careful assessment and evaluation of staging and various other prognostic factors during workup is essential to a successful treatment plan. Important factors include stage, histopathology, age, performance status, gender, bulk of disease, number and location of involved sites, and significant laboratory tests.

A complete history and physical examination of the patient should be performed to detect any B symptoms, such as fever, night sweats, and greater than 10% weight loss during the previous 6 months. Other important symptoms to note are alcohol intolerance, pruritus, fatigue, and respiratory problems. Physical examination should be thorough and all accessible nodal sites must be evaluated, including tonsilar and other lymphoid tissue containing sites. Evaluation of the oral cavity including a dental examination by an experienced oral surgeon is essential. If any dental problems exist, they must be evaluated and repaired. This is especially important to any patient who may undergo radiation therapy to a field that includes the oral cavity. Initial laboratory work should include a complete differential blood count, erythrocyte sedimentation rate, serum electrolytes, liver and renal function tests, serum alkaline phosphatase, and β_2-lactate dehydrogenase. Optional blood tests include serum copper, microglobulin, and various cell surface cytogenetic analyses (1–4).

Radiologic studies are critical to identifying the extent of disease and should include a chest x-ray, computed tomography (CT) scans of the chest, abdomen, and pelvis, bipedal lymphogram, gallium-67 scan, and magnetic resonance imaging (MRI) scans. Over 60% of Hodgkin's disease patients present with initial radiographic evidence of intrathoracic disease. However, in some patients the extent of disease as determined by CT is far greater than suspected by routine radiography. Certain blind areas on routine radiography may be very important in designing radiotherapy fields, including the cardiophrenic and retrocrural nodes at the diaphragm. Pleural based masses may also be difficult to detect in the standard two-projection images obtained on routine radiography. In addition, CT scans are able to detect small, unsuspected masses, evaluate the full extent of large masses, and detect involvement of the lung parenchyma (5,6).

The extent of mediastinal disease is important in quantifying the potential for intrathoracic relapse. Patients with large mediastinal masses have a poor prognosis with higher relapses, especially in the intrathoracic area and in the transnodal sites. There are several ways to define a large mediastinal mass. At the University of Minnesota, a large mass is defined as a mass with an MT ratio of greater than 0.35. The MT ratio is defined as the largest transverse diameter of the mediastinal mass divided by the transverse diameter of the thorax at the level of T5-6 (7) (Figure 29.1). Most institutions arbitrarily define a large mediastinal mass

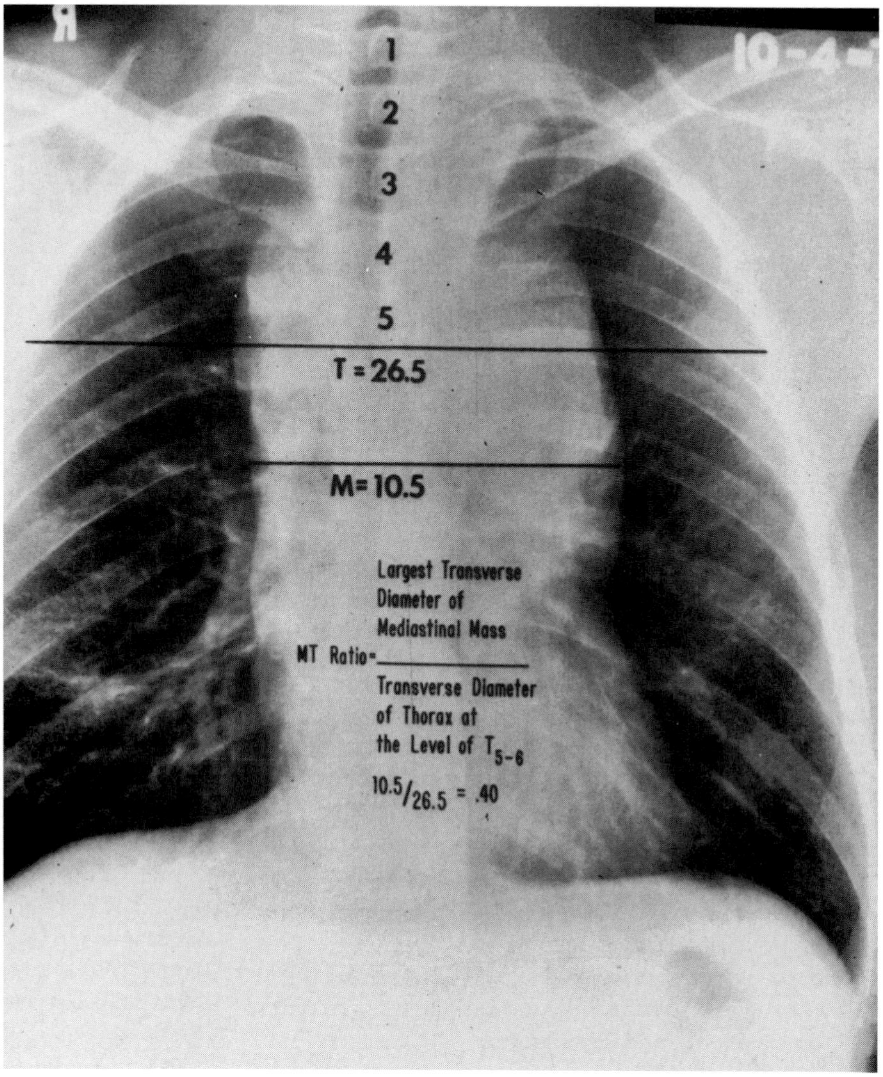

Figure 29.1. The MT ratio is determined by measuring the mediastinal mass on the PA chest film (Definition used at the University of Minnesota). (CANCER [Vol. 46, 1980], 2403–2409. Copyright © (1980) American Cancer Society. Reprinted by permission of Wiley-Liss, Inc., a subsidiary of John Wiley & Sons, Inc.)

as a mass whose greatest diameter is greater than one-third of the largest diameter of the thorax at the diaphragm on an upright posteroanterior chest radiograph (8). Others have used the transverse diameter of the mass and defined a large mass as 5 to 10 cm in size.

The greatest imaging challenge is the detection of disease in the abdominal and pelvic areas. An abdominal and pelvic CT scan may be obtained to evaluate any retroperitoneal, periportal, and celiac lymphadenopathy and involvement of the spleen and liver. However, all imaging studies have limitations with a 20 to 25% false-negative rate. This is primarily due to the inability to detect occult disease in the spleen, which is one of the most common sites of disease below the diaphragm (9,10). Bipedal lymphangiography is rarely practiced in recent years because of diminishing skills in performance and in the interpretation of results. However, it still remains an excellent method to evaluate lymph node size and the internal architecture (11).

The role of ancillary tests, such as MRI, position emission tomography (PET), and gallium scans, is still being defined. Gallium scans may be useful in the assessment of residual masses, especially in the mediastinal area. Its usefulness depends largely on the quality of the study and the site of disease. Higher doses of gallium-67 and better imaging equipment using single photon emission computerized tomography (SPECT) have increased the sensitivity of the tests. There appears to be a high correlation between active disease in a residual mass and a positive gallium scan, although a negative scan does not rule out viable tumor (12). A pretreatment gallium scan is essential in this evaluation as a source for later comparisons. The PET scan is also being explored for similar purposes.

The most precise method of determining abdominal involvement is by surgical staging with laparotomy and splenectomy (9,10). Surgical staging includes inspection, palpation, and biopsy of nodes in the abdomen and pelvis; wedge and needle biopsy of the liver; and the placement of

Table 29.1. Diagnostic and Staging Procedures

Mandatory
- Biopsy of any mass or lymph nodes

History
- Age and gender
- Evaluation of systemic B symptoms: unexplained fever, night sweats, weight loss >10% of body weight in the last 6 months
- Other symptoms: alcohol intolerance, pruritus, respiratory problems, easily fatigued

Physical examination
- Lymphadenopathy (note number, size, location, shape, consistency, and mobility of nodes)
- Palpable liver, spleen, and other masses

Laboratory studies
- Standard
  - Complete blood count
  - Platelet count
  - Liver and renal function
  - Blood chemistries
  - Erythrocyte sedimentation rate
- Optional
  - Serum copper
  - β_2 microglobulin

Radiographic studies
- Standard
  - Chest radiograph: PA and lateral
  - Thoracic computerized tomography (CT)
  - Abdominal and pelvic computerized tomography
- Optional
  - Bipedal lymphogram
  - Gallium scan-67 (with high dose SPECT)
  - Technicium-99 bone scan, magnetic resonance imaging echocardiography

Special tests
- Standard
  - Cytologic examination of effusions, if present
  - Bone marrow, needle biopsy (especially subdiaphragmatic disease of B symptoms)
- Optional
  - Percutaneous or CT-guided liver biopsy
  - Peritoneoscopy
  - Staging laparotomy with splenectomy, liver biopsy, selected lymph node biopsies, and open bone marrow biopsy

(Modified from Hoppe RT. Hodgkin's Disease. In: Perez CA, Brady LW. Principles and Practice of Radiation Oncology. 3rd ed. Philadelphia: Lippincott–Raven Publishers, 1997:1964.)

splenic pedicle clips. Premenopausal women also usually undergo a bilateral midline oophoropexy in anticipation of pelvic irradiation. Staging laparotomy allows for the selection of early stage patients who can be treated with radiation alone and has helped identify the selective criteria for determining a low incidence of abdominal disease. These criteria include clinical Stage (CS) I_A and II_A female patients, patients younger than 26 years of age, and CS IA male patients with lymphocyte predominance (LP) histology.

Routine staging laparotomy in Hodgkin's disease also has resulted in better understanding of the natural evolution of the disease. The disease appears to spread contiguously to adjacent lymph nodes first and extends frequently to the spleen during the early course of disease before spreading to other visceral organs such as the liver. In 20 to 30% of CS IA-IIA patients and 35% of CS IB—IIB patients, occult splenic or upper abdominal disease may be identified at staging laparotomy that was not detected on presurgical clinical staging studies (9–15). By removing the spleen during staging laparotomy, the volume of irradiation is reduced significantly and radiation to the left kidney can be avoided. In patients with negative laparotomy and other favorable prognostic factors, the radiation field can be confined to above the diaphragm (16–20). Table 29.1 summarizes the procedures recommended for proper workup and staging of Hodgkin's disease.

Staging laparotomy is associated with potential morbidity and mortality. Small bowel obstruction, development of wound or subdiaphragmatic abscess, and postoperative bleeding are the major complications but are as low as 3% (21). Following splenectomy, patients are also at increased risk for infection with encapsulated bacteria (22,23). Vaccinations against pneumococcus and meningococcus or prophylactic antibiotics should be used to decrease risk. An approximately twofold increased risk of leukemia following splenectomy has been reported in some studies, especially in those who had received chemotherapy following splenectomy (24). However, the mechanisms for this finding are poorly understood, and the increase is not recognized by all observers.

Table 29.2. Hodgkin's Disease Staging Classification[a]

Stage	Definition
I	Involvement of a single lymph node region (I) or of a single extralymphatic organ (I_E)
II	Involvement of two or more lymphatic regions on the same side of the diaphragm (II), or localized extralymphatic involvement as well as involvement of one or more regional lymphatic sites on the same side of the diaphragm
III	Involvement of lymphatic regions on both sides of the diaphragm (III); such involvement may include splenic involvement (III_S), localized extra lymphatic disease (III_E), or both (III_{SE})
IV	Diffuse or disseminated involvement of one or more extralymphatic organs or tissues, with or without nodal involvement
	The absence or presence of unexplained fever, night sweats, or loss of 10% or more of body weight in the 6 months preceding diagnosis are designated by the suffix letters A or B, respectively. Biopsy-proven involvement of extralymphatic sites is designated by letter suffixes: bone marrow, M+; lung, L+; liver, H+; pleura, P+; bone, O+; skin and subcutaneous tissue, D+

[a] Adopted at the workshop on the staging of Hodgkin's disease held at Ann Arbor, MI in April, 1971. (Reprinted with permission from Carbone PP, et al. Report of the Comittee on Hodgkin's disease. Cancer Res. 1971;31:1860.)

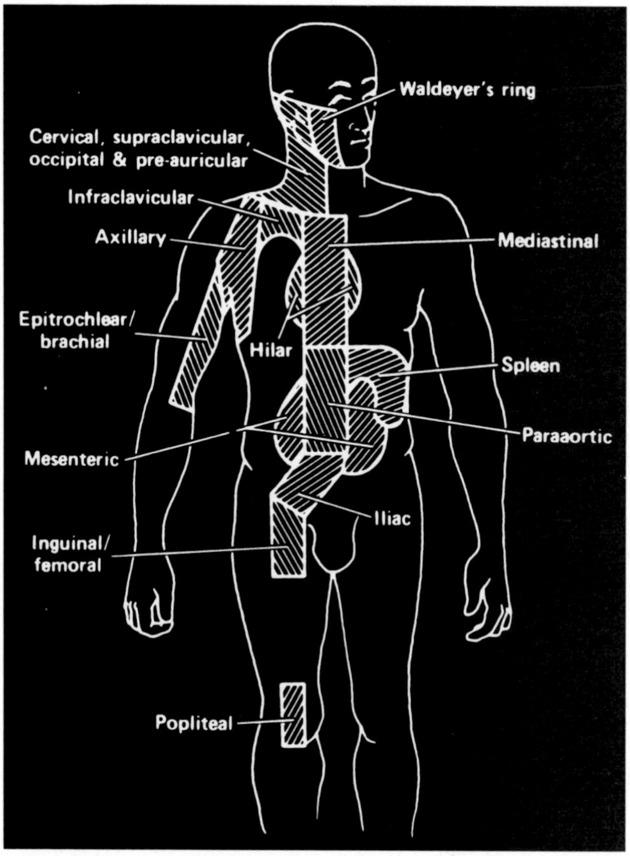

Figure 29.2. Clinical lymphoid regions as defined by the Ann Arbor Staging System.

Table 29.3. Cotswold Modifications to Ann Arbor Staging Classification

(i)	Suffix "X" to designate bulky disease as >⅓ widening of the mediastinum or >10 cm maximum dimension of nodal mass.
(ii)	The number of anatomical regions involved should be indicated by a subscript (e.g., II_3).
(iii)	Stage III may be subdivided into: III_1: with or without splenic, hilar, celiac, or portal nodes III_2: with para-aortic, iliac, mesenteric nodes
(iv)	Staging should be identified as clinical stage (CS) or pathologic stage (PS).
(v)	A new category of response to therapy, unconfirmed/uncertain complete remission ($CR_{(U)}$) be introduced because of the persistent radiologic abnormalities of uncertain significance.

(From CA-A Cancer Journal for Clinicians. 1993;43:333.)

In 1971, the Ann Arbor classification for Hodgkin's disease was established (25) (Table 29.2). This staging system was used for over 2 decades for both clinical and pathologic staging of Hodgkin's and non-Hodgkin's lymphoma. However, inadequacies to the Ann Arbor staging system, including failure to account for bulk and extent of disease and to precisely define extralymphatic involvement, led to a modified classification system proposed at a 1989 international meeting at Cotswolds, England. The new classification relied on anatomic regions based on the knowledge that Hodgkin's disease spreads along the lymphatic channel in an orderly fashion (Figure 29.2). The modifications incorporated some important prognostic factors, such as bulk of disease and a more precise definition of extralymphatic involvement (26) (Table 29.3).

HISTOPATHOLOGIC CLASSIFICATION

There are four histologic subtypes of Hodgkin's disease as defined by the Rye modification of Lukes and Butler system: 1) Lymphocyte predominance (LP), 2) Nodular sclerosis (NS), 3) Mixed cellularity (MC), and 4) Lymphocyte depletion (LD) Hodgkin's disease (27).

Lymphocyte predominance Hodgkin's disease comprises 5 to 10% of all Hodgkin's disease and is often localized to a single peripheral nodal region. Only 8% of these patients have mediastinal and abdominal involvement in early stage disease (28). This subtype is found most often in male patients younger than 15 years of age or older than 40. It contains an abundance of benign-appearing cells and frequent variant lymphocytic and histiocytic cells with multilobulated nuclei (popcorn cells). Some investigators have proposed classifying nodular LP histology as a separate clinically and histologically distinct entity (29).

Nodular sclerosis Hodgkin's disease is the most common histology and accounts for 40 to 60% of all cases. It usually affects patients between the age of 15 and 40, and affects males and females equally. It presents with central nodal regional involvement in 80 to 90% of cases (27).

Approximately 25% of Hodgkin's disease cases have MC histology. Patients with MC Hodgkin's disease are older and more likely to present with systemic symptoms and advanced stages with malignant Reed-Sternberg cells and pleomorphic variant cells in an inflammatory background (30).

Only 5% of Hodgkin's disease patients have LD histology. Generally these patients have advanced stage disease with systemic symptoms (31).

In addition to the above four major subtypes of histopathology, interfollicular Hodgkin's disease presents with an uncommon pattern of focal involvement of a lymph node in the interfollicular zone. It may be easily confused with reactive hyperplasia (32).

GENERAL TREATMENT CONSIDERATIONS

The aim of Hodgkin's disease treatment is to treat all involved and potentially involved lymphatic chains with adequate dose levels in order to increase the probability of tumor eradication. Treatment is guided by the stage and prognostic factors for each patient. A suggested schematic model for management of Hodgkin's disease is shown in Figure 29.3.

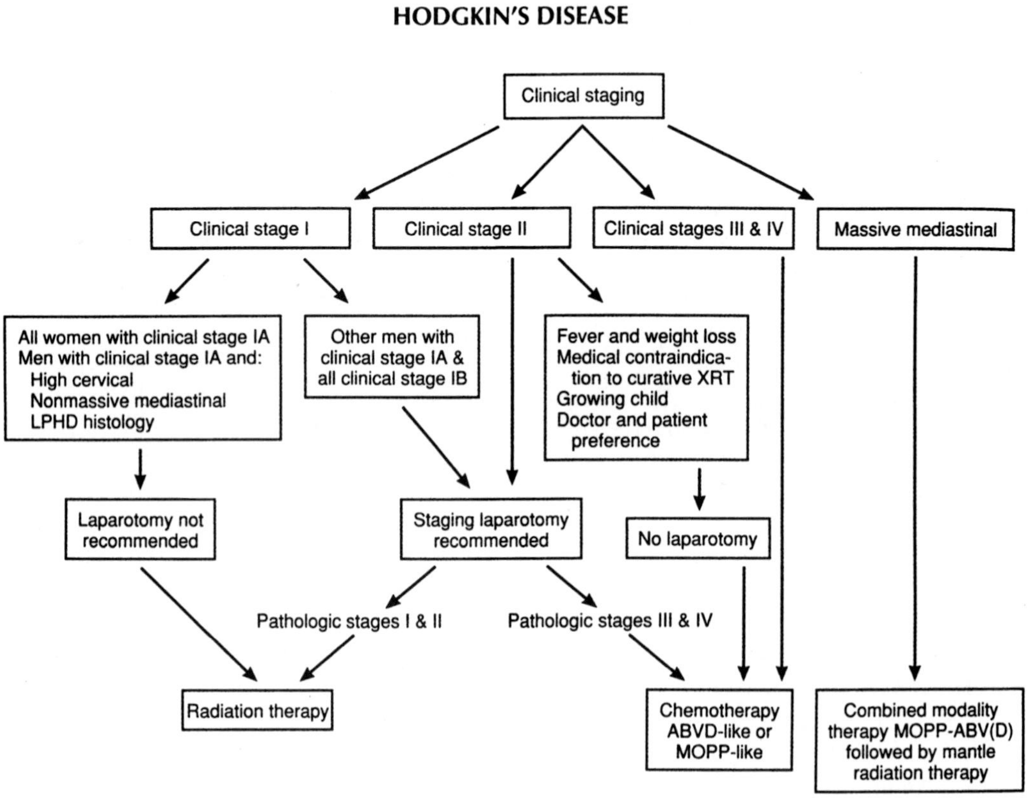

Figure 29.3. Suggested schematic tree for treatment decision making for Hodgkin's disease.

Radiation Therapy Alone

Radiation therapy alone, either by mantle field or extended field (mantle and para-aortic) and spleen, is generally used to treat Stage I and II_A patients who have the most favorable prognostic factors. Prognostic factors reported to be significant are stage of disease, large mediastinal mass with or without hilar disease, bulky disease, systemic symptoms, four or more sites of involvement, male gender, advanced age, elevated sedimentation rate, and poor histologic classification of lymphocytic depletion and mixed cellularity (1,8,33–39). Lymphocyte depletion and MC histology are often associated with other adverse prognostic factors such as older age and advanced stage patients with systemic symptoms.

In general, patients with pathologic Stage I or II_A supradiaphragmatic disease are treated effectively with sequential treatment to the mantle and para-aortic fields with expected long-term relapse-free rate of 75 to 80%. If laparotomy has not been performed, the entire spleen should be included in the radiation field. If the laparotomy is performed and is negative, patients who have certain favorable characteristics (lymphocyte predominance or nodular sclerosing histology, age under 40 years, and erythrocyte sedimentation rate (ESR) under 70) may be treated safely and effectively with only a mantle field (8). The remaining patients are treated with mantle fields, para-aortic, and splenic pedicle irradiation.

In patients that are staged by laparotomy and treated with radiation therapy, several large series have reported a 10-year survival rate of nearly 90% and 10-year relapse-free survival rate of 75 to 80% (33,38,44–46). Most relapses occur within the first 3 years after completing therapy, though late relapses of more than 3 years after remission induced by irradiation can occur in up to 10% of patients at risk (33). Very late relapses are uncommon. Following subtotal nodal irradiation (mantle and para-aortic fields) about 5 to 15% of patients recurred in the pelvis and inguinofemoral lymph nodes region. Using total nodal irradiation (TNI) does not improve these survival rates. This excellent overall survival relates to the high cure rate with primary radiation therapy and salvage combination chemotherapy (33).

In the past, the standard approach of most centers in the United States was to require pathologic staging of Hodgkin's disease prior to recommending radiotherapy alone. However, both Canadian and European studies have shown excellent overall survival for patients who were selected for radiotherapy alone based simply on clinical prognostic factors. Therefore, clinically staged patients with favorable prognostic factors may be treated with radiation alone. The following subgroups have less than 10%

risk of abdominal involvement: clinical Stage I females (6%); patients with involvement of the mediastinum alone (0%), Stage I males with lymphocyte-predominant histology (4%), young (less than 27 years) females with limited (three or less supradiaphragmatic sites) Stage II disease (9%) (35).

Influence of pathologic staging (PS) and clinical staging (CS) on the outcome of Stage I and II HD patients following radiotherapy has been studied by the European Organization for Research and Treatment of Cancer (EORTC) lymphoma cooperative group (H2 study). Both groups were treated with extended field irradiation with the spleen being included in clinically staged patients. At 10 years, there was no difference in recurrence-free survival (CS 68% versus PS 76%), however a higher number of patients with positive findings at laparotomy relapsed compared with those with negative laparotomy (56% versus 83%, $P<.001$) (1).

Treatment for Stage I and II subdiaphragmatic Hodgkin's disease is less well studied. Approximately 10% of these patients present with disease limited to the subdiaphragmatic area. The prognosis of patients with para-aortic lymph node involvement (Stage II) is probably worse than those with a single site of peripheral nodal disease (Stage I). These patients are more likely to present with B symptoms, mixed cellularity, or lymphocytic depleted histology. Staging laparotomy is recommended if the patient is going to be treated with radiation. Pathologic Stage I patients can be treated with an inverted "Y" only (43–46).

Randomized trials conducted to define the proper fields for early stage Hodgkin's disease have shown better relapse-free survival for patients treated with extended field radiotherapy compared to involved field radiotherapy (47–49). Results of mantle or limited irradiation alone in early stage Hodgkin's disease have been disappointing with increasing risk of relapse in the abdomen unless patients present with favorable prognostic factors (35). Furthermore, careful evaluation of the abdomen after completion of treatment can be difficult. Recent clinical trials have suggested using prognostic factors to determine treatment modalities for clinically Staged I and II patients. While radiation alone (including spleen) is recommended for patients with favorable prognostic factors, combined modality treatments are suggested for patients with nonfavorable prognostic factors.

Combined Modality Therapy

Combined modality therapy (CMT) with chemotherapy and radiation therapy is used to treat patients with less favorable prognostic factors, including massive mediastinal disease, nominal Stage III_A disease (extensive splenic involvement or Stage III_{A2}), and Stage $III_{B\text{-}IV}$ disease. In patients who receive combined modality therapy, special consideration is given to the extent of staging, identification of prognostic factors, sequence of treatment, number of cycles of chemotherapy, volume of radiation port, and total dose of radiation.

In general, patients with early stage disease who receive CMT do not undergo staging laparotomy and the extent of volumes irradiated and the total dose of radiation delivered are less aggressive. However, adequate field size and total dose for these patients have yet to be determined. Several studies have shown comparable outcomes between the use of extended field and involved field irradiation when combined with chemotherapy (50–54). More recent data from a systematic overview of randomized trials of more versus less extensive radiotherapy with or without chemotherapy suggest the use of less extensive radiation fields because of similar survival rates achieved with more intensive treatment (55). More randomized studies are needed to confirm this finding. Similarly, more evidence is needed on the appropriate radiation dose for patients treated primarily with chemotherapy.

Patients with Stage III_A disease are a more complex group of patients to treat and require substage analysis. Stein et al. proposed an anatomic substaging of these patients: Stage III_{1A} and III_{2A}. Stage III_{1A} patients have intra-abdominal disease restricted to the upper abdomen above the renal hilar area. Stage III_{2A} patients have intra-abdominal disease in the lower abdomen and/or pelvis (56). Although a staging laparotomy is essential to identify these groups, the medical community has increasingly resisted performing staging laparotomies, and thus, these subgroups are difficult to identify.

Overall disease-free survival of pathologic Stage IIIA patients is reported to be 40 to 78% with radiation treatment alone (57–60). Stein et al. analyzed 130 patients with pathologic Stage III_A disease and found increased overall disease-free survival rates in the 74 Stage III_{1A} patients with a 5-year disease-free survival rate of 63% and an overall survival rate of 91%, compared to 32% and 56%, respectively, for patients with Stage III_{2A} disease (61,62). These results may justify staging laparotomy to identify the Stage III_{1A} patients who can be treated with radiation alone and with limited radiation fields to avoid possible long-term complications. In contrast, the report from the Joint Center suggests that long-term results of combined modality therapy are superior to the results for patients who were treated by radiation alone on both Stage III_{2A} and pathologic Stage III_{1A} diseases (60).

Other prognostic factors, such as the extent of splenic involvement, have been proposed to help define a subgroup of patients with Stage III_A disease. Low dose liver irradiation has been used for Stage III_{1A} patients with splenic disease with improved results (57,59). Nevertheless, in current clinical practice, any clinical Stage III_A patient with clinical evidence of infradiaphragmatic disease is often treated with combined-modality treatment without undergoing staging laparotomy. Most of the combined mo-

dality treatment studies of these patients report 5-year disease-free survival rates of 80 to 90% (59,60,63). Several small series have reported that additional radiation given to Stage III_A patients may lead to superior complete response rates compared to chemotherapy alone (64–66). Evidence from a recent meta-analysis of trials comparing chemotherapy with or without radiotherapy found that the addition of radiotherapy significantly improved long-term remission in patients with intermediate Stage II-III disease, NS histology, and large mediastinal mass. No benefit was found for Stage IV patients (67).

Since combined modality therapy increases the risk of morbidity, including leukemogenesis, careful consideration of the benefits and morbidity of treatment is essential prior to treatment.

Special Consideration: Large Mediastinal Mass (LMM)

Patients with a large mediastinal mass, which is considered the most universally accepted poor prognostic factor, require special treatment consideration. Although the definition of large or bulky mediastinal disease varies, usually it is defined as a mass measuring greater than one-third of the largest transverse chest diameter (68) or the transverse diameter of the mass at T5-6 level divided by the largest transverse diameter of the chest (44) (Figure 29.1).

In patients treated with mantle field irradiation, the majority of failures occur outside or at the edge of the radiation port in the intrathoracic region (8). This suggests that there are geometric difficulties in treatment volume when trying to shield the lung parenchyma. This problem has led to modifications in radiation treatment techniques, including the concept of low-dose lung irradiation to treat microscopic disease and also to reduce the size of the mass to apply appropriately sized lung shielding. The addition of low dose irradiation (15 to 18 Gy) to whole or hemi-lung fields along with mantle field irradiation has resulted in excellent clinical outcomes (8,43,44,68,69).

With the gain in popularity of chemotherapy in the treatment of HD coupled with the greater risk of relapse experienced after standard mantle field irradiation, the use of combined modality has become more widely accepted in the treatment of large mediastinal mass. The combination of radiotherapy and chemotherapy has lowered the relapse rate but has not significantly increased the overall survival rate because of its increased toxicity (70–72). The best combination of chemotherapy and/or radiation therapy to maximize the response rate and minimize toxicity has not been determined. Chemotherapy should be used initially to treat subclinical disease as well as to decrease the bulk of disease. This may allow for the use of lung blocks that are reasonable and adequately sized. Chemotherapy as the sole treatment for this group of patients frequently fails to achieve complete remission and results in greater relapse than when radiation therapy is used alone (50,71). With the development and improvement of CT-guided treatment planning, selected patients with a bulky mass in the upper mediastinal region can be treated effectively with radiation alone (51,52).

RADIATION THERAPY TECHNIQUES

There has been a gradual evolution in concept and application in the use of radiation therapy to treat Hodgkin's disease since Gilbert proposed "segmental roentgen therapy" in 1939 (73) and Peters proposed "radical radiation" in 1950 (74). Knowledge of the predictable patterns of relapse, the contiguous character of regional lymph node involvement, and the availability of megavoltage beam techniques have led to the development of current techniques and reasonably standardized radiation fields for the treatment of Hodgkin's disease (75). Rosenberg and Kaplan demonstrated in 1966 that in the vast majority of untreated patients with disease limited to lymph nodes only contiguous areas were involved, which proved the orderly progression in which Hodgkin's disease spreads (47).

Widely accepted terms to denote treatment fields—such as mantle, para-aortic, inverted Y field, pelvic field, Waldeyer's ring, preauricular field, spade shape field, extended field (mantle and para-aortic fields), total nodal irradiation (mantle and inverted Y fields), involved field—reflect the variation and growing standardization of these fields. Despite this apparent standardization, differences exist in the actual techniques used by different institutions. An example of the techniques used at the University of Minnesota for extended field and total nodal field with liver irradiation are shown in Figures 29.4 and 29.5. Differences in treatment technique may account for different outcomes reported in the literature. A Pattern of Care survey of 163 treatment facilities found that recurrence significantly correlated with technique (involved field versus extended field), treatment machine (less than 80 cm cobalt-60 [^{60}Co] versus greater than 80 cm ^{60}Co, linear accelerator), simulation, and presence of splenic pedicle clips (76).

One way to ensure quality control in the treatment of Hodgkin's disease is by routine field simulation and frequent film verification to verify that involved tissues are adequately treated and sensitive structures properly shielded. Portal films examined in the Patterns of Care Study demonstrated an increased overall recurrence rate (54% versus 14%, $P<.001$) and an infield or marginal recurrence rate (33% vs 7%, $P<.001$) between patients treated with inadequate margins between the protective lung and cardiac blocks and the tumor and patients treated with adequate margins, respectively.

Long-term follow-up of treated patients also provides important information on outcomes and complications of treatment, which allow for modification of irradiation techniques to improve results. Careful follow-up of patients in

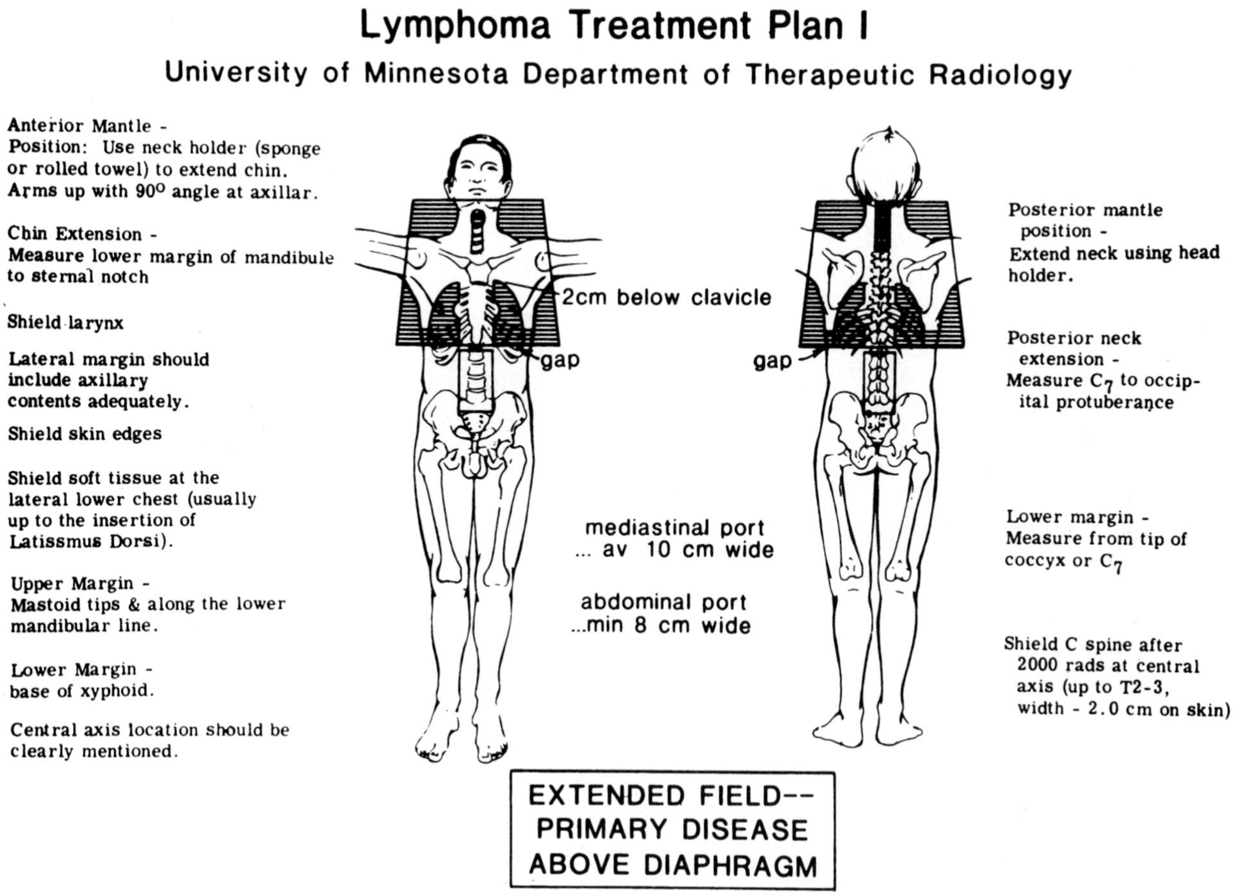
Lymphoma Treatment Plan I
University of Minnesota Department of Therapeutic Radiology
Anterior Mantle -
Position: Use neck holder (sponge or rolled towel) to extend chin.
Arms up with 90° angle at axillar.
Chin Extension -
Measure lower margin of mandibule to sternal notch
Shield larynx
Lateral margin should include axillary contents adequately.
Shield skin edges
Shield soft tissue at the lateral lower chest (usually up to the insertion of Latissmus Dorsi).
Upper Margin -
Mastoid tips & along the lower mandibular line.
Lower Margin -
base of xyphoid.
Central axis location should be clearly mentioned.
2cm below clavicle
gap
gap
mediastinal port
... av 10 cm wide
abdominal port
...min 8 cm wide
Posterior mantle position -
Extend neck using head holder.
Posterior neck extension -
Measure C_7 to occipital protuberance
Lower margin -
Measure from tip of coccyx or C_7
Shield C spine after 2000 rads at central axis (up to T2-3, width - 2.0 cm on skin)
EXTENDED FIELD--
PRIMARY DISEASE
ABOVE DIAPHRAGM

Figure 29.4. View of extended field treatment area, including mantle and para-aortic fields. (University of Minnesota treatment plan.)

large scale clinical trials has permitted a rapid advance in our knowledge and optimal treatment of Hodgkin's disease.

Mantle Fields (Figures 29.6A, 29.6B, and 29.7)

Mantle fields were first used at Stanford in 1956 and since then modifications to mantle fields have been adopted by various institutions. Typical mantle fields will include all the major lymph node bearing areas above the diaphragm, neck, axilla, mediastinal, and occipital preauricular lymph nodes and Waldeyer's ring area. The mantle field is used to treat the major supradiaphragmatic nodal chains that are at a high risk for the involvement of Hodgkin's disease, while maximally shielding the lungs. Preauricular lymph nodes will be treated when there is high neck disease. Optimal design of the mantle field relies on imaging studies. A chest CT scan for patients with significant mediastinal adenopathy provides important information on disease extension to the lung, pericardium, and chest wall as well as internal mammary or pericardial lymph node involvement that may affect field design. Incorporation of the CT scan into treatment planning decisions for patients treated with radiotherapy alone results in treatment field changes in about 15% of patients (33).

Simulation of Mantle Field

The following techniques are used at the University of Minnesota to simulate mantle fields. All patients are treated on a linear accelerator with opposed anteroposterior fields using 6- to 10-MV x-rays.

Anterior Fields

1. Patients are placed in a supine position with arms above the shoulder. The arm position is 90° from the axillae and should eliminate any skin folds of the axillae (Figure 29.8C). Others have used various arm positions as shown in Figure 29.8. Different arm positions may be used but attention must be paid to how the lymph nodes move in relation to the arm position for a given situation. Upper extremity lymphangiograms show that the elevation of the arms results in changes to the location of the axillary lymph nodes (34,77,78). When the hands are over the head with a greater than 90° angle at the axillae, axillary lymph nodes are

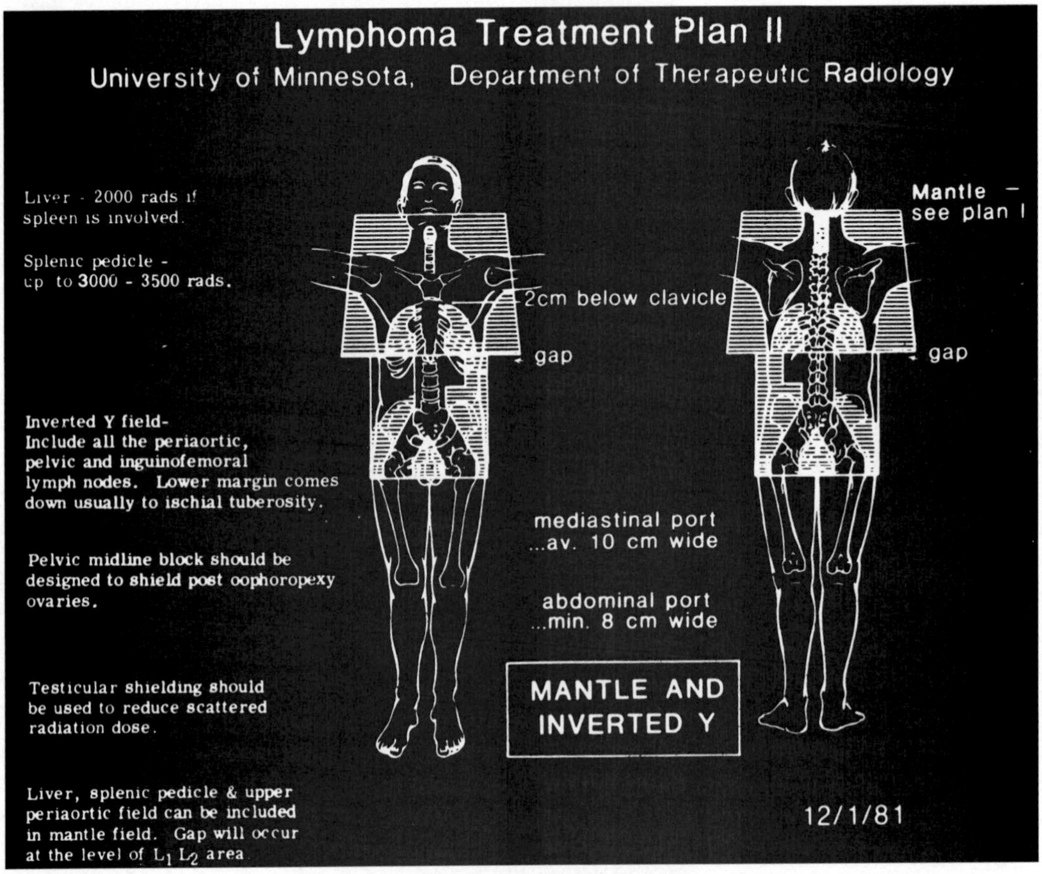

Figure 29.5. View of the mantle and inverted Y treatment field areas, including liver and spleen pedicle. (University of Minnesota treatment plan.)

moved away from the lung area which allows for the design of lung and shoulder shielding.

2. The head position should allow the mandible to be perpendicular to the table top to avoid the possibility of unnecessary radiation through the oral cavity and mandible (Figure 29.9).
3. Palpable lymph nodes can be outlined with a thin wire at the time of simulation to help design the field.
4. Field boundaries are placed superiorly to the level of mastoid tip through the chin line and inferiorly T9-10 or T10-11 vertebral interspace. Inferior border should be extended as needed to the level of T11-12, to include the mediastinum. In patients with an intact spleen, special consideration should be given to the inferior border of the mantle because the spleen is usually included in the para-aortic field. In this situation, lung and diaphragmatic movement by respiration should be watched. In patients who receive whole lung irradiation, lower margins of the mantle field are inferior to the diaphragm to include the lung parenchyma.
5. Laterally, the field includes the axillae as determined clinically.
6. The central axis is defined at the center of the treatment and lies usually close to or at the sternal notch. Simulation radiographs are taken including all borders. This will often require two radiographs to show all the field margins. If the field size to cover the treatment area is too large, an extended source-skin distance (SSD) may be used.
7. Mark the field boundaries and central axis on the patient. A tattoo may be placed at the central axis and inferior border to help daily setup and for future reference when the infraradiodiaphragmatic field is setup. Tattoos may also be placed about 10 cm lateral to the right and left of the central axis line, which helps to confirm the arm position relative to the central axis line.
8. When all the field borders and the central axis positions have been determined, a mantle measurement

Figure 29.6. Techniques used at the University of Minnesota. **A.** Anterior mantle field. **B.** Posterior mantle field.

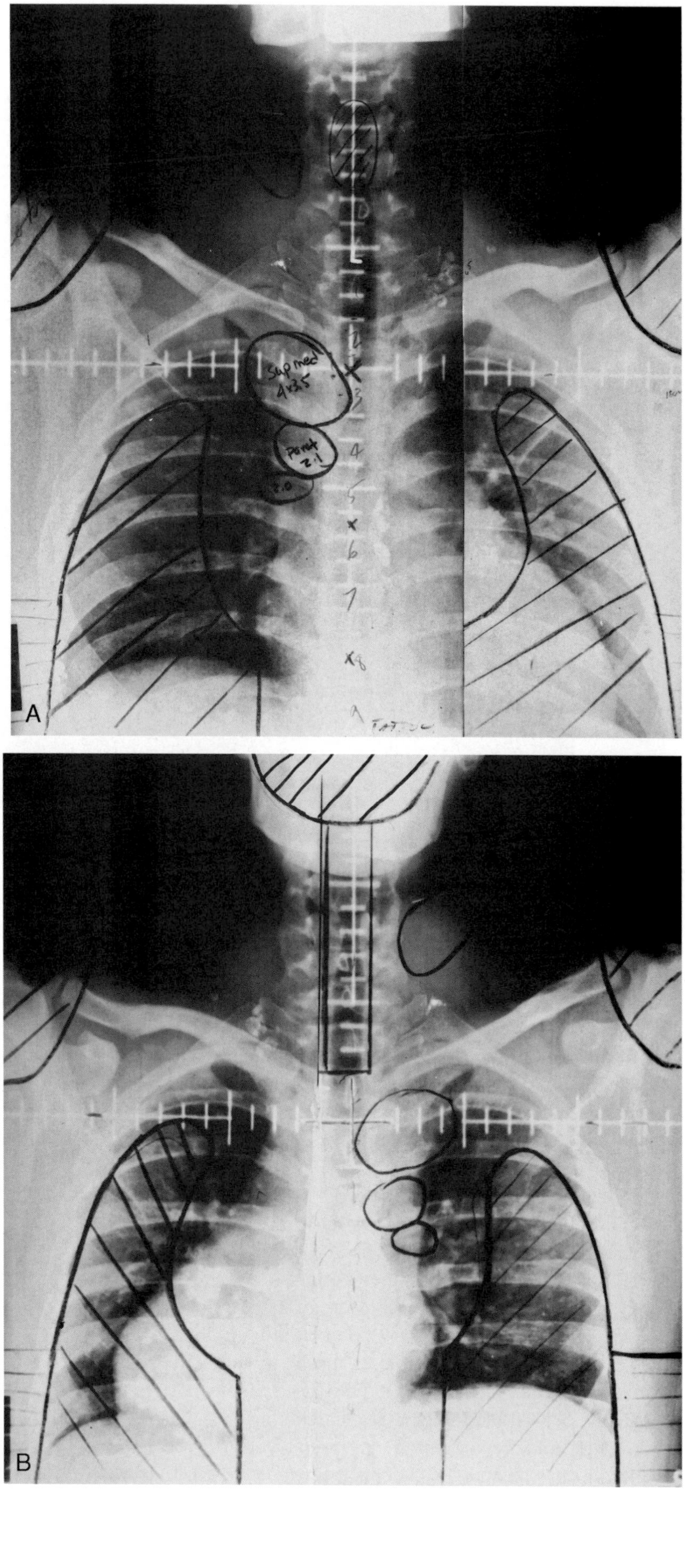

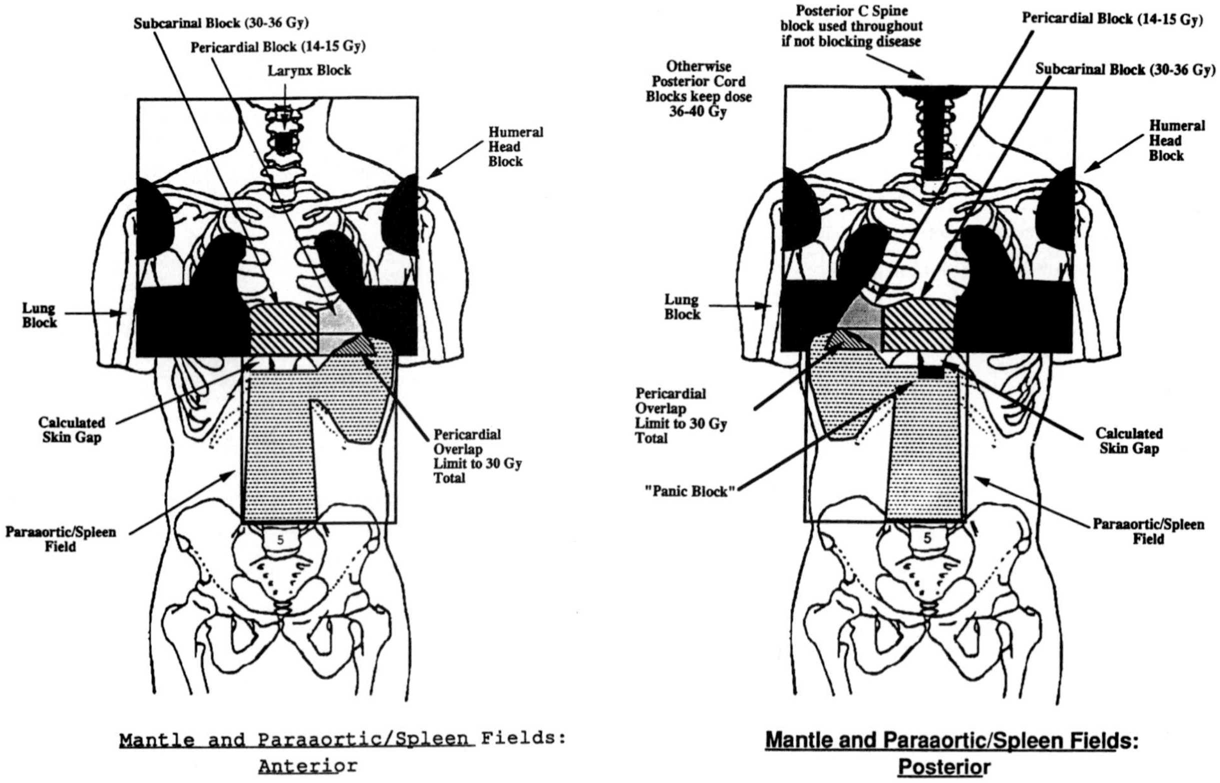

Figure 29.7. Example of modified mantle and para-aortic spleen fields used in CALGB #9497 and SWOG #9133.

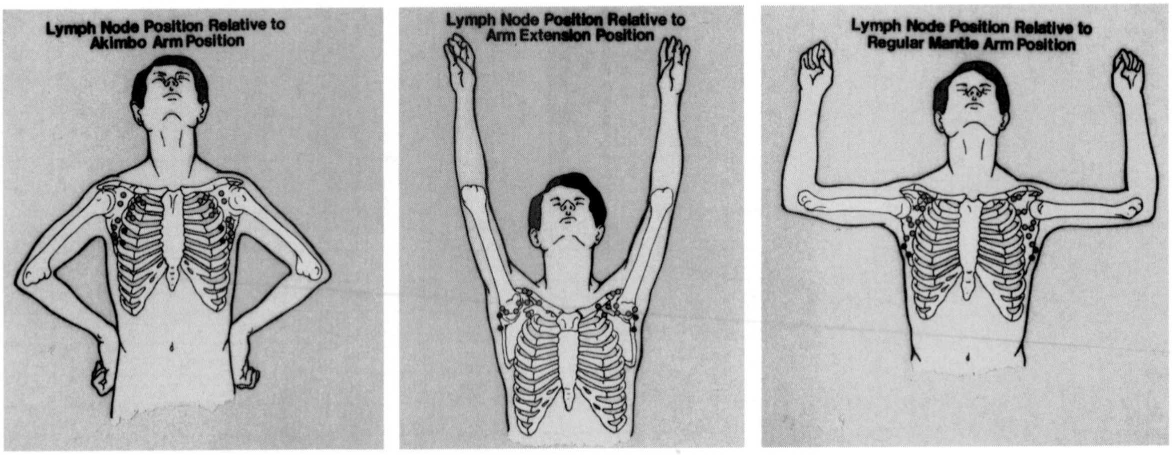

Figure 29.8. Arm positions for mantle fields. **A.** Arm position brings axillary lymph node medially close to the lateral part of the lung. Shielding the lung properly can be difficult. **B.** Arm extension position makes the lymph nodes move over the shoulder area. Shielding the humeral head and shoulder joint can be difficult. **C.** Right angle position gives reasonable room to shield the shoulder and place the lung block without including too much lateral strip of lung.

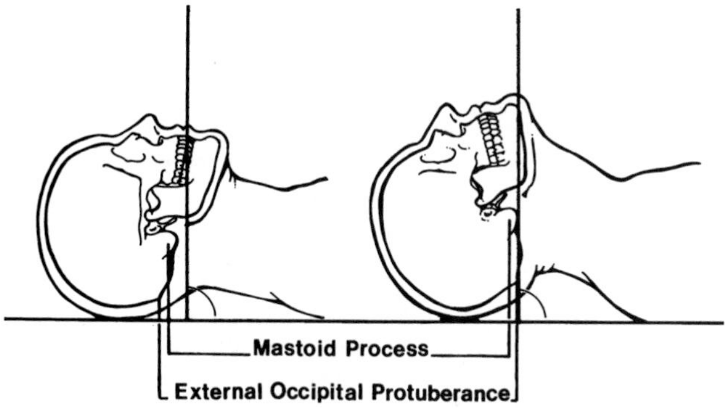

Figure 29.9. Proper chin extension prevents excess dose to the oral cavity and mandible.

sheet for irregular field calculations is prepared. Patient separation is taken at the central axis, axillae, midneck, supraclavicular, midmediastinum, and low mediastinum, about 3 cm above the bottom of the field (Figure 29.10). An irregular field point dose calculation is performed at midseparation for each point using a computerized Clarkson method. These point dose calculations help to achieve the desired cumulative dose to all areas of interest (Figure 29.11).

Posterior Fields

If the treatment machine and table permit, anterior and posterior treatments should be delivered in the same posi-

Figure 29.10. Measurement sheet for mantle fields for various calculations is completed at the time of simulation.

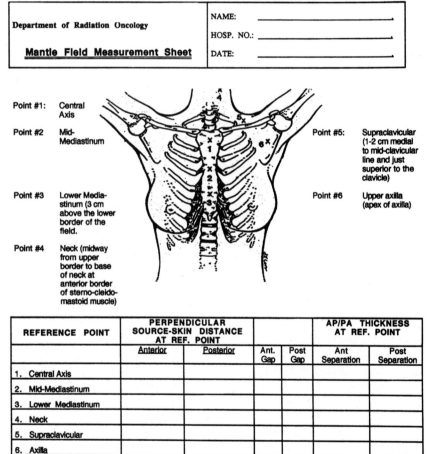

Department of Radiation Oncology **Mantle Field Measurement Sheet**	NAME: ______ HOSP. NO.: ______ DATE: ______

Point #1: Central Axis

Point #2 Mid-Mediastinum

Point #3 Lower Mediastinum (3 cm above the lower border of the field.

Point #4 Neck (midway from upper border to base of neck at anterior border of sterno-cleido-mastoid muscle)

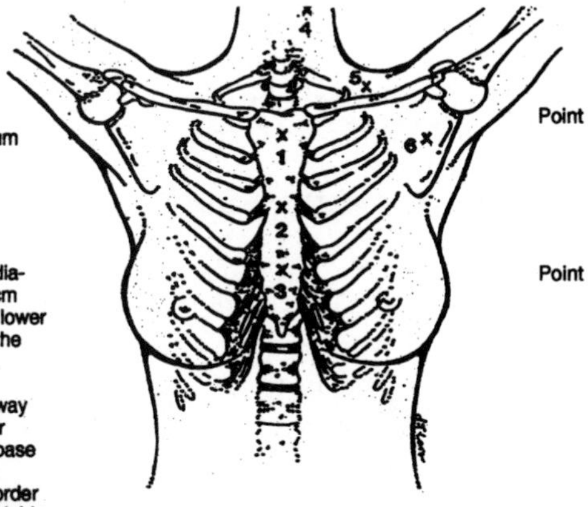

Point #5: Supraclavicular (1-2 cm medial to mid-clavicular line and just superior to the clavicle)

Point #6 Upper axilla (apex of axilla)

REFERENCE POINT	PERPENDICULAR SOURCE-SKIN DISTANCE AT REF. POINT				AP/PA THICKNESS AT REF. POINT	
	Anterior	Posterior	Ant. Gap	Post Gap	Ant Separation	Post Separation
1. Central Axis						
2. Mid-Mediastinum						
3. Lower Mediastinum						
4. Neck						
5. Supraclavicular						
6. Axilla						

OVERALL FIELD SIZE AT SURFACE = ______

SOURCE-FILM DISTANCE: Anterior = ______

Posterior = ______

SOURCE-TRAY DISTANCE: Anterior = ______

Posterior = ______

(Mantle Field Measurement (10/97)

Irregular Field Daily Dose, Output for: on: 3-APR-90

Point #	1	2	3	4	5	6
PDD=	75.6%	72.5%	69.2%	87.3%	79.0%	75.1%
	CA	MID MEDIA	LOW MEDIA	NECK	S CLAV	AXILLA
Rx #						
1	150.	144.	137.	173.	157.	149.
2	300.	283.	275.	346.	313.	298.
3	450.	432.	412.	520.	470.	447.
4	600.	575.	549.	693.	627.	596.
5	750.	719.	687.	866.	784.	745.
6	900.	863.	824.	1039.	940.	894.
7	1050.	1007.	961.	1213.	1097.	1043.
8	1200.	1151.	1098.	1386.	1254.	1192.
9	1350.	1295.	1236.	1559.	1411.	1341.
10	1500.	1438.	1373.	1732.	1567.	1490.
11	1650.	1582.	1510.	1905.	1724.	1639.
12	1800.	1726.	1648.	2079.	1881.	1788.
13	1950.	1870.	1785.	2252.	2038.	1937.
14	2100.	2014.	1922.	2425.	2194.	2086.
15	2250.	2158.	2060.	2598.	2351.	2235.
16	2400.	2302.	2197.	2771.	2508.	2384.
17	2550.	2445.	2334.	2945.	2665.	2533.
18	2700.	2589.	2471.	3118	2821.	2682.
19	2850.	2733.	2609.	3291 upper	2978.	2831.
20	3000.	2877.	2746.	3464 Neck	3135.	2980.
21	3150.	3021.	2883.	3687	3292.	3129.
22	3300.	3165.	3021.	3860	3448.	3278.
23	3450.	3309.	3158.	3984.	3605.	3427.
24	3600.	3452.	3295.	4157.	3762.	3576.
25	3750.	3596.	3433.	4330.	3919.	3725.
26	3900.	3740.	3570.	4504.	4075.	3874.
27	4050.	3884.	3707.	4677.	4232.	4023.
28	4200.	4028.	3844.	4850.	4389.	4172.
29	4350.	4172.	3982.	5023.	4546.	4321.
30	4500.	4315.	4119.	5196.	4702.	4470.
31	4650.	4459.	4256.	5370.	4859.	4619.

Figure 29.11. Computer output sheet showing cumulative midthickness doses for mantle fields.

tions. The patient should remain in the supine position and the beam rotated 180° from the anterior field to set up the posterior field. In this case, a posteroanterior Beam's eye view will include more of the oral cavity, which requires special attention to shield the excess oral cavity in the field (Figure 29.6B). Treating the patient in the supine position, however, makes it difficult to evaluate posterior neck nodes and posterior beam exit. Using the same superior border for the posterior field as in the anterior radiograph may miss the posterior neck node.

If simulation is done in the prone position for the posterior field, the same steps are followed as described above. Since the junction point for the anterior and posterior field is at the midthickness point, the posterior field border in the prone position will usually fall at one vertebrae higher than the anterior field as seen in the simulation radiograph because the spine is located in the posterior part of the body relative to the middle of the anteroposterior thickness.

Design Shielding

The key to good mantle field setup is in the placement of lung blocks. Lung blocks must protect as much lung and heart as possible while irradiating macroscopic and microscopic disease to minimize the risk of treatment failure. The most important aspect of the mantle field design is the individualization that is needed in shaping lung blocks to conform to the specific contours of a given patient. Careful design and placement of shielding blocks protects the pulmonary parenchyma from the effects of excessive dose.

On simulation film, or port film, individualized diversion blocks should be designed for both anterior and posterior films that are not necessarily identical but that include identical nodal groups. The actual blocks are custom designed by following the outline of the block as drawn on the simulation film as well as by the additional use of thoracic CT scans. For uncomplicated cases, the anterior field lung blocks should allow about 2 cm below the medial end of the clavicle to include the infraclavicular lymph node and leave the strip of the lateral part of the lung to include the axillary lymph node with adequate margins. To include the axillary lymph node in the strip, one should pay attention to the patient's arm position (77). Posteriorly, the lung block can be higher than the anterior field and leaves less strip of lung in the infraclavicular area since the lymph nodes in this area are anteriorly located. Falloff area of the lower lateral chest wall as well as shielding below

the line of the fourth intercostal space unless low axillary lymph node is involved are recommended.

In the design of lung blocks, medially at least a 1 to 1.5 cm margin should be allowed for any mediastinal shadow, except for the heart, or any mass shadow. The hilum is hard to define radiographically as is anatomical designation of the lung. Therefore, medial edge of the lung blocks can be a source variation in results among different institutions. Stanford advocates whole pericardial irradiation to the lower prophylactic doses (15 Gy) for mediastinal disease (79,80). This practice is not universally followed.

If there is no gross midline neck disease, trapezoidal or ovoid anterior larynx and posterior cervical spine blocks in addition to lung blocks are recommended. Stanford also recommends an entire posterior thoracic spine block after the delivery of 2000 to 2500 cGy, as well as a subcarinal block. At the University of Minnesota, we use a 2-cm wide posterior cervical block placed above the level of the thoracic inlet after the delivery of 2000 cGy to the central axis (Figure 29.12). If there is no presence of subcarinal disease, the subcarinal block can be used after the delivery of 3000 cGy. Radiation dose at each off axis point will provide information on when to shield each necessary region. The block is placed at the lower edge of the field extending cephalad to within 6 cm of the carina. This appears to significantly reduce the risk of radiation induced heart disease. The humeral head should also be shielded with caution in patients with axillary disease.

After all of the blocks have been drawn, dosimetric calculations should be made at the multiple points of interest. Doses received in these areas can vary considerably because of varying patient thickness in the large field and in the different scatter contributions from the blocks. For example, nodes in the axilla and the high neck receive a greater dose than nodes in the lower mediastinum. Therefore, the dose differences at each site should be calculated (Fig. 29.10) and compensation should be provided by placing the shielding block earlier for the particular anatomic area or by using compensators (Figure 29.13).

In the presence of inferior mediastinal disease or pericardial extension, the entire cardiac silhouette is irradiated to 15 Gy, and then changed to shield the apex of the heart. After a dose of 30 to 35 Gy is delivered, a block is placed about 5 cm below the carina to provide more cardiac and pericardial protection. However, in no instance do we treat areas of clinical involvement of Hodgkin's disease with

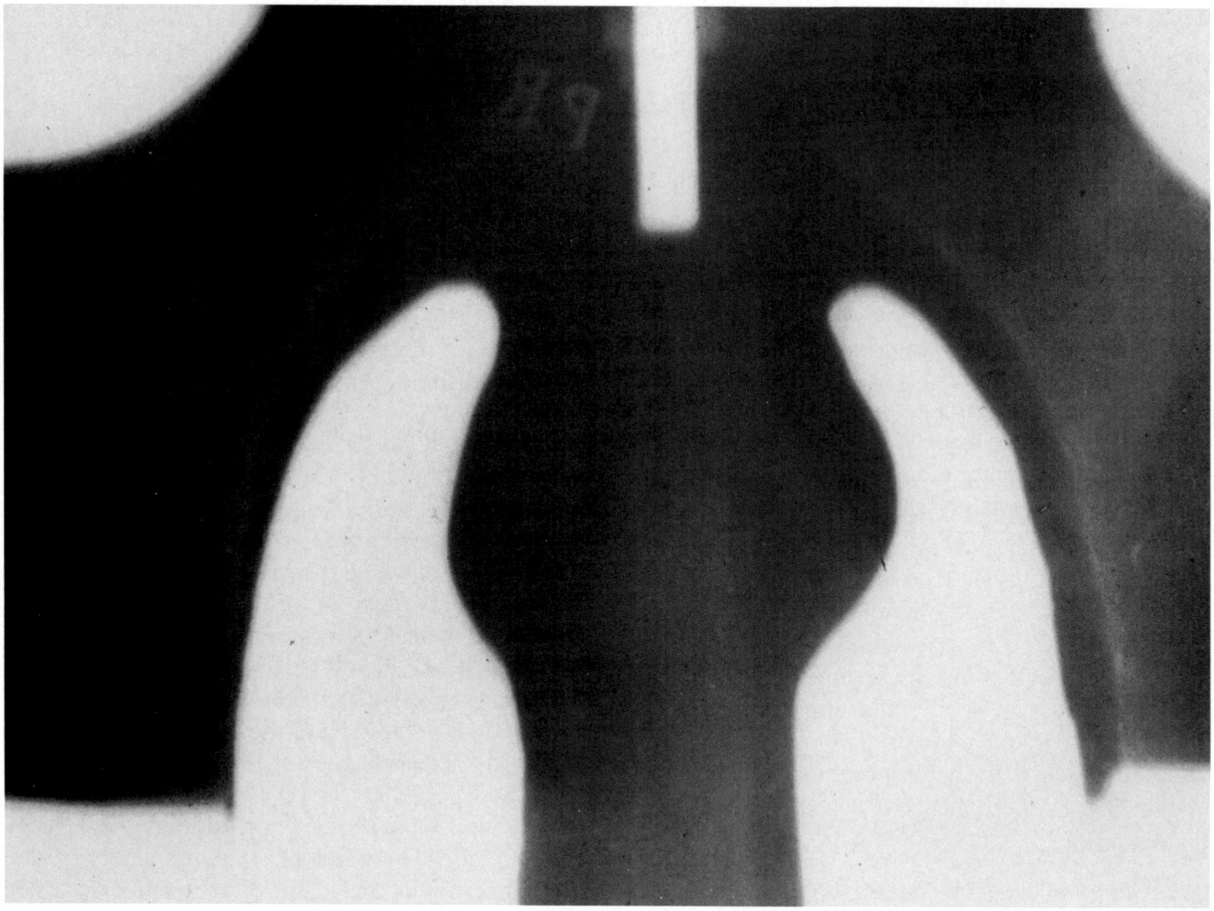

Figure 29.12. Posterior mantle field port film with posterior cervical spine block.

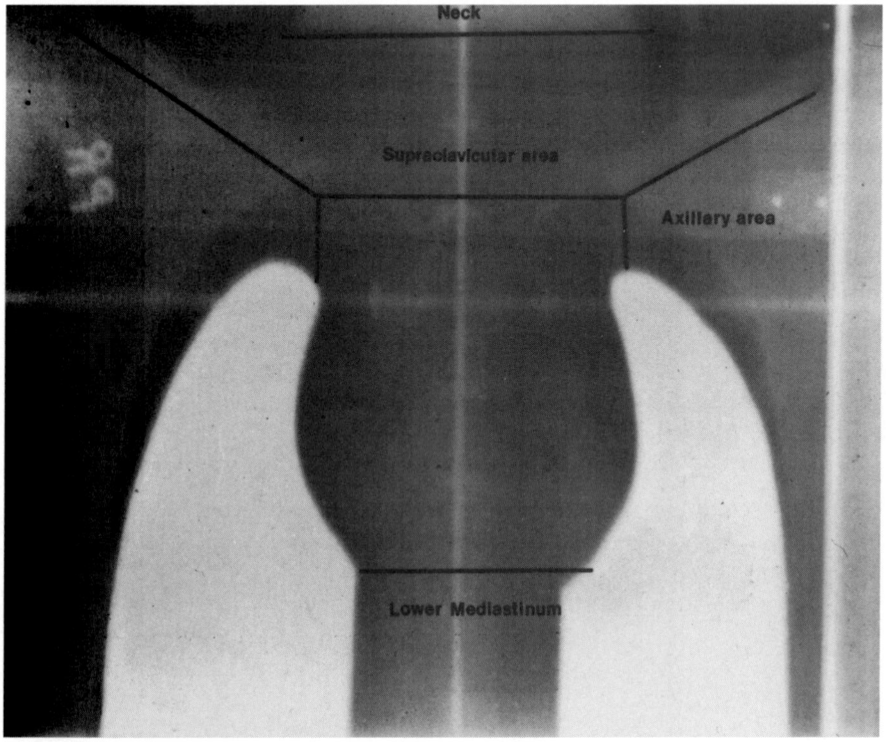

Figure 29.13. Schematic figure for the shielding of the off axis areas according to cumulative dose output.

doses of less than 36 Gy if radiotherapy alone is planned. Figure 29.7 represents examples of field modifications of original mantle fields used in two current clinical trials.

Patients with massive mediastinal disease and/or hilar disease who are treated with radiation alone require further modifications to the lung blocks.

When hilar adenopathy is present, there is substantial risk of subclinical Hodgkin's disease in the lung. There is also an increased risk of subsequent pulmonary relapse and low dose lung irradiation has been recommended using thin lung blocks that transmit 37% of the total 1650 cGy dose delivered to the central axis (80,81).

In patients with a large mediastinal mass, locoregional recurrence is the major cause of failure (7). We treat these patients with low dose bilateral or unilateral lung irradiation (Figure 29.14). Total dose to the lung parenchyma is usually 1000 to 1600 cGy in daily doses of 100 cGy to eliminate microscopic lung disease as well as to shrink the tumor mass to add proper lung blocks (82). The shrinking field technique should be used several times during the treatment course. One can consider a 10- to 14-day treatment break during the course of radiation treatment to allow for tumor shrinkage as Stanford originally introduced (83) (Figure 29.15). The technique of reshaping and enlarging lung blocks as the mass responds to treatment reduces the risk of pulmonary toxicity.

Although historically, whole lung irradiation (WLI) was the best radiation treatment to provide optimal survival rates for patients with LMM, most patients with LMM currently receive combined modality therapy (CMT) with modifications to the radiation fields and dose to deliver less aggressive treatment (84).

An unresolved issue is what volume should be treated in patients with LMM who received CMT—the volume of postchemotherapy disease or the original volume of disease. A possible solution is to treat the prechemotherapy volume with a low dose (18 to 20 cGy) followed by a boost to residual disease from 36 to 40 cGy.

Subdiaphragmatic Fields

The para-aortic field encompasses the para-aortic nodes and splenic pedicle as well as the spleen in clinically staged patients (Fig. 29.16). Treatment of the splenic pedicle is optional in patients who have a negative staging laparotomy. At the time of splenectomy, or staging laparotomy, surgical clips should be placed to mark the splenic pedicle. The splenic tag portion of the para-aortic field should have a 2.5- to 3-cm margin around the clips. The para-aortic field should be wide enough to include other lymph node chains. In patients who did not have a splenectomy but who are receiving subtotal nodal irradiation using mantle and para-aortic fields, the spleen needs to be included in the field. An ultrasound or CT scan of the abdomen should be used to localize the spleen and to allow blocking of the left kidney as much as possible.

The lower margin of the para-aortic field usually extends down to the L4-L5 interface. In some cases it can

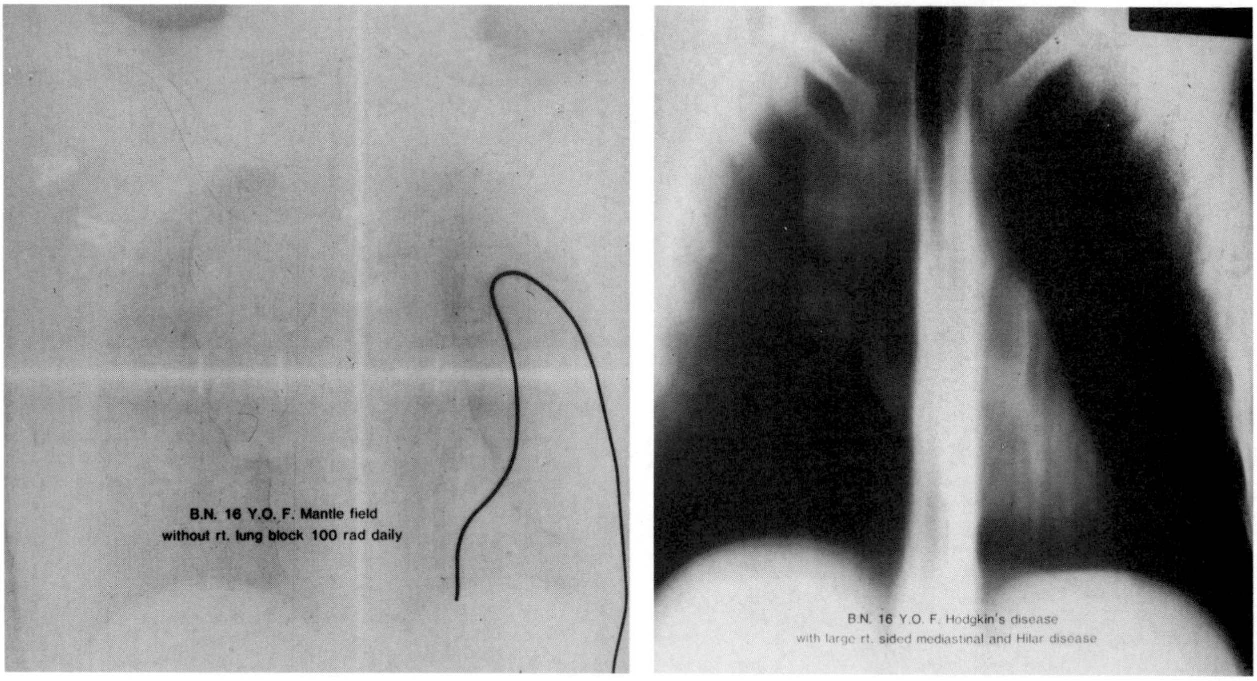

Figure 29.14. Unilateral lung irradiation for a patient with protruding mediastinal disease on the right side.

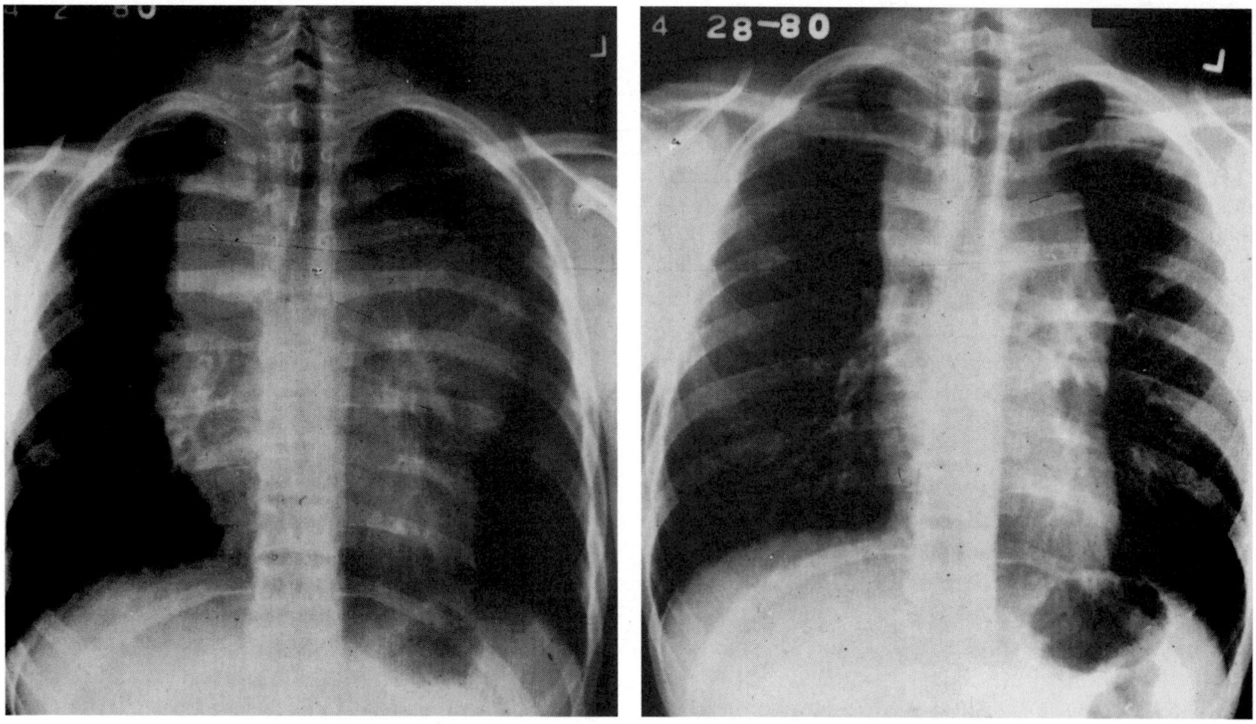

Figure 29.15. Reduction in size of large mediastinal mass after 1500 cGy to the whole lung using 100 cGy daily fractions.

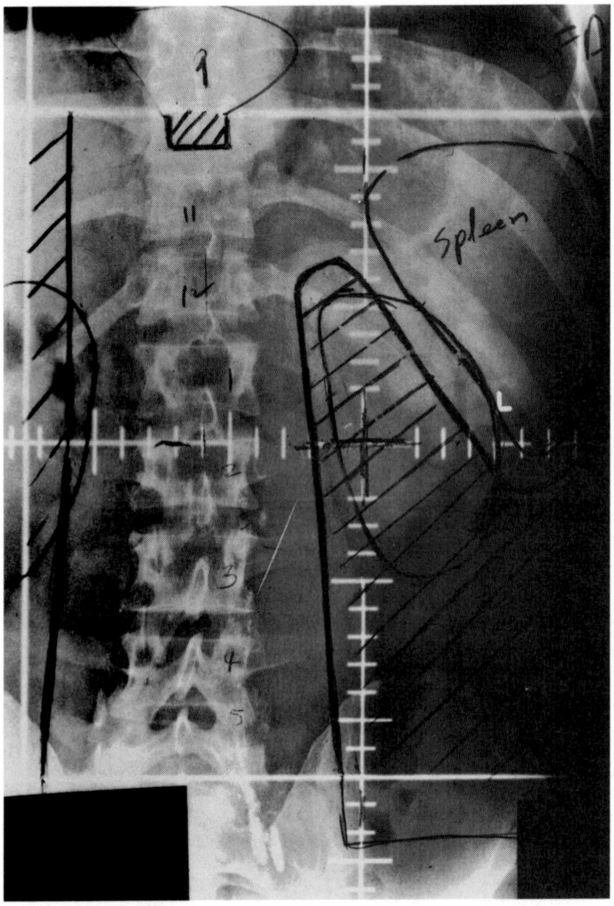

Figure 29.16. View of a para-aortic field that includes the spleen. University of Minnesota technique.

extend below the bifurcation of the aorta to include the common iliac nodes (spade shape field).

The inverted-Y field is used when the patient has indications for total nodal irradiation. This field includes the para-aortic field and pelvic and inguinal femoral lymph nodes. With the development of combined modality treatment, the total nodal field is rarely used. In some situations, the pelvic nodal field is treated separately.

Low dose irradiation to the liver is rarely considered with inverted-Y field in patients who may have a potential for liver disease as previously described. Both Stanford and the University of Minnesota have reported excellent results of liver irradiation in PS IIIA patients (57,59) (Figure 29.5). In recent practice, this is almost historic since most of these patients will receive combined modality treatment and liver irradiation would not be considered.

Careful blocking is required when the pelvic region is treated. The fields must be shaped carefully to minimize the amount of marrow treated. If a lymphogram has been performed, a more precise delineation of the pelvic field is possible and more bone marrow can be spared. Gonadal toxicity may also be an issue. In women, since the ovaries normally overlie the iliac lymph nodes, an oophoropexy must be performed to avoid irradiation-induced amenorrhea (85). This procedure is done by medial transposition of the ovaries and is accomplished most readily at the time of staging laparotomy. The surgeon marks the ovaries with radiopaque sutures or clips and places them medially and as low as possible behind the uterine body. A double thickness (10 half-value layer [HVL]) midline block is then recommended and its location is guided by the position of the opacified nodes and transposed ovaries. When the ovaries are at least 2 cm from the edge of this block, the dose is decreased to 8% of that delivered to the iliac nodes (85).

In males, the testicular dose may be as high as 10% of the dose delivered to the inguinal femoral nodes if no special blocking is provided for the testes. Use of a double thickness midline block and a specially constructed testicular shield can reduce this dose to 0.75% to 3.0%, largely from internal scatter due to the proximity of the position of the testes in relation to the inferior margin of the inguinal femoral field (86).

Preauricular and Waldeyer's Ring Fields

The preauricular lymph nodes are treated either when there is involvement of the preauricular nodes or of the high cervical lymph nodes above the level of the thyroid notch. The superior border is placed at the top of the zygomatic arch such that the sphenoid sinus is included in the field. The posterior border is at the external auditory canal and anteriorly the field extends up to the third molar. The inferior border is matched, on skin, to the divergence of the mantle field. Most commonly, this area is treated with about 9 MeV unilateral electron field to spare the parotid in the uninvolved side.

Waldeyer's Ring is treated in patients with involvement of this region or with bulky superior cervical lymph nodes. This volume is treated with opposed lateral photon beams. The treatment volume is treated with opposed lateral occipital, preauricular, and submandibular lymph nodes as well as the nasopharynx, tonsillar fossa, and base of the tongue. The superior border is placed at the top of the zygomatic arch, the anterior border includes the submandibular triangle, and the posterior border extends beyond the spinous processes. The inferior border is a direct match to the superior border of the mantle field. The match line is placed inferior to any palpable cervical disease to avoid underdosing of involved cervical nodes. If this is not possible, the match line has to be feathered to avoid underdosing the disease or overdosing the spinal cord (Figure 29.17). With disease regression after 2,500 to 3,000 cGy, the Waldeyer's field is discontinued at some institutions. The treatment volume is changed to a mantle with a high superior border and matched to a unilateral preauricular field, thereby decreasing the risk of xerostomia.

Limited Field (Involved Field/Regional Field)

In recent years, limited or regional irradiation has been used with combined modality treatment. No clear guidelines are yet established on the size of the field. Figure 29.18 shows an example of local and regional fields used in a British National Lymphoma study (17). Involved fields usually allow 3- to 5-cm margins around the tumor sites. Regional fields include lymphatic chain of the tumor site.

Gap of Matching Fields

When two fields are matching on the skin, a potential overlap area will be created in between the fields. With sequential treatment of separate mantle para-aortic or inverted Y fields, calculation of the gap between mantle and subdiaphragmatic fields is very important. Beam diversion from supra- and infradiaphragmatic fields creates the potential for field overlap and subsequent radiation doses that exceed spinal cord tolerance. A well-planned matching technique is essential and appropriate gap calculations should be applied. If the patient is being treated in the supine and prone positions, a four-field match can be created at the patient's midseparation.

A number of different matching techniques have been published (87,88). The gap can be calculated at the midline of the body or at the spine to create a junction at the same

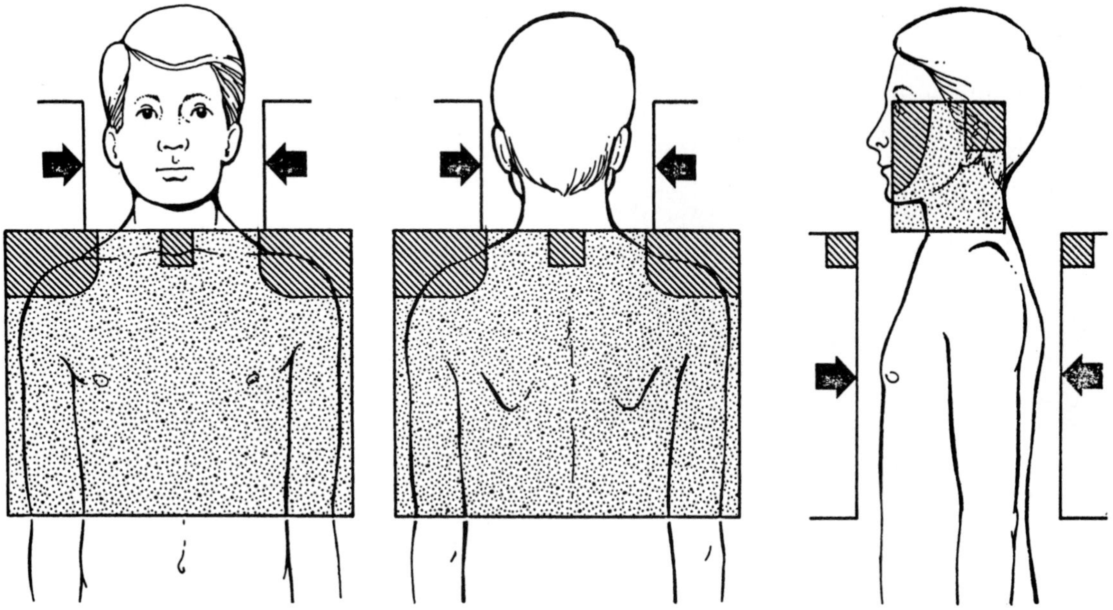

Figure 29.17. Matching for head and neck and mini-mantle fields.

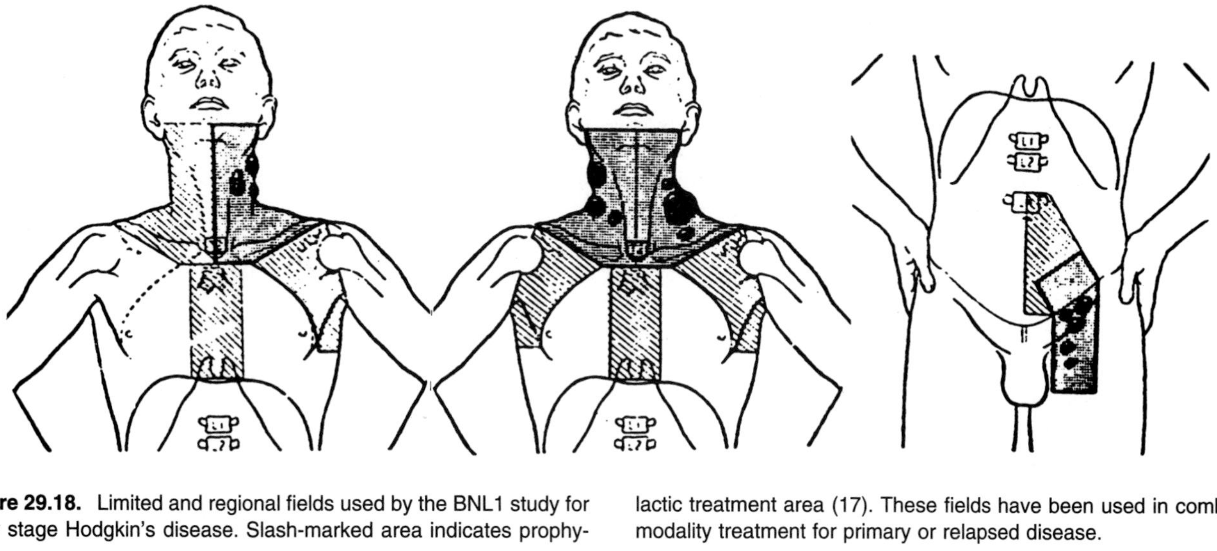

Figure 29.18. Limited and regional fields used by the BNL1 study for early stage Hodgkin's disease. Slash-marked area indicates prophylactic treatment area (17). These fields have been used in combined modality treatment for primary or relapsed disease.

vertebrae. The depth of the matching point length of SSD or source-axis distance (SAD) and field sizes (both mantle and subdiaphragmatic fields) will dictate the divergence of the beam and will show the different levels of vertebrae between the anterior and posterior radiographic fields.

When mantle (AP/PA) and subdiaphragmatic fields are treated sequentially and field length of upper and lower fields is often different, longer fields diverge into the opposing smaller fields. When four fields meet, three fields can be overlapped and total dose of the overlapped area may exceed the central axis dose and it can be in the middle of the body thickness or at the vertebra. This is a concern especially if the overlapped area is the spinal cord. Therefore, it is important to use small blocks to shield the spinal cord area for the second pair of the fields in addition to calculating the proper skin gap using the formula in Figure 29.19. This formula shows the geometry of adjacent beams that join at a given depth to calculate skin gap. Isodose distribution at the midline is almost uniform but cold spots are created anterior and posterior at the junction point (Figure 29.20).

The tattoo at the inferior margin of the mantle field usually helps to show where the skin gap should be given when subdiaphragmatic fields are simulated with a gap. It is very important to verify the inferior margin of the mantle fields at the time of simulation.

Actual treatment of the patient is an important factor after precise simulation plans are completed. In a review of portal films from five major universities in the United States, the Patterns of Care study showed an 11% variation

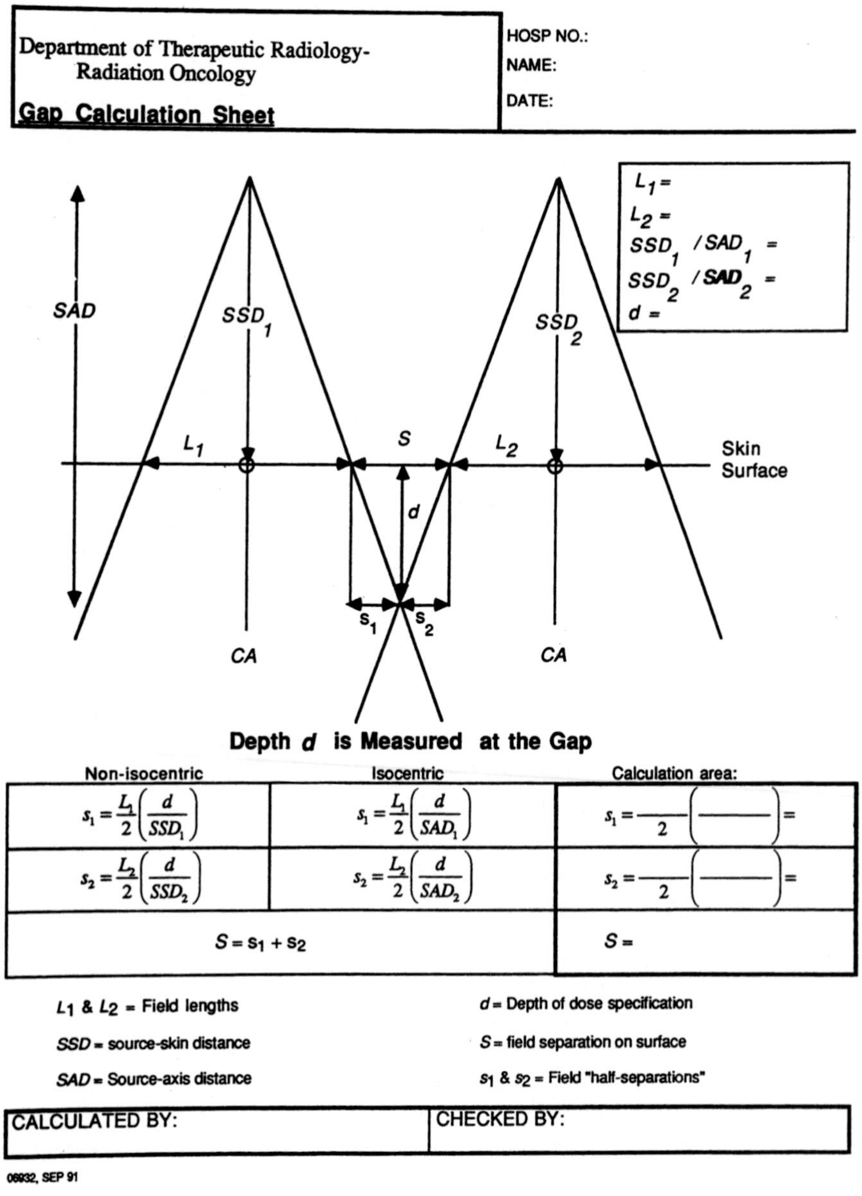

Department of Therapeutic Radiology-
Radiation Oncology
Gap Calculation Sheet
HOSP NO.:
NAME:
DATE:
L1 =
L2 =
SSD1 / SAD1 =
SSD2 / SAD2 =
d =
SAD
SSD1
SSD2
L1
S
L2
Skin Surface
d
s1
s2
CA
CA
Depth d is Measured at the Gap
Non-isocentric
Isocentric
Calculation area:
s1 = L1/2 (d/SSD1)
s1 = L1/2 (d/SAD1)
s1 = —/2 (—) =
s2 = L2/2 (d/SSD2)
s2 = L2/2 (d/SAD2)
s2 = —/2 (—) =
S = s1 + s2
S =
L1 & L2 = Field lengths
SSD = source-skin distance
SAD = Source-axis distance
d = Depth of dose specification
S = field separation on surface
s1 & s2 = Field "half-separations"
CALCULATED BY:
CHECKED BY:
06932, SEP 91

Figure 29.19. Gap calculation measurement sheet.

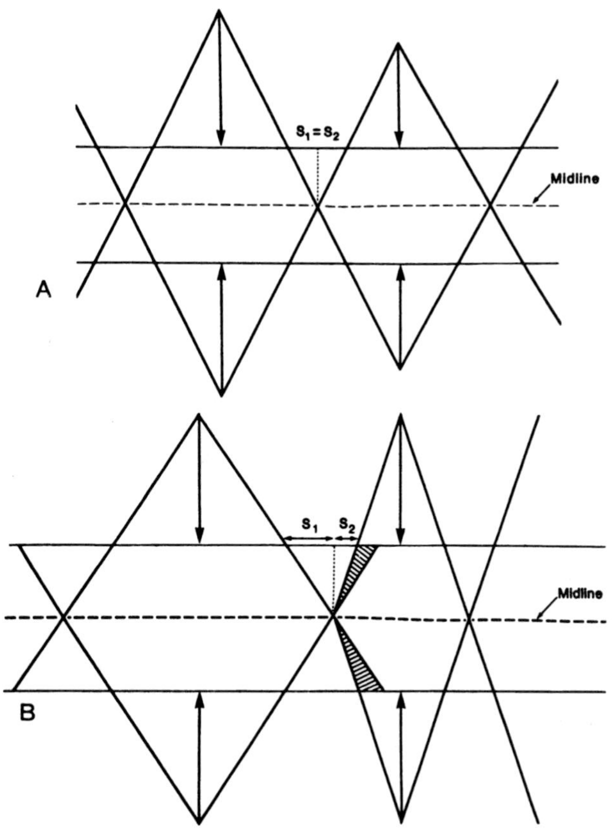

Figure 29.20. Two pairs of parallel opposed fields. Adjacent fields are separated on the surface so that they all join at a point on the midline. **A.** Ideal geometry in which there is no three-field overlap. **B.** arrangement in which there are two regions (shaded) of three-field overlap. (From Khan FM. The Physics of Radiation Therapy. 2nd ed. Baltimore: Williams & Wilkins, 1994:335.)

among the institutions (89). The most frequent inadequate margins were the mediastinum, the hilum, and the axillae. Infield or marginal recurrence was 8% in patients with adequate margins and 32% in patients with inadequate margins.

RADIATION DOSE AND FRACTIONATION

An optimal radiation dose results in a high rate of local disease control and acceptable side effects. Several factors are involved in determining radiation dose including disease extent (macroscopic or microscopic), treatment modality (radiation alone or combined with chemotherapy), total dose delivered, and number of daily fractions.

Radiation Therapy Alone

Historically, the curative doses to treat Hodgkin's disease have been controversial (90–92). Early studies by Peters showed that improvement in 5-year survival in 319 Stage I patients treated with prophylactic irradiation to the subclinical area depended on the dose delivered and the extent of treatment (93). Involved areas received more than 2500 cGy and the adjacent area that received prophylactic irradiation received less than 2500 cGy. A review of the literature in 1966 by Kaplan confirmed that local control for Hodgkin's disease patients by radiation therapy were dose dependent (48,94). Doses of at least 4400 cGy over 4 to 5 weeks achieved 98.6% infield control and doses of 3500 to 4000 cGy resulted in a recurrence rate of 4.4%. Subsequent analysis of most of the same data by Fletcher and Shukovsky, which showed a 93% control rate for 3000 cGy or less and 97% control rate for 3100 to 4000 cGy, concluded that a total dose of 3500 cGy up to 6 weeks is needed to control Hodgkin's disease (95).

A recent compilation of dose-response data by Vijayakumar from a megavoltage series demonstrated a 90% control rate of subclinical disease with 22.1 Gy and 95% control for 27 Gy (96). In patients with lymph nodes smaller than 6 cm, the corresponding doses for 50%, 90%, and 95% control were 26.7 Gy, 33.4 Gy, and 35.2 Gy. For nodes larger than 6 cm, the majority of patients received doses of more than 36 Gy. This retrospective analysis of patients treated at the University of Chicago was performed to assess the dose response in patients treated in a more uniform manner in a single institution (97). Local control of subclinical disease was 100% with 25 to 35 Gy. For gross disease, there was also no dose dependence in the range of 35 to 55 Gy. Local control was 98.3% with 35 to 45 Gy. A recent trial from the German Hodgkin's Lymphoma Study Group randomized early stage Hodgkin's disease patients to 40 Gy extended field irradiation versus 30 Gy extended field plus 10 Gy involved field irradiation (98). No infield relapses were noted in the extended field volumes, and there was no significant difference in overall survival or freedom from failure. Patients with bulky disease (mass of greater than 6 cm or LMM) commonly receive more than 36 Gy, although the need for a higher dose has not been well studied.

In summary, based on available data on the treatment of Hodgkin's disease with radiation, the American College of Radiology in their Patterns of Care Study recommended that optimal doses for local control were 36 to 44 cGy for treatment of involved portions of the field and 30 to 36 cGy for prophylactic portions of the fields (99).

Radiation Dose in Combined Modality Therapy

The doses recommended for patients undergoing combined modality therapy are not as specific and well established. Most of the dose-response data with combined modality therapy are from data on pediatric and advanced Hodgkin's disease. Based on the experience of the German Austrian Pediatric Study Group, 18 to 20 Gy to subclinical sites after chemotherapy was as effective as high dose radiation (100). Dose response data from this cooperative group for childhood Hodgkin's disease show about a 95

to 97% control rate with 15 to 25 Gy to gross disease sites in patients treated with combined modality therapy (101–103). When treated with combined modality therapy, patients who respond poorly to initial chemotherapy show a poor rate of control using 25 Gy. In adults, it is general practice to use 25 to 30 Gy for a completely responded area of previous bulky disease and 36 to 40 Gy to gross disease despite previous chemotherapy.

Radiation Dose in Salvage Treatment

For patients who relapse after primary treatment (either chemotherapy or radiation therapy) and who are treated with salvage chemotherapy, low doses of radiation can be used to sites previously irradiated if maximum tissue tolerance has not been exceeded. Higher doses of radiation should be considered if no previous radiation therapy was given to the involved sites. The radiation field size is usually confined to the loco-regional area (Figure 29.18). Total dose of radiation for these patients is similar to the total dose used for patients treated with primary chemotherapy (104–105).

NORMAL TISSUE TOLERANCE AND COMPLICATIONS

Lung

The lungs parenchyma are the most sensitive organ in the thorax to irradiation. Doses as low as 15 Gy can cause acute pulmonary reactions. Areas of lung treated with 35 to 44 cGy often show fibrosis during long-term follow-up, with varying degrees of severity depending on the volume treated, total dose used, and fraction size. Both lungs may be treated safely with a dose as high as 15 to 16 cGy, especially if partial transmission lung blocks are used or open fields at a 75 to 100 cGy daily dose rate (37,81,82). When patients received 1650 cGy in 10 fractions, 35% developed pulmonary symptoms whereas only 15% developed these symptoms after the same dose in 20 fractions.

Radiation pneumonitis may develop 6 to 12 weeks after completion of mantle irradiation (79). The likelihood of radiation related pulmonary complications may increase with the additional use of chemotherapy, such as Bleomycin (106).

Heart

Symptomatic pericarditis is rare with entire pericardium doses of 30 cGy or less. However, subclinical injury to the pericardium may occur at lower doses. Partial field blocking (apical portion of heart at 15 cGy, subcarinal portion of heart at 30 cGy) is associated with a decreased risk of pericarditis. The myocardium is slightly more resistant than the pericardium, but doses of 35 cGy can cause a higher risk of coronary heart disease.

Heart irradiation modestly increases the relative risk (RR) of coronary artery disease and myocardial infarction. To modify the risk, attention should be paid to the total dose, the radiation port used, the size of the left ventricular block, and the fraction size. Long-term cardiovascular complications include coronary artery disease, pericarditis, pancarditis, and valvular disease (107,108). In an analysis of factors affecting the risk of cardiac related deaths with long-term follow-up, patients who received a dose 30 Gy to the mediastinum had a 3.5 relative risk of cardiac related mortality compared to a 2.6 relative risk in patients who received less than 30 Gy (107). The risk of coronary artery disease appears to be primarily related to mediastinal irradiation; however, the chemotherapeutic agent such as anthrocycliners are also potential cardiotoxic agents. Therefore, it is a concern when combined modality is considered that includes cardiotoxic chemotherapy and radiation.

Central Nervous System

The Lhermitte sign develops in about 10 to 20% of patients after mantle field irradiation. It may be related to transient demyelinization of the spinal cord occurring 1 to 2 months after completion of treatment and usually resolves completely 2 to 6 months after.

Spinal cord tolerance is reported to be reached at dose levels of 45 to 50 Gy and above, with the length and location of the area involved affecting total dose tolerance. Although spinal cord tolerance should not be an issue with standard lymphoma therapy, extreme attention to treatment details should be followed. These details include attention to the length of the spinal cord included in the field, the expected success of treatment, a long follow-up, and the use of contiguous fields that overlap the spinal cord all demand conservative dose guidelines. Lateral simulator radiographs or treatment planning CT scans may be used to determine the doses at key points along the length of the spinal cord. The cord dose should be limited to not more than 40 cGy in posterior spinal cord blocking.

Thyroid

Thyroid glands are usually included when the neck is treated. Subclinical hypothyroidism develops in about half of the patients who receive regular mantle fields (108). It is important to check the long-term thyroid function after mantle field treatment.

Liver

A portion of the left lobe of the liver is included in the para-aortic field. This may cause a transient elevation of the serum alkaline phosphatase but it is not associated with long-term sequelae. If necessary, the entire liver may be treated safely with a dose up to 25 cGy using protracted fractionation; higher doses should be avoided.

Gastrointestinal Tract

The gastrointestinal (GI) tract generally tolerates doses up to 44 Gy. After doses of 35 Gy or more there is some risk. Small bowel obstruction could occur where intra-abdominal adhesions have formed after a staging laparotomy. The Patterns of Care review on complications after intradiaphragmatic field irradiation reported 6% of major bowel complications occurred after 4000 to 4500 cGy (109). Incidence of GI complications was especially high in patients with previous GI problems (19%).

Head and Neck

Xerostomia may develop after mantle or head and neck field irradiation and prophylaxis including daily fluoride treatments are recommended. A dental examination before irradiation should be done on all patients who receive mantle field and Waldeyer's field irradiation to minimize long-term complications.

Reproductive Organs

The ovaries are the most sensitive organ in the pelvis. The gonads are also sensitive. Women over the age of 30 are especially sensitive. Even with oophoropexy and shielding for the relocated ovaries, and testicular shielding, the scattered dose of irradiation may be sufficient to develop menopause and aspermia. Mantle field irradiation delivers 0.2 to 0.5% of the prescribed dose to the testis, 0.5 to 1.0% from the para-aortic field and 5 to 10% from the pelvic field (110). Alkylating agents of chemotherapy also effect the gonads, especially in women older than 30 (111). Combined modality with chemotherapy and pelvic irradiation should be cautiously designed and used because of possible further damage to the gonads as well as to bone marrow reservation.

Secondary Neoplasms

One of the long-term sequelae of radiation is the development of secondary cancers, including solid tumors and leukemia-lymphoma. Overall, there is a 6.4 relative risk of developing a second malignancy after treatment for Hodgkin's disease and an 84% absolute risk (108). Breast cancer in female patients has been increasing after mantle irradiation. Secondary solid tumors, such as lung, breast, and GI cancers, are most likely related primarily to radiation therapy and develop with longer latent period of 7 to 10 years than soft cancer, such as lymphoma or leukemia (112–115).

Long-term follow-up is very important to detect late long-term complications of treatment (108). Continual attempts should be made to reduce any life-threatening consequences of treatment and to balance complications with the benefits of treatment.

References

1. Friedman S, Henry-Amar M, Casset JM, et al. Evolution of erythrocyte sedimentation rate as predictor of early relapse in post-therapy early-stage Hodgkin's disease. J Clin Oncol 1988;6:596.
2. Ray GR, Wolf PH, Kaplan HS. Value of laboratory indicators in Hodgkin's disease: Preliminary results. NCI Monogr 1973;36:315.
3. Tubiana M, Henry-Amar M, Burgers MV, Van Der Werf-Messing B, Hayat M. Prognostic significance of erythrocyte sedimentation rate in clinical stages I-II of Hodgkin's disease. J Clin Oncol 1984;2:194.
4. Agnarsson BA, Kadin ME. The immunophenotype of Reed-Sternberg cells: a study of 50 cases of Hodgkin's disease using fixed frozen tissues. Cancer 1989;63:2083–2087.
5. Castellino RA, Blank N, Hoppe RT, et al. Hodgkin's disease: contributions of chest CT in the initial staging evaluation. Radiology 1986; 160:603–605.
6. Rostock RA, Siegelman SS, Lenhard RE, et al. Thoracic CT scanning for mediastinal Hodgkin's disease. Results and therapeutic implications. Int J Radiat Oncol Biol Phys 1983;9:1451–1457.
7. Lee CK, Bloomfield CD, Goldman AJ, Levitt SH. Prognostic significance of mediastinal involvement in Hodgkin's disease treated with curative radiotherapy. Cancer 1980;46:2403–2409.
8. Mauch P, Tarbell N, Weinstein H, et al. Stage IA and IIA supradiaphragmatic Hodgkin's disease. Prognostic factors in surgically staged patients treated with mantle and paraaortic irradiation. J Clin Oncol 1988;6:1576–1583.
9. Leibenhaut M, Hoppe R, Efron B, et al. Prognostic indicators of laparotomy findings in clinical stage I-II supradiaphragmatic Hodgkin's disease. J Clin Oncol 1989;7:81–91.
10. Mauch P, Larson D, Osteen R, et al. Prognostic factors for positive surgical staging in patients with Hodgkin's disease. J Clin Oncol 1990;8:257–265.
11. Castellino RA, Hoppe RT, Blank N, et al. Computed tomography, lymphography, and staging laparotomy: correlations in initial staging of Hodgkin's disease. Am J Radiol 1984;143:37–41.
12. Front D, Israel O. The role of Ga-67 scintigraphy in evaluating the results of therapy of lymphoma patients. Semin Nucl Med 1995; 60–71.
13. Brada M, Easton D, Horwich A, et al. Clinical presentation as a predictor of laparotomy findings in supradiaphragmatic stage I and II Hodgkin's disease. Radiother Oncol 1986;5:15–22.
14. Rutherford C, Desforges J, Davies B, et al. The decision to perform staging laparotomy in symptomatic Hodgkin's disease. Br J Haematol 1980;44:347–358.
15. Aragon de la Cruz G, Cardenes H, Otero J, et al. Individual risk of abdominal disease in patients with stages I and II supradiaphragmatic Hodgkin's disease. Cancer 1989;63:1799–1803.
16. Tubiana M, Henry-Amar M, Carde P, et al. Toward comprehensive management tailored to prognostic factors of patients with clinical stages I and II Hodgkin's disease. The EORTC Lymphoma Group controlled clinical trials: 1964-1987. Blood 1989;73:47–56.
17. Haybittle J, Easterling M, Bennett M, et al. Review of British National Lymphoma Investigation studies of Hodgkin's disease and development of prognostic index. Lancet 1985;1:967–972.
18. Sutcliff S, Gospodarowicz M, Bergsagel D, et al. Prognostic groups for management of localized Hodgkin's disease. J Clin Oncol 1985; 3:393–401.
19. Mandelli F, Anselmo A, Cartoni C, et al. Evaluation of therapeutic modalities in the control of Hodgkin's disease. Int J Radiat Oncol Biol Phys 1986;12:1617–1620.
20. Mauch P, Canellos G, Shulman L, et al. Mantle irradiation alone for selected patients with laparotomy-staged IA to IIA Hodgkin's disease: preliminary results of a prospective trial. J Clin Oncol 1995; 13:947–952.
21. Taylor M, Kaplan H, Nelsen T. Staging laparotomy with splenectomy for Hodgkin's disease: the Stanford experience. World J Surg 1985; 9:449–460.
22. Molrine D, George S, Tarbell N, et al. Antibody responses to polysaccharide-conjugate vaccines following treatment for Hodgkin's disease. Ann Intern Med 1995;123:824–828.
23. Siber G, Gorham C, Martin P, et al. Antibody response to pretreatment immunization and posttreatment boosting with bacterial poly-

saccharide vaccines in patients with Hodgkin's disease. Ann Intern Med 1986;104:467–475.
24. van der Velden JW, van Putten WLJ, Guinee VF, et al. Subsequent development of acute non-lymphocytic leukemia in patients treated for Hodgkin's disease. Int J Cancer 1988;42:252–255.
25. Carbone PP, Kaplan HS, Musshoff K, Smithers DW, Tubiana M. Report of the committee on Hodgkin's staging classification. Cancer Res 1971;31:1860.
26. Lister T, Crowther D, Sutcliffe S, et al. Report of a committee convened to discuss the evaluation and staging of patients with Hodgkin's disease: Cotswolds meeting. J Clin Oncol 1989;7:1630–1636.
27. Lukes RJ, Butler JJ. The pathology and nomenclature of Hodgkin's disease. Cancer Res 1966;26:1063–1081.
28. Mauch P, Kalish L, Kadin M, et al. Patterns of presentation of Hodgkin's disease. Cancer 1993;71:2062–2071.
29. Mason D, Banks P, Chan J, et al. Nodular lymphocyte predominance Hodgkin's disease: a distinct clinicopathologic entity. Am J Surg Pathol 1994;18:526–530.
30. Lukes R. Criteria for involvement of lymph node, bone marrow, spleen, and liver in Hodgkin' s disease. Cancer Res 1971;31:1755.
31. Neiman RR, Rosen PJ, Lukes RJ. Lymphocyte-depletion Hodgkin's disease. N Engl J Med 1973;288:751–755.
32. Doggett RS, Colby TV, Dorfman RF. Interfollicular Hodgkin's disease. Am J Surg Path 1983;7:145–149.
33. Somers R, Tubiana M, Henry-Amar M. EORTC Lymphoma Cooperative Group Studies in clinical stage I-II Hodgkin's disease 1963-1987. Recent Res in Cancer Res 1989;117:175–181.
34. Crnkovich MJ, Leopold K, Hoppe RT, et al. Stage I to IIB Hodgkin's disease: the combined experience at Stanford and the Joint Center for Radiation Therapy. J Clin Oncol 1987;5:1041–1049.
35. Specht L, Nissen NI. Hodgkin 's disease stages I and II with infradiaphragmatic presentation: a rare and prognostically unfavorable combination. Eur J Haematol 1988;40:396–402.
36. Lee CKK, Aeppli DM, Bloomfield CD, et al. Curative radiotherapy for laparotomy-staged IA, IIA, IIIA Hodgkin's disease. An evaluation of the gains achieved with radical radiotherapy. Int J Radiat Oncol Biol Phys 1990;19:547–549.
37. Henry-Amar M, Friedman S, Hayat M, et al. Erythrocyte sedimentation rate predicts early and survival in early-stage Hodgkin's disease. The EORTC Lymphoma Cooperative Group. Ann Intern Med 1991; 114:361–365.
38. Tubiana M, Henry-Amar M, Hayat M et al. Prognostic significance of the number of involved areas in the early stages of Hodgkin 's disease. Cancer 1982;54:95–104.
39. Hoppe RT, Coleman CN, Cox RS, et al. The management of stage I-II Hodgkin's disease with irradiation alone or combined modality therapy: The Stanford experience. Blood 1982;59:455–465.
40. Farah R, Ultmann J, Griem M, et al. Extended mantle radiation for pathologic stage I and II Hodgkin's disease. J Clin Oncol 1988;6: 1047–1052.
41. Wasserman TH, Trenkner DA, Fineberg B, et al. Cure of early stage Hodgkin's disease with subtotal nodal irradiation. Cancer 1991;68: 1208–1215.
42. Mendenhall NP, Taylor BW, Marcus RB, et al. The impact of pelvic recurrence and elective pelvic irradiation on survival and treatment morbidity in early-stage Hodgkin's disease. Int J Radiat Oncol Biol Phys 1991;21:1157–1165.
43. Mauch P, Greenberg H, Lewin A, et al. Prognostic factors in patients with subdiaphragmatic Hodgkin's disease. Hematol Oncol 1983;1: 205–214.
44. Mai DHW, Peschel RE, Portlock C, et al. Stage I and II subdiaphragmatic Hodgkin's disease. Cancer 1991;68:1476–1481.
45. Krikorian JG, Portlock CS, Mauch PM. Hodgkin's disease presenting below the diaphragm: a review. J Clin Oncol 1986;4:1551–1552.
46. Leibenhaut MH, Hoppe RT, Varaghese A, et al. Subdiaphragmatic Hodgkin's disease: laparotomy and treatment results in 49 patients. J Clin Oncol 1987;5:1050–1055.
47. Rosenberg SA, Kaplan HS. Evidence for an orderly progression in the spread of Hodgkin's disease. Cancer Res 1966;26:1225–1231.
48. Kaplan HS. Hodgkin's disease. 2nd ed. Cambridge, MA: Harvard University Press, 1980.
49. Fuller L, Hutchison G. Collaborative clinical trial for stage I and II Hodgkin's disease: significance of mediastinal and nonmediastinal disease in laparotomy and nonlaparotomy staged patients. Cancer Treat Rep 1982;66:775–787.
50. Zittoun R, Audebert A, Hoerni B, et al. Extended field versus involved field irradiation combined with MOPP chemotherapy in early clinical stages of Hodgkin's disease. J Clin Oncol 1985;3:207–214.
51. Cosset JM, Henry-Amar M, Meerwaldt JH, et al. The E.O.R.T.C. trials for limited stage Hodgkin's disease. Eur J Cancer 1992;11: 1847–1850.
52. Bonadonna G. Modern treatment of malignant lymphomas: a multidisciplinary approach? Ann Oncol 1994;5(suppl 2):5–16.
53. Fuller L, Hagemeister F, North L, et al. The adjuvant role of two cycles of MOPP and low-dose lung irradiation in stage IA through IIB Hodgkin's disease: preliminary results. Int J Radiat Oncol Biol Phys 1988;14:683–692.
54. Straus D, Yahalom J, Gaynor J, et al. Four cycles of chemotherapy and regional radiation therapy for clinical early-stage and intermediate-stage Hodgkin's disease. Cancer 1992;69:1052–1060.
55. Specht L, Gray RG, Clarke MJ, et al. Influence of more extensive radiotherapy and adjuvant chemotherapy on long-term outcome of early-stage Hodgkin's disease: a meta-analysis of 23 randomized trials involving 3,888 patients. J Clin Oncol 1998;16:830–843.
56. Stein RS, Hilborn RM, Flexner JM, et al. Anatomical substages of stage III Hodgkin's disease: Implications for staging, therapy, and experimental design. Cancer 1978;42:429–436.
57. Hoppe RT, Rosenberg SA, Kaplan HS, Cox RS. Prognostic factors in pathological stage IIIA Hodgkin's diseases. Cancer 1980;46: 1240–1246.
58. Hoppe RT, Cox RS, Rosenberg SA, et al. Prognostic factors in pathologic stage III Hodgkin's disease. Cancer Treat Rep 1982;66: 743–749.
59. Lee CKK, Bloomfield CD, Goldman A, et al. Liver irradiation in stage IIIA Hodgkin's disease patients with splenic involvement. Am J Clin Oncol 1984;7:149–157.
60. Mauch P, Goffman T, Rosenthal DS, et al. Stage III Hodgkin's disease: improved survival with combined modality therapy as compared with radiation therapy alone. J Clin Oncol 1985;3:1166–1173.
61. Stein RS, Golomb HM, Diggs CH, et al. Anatomic substages of stage III-A Hodgkin's disease: a collaborative study. Ann Intern Med 1980; 92:159.
62. Stein RS, Golomb HM, Wiernik PH, et al. Anatomic substages of stage IIIA Hodgkin's disease: follow-up of a collaborative study. Cancer Treat Rep 1982;66:733–741.
63. Marcus KC, Kalish LA, Coleman CN, et al. Improved survival in patients with limited stage IIIA Hodgkin's disease treated with combined radiation therapy and chemotherapy. J Clin Oncol 1994;12: 2567–2572.
64. Lister TA, Doreen MS, Faux M, et al. The treatment of stage IIIA Hodgkin's disease. J Clin Oncol 1983;745–749.
65. Longo DL, Young RC, Wesley M, et al. Twenty years of MOPP therapy for Hodgkin's disease. J Clin Oncol 1986;4:1295–1306.
66. Drowther D, Wagstaff J, Deakin D, et al. A randomized study comparing chemotherapy along with chemotherapy followed by radiotherapy in patients with pathologically staged IIIA Hodgkin's disease. J Clin Oncol 1984;2:892–897.
67. Loeffler M, Brosteanu O, Hasenclever D, et al. Meta-analysis of chemotherapy versus combined modality treatment trials in Hodgkin's disease. J Clin Oncol 1998;16:818–829.
68. Mauch PM, Controversies in the management of early stage Hodgkin's disease. Blood 1994;2:318–329.
69. Rosenberg SA, Kaplan HS. The evolution and summary results of the Stanford randomized clinical trials of the management of Hodgkin's disease: 1962–1984. Int J Radiat Oncol Biol Phys 1985;11:5–22.
70. Pavlovsky S, Maschio M, Santarelli MT, et al. Randomized trial of chemotherapy versus chemotherapy plus radiotherapy for stage I-II Hodgkin's disease. J Natl Cancer Inst 1988;80:1466–1473.
71. Biti GA, Cimino G, Cartoni C, et al. Extended-field radiotherapy is superior to MOPP chemotherapy for the treatment of pathologic stage I-II A Hodgkin's disease: Eight-year update of an Italian prospective randomized study. J Clin Oncol 1992;10:378–382.
72. Longo D, Glatstein D, Duffey P, et al. Radiation therapy versus combination chemotherapy in the treatment of early-stage Hodgkin's disease: seven-year results of a prospective randomized trial. J Clin Oncol 1991;9:906–917.
73. Gilbert R. Radiotherapy in Hodgkin's disease (malignant granulomatosis). Am J Roentgenol 1939;41:198–241.

74. Peters M. A study of survival in Hodgkin's disease treated radiologically. Am J Roentgenol 1950;63:299–311.
75. Kaplan HS. The radical radiotherapy of regionally localized Hodgkin's disease. Radiology 1962;89:553–561.
76. Hanks GE, Kinzie JJ, White RL, et al. Patterns of Care Outcome Studies: Results of the National Practice in Hodgkin's disease. Cancer 1983;51:569–573.
77. Grant L, Jackson W. An investigation of the mantle technique. Clin Radiol 1973;24:254–262.
78. Weisenberger TH, Juillard GJF. Upper extremity lymphangiography in the radiation therapy of lymphomas and carcinoma of the breast. Radiology 1977;122:227–230.
79. Carmel RJ, Kaplan HS. Mantle irradiation in Hodgkin's disease. An analysis of technique, tumor eradication and complications. Cancer 1976;37:2813–2825.
80. Page V, Gardner A, Karzmark CJ. Physical and dosimetric aspects of the radiotherapy of malignant lymphomas. I. The mantle technique. Radiology 1970;96:609–626.
81. Palos B, Kaplan HS, Karzmark CJ. The use of thin lung shields to deliver limited whole-lung irradiation during mantle-field treatment of Hodgkin's disease. Radiology 1971;101:441–442.
82. Lee CKK, Bloomfield CD, Levitt SH. Prophylactic whole lung irradiation for extensive mediastinal Hodgkin's disease. Proc Am Soc Clin Oncol 1979;20:4411.
83. Johnson RE, Ruhl U, Johnson SK, Glover M. Split-course radiotherapy of Hodgkin's disease. Local tumor control and normal tissue reactions. Cancer 1976;37:1713–1717.
84. Leopold KA, Canellos GP, Rosenthal D, et al. Stage IA-IIB Hodgkin's disease: Staging and treatment of patients with large mediastinal adenopathy. J Clin Oncol 1989;7:1059–1065.
85. LeFloch O, Donaldson SS, Kaplan HS. Pregnancy following oophoropexy and total nodal irradiation in women with Hodgkin's disease. Cancer 1976;38:2263–2268.
86. Carmel RJ, Palos BB, Duggan JP, et al. Testicular shielding of patients receiving inverted-Y irradiation. Int J Radiat Oncol Biol Phys 1976; 1(supp l1):61.
87. Lutz W, Larsen R. Technique to match mantle and para-aortic fields. Int J Radiat Oncol Biol Phys 1983;9:1753.
88. Fraass B, Tepper J, Glatstein E, van de Geijn J. Clinical use of matchline wedge for adjacent megavoltage radiation field matching. Int J Radiat Oncol Biol Phys 1983;9:209.
89. Kinzie JJ, Hanks GE, Maclean GJ, et al. Patterns of Care Study: Hodgkin's disease relapse rates and adequacy of portals. Cancer 1983; 52:2223–2226.
90. Schewe KL, Kun L, Cox J. A step toward ending the controversies in Hodgkin's disease. Int J Radiat Oncol Biol Phys 1989;17:1123–1124.
91. Raubitschek A, Glatstein E. The never-ending controversies in Hodgkin's disease. Int J Radiat Oncol Biol Phys 1989;17:1115–1117.
92. Vijayakumar S, Rosenberg I, Brandt T, et al. The effect of posterior midline spinal cord block (PMSB) on Hodgkin's disease therapeutic dose estimates: a dosimetric study [abstract]. Int J Radiat Oncol Biol Phys 1989;17:170.
93. Peters MV. Prophylactic treatment of adjacent areas in Hodgkin's disease. Cancer Res 1966;26:1232–1243.
94. Kaplan HS. Evidence for a tumoricidal dose level in the radiotherapy of Hodgkin's disease. Cancer Res 1966;26:1221–1224.
95. Fletcher GH, Shukovsky LJ. The interplay of radio-curability and tolerance in the irradiation of human cancers. J Radiol Electro 1975; 56:383–400.
96. Vijayakumar S, Myrianthopolos LC. An updated dose-response analysis in Hodgkin's disease. Radiother Oncol 1992;24:1–13.
97. Myrianthopoulos L, Nautiyal J, Powers C, et al. A re-evaluation of dose response in Hodgkin's Disease [abstract]. Radiology 1995;197: 359.
98. Duehmke E, Diehl V, Loeffler M, et al. Randomized trial with early stage Hodgkin's disease testing 30 Gy vs. 40 Gy extended field radiotherapy alone [abstract]. Int J Radiat Oncol Biol Phys 1995;32(suppl 1):213.
99. Hoppe RT. Hodgkin's disease. Patterns of Care Study Newsletter No. 3. Philadelphia: American College of Radiology, 1990–1991.
100. Schellong G, Brämswig JH, Schwarze EW, et al. An approach to reduce treatment and invasive strategy in childhood Hodgkin's disease. The sequence of the German DAL multi-center studies. Bull Cancer 1988;75:41–51.
101. Schellong G, Brämswig JH, Hörnig-Franz I, et al. Hodgkin's disease in children: combined modality treatment for stages IA, IB, and IIA. Results in 356 patients of the German/Austrian Pediatric Study Group. Ann Oncol 1994;5(suppl 2):113–115.
102. Donaldson SS, Link MP. Combined modality treatment with low-dose radiation and MOPP chemotherapy for children with Hodgkin's disease. J Clin Oncol 1987;5:742–749.
103. Oberlin O, Leverger G, Pacquement H, et al. Low-dose radiation therapy and reduced chemotherapy in childhood Hodgkin's disease: the experience of the French Society of Pediatric Oncology. J Clin Oncol 1992;10:1602–1608.
104. Prosnitz LR. Hodgkin's disease: the right dose. Int J Radiat Oncol Biol Phys 1990;19:803–804.
105. Noordijk EM, Carde P, Mandard AM, et al. Preliminary results of the EORTC-GPMC controlled clinical trial H7 in early stage Hodgkin's disease. Ann Oncol 1994;5(suppl 2):S107–S112.
106. Cosset JM, Henry-Amar M, Meerwaldt JH: Long-term toxicity of early stages of Hodgkin's disease therapy: The EORTC experience. EORTC Lymphoma Cooperative Group. Ann Oncol 1991;2:77–82.
107. Hancock SL, Tucker MA, Hoppe RT. Factors affecting late mortality from heart disease after treatment of Hodgkin's disease. JAMA 1993; 270:1949–1955.
108. Hancock SL, Hoppe RT. Long-term complications of treatment and causes of mortality after Hodgkin's disease. Semin Radiat Oncol 1996;6:225–242.
109. Coia LR, Hanks GE. Complications from large field intermediate dose infradiaphragmatic radiation: an analysis of the Patterns of Care Outcomes Studies for Hodgkin's disease and seminoma. Int J Radiat Oncol Biol Phys 1988;15:29–35.
110. Miller RW, Van de Geijn J, Raubitschek AA, et al. Dosimetric considerations in treating mediastinal disease with mantle fields: characterization of the dose under mantle blocks. Int J Radiat Oncol Biol Phys 1995;32:1083–1095.
111. Horning SJ, Hoppe RT, Hancock SL, et al. Vinblastine, bleomycin, and methotrexate: an effective adjuvant in favorable Hodgkin's disease. J Clin Oncol 1988;6:1822–1831.
112. Hancock SL, Tucker MA, Hoppe RT. Breast cancer after treatment of Hodgkin's disease. J Natl Cancer Inst 1993;85:25–31.
113. Birdwell SH, Hancock SL, Varghese A, et al. Gastrointestinal cancer after treatment of Hodgkin's disease. Int J Radiat Oncol Biol Phys 1995;37:67–73.
114. van Leeuwen FD, Klokman WJ, Stovall M, et al. Roles of radiotherapy and smoking in lung cancer following Hodgkin's disease. J Natl Cancer Inst 1995;87:1530–1537.
115. Mauch P, Kalish LA, Marcus KC, et al. Long-term survival in Hodgkin's disease: relative impact of mortality, second tumors infection, and cardiovascular disease. Cancer J Sci Am 1995;1:33–42.

Index

Page numbers in *italics* denote figures; those followed by a "t" denote tables.

AAPM (*see* American Association of Physicists in Medicine)
Abdomen
  cancer of
    bulky retroperitoneal metastasis, 474t–475, 523
    conformal radiation therapy, 123–124
  whole irradiation of, 398–*399*
Acetic acid, 409
Acoustic tumors, 152–*153,* 170
Adjacent fields
  dose distribution factors, 67–70, *68–69,* 77–*79*
  hot spots in, 78
  normal tissue factors, 68, 70
  radiation therapy guidelines, 70
  separation guidelines, 68–*70,* 78–79, 131
AFP (alpha feto-protein), 471
AIDS (acquired immunodeficiency syndrome), 336
Air kerma rates and references, 179, 205, 380
AJCC (*see* American Joint Committee on Cancer)
Alanine detectors, 140
ALARA (as-low-as-reasonably-achievable), 214
Algorithms (*see also* Computer software)
  dosimetry
    conformal radiation therapy, 113–115
    HDR brachytherapy, 202–205, *203*
    intensity modulated therapy, 128, 130–131, 137
    stereotactic radiation, 166
  patient selection, *452*
  reconstruction, 105
  in treatment planning, 33, 45–46, 60
Allis clamp, *369*
Alpha cradle, 106–*107,* 353, 450, *490*
Alpha feto-protein (AFP), 471
^{241}Am (*see* Americium)
American Association of Physicists in Medicine (AAPM), 202, 205–206, 453, 506
American Joint Committee on Cancer (AJCC)
  esophageal cancer stages per, 327t
  esophagus divisions per, *326*
  lung cancer stages, survival projections per, 317t
  soft tissue sarcoma stages per, 484–485t
  testicular cancer stages per, 470t
  urinary bladder cancer stages per, 351
  vulvar cancer stages per, 405–406
Americium (^{241}Am), for vaginal cancer, 423
Anal cancer
  chemoirradiation, 17t, 342–344
  diagnostic evaluation, 336
  pathways of spread, 337
  primary treatment, 342–*345*
  radiation therapy
    complications when postoperative, 345
    dose factors, 343–*345*
    field design, 343–*344*
    therapeutic ratio optimization, 344–345
  recurrence after resection, 337–338
Angiographically occult vascular malformations (AOVM), 154
Angiography, in stereotactic radiosurgery, 154, 158, 160, 162, 169
Angiomas, venous, 154
Anisotropy, 202
Ann Arbor classification, for Hodgkin's disease, 521t, 522–*523*
  Cotwold modifications, 522t
AOVM (angiographically occult vascular malformations), 154
Apoptosis, 186–*187*
Applicators, intracavitary brachytherapy
  afterloading
    computer-controlled remote, 200–201, 210, 212–214, 366, 431
    emergency procedures for, 207
    high dose, 200–201, 212–214, 366, 431
    low dose, 210, 212–214, 366
    manual, 366–367, *390*
  Bloedorn, 421, 424
  Burnett, 421
  cervical, 178, 181, 210–214, 366t–*369*
  components, 178, 181, 201
  Delclos, *419,* 421
  for high dose therapy, 200–201, 205–206, 431
  intrauterine afterloading
    cylinder mounted on, *430*
    high dose, 389, *391*
    instruments for inserting, 428, *431*
    low dose, 388–*389*
  for low dose therapy, 366–367, *390*
  MIRALVA, 421, 423–424, *428–429*
  positioning of, 200–201, 205, 211
  quality assurance, 205–206
  safety systems for, 201
  size evolution, 211–212
  vaginal afterloading, *419,* 421, *423–428*
Aquaphor, 341
Aquaplast aids
  cast, 450
  frame, *88*
  head mold, *514*
  immobilizer, *96*
  masks, *92, 290, 515*
Arteriovenous malformations (AVM), 153–154, 157, 169–170
Astrocytomas
  grading systems, 223–224t
  incidence, 224t
  stereotactic radiosurgery, 156–157, *248*
  treatment guidelines, 230t, 253, *256,* 257, *259*
  volume determinations, *228*
^{192}Au (*see* Gold)
Away tables, 375
Axilla
  anatomy, 301–*302*
  irradiation of
    indications, 306
    techniques, 306–*307*

Bacillus Calmette-Guérin (BCG), 23, 349, 352, 358
Barium enema study, value of, 335
BD (*see* Doses, basal)

Beam design *(see also* Field blocks; *specific beam or therapy; specific beams)*
adjacent field guidelines (*see* Adjacent fields)
3-D simulation techniques, 111–*112*
geometric principles, 68–*70*
intensity factors, 128–130, 135
isocentric orientation, 55–56
modification (*see* Beam-modifying devices)
per therapies *(see specific therapy)*
quality factors
contamination, 65, 112, 130, 142
treatment planning, 38
quantity factors, 64
Beam spoiler, *100,* 508
Beam-modifying devices
dose distribution alteration, 86, *89–91*
therapy techniques (*see* Conformal radiation therapy)
treatment planning and, 37–38, 43–45
Beams
electrons (*see* Electron beam therapy)
neutron (*see* Neutron beam therapy)
photon (*see* Photon beam therapy)
protons (*see* Proton beam therapy)
Beam's eye view (BEV)
CT considerations, 60, 106, 111–*112*
lung cancer planning, 320, 322–*323*
in treatment planning, 40–*41,* 46
BED (*see* Doses, biologic effective)
Biliary tree tumors
conformal radiation therapy, 123–124
HDR brachytherapy, 216
Bladder cancer (*see* Urinary bladder)
Blocks
bite, 32, *93,* 160–*161*
cerrobend™
custom, *90*
electron cutouts, *90*
for field shaping, 57, *66,* 77
half-beam, 70
multileaf collimators versus, 66–*67*
standard, *90*
eye, *91*
field (*see* Field blocks)
lead, 64–65, 77–*78*
Lipowitz's metal, *271, 293*
styrofoam, 66
trays as
floor-mounted, *90*
table-mounted, *89*
Block-to-surface distance (BSD), 64–65
BMT (*see* Bone marrow transplantation)
Boards
angle, *97*
arm, *98*
breast, *97*
mantle, *97*
window, *96*
Body brace, *102*
Bolusing
indications, 78
materials, 78, *91*
wax, *84*–85
Bone marrow, chemoirradiation toxicity, 25
Bone marrow transplantation (BMT)
diseases treated by, 499–500t
graft failures per dose fractionation, 502t
histocompatibility tests for, 499
irradiation conditioning for, 499–500t
types of, 499
Bowel tumors (*see* Colon cancer)
Brachytherapy
clinical applications
high dose (*see* High dose-rate brachytherapy)
low dose (*see* Low dose-rate brachytherapy)
nasal vestibule cancer, 292, *294*
oral cavity cancer, 282, *285–286*
parotid gland tumors, 294–*295*
prostate cancer, 451–*452*
tongue cancer, *287–288*
vaginal cuff (*see* Vaginal cuff irradiation)
vulvar cancer, 410–411
computed tomography in, 213
dose distribution
high dose, 202–205
high versus low dose, 215
low dose, 194
rules for, 174–175t
dose optimization, 211, 213, 215
high dose algorithms, 202–205
high versus lose dose, 197–198
dose-rate effect data, *188–193*
inverse, *190*–191
high dose (*see* High dose-rate brachytherapy)
interstitial
activity per implant dimensions, 176
computer system, 175t, *177*
dose calculations, 173–174
dose specification rules, 174–177, 192
Memorial system, 175t, 176
Paris system, 175t, *176*–177, 192, 203, 215
Paterson-Parker system, 174–175t, 192
permanent, 176
Quimby system, 174–176
source distribution rules, 174–175t, 200
target volumes, 176–177
intracavitary (*see also* Cervical cancer, brachytherapy)
applicators for (*see* Applicators)
dosimetry, 136, 178, 213
target volumes, 178–*180,* 213
time-dose pattern in, 181
treatment volumes, 178–*180*
tumor volume, 213
isodose distribution
high dose, *203–204*
interstitial, 173, *176–177*
intracavitary, 178–181
low dose (*see* Low dose-rate Brachytherapy)
magnetic resonance imaging in, 213
principles, 173–*174*
pulsed (PDR)
clinical schedules, 196t
experimental validation, 195–196
principles, *194–195*
stepping source positioning method, 194–195
quality assurance, 215
radioactive source choices, 173–174t
radiobiology
absorption, 184–*185*
cell survival curves, 186–*188*
chromosomal aberrations, 184–*186, 188*
DNA damage, 184–*185*
dose-rate effect, *188–193*
early and late responses, *191*–194
inverse dose-rate effect, *190*–191
stereotactic radiosurgery versus, 157
treatment planning, 38
verification techniques, 205–207, 213–215
Bragg peak radiation, 154–155, 158
Brain
anatomical divisions, 224–*225*
shielding, in total body irradiation, 503
tumors of (*see* Brain tumors)
whole irradiation of, 224, 237–*239*

Brain tumors *(see also specific tumor)*
  benign, 147
  conformal radiation therapy, 122–123
  custom field planning, 238, *240–241*
  external beam therapy, 157, 170
  functional mapping, 225–*226*
  intensity modulated therapy, 139
  malignant, 147
  metastatic
    prophylactic irradiation, 325
    stereotactic radiosurgery, *156*
  radiosurgery for (*see* Stereotactic radiosurgery)
  staging systems, 223–224t, 226
  treatment aids, 97, 100–*101,* 151
  treatment approach examples
    central lesions, *253–254*
    frontal lesions, *248–252*
    parietal lesions, *248–252*
    posterior fossa tumors, 253, *255–258*
    temporal lobe lesions, 246–*247*
    thalamic lesions, *253–254*
    whole brain irradiation, 224, *237–239*
  treatment guidelines, 230t
    tolerance doses, 231t–232t
    volume and dose determinations, 228t–231, *229–230*
  treatment planning
    general principles, 237–241
    imaging modalities, *235–236*
    positioning and immobilization, 232–235, *233–234*
Breast
  anatomy, 301–*302*
    axilla, 301–*302*
    internal mammary nodes, 301, *303*
  immobilization devices, *97–98*
  tumors of (*see* Breast cancer)
Breast cancer (*see also* Chest wall irradiation)
  chemoirradiation, 24
  dissociation effects example, *4*
  electron beam therapy, 83–85, 303
  external beam therapy, *97–98*
  local-regional failures, 10t
  postmastectomy irradiation
    axillary fields, 305–307
    chest wall fields, 305–*307*
    dosing, 305–307
    electron beam techniques, 305
    energy requirements, *304*–305
    indications, 303–*304*
    internal mammary fields, *304*–305
    photon fields, 305–307
    supraclavicular nodal irradiation, 305
  treatment planning, 11–12, 59, 305, 307
  treatment to breast, internal mammary nodes, and supraclavicular areas, 312
  treatment to intact breast
    boost to primary site, *311*–312
    custom blocking, 310
    dose, 311
    indications, 307
    infraclavicular field, 310
    limited to breast, 307–308
    setup parameters, 309–*311*
    simulation techniques, 59, *308*–309
    tangential field formulas, 309–*311*
Bremsstrahlung interactions, 68, 72, 75, 77
BRW (*see* Headrings, Brown-Roberts-Wells)
BSD (block-to-surface distance), 64–65
Bulky abdominal disease, 474t–475, 523
Busulfan, 500

Californium (^{252}Cf), for vaginal cancer, 423
Calipers, in treatment planning, *87*
Camptothecins, 15t–16
Capsules, lateral (*see* Colpostats)
Carboplatin, 22, 322
Carcinoembryonic antigen (CEA), 335
Carcinoma *(see specific anatomical cancer or tumor)*
Cardboard cutouts, *94–95*
Casts
  aquaplast, 450
  immobilization, 54–55, 59, 305
  Vaculock, 305
Catheters
  afterloading, *235,* 398
  Flexiguide, 398
  intraperitoneal, 398
CCRT (*see* Conformal radiation therapy, computer-controlled)
CEA (carcinoembryonic antigen), 335
Cell kill
  acute reactions, *4–6*
  DNA role, 184–186
  dose-rate effect, 188–194
    inverse, *190*–191
  early responding, 147, 191
  fractionated, 147, 151
  late effects, 4–*6,* 147, 191–192
  mitotic, 186
  multihit, 3–4
  programmed, 186–*187*
  recovery factors, *4*–6, 8
  reproductive, 186
  single-hit, 3–5, 147
  therapeutic ratio and, 212–*213*
  tolerance in (*see* Tolerance)
Cell loss factor (CLF), 7–8
Cell survival curves (*see* Survival fraction curves)
Central nervous system
  anatomy, 223–*226*
  normal tissue tolerance, 539
  tumors of (*see* Central nervous system tumors)
Central nervous system tumors *(see also specific segment or tumor)*
  craniospinal axis irradiation, 257, *261–266*
  dose determinations, 228t–231, 242–243
    tolerance doses, 231t–232t
  grading systems, 223–224t, 226
  incidence and epidemiology, 223–224t
  target volumes, 228t–231, 242–243
  treatment planning
    criteria for evaluating, 242–243
    general principles, *237–242*
    imaging modalities, 226–*227, 229–230, 235–236*
    positioning and immobilization, 232–235, *233–234*
Cervical cancer
  brachytherapy
    applicators, 178, 181, 210–214, 366t–*369*
    clinical trials, 210–211
    complications, 181t, *182*
    data needed for reporting, 179t
    dose rate and implant duration, 181–*182,* 212–*231*
    dose specification rules, 178–181
    Fletcher guidelines, 181
    high dose (*see* Cervical cancer, HDR brachytherapy)
    ICRU system, 178–181
    low dose (*see* Cervical cancer, LDR brachytherapy)
    Manchester system, *178*
    principles and techniques, 177–182
    reference point doses, *180–181,* 203, 215, 376–378, 380–381t
    time-dose pattern, 181
  chemoirradiation, 21
  electron beam therapy, 79–80t
  external beam therapy, 181, 198
    box technique, 7
    dose factors, 217–218
    field design, 364–366, *365*
    split pelvis, 382t
    whole pelvis, 382t

Cervical cancer *(Continued)*
HDR brachytherapy
advantages, 363–364t
dose factors, 217–218
guidelines, 198
results and complications, 197–198, 218
LDR brachytherapy
advantages of, 363–364t
application types and performance, 366t, 385
applicator loading determination, 375–*377*
clinical results, 384t
dose calculations, 376–*378*
dose to bladder and rectum, 382–383
equipment, 366–*369, 371*
failure rates, 384t
general procedure, 367, 369–375
ICRU reporting data, 380t
implant duration, 379–383
implant removal, 383–384
milligram hour factors, 379–380
optimizing the geometry of, 370–374
patient care during, 383
patient evaluation, 366
Point A dose factor, *379*–380
Point B dose factors, *379*–380
quality assurance, 384–385t
reference points for dosing, 376–*378,* 380
reference volume determination, 380–381t
sequelae, 384
simulation, 375
surface dose rates, 375t
survival rates, 384t
University of Minnesota dose guidelines, 381–383
written directive completion, *374*–375
lymphatic involvement, *364*–366
treatment planning, *12,* 363–364
Cervix
anatomy, 363
tumors of (*see* Cervical cancer)
Cesium (^{137}Cs)
in brachytherapy, 173–174t, 175, 212
low dose cervical, 367, *369,* 374, 383
for lip cancer, 280
for mouth floor cancer, 282, *285*
for nasal vestibule cancer, 292
for tongue cancer, *287–288*
transport card, 375–*376*
for vaginal cancer, *419,* 421, 423, *425,* 426t–427t, 428, *430*
dummy sources, 424, *426–427*
^{252}Cf (*see* Californium)
CHART (continuous accelerated hyperfractionation radiation therapy), 322
Chemoirradiation
agents used for, 14–16
biological basis, 14–15t
clinical applications
anal cancer, 17t, 342–344
breast cancer, 24
cervical cancer, 21
colon cancer, 335–336
esophageal cancer, 18t–19, 327–328t, 330
gastrointestinal tract tumors, 17–20, 327–330, 335–338, 342–344
gynecologic tumors, 21, 408–409, 413–414
head and neck cancer, 20–21
Hodgkin's disease, 524–525, 533, 538–539
liver cancer, 20
lung cancer, 21–22, 322–324, 326
pancreatic cancer, 19–20
rectal cancer, 17–18, 335–336, 338
soft-tissue sarcoma, 24–25
urinary bladder cancer, 22–24, 349, 352, 354, 358t–359
vulvar cancer, 408–409, 413–414
normal tissue effects, 31
toxicity from, 25
Chemotherapy
clinical applications
leukemias, 500
lung cancer, 321–322
soft tissue sarcomas, 487–488t
urinary bladder cancer, 352, 356, 358t, 359
vulvar cancer, 408–409, 413–414
with irradiation (*see* Chemoirradiation)
resistance to, 500
Chest wall irradiation
beam obliquity challenges, 75–*76,* 83
dosimetry, 83
electron beam therapy, 79–80t, 83–*84*
Cholestyramine, 345
Choline:creatine ratio, *227*
Chondrosarcomas, 157
Chordomas, 157
Choriocarcinomas, 468, 470–471
Chromosomes (*see* DNA)
Cisplatinum, 14–15t, 408
Cisternography, 152
Clarkson scatter-air ratios, 321–322
CLDR (*see* Low dose-rate brachytherapy, continuous)
CLF (cell loss factor), 7–8
Clinical parameters, basic
fractionation, 5–7
survival fraction curve, 3–6, *4*
tolerance, *7,* 9, 30–32
treatment planning (*see* Treatment planning)
tumor dose, 9t–11, *10,* 30
tumor kinetics, 7–*8*
Clonogenic cells, 186
CMT (*see* Combined modality therapy)
Cobalt (^{60}Co)
in brachytherapy, 200–201t
for glottic tumors, 270, 272
for Hodgkin's disease, 525
for mouth floor cancer, *284*
for vaginal cancer, 420, *422*
Cold spots
defined, 242
dose considerations, 45, 113
in nasal vestibule, 80–*81*
Collimators
jaws, for field shaping, 66, 70, 131
multileaf (MLC)
arc-based fan-beam, 132
cerrobend® blocks versus, 66–*67*
in conformal radiation therapy, 116–*117*
for field shaping, 66–*67*
fixed portal cone-beam dynamic, 132
in intensity modulated therapy, 128, 130–132
for simulation, *57,* 59
in treatment planning, 37–38, 43–44
multileaf intensity modulating (MIMIC), 44
stereotactic radiation associated, 160, 162, *164*
tertiary system, *101*
Colon
anatomy, 336
tumors of (*see* Colon cancer)
Colon cancer (*see also* Rectal cancer)
conformal radiation therapy, 123–124
diagnostic evaluation, 335–336
external beam therapy, 341–*342*
pathways of spread, 336–337
recurrence, 10, 341–342
after resection, 337
sacral canal importance, 341
therapeutic ratio optimization, 344–345
Color wash, 114

Colpostats
in cervical brachytherapy, 178, 366t–374
dosing influence, 181, 201, 212, 215, 217
tandem orientation, *372*
in endometrial brachytherapy
postoperative high dose, *393–394*
postoperative low dose, 391
postoperative step-wedge, 395–*396*
preoperative low dose, 388–*389*
Fletcher-Suit, 388–*389, 391, 393–394, 427*
Fletcher-Suit-Delclos, 367, 392–*393*
instruments for inserting, 428, *431*
Simon-Heyman, 388, *389–391*
in vaginal brachytherapy, *425*
Combined modality therapy (CMT)
biological basis, 14–15t
per tumor *(see specific anatomical cancer or tumor)*
toxicity, 25
types of, 14
Compensating filters (*see* Compensators)
Compensators
fixed-portal x-ray, 132
for missing tissue, 56–57, *91,* 128, 132
stacking devices for, 132
for total body irradiation, 97, *99*
trays as, *89*
Compton scattering, 105
Computed tomography (CT)
clinical applications *(see specific disease or therapy)*
electron density relationship, *105,* 108
scanners, 37, 40
single photon emission (SPECT), 45–46, 226
spiral, 108
technical aspects, 105–106
in treatment planning (*see* Treatment planning, 3-D)
Computer implant system, 177
Computer software (*see also* Algorithms)
applicator afterloading (*see* Applicators)
brachytherapy, 173–174, *177*–178, 203–204
intensity modulated therapy, 128, 137
stereotactic radiation, 158–159, 163, 166–168
treatment planning
evolution, 45–46
portal imaging, 33, 38, 46
simulation techniques, 59–61
Cone holder and periscope, intraoral, *94*
Cone output, in stereotactic radiation, *166*–167
Conformal radiation therapy (3-D CRT)
clinical applications
biliary tree cancer, 123–124
central nervous system tumors, 122–123
colon cancer, 123–124
gastrointestinal tract tumors, 123–124
kidney cancer, 123–124
lung cancer, 120t–122t
pancreatic cancer, 123–124
pineal gland tumors, 122
pituitary adenomas, 123
prostate cancer, 118t–120t, *119,* 447–450t, *448–449,* 454–455
upper abdominal malignancies, 123–124
urinary bladder cancer, 355, *357*
computer-controlled (CCRT), 116–*117*
dynamic, 117
segmental, 117
cost-benefit studies, 40–41
developing definitions, 128
dose escalation cautions, 39
intensity modulated (*see* Intensity modulated radiation therapy)
principles, 39–40, 128
research categories, 40
treatment planning (*see* Treatment planning, 3-D)
tumors benefiting from, 39–40, 355
Contrast materials, in treatment planning, *89*
Convolution energy deposition kernels, 45, 113
Cork and tongue blade, *93, 284, 292*
Craniopharyngiomas
incidence, 224t
stereotactic radiosurgery, 156–157
treatment guidelines, 230t
Craniospinal axis irradiation
treatment aids, 97, 100, *101*
treatment field planning, 261, *262–266*
treatment guidelines, 257, *261*
x-ray therapy in, 100
Cranium
irradiation of
for cancer (*see* Brain tumors; Craniospinal axis irradiation)
prophylactic (PCI), 325
tumors of (*see* Brain tumors)
Critical structures (*see* Organs at risk)
Cryptorchidism, 467
^{137}Cs (*see* Cesium)
CT (*see* Computed tomography)
CTV (*see* Target volumes, clinical)
Cumulative radiation effect (CRE), 6
Cyclophosphamide, 24–25
Cylinders, vaginal
cervical cancer, 367–*368,* 374–375
domed, 421, 424–*425*
endometrial cancer, 393
vaginal cancer, 421, *423–431*
Cystectomy, 349, 352, 356–357, 359

Deep vein thrombosis (DVT), prophylaxis, 369, 388
Depth helmet, *158*
Desmoid tumors, 488–489
Digitally reconstructed radiographs (DRR)
clinical applications
in treatment planning, 37, 40, 46, 59–*61,* 108
for esophageal cancer, *329*
in treatment verification, *116,* 136–*137*
Dilatation and curettage tray, *369*
Dixon & Moore Groups, of testicular cancer, 467–468
DNA
aberrations
anaphase bridge, 185
cell survival and, 187–*188*
chromatid, 185
chromosome, 185
dicentric, 185–*186*
dose-rate effect, *188–191*
inverse dose-rate effect, *190*–191
ring, 185–*186*
laddering, *186*
strand breaks
double (DSB), 184–*185*
repair patterns, 184–185, 189, 191
single, 184–*185*
strand composition, 184
Dose clouds, *115*
Dose-rate effect
in cell kill (*see* Survival fraction curves)
per therapies *(see specific therapy)*
Dose-response curves (*see* Tumor control probability)
Doses
basal (BD), 174, *176*–177, 215
biologic effective (BED), 501
calculation of (*see* Dosimetry)
distribution of (*see* Dosimetry)
fractionation of (*see* Fractionation)
Gaussian profiles, 78
matched peripheral (MPD), 453
maximum permissible (MPD), 214
maximum tolerable (MTD), 148–*149*
nominal single (NSD), 6
optimization of (*see* Dosimetry)

Doses *(Continued)*
surface
field shaping considerations, 65
physics, 72–*74*
transit, 202
tumor
gross cancer, 9
postoperative, 9–11, *10*
response analysis, 30–33
subclinical disease, 9t
Dose-volume histograms (DVH)
intensity modulated therapy, 143
reporting recommendations, 110–111
stereotactic radiosurgery, 147–*149*
treatment planning, 37, 40, *42,* 46, *114*–115
Dosimeters
BANG® gel, 134–135, *168*
cone output detector types, 167
electronic point, 132
Fricke solution, *168*
planar, 133
real-time, 132
Dosimetry
calculation
advanced algorithms, 113, 115, 130–131
2-D planning techniques, 112, 114
3-D planning techniques, 112–113
Fermi-Eyges model, 45
Monte Carlo method, 45–46, 113, 202
tumor parameters, 9t–11, *10,* 30
clinical applications *(see specific anatomy, disease, or therapy)*
distribution (*see also* Isodose distribution)
adjacent field factors, 68–70, *69,* 78–79
beamlet-generated, *129*–130
Cartesian coordinate localization system, 133
3-D planning techniques, 114–115, 168
inverse square law, 173–*174*
for field shaping, 69–70
normal tissue parameters, 30, *32*
optimization
criterion specification, 130–131, 140–141
CT algorithms, 60, 114–115, 130
geometric method, 204
inverse method, 115, 128–131, *129,* 143
treatment planning, 38–39, 46
phantoms for, 133–*135,* 137, *140,* 143, 506
quality assurance, 47
thermoluminescent (TLD), 132–*135, 140,* 167–167
lithium fluoride, 509, 513t
in treatment planning, 33, 35, 104
Doxorubicin, 14–15t, 16, 25, 488
DRR (*see* Digitally reconstructed radiographs)
DSB (double strand breaks, DNA), 184–*185*
DVH (*see* Dose-volume histograms)
DVT (*see* Deep vein thrombosis)

EBRT (*see* External beam therapy)
Electron backscatter (EBS), *68,* 77–*78, 100*
Electron beam therapy
biologic absorption, 184
clinical applications
breast cancer, 83–85, 303–305, *304*
cervical cancer, 79–80t
chest wall, 79–80t, 83–*84,* 305
eyelid cancer, 79–*81*
head and neck cancer, 79–*83,* 80t, 275, *277*
lip cancer, 79–80t
miscellaneous, *84*–85
nasal vestibule cancer, 80–*82, 292*–294
oral cavity cancer, 79–80t
parotid gland tumors, 79, 81, *83*
skin cancer, 79–80t
soft tissue sarcomas, 487
superiority for certain cancers, 79–80t
total body irradiation, 503, 510–*511*
vulvar cancer, 410–*412,* 414
contamination by, 65, 112
dose distribution
adjacent fields, 67–*68,* 77–*79*
air gaps, 77–78
beam obliquity, 75–*76*
bolusing, 78
tissue heterogeneities, 45, 76–77, 112–113
uniformity, *75*
energy characteristics
depth dose distribution, 38, 72–*74,* 76
dose gradient, 38, 73, 75
physics, 72–*74*
reduce dose gradient, *73,* 75
surface dose, 72–*74*
x-ray background, *72,* 75
field shaping techniques
filters, *65*–66
shielding, 67–*68,* 77
secondary ranges, 130
Electronic portal imaging devices (EPID)
in treatment planning, 38, 46, 61
verification techniques, 33–34t, 38, 61, 116
Embryonal cancers, 468, 470
Endometrial cancer
external pelvic irradiation, 397
postoperative, *395–396*
preoperative, 391–*392*
HDR brachytherapy, 216–217, 397
postoperative, 392–*394*
preoperative, 389–391
incidence, 387
LDR brachytherapy, 397
postoperative, 391–*393*
preoperative, 387–389t
reference points for dosing, 389
patient evaluation, 387
radiation therapy
preoperative, 400–401
prescription, 396–*397*
recurrence, local
intraperitoneal P-32 irradiation, 399–*400*
palliative irradiation, 400
therapy goals, 397, 400
therapy techniques, 397–400
whole abdominal irradiation, 398–*399*
Endometrium
anatomy, 387–*388*
tumors of (*see* Endometrial cancer)
Endoscopy, value of, 335
Ependymomas
grading systems, 224t
incidence, 226
spread, 226
treatment guidelines, 230t
EPID (*see* Electronic portal imaging devices)
Epilepsy, 152
Esophageal cancer
chemoirradiation, 18t–19, 327–328t, 330
definitive treatment
nonsurgical, 327–328t
sequelae, 330
surgical, 327–328t
dosing factors, *329*–330
external beam therapy, 216
general management, 327
HDR brachytherapy, 203, 216
pathologic features, 326–327
portal design, *328–329,* 330
radiation techniques, 328–330
staging, 327t

Esophagus
anatomy, 326
regional divisions, *326*
tumors of (*see* Esophageal cancer)
Etoposide, 322
Ewing's sarcoma, *84–85*
Examination under anesthesia (EUA)
for cervical cancer, 364
for endometrial cancer, 388
Exposure
as-low-as-reasonably-achievable, 214
with brachytherapy
health care providers, 210, 212, 214
patients, 214
External beam therapy (EBRT)
clinical applications
brain tumors, 157, 170
breast cancer, *97–98*
cervical cancer, 7, 181, 198, 217–218, 363–366, *365,* 382t
colon cancer, 341–*342*
esophageal cancer, 216
lip cancer, 280
lung cancer, *97–98,* 323
nasal vestibule cancer, 289–*290*
oral cavity cancer, *93–94,* 280, 282, *283–289,* 296–298
paranasal sinuses cancer, 289, *291*
parotid gland tumors, 293–*294*
pelvic tumors, 86, *95*–97, 107, 363–366, 382t
prostate cancer, 440–447t, *442–443, 445–446*
rectal cancer, 342
tongue cancer, 275, *278,* 284–285, *287*
urinary bladder cancer, 352–354, 356, 359
vaginal cancer, 418, 420–*422,* 421t
HDR brachytherapy with, 197–198, 211, 214–218
immobilization for (*see* Immobilization devices)
with intraperitoneal P-32, 399
Eye shields, *91, 100*
Eyelid cancer, electron beam therapy, 79–*81*

Farmer-type chambers, for calibration, 205
Fermi-Eyges multiple scattering model, 45
Field blocks (*see also* Beam design; *specific device)*
adjacent field separation
compensating wedges, 70
dosimetric, 69–70
geometric, 68–*70*
guidelines for, 70, 78–79
half-beam block, 70
independent jaw, 70, 131
junction shift, 70
collimators for (*see* Collimators, multileaf)
custom, 57–59, *58,* 66
electron-beam shielding, 67–*68,* 77
evolution, 64
half-value layer (HVL), 64, 418, 502–503, 535
standardized
divergence, 64–65
shadow tray, *65*–66
skin sparing, *65*–66
thickness, 64, 77
total body irradiation shielding, 501–503, 510–*512, 514–515*
Fields
adjacent (*see* Adjacent fields)
inverted-Y
in Hodgkin's disease, 524–525, *527,* 535
separation factors, 68–*69*
mantle
arm positions for, *529*
custom blocks for, *66*
in external beam treatment, *97–98*
field separation factors, 68–*69*
in Hodgkin's disease, 523–525, *526–533*
immobilization aids, *97–98*
multiple boost
in intensity modulated therapy, 142
lymphadenopathy, *85*
placement of
adjacent separation guidelines, 68–*70,* 78–79, 131
errors per verification films, 31–33t
fixed, 55
isocentric, 55
localization and documentation of, *55*–56, 62, 106–110 (*see also* Simulation)
shaping of (*see* Beam design; Field blocks)
source-skin distance, 55
FIGO (*see* International Federation of Gynecology and Obstetrics)
Filters
compensating (*see* Compensators)
electron beam, *65*–66
tin, *65*–66
Fletcher Lymphatic Trapezoid reference points, 377–*378*
Fluence (*see* Beam design, intensity factors)
5-fluorouracil
for anal cancer, 342–344
for colorectal cancer, 335–336, 338, 341
properties, 14–15t
toxicity from, 25
for vulvar cancer, 408
5-fluro-2'-deoxyuridine, 20
fMRI (*see* Magnetic resonance imaging, functional)
Fractionation
accelerated (*see* Hyperfractionation)
conventional, 5–7
unconventional, 7
Free radicals, 184
FSU (multiple functional subunits), 37

Gamma Knife radiosurgery unit, 147–148, 152, 154–158
Gammathalamotomy, 152
Gantry angles *(see specific therapy)*
Gastrointestinal tract
normal tissue tolerance, 540
tumors of (*see* Gastrointestinal tract tumors)
Gastrointestinal tract tumors *(see also specific segment)*
chemoirradiation, 17t–20, 327–330, 335–338, 342–344
toxicity from, 25
conformal radiation therapy, 123–124
recurrence, 8, 10
tumor control probability, 9t
Gaussian dose profiles, 78
Gemcitobine, 20
Germ cell tumors
grading systems, 224t
spread of, 226
testicular (*see* Testicular cancer)
Gimbal bearing assembly, 162, *164*
Glioblastoma multiforme
grading systems, 223–224t
incidence, 224t
recurrent, *227*
stereotactic radiosurgery, 157, 229, *247, 249*
treatment guidelines, 230t
volume determinations, *229*
Gliomas
grading systems, 223–224t, 228
incidence, 223–224t
resection mapping, *226*
stereotactic radiosurgery, 157, 169
Glomus jugulare tumors, 157
Gold (^{192}Au), in brachytherapy, 174t
Gonadoblastomas, 467
Graticule, *102*
Gross tumor volume (GTV)
ICRU recommendations, 108, 110–111
in presimulation planning, *53*
in treatment planning, 34, 36

Gynecologic tumors *(see also specific anatomical cancer or tumor)*
chemoirradiation, 21, 413–414, 4089–409
HDR brachytherapy, 216–217

Half-value layers (HVL) (*see* Field blocks, half-value layer)
β-HCG (human chorionic gonadotropin), 471
HDR (*see* High dose-rate brachytherapy)
Head and neck tumors
chemoirradiation, 20–21
electron beam therapy, 79–*83,* 80t
growth characteristics, 8
immobilization devices
bite block, *93*
cardboard cutout, *94–95*
cork and tongue blade, *93, 284, 292*
cradles, 107
for external beam treatment, 86, *92–95,* 107
eye shields, *100*
headrings, 100–*101*
holders, *92–93*
intraoral cone holder and periscope, *94*
intraoral stent, *94*
masks, *92,* 107, 137
shoulder swing, *95*
supports, *92*
intensity modulated therapy, 137–*141*
ipsilateral irradiation, 82–83t
normal tissue tolerance, 540
photon beam therapy, 82
postoperative irradiation, 272, *274, 289*
recurrence, 9–10t, *11–12*
treatment field designs
definitions, 269
hypopharnyx, 271–*273*
larnyx, 269–271
low neck, *296*–298
lymph nodes, 269, 295–298, *297*
nasal vestibule, *289–294*
nasopharynx, 279–280, *281–282,* 296–298
oral cavity, 280, 282, *283–289,* 296–298
oropharynx, 273–279, 296–298
paranasal sinuses, *289–294*
parotid gland, *293–295*
salivary glands, 293–*295*
submandibular gland, 294–295
unknown primary, *295*–296
treatment planning, 11
treatment verification, 136–*137*
Headrings
Brown-Roberts-Wells (BRW), 158, 160–*162*
Gill-Thomas-Cosman (GTC), 160–*161*
for magnetic resonance scanning, 158–160, *162*
mounted light on, *101*
Heart
chemoirradiation toxicity, 25
normal tissue tolerance, 539
Hegar dilators, *369*
Helium ion radiation, 154–155, 158
Hemangioblastomas, 157
Hemangiopericytomas
meningeal, 253, *255*
soft tissue, *491*
Hemolytic uremic syndrome (HUS), 16
HFX (*see* Hyperfractionation)
High dose-rate brachytherapy (HDR)
advantages, 210–212
clinical applications
bile duct tumors, 216
cervical cancer (*see* Cervical cancer)
endobronchial tumors, 215–216
endometrial cancer, 216–217, 389–*394,* 397
esophageal cancer, 203, 216
intraluminal, 216
prostate cancer, 216, 452–461t
vaginal cancer (*see* Vaginal cancer)
commitment costs
personnel, 206t–207
situations warranting, 197
time, 207
disadvantages, 210, 212–215
emergency procedures, 207
evolution, 210–211, 218–219
external beam treatments with, 197–198, 211, 214–218
low dose versus, 197–*198*
physics, 200–207, 215
quality assurance
devices, 205–206t
procedures, 206–207
radiation injuries from, 212–214, *213*
radiobiology, 184–194
clinical data on, *192–193*
dose-rate effect, *188–191*
early and late responses, *191*–194
inverse dose-rate effect, *190*–191
tumor size bias, 193–194
schedule survey, 197t
source considerations
applicators, 201
facility development, 201
models for, 202
positioning systems, 200–201, 205
remote afterloading units, 200–201
selection per half-life, 200–201t
shielding requirements, 200–201
stepping source positioning method, 200–202
therapeutic ratio, 197, 212–*213,* 218
treatment delivery
concerns, 213–214
guidelines, 211
treatment planning
dose calculation models, 202
dose distribution optimization, 202–205
dwell time optimization, 200, 202–205
transit dose, 202
Histiocytoma, *483, 494*
HIV (human immunodeficiency virus), 336
HLA (human lymphocyte antigen), 499
Hodgkin's disease
chemoirradiation, 524–525, 533, 538–539
diagnostic evaluation, 519–520
imaging studies, 520–521t
histopathologic classifications, 522–523
lymphocyte depletion (LD), 522–523
lymphocyte predominance type, 522
mediastinal masses in, 519–520, 525, 532–*534*
mixed cellularity (MC), 522–523
nodular sclerosis (NS), 522–523
radiation therapy
anterior field simulation, 526–527, *529–530*
blocks for shielding, 531–533, 535
complications, 539–540
dose considerations, 531t–533, 535, 538–539
extended field technique, 523–*526*
gaps of matching fields, 536, *537–538*
indications per stage, 523–524
inverted-Y fields, 524–525, *527,* 535
limited field technique, *536*
mantle field technique, 523–525, *526–533*
para-aortic field technique, 523, 525–*526, 529,* 533, *535*
posterior field simulation, *528,* 530–533, *532*
preauricular field, 525–526, 535
spade shape field, 525
subdiaphragmatic field technique, 523, 525–*526, 529,* 533, *535*
techniques overview, 525–526
total nodal, 523, 525
Waldeyer's ring, 525–526, 535–*536*

Hodgkin's disease *(Continued)*
simulation techniques, 62
staging
classifications, 521t–522t, *523*
procedures, 520–521t
treatment complications
per normal tissue tolerance, 539–540
secondary neoplasms, 540
treatment options
combined modalities, 524–525, 533, 538–539
decision making tree, *522*
with large mediastinal mass, 525, 532–*534*
radiation therapy alone, 523–530, 536–538
salvage, 539
Holders
head and face, *92*
off treatment table head, *93*
Hot spots
in adjacent fields, 78
in chest wall, 83–*84*
defined, 242
electron dose considerations, 45, 77, 113
Human chorionic gonadotropin (β-HCG), 471
Human lymphocyte antigen (HLA), 499
HUS (hemolytic uremic syndrome), 16
HVL (*see* Field blocks, half-value layer)
Hydroxyl radical (OH), 184
Hydroxyurea, 15t–16
Hyperbaric tanks, 3
Hyperfractionation (HFX), 7
with chemotherapy, for lung cancer, 321–322
continuous accelerated (CHART), 322
Hyperthermia, 14
Hypopharyngeal tumors
pharyngeal wall, 271–*273*
postoperative irradiation, 272, *274*
pyriform sinus, 271–*272*
treatment field designs, 271–*273*

^{125}I (*see* Iodine)
ICRU (*see* International Commission of Radiation Units and Measurements)
Ifosfamide, 488
Imaging studies *(see specific study)*
Immobilization devices *(see also specific device or therapy)*
arm, *98*
breast, *97–98*
feet, 107
head and neck, 86, *92–95,* 100–*101,* 107
mantle field, *97–98*
oral cavity, *93–94*
pelvic, 86, *95–96,* 97, 107
thorax, *97–98,* 107
in treatment planning
importance, 31, 34–35, 37, 106–107
for positioning and setup, 100, *102–103*
during simulation, 54–55
Implant systems
for brachytherapy (*see* Brachytherapy, interstitial)
computer, 177
Memorial, 176
Paris (*see* Paris implant system)
Paterson-Parker, 174–175t, 192
Quimby, 175–176
IMRT (*see* Intensity modulated radiation therapy)
Independent jaws (*see* Collimators, jaws)
Independent support stand (ISS)
accuracy checks, 162–164t, *165*
for stereotactic process, *159*–160, 162, *164–165*
Inserts, couch
acrylic, *96*
alpha cradle (*see* Alpha cradle)
mylar window, *95*
Intensity modulated radiation therapy (IMRT)
algorithms, 128, 130–131, 137
average monitor units, 142t
beam design, 128–130, 135, 139–*141*
clinical applications
experience summary, 136–143
nasopharyngeal cancer, 137–140
parotid gland tumors, 141–142
procedures for, 136
spinal cord tumors, 139
compensating filters, 132
current state of, 128–129
delivery systems
arc-based fan-beam dynamic MLC, 132
fixed portal cone-beam dynamic MLC, 132
fixed portal x-ray compensating filter, 132
historical review, 131–132
dose factors
distribution, *129*–130, 133, 135
isodose distribution, 132, *138–141*
optimization, 130–131, 140–142
outside the treatment volume, 142t–143
fan-beam delivery, 130
masks for, 137
medical linear accelerators, 131–132
organs at risk, 143
patient positioning, 135–136
photon beams, 130, *140–141*
principles, 117, 128–130
quality assurance
basis for, 132–133
clinical, 135–136
commissioning, 135
delivery system, 135–136
dosimetry system, 131–135, 143
static beam-intensity, 139
treatment planning
target volumes, 136, 143
techniques, 43–45, 54
verification techniques, 131–136
International Commission of Radiation Units and Measurements (ICRU)
brachytherapy regime per
cervical cancer, 178–181
high dose rate, 200
low dose rate, 380–381t
dose delivery accuracy recommendations, 31, 104
organs at risk per, 36–37, 110
Reference Point recommendations, 110, 377–*378, 380*
volumes of interest per, 36, 53, 108, 110–111
International Federation of Gynecology and Obstetrics (FIGO)
cervical cancer stages, 384t
vaginal cancer stages, 421t
vulvar cancer stages, 405t–406
Intractable pain, 152
Intraoral cone irradiation
for floor of mouth, 282, 284, *286*
immobilization devices for, *94*
for tongue cancers, 289
Intraperitoneal P-32 irradiation, 399–*400*
Inverse square law, 173–*174*
Inverted-Y fields (*see* Fields, inverted-Y)
Iodine (^{125}I)
in brachytherapy, 173–174t, 176
for prostate tumors, 451–456
Ionization chambers
for calibration, 205
in dosimetry, 133–*135*
Iridium (^{192}Ir)
in brachytherapy, 173–174t
high dose, 200–202, 211, 216
interstitial, 175–*177,* 192
low dose, 211
pulsed, 194–195
for lip cancer, 280
for nasal vestibule cancer, 292
for prostate cancer, 457–460
for tongue cancer, 274, *288*
for vaginal cancer, 423, 428, *430,* 432

Irradiated volume
defined, 53, 110
dose adjustment postoperative per, 10–11
single versus fractionated brain dose, 147–*148*
tolerance per, *7,* 9
Isodose distribution
adjacent fields, 67–*68,* 77–*79*
air gaps, 77–78
beam obliquity, 75–76
bolusing, 78
clinical applications *(see specific disease or therapy)*
field shaping, 77 (*see also* Field blocks)
formulas for, 6
reference, 176–177, 181, 215, 380–*381*
tissue heterogeneities, 76–77
uniformity, *75*
ISS (*see* Independent support stand)

Jewett-Strong classification
Marshall modification, 351t
of urinary bladder cancer, 351t

Karnofsky performance status, 156
Kidneys
shielding, in total body irradiation, 502–503
tumors, conformal radiation therapy, 123–124
Kilovoltage reactions, 4, 7

Larnygeal tumors
glottic
stage T3, 270–*271*
stage T1-T2, 269–*270*
postoperative irradiation, 272, *274*
supraglottic, 271
treatment field designs, 269–271
Laser beam simulation, *54, 308*–309
LD (*see* Hodgkin's disease, lymphocyte depletion)
LDR (*see* Low dose-rate brachytherapy)
LET (linear energy transfer radiation), 14, 184
Leukemias, total body irradiation, 499–500t
Levamisole, 341
Leydig cell tumors, 467
Linacs (*see* Medical linear accelerators)
Linear attenuation coefficient, 105
Linear Energy Transfer radiation (LET), 14, 184
Lip cancer
electron beam therapy, 79–80t
treatment field design, 280, *283*
Lipomas, 482
Liver
normal tissue tolerance, 539
tumors, chemoirradiation, 20
LMM (*see* Mediastinal mass, large)
Low dose-rate brachytherapy (LDR)
advantages, 212
clinical applications
cervical cancer (*see* Cervical cancer)
endometrial cancer, 387–389t, 391–*393,* 397
vaginal cancer (*see* Vaginal cancer; Vaginal cuff irradiation)
continuous (CLDR), 188, *190, 194–195,* 197
high dose versus, 197–*198*
physics, 215
radiobiology, 184–194
cell kill by, *192*–194
dose-rate effect, *188–191*
inverse dose-rate effect, *190*–191
rationale, 194
source handling evolution, 210–211
Lugol's iodine, 409
Lung cancer
brachytherapy for obstruction from, 215–216
bronchogenic
incidence, 315
lymphatic spread, 315–*316,* 316t
pathologic features, 315–*316*
staging, 316–317t
chemoirradiation
integration factors, 322–323
non-small cell, 21–22, 322
patterns of failure, 323
small cell, 22, 324, 326
conformal radiation therapy
clinical results, 121–122t
technical innovations, 120t–121
continuous hyperfractionated accelerated therapy, 322
external beam treatment
immobolization for, *97–98*
postoperative, 323
preoperative, 323
multimodality treatment sequelae, 326
non-oat cell
first failure site, 323t
portals for, *322*
non-small cell (NSCLCA)
CHART regimen, 322
definitive radiation therapy, 317–322
fractionation trials, 321–322
left lower lobe plan, 319–*320*
patient selection for treatment, 318
right lower lobe plan, 319–*320*
treatment options by stage, 317–318t
treatment planning, 318–322
tumor dosing, 321
volume considerations, 322–*323*
small cell (SCLC)
dose trials, 324
fractionation trials, 324
prophylactic cranial irradiation, 325
radiation therapy role, 323
systemic therapy coordination, 324t–325
thoracic radiotherapy, 324t–325
traditional portal, *325*
whole irradiation of, 533
Lungs
anatomy, 315–*316*
blocks, for total body irradiation, 502, 510–*512*
immobilization devices, *97–98*
normal tissue tolerance, 539
tumors of (*see* Lung cancer)
Lymphangiography, pedal, *469,* 471, *476*
Lymphatic trapezoid of Fletcher, *180*
Lymphatics
axillary node anatomical levels, 301–*302,* 303t
cancer involvement
with cervical cancer, *364*–366
electron beam therapy, 7, 79–80t, 83–*85*
inguinal nodes, 405, 408
internal mammary nodes, 301, *303*–305, 312
with lung cancer, 315–*316*
neck nodes, 269, *276,* 295–298, *297*
pelvic nodes, 337, 353, 417405
with prostate cancer, 438t–439t, 441–*442, 445*
with testicular cancer, 468–*469,* 472–474t, 475–477
treatment planning factors, 11
with urinary bladder cancer, 350–355
with vaginal cancer, 417, 420–*422*
with vulvar cancer, 403–405, 407
cancer of (*see* Hodgkin's disease; Lymphomas)
Lymphomas
diffuse large cell, 467
malignant (*see* Hodgkin's disease)
non-Hodgkin's, 500t
Lymphoscintigraphy, 303

Magnetic resonance imaging (MRI)
clinical applications *(see specific disease or therapy)*
functional (fMRI), 225–226
spectroscopy, 226–*227*
in treatment planning, 45–46, 52, 59–61, *87–88*
for CNS tumors, 226–*230,* 235–*236*
Magnetoencephalography (MEG), 225
Mantle fields (*see* Fields, mantle)
Masks
aquaplast, *92, 290, 515*
thermoplastic, 107
MC (*see* Hodgkin's disease, mixed cellularity)
MCL (*see* Collimators, multileaf)
Mediastinal mass, large (LMM), 519–520, 525, 532–*534*
Medical linear accelerators
block-to-surface distance, 65
computer-controlled, *117,* 131
in intensity modulated therapy, 131–132
quality assurance, 135–136
stereotactic systems
clinical applications, 147–148, 154–155, 157, 170
mechanics, 160, 162, *164*
Medulloblastomas
grading systems, 224t
incidence, 224t
treatment guidelines, 230t, 257, *261*
MEG (magnetoencephalography), 225
Megavoltage reactions, 4, 7, 65
Melanomas, 5, 467
Memorial implant system, 176
Meningiomas
grading systems, 224t
incidence, 224t
stereotactic radiosurgery, 154–155, 157, 169–170
treatment examples, 253, *255*
treatment guidelines, 230t
Methotrexate, 24
Methyl-CCNU, 18
MIMIC (multileaf intensity modulating collimators), 44
Misonidazole compounds, 14
Mitomycin, 14–16, 342–344, 408
Mixed lymphocyte cultures (MLC), 499
Monitor units (MU)
average
conventional therapy, 142t
intensity modulated therapy, 142t
in total body irradiation, 507
use in quality assurance, 133
Monte Carlo dosing method, 45–46, 113, 202
MPD (*see* Doses, matched peripheral; Doses, maximum permissible)
MRI (*see* Magnetic resonance imaging)
MT ratio, 519–*520*
MTD (*see* Doses, maximum tolerable)
Mucositis, degrees of, 4
Multi-hit mechanism, 3–4
Multiple boost fields (*see* Fields, multiple boost)
Multiple functional subunits (FSU), 37
Musculo-Skeletal Tumor Society, soft tissue sarcoma stages per, 484–485t

Nasal vestibule tumors
dosimetry, 80, *82*
electron beam therapy, 80–*82, 292*–294
external beam therapy, 289–*290*
treatment field designs, *289–294*
Nasopharyngeal tumors
intensity modulated therapy, 137–140
portal films
for correlation with tumor control, 32–34t
for treatment verification, *137*
treatment field designs, 279–280, *280–282,* 296–298
four-field versus two-field, *281*
National Marrow Donor Program (NMDP), 499
Nerve tolerance, cranial, 150t–151, 158
Neutron beam therapy
contamination by, 130, 142
fast, for soft tissue sarcomas, 488
Nonseminomatous tumors, 467, *469,* 477
Normal tissue
brachytherapy therapeutic ratio and, 212–*213*
shielding
techniques (*see* Conformal radiation therapy; Field blocks)
in total body irradiation, 501–503, 510–512, *514–515*
tolerance of radiation
central nervous system, 539
cranial nerves, 150t–151, 158
dependent factors, 231
dosimetry parameters, 30–*32,* 37, 192
gastrointestinal tract, 540
head and neck, 540
heart, 539
with Hodgkin's disease treatment, 539–540
liver, 539
lung, 539
maximum, 192
minimal dose risks, 37
reproductive organs, 540
thyroid, 539
urinary bladder, 355
treatment planning and
adjacent field factors, 68, 70
CT techniques, 108–110, *109*
definition importance, 36–37, 104
impact outcomes per, 43
Normal tissue complication probability (NTCP)
Lyman model, 243
pneumonitis and lung cancer, 318
in treatment planning, 37, 46, 114–115
NSCLCA (*see* Lung cancer, non-small cell)
NSD (*see* Doses, nominal single)
Nuclear Regulatory Commission, U.S. (NRC), 196, 206, 375

Off-axis ratio (OAR), *167*–169
OH (hydroxyl radical), 184
Olsalazine, 345
Oral cavity tumors
electron beam therapy, 79–80t
external beam therapy, *93–94*
treatment field designs, 280–282, *283–289,* 296–298
floor of mouth
custom-made implant device, 282, *285*
external beam irradiation, 282, *284*
interstitial irradiation, 282, *285–286*
intraoral cone irradiation, 282, 284, *286*
immobilization devices, *93–94*
incurable, 9
lip (*see* Lip cancer)
postoperative, 289
tongue (*see* Tongue cancer)
Organs at risk
CT simulation techniques, 108–*109*
defined, 110
in intensity modulated therapy, 143
per ICRU, 36–37
Oropharyngeal tumors
base of tongue, 274–*276*
postoperative irradiation, 289
soft palate, 275, *278–279*
tonsillar area, 275, *277–278*
treatment field designs, 273–279, 296–298
Overhead arm positioner, *98*
Ovoids (*see* Colpostats)

p53 mutations, 440
Paclitaxel, 14–15t, 16
Palladium (^{103}Pd)
in brachytherapy, 173
for prostate tumors, 451–454

Pancreatic cancer
  chemoirradiation, 19–20
  conformal radiation therapy, 123–124
Pantograph device, 56, 59, *87*
Parallel opposed film check, 58–59
Paranasal sinus tumors, *289–294*
Paris implant system, *176*–177, 192, 203, 215
Parkinson's disease, 152
Parotid gland tumors
  electron beam therapy, 79, 81, *83*
  external beam therapy, 293–*294*
  intensity modulated therapy, 141–142
  interstitial irradiation, 294–*295*
  treatment field designs, 293–*295*
Paterson-Parker implant system, 174–175t, 192
Patient contour simulation
  for stereotactic radiation, 159
  in treatment planning, 56, 59, 108–*109*
Patient positioning
  aids for (*see* Treatment aids)
  simulation of (*see* Simulation)
Patient room survey form, 376–*377*
PCI (prohylactic cranial irradiation), 325
^{103}Pd (*see* Palladium)
PDR (*see* Brachytherapy, pulsed)
Pelvic tumors *(see also specific anatomy or tumor)*
  external beam therapy
    megavoltage, 363–366
    split fields, 364, 366, 382t
  immobilization devices and aids, 86, *95*–97, 107
  treatment planning, 12
Pelvis
  immobilization devices, 86, *95*–97, 107
  irradiation of
    box technique, 7
    whole, 217, 353–*354,* 364, 391, 395, 420, *422,* 428
  skin mark reliability, 97
  wall reference points, 180–*181, 378*
Pencil beam planning method, 45
Penumbra
  from air gaps, 78
  in field shaping, 65, *67*
  planning considerations, 31, 53, 166
PET (*see* Positron emission tomography)
Phantom base
  BRW coordinates, 162–163, 166t
  for stereotactic process, *159*–160
  test device for, *160,* 162
Photon beam therapy
  air gaps in, 65
  biologic absorption, 184
  clinical applications, 306
    anal cancer, 343–*344*
    breast cancer, 305–307
    head and neck cancer, 82, 270, *273, 276,* 292, 294, *297*
    lung cancer, 319
    prostate cancer, 445, 447t
    total body irradiation, 503, 514–515
    urinary bladder cancer, 355
    vaginal cancer, 420, *422,* 423
    vulvar cancer, *409–413,* 414
  dose calculation considerations, 112–113
  electron contamination of, 65, 112
  field shaping techniques, 64–67
  in intensity modulated therapy, 130, *140–141*
  in stereotactic radiosurgery, 148–*149*
  treatment planning factors, 3, 38, 43–45, 79, 105
Pineal gland tumors
  conformal radiation therapy, 122
  stereotactic radiosurgery, 157
Pineoblastomas, 223–224t, 226
Pituitary adenomas
  conformal radiation therapy, 123
  incidence, 224t
  radiograph view, *233*
  stereotactic radiosurgery, 155–156
  treatment approach examples, 243, *244–246*
  treatment guidelines, 230t
Platinum, 379
Poor man's wedge, 319
Portal films
  graticule aid, *102*
  holders, *103*
  in treatment planning, 31–33t, 38
  in treatment verification, 61, 116
    head and neck tumors, 136–*137*
Positron emission tomography (PET)
  brain mapping by, 225–226
  portal volume determination via, 330
  in treatment planning, 45–46, *109*
Preoperative studies
  per disease *(see specific disease or therapy)*
  value of, 335
Prostate cancer
  anatomical features
    apex versus pelvis, 441, *444*
    bladder and urethra relationship, 435, *436–437*
    pubic arch interference, 451–*452*
  brachytherapy
    conformal high dose rate, 460t–461t, 460–462
    dose factors, 452t, 452–*455,* 457
    dose fractionation, 460–461t
    dose optimization, 460t–462
    high dose rate, 216
    interstitial implant procedure, 455–457
    interstitial implant removal, 457–*459*
    interstitial implants, permanent, 451
    isotope selection, 452t–453, 457
    patient selection, 451–*452*
    pattern optimization, 460
    perioperative management, 457
    postimplant dosimetry, 457–*458*
    preimplant dosimetry, 454–*455*
    quality assessment, 457
    relative dwell time factors, 460–461
    relative volume factors, 461
    retropubic technique, 453
    Syed's technique, 457–459, *458*
    transperineal technique, 453–*454*
    treatment planning, 454–*456*
  combined modality treatment, 451, 454
  conformal radiation therapy
    acute toxicity results, 119–120t
    chemical disease-free survival results, 118–*119*
    dose-volume histograms, 447, *449*
    dosimetric analysis, 118t
    field simulation, *448*–449
    immobilization aids, 450
    internal motion factors, 449–450t
    patient positioning variability, 449–450
    rectal block morbidity correlation, 450–451t
    seed-loading techniques, 454–455
    setup error detection, 450–451
    time and effort studies, 118
    treatment planning, 447–451
    volumes for, 447–448t
  external beam therapy
    beam energy, 445–446
    box technique, 441–*442,* 445–446
    dose distribution, 445–*446*
    dose standards, 445–447t
    extended field technique, 445
    lateral field technique, 441–*442*
    overview, 440–441
    periaortic lymph node treatment, *445*
    simulation techniques, 441, *443*–444
    volume treated factors, 441–445

Prostate cancer *(Continued)*
Gleason scores, 437t–439
growth patterns
distant metastases, 439
local, 435, 437–438
regional lymph node involvement, 438t–439t, 441–*442, 445*
seminal vesicle invasion, 435, 437t–438t, 441, *444*
immobilization devices, 107, 450
prognostic factors, 439–440
PSA level factors, 437t, 439
staging, 437t–439, 447t, 459
volumes
for conformal radiation therapy, 447–448t
defined by CT slice, *109,* 441, *443*
relative optimization, 461–462
Prostate-specific antigen (PSA), 437t
Proton beam therapy
in stereotactic radiosurgery, 148, 155
treatment planning considerations, 38
Psychiatric disease, 152
PTV (*see* Target volumes, planning)

Quality assurance (QA)
for brachytherapy, 215
high dose, 205–207
low dose, 384–385t
in prostate tumors, 457
cost per patient, 43
for intensity modulated radiation therapy, 132–136
for stereotactic radiation, 169
in treatment planning, 46–48, *111*
Quimby implant system, 175–176

^{226}Ra (*see* Radium)
Radiation necrosis, 147–*149,* 157–158, 170
Radiation oncologist, qualifications, 33, 37
Radiation therapy *(see also specific modality or type)*
actions
direct, 184–*185*
indirect, 184–*185*
biologic absorption, 184
chronologic effect subdivisions, 37
devices for (*see* Treatment aids; *specific device)*
DNA damage from (*see* DNA)
failure factors (*see* Tumors, recurrence of)
"4 Rs" principles, 147
goal of, 52
unintended exposure to (*see* Exposure)
Radiographs
for dosimetry
in intensity modulated therapy, 133–*134,* 136
phantoms, 133–*134*
parallel opposed film check, 58–59
Rando phantoms, 506
reconstruction with (*see* Digitally reconstructed radiographs)
simulation with (*see* Simulation, films for)
for verification (*see also* Portal films)
intensity modulated therapy, 136
stereotactic radiation, 160, 162–164t, *165*
in treatment planning, 31–33t, 38
Radioisotope labeling, of tumor growth, 8t
Radioisotopes *(see specific radioisotope)*
Radionuclides, physical characteristics, 174t
Radium (^{226}Ra)
in brachytherapy, 174t–175, 179, 367, 379
for mouth floor cancer, *286*
platinum filtration of, 379
for tongue cancer, *278*
for vaginal cancer, 423–424, 426t–427t, *430*
dummy sources, 424, *426–427*
Record and verify systems, 61
Rectal cancer (*see also* Anal cancer)
adjuvant irradiation
dose factors, *339,* 341, *341*
field techniques, *338–340*
brachytherapy
complications, 181–*182,* 210, 218
reference points, 180, 377–*378*
chemoirradiation, 17–18, 335–336, 338
diagnostic evaluation, 335–336
external beam therapy field design, 342
pathways of spread, 336–337
recurrence, 10, 341–342
after resection, 337
sacral canal importance, 341
therapeutic ratio optimization, 344–345
Rectum
anatomy, 336
reference points, 180, 377–*378*
tumors of (*see* Rectal cancer)
Reference isodose (*see* Isodose distribution, reference)
Reference points
for brachytherapy
cervical, 376–*378*
dose factors, 180–181, 203
landmarks, *180–181*
ICRU recommendations, 110, 377–*378, 380*
for total body irradiation, 504
Reference volume
in brachytherapy
cervical, 380–*381*
determination factors, 179–181, *180*
Remote afterloaders (*see* Applicators)
Repositioning techniques
aids for (*see* Immobilization devices; Treatment aids)
in treatment planning
devices for, 37–38
as failure factor, 34–35
registration system, 106–107
reproducible components, 31
during simulation, 54–55
for stereotactic radiation, 158–159
Reproductive organs
normal tissue tolerance, 540
tumors of *(see specific organ)*
Respiration, planning considerations, 59, 104
Retractors
cervical, 211
testicular, *95*
Rhabdomyosarcomas, 467
Room-view display tools
3-D isodose surface displays, 114–*115*
in treatment planning, 40–*41,* 46, 111–*113*
Royal Marsden staging system, for testicular cancer, 470t

SAD (source-axis distance), 65
Sarcomas
cartilage, 157
Ewing's, *84*–85
soft tissue (*see* Soft tissue sarcomas)
striated muscle, 467
synovial, *492*
Schwannomas, nonacoustic, 153
SCLC (*see* Lung cancer, small cell)
Seminomas (*see also* Nonseminomatous tumors)
anaplastic, 468
classic, 468
classification systems, 467–468
lymph node metastases patterns, 473–474t
orchiectomy results, 472t
pathology, 467
permatocytic, 468
pure, 472
radiation therapy results, 472t
radiation therapy techniques
dose factors, 477

- Seminomas *(Continued)*
    - field films, *475–477*
    - per stages, 475–476
    - portal design, 476
    - summary, *478*
  - recurrence rates, 473–474t
  - treatment options
    - elective irradiation of nodes, 473–474
    - portal design for stage I-II, 473
    - surveillance for stage I, 472–473
- Seromas, 495–*496*
- Sertoli cell tumors, 467
- SFD (source-film distance), 58
- Shadow tray, in field shaping, *65*–66
- Shields
  - beeswax, *283, 287*
  - nail, *100*
  - testicular, *95*
  - tungsten, 367–*368*
- Shoulder swing, *95*
- Shrinking field technique, *9*
- Simon-Heyman capsules, 388–*389*
- Simulated annealing, 131
- Simulation
  - computed tomography (*see* Treatment planning, 3-D)
  - contrast materials for, *89*
  - conventional, 106
  - evolution, 52, 106
  - films for
    - in treatment planning, 52–53, 55, 58
    - in treatment verification, 31, 61, *116,* 136
  - optimal device elements, 37
  - of patient contours, 56, 59, 108–*109,* 159
  - specialists involved in, 52–53
  - steps in, 60–*61,* 116
    - beam orientation, 55–56
    - compensating filters, 56–57
    - custom field blocking, *57*–59
    - documentation of treatment field, 56
    - external patient contours, 56
    - internal patient contours, 108–110, *109*
    - patient positioning, 54–55, 106
    - presimulation planning, 53–54
    - treatment field localization, *55*–56, 62, 108–110
  - in treatment planning, 37, 52–62, 106–110
  - virtual (*see* Treatment planning, 3-D)
- Single-hit mechanism, 3–5
- Skin cancer
  - electron beam therapy, 79–80t
  - total irradiation, 97, *100*
- Skin marks
  - pelvic reliability, 97
  - in treatment planning, 56, 59, 62, 108
- Skip lesions, 272, 326, 337
- Soft tissue sarcomas
  - aggressive fibromatosis type, 488–489
  - brachytherapy
    - dose fractionation, 493–495, *494*
    - overview and clinical results, 487
    - techniques description, 493–*494*
  - chemoirradiation, 24–25
  - chemotherapy, adjuvant, 487–488t
  - diagnostic factors
    - biopsy techniques, 482, *484*
    - histologic, 484–486
    - imaging characteristics, 482–*483*
  - electron beam therapy, intraoperative, 487
  - incidence, 481
  - neutron beam therapy, fast, 488
  - radiation therapy
    - beam energy, 492
    - custom shaped fields, 490–491
    - dose factors, 490, *492–493,* 495
    - field sizes, 490
    - imaging for simulation, *489–493*
    - immobilization for, 490
    - postoperative, 492–493
    - preoperative, 493
    - with surgery, 486–487
    - target volume design, 489–490, *491–492*
    - time-dose fractionation, 492–495
  - seromas versus, *495*–496
  - staging systems, 484–486
  - surgical resection, 486–487
  - team management of, 481–482
  - treatment options and results, 481–482t
    - chemotherapy, 24–25, 487–488t
    - combined modality treatment, 24–25, 486–488
    - innovative, 488
    - patient care recommendations, 495
    - radiation, 486–495
    - sequelae, *495*–496
    - surgical, 486–487
- Solder wire, 59
- Somnolence syndrome, 231
- Source-axis distance (SAD), 65
- Source-film distance (SFD), 58
- Source-skin distance fields (SSD), 55
- Source-surface distance (SSD), 72, *74–75*
  - air gap impact, 77–78
- Source-tray distance (STD), 58
- Special particles, 45
- SPECT (*see* Computed tomography, single photon emission)
- Speculum, weighted, *369*
- S-phase fraction, in prostate tumors, 440
- Spinal column, 139
- Spinal cord tumors
  - intensity modulated therapy, 139
  - treatment guidelines, 230t
    - general principles, *241–242*
    - tolerance doses, 231t–232t
- Spine, irradiation of, 97, 100–*101*
- Sponges, *102*
- SRS (*see* Stereotactic radiosurgery)
- SRT (*see* Stereotactic radiation therapy)
- SSD (*see* Source-surface distance)
- Static light field check, 58–59
- STD (source-tray distance), 58
- Stents, intraoral, *94*
- Stepping source positioning method
  - HDR brachytherapy, 200–202
  - pulsed brachytherapy, 194–195
- Stereotactic radiation therapy (SRT)
  - computer software, 158–159, 163, 166–168
  - dosimetry
    - cone output factors, *166*–167
    - distribution factors, 167–169, *168*
    - fractionated, 147, 151
    - off-axis ratio, *167*–169
    - tissue maximum ratio, 167
  - helium ion Bragg peak, 154, 158
  - immobilization for, *158–162,* 232, *234*
  - patient contour simulation, 159
  - patient positioning, 158–159
    - treatment couch for, 159, 162, 164t
  - quality assurance, 169
  - surgery with (*see* Stereotactic radiosurgery)
  - technical aspects
    - beam design, 159, 166–167
    - collimators associated with, 160, 162, *164*
    - gantry angles for, 162, 164t–165t
    - medical linear accelerators in, 147–148, 154–157, 160, 162, *164,* 170
  - verification techniques, 160, 162–*165,* 164t

Stereotactic radiosurgery (SRS)
achievable accuracies, 169t
angiography role, 154, 158, 160, 162, 169
brachytherapy versus, 157
Bragg peak radiation, 154–155, 158
clinical applications
acoustic tumors, 152–*153,* 170
angiographically occult vascular malformations, 154
angiomas, venous, 154
arteriovenous malformations, 153–154, 157, 169–170
astrocytomas, 156–157, *248*
brain tumors, 147, *156*
chondrosarcomas, 157
chordomas, 157
craniopharyngiomas, 155–157
epilepsy, 152
functional, 152
glioblastoma multiforme, 157, 229, *247, 249*
gliomas, 157, 169
glomus jugulare tumors, 157
hemangioblastomas, 157
intractable pain, 152
meningiomas, 154–155, 157, 169–170
metastatic tumors, *156*
miscellaneous tumors, 157
nonfunctional, 152–157
Parkinson's disease, 152
pineal gland tumors, 157
pituitary adenomas, 155–156
psychiatric disease, 152
trigeminal neuralgia, 152
complications, 151, 154, 157–158
computed tomography in
clinical applications, 151, 154, 156
localizer frames, 160, *162–163*
planning techniques, 158–160, 162–163, 166–169
cost comparisons, 170
cranial nerve tolerance, 150t–151, 158
dosimetry
calculations, 158, 166–169, *168*
cone output factors, *166*–167
data needed, 166
dose-volume histograms, 147–*149*
off-axis ratio data, *167*–169
target composition, 149t–150
tissue maximum ratio determination, 167
tissue response, 147–*148*
evolution, 147
fractionated stereotactic radiotherapy versus, 147–*148,* 151
frameless, 170
future directions, 169–170
helium ion radiation, 154–155, 158
magnetic resonance imaging in
clinical applications, 148, 151, 153, 156
localizer frames, 160, *162*–163
planning techniques, 158–160, 162–163, 166–169
photon beam therapy, 148–*149*
principle basis of, 147–148
proton beam therapy, 148, 155
quality assurance, 169
technical aspects
equipment, *159–162*
Gamma Knife radiosurgery unit, 147–148, 152, 154–155, 157–158
imaging accuracy tests, 163, *166*
mechanical accuracy tests, 162–*165,* 164t, 166t
phantom base, *159*–163, *160,* 166t
steps in, 158–159
treatment aids, 97, 100, *101, 158–162*
independent support stand, *159*–160, 162–164t, *164–165*
treatment planning, 158–169
target volume factors, 149t–150, 158–159, 169–170
tumor definition factors, 169
Stirrups, *102*
Stomach tumors, 123–124
Strandqvist formula, 6
Streptozotocin, 19
Subclinical disease
defined, 9
microscopic tumor evidence versus, 30
Submandibular gland tumors, 294–295
Supports
head and neck, *92*
for lying (*see* Treatment couch)
for sitting, *98–99*
for standing, *99, 512* (*see also* Independent support stand)
Survival fraction curves
acute reactions, 4
α/β ratios, *4*–6, 188, *191*–192, 197
defined, 186
dissociation of acute reactions and late effects, *5–6*
dose-rate effect
inverse, *190*–191
principles, *188–191*
tumor size bias, 193–194
early responses, 191
isoeffect formulas, 6
late effects, 4–5, 191–192
linear quadratic model, 3–6, *4,* 187–*188*
models and origins, 187–*188*
shape after radiation exposure, 187–*188*
two-component, 3, *4,* 6

Tandems
for brachytherapy
cervical, 217, 366t–375t, *370–372*
guidelines, 178, 181
high dose rate, 201
Fletcher-Suit, 388, *389–391, 423*
Fletcher-Suit-Delclos, *367,* 369–374
hanging, 371
intrauterine, 374–375, *423–424, 426, 428*
Target volumes
clinical (CTV)
ICRU recommendations, 110–111
importance, 32, 34, 36, 46, 108
in simulation planning, *53,* 108
CT versus portal determination, 108
per therapies *(see specific therapy)*
planning (PTV)
ICRU recommendations, 110–111
importance, 31, 34, 36
in simulation planning, *53,* 55–56, 60, 108, 110
TBI (*see* Total body irradiation)
TCP (*see* Tumor control probability)
TDF (time dose factor), 6, 181
Templates
interstitial implant, 428, 431–*432,* 458
Martinez Universal Perineal, *432*
perineal, 459
Syed, 398
transperineal, 453
Teratocarcinomas, 468, 470
Teratomas, 468
Testicles
immobilization devices, *95*
lymphatic drainage system, *469*
tumors of (*see* Testicular cancer)
Testicular cancer
bulky abdominal disease, 474t–475
choriocarcinoma, 468
clinical evaluation, 470–471
Dixon & Moore Groups, 467–468
germ cell pathology, 467–468
imaging evaluation
abdominal view, 471
computed tomography, 471
lymphangiography, *469,* 471

Testicular cancer *(Continued)*
incidence, 467
metastasis of
hematogenous, 470
local, 468
lymphatic, 468–*469,* 472–474t, 475–477
mixed tumors, 468
nonseminomatous, 477
portal design, *476–478*
radiation therapy per stages, *475*–476
seminomas, 467–468, 472–474
staging systems, 470t
teratoma, 468
tumor markers for, 471
TG-43 formalism dosing method, 202
Thalamotomies, 152
Therapeutic gain factor (TGF), 38
Therapeutic ratio
defined, 212
dose rate effect on, 212–*213*
Thoracic radiation therapy (TRT), 324t–325, 328t (*see also* Chest wall irradiation)
Thoracic tumors, *97–98,* 107
Three-D CRT (*see* Conformal radiation therapy)
Three-D RTP (*see* Treatment planning, 3-D)
Thyroid
cancer, 139
normal tissue tolerance, 539
Time dose factor (TDF), 6, 181
Tissue
generic types, 3
irradiated (*see* Irradiated volume)
missing
bolus for (*see* Bolusing)
compensators for (*see* Compensators)
normal (*see* Normal tissue)
Tissue maximum ratio (TMR)
as stereotactic radiation factor, 167
in total body irradiation, 507–508
TNI (total nodal irradiation), 523, 525
TNM classifications
esophageal cancer, 327t
lung cancer, 316–317t
soft tissue sarcomas, 484–485t
testicular cancer, 470t
Tolerance
as basic parameter, 30–32
of normal tissue (*see* Normal tissue)
per tissue volume irradiated, *7,* 9
Tomotherapy, 132, 139
Tongue cancer
in base, 274–*276*
external beam therapy, 275, *278,* 284–285, *287*
interstitial irradiation, *287–288*
intraoral cone irradiation, 289
treatment field design, *284*
submental boost technique, 274, *276*
Total body irradiation (TBI)
anteroposterior technique
brain blocks, *514–515*
chest wall boosts, 513–*513*
dose factors, 509–*511,* 515
dose verification, 513t
in infants, 512–*513*
lung blocks, 510–*512*
patient position factors, *510, 512–513*
patient treatment, 511–513
schedule summary, 510t
simulation and patient measurements, 510
testicular boosts, 512
brain sparing technique, *514–515*
children considerations, 515–516
complications, 501t–502t, 516
for conditioning
diseases indicating, 500t, 503
dose fractionation and rate, 500–502t
goals of, 499–500
normal tissue shielding, 501–503
regimen overview, 499–500
sequencing, 501
techniques overview, 503
general anesthesia for, 515–*516*
right and left lateral technique
compensator design, 506–*508*
compensator thickness determination, *505*–506t
dose verification, 509
machine calibration and treatment calculation, 507–*508*
patient position documentation, *504–505, 507*
patient treatment, 509
reference points, 504
schedule summary, 509t
simulation and patient measurements, 503–*506*
x-ray buildup in, *508*
shielding field blocks, 501–503, 510–512, *514–515*
television monitoring system, 515–*516*
treatment aids, 97, *99, 513*
Total nodal irradiation (TNI), 523, 525
Total skin irradiation, 97, *100*
Total source strength, 179
Tracking Cobalt Project, 131
Transfer pointer assembly, *159,* 162–163, *165*
Transurethral bladder resection (TUR), 349, 352, 356–359
Transurethral resection of prostate (TURP), 440–441, 452
Treatment aids
beam modifiers (*see* Beam-modifying devices)
for brain tumors, 97, 100–*101,* 151
for craniospinal irradiation, 97, 100, *101*
evaluation in treatment planning, 37–38, 54–55
importance, 86
patient data acquisiton and registration devices, 86–*89*
for patient immobilization and positioning (*see* Immobilization devices)
for setup verification, 100, *102–103*
for stereotactic treatment
radiosurgery, 97, 100, *101, 158–162*
radiotherapy, 151
for total body irradiation, 97, *99, 513*
for total skin irradiation, 97, *100*
Treatment chair, *99*
Treatment couch
inserts for immobilization, *95–96,* 106–*107*
for intensity modulated therapy, 136
for stereotactic radiation, 159, 162, 164t
for total body irradiation, *513*
in treatment planning
CT scanner considerations, *59*
indexing of, 44, 106–*107,* 135
simulation, 54
Treatment fields (*see* Fields)
Treatment planning
algorithms for (*see* Algorithms)
clinical versus physical, 11, 35
computer software in (*see* Computer software)
3-D (3-D RTP)
clinical applications *(see specific anatomy or tumor)*
components, 62
conclusions regarding, 124–125
evolution, 104
immobilization devices, 106–108
implementation and verification, 116
limitations, 110–111
multimodality imaging techniques, 45–46, 59–61
optimization and evaluation, 60, 113–116, 130
patient data acquisition aids, 86–*88*
quality assurance, 48, *111*
steps in, 52–62, 104–106t